VITAL STATISTICS OF THE UNITED STATES

VITAL STATISTICS OF THE UNITED STATES

Births, Life Expectancy, Deaths, and Selected Health Data

Eighth Edition
2018

Edited by Shana Hertz Hattis

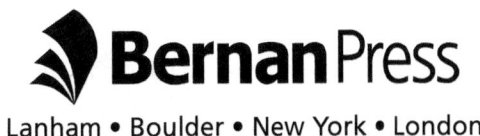

Lanham • Boulder • New York • London

Published by Bernan Press
An imprint of The Rowman & Littlefield Publishing Group, Inc.
4501 Forbes Boulevard, Suite 200, Lanham, Maryland 20706
www.rowman.com
800-865-3457

Unit A, Whitacre Mews, 26-34 Stannary Street, London SE11 4AB

ISBN: 978-159888-992-5
E-ISBN: 978-159888-993-2
ISSN: 1549-8603

♾™ The paper used in this publication meets the minimum requirements of
American National Standard for Information Sciences—Permanence of Paper for
Printed Library Materials, ANSI/NISO Z39.48-1992.

Printed in the United States of America

CONTENTS

LIST OF TABLES

PART II: MORTALITY

PART III: HEALTH

Determinants and Measures of Health

Use of Addictive Substances

Ambulatory Care

Inpatient Care

LIST OF FIGURES

INTRODUCTION

Bernan Press is pleased to present a comprehensive collection of birth, mortality, and health data in the eighth edition of *Vital Statistics of the United States: Births, Life Expectancy, Deaths, and Selected Health Data.* This volume provides valuable information compiled by various government agencies including the Centers for Disease Control (CDC) and its National Center for Health Statistics (NCHS) and National Vital Statistics System (NVSS), the U.S. Census Bureau, and the Bureau of Labor Statistics (BLS).

Until 1993, the federal government published *Vital Statistics of the United States* in several thick-bound volumes. However, between the last publication of the federal volume and the first *Vital Statistics* edition from Bernan Press, nothing comparable was offered. During this time, the CDC continued to compile its information as periodical reports and news releases, and Bernan took this opportunity to streamline this information into a cohesive, inclusive volume.

This edition builds upon the groundwork laid by previous editions in the areas of birth, mortality, health, and marriage and divorce. Each part is preceded by highlights of salient data. These sections also contain a diverse array of information about their tables and figures. Notes and definitions and source information are also provided for all four parts.

The Birth section, in many instances, provides final data through 2015. This section covers many aspects of natality, including birth and fertility rates, number of children, births to unmarried women, methods of delivery, and demographic characteristics of mothers.

The Mortality section focuses on deaths and death rates as told through various medical, demographic, and social characteristics. Especially detailed are the tables on causes of death, which are shown by leading causes of death, age, sex, Hispanic origin, race, and (to a lesser extent) state of residence. Death rates are also given by marital status and level of educational attainment, and special tables are provided for infant mortality.

The Health section, the largest in the book, offers a collection of statistics concerning health and disease. While health is not a traditional component of vital statistics, its importance to this volume cannot be overstated. Health data provides the user with an even deeper picture of births and deaths in the United States. For example, a user interested in cerebrovascular disease mortality may glean useful information from tables about incidence and survival rates. This chapter shows selected data on several topics, including determinants and measures of health, use of addictive substances, ambulatory care, inpatient care, health personnel, health expenditures, and health insurance.

The Marriage and Divorce section provides marriage and divorce rates by state and demographic characteristics. This chapter also provides statistics on multiple marriages, marriages ending in widowhood, and number of marriages for U.S. residents.

About the Editor

Shana Hertz Hattis is an editor with over a decade of experience in statistical and government research publications. Past titles include *State Profiles: The Population and Economy of Each U.S. State, Housing Statistics of the United States,* and *Justice Statistics: An Extended Look at Crime in the United States.* She earned her bachelor of science in journalism and master of science in education degrees from Northwestern University.

PART I: BIRTH

PART I: BIRTHS

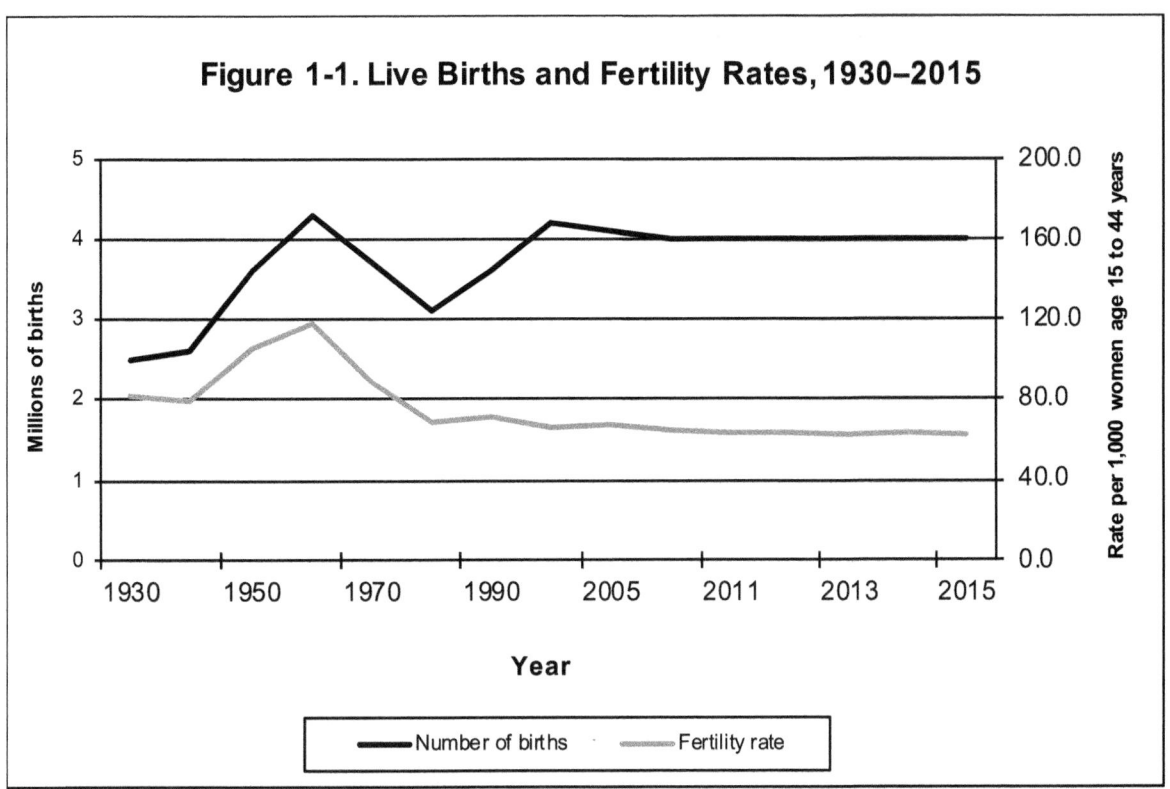

Figure 1-1. Live Births and Fertility Rates, 1930–2015

HIGHLIGHTS

- There were 3,978,497 births in the United States in 2015, down from 3,988,076 in 2014. Births declined for all racial and ethnic groups. The number of births increased for non-Hispanic Blacks and Asian or Pacific Islanders; the number also increased for those of Hispanic ethnicity. (Table 1-1)

- The preliminary birth rate for teenagers age 15 to 19 years fell to 22.3 births per 1,000 females. From 2007 to 2015, this rate declined 46.38 percent. (Table 1-6)

- In 2015, 40.3 percent of all births were to unmarried women, down from 41.0 percent in 2009. The numbers varied significantly by state. Utah had the lowest number of births to unmarried woman at 18.8 percent, followed by Colorado at 22.7 percent. Mississippi had the highest percentage of births to unmarried women of any state at 53.5 percent, followed by Louisiana at 52.9 percent and New Mexico at 52.1 percent. No other state topped 50 percent. The Northern Marianas had the highest percentage of births to unmarried women of any state or territory at 81.3 percent. (Table 1-39)

Table 1-1. Selected Characteristics, by Race and Hispanic Origin of Mother, 2014 and 2015

(Number, rate, percent.)

Race and Hispanic origin of mother	Number		Birth rate		Fertility rate		Total fertility rate		Percent of births to unmarried women	
	2014	2015	2014	2015	2014	2015	2014	2015	2014	2015
All Races and Origins[1]	3,988,076	3,978,497	12.5	12.4	62.9	60.2	1,862.5	1,843.5	40.2	40.3
Non-Hispanic White[2]	2,149,302	2,130,279	10.8	10.7	59.5	59.3	1,762.5	1,746.0	29.2	29.2
Non-Hispanic Black[2]	588,891	589,047	14.4	14.2	64.5	64.1	1,873.5	1,857.0	70.9	70.6
American Indian or Alaska Native total[2,3]	44,928	44,299	9.9	9.7	44.8	43.9	1,288.5	1,262.5	65.7	65.8
Asian or Pacific Islander total[2,3]	272,949	281,264	14.6	14.0	60.7	58.5	1,715.5	1,646.0	16.4	16.4
Hispanic[4]	914,065	924,048	16.5	16.3	72.1	71.7	2,130.5	1,843.5	52.9	53.0

[1]Includes origin not stated.
[2]Race and Hispanic origin are reported separately on birth certificates. Persons of Hispanic origin may be of any race. Forty-nine states and the District of Columbia reported multiple-race data for 2015 bridged to single-race categories in order to maintain comparability among all reported areas.
[3]Includes persons of Hispanic origin, and origin not stated, according to the mother's reported race.
[4]Persons of Hispanic origin may be of any race.

Table 1-2. Births and Birth Rates, by Age, Race, and Hispanic Origin of Mother, 2014 and 2015

(Number, rate per 1,000 women in specified age group.)

Age, race, and Hispanic origin of mother	2014		2015	
	Number	Rate	Number	Rate
All Races and Origins				
Total	3,988,076	62.9	3,978,497	62.5
10 to 14 years	2,769	0.3	2,500	0.2
15 to 19 years	249,078	24.2	229,715	22.3
20 to 24 years	882,567	79.0	850,509	76.8
25 to 29 years	1,145,392	105.8	1,152,311	104.3
30 to 34 years	1,081,058	100.8	1,094,693	101.5
35 to 39 years	508,748	51.0	527,996	51.8
40 to 44 years	110,021	10.6	111,848	11.0
45 to 49 years	7,700	0.8	8,171	0.8
50 to 54 years	743	NA	754	NA
Non-Hispanic White				
Total	2,149,302	59.5	2,130,279	59.3
10 to 14 years	679	0.1	582	0.1
15 to 19 years	99,220	17.3	90,833	16.0
20 to 24 years	420,224	67.1	399,373	65.0
25 to 29 years	646,907	103.9	642,150	102.3
30 to 34 years	642,219	104.7	646,767	105.1
35 to 39 years	280,788	49.6	290,877	50.6
40 to 44 years	55,609	9.1	55,040	9.4
45 to 49 years	4,123	0.7	4,323	0.7
50 to 54 years	343	NA	334	NA
Non-Hispanic Black				
Total	588,891	64.5	589,047	64.1
10 to 14 years	955	0.6	845	0.6
15 to 19 years	54,819	34.9	50,039	31.8
20 to 24 years	182,435	102.8	175,597	100.2
25 to 29 years	160,935	103.3	165,895	102.0
30 to 34 years	116,939	79.6	119,976	81.6
35 to 39 years	57,647	42.5	60,863	43.6
40 to 44 years	14,000	10.1	14,592	10.7
45 to 49 years	1,043	0.9	1,104	0.9
50 to 54 years	118	NA	136	NA
American Indian or Alaska Native Total				
Total	44,928	47.0	44,299	43.9
10 to 14 years	55	0.5	53	0.3
15 to 19 years	5,001	34.9	4,738	25.7
20 to 24 years	14,099	81.7	13,458	70.2
25 to 29 years	12,784	73.9	12,842	73.2
30 to 34 years	8,592	49.7	8,506	51.7
35 to 39 years	3,576	22.3	3,824	25.2
40 to 44 years	784	5.5	824	5.8
45 to 49 years	35	0.5	51	0.4
50 to 54 years	2	NA	3	NA
Asian or Pacific Islander Total				
Total	282,723	44.8	281,264	58.5
10 to 14 years	40	0.3	37	0.1
15 to 19 years	4,637	27.3	4,297	6.9
20 to 24 years	27,003	37.5	26,174	35.6
25 to 29 years	74,950	90.0	73,386	84.1
30 to 34 years	105,442	121.3	105,490	117.4
35 to 39 years	56,449	68.9	57,400	67.6
40 to 44 years	13,157	16.1	13,299	15.9
45 to 49 years	911	1.5	1,067	1.6
50 to 54 years	134	NA	114	NA
Hispanic				
Total	914,065	72.1	924,048	71.7
10 to 14 years	1,037	0.4	986	0.4
15 to 19 years	85,970	38.0	80,634	34.9
20 to 24 years	239,121	104.5	236,264	102.1
25 to 29 years	248,171	118.7	256,106	119.3
30 to 34 years	204,232	96.5	209,647	98.6
35 to 39 years	107,644	53.6	112,045	54.5
40 to 44 years	25,636	13.5	27,117	14.0
45 to 49 years	1,374	0.9	1,433	0.9
50 to 54 years	80	NA	86	NA

Note: Race and Hispanic origin are reported separately on birth certificates. Race categories are consistent with 1977 Office of Management and Budget standards. Forty-nine states and the District of Columbia reported multiple-race data for 2015 that were bridged to single-race categories for comparability with other states. Multiple-race reporting areas vary for 2003–2015. Includes births to women of all ages. The rate shown for all ages is the fertility rate, which is defined as the total number of births (regardless of the age of the mother) per 1,000 women age 15 to 44 years. The birth rate for women age 45 to 49 years is computed by relating the number of births to women age 45 and over to women age 45 to 49 years, as most of the births are to women age 45 to 49 years.
NA = Not applicable.

Table 1-3. Live Births, by Age of Mother, Live-Birth Order, and Race and Hispanic Origin of Mother, 2015

(Number.)

Live-birth order and race and Hispanic origin of mother	All ages	Under 15 years	15 to 19 years	20 to 24 years	25 to 29 years	30 to 34 years	35 to 39 years	40 to 44 years	45 to 49 years	50 to 54 years
All Races and Origins	3,978,497	2,500	229,715	850,509	1,152,311	1,094,693	527,996	111,848	8,171	754
1st child	1,525,594	2,474	190,538	431,994	427,498	327,605	118,881	23,976	2,396	232
2nd child	1,270,034	16	33,353	278,360	381,675	373,560	170,125	30,784	1,996	165
3rd child	671,884	3	4,405	100,438	209,268	216,642	116,648	23,048	1,317	115
4th child	288,766	1	481	27,457	84,359	99,450	61,592	14,431	907	88
5th child	112,207	–	62	6,539	28,778	40,288	28,101	7,846	541	52
6th child	46,100	–	9	1,394	9,747	17,079	13,422	4,117	305	27
7th child	21,247	–	4	324	3,265	7,736	7,252	2,436	198	32
8th child and over	22,245	–	10	308	1,753	6,279	8,942	4,473	447	33
Not stated	20,420	6	853	3,695	5,968	6,054	3,033	737	64	10
Non-Hispanic White	2,130,279	582	90,833	399,373	642,150	646,767	290,877	55,040	4,323	334
1st child	855,738	578	77,564	214,704	265,180	210,258	72,352	13,580	1,412	110
2nd child	709,069	2	11,576	129,850	217,327	233,048	99,881	16,198	1,104	83
3rd child	339,155	–	1,278	41,233	103,301	119,822	62,068	10,751	653	49
4th child	130,385	–	99	9,641	37,170	48,678	28,532	5,853	382	30
5th child	46,732	–	18	1,873	11,302	18,019	12,289	2,990	219	22
6th child	18,947	–	1	331	3,353	7,542	5,976	1,604	133	7
7th child	9,172	–	2	70	1,014	3,467	3,431	1,081	91	16
8th child and over	11,134	–	4	140	541	2,659	4,831	2,653	294	12
Not stated	9,947	2	291	1,531	2,962	3,274	1,517	330	35	5
Non-Hispanic Black	589,047	845	50,039	175,597	165,895	119,976	60,863	14,592	1,104	136
1st child	214,195	838	40,901	84,422	46,747	26,951	11,315	2,690	283	48
2nd child	168,767	5	7,553	54,961	52,024	34,643	15,849	3,458	250	24
3rd child	105,219	2	1,174	23,918	35,447	27,177	14,162	3,128	186	25
4th child	51,857	–	141	8,081	17,825	14,958	8,649	2,063	129	11
5th child	23,378	–	18	2,320	7,580	7,623	4,506	1,235	88	8
6th child	10,538	–	5	567	3,116	3,700	2,406	682	58	4
7th child	5,104	–	–	145	1,197	1,891	1,416	413	38	4
8th child and over	5,458	–	3	104	668	1,919	1,933	764	60	7
Not stated	4,531	–	244	1,079	1,291	1,114	627	159	12	5
American Indian or Alaska Native	44,299	53	4,738	13,458	12,842	8,506	3,824	824	51	3
1st child	14,233	53	3,853	5,593	2,824	1,306	480	116	8	–
2nd child	12,032	–	745	4,619	3,791	1,987	745	135	9	1
3rd child	8,299	–	108	2,208	3,023	2,005	793	152	9	1
4th child	4,761	–	13	743	1,780	1,405	681	132	7	–
5th child	2,451	–	1	195	843	855	450	102	5	–
6th child	1,236	–	–	38	365	477	282	67	6	1
7th child	613	–	1	14	126	250	179	43	–	–
8th child and over	511	–	–	5	44	188	194	73	7	–
Not stated	163	–	17	43	46	33	20	4	–	–
Asian or Pacific Islander	281,264	37	4,297	26,174	73,386	105,490	57,400	13,299	1,067	114
1st child	125,015	36	3,573	16,043	40,792	44,232	16,404	3,540	358	37
2nd child	101,583	1	608	7,135	21,435	42,004	24,963	5,086	325	26
3rd child	34,504	–	88	2,133	7,035	12,242	10,159	2,654	174	19
4th child	11,443	–	9	565	2,371	3,983	3,328	1,071	96	20
5th child	4,073	–	–	137	852	1,401	1,213	421	45	4
6th child	1,652	–	–	20	293	611	502	196	27	3
7th child	761	–	–	10	102	244	264	124	15	2
8th child and over	742	–	–	3	59	222	291	141	23	3
Not stated	1,491	–	19	128	447	551	276	66	4	–
Hispanic[1]	924,048	986	80,364	236,264	256,106	209,647	112,045	27,117	1,433	86
1st child	312,163	973	65,109	111,257	70,850	42,661	17,248	3,745	292	28
2nd child	275,951	8	12,970	82,071	86,689	60,604	27,724	5,595	272	18
3rd child	183,861	1	1,780	31,068	60,423	55,071	29,029	6,216	267	6
4th child	90,009	1	218	8,496	25,166	30,323	20,285	5,250	261	9
5th child	35,427	–	26	2,025	8,185	12,359	9,574	3,084	164	10
6th child	13,569	–	2	438	2,608	4,688	4,207	1,545	75	6
7th child	5,482	–	1	85	818	1,840	1,923	765	45	5
8th child and over	4,150	–	3	56	429	1,239	1,586	782	51	4
Not stated	3,436	3	255	768	938	862	469	135	6	–

Note: Race and Hispanic origin are reported separately on birth certificates. Race categories are consistent with 1977 Office of Management and Budget standards. Forty-nine states and the District of Columbia reported multiple-race data for 2015 that were bridged to single-race categories for comparability with other states.
- = Quantity zero.
[1]Persons of Hispanic origin may be of any race.

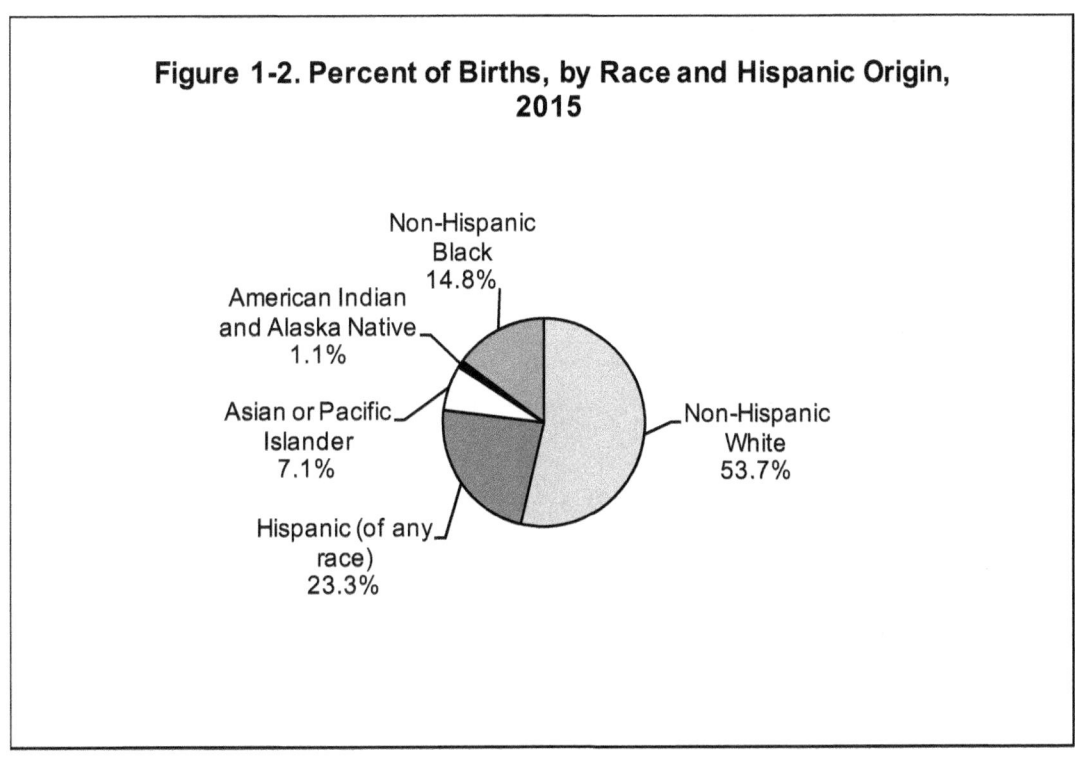

Figure 1-2. Percent of Births, by Race and Hispanic Origin, 2015

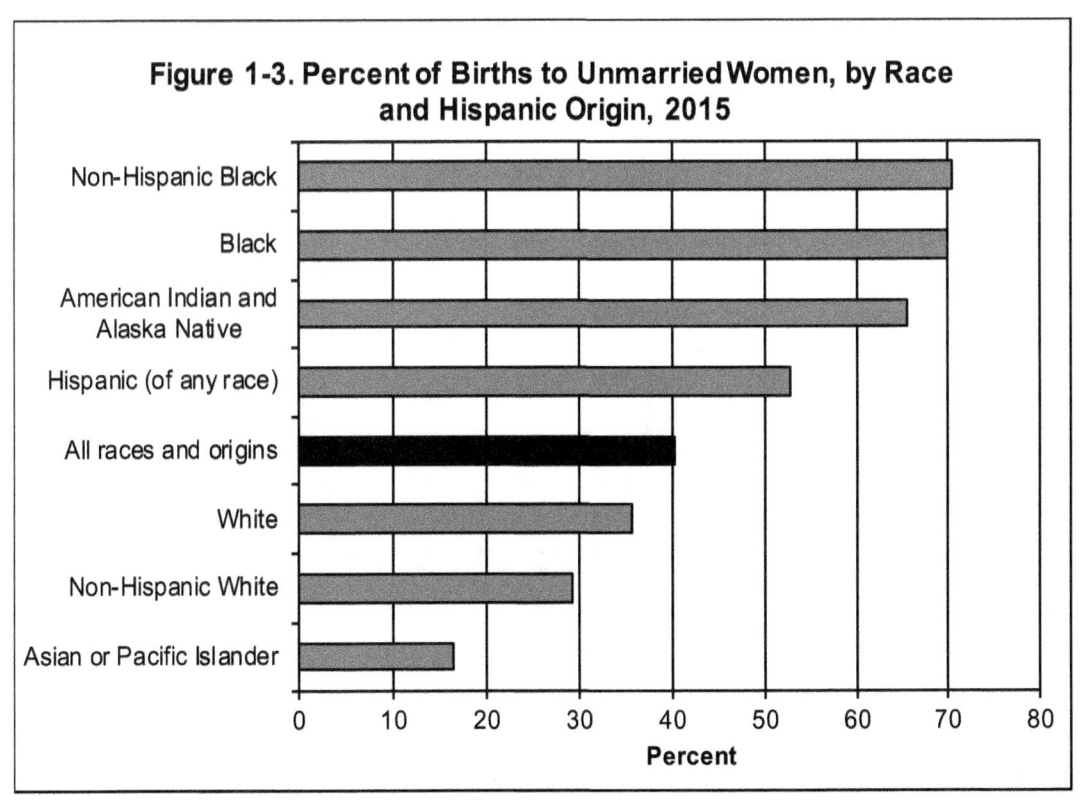

Figure 1-3. Percent of Births to Unmarried Women, by Race and Hispanic Origin, 2015

Table 1-4. Live Births, by Age of Mother, Live-Birth Order, and Race and Hispanic Origin of Mother, 2015

(Number.)

Live-birth order and race and Hispanic origin of mother	All ages	Under 15 years	15 to 19 years	20 to 24 years	25 to 29 years	30 to 34 years	35 to 39 years	40 to 44 years	45 to 49 years	50 to 54 years
All Races and Origins	3,978,497	2,500	229,715	850,509	1,152,311	1,094,693	527,996	111,848	8,171	754
1st child	1,525,594	2,474	190,538	431,994	427,498	327,605	118,881	23,976	2,396	232
2nd child	1,270,034	16	33,353	278,360	381,675	373,560	170,125	30,784	1,996	165
3rd child	671,884	3	4,405	100,438	209,268	216,642	116,648	23,048	1,317	115
4th child	288,766	1	481	27,457	84,359	99,450	61,592	14,431	907	88
5th child	112,207	–	62	6,539	28,778	40,288	28,101	7,846	541	52
6th child	46,100	–	9	1,394	9,747	17,079	13,422	4,117	305	27
7th child	21,247	–	4	324	3,265	7,736	7,252	2,436	198	32
8th child and over	22,245	–	10	308	1,753	6,279	8,942	4,473	447	33
Not stated	20,420	6	853	3,695	5,968	6,054	3,033	737	64	10
Non-Hispanic White	2,130,279	582	90,833	399,373	642,150	646,767	290,877	55,040	4,323	334
1st child	855,738	578	77,564	214,704	265,180	210,258	72,352	13,580	1,412	110
2nd child	709,069	2	11,576	129,850	217,327	233,048	99,881	16,198	1,104	83
3rd child	339,155	–	1,278	41,233	103,301	119,822	62,068	10,751	653	49
4th child	130,385	–	99	9,641	37,170	48,678	28,532	5,853	382	30
5th child	46,732	–	18	1,873	11,302	18,019	12,289	2,990	219	22
6th child	18,947	–	1	331	3,353	7,542	5,976	1,604	133	7
7th child	9,172	–	2	70	1,014	3,467	3,431	1,081	91	16
8th child and over	11,134	–	4	140	541	2,659	4,831	2,653	294	12
Not stated	9,947	2	291	1,531	2,962	3,274	1,517	330	35	5
Non-Hispanic Black	589,047	845	50,039	175,597	165,895	119,976	60,863	14,592	1,104	136
1st child	214,195	838	40,901	84,422	46,747	26,951	11,315	2,690	283	48
2nd child	168,767	5	7,553	54,961	52,024	34,643	15,849	3,458	250	24
3rd child	105,219	2	1,174	23,918	35,447	27,177	14,162	3,128	186	25
4th child	51,857	–	141	8,081	17,825	14,958	8,649	2,063	129	11
5th child	23,378	–	18	2,320	7,580	7,623	4,506	1,235	88	8
6th child	10,538	–	5	567	3,116	3,700	2,406	682	58	4
7th child	5,104	–	–	145	1,197	1,891	1,416	413	38	4
8th child and over	5,458	–	3	104	668	1,919	1,933	764	60	7
Not stated	4,531	–	244	1,079	1,291	1,114	627	159	12	5
American Indian or Alaska Native	44,299	53	4,738	13,458	12,842	8,506	3,824	824	51	3
1st child	14,233	53	3,853	5,593	2,824	1,306	480	116	8	–
2nd child	12,032	–	745	4,619	3,791	1,987	745	135	9	1
3rd child	8,299	–	108	2,208	3,023	2,005	793	152	9	1
4th child	4,761	–	13	743	1,780	1,405	681	132	7	–
5th child	2,451	–	1	195	843	855	450	102	5	–
6th child	1,236	–	–	38	365	477	282	67	6	1
7th child	613	–	1	14	126	250	179	43	–	–
8th child and over	511	–	–	5	44	188	194	73	7	–
Not stated	163	–	17	43	46	33	20	4	–	–
Asian or Pacific Islander	281,264	37	4,297	26,174	73,386	105,490	57,400	13,299	1,067	114
1st child	125,015	36	3,573	16,043	40,792	44,232	16,404	3,540	358	37
2nd child	101,583	1	608	7,135	21,435	42,004	24,963	5,086	325	26
3rd child	34,504	–	88	2,133	7,035	12,242	10,159	2,654	174	19
4th child	11,443	–	9	565	2,371	3,983	3,328	1,071	96	20
5th child	4,073	–	–	137	852	1,401	1,213	421	45	4
6th child	1,652	–	–	20	293	611	502	196	27	3
7th child	761	–	–	10	102	244	264	124	15	2
8th child and over	742	–	–	3	59	222	291	141	23	3
Not stated	1,491	–	19	128	447	551	276	66	4	–
Hispanic[1]	924,048	986	80,364	236,264	256,106	209,647	112,045	27,117	1,433	86
1st child	312,163	973	65,109	111,257	70,850	42,661	17,248	3,745	292	28
2nd child	275,951	8	12,970	82,071	86,689	60,604	27,724	5,595	272	18
3rd child	183,861	1	1,780	31,068	60,423	55,071	29,029	6,216	267	6
4th child	90,009	1	218	8,496	25,166	30,323	20,285	5,250	261	9
5th child	35,427	–	26	2,025	8,185	12,359	9,574	3,084	164	10
6th child	13,569	–	2	438	2,608	4,688	4,207	1,545	75	6
7th child	5,482	–	1	85	818	1,840	1,923	765	45	5
8th child and over	4,150	–	3	56	429	1,239	1,586	782	51	4
Not stated	3,436	3	255	768	938	862	469	135	6	–

Note: Race and Hispanic origin are reported separately on birth certificates. Race categories are consistent with 1977 Office of Management and Budget standards. Forty-nine states and the District of Columbia reported multiple-race data for 2015 that were bridged to single-race categories for comparability with other states.
- = Quantity zero.
[1]Persons of Hispanic origin may be of any race.

Table 1-5. Birth Rates for Women Under 20 Years of Age, by Age and Race and Hispanic Origin of Mother, Selected Years, 1991–2015

(Rates per 1,000 women in specified group.)

Age, race, and Hispanic origin of mother	Year					Percent change		
	1991	2007	2010	2014	2015	1991–2015	2007–2015	2014–2015
10 to 14 Years								
All races and origins	1.4	0.6	0.4	0.3	0.2	-85.7	-66.7	-33.3
Non-Hispanic White	0.5	0.2	0.2	0.1	0.1	20.0	-50.0	†
Non-Hispanic Black	4.9	1.4	1.0	0.6	0.6	-93.9	-78.6	†
American Indian or Alaska Native total	1.6	0.7	0.5	0.3	0.3	-81.3	-57.1	†
Asian or Pacific Islander total	0.8	0.2	0.1	0.1	0.1	-87.5	-50.0	†
Hispanic	2.4	1.2	0.8	0.4	0.4	-83.3	-66.7	†
15 to 19 Years								
All races and origins	61.8	41.5	34.2	24.2	22.3	-63.9	-46.3	-7.9
Non-Hispanic White	43.4	27.2	23.5	17.3	16.0	-63.1	-41.2	-7.5
Non-Hispanic Black	118.2	62.0	51.5	34.9	31.8	-73.1	-48.7	-8.9
American Indian or Alaska Native total	84.1	49.3	38.7	27.3	25.7	-69.4	-47.9	-5.9
Asian or Pacific Islander total	27.3	14.8	10.9	7.7	6.9	-74.7	-53.4	-10.4
Hispanic	104.6	75.3	55.7	38.0	34.9	-66.6	-53.7	-8.2
15 to 17 Years								
All races and origins	38.6	21.7	17.3	10.9	9.9	-74.4	-54.4	-9.2
Non-Hispanic White	23.6	11.9	10.0	6.7	6.0	-74.6	-49.6	-10.4
Non-Hispanic Black	86.1	34.6	27.4	16.6	15.3	-82.2	-55.8	-7.8
American Indian or Alaska Native total	51.9	26.1	20.1	13.2	12.7	-75.5	-51.3	-3.8
Asian or Pacific Islander total	16.3	7.4	5.1	3.3	2.7	-83.4	-63.5	-18.2
Hispanic	69.2	44.4	32.3	19.3	17.4	-74.9	-60.8	-9.8
18 to 19 Years								
All races and origins	94.0	71.7	58.2	43.8	40.7	-56.7	-43.2	-7.1
Non-Hispanic White	70.6	50.4	42.5	32.9	30.6	-56.7	-39.3	-7.0
Non-Hispanic Black	162.2	105.2	85.6	61.5	56.7	-65.0	-46.1	-7.8
American Indian or Alaska Native total	134.2	86.3	66.1	48.6	45.8	-65.9	-46.9	-5.8
Asian or Pacific Islander total	42.2	24.9	18.7	13.9	12.8	-69.7	-48.6	-7.9
Hispanic	155.5	124.7	90.7	66.1	61.9	-60.2	-50.4	-6.4

Note: Race and Hispanic origin are reported separately on birth certificates. Race categories are consistent with 1977 Office of Management and Budget standards. Forty-nine states and the District of Columbia reported multiple-race data for 2015 that were bridged to single-race categories for comparability with other states. Persons of Hispanic origin may be of any race.
† = Difference not statistically significant.

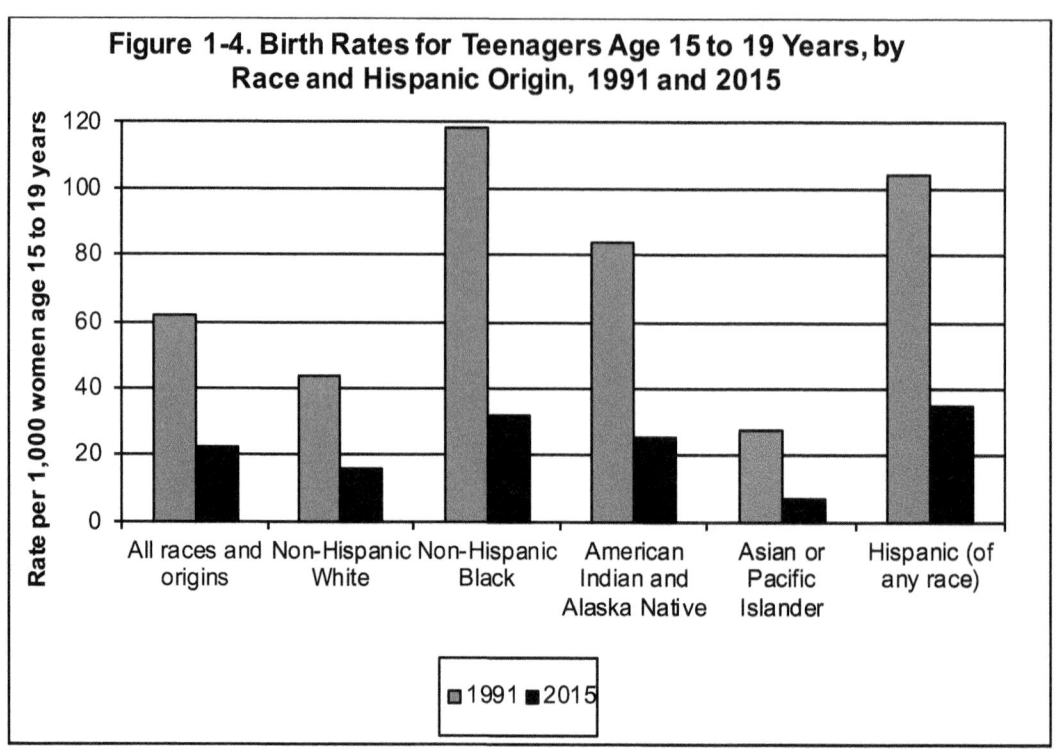

Figure 1-4. Birth Rates for Teenagers Age 15 to 19 Years, by Race and Hispanic Origin, 1991 and 2015

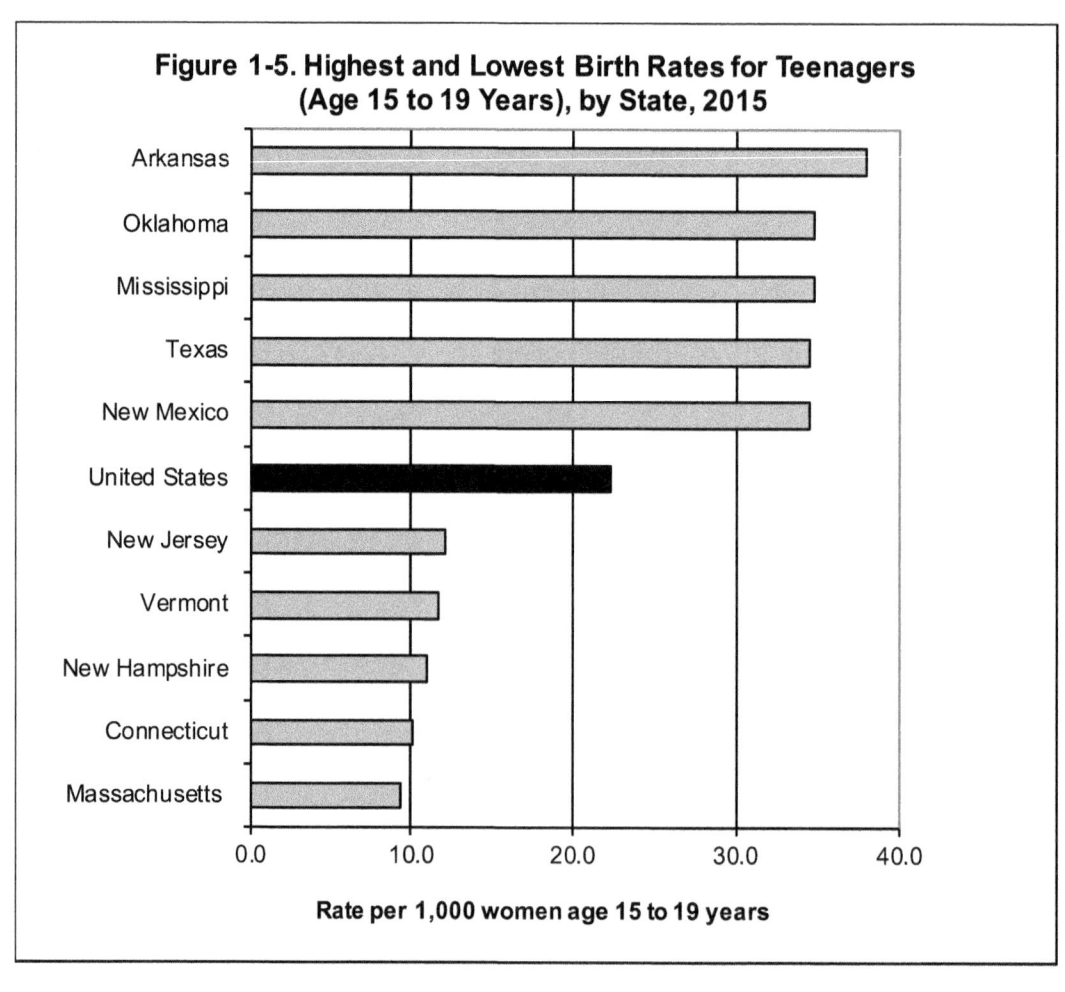

Figure 1-5. Highest and Lowest Birth Rates for Teenagers (Age 15 to 19 Years), by State, 2015

Table 1-6. Birth Rate for Teenagers Age 15 to 19 Years, by State, 2007 and 2015

(Rate per 1,000 female population age 15 to 19 years.)

State	2007	2015	Percent change
United States	41.5	22.3	-46.3
Alabama	52.1	30.1	-42.2
Alaska	42.9	29.3	-31.7
Arizona	59.6	26.3	-55.9
Arkansas	60.1	38.0	-36.8
California	39.6	19.0	-52.0
Colorado	41.6	19.3	-53.6
Connecticut	23.0	10.1	-56.1
Delaware	39.2	18.1	-53.8
District of Columbia	50.4	25.6	-49.2
Florida	43.0	20.8	-51.6
Georgia	53.4	25.6	-52.1
Hawaii	38.7	20.6	-46.8
Idaho	39.9	22.5	-43.6
Illinois	40.2	21.1	-47.5
Indiana	43.0	26.0	-39.5
Iowa	32.8	18.6	-43.3
Kansas	42.5	25.5	-40.0
Kentucky	52.6	32.4	-38.4
Louisiana	55.2	34.1	-38.2
Maine	26.0	15.4	-40.8
Maryland	34.3	17.0	-50.4
Massachusetts	21.4	9.4	-56.1
Michigan	33.5	19.4	-42.1
Minnesota	27.9	13.7	-50.9
Mississippi	70.1	34.8	-50.4
Missouri	44.0	25.0	-43.2
Montana	35.3	25.3	-28.3
Nebraska	35.5	22.0	-38.0
Nevada	51.7	27.6	-46.6
New Hampshire	19.3	10.9	-43.5
New Jersey	24.9	12.1	-51.4
New Mexico	63.9	34.6	-45.9
New York	26.0	14.6	-43.8
North Carolina	48.0	23.6	-50.8
North Dakota	29.2	22.2	-24.0
Ohio	39.9	23.2	-41.9
Oklahoma	58.5	34.8	-40.5
Oregon	34.5	19	-44.9
Pennsylvania	30.7	17.7	-42.3
Rhode Island	29.2	14.3	-51.0
South Carolina	51.9	26.2	-49.5
South Dakota	41.3	26.4	-36.1
Tennessee	53.4	30.5	-42.9
Texas	61.8	34.6	-44.0
Utah	35.4	17.6	-50.3
Vermont	21.0	11.6	-44.8
Virginia	34.2	17.1	-50.0
Washington	33.3	17.6	-47.1
West Virginia	45.8	31.9	-30.3
Wisconsin	31.1	16.2	-47.9
Wyoming	49.9	29.2	-41.5

Table 1-7. Selected Characteristics of Births, by Race and Hispanic Origin of Mother, 2011 and 2015

(Number; percent.)

Race and Hispanic origin of mother	Number		Cesarean[1]		Preterm				Low birthweight			
					Total[2]		Late[3]		Total[4]		Very low birthweight[5]	
	2011	2015	2011	2015	2011	2015	2011	2015	2011	2015	2011	2015
All Races and Origins[6]	3,953,590	3,988,076	32.8	32.0	11.7	9.6	8.3	8.1	8.1	8.1	1.4	1.4
Non-Hispanic White[7]	2,146,566	2,149,302	32.4	31.1	10.5	8.9	7.6	6.5	7.1	6.9	1.1	1.1
Non-Hispanic Black[7]	582,345	588,891	35.5	35.5	16.8	13.4	10.7	6.5	13.3	13.3	3.0	2.9
American Indian or Alaska Native total[7]	46,419	44,928	28.4	28.3	13.5	10.5	9.6	7.7	7.6	7.5	1.3	1.3
Asian or Pacific Islander total[7]	253,915	272,949	33.2	33.0	10.4	8.6	7.6	6.4	8.4	8.4	1.2	1.3
Hispanic[8]	918,129	914,065	32.0	31.7	11.7	9.1	8.4	6.8	7.0	7.2	1.2	1.1

[1]Percentage of all live births by cesarean delivery.
[2]Born prior to 37 completed weeks of gestation.
[3]Born between 34 and 36 completed weeks of gestation.
[4]Birthweight of less than 2,500 grams (5 lb 8 oz).
[5]Birthweight of less than 1,500 grams (3 lb 4 oz).
[6]Includes births to White Hispanic and Black Hispanic women and births with origin not stated, not shown separately.
[7]Race and Hispanic origin are reported separately on birth certificates. Persons of Hispanic origin may be of any race. Race categories are consistent with 1977 Office of Management and Budget standards. Forty-nine states and the District of Columbia reported multiple-race data for 2015 that were bridged to single-race categories for comparability with other states.
[8]Persons of Hispanic origin may be of any race.

Table 1-8. Low Birthweight Births, by Race and Hispanic Origin of Mother and State and Territory of Residence, 2015

(Number, percent. Low birthweight is birthweight of less than 2,500 grams [5 lb. 8 oz.])

State and territory	Number All races[1]	Number Non-Hispanic White[2]	Number Non-Hispanic Black[2]	Number Hispanic[3]	Percent All races[1]	Percent Non-Hispanic White[2]	Percent Non-Hispanic Black[2]	Percent Hispanic[3]
United States[4]	320,869	147,479	78,514	66,623	8.1	6.9	13.3	7.2
Alabama	6,218	2,892	2,898	305	10.4	8.1	15.9	7.1
Alaska	653	341	37	52	5.8	5.2	8.7	6.4
Arizona	6,128	2,442	557	2,454	7.2	6.6	12.2	7.0
Arkansas	3,564	1,990	1,169	267	9.2	7.7	15.4	6.7
California	33,666	8,369	3,112	15,246	6.8	5.9	11.5	6.5
Colorado	6,001	3,459	456	1,611	9.0	8.5	13.2	8.9
Connecticut	2,836	1,332	563	702	7.9	6.5	12.7	8.5
Delaware	1,036	457	394	133	9.3	7.7	13.2	8.7
District of Columbia	959	207	635	87	10.0	7.0	13.2	6.6
Florida	19,306	7,328	6,547	4,666	8.6	7.1	13.2	7.3
Georgia	12,464	4,278	6,270	1,235	9.5	7.1	13.8	6.9
Hawaii	1,531	276	64	232	8.3	5.8	11.1	8.4
Idaho	1,501	1,157	27	252	6.6	6.4	11.3	6.9
Illinois	13,069	5,834	3,727	2,407	8.3	6.8	13.7	7.1
Indiana	6,725	4,709	1,283	538	8.0	7.4	12.4	7.1
Iowa	2,663	2,073	252	219	6.7	6.5	10.1	6.4
Kansas	2,672	1,844	337	369	6.8	6.5	11.6	5.9
Kentucky	4,846	3,813	730	195	8.7	8.2	13.9	6.5
Louisiana	6,839	2,708	3,618	346	10.6	8.0	15.0	7.2
Maine	871	782	47	17	6.9	6.8	10.2	*
Maryland	6,297	2,164	2,796	841	8.6	6.7	11.8	7.2
Massachusetts	5,312	2,816	743	1,071	7.5	6.5	10.6	8.3
Michigan	9,612	5,486	3,119	555	8.5	7.0	14.3	7.5
Minnesota	4,494	2,881	754	293	6.4	5.8	9.4	6.0
Mississippi	4,387	1,533	2,704	91	11.4	7.8	16.5	5.6
Missouri	6,248	4,114	1,628	290	8.3	7.2	14.4	7.2
Montana	887	702	11	42	7.1	6.8	*	7.3
Nebraska	1,893	1,242	255	290	7.1	6.5	13.6	6.8
Nevada	3,093	1,168	605	970	8.5	7.8	13.6	7.3
New Hampshire	852	732	23	44	6.9	6.7	9.7	6.9
New Jersey	8,345	3,220	1,817	2,141	8.1	6.8	12.2	7.7
New Mexico	2,244	605	66	1,275	8.7	8.5	14.0	8.9
New York	18,507	7,277	4,359	4,335	7.8	6.4	12.0	7.8
North Carolina	11,023	4,998	4,142	1,252	9.1	7.5	14.4	6.9
North Dakota	700	531	41	42	6.2	6.0	7.2	7.2
Ohio	11,807	7,514	3,296	535	8.5	7.3	13.9	7.7
Oklahoma	4,172	2,429	675	540	7.9	7.3	13.5	7.3
Oregon	2,919	1,935	125	571	6.4	6.0	9.4	6.7
Pennsylvania	11,453	6,751	2,631	1,300	8.2	6.9	13.2	8.7
Rhode Island	833	460	104	205	7.6	6.9	10.9	7.8
South Carolina	5,535	2,485	2,579	315	9.5	7.3	14.5	6.4
South Dakota	754	525	19	31	6.1	5.8	*	5.5
Tennessee	7,460	4,312	2,452	490	9.2	7.8	14.7	6.8
Texas	33,275	10,016	6,526	14,676	8.2	7.1	13.1	7.7
Utah	3,561	2,547	60	652	7.0	6.6	9.3	8.3
Vermont	390	340	14	13	6.6	6.3	*	*
Virginia	8,111	3,881	2,654	891	7.9	6.6	12.2	6.4
Washington	5,730	3,228	453	980	6.4	5.8	9.8	6.1
West Virginia	1,891	1,735	95	26	9.6	9.4	13.6	7.9
Wisconsin	4,870	3,059	1,037	442	7.3	6.2	14.6	6.7
Wyoming	666	502	8	91	8.6	8.1	*	9.5
Puerto Rico	3,282	176	13	3,082	10.5	12.1	*	10.5
Virgin Islands	114	12	82	16	9.2	*	9	*
Guam	307	5	-	1	9.2	*	*	*
American Samoa	34	NA	NA	NA	3,2	NA	NA	NA
Northern Marianas	33	-	-	-	7.8	*	*	*

NA = Not available.
- = Quantity zero.
* = Figure does not meet standards of reliability or precision; based on fewer than 20 births in the numerator.
[1]Includes races other than White and Black and origin not stated.
[2]Race and Hispanic origin are reported separately on birth certificates. Persons of Hispanic origin may be of any race. Race categories are consistent with 1977 Office of Management and Budget standards. Forty-nine states and the District of Columbia reported multiple-race data for 2015 that were bridged to single-race categories for comparability with other states.
[3]Includes all persons of Hispanic origin of any race.
[4]Excludes data for the territories.

Table 1-9. Preterm Births, 2007–2015

(Percent.)

Year	Total preterm[1]	Late preterm[2]	Early preterm (less than 34 weeks)		
			Total	32–33 weeks	Less than 32 weeks
	Percentage				
2007	10.4	7.5	2.9	1.2	1.7
2008	10.4	7.5	2.9	1.2	1.7
2009	10.1	7.2	2.8	1.2	1.7
2010	10.0	7.2	2.8	1.2	1.7
2011	9.8	7.0	2.8	1.2	1.6
2012	9.8	7.0	2.8	1.2	1.6
2013	9.6	6.8	2.8	1.2	1.6
2014	9.6	6.8	2.7	1.1	1.6
2015	9.6	6.9		1.2	1.6

[1]Preterm is less than 37 completed weeks of gestation.
[2]Late preterm is 34 to 36 completed weeks of gestation.

Table 1-10. Preterm Births, by Race and Hispanic Origin of Mother and State and Territory of Residence, 2015

(Number, percent. Preterm is under 37 completed weeks of gestation based on the obstetric estimate.)

State and territory	Number All races[1]	Non-Hispanic White[2]	Non-Hispanic Black[2]	Hispanic[3]	Percent All races[1]	Non-Hispanic White[2]	Non-Hispanic Black[2]	Hispanic[3]
United States[4]	382,786	189,146	78,911	84,418	9.6	8.9	13.4	9.1
Alabama	6,999	3,666	2,818	395	11.7	10.2	15.4	9.2
Alaska	1,008	505	40	59	9.0	7.7	9.5	7.3
Arizona	7,724	3,132	573	3,208	9.1	8.5	12.5	9.1
Arkansas	4,207	2,554	1,147	355	10.8	9.9	15.1	8.9
California	41,600	10,835	3,180	20,075	8.5	7.7	11.8	8.6
Colorado	5,770	3,348	389	1,613	8.7	8.2	11.3	8.9
Connecticut	3,340	1,674	555	869	9.4	8.2	12.5	10.5
Delaware	1,101	565	348	140	9.9	9.5	11.7	9.1
District of Columbia	984	227	605	108	10.3	7.6	12.6	8.1
Florida	22,407	9,175	6,696	5,764	10.0	9.0	13.5	9.0
Georgia	14,133	5,708	6,189	1,579	10.8	9.5	13.6	8.9
Hawaii	1,861	363	75	297	10.1	7.6	13.0	10.7
Idaho	1,859	1,436	25	319	8.2	7.9	10.4	8.8
Illinois	16,048	7,880	3,822	3,243	10.2	9.2	14.1	9.6
Indiana	8,061	5,828	1,326	707	9.6	9.2	12.8	9.3
Iowa	3,565	2,853	257	305	9.0	8.9	10.3	8.9
Kansas	3,426	2,410	332	522	8.8	8.5	11.4	8.3
Kentucky	6,026	4,950	700	266	10.8	10.7	13.3	8.9
Louisiana	7,964	3,575	3,735	466	12.3	10.5	15.5	9.7
Maine	1,065	977	44	21	8.5	8.5	9.5	8.4
Maryland	7,380	2,831	2,964	1,076	10.0	8.7	12.6	9.2
Massachusetts	6,002	3,394	734	1,199	8.4	7.8	10.5	9.2
Michigan	11,200	7,039	3,033	669	9.9	8.9	13.9	9.0
Minnesota	5,906	4,096	756	392	8.5	8.3	9.4	8.1
Mississippi	5,008	2,146	2,642	144	13.1	10.9	16.1	8.9
Missouri	7,504	5,353	1,572	358	10.0	9.4	13.9	8.9
Montana	1,059	799	7	54	8.4	7.8	*	9.4
Nebraska	2,629	1,830	242	430	9.9	9.5	13.0	10.1
Nevada	3,609	1,396	591	1,218	10.0	9.4	13.3	9.2
New Hampshire	981	851	22	58	7.9	7.8	9.4	9.1
New Jersey	10,064	4,151	1,977	2,729	9.8	8.8	13.3	9.8
New Mexico	2,462	685	55	1,358	9.5	9.6	11.7	9.4
New York	20,531	8,658	4,365	5,040	8.7	7.6	12.0	9.0
North Carolina	12,297	6,086	4,023	1,566	10.2	9.1	13.9	8.7
North Dakota	955	707	37	54	8.4	8.0	6.5	9.3
Ohio	14,300	9,758	3,341	730	10.3	9.4	14.1	10.5
Oklahoma	5,485	3,355	704	675	10.3	10.1	14.1	9.1
Oregon	3,459	2,363	120	688	7.6	7.4	9.0	8.1
Pennsylvania	13,224	8,470	2,544	1,465	9.4	8.7	12.6	9.8
Rhode Island	947	548	103	237	8.6	8.2	10.8	9.0
South Carolina	6,429	3,197	2,604	460	11.1	9.4	14.6	9.3
South Dakota	1,053	707	23	50	8.5	7.8	7.0	8.9
Tennessee	8,959	5,617	2,485	668	11.0	10.2	14.8	9.2
Texas	41,019	13,494	6,717	18,797	10.2	9.6	13.5	9.8
Utah	4,722	3,451	58	822	9.3	9.0	9.0	10.4
Vermont	429	386	10	12	7.3	7.2	*	*
Virginia	9,549	4,913	2,750	1,174	9.3	8.3	12.6	8.4
Washington	7,216	4,247	475	1,270	8.1	7.7	10.3	7.9
West Virginia	2,227	2,058	101	26	11.3	11.2	14.5	7.9
Wisconsin	6,271	4,314	996	585	9.4	8.8	14.1	8.9
Wyoming	762	585	4	103	9.8	9.4	*	10.7
Puerto Rico	3,547	163	14	3,360	11.4	11.2	*	11.4
Virgin Islands	110	10	81	16	10.6	*	10.8	*
Guam	335	10	-	1	10.0	*	*	*
American Samoa	NA	NA	NA	NA	NA	NA	NA	NA
Northern Marianas	41	-	-	-	9.7	*	*	*

NA = Not available.
- = Quantity zero.
* = Figure does not meet standards of reliability or precision; based on fewer than 20 births in the numerator.
[1]Includes races other than White and Black and origin not stated.
[2]Race and Hispanic origin are reported separately on birth certificates. Persons of Hispanic origin may be of any race. Race categories are consistent with 1977 Office of Management and Budget standards. Forty-nine states and the District of Columbia reported multiple-race data for 2015 that were bridged to single-race categories for comparability with other states.
[3]Includes all persons of Hispanic origin of any race.
[4]Excludes data for the territories.

Table 1-11. Total Cesarean Delivery and Low-Risk Cesarean Delivery, by Race and Hispanic Origin of Mother and State and Territory of Residence, 2015

(Percent.)

State and territory	Total cesarean delivery rate[1]				Low-risk cesarean delivery rate[2]			
	All races[3]	Non-Hispanic		Hispanic[5]	All races[3]	Non-Hispanic		Hispanic[5]
		White[4]	Black[4]			White[4]	Black[4]	
United States[6]	32.0	31.1	35.5	31.7	25.8	24.8	29.7	25.2
Alabama	35.2	35.4	37.3	26.0	28.5	27.8	30.8	23.4
Alaska	22.9	24.8	32.9	28.1	20.2	21.2	34.3	21.1
Arizona	27.6	28.2	32.4	26.4	22.5	22.7	28.3	21.5
Arkansas	32.3	32.4	32.8	30.3	24.8	24.9	25.0	23.5
California	32.3	31.1	37.3	32.1	25.3	24.6	29.5	25.1
Colorado	25.9	26.4	29.8	23.6	20.6	21.1	25.2	18.0
Connecticut	34.0	33.5	36.6	33.1	28.3	27.6	31.9	26.9
Delaware	31.9	31.8	33.3	29.4	25.3	25.0	27.7	21.9
District of Columbia	31.9	30.2	34.3	26.1	27.1	25.0	29.5	23.9
Florida	37.3	34.4	38.6	41.2	31.0	27.9	31.8	36.1
Georgia	33.6	33.5	35.5	29.1	27.7	26.9	30.0	23.3
Hawaii	25.9	24.5	28.3	25.6	20.3	16.6	20.4	21.1
Idaho	24.4	23.9	25.9	26.3	19.5	19.2	*	20.1
Illinois	31.0	31.0	31.7	29.2	24.2	24.0	25.0	22.8
Indiana	29.6	29.5	32.2	27.3	22.9	22.6	26.0	19.0
Iowa	29.8	29.7	30.4	29.8	23.8	23.7	26.0	22.8
Kansas	29.6	30.2	31.7	26.2	23.8	23.8	25.0	21.6
Kentucky	34.4	34.4	36.6	31.3	27.4	27.0	29.9	27.2
Louisiana	37.5	38.5	37.2	32.9	30.8	31.0	30.8	29.2
Maine	29.4	29.4	29.6	29.5	22.9	22.7	25.0	24.1
Maryland	34.9	32.7	39.6	30.7	29.9	26.9	35.2	25.8
Massachusetts	31.4	31.5	35.3	30.4	24.0	24.1	29.2	22.1
Michigan	31.9	31.9	32.1	30.6	26.3	25.8	27.8	26.0
Minnesota	26.5	27.0	28.3	25.0	21.6	21.3	25.9	19.5
Mississippi	38.0	38.1	38.7	32.0	31.2	30.7	31.8	31.3
Missouri	30.3	30.0	31.8	28.5	23.6	22.9	27.0	20.6
Montana	29.7	29.0	33.7	30.5	23.7	23.5	*	21.8
Nebraska	31.1	31.6	32.8	28.2	24.4	24.7	29.1	21.7
Nevada	34.6	33.9	41.3	32.0	29.7	28.0	34.0	29.0
New Hampshire	30.8	30.6	32.1	33.9	24.6	24.7	*	24.5
New Jersey	36.8	35.5	39.2	36.8	30.9	30.1	32.3	30.5
New Mexico	24.3	24.7	25.6	24.6	18.0	17.6	20.8	18.2
New York	33.8	32.0	38.3	34.6	28.5	27.1	32.7	28.5
North Carolina	29.3	29.7	32.2	23.3	22.7	22.2	26.2	18.6
North Dakota	27.5	26.7	27.9	30.0	20.6	19.5	31.8	18.7
Ohio	30.4	30.2	31.9	27.5	24.2	23.7	27.3	20.7
Oklahoma	32.4	32.6	35.8	30.1	24.4	24.2	29.4	22.9
Oregon	27.1	26.9	30.6	26.4	21.7	21.5	26.5	20.7
Pennsylvania	30.1	29.9	30.4	29.7	24.7	24.5	25.9	23.0
Rhode Island	30.6	31.6	30.1	29.3	23.5	25.1	22.6	19.4
South Carolina	33.7	33.0	36.9	28.1	26.9	25.6	30.6	23.4
South Dakota	25.7	25.0	25.3	25.9	18.5	18.4	24.1	21.6
Tennessee	33.2	33.0	35.2	29.2	27.6	27.1	30.4	24.2
Texas	34.4	34.3	38.4	33.2	27.0	27.5	32.3	24.7
Utah	22.8	22.1	27.2	24.0	18.0	17.2	23.9	18.8
Vermont	25.5	24.9	27.5	37.4	20.2	19.7	*	*
Virginia	32.9	31.6	36.3	30.1	25.1	23.4	28.6	22.8
Washington	27.5	26.4	34.4	26.3	22.8	21.6	30.2	21.1
West Virginia	34.9	34.9	36.0	31.1	27.2	27.1	26.8	32.0
Wisconsin	26.2	26.4	26.7	25.6	21.3	21.0	23.1	20.1
Wyoming	27.3	26.4	29.9	31.8	17.8	17.5	*	18.0
Puerto Rico	46.7	45.9	49.3	46.8	41.4	39.3	*	41.5
Virgin Islands	31.5	26.7	31.8	31.6	25.5	*	25.0	*
Guam	26.4	21.3	*	*	11.6	*	*	*
American Samoa	NA	NA	NA	NA	NA	NA	NA	NA
Northern Marianas	28.8	*	*	*	27.9	*	*	*

NA = Not available.

* = Figure does not meet standards of reliability or precision; based on fewer than 20 births in the numerator.

[1]Percentage of all live births by cesarean delivery.

[2]Low-risk cesarean is defined as singleton, term (37 weeks or more of gestation), vertex (not breech) cesarean deliveries to women having a first birth per 100 women delivering singleton, term, vertex first births.

[3]Includes races other than White and Black and origin not stated.

[4]Race and Hispanic origin are reported separately on birth certificates. Persons of Hispanic origin may be of any race. Race categories are consistent with 1977 Office of Management and Budget standards. Forty-nine states and the District of Columbia reported multiple-race data for 2015 that were bridged to single-race categories for comparability with other states.

[5]Includes all persons of Hispanic origin of any race.

[6]Excludes data for the territories.

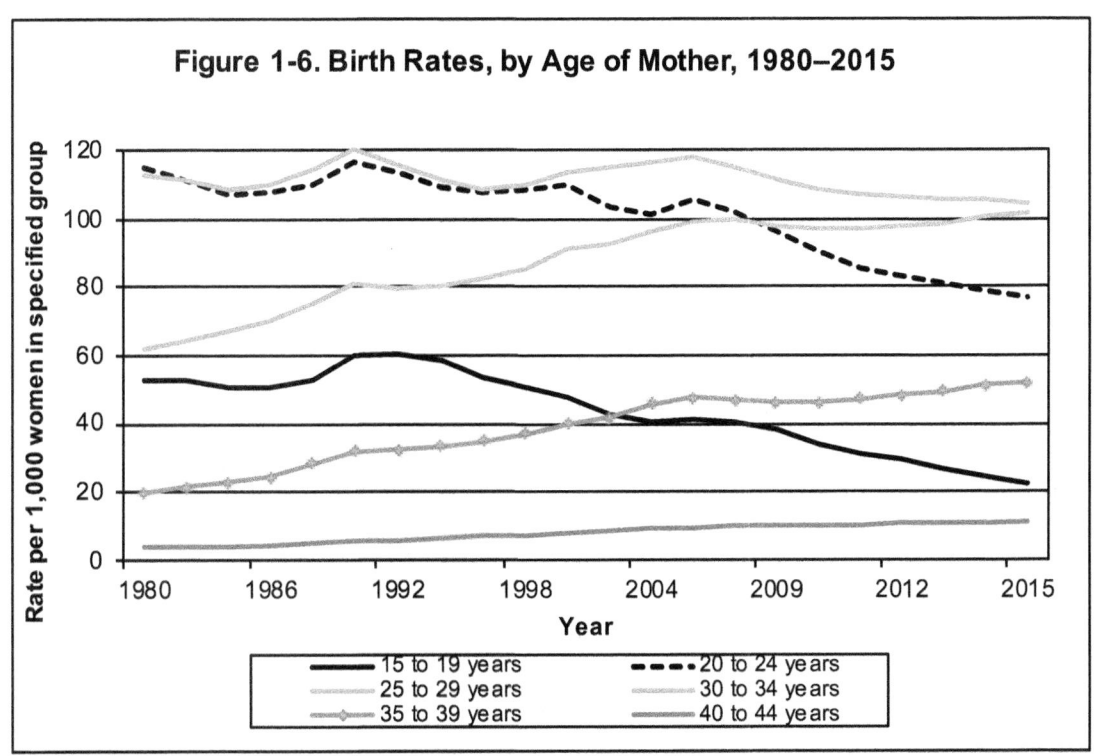

Figure 1-6. Birth Rates, by Age of Mother, 1980–2015

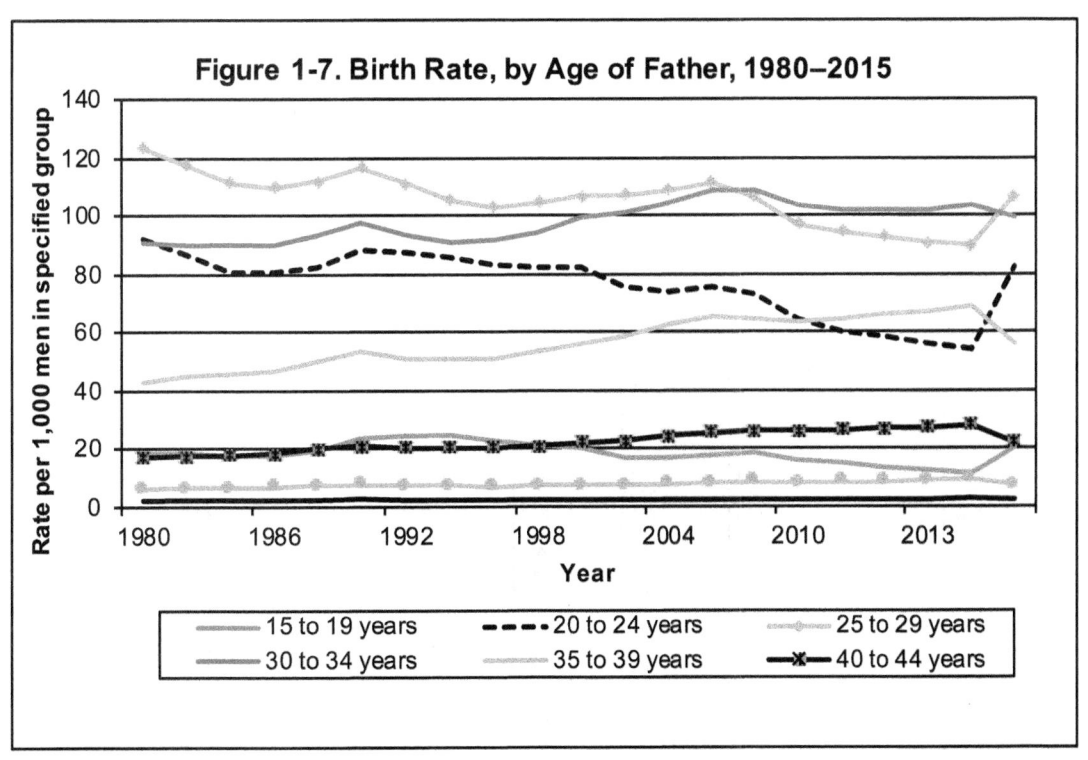

Figure 1-7. Birth Rate, by Age of Father, 1980–2015

Table 1-12. Birth Rates, by Age and Race and Hispanic Origin of Mother, 2000–2015

(Total fertility rates are sums of birth rates for 5-year age groups multiplied by 5; percent.)

| Race, origin, and year | Total fertility rate | 10 to 14 years | 15 to 19 years | | | 20 to 24 years | 25 to 29 years | 30 to 34 years | 35 to 39 years | 40 to 44 years | 45 to 49 years[1] |
			Total	15 to 17 years	18 to 19 years						
All Races and Origins											
2000	2,056.0	0.9	47.7	26.9	78.1	109.7	113.5	91.2	39.7	8.0	0.5
2001	2,030.5	0.8	45.0	24.5	75.5	105.6	113.8	91.8	40.5	8.1	0.5
2002	2,020.5	0.7	42.6	23.1	72.2	103.1	114.7	92.6	41.6	8.3	0.5
2003	2,047.5	0.6	41.1	22.2	69.6	102.3	116.7	95.7	43.9	8.7	0.5
2004	2,051.5	0.6	40.5	21.8	68.7	101.5	116.5	96.2	45.5	9.0	0.5
2005	2,057.0	0.6	39.7	21.1	68.4	101.8	116.5	96.7	46.4	9.1	0.6
2006	2,108.0	0.6	41.1	21.6	71.2	105.5	118.0	98.9	47.5	9.4	0.6
2007	2,120.0	0.6	41.5	21.7	71.7	105.4	118.1	100.6	47.6	9.6	0.6
2008	2,072.0	0.6	40.2	21.1	68.2	101.8	115.0	99.4	46.8	9.9	0.7
2009	2,002.0	0.5	37.9	19.6	64.0	96.2	111.5	97.5	46.1	10.0	0.7
2010	1,931.0	0.4	34.2	17.3	58.2	90.0	108.3	96.5	45.9	10.2	0.7
2011	1,894.5	0.4	31.3	15.4	54.1	85.3	107.2	96.5	47.2	10.3	0.7
2012	1,880.5	0.4	29.4	14.1	51.4	83.1	106.5	97.3	48.3	10.4	0.7
2013	1,857.5	0.3	26.5	12.3	47.1	80.7	105.5	98.0	49.3	10.4	0.8
2014	1,862.5	0.3	24.2	10.9	43.8	79.0	105.8	100.8	51.0	10.6	0.8
2015	1,843.5	0.2	22.3	9.9	40.7	76.8	104.3	101.5	51.8	11.0	0.8
Non-Hispanic White											
2000	1,866.0	0.3	32.6	15.8	57.5	91.2	109.4	93.2	38.8	7.3	0.4
2001	1,846.0	0.3	30.3	14.0	54.7	87.0	109.6	94.3	39.8	7.5	0.4
2002	1,840.0	0.2	28.6	13.1	52.0	84.7	110.4	95.0	40.9	7.7	0.5
2003	1,874.5	0.2	27.4	12.4	50.0	84.1	112.7	98.4	43.5	8.1	0.5
2004	1,871.0	0.2	26.7	12.0	48.6	83.0	112.2	98.3	45.1	8.3	0.5
2005	1,869.0	0.2	26.0	11.5	48.0	82.7	111.7	98.4	46.0	8.3	0.5
2006	1,900.5	0.2	26.7	11.8	49.4	85.1	112.2	100.0	46.8	8.5	0.6
2007	1,908.0	0.2	27.2	11.9	50.4	85.1	112.0	101.5	46.3	8.7	0.6
2008	1,874.5	0.2	26.7	11.6	48.6	82.8	109.7	100.8	45.2	8.9	0.6
2009	1,830.0	0.2	25.7	11.0	46.2	79.2	107.1	99.7	44.4	9.1	0.6
2010	1,791.0	0.2	23.5	10.0	42.5	74.9	105.8	99.9	44.1	9.2	0.6
2011	1,773.5	0.2	21.7	9.0	39.9	71.8	105.2	100.1	45.8	9.3	0.6
2012	1,761.5	0.2	20.5	8.4	37.9	70.2	104.4	100.5	46.8	9.1	0.6
2013	1,751.0	0.1	18.6	7.4	35.0	68.3	103.5	101.9	48.0	9.1	0.7
2014	1,762.5	0.1	20.5	6.7	32.9	67.1	103.9	104.7	49.6	9.1	0.7
2015	1,746.0	0.1	16.0	6.0	30.6	65.0	102.3	105.1	50.6	9.4	0.7
Non-Hispanic Black											
2000	2,178.5	2.4	79.2	50.1	121.9	145.4	102.8	66.5	31.8	7.2	0.4
2001	2,106.5	2.1	73.1	44.8	115.8	137.3	102.8	66.4	32.0	7.3	0.4
2002	2,053.0	1.9	67.7	40.6	109.5	131.4	103.1	66.5	32.1	7.5	0.4
2003	2,037.5	1.6	63.8	38.2	103.4	128.8	104.0	67.7	33.4	7.7	0.5
2004	2,030.5	1.6	61.9	36.4	101.6	127.9	105.0	67.8	33.6	7.8	0.5
2005	2,030.5	1.6	59.4	34.1	100.2	127.9	105.5	68.8	34.2	8.2	0.5
2006	2,128.5	1.5	61.9	35.2	105.0	134.4	110.0	73.2	35.9	8.3	0.5
2007	2,142.0	1.4	62.0	34.6	105.2	134.5	110.5	74.7	36.2	8.5	0.6
2008	2,115.0	1.4	60.4	33.6	100.0	131.5	108.8	75.3	36.3	8.7	0.6
2009	2,046.5	1.1	56.8	31.0	93.5	125.9	106.0	73.9	36.1	8.9	0.6
2010	1,971.5	1.0	51.5	27.4	85.6	119.4	102.5	73.6	36.4	9.2	0.7
2011	1,919.5	0.9	47.3	24.6	78.8	112.3	101.7	73.9	37.8	9.3	0.7
2012	1,898.5	0.8	43.9	21.9	74.1	109.0	101.7	75.1	38.9	9.6	0.7
2013	1,881.5	0.7	39.0	18.9	67.0	105.6	102.7	77.3	40.3	9.9	0.8
2014	1,873.5	0.6	34.9	16.6	61.5	102.8	103.3	79.6	42.5	10.1	0.9
2015	1,857.0	0.6	31.8	15.3	56.7	100.2	102.0	81.6	43.6	10.7	0.9
American Indian or Alaska Native											
2000	1,772.5	1.1	58.3	34.1	97.1	117.2	91.8	55.5	24.6	5.7	0.3
2001	1,712.5	0.9	54.5	30.2	92.7	113.8	89.2	54.2	24.0	5.6	0.3
2002	1,675.5	0.8	50.9	28.8	85.3	110.7	88.9	53.7	24.1	5.7	0.3
2003	1,629.5	0.9	49.0	27.9	82.1	107.0	89.3	52.8	23.3	5.2	0.4
2004	1,610.5	0.8	47.2	26.7	79.9	105.4	87.1	51.9	23.9	5.6	0.2
2005	1,584.0	0.8	46.0	26.3	78.0	102.9	86.3	51.8	23.3	5.4	0.3
2006	1,625.0	0.7	46.9	25.9	80.8	106.8	89.0	52.0	23.9	5.4	0.3
2007	1,621.5	0.7	49.3	26.1	86.3	105.8	86.2	52.5	24.3	5.2	0.3
2008	1,569.0	0.7	47.3	25.8	80.2	102.7	83.2	51.2	23.1	5.3	0.3
2009	1,494.0	0.6	43.7	23.6	73.5	96.3	79.3	50.7	22.6	5.3	0.3
2010	1,404.0	0.5	38.7	20.1	66.1	91.0	74.4	48.4	22.3	5.2	0.3
2011	1,373.5	0.5	36.1	18.2	61.6	86.6	75.4	47.3	23.1	5.5	0.2
2012	1,350.0	0.5	34.9	17.0	60.5	81.7	73.9	49.7	23.3	5.5	0.5
2013	1,334.5	0.4	31.1	15.9	53.3	78.9	75.6	50.4	24.7	5.5	0.3
2014	1,288.5	0.3	27.3	13.2	48.6	73.2	74.7	52.3	24.1	5.5	0.3
2015	1,262.5	0.3	25.7	12.7	45.8	70.2	73.2	51.7	25.2	5.8	0.4

Note: Race and Hispanic origin are reported separately on birth certificates. Race categories are consistent with 1977 Office of Management and Budget standards. Forty-nine states and the District of Columbia reported multiple-race data for 2015 that were bridged to single-race categories for comparability with other states. Multiple-race reporting areas vary for 2003–2015. Persons of Hispanic origin may be of any race.
[1]Rates are computed by relating births to women age 45 years and over to women age 45 to 49.

Table 1-12. Birth Rates, by Age and Race and Hispanic Origin of Mother, 2000–2015—*Continued*

(Total fertility rates are sums of birth rates for 5-year age groups multiplied by 5; percent.)

Race, origin, and year	Total fertility rate	10 to 14 years	15 to 19 years			20 to 24 years	25 to 29 years	30 to 34 years	35 to 39 years	40 to 44 years	45 to 49 years[1]
			Total	15 to 17 years	18 to 19 years						
Asian or Pacific Islander											
2000	1,892.0	0.3	20.5	11.6	32.6	60.3	108.4	116.5	59.0	12.6	0.8
2001	1,785.5	0.2	19.3	10.1	32.0	56.0	102.3	109.9	56.2	12.2	0.9
2002	1,798.5	0.3	17.7	8.8	29.9	55.5	102.4	112.5	57.8	12.6	0.9
2003	1,819.0	0.2	16.4	8.5	27.3	54.3	102.7	115.9	60.0	13.4	0.9
2004	1,825.0	0.2	16.0	8.4	26.6	53.3	100.4	118.3	62.2	13.6	1.0
2005	1,784.5	0.2	15.4	7.7	26.4	52.9	96.6	115.3	61.8	13.7	1.0
2006	1,803.0	0.1	15.3	8.2	25.4	53.8	95.7	117.3	63.4	14.0	1.0
2007	1,850.5	0.2	14.8	7.4	24.9	53.2	99.2	121.6	65.8	14.2	1.1
2008	1,797.5	0.2	13.8	7.0	23.0	50.4	96.6	117.6	64.9	14.7	1.2
2009	1,743.0	0.1	12.6	6.3	20.9	46.4	94.6	115.1	63.8	14.9	1.1
2010	1,689.0	0.1	10.9	5.1	18.7	42.6	91.5	113.6	62.8	15.1	1.2
2011	1,706.5	0.1	10.2	4.6	18.1	41.9	93.7	114.9	64.1	15.2	1.2
2012	1,769.5	0.1	9.7	4.1	17.7	41.4	95.8	121.3	68.1	16.1	1.4
2013	1,681.0	0.1	8.7	3.7	16.1	39.1	89.5	114.6	66.6	16.1	1.5
2014	1,715.1	0.1	7.7	3.3	13.9	37.5	90.0	121.3	68.9	16.1	1.5
2015	1,646.0	0.1	6.9	2.7	12.8	35.6	84.1	117.4	67.6	15.9	1.6
Hispanic											
2000	2,730.0	1.7	87.3	55.5	132.6	161.3	139.9	97.1	46.6	11.5	0.6
2001	2,726.0	1.5	84.4	51.9	131.3	160.5	140.8	97.8	47.9	11.6	0.7
2002	2,711.0	1.4	80.6	49.3	127.1	159.0	141.6	98.3	48.8	11.7	0.8
2003	2,736.0	1.3	78.4	47.6	124.8	159.1	144.0	101.5	50.1	12.1	0.7
2004	2,759.0	1.2	78.1	47.3	124.8	159.2	144.7	103.4	52.2	12.3	0.7
2005	2,792.0	1.3	76.5	45.8	124.4	161.1	147.0	105.6	53.3	12.8	0.8
2006	2,856.0	1.2	77.4	45.1	128.7	166.7	149.9	107.5	54.6	13.1	0.8
2007	2,840.0	1.2	75.3	44.4	124.7	164.6	149.5	108.5	55.0	13.1	0.8
2008	2,706.0	1.1	70.3	42.2	114.0	154.1	142.3	105.3	54.0	13.3	0.8
2009	2,531.5	1.0	63.6	37.3	103.3	140.1	134.3	100.8	52.5	13.2	0.8
2010	2,350.0	0.8	55.7	32.3	90.7	126.1	125.3	96.6	51.7	13.0	0.8
2011	2,240.0	0.7	49.6	28.0	81.5	116.0	121.3	95.2	51.3	13.1	0.8
2012	2,189.5	0.6	46.3	25.5	77.2	111.5	119.6	94.3	51.6	13.2	0.8
2013	2,149.0	0.5	41.7	22.0	70.8	107.2	119.1	94.8	52.4	13.3	0.8
2014	2,130.5	0.4	38.0	19.3	66.1	104.5	118.7	96.5	53.6	13.5	0.9
2015	1,843.5	0.2	22.3	9.9	40.7	76.8	104.3	101.1	51.8	11.0	0.8

Note: Race and Hispanic origin are reported separately on birth certificates. Race categories are consistent with 1977 Office of Management and Budget standards. Forty-nine states and the District of Columbia reported multiple-race data for 2015 that were bridged to single-race categories for comparability with other states. Multiple-race reporting areas vary for 2003–2015. Persons of Hispanic origin may be of any race.
[1] Rates are computed by relating births to women age 45 years and over to women age 45 to 49.

Table 1-12A. Birth Rates, by Age and Race and Hispanic Origin of Father, 2000–2015

(Rates are births per 1,000 men in specified group. Populations based on counts enumerated as of April 1 for census years and estimated as of July 1 for all other years.)

Race, origin, and year	15 to 54 years	15 to 19 years	20 to 24 years	25 to 29 years	30 to 34 years	35 to 39 years	40 to 44 years	45 to 49 years[1]	50 to 54 years	55 years and over
All Races and Origins										
2000	50.0	19.8	82.1	106.5	99.5	56.3	22.2	7.3	2.5	0.3
2001	48.9	18.3	78.3	106.7	99.9	57.1	22.3	7.3	2.4	0.3
2002	48.7	17.2	75.7	107.1	100.7	58.3	22.7	7.4	2.4	0.3
2003	49.3	16.6	74.7	109.1	104.0	60.9	23.6	7.6	2.5	0.3
2004	49.3	16.6	73.4	108.9	104.7	62.5	24.1	7.7	2.4	0.3
2005	49.3	16.4	72.7	109.4	105.9	63.4	24.5	7.9	2.5	0.2
2006	50.4	17.3	75.3	111.4	108.6	65.2	25.3	8.1	2.6	0.2
2007	50.8	18.2	75.6	110.4	110.3	65.6	25.7	8.2	2.6	0.3
2008	49.8	18.4	73.2	106.4	108.3	64.8	25.8	8.3	2.6	0.3
2009	48.3	17.7	69.5	101.5	105.5	63.8	25.9	8.2	2.6	0.3
2010	46.8	16.1	64.6	97.1	103.6	63.4	25.9	8.2	2.6	0.3
2011	46.1	14.7	60.5	94.4	102.2	64.6	26.4	8.3	2.6	0.3
2012	46.1	13.8	58.3	92.5	102.0	65.9	26.8	8.6	2.6	0.3
2013	45.8	12.3	55.7	90.6	101.8	66.6	27.0	8.8	2.7	0.3
2014	46.3	11.3	53.9	89.7	103.9	68.8	27.9	9.3	2.8	0.4
2015	46.1	10.4	51.6	87.4	103.8	69.1	28.6	9.6	2.9	0.4
Non-Hispanic White										
2000	0.3			109.4	93.2	38.8	7.3	0.4		
2001	0.3			109.6	94.3	39.8	7.5	0.4		
2002	0.2			110.4	95.0	40.9	7.7	0.5		
2003	0.2			112.7	98.4	43.5	8.1	0.5		
2004	0.2			112.2	98.3	45.1	8.3	0.5		
2005	0.2			111.7	98.4	46.0	8.3	0.5		
2006	0.2			112.2	100.0	46.8	8.5	0.6		
2007	0.2			112.0	101.5	46.3	8.7	0.6		
2008	0.2			109.7	100.8	45.2	8.9	0.6		
2009	0.2			107.1	99.7	44.4	9.1	0.6		
2010	0.2			105.8	99.9	44.1	9.2	0.6		
2011	0.2			105.2	100.1	45.8	9.3	0.6		
2012	0.2			104.4	100.5	46.8	9.1	0.6		
2013	0.1			103.5	101.9	48.0	9.1	0.7		
2014	0.1			103.9	104.7	49.6	9.1	0.7		
2015	0.1			102.3	105.1	50.6	9.4	0.7		
Non-Hispanic Black										
2000	2.4			102.8	66.5	31.8	7.2	0.4		
2001	2.1			102.8	66.4	32.0	7.3	0.4		
2002	1.9			103.1	66.5	32.1	7.5	0.4		
2003	1.6			104.0	67.7	33.4	7.7	0.5		
2004	1.6			105.0	67.8	33.6	7.8	0.5		
2005	1.6			105.5	68.8	34.2	8.2	0.5		
2006	1.5			110.0	73.2	35.9	8.3	0.5		
2007	1.4			110.5	74.7	36.2	8.5	0.6		
2008	1.4			108.8	75.3	36.3	8.7	0.6		
2009	1.1			106.0	73.9	36.1	8.9	0.6		
2010	1.0			102.5	73.6	36.4	9.2	0.7		
2011	0.9			101.7	73.9	37.8	9.3	0.7		
2012	0.8			101.7	75.1	38.9	9.6	0.7		
2013	0.7			102.7	77.3	40.3	9.9	0.8		
2014	0.6			103.3	79.6	42.5	10.1	0.9		
2015	0.6			102.0	81.6	43.6	10.7	0.9		
American Indian or Alaska Native										
2000	1.1			91.8	55.5	24.6	5.7	0.3		
2001	0.9			89.2	54.2	24.0	5.6	0.3		
2002	0.8			88.9	53.7	24.1	5.7	0.3		
2003	0.9			89.3	52.8	23.3	5.2	0.4		
2004	0.8			87.1	51.9	23.9	5.6	0.2		
2005	0.8			86.3	51.8	23.3	5.4	0.3		
2006	0.7			89.0	52.0	23.9	5.4	0.3		
2007	0.7			86.2	52.5	24.3	5.2	0.3		
2008	0.7			83.2	51.2	23.1	5.3	0.3		
2009	0.6			79.3	50.7	22.6	5.3	0.3		
2010	0.5			74.4	48.4	22.3	5.2	0.3		
2011	0.5			75.4	47.3	23.1	5.5	0.2		
2012	0.5			73.9	49.7	23.3	5.5	0.5		
2013	0.4			75.6	50.4	24.7	5.5	0.3		
2014	0.3			74.7	52.3	24.1	5.5	0.3		
2015	0.3			73.2	51.7	25.2	5.8	0.4		

Note: Race and Hispanic origin are reported separately on birth certificates. Race categories are consistent with 1977 Office of Management and Budget standards. Forty-nine states and the District of Columbia reported multiple-race data for 2015 that were bridged to single-race categories for comparability with other states. Multiple-race reporting areas vary for 2003–2015. Persons of Hispanic origin may be of any race.
[1] Rates are computed by relating births to women age 45 years and over to women age 45 to 49.

Table 1-12A. Birth Rates, by Age and Race and Hispanic Origin of Father, 2000–2015—*Continued*

(Rates are births per 1,000 men in specified group. Populations based on counts enumerated as of April 1 for census years and estimated as of July 1 for all other years.)

Race, origin, and year	15 to 54 years	15 to 19 years	20 to 24 years	25 to 29 years	30 to 34 years	35 to 39 years	40 to 44 years
Asian or Pacific Islander							
2000..	0.3		108.4	116.5	59.0	12.6	0.8
2001..	0.2		102.3	109.9	56.2	12.2	0.9
2002..	0.3		102.4	112.5	57.8	12.6	0.9
2003..	0.2		102.7	115.9	60.0	13.4	0.9
2004..	0.2		100.4	118.3	62.2	13.6	1.0
2005..	0.2		96.6	115.3	61.8	13.7	1.0
2006..	0.1		95.7	117.3	63.4	14.0	1.0
2007..	0.2		99.2	121.6	65.8	14.2	1.1
2008..	0.2		96.6	117.6	64.9	14.7	1.2
2009..	0.1		94.6	115.1	63.8	14.9	1.1
2010..	0.1		91.5	113.6	62.8	15.1	1.2
2011..	0.1		93.7	114.9	64.1	15.2	1.2
2012..	0.1		95.8	121.3	68.1	16.1	1.4
2013..	0.1		89.5	114.6	66.6	16.1	1.5
2014..	0.1		90.0	121.3	68.9	16.1	1.5
2015..	0.1		84.1	117.4	67.6	15.9	1.6
Hispanic							
2000..	1.7		139.9	97.1	46.6	11.5	0.6
2001..	1.5		140.8	97.8	47.9	11.6	0.7
2002..	1.4		141.6	98.3	48.8	11.7	0.8
2003..	1.3		144.0	101.5	50.1	12.1	0.7
2004..	1.2		144.7	103.4	52.2	12.3	0.7
2005..	1.3		147.0	105.6	53.3	12.8	0.8
2006..	1.2		149.9	107.5	54.6	13.1	0.8
2007..	1.2		149.5	108.5	55.0	13.1	0.8
2008..	1.1		142.3	105.3	54.0	13.3	0.8
2009..	1.0		134.3	100.8	52.5	13.2	0.8
2010..	0.8		125.3	96.6	51.7	13.0	0.8
2011..	0.7		121.3	95.2	51.3	13.1	0.8
2012..	0.6		119.6	94.3	51.6	13.2	0.8
2013..	0.5		119.1	94.8	52.4	13.3	0.8
2014..	0.4		118.7	96.5	53.6	13.5	0.9
2015..	0.2		104.3	101.1	51.8	11.0	0.8

Note: Race and Hispanic origin are reported separately on birth certificates. Race categories are consistent with 1977 Office of Management and Budget standards. Forty-nine states and the District of Columbia reported multiple-race data for 2015 that were bridged to single-race categories for comparability with other states. Multiple-race reporting areas vary for 2003–2015. Persons of Hispanic origin may be of any race.

Table 1-13. Birth Rates, by Live-Birth Order and by Race and Hispanic Origin of Mother, 2000–2015

(Rates are live births per 1,000 women age 15 to 44 years.)

Year, race, and Hispanic origin of mother	Fertility rate	Live-birth order						
		1st child	2nd child	3rd child	4th child	5th child	6th and 7th child	8th child and over
All Races and Origins[1,2]								
2000	65.9	26.5	21.4	11.0	4.2	1.6	0.9	0.3
2001	65.1	25.9	21.3	11.0	4.3	1.6	0.9	0.3
2002	65.0	25.8	21.2	10.9	4.3	1.6	0.9	0.3
2003	66.1	26.5	21.4	11.1	4.3	1.6	0.9	0.3
2004	66.4	26.4	21.4	11.2	4.4	1.6	0.9	0.3
2005	66.7	26.5	21.5	11.3	4.5	1.6	0.9	0.3
2006	68.6	27.4	21.9	11.6	4.7	1.7	1.0	0.3
2007	69.3	27.8	22.0	11.7	4.7	1.8	1.0	0.3
2008	68.1	27.5	21.5	11.4	4.7	1.7	1.0	0.3
2009	66.2	26.8	20.8	11.0	4.6	1.7	1.0	0.3
2010	64.1	25.9	20.2	10.6	4.4	1.7	1.0	0.3
2011	63.2	25.4	20.0	10.4	4.4	1.7	1.0	0.3
2012	63.0	25.2	19.9	10.4	4.4	1.7	1.0	0.3
2013	62.5	24.7	19.9	10.4	4.4	1.7	1.0	0.3
2014	62.9	24.6	20.1	10.6	4.5	1.8	1.1	0.3
2015	62.5	24.1	20.1	10.6	4.6	1.8	1.1	0.4
Non-Hispanic White[2,3]								
2000	58.5	24.2	19.8	9.4	3.3	1.1	0.6	0.2
2001	57.7	23.6	19.7	9.4	3.3	1.1	0.6	0.2
2002	57.6	23.6	19.6	9.3	3.3	1.1	0.6	0.2
2003	58.9	24.5	19.8	9.4	3.3	1.1	0.6	0.2
2004	58.9	24.4	19.8	9.5	3.3	1.1	0.6	0.2
2005	59.0	24.4	19.8	9.5	3.4	1.1	0.6	0.2
2006	60.3	25.1	20.0	9.6	3.5	1.1	0.6	0.2
2007	61.0	25.6	20.1	9.7	3.5	1.2	0.6	0.2
2008	60.5	25.5	19.8	9.5	3.5	1.2	0.7	0.2
2009	59.6	25.3	19.5	9.2	3.4	1.2	0.7	0.3
2010	58.7	25.0	19.2	9.1	3.4	1.2	0.7	0.3
2011	58.7	24.9	19.2	9.0	3.4	1.2	0.7	0.3
2012	58.6	24.7	19.2	9.1	3.4	1.2	0.7	0.3
2013	58.7	24.4	19.3	9.2	3.5	1.2	0.7	0.3
2014	59.5	24.5	19.7	9.4	3.6	1.3	0.8	0.3
2015	59.3	23.9	19.8	9.5	3.7	1.3	0.8	0.3
Non-Hispanic Black[2,3]								
2000	71.4	26.7	21.2	12.8	5.9	2.6	1.8	0.6
2001	69.1	25.9	20.4	12.4	5.8	2.5	1.7	0.6
2002	67.5	25.4	19.7	12.1	5.7	2.5	1.7	0.6
2003	67.1	25.4	19.6	11.9	5.6	2.4	1.6	0.5
2004	67.1	25.5	19.4	11.9	5.6	2.4	1.7	0.5
2005	67.2	25.8	19.3	11.8	5.6	2.5	1.7	0.5
2006	70.7	27.5	20.3	12.3	5.8	2.5	1.7	0.5
2007	71.4	27.9	20.4	12.3	5.9	2.6	1.7	0.5
2008	70.8	28.1	20.0	12.1	5.8	2.6	1.7	0.5
2009	68.9	27.3	19.4	11.7	5.7	2.5	1.7	0.6
2010	66.6	26.3	18.9	11.3	5.4	2.5	1.7	0.5
2011	65.4	25.6	18.5	11.1	5.4	2.4	1.7	0.6
2012	65.0	25.1	18.6	11.2	5.5	2.4	1.7	0.5
2013	64.6	24.4	18.6	11.3	5.5	2.5	1.7	0.6
2014	64.5	23.9	18.6	11.5	5.6	2.5	1.7	0.6
2015	64.1	23.5	18.5	11.5	5.7	2.6	1.7	0.6
Hispanic[4]								
2000	95.9	35.8	29.2	18.0	5.9	2.6	1.8	0.6
2001	95.4	35.2	29.3	18.0	5.8	2.5	1.7	0.6
2002	94.7	34.7	29.1	18.0	5.7	2.5	1.7	
2003	95.2	34.5	29.4	18.3	5.6	2.5	1.6	0.5
2004	95.7	34.4	29.3	18.7	5.6	2.5	1.7	0.5
2005	96.4	34.4	29.6	19.0	5.6	2.5	1.7	0.5
2006	98.3	35.1	29.9	19.3	5.8	2.6	1.7	0.5
2007	97.4	34.7	29.4	19.3	5.9	2.6	1.7	0.5
2008	92.7	33.0	27.8	18.3	5.8	2.5	1.7	0.5
2009	86.5	30.6	25.9	17.0	5.7	2.5	1.7	0.6
2010	80.2	28.0	24.0	15.9	5.4		1.7	0.5
2011	76.2	26.3	22.9	15.2	5.4	2.4	1.7	0.6
2012	74.4	25.5	22.3	14.9	5.5	2.4	1.7	0.5
2013	72.9	24.9	21.8	14.6	5.5	2.5	1.7	0.6
2014	72.1	24.5	21.6	14.4	5.6	2.5	1.7	0.6
2015	64.1	23.5	18.5	11.5	5.7	2.6	1.7	0.6

[1]Includes births to races other than White and Black.
[2]Includes origin not stated.
[3]Race and Hispanic origin are reported separately on birth certificates. Persons of Hispanic origin may be of any race. Race categories are consistent with 1977 Office of Management and Budget standards. Forty-nine states and the District of Columbia reported multiple-race data for 2015 that were bridged to single-race categories for comparability with other states. Multiple-race reporting areas vary for 2003–2015.
[4]Includes all persons of Hispanic origin of any race.

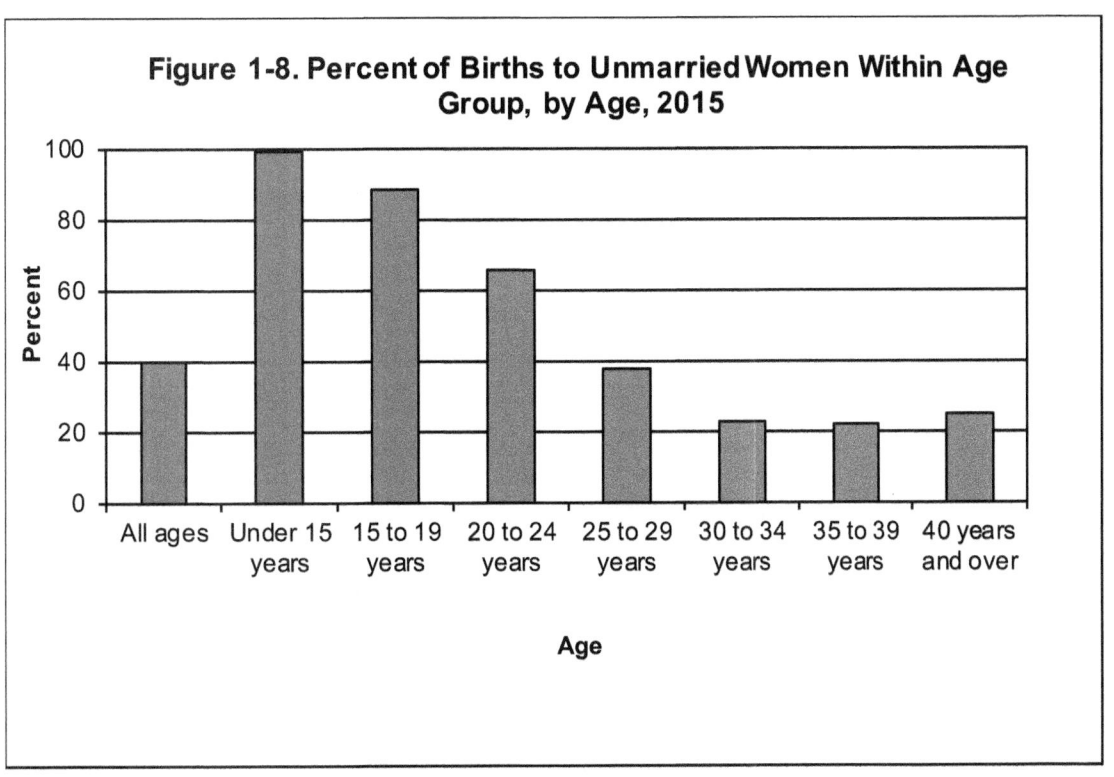

Figure 1-8. Percent of Births to Unmarried Women Within Age Group, by Age, 2015
100
80
60
40
20
0
Percent
All ages
Under 15 years
15 to 19 years
20 to 24 years
25 to 29 years
30 to 34 years
35 to 39 years
40 years and over
Age

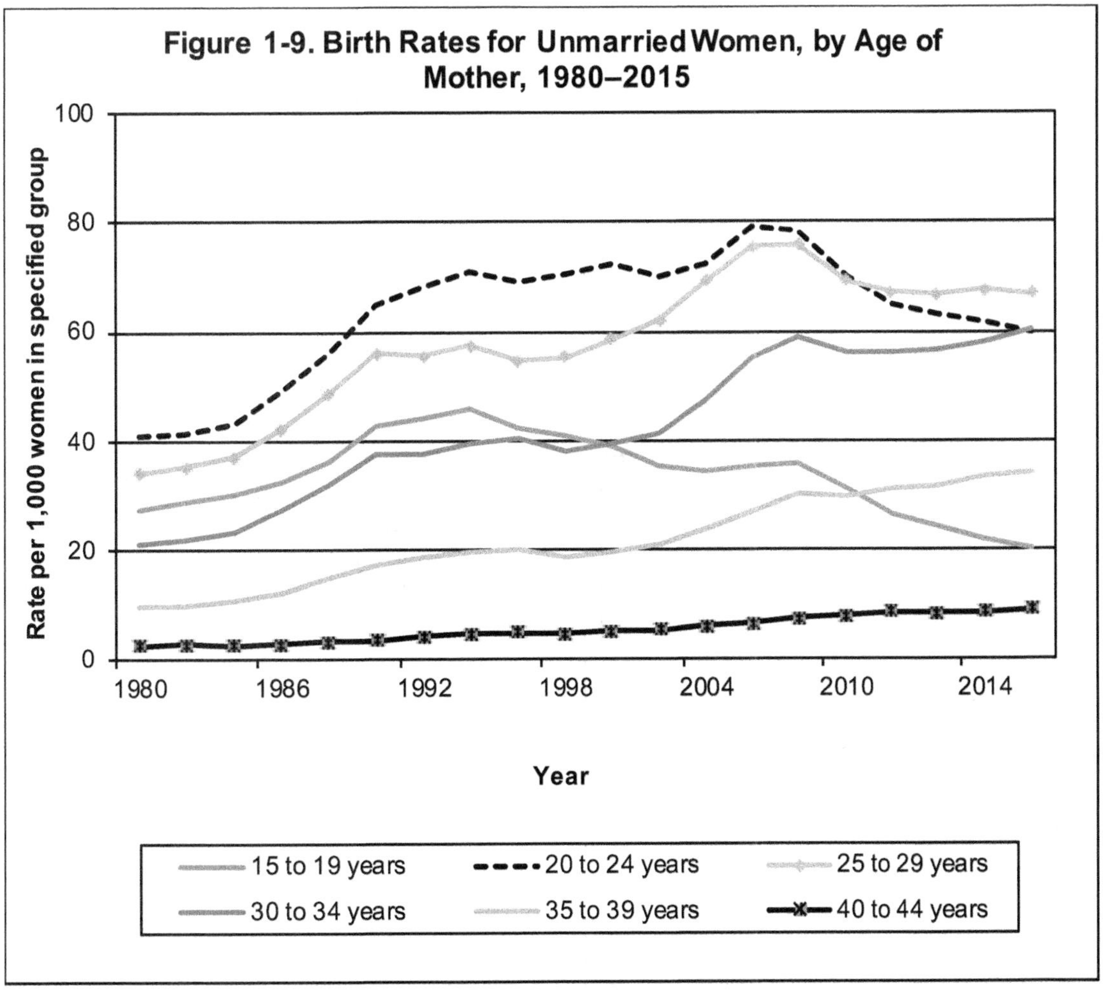

Figure 1-9. Birth Rates for Unmarried Women, by Age of Mother, 1980–2015
100
80
60
40
20
0
Rate per 1,000 women in specified group
1980
1986
1992
1998
2004
2010
2014
Year
15 to 19 years
20 to 24 years
25 to 29 years
30 to 34 years
35 to 39 years
40 to 44 years

Table 1-14. Births to Unmarried Mothers, by Race and Hispanic Origin of Mother and State and Territory of Residence, 2016

(Number; percent.)

State and territory	Number				Percent			
		Non-Hispanic				Non-Hispanic		
	All races[1]	White[2]	Black[2]	Hispanic[3]	All races[1]	White[2]	Black[2]	Hispanic[3]
United States[4]	15,69,796	5,85,059	3,89,780	4,83,527	39.8	28.5	69.8	52.6
Alabama	26,450	10,302	13,735	1,762	44.7	29.5	xs	38.5
Alaska	4,052	1,248	110	262	36.1	21.6	34.5	32.3
Arizona	38,053	10,724	2,460	19,676	45.0	30.4	60.4	56.3
Arkansas	17,036	8,440	5,654	2,021	44.5	33.8	79.7	49.7
California	1,86,851	29,961	15,610	1,20,443	38.2	22.6	65.2	52.6
Colorado	14,981	6,548	1,094	6,247	22.5	16.5	36.4	33.7
Connecticut	13,288	4,485	2,859	5,356	36.9	22.9	64.2	62.1
Delaware	5,037	2,030	1,950	858	45.8	34.8	68.9	59.9
District of Columbia	4,771	186	3,705	773	48.4	6.1	77.1	57.3
Florida	1,05,537	36,265	33,037	33,295	46.9	36.5	67.5	50.5
Georgia	58,395	16,287	30,911	8,878	44.9	28.1	69.6	49.4
Hawaii	6,680	624	64	1,263	37.0	17.1	13.8	45.7
Idaho	6,206	4,159	53	1,577	27.6	23.7	24.4	43.6
Illinois	61,292	21,448	20,192	17,219	39.7	26.1	78.8	52.8
Indiana	35,448	22,608	7,613	4,092	42.7	36.4	77.9	55.0
Iowa	13,801	9,608	1,661	1,797	35.0	30.6	67.3	51.7
Kansas	13,696	7,957	1,734	3,307	36.0	29.5	68.2	52.5
Kentucky	22,933	16,893	3,597	1,638	41.4	37.4	73.4	52.2
Louisiana	32,883	11,279	18,259	2,572	52.0	34.2	78.9	54.8
Maine	5,047	4,546	116	111	39.7	39.6	28.2	46.6
Maryland	29,006	7,457	13,854	6,366	39.7	23.8	60.7	53.6
Massachusetts	23,535	10,355	3,613	7,813	33.0	24.6	52.6	59.3
Michigan	46,500	24,086	16,397	3,848	41.0	31.0	79.7	51.4
Minnesota	22,487	11,693	3,936	2,652	32.2	24.1	50.6	54.4
Mississippi	20,173	6,247	12,647	882	53.2	32.2	79.6	53.0
Missouri	29,753	18,056	7,831	2,071	39.8	32.6	75.0	50.1
Montana	4,466	2,875	22	270	36.4	29.5	38.6	49.3
Nebraska	8,583	4,591	1,083	2,136	32.3	24.5	64.3	49.9
Nevada	17,323	4,872	3,111	7,446	47.8	35.0	74.0	55.6
New Hampshire	4,130	3,603	68	338	33.7	33.9	32.7	48.5
New Jersey	35,504	8,333	9,234	16,303	34.6	18.1	66.6	58.1
New Mexico	12,621	2,176	199	7,840	51.1	31.1	56.2	57.5
New York	90,140	27,592	22,614	33,437	38.5	24.8	66.2	61.7
North Carolina	48,835	17,092	19,556	9,275	40.4	26.0	71.3	50.5
North Dakota	3,599	2,069	255	286	31.6	24.4	41.7	49.0
Ohio	59,320	34,914	17,156	4,453	43.0	34.8	76.8	60.0
Oklahoma	22,225	10,310	3,226	3,738	42.3	33.8	73.4	49.5
Oregon	16,297	9,877	520	4,216	35.8	31.8	55.1	49.8
Pennsylvania	56,680	29,039	14,055	9,916	40.7	30.7	76.6	64.6
Rhode Island	4,850	2,248	484	1,665	44.9	35.5	61.7	62.0
South Carolina	25,965	9,684	12,633	2,569	45.3	29.4	76.4	50.0
South Dakota	4,526	2,212	158	350	36.9	25.0	43.5	55.2
Tennessee	35,228	18,048	12,154	3,919	43.6	33.5	76.5	51.4
Texas	1,64,551	35,137	29,514	95,942	41.3	26.2	60.8	50.9
Utah	9,390	5,037	195	3,178	18.6	13.3	37.3	39.9
Vermont	2,266	2,069	31	50	39.4	39.7	44.3	36.8
Virginia	34,851	13,309	13,117	7,077	34.0	23.2	63.1	49.7
Washington	28,735	13,906	1,751	8,031	31.7	26.1	45.3	48.6
West Virginia	8,584	7,682	403	178	45.0	44.0	68.7	47.1
Wisconsin	24,811	13,238	5,536	3,653	37.2	27.6	84.3	56.2
Wyoming	2,425	1,654	13	482	32.8	28.7	*	49.5
Puerto Rico	19,263	426	49	18,733	68.2	62.6	69.0	68.4
Virgin Islands	852	44	621	141	71.8	40.7	74.7	76.6
Guam	2,049	18	5	4	59.7	*	*	*
American Samoa	411	NA	NA	NA	40.6	NA	NA	NA
Northern Marianas	341	-	-	-	82.0	*	*	*

NA = Not available.

'- = Quantity zero.

* = Figure does not meet standards of reliability or precision; based on fewer than 20 births in the numerator.

[1] Includes births to race and origin groups not shown separately, such as Hispanic single-race white, Hispanic single-race black, and non-Hispanic multiple-race women, as well as births with origin not stated.

[2] Race and Hispanic origin are reported separately on birth certificates; persons of Hispanic origin may be of any race. In this table, non-Hispanic women are classified by race. Race categories are consistent with 1997 Office of Management and Budget standards. Single race is defined as only one race reported on the birth certificate.

[3] Includes all persons of Hispanic origin of any race.

[4] Excludes data for the territories.

Table 1-15. Birth Rates for Teenagers Age 15 to 19 Years, by State and Territory of Residence, Selected Years, 1991–2015

(Birth rates per 1,000 estimated female population age 15 to 19 years in each area, percent)

State and territory	1991	2007	2009	2010	2015	Percent change, 1991–2015	Percent change, 2007–2015	Percent change, 2009–2015	Percent change, 2010–2015
United States[1]	61.8	41.5	39.1	34.2	22.3	-63.9	-46.3	-43.0	-34.8
Alabama	73.6	52.1	50.7	43.6	30.1	-59.1	-42.2	-40.6	-31.0
Alaska	66.0	42.9	44.5	38.3	29.3	-55.6	-31.7	-34.2	-23.5
Arizona	79.7	59.6	50.6	41.9	26.3	-67.0	-55.9	-48.0	-37.2
Arkansas	79.5	60.1	59.2	52.5	38.0	-52.2	-36.8	-35.8	-27.6
California	73.8	39.6	36.6	31.5	19.0	-74.3	-52.0	-48.1	-39.7
Colorado	58.3	41.6	38.5	33.4	19.3	-66.9	-53.6	-49.9	-42.2
Connecticut	40.1	23.0	21.0	18.7	10.1	-74.8	-56.1	-51.9	-46.0
Delaware	60.4	39.2	35.3	30.5	18.1	-70.0	-53.8	-48.7	-40.7
District of Columbia	109.6	50.4	47.7	45.4	25.6	-76.6	-49.2	-46.3	-43.6
Florida	67.9	43.0	39.0	32.0	20.8	-69.4	-51.6	-46.7	-35.0
Georgia	76.0	53.4	47.7	41.4	25.6	-66.3	-52.1	-46.3	-38.2
Hawaii	59.2	38.7	40.9	32.5	20.6	-65.2	-46.8	-49.6	-36.6
Idaho	53.9	39.9	35.9	33.0	22.5	-58.3	-43.6	-37.3	-31.8
Illinois	64.5	40.2	36.1	33.0	21.2	-67.1	-47.3	-41.3	-35.8
Indiana	60.4	43.0	42.5	37.3	26.0	-57.0	-39.5	-38.8	-30.3
Iowa	42.5	32.8	32.1	28.6	18.6	-56.2	-43.3	-42.1	-35.0
Kansas	55.4	42.5	43.8	39.3	25.5	-54.0	-40.0	-41.8	-35.1
Kentucky	68.8	52.6	51.3	46.2	32.4	-52.9	-38.4	-36.8	-29.9
Louisiana	76.0	55.2	52.7	47.7	34.1	-55.1	-38.2	-35.3	-28.5
Maine	43.5	36.0	24.4	21.4	15.4	-64.6	-57.2	-36.9	-28.0
Maryland	54.1	34.3	31.3	27.3	17.0	-68.6	-50.4	-45.7	-37.7
Massachusetts	37.5	21.4	19.6	17.2	9.4	-74.9	-56.1	-52.0	-45.3
Michigan	58.9	33.5	32.7	30.1	19.4	-67.1	-42.1	-40.7	-35.5
Minnesota	37.3	27.9	24.3	22.5	13.7	-63.3	-50.9	-43.6	-39.1
Mississippi	85.3	70.1	64.2	55.0	34.8	-59.2	-50.4	-45.8	-36.7
Missouri	64.4	44.0	41.6	37.1	25.0	-61.2	-43.2	-39.9	-32.6
Montana	46.8	35.3	38.5	35.0	25.3	-45.9	-28.3	-34.3	-27.7
Nebraska	42.4	35.5	34.6	31.1	22.0	-48.1	-38.0	-36.4	-29.3
Nevada	74.5	51.7	47.4	38.6	27.6	-63.0	-46.6	-41.8	-28.5
New Hampshire	33.1	19.3	16.4	15.7	10.9	-67.1	-43.5	-33.5	-30.6
New Jersey	41.3	24.9	22.7	20.1	12.1	-70.7	-51.4	-46.7	-39.8
New Mexico	79.5	63.9	63.9	53.0	34.6	-56.5	-45.9	-45.9	-34.7
New York	45.5	26.0	24.4	22.7	14.6	-67.9	-43.8	-40.2	-35.7
North Carolina	70.0	48.0	44.9	38.3	23.6	-66.3	-50.8	-47.4	-38.4
North Dakota	35.5	29.2	27.9	28.8	22.2	-37.5	-24.0	-20.4	-22.9
Ohio	60.5	39.9	38.9	34.1	23.2	-61.7	-41.9	-40.4	-32.0
Oklahoma	72.1	58.5	60.1	50.4	34.8	-51.7	-40.5	-42.1	-31.0
Oregon	54.8	34.5	33.1	28.2	19.0	-65.3	-44.9	-42.6	-32.6
Pennsylvania	46.7	30.7	29.3	27.0	17.7	-62.1	-42.3	-39.6	-34.4
Rhode Island	44.7	29.2	26.8	22.3	14.3	-68.0	-51.0	-46.6	-35.9
South Carolina	72.5	51.9	49.1	42.6	26.2	-63.9	-49.5	-46.6	-38.5
South Dakota	47.6	41.3	38.4	34.9	26.4	-44.5	-36.1	-31.3	-24.4
Tennessee	74.8	53.4	50.6	43.2	30.5	-59.2	-42.9	-39.7	-29.4
Texas	78.4	61.8	60.7	52.2	34.6	-55.9	-44.0	-43.0	-33.7
Utah	48.0	35.4	30.7	27.9	17.6	-63.3	-50.3	-42.7	-36.9
Vermont	39.2	21.0	17.4	17.9	11.6	-70.4	-44.8	-33.3	-35.2
Virginia	53.4	34.2	31.0	27.4	17.1	-68.0	-50.0	-44.8	-37.6
Washington	53.7	33.3	31.9	26.7	17.6	-67.2	-47.1	-44.8	-34.1
West Virginia	58.0	45.8	49.8	44.8	31.9	-45.0	-30.3	-35.9	-28.8
Wisconsin	43.7	31.1	29.4	26.2	16.2	-62.9	-47.9	-44.9	-38.2
Wyoming	54.3	49.9	45.0	39.0	29.2	-46.2	-41.5	-35.1	-25.1
Puerto Rico	72.4	NA	54.7	51.4	NA	NA	NA	NA	NA
Virgin Islands	77.9	NA	51.5	50.5	NA	NA	NA	NA	NA
Guam	95.7	NA	50.8	60.1	NA	NA	NA	NA	NA
America Samoa	NA	NA	35.2	34.1	NA	NA	NA	NA	NA
Northern Marinas	NA	NA	50.2	53.4	NA	NA	NA	NA	NA

Note: Comparisons are made with 2007 and 1991 because these years represent recent and longer-term highs in teenage birth rates. Birth rates by state are based on population estimates provided by the U.S. Census Bureau and, therefore, the rates shown here may differ from rates computed on the basis of other population estimates. Rates by race and Hispanic origin cannot be computed for the territories because populations by race and Hispanic origin are not available for these areas. Data includes births to race and Hispanic-origin groups not shown separately, such as White Hispanic and Black Hispanic women, and births with origin not stated.
NA = Not available.
[1]Excludes data for the territories.

Table 1-16. Responses to the Statement, "If You Got Pregnant Now/Got a Female Pregnant Now, How Would You Feel?" for Never-Married Females and Males Age 15 to 19 Years, 2011–2015

(Numbers in thousands; percent.)

Characteristic	Number of respondents	Percent surveyed[1]	Very upset		A little upset		A little pleased		Very pleased	
			Percent	Standard error	Percent	Standard error	Percent	Standard error	Percent	Standard error
FEMALE										
Total[2]	9,128	100.0	60.5	1.8	28.0	1.5	7.3	0.8	4.0	0.8
Hispanic Origin and Race										
Hispanic or Latina	2,057	100.0	51.8	3.1	34.0	2.9	9.8	1.5	4.2	0.9
Non-Hispanic										
White, single race	4,761	100.0	65.6	2.3	26.1	2.1	5.8	0.9	2.3	0.7
Black, single race	1,307	100.0	59.2	4.1	26.7	3.1	10.0	2.9	3.7	1.1
Age										
15–17 years	5,394	100.0	65.5	2.3	25.8	2.1	6.3	1.0	2.1	0.9
18–19 years	3,734	100.0	53.4	2.5	31.2	2.1	8.8	1.1	6.7	1.5
Ever Had Sex										
Yes	3,749	100.0	49.4	2.4	32.7	2.2	12.6	1.6	5.2	0.9
No	5,379	100.0	68.3	2.4	24.7	2.0	3.7	0.7	3.1	1.2
Family Structure at Age 14										
Both biological or adoptive parents.....	5,463	100.0	65.0	2.3	25.9	2.0	4.8	0.7	4.3	1.2
Other[3]	3,665	100.0	53.9	2.7	31.1	2.6	11.1	1.6	3.6	0.7
MALE										
Total[2]	9,644	100.0	46.1	1.7	33.7	1.5	13.6	0.9	6.0	0.8
Hispanic Origin and Race										
Hispanic or Latino	2,197	100.0	30.0	2.5	36.3	2.3	22.8	2.7	9.9	1.4
Non-Hispanic										
White, single race	4,993	100.0	54.7	2.5	32.0	2.2	8.3	1.1	4.7	1.3
Black, single race	1,353	100.0	32.0	3.0	40.4	3.3	19.7	2.2	7.5	1.6
Age										
15–17 years	5,924	100.0	51.1	2.2	31.9	1.8	11.3	1.0	5.1	1.0
18–19 years	3,720	100.0	38.2	2.5	36.5	2.7	17.4	1.9	7.6	1.4
Ever Had Sex										
Yes	4,271	100.0	36.0	2.0	36.9	2.1	18.6	1.6	7.9	1.0
No	5,373	100.0	54.2	2.5	31.2	2.1	9.7	1.0	4.6	1.2
Family Structure at Age 14										
Both biological or adoptive parents.....	5,960	100.0	48.0	2.2	34.0	2.0	11.8	1.3	6.0	1.1
Other[3]	3,684	100.0	43.1	2.5	33.1	2.3	16.6	1.6	6.3	1.1

[1]Percentages may not add to 100 because responses of "would not care" (coded only if respondent insisted) are not shown separately.
[2]Includes persons of other or unknown origin and race groups, not shown separately.
[3]Refers to anything other than two biological or adoptive parents or biological mother and stepfather, including one biological parent and no other parents(s)/parent figures or no parent(s)/parent figures.

Table 1-17. Birth Rates for Women Age 10 to 19 Years, by Age, Race, and Hispanic Origin of Mother, Selected Years, 1991–2015

(Rates per 1,000 women in specified age, race, and Hispanic origin groups; percent.)

Age, race, and Hispanic origin of mother	1991	2007	2014	2015	Percent change, 1991–2015	Percent change, 2007–2015	Percent change, 2014–2015
10 to 14 Years							
All races and origins[1]	1.4	0.6	0.3	0.2	-86	-67	-33
Non-Hispanic White[2]	0.5	0.2	0.1	0.1	-80	-50	†
Non-Hispanic Black[2]	4.9	1.4	0.6	0.6	-88	-57	†
American Indian or Alaska Native total[2,3]	1.6	0.7	0.3	0.3	-81	-57	†
Asian or Pacific Islander total[2,3]	0.8	0.2	0.1	0.1	-88	-50	†
Hispanic[4]	2.4	1.2	0.4	0.4	-83	-67	†
15 to 19 Years							
All races and origins[1]	61.8	41.5	24.2	22.3	-64	-46	-8
Non-Hispanic White[2]	43.4	27.2	17.3	16.0	-63	-41	-8
Non-Hispanic Black[2]	118.2	62.0	34.9	31.8	-73	-49	-9
American Indian or Alaska Native total[2,3]	84.1	49.3	27.3	25.7	-69	-48	-6
Asian or Pacific Islander total[2,3]	27.3	14.8	7.7	6.9	-75	-53	-10
Hispanic[4]	104.6	75.3	38.0	34.9	-67	-54	-8
15 to 17 Years							
All races and origins[1]	38.6	21.7	10.9	9.9	-74	-54	-9
Non-Hispanic White[2]	23.6	11.9	6.7	6.0	-75	-50	-10
Non-Hispanic Black[2]	86.1	34.6	16.6	15.3	-82	-56	-8
American Indian or Alaska Native total[2,3]	51.9	26.1	13.2	12.7	-76	-51	†
Asian or Pacific Islander total[2,3]	16.3	7.4	3.3	2.7	-83	-64	-18
Hispanic[4]	69.2	44.4	19.3	17.4	-75	-61	-10
18 to 19 Years							
All races and origins[1]	94.0	71.7	43.8	40.7	-57	-43	-7
Non-Hispanic White[2]	70.6	50.4	32.9	30.6	-57	-39	-7
Non-Hispanic Black[2]	162.2	105.2	61.5	56.7	-65	-46	-8
American Indian or Alaska Native total[2,3]	134.2	86.3	48.6	45.8	-66	-47	-6
Asian or Pacific Islander total[2,3]	42.2	24.9	13.9	12.8	-70	-48	-8
Hispanic[4]	155.5	124.7	66.1	61.9	-60	-50	-6

Note: 1991 excludes data for New Hampshire, which did not report Hispanic origin.

† = Difference not statistically significant.

[1]Includes births to race and origin groups not shown separately, such as White Hispanic and Black Hispanic women, and births with origin not stated.

[2]Race and Hispanic origin are reported separately on birth certificates. Persons of Hispanic origin may be of any race. Race categories are consistent with the 1977 Office of Management and Budget (OMB) standards. Forty-nine states and the District of Columbia reported multiple-race data in 2015 that were bridged to the single-race categories of the 1977 OMB standards for comparability with other states. Multiple-race reporting areas vary for 2007, 2014, and 2015.

[3]Includes persons of Hispanic origin, and origin not stated, according to the mother's reported race.

[4]Includes all persons of Hispanic origin of any race.

Table 1-18. Mean Age of Mother, by Live-Birth Order and Race and Hispanic Origin of Mother, Selected Years, 1980–2015

(Arithmetic average of the age of mothers at the times of births.)

Year, race, and, Hispanic origin of mother	Total	Live-birth order								Unknown or not stated
		1	2	3	4	5	6 and 7	8 and over	
All Races[1]									
1980[2]	25.0	22.7	25.4	27.3	29.0	30.6	32.7	36.0	23.9
1985	25.8	23.7	26.3	27.9	29.3	30.6	32.5	35.7	26.1
1990	26.4	24.2	26.9	28.3	29.4	30.6	32.1	35.1	27.4
1995	26.9	24.5	27.5	29.1	30.1	31.2	32.6	35.4	27.1
2000	27.2	24.9	27.7	29.2	30.3	31.4	32.9	35.8	27.4
2001	27.3	25.0	27.8	29.2	30.3	31.4	32.9	35.9	27.0
2002	27.3	25.1	27.9	29.2	30.3	31.4	32.9	35.9	27.7
2003	27.4	25.2	28.0	29.3	30.4	31.4	33.0	35.8	27.9
2004	27.5	25.2	28.0	29.4	30.4	31.4	32.9	35.9	27.6
2005	27.4	25.2	28.0	29.4	30.4	31.4	32.9	35.9	28.0
2006	27.4	25.0	27.9	29.3	30.4	31.4	33.0	35.8	28.0
2007	27.4	25.0	27.9	29.3	30.4	31.5	32.9	35.7	27.9
2008	27.4	25.1	27.9	29.4	30.5	31.5	32.9	35.7	27.7
2009	27.5	25.2	28.0	29.5	30.6	31.6	32.9	35.7	27.6
2010	27.7	25.4	28.2	29.6	30.7	31.7	33.0	35.7	27.7
2011	27.9	25.6	28.3	29.7	30.8	31.8	33.1	35.5	28.2
2012	28.0	25.8	28.4	29.8	30.9	31.9	33.2	35.7	27.9
2013	28.2	26.0	28.6	29.9	31.1	32.0	33.3	35.7	28.3
2014	28.3	26.3	28.7	30.0	31.0	32.0	33.4	35.7	28.7
2015	28.5	26.4	28.8	30.1	31.2	32.2	33.4	35.8	29.3
Non-Hispanic White[3]									
1990[4]	27.1	25.0	27.6	29.1	30.3	31.6	33.2	36.2	28.5
1995	27.6	25.4	28.3	29.9	31.2	32.4	33.9	36.7	28.5
2000	28.0	25.9	28.6	30.0	31.3	32.4	34.0	37.0	28.9
2001	28.1	26.0	28.6	30.1	31.3	32.4	33.9	37.0	28.2
2002	28.2	26.1	28.7	30.1	31.2	32.3	33.9	37.1	28.6
2003	28.2	26.2	28.8	30.1	31.2	32.3	33.9	37.0	28.8
2004	28.2	26.2	28.8	30.2	31.2	32.2	33.8	36.9	28.7
2005	28.2	26.2	28.8	30.1	31.2	32.2	33.8	36.9	29.1
2006	28.1	26.0	28.8	30.1	31.1	32.1	33.7	36.7	29.1
2007	28.1	26.0	28.7	30.0	31.1	32.1	33.7	36.7	28.8
2008	28.1	26.0	28.7	30.1	31.1	32.1	33.6	36.7	28.7
2009	28.1	26.1	28.8	30.1	31.1	32.1	33.6	36.7	28.6
2010	28.3	26.3	28.9	30.2	31.1	32.2	33.6	36.6	28.7
2011	28.4	26.5	29.0	30.2	31.2	32.2	33.7	36.4	29.0
2012	28.5	26.6	29.0	30.2	31.3	32.2	33.7	36.5	28.6
2013	28.6	26.8	29.1	30.3	31.3	32.3	33.7	36.6	29.0
2014	28.8	27.0	29.2	30.4		32.3	33.8	36.6	29.3
2015	28.9	27.2	29.3	30.5	31.4	32.4	33.8	36.6	29.7
Non-Hispanic Black[3]									
1990[4]	24.4	21.7	24.6	26.3	27.4	28.7	30.3	33.3	26.0
1995	24.8	21.9	25.3	27.0	28.0	29.3	30.8	33.2	25.4
2000	25.2	22.3	25.5	27.1	28.2	29.5	31.0	33.9	26.0
2001	25.3	22.4	25.7	27.2	28.3	29.6	31.2	34.1	26.4
2002	25.4	22.6	25.8	27.3	28.5	29.6	31.2	34.1	26.5
2003	25.6	22.7	25.9	27.5	28.6	29.7	31.3	34.0	26.3
2004	25.6	22.7	25.9	27.5	28.6	29.8	31.2	34.1	25.7
2005	25.6	22.7	26.0	27.6	28.8	29.8	31.3	34.2	25.8
2006	25.6	22.7	26.0	27.7	28.8	29.9	31.4	34.1	25.9
2007	25.6	22.7	26.0	27.7	28.9	30.0	31.4	34.2	26.1
2008	25.6	22.8	26.0	27.8	29.0	30.0	31.5	34.2	26.2
2009	25.7	22.9	26.1	27.9	29.1	30.2	31.5	34.3	26.2
2010	25.9	23.1	26.3	28.0	29.3	30.3	31.7	34.2	26.5
2011	26.1	23.4	26.4	28.2	29.4	30.5	31.8	34.2	26.6
2012	26.3	23.6	26.6	28.3	29.5	30.5	31.9	34.2	26.5
2013	26.6	23.9	26.8	28.5	29.6	30.6	31.9	34.4	27.1
2014	26.9	24.2	27.0	28.6	29.8	30.7	32.1	34.3	17.7
2015	27.1	24.4	27.2	28.9	30.0	30.9	32.2	34.6	28.5
Hispanic[5]									
1990[4]	25.3	22.4	25.2	27.4	29.1	30.6	32.3	35.3	26.1
1995	25.4	22.4	25.5	27.8	29.6	31.1	32.8	35.5	24.2

[1]Includes races other than White and Black and origin not stated.
[2]Based on 100 percent of births in selected states and on a 50-percent sample of births in all other states.
[3]Race and Hispanic origin are reported separately on birth certificates. Persons of Hispanic origin may be of any race. Multiple-race data, when reported, were bridged to single-race categories in order to maintain comparability among all reported areas. Forty-nine states and the District of Columbia reported multiple-race data for 2015 that were bridged to single-race categories for comparability with other states. Multiple-race reporting areas vary for 2003–2015.
[4]Excludes data for New Hampshire and Oklahoma, which did not report Hispanic origin.
[5]Includes all persons of Hispanic origin of any race.

Table 1-18. Mean Age of Mother, by Live-Birth Order and Race and Hispanic Origin of Mother, Selected Years, 1980–2015—*Continued*

(Arithmetic average of the age of mothers at the times of births.)

Year, race, and, Hispanic origin of mother	Total	Live-birth order							
		1	2	3	4	5	6 and 7	8 and over	Unknown or not stated
2000..	25.7	22.7	25.8	28.1	29.8	31.3	33.0	35.5	24.2
2001..	25.9	22.8	25.9	28.2	29.9	31.4	33.1	35.7	24.4
2002..	26.0	23.0	26.0	28.3	29.9	31.4	33.1	35.7	25.7
2003..	26.1	23.1	26.1	28.4	30.0	31.4	33.1	35.4	25.8
2004..	26.2	23.1	26.2	28.5	30.1	31.5	33.1	35.5	25.8
2005..	26.2	23.1	26.2	28.5	30.1	31.4	33.2	35.6	26.5
2006..	26.2	23.1	26.2	28.6	30.2	31.5	33.2	35.5	26.6
2007..	26.3	23.1	26.3	28.6	30.3	31.6	33.1	35.3	26.7
2008..	26.4	23.1	26.4	28.7	30.4	31.6	33.2	35.3	26.7
2009..	26.5	23.3	26.5	28.9	30.5	31.8	33.1	35.3	26.8
2010..	26.8	23.4	26.7	29.0	30.7	32.0	33.3	35.3	27.2
2011..	27.0	23.7	26.9	29.2	30.9	32.1	33.3	35.0	28.0
2012..	27.1	23.8	27.0	29.3	31.0	32.2	33.5	35.1	27.6
2013..	27.3	24.0	27.2	29.4	31.1	32.3	33.6	35.2	27.9
2014..	27.5	24.3	27.3	29.5	31.2	32.4	33.7	35.2	28.1
2015..	27.7	24.5	27.5	29.7	31.4	32.6	33.8	35.3	28.4

Table 1-19. Live Births, Birth Rates, and Fertility Rates, by Race, Selected Years, 1940–2015

(Number, rate per 1,000 population in specified group.)

Characteristic and year	Number All races[1]	Number White	Number Black	Number American Indian or Alaska Native	Number Asian or Pacific Islander	Birth rate All races[1]	Birth rate White	Birth rate Black	Birth rate American Indian or Alaska Native	Birth rate Asian or Pacific Islander	Fertility rate All races[1]	Fertility rate White	Fertility rate Black	Fertility rate American Indian or Alaska Native	Fertility rate Asian or Pacific Islander
Race of Mother															
1980[2]	3,612,258	2,936,351	568,080	29,389	74,355	15.9	15.1	21.3	20.7	19.9	68.4	65.6	84.7	82.7	73.2
1981[2]	3,629,238	2,947,679	564,955	29,688	84,553	15.8	15.0	20.8	20.0	20.1	67.3	64.8	82.0	79.6	73.7
1982[2]	3,680,537	2,984,817	568,506	32,436	93,193	15.9	15.1	20.7	21.1	20.3	67.3	64.8	80.9	83.6	74.8
1983[2]	3,638,933	2,946,468	562,624	32,881	95,713	15.6	14.8	20.2	20.6	19.5	65.7	63.4	78.7	81.8	71.7
1984[2]	3,669,141	2,967,100	568,138	33,256	98,926	15.6	14.8	20.1	20.1	18.8	65.5	63.2	78.2	79.8	69.2
1985	3,760,561	3,037,913	581,824	34,037	104,606	15.8	15.0	20.4	19.8	18.7	66.3	64.1	78.8	78.6	68.4
1986	3,756,547	3,019,175	592,910	34,169	107,797	15.6	14.8	20.5	19.2	18.0	65.4	63.1	78.9	75.9	66.0
1987	3,809,394	3,043,828	611,173	35,322	116,560	15.7	14.9	20.8	19.1	18.4	65.8	63.3	80.1	75.6	67.1
1988	3,909,510	3,102,083	638,562	37,088	129,035	16.0	15.0	21.5	19.3	19.2	67.3	64.5	82.6	76.8	70.2
1989	4,040,958	3,192,355	673,124	39,478	133,075	16.4	15.4	22.3	19.7	18.7	69.2	66.4	86.2	79.0	68.2
1990	4,158,212	3,290,273	684,336	39,051	141,635	16.7	15.8	22.4	18.9	19.0	70.9	68.3	86.8	76.2	69.6
1991	4,110,907	3,241,273	682,602	38,841	145,372	16.2	15.3	21.8	18.3	18.3	69.3	66.7	84.8	73.9	67.1
1992	4,065,014	3,201,678	673,633	39,453	150,250	15.8	15.0	21.1	17.9	17.9	68.4	66.1	82.4	73.1	66.1
1993	4,000,240	3,149,833	658,875	38,732	152,800	15.4	14.6	20.2	17.0	17.3	67.0	64.9	79.6	69.7	64.3
1994	3,952,767	3,121,004	636,391	37,740	157,632	15.0	14.3	19.1	16.0	17.1	65.9	64.2	75.9	65.8	63.9
1995	3,899,589	3,098,885	603,139	37,278	160,287	14.6	14.1	17.8	15.3	16.7	64.6	63.6	71.0	63.0	62.6
1996	3,891,494	3,093,057	594,781	37,880	165,776	14.4	13.9	17.3	14.9	16.5	64.1	63.3	69.2	61.8	62.3
1997	3,880,894	3,072,640	599,913	38,572	169,769	14.2	13.7	17.1	14.7	16.2	63.6	62.8	69.0	60.8	61.3
1998	3,941,553	3,118,727	609,902	40,272	172,652	14.3	13.8	17.1	14.8	15.9	64.3	63.6	69.4	61.3	60.1
1999	3,959,417	3,132,501	605,970	40,170	180,776	14.2	13.7	16.8	14.2	15.9	64.4	64.0	68.5	59.0	60.9
2000	4,058,814	3,194,005	622,598	41,668	200,543	14.4	13.9	17.0	14.0	17.1	65.9	65.3	70.0	58.7	65.8
2001	4,025,933	3,177,626	606,156	41,872	200,279	14.1	13.7	16.3	13.5	16.1	65.1	65.0	67.5	56.8	62.5
2002	4,021,726	3,174,760	593,691	42,368	210,907	14.0	13.6	15.7	13.2	16.3	65.0	65.1	65.7	55.7	63.3
2003	4,089,950	3,225,848	599,847	43,052	221,203	14.1	13.7	15.7	13.0	16.4	66.1	66.4	66.0	54.8	64.2
2004	4,112,052	3,222,928	616,074	43,927	229,123	14.0	13.6	15.9	12.8	16.4	66.4	66.5	67.2	54.2	64.5
2005	4,138,349	3,229,294	633,134	44,813	231,108	14.0	13.6	16.1	12.6	15.9	66.7	66.8	68.5	53.6	63.0
2006	4,265,555	3,310,308	666,481	47,721	241,045	14.3	13.8	16.7	12.9	16.0	68.6	68.7	71.4	55.3	63.7
2007	4,316,233	3,336,626	675,676	49,443	254,488	14.3	13.8	16.7	12.9	16.4	69.3	69.4	71.7	55.5	65.3
2008	4,247,694	3,274,163	670,809	49,537	253,185	14.0	13.5	16.3	12.4	15.7	68.1	68.3	70.6	54.0	63.3
2009	4,130,665	3,173,293	657,618	48,665	251,089	13.5	13.0	15.8	11.8	15.1	66.2	66.4	68.8	51.6	61.3
2010	3,999,386	3,069,315	636,425	46,760	246,886	13.0	12.5	15.1	11.0	14.5	64.1	64.4	66.3	48.6	59.2
2011	3,953,590	3,020,355	632,901	46,419	253,915	12.7	12.2	14.8	10.7	14.5	63.2	63.4	65.5	47.7	59.9
2012	3,952,841	2,999,820	634,126	46,093	272,802	12.6	12.1	14.7	10.5	15.1	63.0	63.0	65.1	47.0	62.2
2013	3,932,181	2,985,757	634,760	45,991	265,673	12.4	12.0	14.5	10.3	14.3	62.5	62.7	64.7	46.4	59.2
2014	3,988,076	3,019,863	640,562	44,928	282,723	12.5	12.0	14.5	9.9	14.6	62.9	63.2	64.6	44.8	60.7
2015	3,978,497	3,012,855	640,070	44,299	281,263	12.4	12.0	14.3	9.7	14.0	62.5	63.1	64.0	43.9	58.5
Race of Child															
1960[3]	4,257,850	3,600,744	602,264	21,114	NA	23.7	22.7	31.9	NA	NA	118.0	113.2	153.5	NA	NA
1961[3]	4,268,326	3,600,864	611,072	21,464	NA	23.3	22.2	NA	NA	NA	117.1	112.3	NA	NA	NA
1962[3,4]	4,167,362	3,394,068	584,610	21,968	NA	22.4	21.4	NA	NA	NA	112.0	107.5	NA	NA	NA
1963[3]	4,098,020	3,326,344	580,658	22,358	NA	21.7	20.7	NA	NA	NA	108.3	103.6	NA	NA	NA
1964[3]	4,027,490	3,369,160	607,556	24,382	NA	21.1	20.0	29.5	NA	NA	104.7	99.8	142.6	NA	NA
1965[3]	3,760,358	3,123,860	581,126	24,066	NA	19.4	18.3	27.7	NA	NA	96.3	91.3	133.2	NA	NA
1966[3]	3,606,274	2,993,230	558,244	23,014	NA	18.4	17.4	26.2	NA	NA	90.8	86.2	124.7	NA	NA
1967[5]	3,520,959	2,922,502	543,976	22,665	NA	17.8	16.8	25.1	NA	NA	87.2	82.8	118.5	NA	NA
1968[3]	3,501,564	2,912,224	531,152	24,156	NA	17.6	16.6	24.2	NA	NA	85.2	81.3	112.7	NA	NA
1969[3]	3,600,206	2,993,614	543,132	24,008	NA	17.9	16.9	24.4	NA	NA	86.1	82.2	112.1	NA	NA
1970[3]	3,731,386	3,091,264	572,362	25,864	NA	18.4	17.4	25.3	NA	NA	87.9	84.1	115.4	NA	NA
1971[3]	3,555,970	2,919,746	564,960	27,148	NA	17.2	16.1	24.4	NA	NA	81.6	77.3	109.7	NA	NA
1972[2]	3,258,411	2,655,558	531,329	27,368	NA	15.6	14.5	22.5	NA	NA	73.1	68.9	99.9	NA	NA
1973[2]	3,136,965	2,551,030	512,597	26,464	NA	14.8	13.8	21.4	NA	NA	68.8	64.9	93.6	NA	NA
1974[2]	3,159,958	2,575,792	507,162	26,631	NA	14.8	13.9	20.8	NA	NA	67.8	64.2	89.7	NA	NA
1975[2]	3,144,198	2,551,996	511,581	27,546	NA	14.6	13.6	20.7	NA	NA	66.0	62.5	87.9	NA	NA
1976[2]	3,167,788	2,567,614	514,479	29,009	NA	14.6	13.6	20.5	NA	NA	65.0	61.5	85.8	NA	NA
1977[2]	3,326,632	2,691,070	544,221	30,500	NA	15.1	14.1	21.4	NA	NA	66.8	63.2	88.1	NA	NA
1978[2]	3,333,279	2,681,116	551,540	33,160	NA	15.0	14.0	21.3	NA	NA	65.5	61.7	86.7	NA	NA
1979[2]	3,494,398	2,808,420	577,855	34,269	NA	15.6	14.5	22.0	NA	NA	67.2	63.4	88.3	NA	NA
1980[2]	3,612,258	2,898,732	589,616	36,797	NA	15.9	14.9	22.1	NA	NA	68.4	64.7	88.1	NA	NA
Births adjusted for underregistration															
Race of Child															
1940	2,559,000	2,199,000	NA	NA	NA	19.4	18.6	NA	NA	NA	79.9	77.1	NA	NA	NA
1945	2,858,000	2,471,000	NA	NA	NA	20.4	19.7	NA	NA	NA	85.9	83.4	NA	NA	NA
1950	3,632,000	3,108,000	NA	NA	NA	24.1	23.0	NA	NA	NA	106.2	102.3	NA	NA	NA
1955	4,097,000	3,485,000	NA	NA	NA	25.0	23.8	NA	NA	NA	118.3	113.7	NA	NA	NA

Note: Race and Hispanic origin are reported separately on birth certificates. Race categories are consistent with 1977 Office of Management and Budget standards. Forty-nine states and the District of Columbia reported multiple-race data for 2015 that were bridged to single-race categories for comparability with other states. Multiple-race reporting areas vary for 2003–2015;. In this table, all women, including Hispanic women, are classified only according to their race.
NA = Not available.
[1]Data for 1960–1991 includes births to races not shown separately. For 1992 and later years, unknown race of mother is imputed.
[2]Based on 100 percent of births in selected states and on a 50 percent sample of births in all other states.
[3]Based on a 50 percent sample of births.
[4]Figures by race exclude New Jersey.
[5]Based on a 20 to 50 percent sample of births.

Table 1-20. Births and Birth Rates, by Hispanic Origin of Mother and by Race for Mothers of Non-Hispanic Origin, 1989–2015

(Birth rates are live births per 1,000 population in specified group; fertility rates are live births per 1,000 women age 15 to 44 years in specified group.)

Measure and year	All origins[1]	Hispanic (may be of any race)						Non-Hispanic		
		Total	Mexican	Puerto Rican	Cuban	Central and South American	Other and unknown Hispanic	Total[2]	White	Black
Number										
1989[3]	3,903,012	532,249	327,233	56,229	10,842	72,443	65,502	3,297,493	2,526,367	611,269
1990[4]	4,092,994	595,073	385,640	58,807	11,311	83,008	56,307	3,457,417	2,626,500	661,701
1991[5]	4,094,566	623,085	411,233	59,833	11,058	86,908	54,053	3,434,464	2,589,878	666,758
1992[5]	4,049,024	643,271	432,047	59,569	11,472	89,031	51,152	3,365,862	2,527,207	657,450
1993	4,000,240	654,418	443,733	58,102	11,916	92,371	48,296	3,295,345	2,472,031	641,273
1994	3,952,767	665,026	454,536	57,240	11,889	93,485	47,876	3,245,115	2,438,855	619,198
1995	3,899,589	679,768	469,615	54,824	12,473	94,996	47,860	3,160,495	2,382,638	587,781
1996	3,891,494	701,339	489,666	54,863	12,613	97,888	46,309	3,133,484	2,358,989	578,099
1997	3,880,894	709,767	499,024	55,450	12,887	97,405	45,001	3,115,174	2,333,363	581,431
1998	3,941,553	734,661	516,011	57,349	13,226	98,226	49,849	3,158,975	2,361,462	593,127
1999	3,959,417	764,339	540,674	57,138	13,088	103,307	50,132	3,147,580	2,346,450	588,981
2000	4,058,814	815,868	581,915	58,124	13,429	113,344	49,056	3,199,994	2,362,968	604,346
2001	4,025,933	851,851	611,000	57,568	14,017	121,365	47,901	3,149,572	2,326,578	589,917
2002	4,021,726	876,642	627,505	57,465	14,232	125,981	51,459	3,119,944	2,298,156	578,335
2003	4,089,950	912,329	654,504	58,400	14,867	135,586	48,972	3,149,034	2,321,904	576,033
2004	4,112,052	946,349	677,621	61,221	14,943	143,520	49,044	3,133,125	2,296,683	578,772
2005	4,138,349	985,505	693,197	63,340	16,064	151,201	61,703	3,123,005	2,279,768	583,759
2006	4,265,555	1,039,077	718,146	66,932	16,936	165,321	71,742	3,196,082	2,308,640	617,247
2007	4,316,233	1,062,779	722,055	68,488	16,981	169,851	85,404	3,222,460	2,310,333	627,191
2008	4,247,694	1,041,239	684,883	69,015	16,718	155,578	115,045	3,173,629	2,267,817	623,029
2009	4,130,665	999,548	645,297	68,486	16,641	148,647	120,477	3,101,330	2,212,552	609,584
2010	3,999,396	945,180	598,317	66,368	16,882	142,692	120,921	3,026,314	2,162,406	589,808
2011	3,953,590	918,129	566,699	67,018	17,131	136,221	131,060	3,008,200	2,146,566	582,345
2012	3,952,841	907,677	555,823	67,182	17,396	131,794	135,482	3,014,304	2,134,044	583,489
2013	3,932,181	901,033	545,303	68,302	18,854	131,305	137,370	3,003,556	2,129,196	583,834
2014	3,988,076	914,065	545,977	69,879	20,163	136,656	141,390	3,043,519	2,149,302	588,891
2015	3,978,497	924,048	546,169	70,987	21,107	142,249	143,536	3,021,999	2,130,379	589,047
Birth Rate										
1989[3,6]	16.3	26.2	25.7	23.7	10.0	28.3	(6)	15.4	14.2	22.8
1990[4,6]	16.7	26.7	28.7	21.6	10.9	27.5	(6)	15.7	14.4	23.0
1991[5,6]	16.2	26.5	27.6	23.3	9.8	28.3	(6)	15.2	13.9	22.4
1992[5,6]	15.8	26.1	27.4	22.9	10.1	27.5	(6)	14.8	13.4	21.6
1993[6]	15.4	25.4	26.8	21.5	10.5	26.3	(6)	14.3	13.1	20.7
1994[6]	15.0	24.7	26.1	20.8	10.7	24.9	(6)	13.9	12.8	19.5
1995[6]	14.6	24.1	25.8	19.0	10.8	24.2	(6)	13.5	12.5	18.2
1996[6]	14.4	23.8	26.2	17.2	10.6	22.5	(6)	13.3	12.3	17.6
1997[6]	14.2	23.0	25.3	17.2	10.0	21.3	(6)	13.1	12.2	17.4
1998[6]	14.3	22.7	24.6	17.9	9.7	21.7	(6)	13.2	12.2	17.5
1999[6]	14.2	22.5	24.2	18.0	9.4	21.7	(6)	13.0	12.1	17.1
2000[6]	14.4	23.1	25.0	18.1	9.7	21.8	(6)	13.2	12.2	17.3
2001[6]	14.1	22.9	24.7	17.7	10.3	21.7	(6)	12.8	11.9	16.6
2002[6]	14.0	22.7	24.3	16.5	10.1	22.5	(6)	12.6	11.7	16.1
2003[6]	14.1	22.8	24.6	15.0	10.0	23.0	(6)	12.7	11.8	15.9
2004[6]	14.0	22.8	24.8	16.0	9.3	22.1	(6)	12.6	11.7	15.8
2005[6]	14.0	22.9	24.5	17.0	10.2	22.7	(6)	12.5	11.6	15.8
2006[6]	14.3	23.3	24.6	17.5	10.4	23.8	(6)	12.7	11.7	16.5
2007[6]	14.3	23.0	23.9	17.1	10.2	24.6	(6)	12.8	11.7	16.6
2008[6]	14.0	21.8	21.7	16.4	10.1	26.1	(6)	12.5	11.5	16.3
2009[6]	13.5	20.3	19.8	15.5	9.5	25.5	(6)	12.2	11.2	15.7
2010[6]	13.0	18.7	18.2	14.1	9.0	23.4	(6)	11.8	10.9	15.1
2011[6]	12.7	17.6	16.9	13.7	9.1	23.0	(6)	11.7	10.8	14.7
2012[6]	12.6	17.1	16.3	16.3	13.5	8.9	(6)	11.7	10.7	14.6
2013[6]	12.4	16.7	15.8	15.8	13.3	9.4	(6)	11.6	10.7	14.4
2014[6]	12.5	16.5	NA	NA	NA	NA	(6)	11.7	10.8	14.4
2015[6]	12.4	16.3	NA	NA	NA	NA	(6)	11.5	10.7	14.2
Fertility Rate										
1989[3,6]	69.2	104.9	106.6	86.6	49.8	95.8	(6)	65.7	60.5	84.8
1990[4,6]	71.0	107.7	118.9	82.9	52.6	102.7	(6)	67.1	62.8	89.0
1991[5,6]	69.3	106.9	114.9	87.9	47.6	105.5	(6)	65.2	60.9	87.0
1992[5,6]	68.4	106.1	113.3	87.9	49.4	104.7	(6)	64.2	60.0	84.5
1993[6]	67.0	103.3	110.9	79.8	53.9	101.5	(6)	62.7	58.9	81.5

Note: Race and Hispanic origin are reported separately on birth certificates. Race categories are consistent with 1977 Office of Management and Budget standards. Forty-nine states and the District of Columbia reported multiple-race data for 2015 that were bridged to single-race categories for comparability with other states. Multiple-race reporting areas vary for 2003–2015. Persons of Hispanic origin may be of any race. In this table, Hispanic women are classified only by place of origin; non-Hispanic women are classified by race. NA = Not available.
[1] Includes origin not stated.
[2] Includes races other than White and Black.
[3] Excludes data for Louisiana, New Hampshire, and Oklahoma, which did not report Hispanic origin.
[4] Excludes data for New Hampshire and Oklahoma, which did not report Hispanic origin.
[5] Excludes data for New Hampshire, which did not report Hispanic origin.
[6] Rates for the Central and South American population includes other and unknown Hispanic.

Table 1-20. Births and Birth Rates, by Hispanic Origin of Mother and by Race for Mothers of Non-Hispanic Origin, 1989–2015—*Continued*

(Birth rates are live births per 1,000 population in specified group; fertility rates are live births per 1,000 women age 15 to 44 years in specified group.)

Measure and year	All origins[1]	Hispanic (may be of any race)						Non-Hispanic		
		Total	Mexican	Puerto Rican	Cuban	Central and South American	Other and unknown Hispanic	Total[2]	White	Black
1994[6]	65.9	100.7	109.9	78.2	53.6	93.2	[6]	61.6	58.2	77.5
1995[6]	64.6	98.8	109.9	71.3	52.2	89.1	[6]	60.2	57.5	72.8
1996[6]	64.1	97.5	110.7	66.5	55.1	84.2	[6]	59.6	57.1	70.7
1997[6]	63.6	94.2	106.6	65.8	53.1	80.6	[6]	59.3	56.8	70.3
1998[6]	64.3	93.2	103.2	69.7	46.5	83.5		60.0	57.6	70.9
1999[6]	64.4	93.0	101.5	71.1	47.0	84.8	[6]	60.0	57.7	69.9
2000[6]	65.9	95.9	105.1	73.5	49.3	85.1	[6]	61.1	58.5	71.4
2001[6]	65.1	95.4	105.0	71.7	56.4	82.2	[6]	60.0	57.7	69.1
2002[6]	65.0	94.7	103.0	65.6	59.3	86.5	[6]	59.8	57.6	67.5
2003[6]	66.1	95.2	103.7	60.6	60.8	89.7	[6]	60.7	58.9	67.1
2004[6]	66.4	95.7	104.5	66.8	52.2	87.4	[6]	60.8	58.9	67.1
2005[6]	66.7	96.4	104.5	69.8	49.1	90.5	[6]	60.8	59.0	67.2
2006[6]	68.6	98.3	105.6	71.6	47.9	95.6	[6]	62.5	60.3	70.7
2007[6]	69.3	97.4	102.8	70.3	47.6	100.1	[6]	63.3	61.0	71.4
2008[6]	68.1	92.7	92.6	67.0	50.1	109.1	[6]	62.7	60.5	70.8
2009[6]	66.2	86.5	84.8	63.7	46.0	107.5	[6]	61.6	59.6	68.9
2010[6]	64.1	80.2	78.2	59.7	46.4	97.1	[6]	60.4	58.7	66.6
2011[6]	63.2	76.2	73.0	59.6	46.1	96.3	[6]	60.1	58.7	65.4
2012[6]	63.0	74.4	70.7	58.2	45.4	94.9	[6]	60.3	58.5	65.0
2013[6]	62.5	72.9	68.4	57.8	48.0	94.4	[6]	59.9	58.7	64.6
2014[6]	62.9	72.1	NA	NA	NA	NA	[6]	60.7	59.5	64.5
2015[6]	62.5	71.7	NA	NA	NA	NA	[6]	60.2	59.3	64.1

Note: Race and Hispanic origin are reported separately on birth certificates. Race categories are consistent with 1977 Office of Management and Budget standards. Forty-nine states and the District of Columbia reported multiple-race data for 2015 that were bridged to single-race categories for comparability with other states. Multiple-race reporting areas vary for 2003–2015. Persons of Hispanic origin may be of any race. In this table, Hispanic women are classified only by place of origin; non-Hispanic women are classified by race.
NA = Not available.
[1] Includes origin not stated.
[2] Includes races other than White and Black.
[6] Rates for the Central and South American population includes other and unknown Hispanic.

Table 1-21. Live Births, by Age of Mother, Live-Birth Order, and Race of Mother, 2015

(Number of children born alive to mother.)

Live birth order and race of mother	All ages	Under 15 years	15 to 19 years						20 to 24 years	25 to 29 years	30 to 34 years	35 to 39 years	40 to 44 years	45 to 49 years	50 to 54 years
			Total	15 years	16 years	17 years	18 years	19 years							
All Races	3,978,497	2,500	229,715	7,589	18,430	35,165	63,508	105,023	850,509	1,152,311	1,094,693	527,996	111,848	8,171	754
1st child	1,525,594	2,474	190,538	7,371	17,403	31,540	53,294	80,930	431,994	427,498	327,605	118,881	23,976	2,396	232
2nd child	1,270,034	16	33,353	187	904	3,254	8,916	20,092	278,360	381,675	373,560	170,125	30,784	1,996	165
3rd child	671,884	3	4,405	4	62	231	959	3,149	100,438	209,268	216,642	116,648	23,048	1,317	115
4th child	288,766	1	481	3	6	22	90	360	27,457	84,359	99,450	61,592	14,431	907	88
5th child	112,207	–	62	–	–	5	12	45	6,539	28,778	40,288	28,101	7,846	541	52
6th child	46,100	–	9	–	–	1	4	4	1,394	9,747	17,079	13,422	4,117	305	27
7th child	21,247	–	4	–	1	–	1	2	324	3,265	7,736	7,252	2,436	198	32
8th child and over	22,245	–	10	–	–	2	2	6	308	1,753	6,279	8,942	4,473	447	33
Not stated	20,420	6	853	24	54	110	230	435	3,695	5,968	6,054	3,033	737	64	10
White	3,012,855	1,512	165,934	5,043	12,843	25,135	46,262	76,651	620,891	885,936	850,028	400,342	81,865	5,858	489
1st child	1,153,172	1,496	138,307	4,905	12,185	22,688	39,008	59,521	318,477	333,018	252,800	89,770	17,434	1,728	142
2nd child	972,598	10	23,778	120	576	2,217	6,394	14,471	207,140	299,508	291,783	127,061	21,814	1,392	112
3rd child	514,784	–	2,944	3	42	141	651	2,107	70,507	160,723	172,587	90,206	16,819	929	69
4th child	216,297	1	312	2	3	16	59	232	17,582	61,061	77,694	47,998	10,937	657	55
5th child	80,600	–	41	–	–	2	9	30	3,773	19,059	29,810	21,504	5,976	397	40
6th child	31,949	–	3	–	–	–	1	2	740	12,029	10,038	3,123	211	19	
7th child	14,459	–	3	–	1	–	–	2	150	1,788	5,233	5,298	1,819	143	25
8th child and over	15,247	–	7	–	–	2	1	4	190	944	3,856	6,421	3,454	353	22
Not stated	13,749	5	539	13	36	69	139	282	2,332	4,049	4,236	2,046	489	48	5
Black	640,079	898	54,746	2,255	4,883	8,625	14,794	24,189	189,986	180,147	130,669	66,430	15,860	1,195	148
1st child	233,174	889	44,805	2,182	4,556	7,601	12,224	18,242	91,881	50,864	29,267	12,227	2,886	302	53
2nd child	183,821	5	8,222	60	290	900	2,191	4,781	59,466	56,941	37,786	17,356	3,749	270	26
3rd child	114,297	3	1,265	1	17	83	260	904	25,590	38,487	29,808	15,490	3,423	205	26
4th child	56,265	–	147	1	3	3	29	111	8,567	19,147	16,368	9,585	2,291	147	13
5th child	25,083	–	20	–	–	3	3	14	2,434	8,024	8,222	4,934	1,347	94	8
6th child	11,263	–	6	–	–	1	3	2	596	3,303	3,962	2,600	731	61	4
7th child	5,414	–	–	–	–	–	–	–	150	1,249	2,009	1,511	450	40	5
8th child and over	5,745	–	3	–	–	–	1	2	110	706	2,013	2,036	805	64	8
Not stated	5,017	1	278	11	17	34	83	133	1,192	1,426	1,234	691	178	12	5
American Indian or Alaska Native	44,299	53	4,738	168	420	823	1,287	2,040	13,458	12,842	8,506	3,824	824	51	3
1st child	14,233	53	3,853	164	397	737	1,065	1,490	5,593	2,824	1,306	480	116	8	–
2nd child	12,032	–	745	4	19	79	187	456	4,619	3,791	1,987	745	135	9	1
3rd child	8,299	–	108	–	3	1	29	75	2,208	3,023	2,005	793	152	9	1
4th child	4,761	–	13	–	–	2	2	9	743	1,780	1,405	681	132	7	–
5th child	2,451	–	1	–	–	–	–	1	195	843	855	450	102	5	–
6th child	1,236	–	–	–	–	–	–	–	38	365	477	282	67	6	1
7th child	613	–	1	–	–	–	1	–	14	126	250	179	43	–	–
8th child and over	511	–	–	–	–	–	–	–	5	44	188	194	73	7	–
Not stated	163	–	17	–	1	4	3	9	43	46	33	20	4	–	–
Asian or Pacific Islander	281,264	37	4,297	123	284	582	1,165	2,143	26,174	73,386	105,490	57,400	13,299	1,067	114
1st child	125,015	36	3,573	120	265	514	997	1,677	16,043	40,792	44,232	16,404	3,540	358	37
2nd child	101,583	1	608	3	19	58	144	384	7,135	21,435	42,004	24,963	5,086	325	26
3rd child	34,504	–	88	–	–	6	19	63	2,133	7,035	12,242	10,159	2,654	174	19
4th child	11,443	–	9	–	–	1	–	8	565	2,371	3,983	3,328	1,071	96	20
5th child	4,073	–	–	–	–	–	–	–	137	852	1,401	1,213	421	45	4
6th child	1,652	–	–	–	–	–	–	–	20	293	611	502	196	27	3
7th child	761	–	–	–	–	–	–	–	10	102	244	264	124	15	2
8th child and over	742	–	–	–	–	–	–	–	3	59	222	291	141	23	3
Not stated	1,491	–	19	–	–	3	5	11	128	447	551	276	66	4	–

– = Quantity zero.

Table 1-22. Live Births, by Age of Mother, Live-Birth Order, and Hispanic Origin and Selected Race, 2015

(Number of children born alive to mother; includes births with stated origin of mother only.)

Live-birth order and origin of mother	All ages	Under 15 years	Total	15 years	16 years	17 years	18 years	19 years	20 to 24 years	25 to 29 years	30 to 34 years	35 to 39 years	40 to 44 years	45 to 49 years	50 to 54 years
Hispanic,[1] Total	924,048	986	80,364	3,110	7,433	13,644	22,251	33,926	236,264	256,106	209,647	112,045	27,117	1,433	86
1st child	312,163	973	65,109	3,010	6,973	12,019	18,063	25,044	111,257	70,850	42,661	17,248	3,745	292	28
2nd child	275,951	8	12,970	87	400	1,477	3,638	7,368	82,071	86,689	60,604	27,724	5,595	272	18
3rd child	183,861	1	1,780	1	27	98	447	1,207	31,068	60,423	55,071	29,029	6,216	267	6
4th child	90,009	1	218	2	3	11	40	162	8,496	25,166	30,323	20,285	5,250	261	9
5th child	35,427	–	26	–	–	1	2	23	2,025	8,185	12,359	9,574	3,084	164	10
6th child	13,569	–	2	–	–	–	–	2	438	2,608	4,688	4,207	1,545	75	6
7th child	5,482	–	1	–	1	–	–	–	85	818	1,840	1,923	765	45	5
8th child and over	4,150	–	3	–	–	–	–	3	56	429	1,239	1,586	782	51	4
Not stated	3,436	3	255	10	29	38	61	117	768	938	862	469	135	6	–
Mexican	546,169	586	50,305	1,948	4,708	8,642	13,877	21,130	143,962	150,279	120,961	63,524	15,772	749	31
1st child	173,642	582	40,381	1,889	4,399	7,557	11,168	15,368	65,019	37,319	20,564	7,898	1,752	117	10
2nd child	155,993	4	8,381	48	263	987	2,340	4,743	51,066	49,387	31,618	12,846	2,558	126	7
3rd child	114,882	–	1,194	–	20	66	301	807	20,094	38,404	34,447	17,103	3,507	132	1
4th child	60,122	–	162	2	3	9	27	121	5,623	16,661	20,403	13,590	3,529	147	7
5th child	24,000	–	16	–	–	1	1	14	1,342	5,440	8,320	6,579	2,193	107	3
6th child	9,199	–	1	–	–	–	–	1	292	1,732	3,131	2,908	1,081	54	–
7th child	3,708	–	1	–	1	–	–	–	51	562	1,209	1,322	526	35	2
8th child and over	2,637	–	1	–	–	–	–	1	28	252	800	997	532	26	1
Not stated	1,986	–	168	9	22	22	40	75	447	522	469	281	94	5	–
Puerto Rican	70,987	70	6,877	221	604	1,031	1,897	3,124	21,012	20,213	14,246	6,962	1,501	100	6
1st child	26,751	69	5,648	214	578	926	1,562	2,368	10,162	5,806	3,370	1,393	274	26	3
2nd child	22,196	–	1,058	7	25	97	293	636	7,074	7,083	4,475	2,099	388	19	–
3rd child	12,535	1	125	–	–	4	30	91	2,676	4,410	3,305	1,652	349	17	–
4th child	5,386	–	18	–	–	–	3	15	747	1,816	1,662	899	224	20	–
5th child	2,090	–	1	–	–	–	–	1	189	619	727	441	101	11	1
6th child	875	–	–	–	–	–	–	–	42	233	329	205	64	1	1
7th child	395	–	–	–	–	–	–	–	13	65	170	108	37	1	1
8th child and over	353	–	1	–	–	–	–	1	6	54	113	124	50	5	–
Not stated	406	–	26	–	1	4	9	12	103	127	95	41	14	–	–
Cuban	21,107	7	768	14	60	120	216	358	4,115	6,845	5,857	2,772	701	41	1
1st child	9,787	7	689	14	58	108	188	321	2,681	3,270	2,172	774	173	20	1
2nd child	7,516	–	73	–	2	10	25	36	1,080	2,487	2,426	1,157	280	13	–
3rd child	2,557	–	3	–	–	–	3	–	279	733	854	544	140	4	–
4th child	764	–	–	–	–	–	–	–	46	229	238	179	69	3	–
5th child	246	–	1	–	–	–	–	1	11	71	79	66	18	–	–
6th child	94	–	–	–	–	–	–	–	2	23	39	22	8	–	–
7th child	34	–	–	–	–	–	–	–	–	5	10	12	7	–	–
8th child and over	36	–	–	–	–	–	–	–	2	6	9	13	5	1	–
Not stated	73	–	2	–	–	2	–	–	14	21	30	5	1	–	–
Central and South American	142,249	111	8,319	312	726	1,411	2,402	3,468	26,296	38,594	39,047	23,618	5,889	357	18
1st child	48,189	107	6,759	301	680	1,250	1,962	2,566	13,528	12,499	9,748	4,448	1,016	80	4
2nd child	46,100	2	1,356	11	43	143	384	775	9,041	13,958	12,863	7,294	1,505	77	4
3rd child	27,658	–	150	–	–	10	44	96	2,820	7,985	9,271	5,935	1,414	79	4
4th child	12,201	1	15	–	–	2	4	9	625	2,867	4,399	3,302	934	57	1
5th child	4,676	–	2	–	–	–	–	2	120	828	1,713	1,474	509	28	2
6th child	1,644	–	–	–	–	–	–	–	26	189	579	585	250	13	2
7th child	634	–	–	–	–	–	–	–	2	57	172	269	127	6	1
8th child and over	522	–	1	–	–	–	–	1	12	34	117	221	120	17	–
Not stated	625	1	36	–	3	6	8	19	122	177	185	90	14	–	–
Other and Unknown Hispanic	143,536	212	14,095	615	1,335	2,440	3,859	5,846	40,879	40,175	29,536	15,169	3,254	186	30
1st child	53,794	208	11,632	592	1,258	2,178	3,183	4,421	19,867	11,956	6,807	2,735	530	49	10
2nd child	44,146	2	2,102	21	67	240	596	1,178	13,810	13,774	9,222	4,328	864	37	7
3rd child	26,229	–	308	1	7	18	69	213	5,199	8,891	7,194	3,795	806	35	1
4th child	11,536	–	23	–	–	–	6	17	1,455	3,593	3,621	2,315	494	34	1
5th child	4,415	–	6	–	–	–	1	5	363	1,227	1,520	1,014	263	18	4
6th child	1,757	–	1	–	–	–	–	1	76	431	610	487	142	7	3
7th child	711	–	–	–	–	–	–	–	19	129	279	212	68	3	1
8th child and over	602	–	–	–	–	–	–	–	8	83	200	231	75	2	3
Not stated	346	2	23	1	3	4	4	11	82	91	83	52	12	1	–
Non-Hispanic	3,021,999	1,501	148,103	4,440	10,892	21,332	40,917	70,522	609,438	888,135	875,038	409,833	82,943	6,440	568
1st child	1,200,764	1,489	124,412	4,326	10,336	19,353	34,956	55,441	318,302	353,570	281,159	99,835	19,764	2,042	191
2nd child	984,642	8	20,215	98	496	1,762	5,229	12,630	194,826	292,593	310,018	140,523	24,660	1,668	131
3rd child	483,225	2	2,605	3	35	132	509	1,926	68,846	147,583	160,037	86,542	16,524	997	89
4th child	196,431	–	259	1	3	11	48	196	18,813	58,594	68,331	40,780	9,002	595	57
5th child	75,781	–	36	–	–	4	10	22	4,484	20,356	27,597	18,251	4,678	346	33
6th child	32,039	–	6	–	–	1	3	2	946	7,055	12,225	9,062	2,514	218	13
7th child	15,500	–	3	–	–	–	1	2	236	2,420	5,804	5,233	1,639	143	22
8th child and over	17,716	–	7	–	–	2	2	3	252	1,300	4,947	7,196	3,612	380	22
Not stated	15,901	2	560	12	22	67	159	300	2,733	4,664	4,920	2,411	550	51	10

Note: Race and Hispanic origin are reported separately on birth certificates. Race categories are consistent with 1977 Office of Management and Budget standards. Forty-nine states and the District of Columbia reported multiple-race data for 2015 that were bridged to single-race categories for comparability with other states. Persons of Hispanic origin may be of any race. In this table, Hispanic women are classified only by place of origin; non-Hispanic women are classified by race.
– = Quantity zero.
[1] Includes races other than White and Black.

Table 1-22. Live Births, by Age of Mother, Live-Birth Order, and Hispanic Origin and Selected Race, 2015—*Continued*

(Number of children born alive to mother; includes births with stated origin of mother only.)

Live-birth order and origin of mother	All ages	Under 15 years	Total	15 years	16 years	17 years	18 years	19 years	20 to 24 years	25 to 29 years	30 to 34 years	35 to 39 years	40 to 44 years	45 to 49 years	50 to 54 years
Non-Hispanic White	2,130,279	582	90,833	2,135	5,854	12,417	25,426	45,001	399,373	642,150	646,767	290,877	55,040	4,323	334
1st child	855,738	578	77,564	2,093	5,639	11,493	22,102	36,237	214,704	265,180	210,258	72,352	13,580	1,412	110
2nd child	709,069	2	11,576	36	190	829	2,990	7,531	129,850	217,327	233,048	99,881	16,198	1,104	83
3rd child	339,155	–	1,278	2	16	54	232	974	41,233	103,301	119,822	62,068	10,751	653	49
4th child	130,385	–	99	–	–	5	17	77	9,641	37,170	48,678	28,532	5,853	382	30
5th child	46,732	–	18	–	–	1	8	9	1,873	11,302	18,019	12,289	2,990	219	22
6th child	18,947	–	1	–	–	–	1	–	331	3,353	7,542	5,976	1,604	133	7
7th child	9,172	–	2	–	–	–	–	2	70	1,014	3,467	3,431	1,081	91	16
8th child and over	11,134	–	4	–	–	2	1	1	140	541	2,659	4,831	2,653	294	12
Not stated	9,947	2	291	4	9	33	75	170	1,531	2,962	3,274	1,517	330	35	5
Non-Hispanic Black	589,047	845	50,039	2,079	4,486	7,801	13,553	22,120	175,597	165,895	119,976	60,863	14,592	1,104	136
1st child	214,195	838	40,901	2,013	4,179	6,858	11,209	16,642	84,422	46,747	26,951	11,315	2,690	283	48
2nd child	168,767	5	7,553	56	274	832	1,986	4,405	54,961	52,024	34,643	15,849	3,458	250	24
3rd child	105,219	2	1,174	1	17	74	245	837	23,918	35,447	27,177	14,162	3,128	186	25
4th child	51,857	–	141	1	3	3	29	105	8,081	17,825	14,958	8,649	2,063	129	11
5th child	23,378	–	18	–	–	3	2	13	2,320	7,580	7,623	4,506	1,235	88	8
6th child	10,538	–	5	–	–	1	2	2	567	3,116	3,700	2,406	682	58	4
7th child	5,104	–	–	–	–	–	–	–	145	1,197	1,891	1,416	413	38	4
8th child and over	5,458	–	3	–	–	–	1	2	104	668	1,919	1,933	764	60	7
Not stated	4,531	–	244	8	13	30	79	114	1,079	1,291	1,114	627	159	12	5

Note: Race and Hispanic origin are reported separately on birth certificates. Race categories are consistent with 1977 Office of Management and Budget standards. Forty-nine states and the District of Columbia reported multiple-race data for 2015 that were bridged to single-race categories for comparability with other states. Persons of Hispanic origin may be of any race. In this table, Hispanic women are classified only by place of origin; non-Hispanic women are classified by race.
– = Quantity zero.
[1] Includes races other than White and Black.

Table 1-23. Live Births, by Race of Mother, by State and Territory, 2015

(Number.)

State and territory	All races	White	Black	American Indian or Alaska Native	Asian or Pacific Islander
United States[1]	3,978,497	3,012,855	640,079	44,299	281,264
Alabama	59,657	39,845	18,429	190	1,193
Alaska	11,282	7,244	509	2,415	1,114
Arizona	85,351	71,422	5,095	5,316	3,518
Arkansas	38,886	29,532	7,767	353	1,234
California	491,748	377,423	30,546	3,510	80,269
Colorado	66,581	58,756	4,049	803	2,973
Connecticut	35,746	28,164	4,988	97	2,497
Delaware	11,166	7,341	3,134	16	675
District of Columbia	9,578	4,061	5,002	16	499
Florida	224,269	162,594	53,699	373	7,603
Georgia	131,404	76,904	47,734	298	6,468
Hawaii	18,420	6,322	620	35	11,443
Idaho	22,827	21,618	287	406	516
Illinois	158,116	119,630	28,059	205	10,222
Indiana	84,040	70,741	10,656	120	2,523
Iowa	39,482	35,279	2,597	242	1,364
Kansas	39,154	34,251	3,090	330	1,483
Kentucky	55,971	49,061	5,507	88	1,315
Louisiana	64,692	37,801	25,001	392	1,498
Maine	12,607	11,805	473	143	186
Maryland	73,616	42,471	25,017	279	5,849
Massachusetts	71,492	55,350	9,288	141	6,713
Michigan	113,312	85,838	22,394	786	4,294
Minnesota	69,834	54,407	8,353	1,415	5,659
Mississippi	38,394	20,730	16,846	259	559
Missouri	75,061	60,913	11,660	359	2,129
Montana	12,583	10,768	103	1,560	152
Nebraska	26,679	23,126	2,009	557	987
Nevada	36,298	27,648	4,803	510	3,337
New Hampshire	12,433	11,600	280	26	527
New Jersey	103,127	72,400	18,363	172	12,192
New Mexico	25,816	21,183	664	3,452	517
New York	237,274	163,871	46,109	738	26,556
North Carolina	120,843	81,154	31,864	1,964	5,861
North Dakota	11,314	9,345	640	985	344
Ohio	139,264	109,566	25,078	253	4,367
Oklahoma	53,122	40,143	5,293	5,924	1,762
Oregon	45,655	40,484	1,463	813	2,895
Pennsylvania	141,047	109,595	24,100	391	6,961
Rhode Island	10,993	8,824	1,392	138	639
South Carolina	58,139	38,056	18,577	217	1,289
South Dakota	12,336	9,504	344	2,166	322
Tennessee	81,685	61,814	17,507	211	2,153
Texas	403,618	327,429	53,144	1,270	21,775
Utah	50,778	47,381	823	699	1,875
Vermont	5,903	5,554	149	25	175
Virginia	103,303	71,485	23,029	254	8,535
Washington	88,990	71,041	5,302	2,036	10,611
West Virginia	19,805	18,814	738	28	225
Wisconsin	67,041	55,350	7,386	1,029	3,276
Wyoming	7,765	7,217	119	294	135
Puerto Rico	31,157	27,691	3,374	40	52
Virgin Islands	1325	129	1180	1	15
Guam	3,366	217	38	13	3,098
American Samoa	1,078	2	1	–	1,075
Northern Marianas	427	3	–	–	424

Note: Race and Hispanic origin are reported separately on birth certificates. Race categories are consistent with the 1977 Office of Management and Budget standards. Forty-nine states and the District of Columbia reported mulitple-race data for 2015 that were bridged to the single-race categories for comparability with other states. In this table, all women, including Hispanic women, are classified only according to their race.
- = Quantity zero.
[1]Excludes data for the territories.

Table 1-24. Live Births, by Hispanic Origin of Mother and by Race for Mothers of Non-Hispanic Origin, by State and Territory, 2015

(Number.)

| State and territory | All origins | Hispanic (may be of any race) | | | | | | Non-Hispanic | | | Not stated |
		Total	Mexican	Puerto Rican	Cuban	Central and South American	Other and unknown Hispanic	Total[1]	White	Black	
United States[2]	3,978,497	924,048	546,169	70,987	21,107	142,249	143,536	3,021,999	2,130,279	589,047	32,450
Alabama	59,657	4,295	2,606	239	51	1,272	127	55,344	35,826	18,261	18
Alaska	11,282	810	411	91	17	119	172	10,290	6,543	423	182
Arizona	85,351	35,247	31,165	548	186	1,195	2,153	49,626	36,976	4,582	478
Arkansas	38,886	4,008	2,928	91	18	693	278	34,762	25,714	7,589	116
California	491,748	234,237	175,341	2,139	770	18,297	37,690	246,400	141,592	27,035	11,111
Colorado	66,581	18,139	11,726	461	116	1,205	4,631	47,592	40,878	3,453	850
Connecticut	35,746	8,275	805	4,282	96	2,869	223	27,377	20,395	4,439	94
Delaware	11,166	1,532	598	328	19	454	133	9,622	5,959	2,986	12
District of Columbia	9,578	1,327	161	40	27	898	201	8,224	2,976	4,802	27
Florida	224,269	64,078	12,102	13,126	13,768	21,124	3,958	159,617	102,549	49,609	574
Georgia	131,404	17,836	11,148	1,200	313	3,939	1,236	111,866	60,328	45,461	1,702
Hawaii	18,420	2,775	807	976	21	125	846	15,628	4,803	579	17
Idaho	22,827	3,645	2,940	56	13	161	475	19,116	18,087	240	66
Illinois	158,116	33,902	27,696	2,526	211	2,504	965	122,761	85,424	27,160	1,453
Indiana	84,040	7,634	5,540	406	54	931	703	76,370	63,472	10,343	36
Iowa	39,482	3,418	2,608	103	16	557	134	36,060	32,028	2,503	4
Kansas	39,154	6,300	4,619	159	41	622	859	32,812	28,236	2,912	42
Kentucky	55,971	3,000	1,661	235	223	611	270	52,900	46,344	5,269	71
Louisiana	64,692	4,826	1,778	200	145	2,164	539	59,791	34,047	24,064	75
Maine	12,607	251	64	74	15	58	40	12,348	11,563	463	8
Maryland	73,616	11,750	1,661	730	139	8,017	1,203	61,662	32,412	23,626	204
Massachusetts	71,492	13,015	513	4,629	137	3,630	4,106	57,268	43,651	7,019	1,209
Michigan	113,312	7,431	4,722	555	118	777	1,259	105,683	78,960	21,822	198
Minnesota	69,834	4,852	3,247	180	62	1,040	323	64,460	49,673	8,030	522
Mississippi	38,394	1,613	904	116	16	427	150	36,776	19,635	16,419	5
Missouri	75,061	4,042	2,478	198	82	737	547	70,720	57,092	11,304	299
Montana	12,583	573	343	27	6	33	164	11,968	10,270	89	42
Nebraska	26,679	4,249	2,994	85	74	860	236	22,415	19,201	1,872	15
Nevada	36,298	13,225	10,325	330	339	1,473	758	22,952	14,937	4,455	121
New Hampshire	12,433	638	104	173	15	123	223	11,698	10,928	237	97
New Jersey	103,127	27,919	5,094	6,113	721	11,814	4,177	73,932	47,425	14,880	1,276
New Mexico	25,816	14,431	5,233	99	51	152	8,896	11,096	7,157	472	289
New York	237,274	55,796	8,529	12,721	676	17,971	15,899	177,387	114,643	36,392	4,091
North Carolina	120,843	18,091	10,297	1,454	316	4,712	1,312	102,695	67,122	28,866	57
North Dakota	11,314	580	384	45	8	40	103	10,586	8,796	573	148
Ohio	139,264	6,974	3,056	1,672	105	1,278	863	131,683	103,586	23,739	607
Oklahoma	53,122	7,406	5,537	199	43	778	849	45,631	33,293	4,995	85
Oregon	45,655	8,518	7,419	140	73	558	328	36,910	32,147	1,335	227
Pennsylvania	141,047	14,950	2,440	7,435	252	1,868	2,955	124,479	97,845	20,160	1,618
Rhode Island	10,993	2,622	164	737	23	777	921	8,289	6,702	952	82
South Carolina	58,139	4,942	2,652	492	99	1,283	416	53,055	33,927	17,801	142
South Dakota	12,336	559	307	45	9	143	55	11,760	9,063	328	17
Tennessee	81,685	7,264	4,641	399	111	1,782	331	74,280	55,420	16,792	141
Texas	403,618	191,157	140,254	2,264	1,063	14,668	32,908	212,089	140,553	49,662	372
Utah	50,778	7,876	5,493	161	35	1,246	941	41,361	38,473	644	1,541
Vermont	5,903	139	37	39	6	30	27	5,683	5,370	131	81
Virginia	103,303	13,930	3,028	1,224	211	4,331	5,136	89,244	59,244	21,777	129
Washington	88,990	16,073	12,062	436	118	1,351	2,106	71,517	55,352	4,619	1,400
West Virginia	19,805	331	132	61	9	61	68	19,354	18,442	698	120
Wisconsin	67,041	6,604	4,761	929	67	428	419	60,195	49,024	7,098	242
Wyoming	7,765	963	654	19	3	63	224	6,665	6,196	87	137
Puerto Rico	31,157	29,464	50	28,548	25	166	675	1,625	1,454	134	68
Virgin Islands	1,325	237	2	14	1	4	216	1,066	104	946	22
Guam	3,366	31	11	5	1	5	9	3,306	197	34	29
American Samoa	1,078	NA	NA	NA	NA	NA	NA	-	-	-	1,078
Northern Marianas	427	-	-	-	-	-	-	422	3	-	5

Note: Race and Hispanic origin are reported separately on birth certificates. Race categories are consistent with 1977 Office of Management and Budget standards. Forty-nine states and the District of Columbia reported multiple-race data for 2015 that were bridged to single-race categories for comparability with other states. In this table, Hispanic women are classified only by place of origin; non-Hispanic women are classified by race.
NA = Not available.
- = Quantity zero.
[1] Includes races other than White and Black.
[2] Excludes data for the territories.

Table 1-25. Birth Rates, by Age of Mother, State, and Territory, 2015

(Fertility rates are births per 1,000 women age 15 to 44 years estimated in each area; total fertility rates are sums of birth rates for 5-year age groups multiplied by 5; birth rates by age are births per 1,000 women in specified age group estimated in each area.)

State and territory	Birth rate	Fertility rate	Total fertility rate	10 to 14 years	15 to 19 years Total	15 to 17 years	18 to 19 years	20 to 24 years	25 to 29 years	30 to 34 years	35 to 39 years	40 to 44 years	45 to 49 years[1]
United States[2]	12.4	62.5	1,843.5	0.2	22.3	9.9	40.7	76.8	104.3	101.5	51.8	11.0	0.8
Alabama	12.3	62.2	1,833.5	0.3	30.1	13.5	55.8	98.2	112.5	84.8	34.6	5.9	0.3
Alaska	15.3	77.0	2,172.0	*	29.3	9.8	63.8	106.1	123.2	108.7	55.1	11.1	*
Arizona	12.5	64.7	1,916.0	0.2	26.3	11.8	48.2	88.1	113.0	96.3	48.2	10.4	0.7
Arkansas	13.1	67.5	1,986.5	0.4	38.0	15.6	72.4	114.1	120.1	83.7	34.5	6.1	0.4
California	12.6	60.8	1,785.5	0.2	19.0	8.5	34.6	63.7	89.4	104.8	63.2	15.4	1.4
Colorado	12.2	60.2	1,748.0	0.2	19.3	8.4	35.9	68.3	94.0	100.9	54.8	11.3	0.8
Connecticut	10.0	52.5	1,609.5	*	10.1	4.6	17.7	43.4	87.0	109.5	58.8	12.0	1.0
Delaware	11.8	61.8	1,812.5	*	18.1	8.2	31.5	74.4	99.2	106.9	52.9	9.7	0.8
District of Columbia	14.2	52.8	1,483.5	*	25.6	18.2	30.5	51.4	46.4	75.9	72.7	21.8	2.5
Florida	11.1	60.0	1,769.0	0.2	20.8	8.8	39.7	75.9	100.3	95.5	49.2	11.1	0.8
Georgia	12.9	62.0	1,854.5	0.3	25.6	11.4	47.4	88.8	106.5	93.2	46.0	9.8	0.7
Hawaii	12.9	68.7	1,969.0	*	20.6	7.8	40.7	84.3	101.7	102.0	66.9	16.6	1.5
Idaho	13.8	71.8	2,134.0	*	22.5	8.5	44.9	108.4	134.9	104.7	45.9	9.5	0.7
Illinois	12.3	61.3	1,813.0	0.2	21.1	9.7	38.5	68.5	98.6	107.1	54.9	11.3	0.9
Indiana	12.7	64.8	1,927.0	0.3	26.0	11.1	48.7	90.0	124.4	97.0	39.7	7.5	0.5
Iowa	12.6	67.1	2,006.0	*	18.6	7.7	33.5	74.7	142.9	110.8	45.9	7.5	0.7
Kansas	13.4	69.9	2,053.0	*	25.5	9.9	48.9	88.7	134.9	106.5	45.6	8.8	0.5
Kentucky	12.6	65.7	1,951.0	0.4	32.4	13.3	61.9	104.7	121.1	88.0	36.6	6.6	0.4
Louisiana	13.9	68.5	1,962.5	0.6	34.1	14.9	65.1	108.4	115.6	87.7	38.2	7.5	0.4
Maine	9.5	54.3	1,640.5	*	15.4	5.3	29.8	69.9	100.7	92.8	42.0	6.8	0.5
Maryland	12.3	61.3	1,803.0	0.2	17.0	8.4	29.6	63.3	96.2	108.6	60.6	13.5	1.2
Massachusetts	10.5	52.0	1,551.0	0.1	9.4	4.4	15.3	36.8	72.5	110.5	66.3	13.6	1.0
Michigan	11.4	60.3	1,808.5	0.2	19.4	7.8	36.8	73.0	112.9	102.9	44.5	8.2	0.6
Minnesota	12.7	66.3	1,934.0	0.1	13.7	5.7	25.7	60.3	121.2	123.2	56.8	10.6	0.9
Mississippi	12.8	64.0	1,876.0	0.7	34.8	16.1	62.8	110.9	115.3	76.3	31.6	5.3	0.3
Missouri	12.3	63.8	1,863.5	0.2	25.0	10.3	47.6	87.4	115.1	96.3	41.2	7.1	0.4
Montana	12.2	67.3	1,957.5	*	25.3	9.9	48.2	81.2	123.6	104.8	46.4	9.4	*
Nebraska	14.1	72.8	2,151.5	*	22.0	10.0	39.1	78.6	146.6	118.9	53.2	10.3	0.6
Nevada	12.6	63.3	1,857.5	*	27.6	11.6	56.0	91.5	100.0	91.2	49.1	11.0	0.9
New Hampshire	9.3	51.3	1,590.5	*	10.9	4.2	19.5	44.3	97.9	106.4	49.3	8.7	0.5
New Jersey	11.5	60.0	1,800.5	0.1	12.1	5.3	23.3	52.5	94.1	119.4	66.2	14.7	1.0
New Mexico	12.4	65.3	1,901.5	0.3	34.6	17.1	61.4	100.0	111.5	83.9	41.2	8.3	0.5
New York	12.0	58.8	1,710.0	0.2	14.6	6.8	25.4	56.8	84.4	103.6	65.0	16.0	1.4
North Carolina	12.0	60.7	1,816.0	0.3	23.6	10.9	42.1	84.4	104.8	95.8	45.1	8.6	0.6
North Dakota	14.9	76.4	2,158.0	*	22.2	10.0	36.6	75.9	153.1	121.1	49.9	9.0	*
Ohio	12.0	63.1	1,872.0	0.3	23.2	10.1	43.4	85.5	112.3	101.3	43.6	7.7	0.5
Oklahoma	13.6	69.1	2,002.5	0.3	34.8	15.9	64.2	107.0	123.5	89.5	37.6	7.3	0.5
Oregon	11.3	58.1	1,696.5	*	19.0	7.9	36.1	67.6	97.2	94.0	49.9	10.7	0.8
Pennsylvania	11.0	58.7	1,739.5	0.2	17.7	8.2	30.3	66.8	98.0	104.9	50.4	9.2	0.7
Rhode Island	10.4	52.5	1,578.5	*	14.3	7.5	21.4	49.5	80.5	104.3	55.4	10.7	0.6
South Carolina	11.9	61.1	1,796.5	0.4	26.2	11.4	47.8	88.0	104.6	90.3	41.6	7.7	0.5
South Dakota	14.4	78.2	2,272.5	*	26.4	9.7	50.2	93.2	156.9	122.2	45.8	9.0	*
Tennessee	12.4	62.8	1,853.0	0.3	30.5	12.6	58.8	95.5	110.2	88.2	38.2	7.3	0.4
Texas	14.7	70.2	2,075.0	0.5	34.6	16.7	63.0	100.3	116.6	101.8	49.6	10.8	0.8
Utah	16.9	78.0	2,290.0	*	17.6	6.9	34.5	86.4	162.3	124.0	55.5	11.3	0.8
Vermont	9.4	51.1	1,581.0	*	11.6	3.9	19.8	46.8	98.7	97.8	53.1	7.5	*
Virginia	12.3	61.3	1,803.0	0.2	17.1	6.9	31.3	68.3	100.1	106.0	56.1	11.9	0.9
Washington	12.4	62.8	1,816.0	0.1	17.6	7.3	33.9	69.0	101.6	105.6	56.2	12.2	0.9
West Virginia	10.7	59.4	1,783.0	*	31.9	12.3	61.6	100.6	111.4	76.1	30.5	5.7	*
Wisconsin	11.6	61.8	1,846.0	0.2	16.2	6.4	30.4	64.0	122.2	109.9	47.7	8.5	0.5
Wyoming	13.2	70.2	2,010.0	*	29.2	9.7	59.2	104.0	124.2	94.2	41.4	7.9	*
Puerto Rico	9	44.8	1,336.5	0.4	33.9	18.1	57.0	85.8	72.0	47.1	22.9	4.7	0.2
Virgin Islands	12.8	69.6	2217.5	*	39.1	14.7	79.5	118.6	137.3	92.9	40.7	13.7	*
Guam	20.8	98.0	2,928.0	*	38.3	16.9	71.6	138.6	161.7	145.7	81.9	17.7	*
American Samoa	19.8	86.3	2,546.5	*	46.9	25.8	71.4	102.9	139.8	116.9	77.2	24.6	*
Northern Marianas	8.2	33.0	1,075.0	*	36.9	*	62.9	87.8	54.1	18.8	13.8	*	*

Note: Population data for computing birth rates were provided by the U.S. Census Bureau. Rates by state may differ from rates computed on the basis of other population estimates.
* = Figure does not meet standards of reliability or percision; birth rates based on fewer than 20 births.
[1]Birth rates computed by relating births to women age 45 years and over to women age 45 to 49 years.
[2]Excludes data for the territories.

Table 1-26. Birth Rates, by Age of Mother, Live-Birth Order, and Race of Mother, 2015

(Live births per 1,000 women in specified age and racial group.)

Live-birth order and race of mother	15 to 44 years	10 to 14 years	15 to 19 years Total	15 to 17 years	18 to 19 years	20 to 24 years	25 to 29 years	30 to 34 years	35 to 39 years	40 to 44 years	45 to 49 years[1]
All Races	62.5	0.2	22.3	9.9	40.7	76.8	104.3	101.5	51.8	11.0	0.8
1st child	24.1	0.2	18.5	9.2	32.5	39.2	38.9	30.5	11.7	2.4	0.3
2nd child	20.1	*	3.2	0.7	7.0	25.3	34.7	34.8	16.8	3.0	0.2
3rd child	10.6	*	0.4	0.0	1.0	9.1	19.0	20.2	11.5	2.3	0.1
4th child	4.6	*	0.0	0.0	0.1	2.5	7.7	9.3	6.1	1.4	0.1
5th child	1.8	*	0.0	*	0.0	0.6	2.6	3.8	2.8	0.8	0.1
6th and 7th child	1.1	*	*	*	*	0.2	1.2	2.3	2.0	0.6	0.1
8th child and over	0.4	*	*	*	*	0.0	0.2	0.6	0.9	0.4	0.0
White	63.1	0.2	21.3	9.2	39.3	75.3	107.6	104.8	52.2	10.6	0.8
1st child	24.2	0.2	17.8	8.5	31.6	38.8	40.6	31.3	11.8	2.3	0.2
2nd child	20.4	*	3.1	0.6	6.7	25.2	36.5	36.2	16.6	2.8	0.2
3rd child	10.8	*	0.4	0.0	0.9	8.6	19.6	21.4	11.8	2.2	0.1
4th child	4.5	*	0.0	0.0	0.1	2.1	7.5	9.6	6.3	1.4	0.1
5th child	1.7	*	0.0	*	0.0	0.5	2.3	3.7	2.8	0.8	0.1
6th and 7th child	1.0	*	*	*	*	0.1	0.9	2.1	2.0	0.6	0.0
8th child and over	0.3	*	*	*	*	0.0	0.1	0.5	0.8	0.4	0.0
Black	64.0	0.5	32.0	15.3	57.1	100.2	101.8	81.0	43.4	10.7	0.9
1st child	23.5	0.5	26.3	14.0	44.8	48.8	29.0	18.3	8.1	2.0	0.2
2nd child	18.5	*	4.8	1.2	10.3	31.6	32.4	23.7	11.5	2.6	0.2
3rd child	11.5	*	0.7	0.1	1.7	13.6	21.9	18.7	10.2	2.3	0.2
4th child	5.7	*	0.1	*	0.2	4.5	10.9	10.2	6.3	1.6	0.1
5th child	2.5	*	0.0	*	*	1.3	4.6	5.1	3.3	0.9	0.1
6th and 7th child	1.7	*	*	*	*	0.4	2.6	3.7	2.7	0.8	0.1
8th child and over	0.6	*	*	*	*	0.1	0.4	1.3	1.3	0.5	0.0
American Indian or Alaska Native	43.9	0.3	25.7	12.7	45.8	70.2	73.2	51.7	25.2	5.8	0.4
1st child	14.1	0.3	21.0	11.7	35.3	29.3	16.2	8.0	3.2	0.8	*
2nd child	12.0	*	4.1	0.9	8.9	24.2	21.7	12.1	4.9	1.0	*
3rd child	8.2	*	0.6	*	1.4	11.6	17.3	12.2	5.3	1.1	*
4th child	4.7	*	*	*	*	3.9	10.2	8.6	4.5	0.9	*
5th child	2.4	*	*	*	*	1.0	4.8	5.2	3.0	0.7	*
6th and 7th child	1.8	*	*	*	*	0.3	2.8	4.4	3.0	0.8	*
8th child and over	0.5	*	*	*	*	*	0.3	1.1	1.3	0.5	*
Asian or Pacific Islander	58.5	0.1	6.9	2.7	12.8	35.6	84.1	117.4	67.6	15.9	1.6
1st child	26.1	0.1	5.8	2.5	10.4	21.9	47.0	49.5	19.4	4.3	0.5
2nd child	21.2	*	1.0	0.2	2.1	9.8	24.7	47.0	29.5	6.1	0.5
3rd child	7.2	*	0.1	*	0.3	2.9	8.1	13.7	12.0	3.2	0.3
4th child	2.4	*	*	*	*	0.8	2.7	4.5	3.9	1.3	0.2
5th child	0.9	*	*	*	*	0.2	1.0	1.6	1.4	0.5	0.1
6th and 7th child	0.5	*	*	*	*	0.0	0.5	1.0	0.9	0.4	0.1
8th child and over	0.2	*	*	*	*	*	0.1	0.2	0.3	0.2	0.0

Note: Race and Hispanic origin are reported separately on birth certificates. Race categories are consistent with 1977 Office of Management and Budget standards. Forty-nine states and the District of Columbia reported multiple-race data for 2015 that were bridged to single-race categories for comparability with other states. In this table, all women, including Hispanic women, are classified only according to their race.
* = Figure does not meet standards of reliability or precision; based on fewer than 20 births in the numerator.
[1]Birth rates computed by relating births to women age 45 years and over to women age 45 to 49 years.

Table 1-27. Total Fertility Rates and Birth Rates, by Age and Race of Mother, 1970–2015

(Live births per 1,000 women in specified group.)

| Year and race | Total fertility rate | 10 to 14 years | Age of mother | | | 20 to 24 years | 25 to 29 years | 30 to 34 years | 35 to 39 years | 40 to 44 years | 45 to 49 years[1] |
| | | | 15 to 19 years | | | | | | | | |
			Total	15 to 17 years	18 to 19 years						
All Races[2]											
1970[3]	2,480.0	1.2	68.3	38.8	114.7	167.8	145.1	73.3	31.7	8.1	0.5
1971[3]	2,266.5	1.1	64.5	38.2	105.3	150.1	134.1	67.3	28.7	7.1	0.4
1972[4]	2,010.0	1.2	61.7	39.0	96.9	130.2	117.7	59.8	24.8	6.2	0.4
1973[4]	1,879.0	1.2	59.3	38.5	91.2	119.7	112.2	55.6	22.1	5.4	0.3
1974[4]	1,835.0	1.2	57.5	37.3	88.7	117.7	111.5	53.8	20.2	4.8	0.3
1975[4]	1,774.0	1.3	55.6	36.1	85.0	113.0	108.2	52.3	19.5	4.6	0.3
1976[4]	1,738.0	1.2	52.8	34.1	80.5	110.3	106.2	53.6	19.0	4.3	0.2
1977[4]	1,789.5	1.2	52.8	33.9	80.9	112.9	111.0	56.4	19.2	4.2	0.2
1978[4]	1,760.0	1.2	51.5	32.2	79.8	109.9	108.5	57.8	19.0	3.9	0.2
1979[4]	1,808.0	1.2	52.3	32.3	81.3	112.8	111.4	60.3	19.5	3.9	0.2
1980[4]	1,839.5	1.1	53.0	32.5	82.1	115.1	112.9	61.9	19.8	3.9	0.2
1981[4]	1,812.0	1.1	52.2	32.0	80.0	112.2	111.5	61.4	20.0	3.8	0.2
1982[4]	1,827.5	1.1	52.4	32.3	79.4	111.6	111.0	64.1	21.2	3.9	0.2
1983[4]	1,799.0	1.1	51.4	31.8	77.4	107.8	108.5	64.9	22.0	3.9	0.2
1984[4]	1,806.5	1.2	50.6	31.0	77.4	106.8	108.7	67.0	22.9	3.9	0.2
1985	1,844.0	1.2	51.0	31.0	79.6	108.3	111.0	69.1	24.0	4.0	0.2
1986	1,837.5	1.3	50.2	30.5	79.6	107.4	109.8	70.1	24.4	4.1	0.2
1987	1,872.0	1.3	50.6	31.7	78.5	107.9	111.6	72.1	26.3	4.4	0.2
1988	1,934.0	1.3	53.0	33.6	79.9	110.2	114.4	74.8	28.1	4.8	0.2
1989	2,014.0	1.4	57.3	36.4	84.2	113.8	117.6	77.4	29.9	5.2	0.2
1990	2,081.0	1.4	59.9	37.5	88.6	116.5	120.2	80.8	31.7	5.5	0.2
1991	2,062.5	1.4	61.8	38.6	94.0	115.3	117.2	79.2	31.9	5.5	0.2
1992	2,046.0	1.4	60.3	37.6	93.6	113.7	115.7	79.6	32.3	5.9	0.3
1993	2,019.5	1.4	59.0	37.5	91.1	111.3	113.2	79.9	32.7	6.1	0.3
1994	2,001.5	1.4	58.2	37.2	90.2	109.2	111.0	80.4	33.4	6.4	0.3
1995	1,978.0	1.3	56.0	35.5	87.7	107.5	108.8	81.1	34.0	6.6	0.3
1996	1,976.0	1.2	53.5	33.3	84.7	107.8	108.6	82.1	34.9	6.8	0.3
1997	1,971.0	1.1	51.3	31.4	82.1	107.3	108.3	83.0	35.7	7.1	0.4
1998	1,999.0	1.0	50.3	29.9	80.9	108.4	110.2	85.2	36.9	7.4	0.4
1999	2,007.5	0.9	48.8	28.2	79.1	107.9	111.2	87.1	37.8	7.4	0.4
2000	2,056.0	0.9	47.7	26.9	78.1	109.7	113.5	91.2	39.7	8.0	0.5
2001	2,030.5	0.8	45.0	24.5	75.5	106.2	113.8	91.8	40.5	8.1	0.5
2002	2,020.5	0.7	42.6	23.1	72.2	103.1	114.7	92.6	41.6	8.3	0.5
2003	2,047.5	0.6	41.1	22.2	69.6	102.3	116.7	95.7	43.9	8.7	0.5
2004	2,051.5	0.6	40.5	21.8	68.7	101.5	116.5	96.2	45.5	9.0	0.5
2005	2,057.0	0.6	39.7	21.1	68.4	101.8	116.5	96.7	46.4	9.1	0.6
2006	2,108.0	0.6	41.1	21.6	71.2	105.5	118.0	98.9	47.5	9.4	0.6
2007	2,120.0	0.6	41.5	21.7	71.7	105.4	118.1	100.6	47.6	9.6	0.6
2008	2,072.0	0.6	40.2	21.1	68.2	101.8	115.0	99.4	46.8	9.9	0.7
2009	2,002.0	0.5	37.9	19.6	64.0	96.2	111.5	97.5	46.1	10.0	0.7
2010	1,931.0	0.4	34.2	17.3	58.2	90.0	108.3	96.5	45.9	10.2	0.7
2011	1,894.5	0.4	31.3	15.4	54.1	85.3	107.2	96.5	47.2	10.3	0.7
2012	1,880.5	0.4	29.4	14.1	51.4	83.1	106.5	97.3	48.3	10.4	0.8
2013	1,857.5	0.3	26.5	12.3	47.1	80.7	105.5	98.0	49.3	10.4	0.8
2014	1,862.5	0.3	24.2	10.9	43.8	79.0	105.8	100.8	51.0	10.0	0.7
2015	1,843.5	0.2	22.3	9.9	40.7	76.8	104.3	101.5	51.8	11.0	0.8
White											
1980[4]	1,773.0	0.6	45.4	25.5	73.2	111.1	113.8	61.2	18.8	3.5	0.2
1981[4]	1,748.0	0.5	44.9	25.4	71.5	108.3	112.3	61.0	19.0	3.4	0.2
1982[4]	1,767.0	0.6	45.0	25.5	70.8	107.7	111.9	64.0	20.4	3.6	0.2
1983[4]	1,740.5	0.6	43.9	25.0	68.8	103.8	109.4	65.3	21.3	3.6	0.2
1984[4]	1,748.5	0.6	42.9	24.3	68.4	102.7	109.8	67.7	22.2	3.6	0.2
1985	1,787.0	0.6	43.3	24.4	70.4	104.1	112.3	69.9	23.3	3.7	0.2
1986	1,776.0	0.6	42.3	23.8	70.1	102.7	110.8	70.9	23.9	3.8	0.2
1987	1,804.5	0.6	42.5	24.6	68.9	102.3	112.3	73.0	25.9	4.1	0.2
1988	1,856.5	0.6	44.4	26.0	69.6	103.7	114.8	75.4	27.7	4.5	0.2
1989	1,931.0	0.7	47.9	28.1	72.9	106.9	117.8	78.1	29.7	4.9	0.2
1990	2,003.0	0.7	50.8	29.5	78.0	109.8	120.7	81.7	31.5	5.2	0.2
1991	1,988.0	0.8	52.6	30.5	83.3	108.8	118.0	80.2	31.8	5.2	0.2
1992	1,978.0	0.8	51.4	29.9	83.2	107.7	116.9	80.8	32.1	5.7	0.2
1993	1,961.5	0.8	50.6	30.0	81.5	106.1	114.7	81.3	32.6	5.9	0.3
1994	1,957.5	0.8	50.5	30.4	81.2	105.0	113.0	82.2	33.5	6.2	0.3
1995	1,954.5	0.8	49.5	29.6	80.2	104.7	111.7	83.3	34.2	6.4	0.3
1996	1,960.5	0.7	47.5	28.0	77.6	105.3	111.7	84.6	35.3	6.7	0.3

Note: Race and Hispanic origin are reported separately on birth certificates. Race categories are consistent with 1977 Office of Management and Budget standards. Forty-nine states and the District of Columbia reported multiple-race data for 2015 that were bridged to single-race categories for comparability with other states. Multiple-race reporting areas vary for 2003–2015. In this table, all women, including Hispanic women, are classified only according to their race.
* = Figure does not meet standards of reliability or precision; based on fewer than 20 births in the numerator.
[1] Beginning in 1997, rates computed by relating births to women age 45 years and over to women age 45 to 49 years.
[2] For 1970 to 1991 includes births to races not shown separately. For 1992 and later years, unknown race of mother is imputed.
[3] Based on a 50 percent sample of births.
[4] Based on 100-percent of births in selected states and on a 50-percent sample of births in all other states.

Table 1-27. Total Fertility Rates and Birth Rates, by Age and Race of Mother, 1970–2015—*Continued*

(Live births per 1,000 women in specified group.)

Year and race	Total fertility rate	10 to 14 years	15 to 19 years			20 to 24 years	25 to 29 years	30 to 34 years	35 to 39 years	40 to 44 years	45 to 49 years[1]
			Total	15 to 17 years	18 to 19 years						
1997............	1,955.0	0.7	45.5	26.6	75.0	104.5	111.3	85.7	36.1	6.9	0.3
1998............	1,991.0	0.6	44.9	25.6	74.1	105.4	113.6	88.5	37.5	7.3	0.4
1999............	2,007.5	0.6	44.0	24.4	73.0	105.0	114.9	90.7	38.5	7.4	0.4
2000............	2,051.0	0.6	43.2	23.3	72.3	106.6	116.7	94.6	40.2	7.9	0.4
2001............	2,042.5	0.5	41.0	21.4	70.4	103.4	117.8	95.9	41.4	8.0	0.5
2002............	2,041.5	0.5	39.2	20.4	67.7	101.6	119.0	96.7	42.6	8.2	0.5
2003............	2,075.0	0.5	38.0	19.6	65.6	100.9	121.3	100.1	45.0	8.7	0.5
2004............	2,074.5	0.5	37.4	19.4	64.4	99.8	120.8	100.3	46.7	8.9	0.5
2005............	2,078.5	0.5	36.7	18.8	64.0	99.9	120.7	100.7	47.6	9.0	0.6
2006............	2,125.0	0.5	37.9	19.2	66.7	103.4	122.0	102.7	48.6	9.3	0.6
2007............	2,137.0	0.5	38.4	19.5	67.2	103.5	122.0	104.4	48.5	9.5	0.6
2008............	2,087.0	0.4	37.3	19.1	64.0	99.8	118.8	103.3	47.5	9.7	0.6
2009............	2,016.5	0.4	35.3	17.8	60.2	94.1	114.9	101.3	46.7	9.9	0.7
2010............	1,947.5	0.3	31.9	15.8	54.8	87.9	111.9	100.5	46.4	10.0	0.6
2011............	1,905.0	0.3	29.1	14.1	50.8	83.0	110.2	100.1	47.6	10.1	0.6
2012............	1,885.5	0.3	27.4	13.0	48.3	80.8	109.2	100.2	48.5	10.0	0.7
2013............	1,868.0	0.2	24.9	11.3	44.7	78.5	108.3	101.3	49.6	10.1	0.7
2014............	1,875.5	0.2	23.0	10.2	42.0	77.3	108.6	103.9	51.2	10.2	0.7
2015............	1,864.0	0.2	21.3	9.2	39.3	75.3	107.6	104.8	52.2	10.6	0.8
Black											
1980[4].........	2,176.5	4.3	97.8	72.5	135.1	140.0	103.9	59.9	23.5	5.6	0.3
1981[4].........	2,117.5	4.0	94.5	69.3	131.0	136.5	102.3	57.4	23.1	5.4	0.3
1982[4].........	2,106.5	4.0	94.3	69.7	128.9	135.4	101.3	57.5	23.3	5.1	0.4
1983[4].........	2,066.0	4.1	93.9	69.6	127.1	131.9	98.4	56.2	23.3	5.1	0.3
1984[4].........	2,070.5	4.4	94.1	69.2	128.1	132.2	98.4	56.7	23.3	4.8	0.2
1985............	2,109.0	4.5	95.4	69.3	132.4	135.0	100.2	57.9	23.9	4.6	0.3
1986............	2,135.5	4.7	95.8	69.3	135.1	137.3	101.1	59.3	23.8	4.8	0.3
1987............	2,198.0	4.8	97.6	72.1	135.8	142.7	104.3	60.6	24.6	4.8	0.2
1988............	2,298.0	4.9	102.7	75.7	142.7	149.7	108.2	63.1	25.6	5.1	0.3
1989............	2,432.5	5.1	111.5	81.9	151.9	156.8	114.4	66.3	26.7	5.4	0.3
1990............	2,480.0	4.9	112.8	82.3	152.9	160.2	115.5	68.7	28.1	5.5	0.3
1991............	2,462.0	4.7	114.8	83.5	157.6	159.7	112.0	67.3	28.2	5.5	0.2
1992............	2,416.0	4.6	111.3	80.5	156.3	156.2	109.7	67.0	28.6	5.6	0.2
1993............	2,351.0	4.5	107.3	78.9	150.2	150.2	106.4	66.6	29.0	5.9	0.3
1994............	2,258.5	4.5	102.9	75.1	146.2	142.9	101.5	65.0	28.7	5.9	0.3
1995............	2,127.5	4.1	94.4	68.5	135.0	133.7	95.6	63.0	28.4	6.0	0.3
1996............	2,088.5	3.5	89.6	63.3	130.5	133.2	94.3	62.0	28.7	6.1	0.3
1997............	2,091.5	3.1	86.3	59.3	127.7	135.2	95.0	62.6	29.3	6.5	0.3
1998............	2,111.5	2.8	83.5	55.4	124.8	138.4	97.5	63.2	30.0	6.6	0.3
1999............	2,082.5	2.5	79.1	50.5	120.6	137.9	97.3	62.7	30.2	6.5	0.3
2000............	2,129.0	2.3	77.4	49.0	118.8	141.3	100.3	65.4	31.5	7.2	0.4
2001............	2,049.5	2.0	71.3	43.7	112.9	132.9	99.6	64.9	31.6	7.2	0.4
2002............	1,990.0	1.8	65.8	39.5	106.3	126.9	99.4	64.7	31.6	7.4	0.4
2003............	1,994.5	1.5	62.5	37.5	101.3	125.9	101.4	66.4	33.1	7.6	0.5
2004............	2,026.0	1.6	61.7	36.3	101.3	127.5	104.4	67.8	33.8	7.9	0.5
2005............	2,062.0	1.6	60.1	34.5	101.2	129.5	107.0	70.2	35.1	8.4	0.5
2006............	2,143.0	1.5	62.2	35.3	105.6	135.2	110.6	73.8	36.3	8.5	0.5
2007............	2,145.5	1.4	62.1	34.7	105.2	134.6	110.4	74.9	36.4	8.7	0.6
2008............	2,102.5	1.3	60.1	33.5	99.5	130.6	107.9	74.8	36.4	8.8	0.6
2009............	2,036.0	1.1	56.5	30.9	92.9	125.1	105.3	73.5	36.2	8.9	0.6
2010............	1,957.0	1.0	51.1	27.3	84.8	118.1	101.8	73.0	36.4	9.3	0.7
2011............	1,920.0	0.9	47.3	24.7	78.8	111.9	101.7	74.1	38.0	9.4	0.7
2012............	1,899.5	0.8	44.0	22.0	74.4	106.7	101.7	75.1	39.2	9.7	0.7
2013............	1,882.5	0.7	39.1	19.0	67.3	105.5	102.6	77.3	40.5	10.0	0.8
2014............	1,872.0	0.6	35.1	16.7	61.9	102.6	103.1	79.4	42.6	10.2	0.8
2015............	1,852.5	0.5	32.0	15.3	57.1	100.2	101.8	81.0	43.4	10.7	0.9
American Indian or Alaska Native											
1980[4].........	2,165.0	1.9	82.2	51.5	129.5	143.7	106.6	61.8	28.1	8.2	*
1981[4].........	2,092.5	2.1	78.4	49.7	121.5	141.2	105.6	58.9	25.2	6.6	*
1982[4].........	2,215.0	1.4	83.5	52.6	127.6	148.1	115.8	60.9	26.9	6.0	*
1983[4].........	2,182.0	1.9	84.2	55.2	121.4	145.5	113.7	58.9	25.5	6.4	*
1984[4].........	2,137.5	1.7	81.5	50.7	124.7	142.4	109.2	60.5	26.3	5.6	*
1985............	2,129.5	1.7	79.2	47.7	124.1	139.1	109.6	62.6	27.4	6.0	*
1986............	2,083.0	1.8	78.1	48.7	125.3	138.8	107.9	60.7	23.8	5.3	*
1987............	2,100.5	1.7	77.2	48.8	122.2	140.0	107.9	63.0	24.4	5.6	*

Note: Race and Hispanic origin are reported separately on birth certificates. Race categories are consistent with 1977 Office of Management and Budget standards. Forty-nine states and the District of Columbia reported multiple-race data for 2015 that were bridged to single-race categories for comparability with other states. Multiple-race reporting areas vary for 2003–2015. In this table, all women, including Hispanic women, are classified only according to their race.
* = Figure does not meet standards of reliability or precision; based on fewer than 20 births in the numerator.
[1]Beginning in 1997, rates computed by relating births to women age 45 years and over to women age 45 to 49 years.
[4]Based on 100-percent of births in selected states and on a 50-percent sample of births in all other states.

Table 1-27. Total Fertility Rates and Birth Rates, by Age and Race of Mother, 1970–2015—*Continued*

(Live births per 1,000 women in specified group.)

Year and race	Total fertility rate	10 to 14 years	15 to 19 years			20 to 24 years	25 to 29 years	30 to 34 years	35 to 39 years	40 to 44 years	45 to 49 years[1]
			Total	15 to 17 years	18 to 19 years						
1988	2,155.0	1.7	77.5	49.7	121.1	145.2	110.9	64.5	25.6	5.3	*
1989	2,248.5	1.5	82.7	51.6	128.9	152.4	114.2	64.8	27.4	6.4	*
1990	2,184.5	1.6	81.1	48.5	129.3	148.7	110.3	61.5	27.5	5.9	*
1991	2,142.5	1.6	84.1	51.9	134.2	143.8	105.6	60.8	26.4	5.8	0.4
1992	2,135.5	1.6	82.4	52.3	130.5	142.3	107.0	61.0	26.7	5.9	*
1993	2,048.5	1.4	79.8	51.5	126.3	134.2	103.5	59.5	25.5	5.6	*
1994	1,950.0	1.8	76.4	48.4	123.7	126.5	98.2	56.6	24.8	5.4	0.3
1995	1,878.5	1.6	72.9	44.6	122.2	123.1	91.6	56.5	24.3	5.5	*
1996	1,855.0	1.6	68.2	42.7	113.3	123.5	91.1	56.5	24.4	5.5	*
1997	1,834.5	1.5	65.2	41.0	107.1	122.5	91.6	56.0	24.4	5.4	0.3
1998	1,851.0	1.5	64.7	39.7	106.9	125.1	92.0	56.8	24.6	5.3	*
1999	1,783.5	1.4	59.9	36.5	98.0	120.7	90.6	53.8	24.3	5.7	0.3
2000	1,772.5	1.1	58.3	34.1	97.1	117.2	91.8	55.5	24.6	5.7	0.3
2001	1,675.5	0.8	50.9	28.8	85.3	110.7	88.9	53.7	24.1	5.7	0.3
2002	1,639.5	0.9	49.0	27.9	82.1	107.0	89.3	52.8	23.3	5.2	0.4
2003	1,610.5	0.8	47.2	26.7	79.9	105.4	87.1	51.9	23.9	5.6	0.2
2004	1,584.0	0.8	46.0	26.3	78.0	102.9	86.3	51.8	23.3	5.4	0.3
2005	1,625.0	0.7	46.9	25.9	80.8	106.8	89.0	52.0	23.9	5.4	0.3
2006	1,621.5	0.7	49.3	26.1	86.3	105.8	86.2	52.5	24.3	5.2	0.3
2007	1,569.0	0.7	47.3	25.8	80.2	102.7	83.2	51.2	23.1	5.3	0.3
2008	1,569.0	0.7	47.3	25.8	80.2	102.7	83.2	51.2	23.1	5.3	0.3
2009	1,494.0	0.6	43.7	23.6	73.5	96.3	79.3	50.7	22.6	5.3	0.3
2010	1,404.0	0.5	38.7	20.1	66.1	91.0	74.4	48.4	22.3	5.2	0.3
2011	1,373.5	0.5	36.1	18.2	61.6	86.6	75.4	47.3	23.1	5.5	0.2
2012	1,350.0	0.5	34.9	17.0	60.5	81.7	73.9	49.7	23.3	5.5	0.5
2013	1,334.5	0.4	31.1	15.9	53.3	78.9	75.6	50.4	24.7	5.5	0.3
2014	1,288.5	0.3	27.3	13.2	48.6	73.2	74.7	52.3	24.1	5.5	0.3
2015	1,262.5	0.3	25.7	12.7	45.8	70.2	73.2	51.7	25.2	5.8	0.4
Asian or Other Pacific Islander											
1980[4]	1,953.5	0.3	26.2	12.0	46.2	93.3	127.4	96.0	38.3	8.5	0.7
1981[4]	1,976.0	0.3	28.5	13.4	49.5	96.4	129.1	93.4	38.0	8.6	0.9
1982[4]	2,015.5	0.4	29.4	14.0	50.8	98.9	130.9	94.4	39.2	8.8	1.1
1983[4]	1,943.5	0.5	26.1	12.9	44.5	94.0	126.2	93.3	39.4	8.2	1.0
1984[4]	1,892.0	0.5	24.2	12.6	40.7	86.7	124.3	92.4	40.6	8.7	1.0
1985	1,885.0	0.4	23.8	12.5	40.8	83.6	123.0	93.6	42.7	8.7	1.2
1986	1,836.0	0.5	22.8	12.1	38.8	79.2	119.9	92.6	41.9	9.3	1.0
1987	1,886.0	0.6	22.4	12.6	37.0	79.7	122.7	97.0	44.2	9.5	1.1
1988	1,983.5	0.6	24.2	13.6	39.6	80.7	128.0	104.4	47.5	10.3	1.0
1989	1,947.5	0.6	25.6	15.0	40.4	78.8	124.0	102.3	47.0	10.2	1.0
1990	2,002.5	0.7	26.4	16.0	40.2	79.2	126.3	106.5	49.6	10.7	1.1
1991	1,928.0	0.8	27.3	16.3	42.2	73.8	118.9	103.3	49.2	11.2	1.1
1992	1,894.5	0.7	26.5	15.4	41.9	71.7	114.6	102.7	50.7	11.1	0.9
1993	1,841.5	0.7	26.5	16.1	41.2	68.1	110.3	101.2	49.4	11.2	0.9
1994	1,834.0	0.7	26.6	16.3	41.3	66.4	108.0	102.2	50.4	11.5	1.0
1995	1,795.5	0.7	25.5	15.6	40.1	64.2	103.7	102.3	50.1	11.8	0.8
1996	1,787.0	0.6	23.5	14.7	36.8	63.5	102.8	104.1	50.2	11.9	0.8
1997	1,757.5	0.5	22.3	14.0	34.9	61.2	101.6	102.5	51.0	11.5	0.9
1998	1,731.5	0.5	22.2	13.8	34.5	59.2	98.7	101.6	51.4	11.8	0.9
1999	1,754.5	0.4	21.4	12.4	33.9	58.9	100.8	104.3	52.9	11.3	0.9
2000	1,892.0	0.3	20.5	11.6	32.6	60.3	108.4	116.5	59.0	12.6	0.8
2001	1,785.0	0.2	19.3	10.1	32.0	56.0	102.3	109.9	56.2	12.2	0.9
2002	1,798.5	0.3	17.7	8.8	29.9	55.5	102.4	112.5	57.8	12.6	0.9
2003	1,819.0	0.2	16.4	8.5	27.3	54.3	102.7	115.9	60.0	13.4	0.9
2004	1,825.0	0.2	16.0	8.4	26.6	53.3	100.4	118.3	62.2	13.6	1.0
2005	1,784.5	0.2	15.4	7.7	26.4	52.9	96.6	115.3	61.8	13.7	1.0
2006	1,803.0	0.1	15.3	8.2	25.4	53.8	95.7	117.3	63.4	14.0	1.0
2007	1,850.5	0.2	14.8	7.4	24.9	53.2	99.2	121.6	65.8	14.2	1.1
2008	1,797.5	0.2	13.8	7.0	23.0	50.4	96.6	117.7	64.9	14.7	1.2
2009	1,743.0	0.1	12.6	6.3	20.9	46.4	94.6	115.1	63.8	14.9	1.1
2010	1,689.0	0.1	10.9	5.1	18.7	42.6	91.5	113.6	62.8	15.1	1.2
2011	1,706.5	0.1	10.2	4.6	18.1	41.9	93.7	114.9	64.1	15.2	1.2
2012	1,769.5	0.1	9.7	4.1	17.7	41.4	95.8	121.3	68.1	16.1	1.4
2013	1,681.0	0.1	8.7	3.7	16.1	39.1	89.5	114.6	66.6	16.1	1.5
2014	1,715.5	0.1	7.7	3.3	13.9	37.5	90.0	121.3	68.9	16.1	1.5
2015	1,646.0	0.1	6.9	2.7	12.8	35.6	84.1	117.4	67.6	15.9	1.4

Note: Race and Hispanic origin are reported separately on birth certificates. Race categories are consistent with 1977 Office of Management and Budget standards. Forty-nine states and the District of Columbia reported multiple-race data for 2015 that were bridged to single-race categories for comparability with other states. Multiple-race reporting areas vary for 2003–2015. In this table, all women, including Hispanic women, are classified only according to their race.
* = Figure does not meet standards of reliability or precision; based on fewer than 20 births in the numerator.
[1]Beginning in 1997, rates computed by relating births to women age 45 years and over to women age 45 to 49 years.
[4]Based on 100-percent of births in selected states and on a 50-percent sample of births in all other states.

Table 1-28. Total Fertility Rates, Fertility Rates, and Birth Rates, by Age and Hispanic Origin of Mother and by Race for Mothers of Non-Hispanic Origin, 1989–2015

(Total fertility rates are sums of birth rates for 5-year age groups multiplied by 5; fertility rates are live births per 1,000 women age 15 to 44 years in specified racial group; birth rates are live births per 1,000 women in specified age group.)

Year, origin, and race of mother	Total fertility rate	Fertility rate[1]	10–14 years	15–19 years Total	15–17 years	18–19 years	20–24 years	25–29 years	30–34 years	35–39 years	40–44 years	45–49 years[2]
ALL ORIGINS												
1989	2,014.0	69.2	1.4	57.3	36.4	84.2	113.8	117.6	77.4	29.9	5.2	0.2
1990	2,081.0	70.9	1.4	59.9	37.5	88.6	116.5	120.2	80.8	31.7	5.5	0.2
1991	2,062.5	69.3	1.4	61.8	38.6	94.0	115.3	117.2	79.2	31.9	5.5	0.2
1992	2,046.0	68.4	1.4	60.3	37.6	93.6	113.7	115.7	79.6	32.3	5.9	0.3
1993	2,019.5	67.0	1.4	59.0	37.5	91.1	111.3	113.2	79.9	32.7	6.1	0.3
1994	2,001.5	65.9	1.4	58.2	37.2	90.2	109.2	111.0	80.4	33.4	6.4	0.3
1995	1,978.0	64.6	1.3	56.0	35.5	87.7	107.5	108.8	81.1	34.0	6.6	0.3
1996	1,976.0	64.1	1.2	53.5	33.3	84.7	107.8	108.6	82.1	34.9	6.8	0.3
1997	1,971.0	63.6	1.1	51.3	31.4	82.1	107.3	108.3	83.0	35.7	7.1	0.4
1998	1,999.0	64.3	1.0	50.3	29.9	80.9	108.4	110.2	85.2	36.9	7.4	0.4
1999	2,007.5	64.4	0.9	48.8	28.2	79.1	107.9	111.2	87.1	37.8	7.4	0.4
2000	2,056.0	65.9	0.9	47.7	26.9	78.1	109.7	113.5	91.2	39.7	8.0	0.5
2001	2,030.5	65.1	0.8	45.0	24.5	75.5	105.6	113.8	91.8	40.5	8.1	0.5
2002	2,020.5	65.0	0.7	42.6	23.1	72.2	103.1	114.7	92.6	41.6	8.3	0.5
2003	2,047.5	66.1	0.6	41.1	22.2	69.6	102.3	116.7	95.7	43.9	8.7	0.5
2004	2,051.5	66.4	0.6	40.5	21.8	68.7	101.5	116.5	96.2	45.5	9.0	0.5
2005	2,057.0	66.7	0.6	39.7	21.1	68.4	101.8	116.5	96.7	46.4	9.1	0.6
2006	2,108.0	68.6	0.6	41.1	21.6	71.2	105.5	118.0	98.9	47.5	9.4	0.6
2007	2,120.0	69.3	0.6	41.5	21.7	71.7	105.4	118.1	100.6	47.6	9.6	0.6
2008	2,072.0	68.1	0.6	40.2	21.1	68.2	101.8	115.0	99.4	46.8	9.9	0.7
2009	2,002.0	66.2	0.5	37.9	19.6	64.0	96.2	111.5	97.5	46.1	10.0	0.7
2010	1,931.0	64.1	0.4	34.2	17.3	58.2	90.0	108.3	96.5	45.9	10.2	0.7
2011	1,894.5	63.2	0.4	31.3	15.4	54.1	85.3	107.2	96.5	47.2	10.3	0.7
2012	1,880.5	63.0	0.4	29.4	14.1	51.4	83.1	106.5	97.3	48.3	10.4	0.8
2013	1,857.5	62.5	0.3	26.5	12.3	47.1	80.7	105.5	98.0	49.3	10.4	0.8
2014	1,862.5	62.9	0.3	24.2	10.9	43.8	79.0	106.5	100.8	51.0	10.0	0.7
2015	1,843.5	62.5	0.2	22.3	9.9	40.7	76.8	104.3	101.5	51.8	11.0	0.8
HISPANIC												
1989[3]	2,903.5	104.9	2.3	100.8	NA	NA	184.4	146.6	92.1	43.5	10.4	0.6
1990[4]	2,959.5	107.7	2.4	100.3	65.9	147.7	181.0	153.0	98.3	45.3	10.9	0.7
1991[5]	2,963.5	106.9	2.4	104.6	69.2	155.5	184.6	150.0	95.1	44.7	10.7	0.6
1992[5]	2,957.5	106.1	2.5	103.3	68.9	153.9	185.2	148.8	94.8	45.3	11.0	0.6
1993	2,894.5	103.3	2.6	101.8	68.5	151.1	180.0	146.0	93.2	44.1	10.6	0.6
1994	2,839.0	100.7	2.6	101.3	69.9	147.5	175.7	142.4	91.1	43.4	10.7	0.6
1995	2,798.5	98.8	2.6	99.3	68.3	145.4	171.9	140.4	90.5	43.7	10.7	0.6
1996	2,772.0	97.5	2.4	94.6	64.2	140.0	170.2	140.7	91.3	43.9	10.7	0.6
1997	2,680.5	94.2	2.1	89.6	61.1	132.4	162.6	137.5	89.6	43.4	10.7	0.6
1998	2,652.5	93.2	1.9	87.9	58.5	131.5	159.3	136.1	90.5	43.4	10.8	0.6
1999	2,649.0	93.0	1.9	86.8	56.9	129.5	157.3	135.8	92.3	44.5	10.6	0.6
2000	2,730.0	95.9	1.7	87.3	55.5	132.6	161.3	139.9	97.1	46.6	11.5	0.6
2001	2,030.5	65.1	0.8	45.0	24.5	75.5	105.6	113.8	91.8	40.5	8.1	0.5
2002	2,020.5	65.0	0.7	42.6	23.1	72.2	103.1	114.7	92.6	41.6	8.3	0.5
2003	2,047.5	66.1	0.6	41.1	22.2	69.6	102.3	116.7	95.7	43.9	8.7	0.5
2004	2,051.5	66.4	0.6	40.5	21.8	68.7	101.5	116.5	96.2	45.5	9.0	0.5
2005	2,057.0	66.7	0.6	39.7	21.1	68.4	101.8	116.5	96.7	46.4	9.1	0.6
2006	2,108.0	68.6	0.6	41.1	21.6	71.2	105.5	118.0	98.9	47.5	9.4	0.6
2007	2,120.0	69.3	0.6	41.5	21.7	71.7	105.4	118.1	100.6	47.6	9.6	0.6
2008	2,072.0	68.1	0.6	40.2	21.1	68.2	101.8	115.0	99.4	46.8	9.9	0.7
2009	2,002.0	66.2	0.5	37.9	19.6	64.0	96.2	111.5	97.5	46.1	10.0	0.7
2010	1,931.0	64.1	0.4	34.2	17.3	58.2	90.0	108.3	96.5	45.9	10.2	0.7
2011	1,894.5	63.2	0.4	31.3	15.4	54.1	85.3	107.2	96.5	47.2	10.3	0.7
2012	2,189.5	74.4	0.6	46.3	22.5	77.2	111.5	119.6	94.3	51.6	13.2	0.8
2013	2,149.5	72.9	0.5	41.7	22.0	70.8	107.2	119.1	94.8	52.4	13.3	0.8
2014	2,130.5	72.1	0.4	38.0	19.3	66.1	104.5	118.7	96.5	53.6	13.5	0.9
2015	2,123.5	71.7	0.4	34.9	17.4	61.9	102.1	119.3	98.6	54.5	14.0	0.9
Mexican												
1989[3]	2,916.5	106.6	2.0	94.5	NA	NA	184.3	153.7	96.1	41.0	11.1	0.6
1990[4]	3,214.0	118.9	2.5	108.0	69.7	162.2	200.3	165.3	104.4	49.1	12.4	0.8
1991[5]	3,103.5	114.9	2.5	108.3	70.0	164.7	192.4	156.1	99.7	49.1	11.9	0.7

Note: Race and Hispanic origin are reported separately on birth certificates. Race categories are consistent with 1977 Office of Management and Budget standards. Forty-nine states and the District of Columbia reported multiple-race data for 2015 that were bridged to single-race categories for comparability with other states. Multiple-race reporting areas vary for 2003–2015. Persons of Hispanic origin may be of any race. In this table, Hispanic women are classified only by place of origin; non-Hispanic women are classified by race.
NA = Not available.
* = Figure does not meet standards of reliability or precision; based on fewer than 20 births in the numerator or, for the Hispanic subgroups, a relative standard error for the rate of 23% or more for the American Community Survey-based rates of 2010–2015 or fewer than 50 women for census years and 75,000 women for noncensus years in the denominator for the Current Population Survey-based rates for 1989–2009.
[1]Fertility rates computed by relating total births, regardless of age of mother, to women aged 15–44.
[2]Beginning in 1997, birth rates computed by relating births to women aged 45 and over to women aged 45–49.
[3]Excludes data for Louisiana, New Hampshire, and Oklahoma, which did not report Hispanic origin.
[4]Excludes data for New Hampshire and Oklahoma, which did not report Hispanic origin.
[5]Excludes data for New Hampshire, which did not report Hispanic origin.

Table 1-28. Total Fertility Rates, Fertility Rates, and Birth Rates, by Age and Hispanic Origin of Mother and by Race for Mothers of Non-Hispanic Origin, 1989–2015—*Continued*

(Total fertility rates are sums of birth rates for 5-year age groups multiplied by 5; fertility rates are live births per 1,000 women age 15 to 44 years in specified racial group; birth rates are live births per 1,000 women in specified age group.)

Year, origin, and race of mother	Total fertility rate	Fertility rate[1]	10–14 years	15–19 years Total	15–17 years	18–19 years	20–24 years	25–29 years	30–34 years	35–39 years	40–44 years	45–49 years[2]
1992[5]	3,107.0	113.3	2.4	105.1	NA	NA	196.6	160.2	97.1	47.4	11.8	0.8
1993	3,041.5	110.9	2.5	103.6	68.4	156.6	187.9	159.5	97.2	45.5	11.3	0.8
1994	3,024.0	109.9	2.7	109.2	73.6	163.3	189.1	153.6	92.5	45.3	11.7	0.7
1995	3,033.5	109.9	2.7	115.9	79.1	170.7	190.4	146.6	93.0	45.5	11.9	0.7
1996	3,052.0	110.7	2.6	112.2	77.7	161.6	185.3	154.7	96.5	46.4	12.0	0.7
1997	2,957.0	106.6	2.3	103.4	71.3	151.6	180.9	150.0	95.3	47.4	11.5	0.6
1998	2,878.0	103.2	2.1	96.4	62.9	149.2	176.5	147.4	94.9	46.9	10.8	0.6
1999	2,823.0	101.5	2.1	94.3	60.8	145.6	170.8	141.4	97.4	47.2	10.7	0.7
2000	2,906.5	105.1	1.9	95.4	60.6	146.7	174.9	144.7	102.3	49.2	12.2	0.7
2001	2,905.0	105.0	1.7	93.2	58.2	142.5	173.8	146.8	102.1	50.1	12.6	0.7
2002	2,869.0	103.0	1.5	91.4	57.0	141.0	171.2	146.8	101.1	48.5	12.5	0.8
2003	2,903.0	103.7	1.4	88.8	54.4	140.7	172.2	151.0	104.2	49.6	12.7	0.7
2004	2,948.5	104.5	1.4	90.3	55.6	142.5	173.4	152.5	105.5	53.5	12.4	0.7
2005	2,954.5	104.5	1.4	87.5	52.3	144.5	173.5	152.1	107.1	55.3	13.2	0.8
2006	2,997.0	105.6	1.3	86.6	50.7	145.4	180.3	152.3	109.0	55.5	13.6	0.8
2007	2,944.5	102.8	1.2	81.7	49.9	130.6	176.0	150.2	110.1	55.4	13.5	0.8
2008	2,663.5	92.6	1.1	71.4	44.4	111.7	154.3	138.4	101.9	51.4	13.4	0.8
2009	2,442.0	84.8	1.0	62.9	37.8	100.5	135.2	129.0	96.0	50.6	13.0	0.7
2010	2,276.5	78.2	0.8	55.3	32.6	89.9	123.3	122.9	91.5	48.1	12.7	0.7
2011	2,143.0	73.0	0.6	47.9	27.7	77.6	111.6	118.2	89.3	47.9	12.4	0.7
2012	2,082.5	70.7	0.6	44.5	24.8	74.2	106.0	113.5	88.3	48.1	12.5	0.8
2013	2,018.5	68.4	0.5	39.5	21.2	66.5	101.6	115.7	87.4	47.7	12.7	0.8
2014	1983,5	67.0	0.4	35.5	18.2	61.2	97.4	111.9	88.8	49.3	12.6	0.8
2015	NA	NA	NA	NA	NA	NA	NA	NA	NA	NA	NA	NA
Puerto Rican												
1989[3]	2,421.0	86.6	3.8	112.7	NA	NA	171.0	98.0	65.2	26.9	6.3	*
1990[4]	2,301.0	82.9	2.9	101.6	71.6	141.6	150.1	109.9	62.8	26.2	6.2	0.5
1991[5]	2,573.5	87.9	2.7	111.0	*	*	193.3	108.9	68.1	23.9	6.5	*
1992[5]	2,568.5	87.9	3.4	106.5	NA	NA	199.1	102.6	65.3	29.9	6.6	*
1993	2,416.0	79.8	3.1	104.9	70.1	*	184.6	102.8	54.4	26.7	6.2	*
1994	2,341.5	78.2	3.1	99.6	68.8	*	169.0	103.8	59.5	27.5	5.6	0.2
1995	2,078.0	71.3	2.9	82.8	57.3	*	138.1	97.9	61.2	26.9	5.5	0.3
1996	1,965.0	66.5	1.9	76.5	48.6	*	133.7	95.6	54.3	25.2	5.6	*
1997	1,931.5	65.8	1.7	68.9	45.0	*	136.0	92.9	54.1	26.1	6.2	0.4
1998	2,043.5	69.7	1.8	76.2	51.7	*	146.7	88.7	61.9	25.8	7.2	0.4
1999	2,104.5	71.1	1.6	74.0	49.4	*	146.0	106.5	58.0	27.3	7.2	0.3
2000	2,178.5	73.5	1.7	82.9	54.7	120.4	149.5	101.6	61.1	32.0	6.6	0.3
2001	2,144.5	71.7	1.7	80.3	*	*	144.5	93.9	70.6	30.8	6.7	0.4
2002	1,937.0	65.6	1.3	59.3	38.6	*	132.2	92.1	63.6	32.0	6.4	0.5
2003	1,805.0	60.6	1.0	57.9	34.4	*	124.5	86.3	55.4	29.2	6.3	0.4
2004	2,005.0	66.8	0.9	59.1	37.0	*	133.9	101.5	66.0	32.4	6.7	0.5
2005	2,065.5	69.8	0.9	59.2	35.1	*	124.1	108.8	76.6	35.3	7.8	0.4
2006	2,088.5	71.6	1.0	64.7	35.8	*	130.7	100.7	72.3	39.2	8.5	0.6
2007	2,101.0	70.3	0.8	61.8	32.8	*	139.2	105.9	65.0	39.8	7.3	0.4
2008	2,004.0	67.0	0.7	56.0	28.8	*	119.3	114.3	65.9	37.3	6.9	0.4
2009	1,922.5	63.7	0.7	50.8	28.2	82.4	118.9	106.6	66.9	32.6	7.4	0.6
2010	1,747.5	59.7	0.6	45.4	25.0	73.4	105.7	90.7	66.0	32.6	7.9	0.6
2011	1,747.5	59.6	0.5	42.8	22.9	69.5	106.0	93.8	64.9	33.2	7.8	0.5
2012	1,688.5	58.2	0.4	40.6	22.0	64.8	96.4	91.3	66.0	34.0	8.4	0.7
2013	1,684.0	57.8	0.5	36.3	18.2	61.8	94.8	91.5	70.6	34.5	8.0	0.5
2014	1,681.0	57.5	0.4	32.8	15.4	58.9	94.8	94.6	69.7	35.2	8.1	0.6
2015	NA	NA	NA	NA	NA	NA	NA	NA	NA	NA	NA	NA
Cuban												
1989[3]	1,479.0	49.8	*	*	NA	NA	*	*	*	*	*	*
1990[4]	1,459.5	52.6	*	30.3	18.2	46.1	64.6	95.4	67.6	28.2	4.9	*
1991[5]	1,352.5	47.6	*	*	*	*	*	*	*	*	*	*
1992[5]	1,453.5	49.4	*	*	NA	NA	*	*	*	*	*	*
1993	1,570.0	53.9	*	*	*	*	*	*	*	*	*	*
1994	1,587.0	53.6	*	*	*	*	*	*	*	*	*	*
1995	1,584.0	52.2	*	*	*	*	*	*	*	*	*	*
1996	1,617.0	55.1	*	*	*	*	*	*	*	*	*	*

Note: Race and Hispanic origin are reported separately on birth certificates. Race categories are consistent with 1977 Office of Management and Budget standards. Forty-nine states and the District of Columbia reported multiple-race data for 2015 that were bridged to single-race categories for comparability with other states. Multiple-race reporting areas vary for 2003–2015. Persons of Hispanic origin may be of any race. In this table, Hispanic women are classified only by place of origin; non-Hispanic women are classified by race.
NA = Not available.
* = Figure does not meet standards of reliability or precision; based on fewer than 20 births in the numerator or, for the Hispanic subgroups, a relative standard error for the rate of 23% or more for the American Community Survey-based rates of 2010–2015 or fewer than 50 women for census years and 75,000 women for noncensus years in the denominator for the Current Population Survey-based rates for 1989–2009.
[1]Fertility rates computed by relating total births, regardless of age of mother, to women aged 15–44.
[2]Beginning in 1997, birth rates computed by relating births to women aged 45 and over to women aged 45–49.
[3]Excludes data for Louisiana, New Hampshire, and Oklahoma, which did not report Hispanic origin.
[4]Excludes data for New Hampshire and Oklahoma, which did not report Hispanic origin.
[5]Excludes data for New Hampshire, which did not report Hispanic origin.

Table 1-28. Total Fertility Rates, Fertility Rates, and Birth Rates, by Age and Hispanic Origin of Mother and by Race for Mothers of Non-Hispanic Origin, 1989–2015—*Continued*

(Total fertility rates are sums of birth rates for 5-year age groups multiplied by 5; fertility rates are live births per 1,000 women age 15 to 44 years in specified racial group; birth rates are live births per 1,000 women in specified age group.)

Year, origin, and race of mother	Total fertility rate	Fertility rate[1]	10–14 years	15–19 years Total	15–17 years	18–19 years	20–24 years	25–29 years	30–34 years	35–39 years	40–44 years	45–49 years[2]
1997	1,619.5	53.1	*	*	*	*	*	*	*	*	*	*
1998	1,402.5	46.5	*	*	*	*	*	*	*	*	*	*
1999	1,388.5	47.0	*	*	*	*	*	*	*	*	*	*
2000	1,528.0	49.3	*	23.5	14.2	43.4	64.2	104.0	68.1	37.3	7.9	*
2001	1,786.0	56.4	*	*	*	*	*	*	*	*	*	*
2002	1,958.5	59.3	*	*	*	*	*	*	*	*	*	*
2003	2,032.5	60.8	*	*	*	*	*	*	*	*	*	*
2004	1,699.5	52.2	*	*	*	*	*	*	*	*	*	*
2005	1,540.5	49.1	*	*	*	*	*	*	*	*	*	*
2006	1,556.5	47.9	*	*	*	*	*	*	*	*	6.8	*
2007	1,542.5	47.6	*	*	*	*	*	*	*	*	6.4	*
2008	1,536.5	50.1	*	*	*	*	*	*	*	*	*	*
2009	1,352.0	46.0	*	*	*	*	*	*	*	*	*	*
2010	1,452.5	46.4	*	17.8	8.0	29.7	61.6	80.6	82.8	39.1	8.0	0.5
2011	1,433.5	46.1	*	15.8	6.7	29.0	54.7	86.1	78.4	42.0	9.1	0.5
2012	1,370.5	45.4	*	15.0	6.6	24.9	57.3	78.7	72.9	40.7	8.8	0.6
2013	1,449.0	48.0	*	14.9	6.0	26.2	58.4	85.2	78.2	44.0	8.5	0.5
2014	1,570.5	52.1	*	14.2	5.2	37.5	66.5	94.5	84.9	43.4	9.8	0.7
2015	NA	NA	NA	NA	NA	NA	NA	NA	NA	NA	NA	NA
Other Hispanic												
1989[3]	2,683.0	95.8	1.7	66.4	NA	NA	159.2	150.4	85.1	60.3	12.7	0.8
1990[4]	2,877.0	102.7	2.1	86.0	57.2	123.8	162.9	155.8	106.9	49.4	11.6	0.7
1991[5]	3,064.5	105.5	2.2	100.7	67.3	145.6	184.1	164.5	100.2	49.2	11.4	0.6
1992[5]	2,989.0	104.7	2.4	108.2	NA	NA	168.0	151.9	104.4	49.9	12.5	0.5
1993	2,914.5	101.5	2.6	102.0	74.7	134.6	167.5	139.4	106.7	51.7	12.5	0.5
1994	2,693.0	93.2	2.5	82.6	62.7	105.0	151.2	137.0	104.4	48.4	11.9	0.6
1995	2,629.5	89.1	2.3	72.1	51.3	99.4	144.3	147.7	97.9	49.4	11.6	0.6
1996	2,516.5	84.2	2.2	64.8	43.4	95.6	149.6	127.9	98.0	49.1	11.0	0.7
1997	2,376.5	80.6	1.8	66.4	44.5	98.0	129.3	125.8	95.6	43.9	11.8	0.7
1998	2,448.5	83.5	1.8	75.0	53.3	100.3	122.7	133.6	97.8	45.4	12.8	0.6
1999	2,517.0	84.8	1.5	75.5	53.1	100.5	130.2	138.4	98.3	46.5	12.3	0.7
2000	2,563.5	85.1	1.2	69.9	44.4	102.0	133.2	143.9	103.6	47.7	12.5	0.7
2001	2,503.5	82.2	1.1	63.8	35.0	111.6	133.6	143.7	95.6	50.4	11.6	0.9
2002	2,612.0	86.5	1.1	60.9	33.7	105.4	138.8	149.5	101.7	57.3	12.3	0.8
2003	2,690.0	89.7	1.0	57.5	34.9	88.0	138.4	152.3	111.8	62.4	13.8	0.8
2004	2,594.0	87.4	1.1	54.6	31.1	90.2	131.1	143.5	113.5	59.2	15.0	0.8
2005	2,737.0	90.5	1.1	58.2	35.0	90.2	148.1	152.3	115.0	57.6	14.3	0.8
2006	2,918.0	95.6	1.1	62.5	36.3	99.7	154.3	172.7	118.0	59.3	14.7	1.0
2007	2,995.0	100.1	1.2	68.1	38.8	113.4	154.5	173.4	124.1	60.7	15.9	1.1
2008	3,278.0	109.1	1.4	80.5	47.9	129.3	180.5	171.1	135.9	69.1	16.0	1.1
2009	3,248.5	107.5	1.3	78.4	44.2	131.3	181.3	169.4	133.5	68.3	16.3	1.2
2010	2,870.0	97.1	1.0	67.4	39.6	105.2	146.6	154.2	120.5	67.0	16.2	1.1
2011	2,847.5	96.3	1.1	62.1	35.1	99.9	142.3	150.3	127.3	68.6	16.7	1.1
2012	2,812.5	94.9	0.9	58.9	33.2	93.4	140.7	153.6	122.3	68.0	17.7	1.1
2013	2,799.5	94.4	0.7	52.2	28.6	84.7	136.3	154.2	125.5	72.2	17.0	1.1
2014	2,805.5	94.9	0.7	51.6	27.9	84.1	134.3	154.5	129.1	71.6	18.0	1.3
2015	NA	NA	NA	NA	NA	NA	NA	NA	NA	NA	NA	NA
NON-HISPANIC												
1989[3]	1,921.0	65.7	1.3	53.4	---	---	107.8	113.4	74.7	28.6	4.8	0.2
1990[4]	1,979.5	67.1	1.3	54.8	33.8	81.4	108.1	116.5	79.2	30.7	5.1	0.2
1991[5]	1,953.0	65.2	1.3	56.1	34.4	86.1	106.5	113.1	77.5	30.8	5.1	0.2
1992[5]	1,929.0	64.2	1.2	54.3	33.2	85.3	104.3	111.4	77.9	31.1	5.4	0.2
1993	1,901.5	62.7	1.2	52.7	32.9	82.3	101.7	108.7	78.4	31.6	5.7	0.3
1994	1,883.5	61.6	1.2	51.7	32.3	81.4	99.5	106.5	79.1	32.4	6.0	0.3
1995	1,856.5	60.2	1.1	49.3	30.5	78.6	97.4	104.1	79.9	33.0	6.2	0.3
1996	1,852.0	59.6	1.0	47.0	28.4	75.8	97.3	103.6	80.8	33.9	6.5	0.3
1997	1,853.0	59.3	0.9	45.0	26.7	73.7	97.4	103.5	82.0	34.8	6.7	0.3
1998	1,887.5	60.0	0.8	44.0	25.2	72.4	98.9	105.8	84.4	36.2	7.0	0.4
1999	1,894.0	60.0	0.8	42.2	23.3	70.2	98.4	106.7	86.2	37.0	7.1	0.4
2000	1,931.5	61.1	0.7	40.7	21.9	68.2	99.5	108.4	90.2	38.8	7.6	0.4
2001	1,898.0	60.0	0.6	37.8	19.6	65.0	94.6	108.1	90.8	39.5	7.7	0.5

Note: Race and Hispanic origin are reported separately on birth certificates. Race categories are consistent with 1977 Office of Management and Budget standards. Forty-nine states and the District of Columbia reported multiple-race data for 2015 that were bridged to single-race categories for comparability with other states. Multiple-race reporting areas vary for 2003–2015. Persons of Hispanic origin may be of any race. In this table, Hispanic women are classified only by place of origin; non-Hispanic women are classified by race. NA = Not available.

* = Figure does not meet standards of reliability or precision; based on fewer than 20 births in the numerator or, for the Hispanic subgroups, a relative standard error for the rate of 23% or more for the American Community Survey-based rates of 2010–2015 or fewer than 50 women for census years and 75,000 women for noncensus years in the denominator for the Current Population Survey-based rates for 1989–2009.

[1]Fertility rates computed by relating total births, regardless of age of mother, to women aged 15–44.
[2]Beginning in 1997, birth rates computed by relating births to women aged 45 and over to women aged 45–49.
[3]Excludes data for Louisiana, New Hampshire, and Oklahoma, which did not report Hispanic origin.
[4]Excludes data for New Hampshire and Oklahoma, which did not report Hispanic origin.
[5]Excludes data for New Hampshire, which did not report Hispanic origin.

Table 1-28. Total Fertility Rates, Fertility Rates, and Birth Rates, by Age and Hispanic Origin of Mother and by Race for Mothers of Non-Hispanic Origin, 1989–2015—*Continued*

(Total fertility rates are sums of birth rates for 5-year age groups multiplied by 5; fertility rates are live births per 1,000 women age 15 to 44 years in specified racial group; birth rates are live births per 1,000 women in specified age group.)

Year, origin, and race of mother	Total fertility rate	Fertility rate[1]	10–14 years	15–19 years			20–24 years	25–29 years	30–34 years	35–39 years	40–44 years	45–49 years[2]
				Total	15–17 years	18–19 years						
2002	1,885.0	59.8	0.6	35.4	18.2	61.6	91.8	108.7	91.6	40.5	7.9	0.5
2003	1,909.0	60.7	0.5	33.9	17.2	58.9	90.6	110.6	94.6	42.8	8.3	0.5
2004	1,906.0	60.8	0.5	33.1	16.7	57.6	89.5	110.1	94.7	44.3	8.5	0.5
2005	1,902.0	60.8	0.5	32.1	15.9	56.9	89.2	109.5	94.7	45.2	8.6	0.6
2006	1,946.0	62.5	0.5	33.2	16.5	59.0	92.3	110.7	96.9	46.2	8.8	0.6
2007	1,959.5	63.3	0.5	33.8	16.4	60.1	92.3	110.9	98.7	46.1	9.0	0.6
2008	1,926.0	62.7	0.4	33.1	16.0	57.8	90.0	108.6	97.9	45.3	9.3	0.6
2009	1,877.5	61.6	0.4	31.6	15.1	54.7	86.0	106.0	96.7	44.7	9.4	0.7
2010	1,831.0	60.4	0.3	28.8	13.4	50.3	81.5	104.2	96.5	44.5	9.7	0.7
2011	1,810.5	60.1	0.3	26.5	12.0	47.0	78.0	103.8	96.8	46.2	9.8	0.7
2012	1,803.0	60.3	0.3	24.8	10.9	44.5	76.2	103.3	98.0	47.5	9.8	0.8
2013	1,784.0	59.9	0.2	22.3	9.5	40.6	74.1	102.3	98.8	48.5	9.8	0.8
2014	1,793.0	60.7	0.2	20.3	8.5	37.6	72.4	102.7	101.9	50.3	10.0	0.7
2015	1,769.5	60.2	0.2	18.6	7.7	34.8	70.1	100.6	102.2	51.1	10.3	0.8
White												
1989[3]	1,770.0	60.5	0.4	39.9	NA	NA	94.7	111.7	75.0	27.8	4.3	0.2
1990[4]	1,850.5	62.8	0.5	42.5	23.2	66.6	97.5	115.3	79.4	30.0	4.7	0.2
1991[5]	1,822.5	60.9	0.5	43.4	23.6	70.6	95.7	112.1	77.7	30.2	4.7	0.2
1992[5]	1,803.5	60.0	0.5	41.7	22.7	69.8	93.9	110.6	78.3	30.4	5.1	0.2
1993	1,786.0	58.9	0.5	40.7	22.7	67.7	92.2	108.2	79.0	31.0	5.4	0.2
1994	1,782.5	58.2	0.5	40.4	22.7	67.6	90.9	106.6	80.2	32.0	5.7	0.2
1995	1,777.5	57.5	0.4	39.3	22.0	66.2	90.2	105.1	81.5	32.8	5.9	0.3
1996	1,781.0	57.1	0.4	37.6	20.6	64.0	90.1	104.9	82.8	33.9	6.2	0.3
1997	1,785.5	56.8	0.4	36.0	19.3	62.1	90.0	104.8	84.3	34.8	6.5	0.3
1998	1,825.0	57.6	0.3	35.3	18.3	60.9	91.2	107.4	87.2	36.4	6.8	0.4
1999	1,838.5	57.7	0.3	34.1	17.1	59.4	90.6	108.6	89.5	37.3	6.9	0.4
2000	1,866.0	58.5	0.3	32.6	15.8	57.5	91.2	109.4	93.2	38.8	7.3	0.4
2001	1,846.0	57.7	0.3	30.3	14.0	54.7	87.0	109.6	94.3	39.8	7.5	0.4
2002	1,840.0	57.6	0.2	28.6	13.1	52.0	84.7	110.4	95.0	40.9	7.7	0.5
2003	1,874.5	58.9	0.2	27.4	12.4	50.0	84.1	112.7	98.4	43.5	8.1	0.5
2004	1,871.0	58.9	0.2	26.7	12.0	48.6	83.0	112.1	98.3	45.1	8.3	0.5
2005	1,869.0	59.0	0.2	26.0	11.5	48.0	82.7	111.7	98.4	46.0	8.3	0.5
2006	1,900.5	60.3	0.2	26.7	11.8	49.4	85.1	112.2	100.0	46.8	8.5	0.6
2007	1,908.0	61.0	0.2	27.2	11.9	50.4	85.1	112.0	101.5	46.3	8.7	0.6
2008	1,874.5	60.5	0.2	26.7	11.6	48.6	82.8	109.7	100.8	45.2	8.9	0.6
2009	1,830.0	59.6	0.2	25.7	11.0	46.2	79.2	107.1	99.7	44.4	9.1	0.6
2010	1,791.0	58.7	0.2	23.5	10.0	42.5	74.9	105.8	99.9	44.1	9.2	0.6
2011	1,773.5	58.7	0.2	21.7	9.0	39.9	71.8	105.2	100.1	45.8	9.3	0.6
2012	1,761.5	58.6	0.2	20.5	8.4	37.9	70.2	104.4	104.7	46.8	9.1	0.6
2013	1,751.0	58.7	0.1	18.6	7.4	35.0	68.3	103.5	101.9	48.0	9.1	0.7
2014	1,762.5	59.5	0.1	17.3	6.7	32.9	67.1	103.9	100.5	49.6	9.1	0.7
2015	1,746.0	59.3	0.1	16.0	6.0	30.6	65.0	102.3	105.1	50.6	9.4	0.7
Black												
1989[3]	2,424.0	84.8	5.2	111.9	NA	NA	156.3	113.8	65.7	26.3	5.3	0.3
1990[4]	2,547.5	89.0	5.0	116.2	84.9	157.5	165.1	118.4	70.2	28.7	5.6	0.3
1991[5]	2,532.0	87.0	4.9	118.2	86.1	162.2	164.8	115.1	68.9	28.7	5.6	0.2
1992[5]	2,482.5	84.5	4.8	114.7	82.9	161.1	160.8	112.8	68.4	29.1	5.7	0.2
1993	2,412.5	81.5	4.6	110.5	81.1	154.6	154.5	109.2	68.1	29.4	5.9	0.3
1994	2,314.5	77.5	4.6	105.7	77.0	150.4	146.8	104.1	66.3	29.1	6.0	0.3
1995	2,186.5	72.8	4.2	97.2	70.4	139.2	137.8	98.5	64.4	28.8	6.1	0.3
1996	2,140.0	70.7	3.6	91.9	64.8	134.1	137.0	96.7	63.2	29.1	6.2	0.3
1997	2,137.5	70.3	3.2	88.3	60.7	131.0	138.8	97.2	63.6	29.6	6.5	0.3
1998	2,164.0	70.9	2.9	85.7	56.8	128.2	142.5	99.9	64.4	30.4	6.7	0.3
1999	2,134.0	69.9	2.6	81.0	51.7	123.9	142.1	99.8	63.9	30.6	6.5	0.3
2000	2,178.5	71.4	2.4	79.2	50.1	121.9	145.4	102.8	66.5	31.8	7.2	0.4
2001	2,107.0	69.1	2.1	73.1	44.8	115.9	137.3	102.8	66.4	32.0	7.3	0.4
2002	2,053.0	67.5	1.9	67.7	40.6	109.5	131.4	103.1	66.5	32.1	7.5	0.4
2003	2,037.5	67.1	1.6	63.8	38.2	103.4	128.8	104.0	67.7	33.4	7.7	0.5
2004	2,030.5	67.1	1.6	61.9	36.4	101.6	127.9	105.0	67.8	33.6	7.8	0.5
2005	2,030.5	67.2	1.6	59.4	34.1	100.2	127.9	105.5	68.8	34.2	8.2	0.5

Note: Race and Hispanic origin are reported separately on birth certificates. Race categories are consistent with 1977 Office of Management and Budget standards. Forty-nine states and the District of Columbia reported multiple-race data for 2015 that were bridged to single-race categories for comparability with other states. Multiple-race reporting areas vary for 2003–2015. Persons of Hispanic origin may be of any race. In this table, Hispanic women are classified only by place of origin; non-Hispanic women are classified by race.
NA = Not available.
* = Figure does not meet standards of reliability or precision; based on fewer than 20 births in the numerator or, for the Hispanic subgroups, a relative standard error for the rate of 23% or more for the American Community Survey-based rates of 2010–2015 or fewer than 50 women for census years and 75,000 women for noncensus years in the denominator for the Current Population Survey-based rates for 1989–2009.
[1]Fertility rates computed by relating total births, regardless of age of mother, to women aged 15–44.
[2]Beginning in 1997, birth rates computed by relating births to women aged 45 and over to women aged 45–49.
[3]Excludes data for Louisiana, New Hampshire, and Oklahoma, which did not report Hispanic origin.
[4]Excludes data for New Hampshire and Oklahoma, which did not report Hispanic origin.
[5]Excludes data for New Hampshire, which did not report Hispanic origin.

Table 1-28. Total Fertility Rates, Fertility Rates, and Birth Rates, by Age and Hispanic Origin of Mother and by Race for Mothers of Non-Hispanic Origin, 1989–2015—*Continued*

(Total fertility rates are sums of birth rates for 5-year age groups multiplied by 5; fertility rates are live births per 1,000 women age 15 to 44 years in specified racial group; birth rates are live births per 1,000 women in specified age group.)

Year, origin, and race of mother	Total fertility rate	Fertility rate[1]	10–14 years	15–19 years			20–24 years	25–29 years	30–34 years	35–39 years	40–44 years	45–49 years[2]
				Total	15–17 years	18–19 years						
2006	2,128.5	70.7	1.5	61.9	35.2	105.1	134.4	110.0	73.2	35.9	8.3	0.5
2007	2,142.0	71.4	1.4	62.0	34.6	105.2	134.5	110.5	74.7	36.2	8.5	0.6
2008	2,115.5	70.8	1.4	60.4	33.6	100.0	131.6	108.8	75.3	36.3	8.7	0.6
2009	2,046.5	68.9	1.1	56.8	31.0	93.5	125.9	106.0	73.9	36.1	8.9	0.6
2010	1,971.5	66.6	1.0	51.5	27.4	85.6	119.4	102.5	73.6	36.4	9.2	0.7
2011	1,919.5	65.4	0.9	47.3	24.6	78.8	112.3	101.7	73.9	37.8	9.3	0.7
2012	1,898.5	65.0	0.8	43.9	21.9	74.1	109.0	101.7	75.1	38.9	9.6	0.7
2013	1,881.5	64.6	0.7	39.0	18.9	67.0	105.6	102.7	77.3	40.3	9.9	0.8
2014	1,873.5	64.5	0.6	34.9	16.6	61.5	102.8	103.3	79.6	42.5	10.1	0.9
2015	1,857.0	64.1	0.6	31.8	15.3	56.7	100.2	102.0	81.6	43.6	10.7	0.9

Note: Race and Hispanic origin are reported separately on birth certificates. Race categories are consistent with 1977 Office of Management and Budget standards. Forty-nine states and the District of Columbia reported multiple-race data for 2015 that were bridged to single-race categories for comparability with other states. Multiple-race reporting areas vary for 2003–2015. Persons of Hispanic origin may be of any race. In this table, Hispanic women are classified only by place of origin; non-Hispanic women are classified by race. NA = Not available.

* = Figure does not meet standards of reliability or precision; based on fewer than 20 births in the numerator or, for the Hispanic subgroups, a relative standard error for the rate of 23% or more for the American Community Survey-based rates of 2010–2015 or fewer than 50 women for census years and 75,000 women for noncensus years in the denominator for the Current Population Survey-based rates for 1989–2009.

[1]Fertility rates computed by relating total births, regardless of age of mother, to women aged 15–44.

[2]Beginning in 1997, birth rates computed by relating births to women aged 45 and over to women aged 45–49.

Table 1-29. Fertility Rates and Birth Rates, by Live-Birth Order and by Race and Hispanic Origin of Mother, 1980–2015

(Births per 1,000 women age 15 to 44 years.)

Year, race, and Hispanic origin of mother	Fertility rate	Live-birth order						
		1	2	3	4	5	6 and 7	8 and over
All Races[1,2]								
1980[3]	68.4	29.5	21.8	10.3	3.9	1.5	1.0	0.4
1981[3]	67.3	29.0	21.6	10.1	3.8	1.5	0.9	0.4
1982[3]	67.3	28.6	22.0	10.2	3.8	1.4	0.9	0.3
1983[3]	65.7	27.8	21.5	10.1	3.7	1.4	0.9	0.3
1984[3]	65.5	27.4	21.7	10.1	3.7	1.4	0.9	0.3
1985	66.3	27.6	22.0	10.4	3.8	1.4	0.8	0.3
1986	65.4	27.2	21.6	10.3	3.8	1.4	0.8	0.3
1987	65.8	27.2	21.6	10.5	3.9	1.4	0.8	0.3
1988	67.3	27.6	22.0	10.9	4.1	1.5	0.9	0.3
1989	69.2	28.4	22.4	11.3	4.3	1.6	0.9	0.3
1990	70.9	29.0	22.8	11.7	4.5	1.7	1.0	0.3
1991	69.3	28.2	22.3	11.4	4.4	1.7	1.0	0.3
1992	68.4	27.6	22.2	11.2	4.4	1.7	1.0	0.3
1993	67.0	27.3	21.7	10.9	4.3	1.6	1.0	0.3
1994	65.9	27.1	21.2	10.6	4.1	1.6	0.9	0.3
1995	64.6	26.9	20.7	10.3	4.0	1.5	0.9	0.3
1996	64.1	26.3	20.7	10.4	4.0	1.5	0.9	0.3
1997	63.6	25.9	20.7	10.4	4.0	1.5	0.9	0.3
1998	64.3	25.9	21.0	10.6	4.1	1.5	0.9	0.3
1999	64.4	26.0	21.0	10.7	4.1	1.5	0.9	0.3
2000	65.9	26.5	21.4	11.0	4.2	1.6	0.9	0.3
2001	65.1	25.9	21.3	11.0	4.3	1.6	0.9	0.3
2002	65.0	25.8	21.2	10.9	4.3	1.6	0.9	0.3
2003	66.1	26.5	21.4	11.1	4.3	1.6	0.9	0.3
2004								
	66.4	26.4	21.4	11.2	4.4	1.6	0.9	0.3
2005	66.7	26.5	21.5	11.3	4.5	1.6	0.9	0.3
2006	68.6	27.4	21.9	11.6	4.7	1.7	1.0	0.3
2007	69.3	27.8	22.0	11.7	4.7	1.8	1.0	0.3
2008	68.1	27.5	21.5	11.4	4.7	1.7	1.0	0.3
2009	66.2	26.8	20.8	11.0	4.6	1.7	1.0	0.3
2010	64.1	25.9	20.2	10.6	4.4	1.7	1.0	0.3
2011	63.2	25.4	20.0	10.4	4.4	1.7	1.0	0.3
2012	63.0	25.2	19.9	10.4	4.4	1.7	1.0	0.3
2013	62.5	24.7	19.9	10.4	4.4	1.7	1.0	0.3
2014	62.9	24.6	20.1	10.6	4.5	1.8	1.1	0.3
2015	62.5	24.1	20.1	10.6	4.6	1.8	1.1	0.4
Non-Hispanic White[2,4]								
1990[5]	62.8	26.7	21.2	9.9	3.3	1.1	0.5	0.2
1991[6]	60.9	25.8	20.6	9.6	3.2	1.0	0.5	0.2
1992[6]	60.0	25.1	20.5	9.5	3.2	1.0	0.5	0.2
1993	58.9	24.8	20.1	9.2	3.1	1.0	0.5	0.2
1994	58.2	24.6	19.7	9.1	3.1	1.0	0.5	0.2
1995	57.5	24.5	19.3	8.9	3.0	1.0	0.5	0.2
1996	57.1	24.1	19.3	8.9	3.0	1.0	0.5	0.2
1997	56.8	23.8	19.3	8.9	3.0	1.0	0.5	0.2
1998	57.6	23.8	19.7	9.2	3.1	1.0	0.6	0.2
1999	57.7	24.0	19.6	9.2	3.2	1.0	0.6	0.2
2000	58.5	24.2	19.8	9.4	3.3	1.1	0.6	0.2
2001	57.7	23.6	19.7	9.4	3.3	1.1	0.6	0.2
2002	57.6	23.6	19.6	9.3	3.3	1.1	0.6	0.2
2003	58.9	24.5	19.8	9.4	3.3	1.1	0.6	0.2
2004								
	58.9	24.4	19.8	9.5	3.3	1.1	0.6	0.2
2005	59.0	24.4	19.8	9.5	3.4	1.1	0.6	0.2
2006	60.3	25.1	20.0	9.6	3.5	1.1	0.6	0.2
2007	61.0	25.6	20.1	9.7	3.5	1.2	0.7	0.2
2008	60.5	25.5	19.8	9.5	3.5	1.2	0.7	0.2
2009	59.6	25.3	19.5	9.2	3.4	1.2	0.7	0.3
2010	58.7	25.0	19.2	9.1	3.4	1.2	0.7	0.3
2011	58.7	24.9	19.2	9.0	3.4	1.2	0.7	0.3
2012	58.6	24.7	19.2	9.1	3.4	1.2	0.7	0.3
2013	58.7	24.4	19.3	9.2	3.5	1.2	0.7	0.3
2014	59.5	24.5	19.7	9.4	3.6	1.3	0.8	0.3
2015	59.3	23.9	19.8	9.5	3.6	1.3	0.8	0.3

[1]Includes races other than White and Black.
[2]Includes origin not stated.
[3]Based on 100 percent of births in selected states and on a 50 percent sample of births in all other states.
[4]Race and Hispanic origin are reported separately on birth certificates. Persons of Hispanic origin may be of any race. Multiple-race data, when reported, were bridged to single-race categories in order to maintain comparability among all reported areas. Forty-nine states and the District of Columbia reported multiple-race data for 2015 that were bridged to single-race categories for comparability with other states.
[5]Excludes data for New Hampshire and Oklahoma, which did not report Hispanic origin.
[6]Excludes data for New Hampshire, which did not report Hispanic origin.

Table 1-29. Fertility Rates and Birth Rates, by Live-Birth Order and by Race and Hispanic Origin of Mother, 1980–2015—Continued

(Births per 1,000 women age 15 to 44 years.)

Year, race, and Hispanic origin of mother	Fertility rate	Live-birth order						
		1	2	3	4	5	6 and 7	8 and over
Non-Hispanic Black[2,4]								
1990[5]	89.0	33.2	26.3	16.0	7.6	3.3	2.0	0.6
1991[6]	87.0	32.1	25.5	15.7	7.5	3.4	2.2	0.6
1992[6]	84.5	31.1	24.8	15.2	7.3	3.4	2.2	0.6
1993	81.5	30.5	23.6	14.3	7.0	3.2	2.2	0.7
1994	77.5	30.0	22.4	13.2	6.3	2.9	2.0	0.6
1995	72.8	28.9	20.9	12.1	5.8	2.7	1.9	0.6
1996	70.7	27.6	20.5	12.0	5.6	2.6	1.8	0.6
1997	70.3	27.2	20.6	12.0	5.7	2.5	1.8	0.6
1998	70.9	27.0	21.0	12.3	5.7	2.6	1.8	0.6
1999	69.9	26.4	20.8	12.3	5.7	2.5	1.7	0.6
2000	71.4	26.7	21.2	12.8	5.9	2.6	1.8	0.6
2001	69.1	25.9	20.4	12.4	5.8	2.5	1.7	0.6
2002	67.5	25.4	19.7	12.1	5.7	2.5	1.7	0.6
2003	67.1	25.4	19.6	11.9	5.6	2.5	1.6	0.5
2004	67.1	25.5	19.4	11.9	5.6	2.5	1.7	0.5
2005	67.2	25.8	19.3	11.8	5.6	2.5	1.7	0.5
2006	70.7	27.5	20.3	12.3	5.8	2.5	1.7	0.5
2007	71.4	27.9	20.4	12.3	5.9	2.6	1.7	0.5
2008	70.8	28.1	20.0	12.1	5.8	2.6	1.7	0.5
2009	68.9	27.3	19.4	11.7	5.7	2.5	1.7	0.6
2010	66.6	26.3	18.9	11.3	5.4	2.5	1.7	0.5
2011	65.4	25.6	18.5	11.1	5.4	2.4	1.7	0.6
2012	65.0	25.1	18.6	11.2	5.5	2.4	1.7	0.5
2013	64.6	24.4	18.6	11.3	5.5	2.5	1.7	0.6
2014	64.5	23.9	18.6	11.5	5.6	2.5	1.7	0.6
2015	64.1	23.5	18.5	11.5	5.7	2.6	1.7	0.6
Hispanic[7]								
1990[5]	107.7	40.7	30.9	19.5	9.3	4.0	2.6	0.8
1991[6]	106.9	40.8	30.6	19.2	9.2	3.9	2.5	0.7
1992[6]	106.1	40.1	30.9	19.0	9.1	3.9	2.5	0.7
1993	103.3	39.3	30.4	18.3	8.6	3.7	2.3	0.6
1994	100.7	39.0	29.7	17.6	8.2	3.4	2.1	0.6
1995	98.8	38.4	29.3	17.4	7.8	3.3	2.0	0.6
1996	97.5	37.2	29.4	17.4	7.8	3.2	1.9	0.5
1997	94.2	35.6	28.6	17.1	7.6	3.0	1.8	0.5
1998	93.2	34.8	28.5	17.2	7.6	3.0	1.7	0.4
1999	93.0	34.6	28.5	17.3	7.5	2.9	1.7	0.4
2000	95.9	35.8	29.2	18.0	7.7	3.0	1.7	0.4
2001	95.4	35.2	29.3	18.0	7.9	3.0	1.7	0.4
2002	94.7	34.7	29.1	18.0	7.9	3.0	1.6	0.4
2003	95.2	34.5	29.4	18.3	8.0	3.0	1.6	0.4
2004	95.7	34.4	29.3	18.7	8.2	3.1	1.6	0.4
2005	96.4	34.4	29.6	19.0	8.4	3.1	1.6	0.4
2006	98.3	35.1	29.9	19.3	8.7	3.3	1.7	0.4
2007	97.4	34.7	29.4	19.3	8.7	3.3	1.7	0.4
2008	92.7	33.0	27.8	18.3	8.4	3.2	1.7	0.3
2009	86.5	30.6	25.9	17.0	8.0	3.0	1.6	0.3
2010	80.2	28.0	24.0	15.9	7.5	2.9	1.5	0.3
2011	76.2	26.3	22.9	15.2	7.2	2.8	1.5	0.3
2012	74.4	25.5	22.3	14.9	7.1	2.8	1.5	0.3
2013	72.9	24.9	21.8	14.6	7.0	2.8	1.5	0.3
2014	72.1	24.5	21.6	14.4	7.0	2.8	1.5	0.3
2015	71.7	24.3	21.5	14.3	7.0	2.8	1.5	0.3

[1]Includes races other than White and Black.
[2]Includes origin not stated.
[3]Based on 100 percent of births in selected states and on a 50 percent sample of births in all other states.
[4]Race and Hispanic origin are reported separately on birth certificates. Persons of Hispanic origin may be of any race. Multiple-race data, when reported, were bridged to single-race categories in order to maintain comparability among all reported areas. Forty-nine states and the District of Columbia reported multiple-race data for 2015 that were bridged to single-race categories for comparability with other states.
[5]Excludes data for New Hampshire and Oklahoma, which did not report Hispanic origin.
[6]Excludes data for New Hampshire, which did not report Hispanic origin.
[7]Includes all persons of Hispanic origin of any race.

Table 1-30. Selected Demographic Characteristics of Births, by Race of Mother, 2015

(Number; rates are live births per 1,000 population; percent.)

Characteristic	All races	White	Black	American Indian or Alaska Native	Asian or Pacific Islander
Number					
Births	3,978,497	3,012,855	640,079	44,299	281,264
Rate					
Birth rate	12.4	12.0	14.3	9.7	14.0
Fertility rate	62.5	63.1	64.0	43.9	58.5
Total fertility rate	1,843.5	1,864.0	1,852.5	1,262.5	1,646.0
Sex ratio[1]	1,048	1,050	1,033	1,052	1,062
Percent, All Births					
Births to mothers under 20 years	5.8	5.6	8.7	10.8	1.5
4th and higher-order births[2]	12.4	12.0	16.3	21.7	6.7
Births to unmarried mothers	40.3	35.8	70.1	65.8	16.4
Mothers born in the 50 states or DC	77.4	81.0	82.6	94.6	23.3
Mean					
Age of mother at first birth (years)	26.4	26.5	24.4	23.2	29.6

Note: Race and Hispanic origin are reported separately on birth certificates. Race categories are consistent with 1977 Office of Management and Budget standards. Forty-nine states and the District of Columbia reported multiple-race data for 2015 that were bridged to single-race categories for comparability with other states. In this table, all women, including Hispanic women, are classified only according to their race.
[1]Male births per 1,000 female births.
[2]Based on live-birth order.

Table 1-31. Births, by Day of Week and Index of Occurrence, by Method of Delivery, 2015

(Number; ratio.)

Day of the week	Average number of births	Index of occurrence[1]		
		Total[2]	Method of delivery	
			Vaginal	Cesarean
Total, All Days	10,900	100.0	100.0	100.0
Sunday	7,398	67.9	77.0	48.5
Monday	11,739	107.7	101.3	121.3
Tuesday	12,586	115.5	111.6	123.7
Wednesday	12,279	112.7	108.4	115.1
Thursday	12,083	110.9	111.1	117.0
Friday	11,835	108.6	104.6	117.0
Saturday	8,357	76.7	85.8	57.3

[1]Index is the ratio of the average number of births by a specified method of delivery on a given day of the week to the average daily number of births by a specified method of delivery for the year, multiplied by 100.
[2]Includes method of delivery not stated.

Table 1-32. Births and Observed and Seasonally Adjusted Birth and Fertility Rates, by Month, 2015

(Rates on an annual basis per 1,000 population for specified month; birth rates are live births per 1,000 total population; fertility rates are births per 1,000 women age 15 to 44 years.)

Month	Number	Observed		Seasonally adjusted[1]	
		Birth rate	Fertility rate	Birth rate	Fertility rate
Total, All Months	3,978,497	12.4	62.5	X	X
January	325,955	12.0	60.5	13.4	65.6
February	298,058	12.1	61.2	13.4	65.6
March	328,923	12.1	61.0	13.3	65.5
April	320,832	12.2	61.4	13.4	65.6
May	327,917	12.0	60.7	13.3	65.6
June	330,541	12.5	63.3	13.4	65.8
July	353,415	12.9	65.4	13.3	65.5
August	351,791	12.9	65.1	13.3	65.5
September	347,516	13.1	66.4	13.2	65.1
October	339,007	12.4	62.7	13.2	65.2
November	318,820	12.0	60.9	13.2	64.9
December	335,722	12.3	62.1	13.2	65.1

Note: Monthly population estimates for 2015 were provided by the U.S. Census Bureau. Available from: https://www.census.gov/popest/data/national/asrh/2015/2015-nat-res.html).
X = Not applicable.
[1]Method of seasonal adjustment developed by the U.S. Census Bureau. For more information, see: http://www.census.gov/ts/papers/ShiskinYoungMusgrave1967.pdf

Table 1-33. Number, Rate, and Percent of Births to Unmarried Women and Birth Rate for Married Women, Selected Years, 1980–2015

(Number, rate per 1,000 women age 15 to 44 years; percent.)

Year	Births to unmarried women			Birth rate for married women[3]
	Number	Rate[1]	Percent[2]	
1980	665,747	29.4	18.4	97.0
1985	828,174	32.8	22.0	93.3
1990	1,165,384	43.8	28.0	93.2
1995	1,253,976	44.3	32.2	82.6
2000	1,347,043	44.1	33.2	87.4
2001	1,349,249	43.7	33.5	86.6
2002	1,365,966	43.6	34.0	86.9
2003	1,415,995	44.7	34.6	88.4
2004	1,470,189	46.0	35.8	88.1
2005	1,527,034	47.2	36.9	87.9
2006	1,641,946	50.3	38.5	88.7
2007	1,715,047	51.8	39.7	89.1
2008	1,726,566	51.8	40.6	86.9
2009	1,693,658	49.9	41.0	85.6
2010	1,633,471	47.5	40.8	84.3
2011	1,607,773	46.0	40.7	85.1
2012	1,609,619	45.3	40.7	86.0
2013	1,595,873	44.4	40.6	86.9
2014	1,604,870	43.9	40.2	88.9
2015	1,601,527	43.4	40.3	88.9

Note: Rates for 2001 to 2009 have been revised using revised intercensal populations based on the 2010 census.
[1]Births to unmarried women per 1,000 unmarried women age 15 to 44 years.
[2]Percentage of all births to unmarried women.
[3]Births to married women per 1,000 married women age 15 to 44 years.

Table 1-34. Birth Rates for Unmarried Women, by Age of Mother, Selected Years, 1970–2015, and by Age, Race, and Hispanic Origin of Mother, Selected Years, 1970–2015

(Births to unmarried women per 1,000 unmarried women.)

| Characteristic | 15 to 44 years[1] | Age of mother | | | 20 to 24 years | 25 to 29 years | 30 to 34 years | 35 to 39 years | 40 to 44 years[2] |
| | | 15 to 19 years | | | | | | | |
		Total	15 to 17 years	18 to 19 years					
All Races[3]									
1970[4,5]	26.4	22.4	17.1	32.9	38.4	37.0	27.1	13.6	3.5
1975[5,6]	24.5	23.9	19.3	32.5	31.2	27.5	17.9	9.1	2.6
1980[5,6]	29.4	27.6	20.6	39.0	40.9	34.0	21.1	9.7	2.6
1980[6,7]	28.4	27.5	20.7	38.7	39.7	31.4	18.5	8.4	2.3
1981[6,7]	29.5	27.9	20.9	39.0	41.1	34.5	20.8	9.8	2.6
1982[6,7]	30.0	28.7	21.5	39.6	41.5	35.1	21.9	10.0	2.7
1983[6,7]	30.3	29.5	22.0	40.7	41.8	35.5	22.4	10.2	2.6
1984[6,7]	31.0	30.0	21.9	42.5	43.0	37.1	23.3	10.9	2.5
1985[7]	32.8	31.4	22.4	45.9	46.5	39.9	25.2	11.6	2.5
1986[7]	34.2	32.3	22.8	48.0	49.3	42.2	27.2	12.2	2.7
1987[7]	36.0	33.8	24.5	48.9	52.6	44.5	29.6	13.5	2.9
1988[7]	38.5	36.4	26.4	51.5	56.0	48.5	32.0	15.0	3.2
1989[7]	41.6	40.1	28.7	56.0	61.2	52.8	34.9	16.0	3.4
1990[7]	43.8	42.5	29.6	60.7	65.1	56.0	37.6	17.3	3.6
1991[7]	45.0	44.6	30.8	65.4	67.8	56.0	37.9	17.9	3.8
1992[7]	44.9	44.2	30.2	66.7	67.9	55.6	37.6	18.8	4.1
1993[7]	44.8	44.0	30.3	66.2	68.5	55.9	38.0	18.9	4.4
1994[7]	46.2	45.8	31.7	69.1	70.9	57.4	39.6	19.7	4.7
1995[7]	44.3	43.8	30.1	66.5	68.7	54.3	38.9	19.3	4.7
1996[7]	43.8	42.2	28.5	64.9	68.9	54.5	40.2	19.9	4.8
1997[7]	42.9	41.4	27.7	63.9	68.9	53.4	37.9	18.7	4.6
1998[7]	43.3	40.9	26.5	63.6	70.4	55.4	38.1	18.7	4.6
1999[7]	43.3	39.7	25.0	62.3	70.8	56.9	38.1	19.0	4.6
2000[7]	44.1	39.0	23.9	62.2	72.2	58.5	39.3	19.7	5.0
2001[7]	43.7	36.8	21.8	60.2	70.8	59.6	40.3	20.4	5.3
2002[7]	43.6	35.1	20.7	58.1	70.0	62.0	41.3	20.9	5.4
2003[7]	44.7	34.3	20.1	56.6	71.0	66.2	44.2	22.3	5.8
2004[7]	46.0	34.2	19.9	56.6	72.3	69.1	47.3	23.5	6.0
2005[7]	47.2	33.9	19.4	57.0	74.5	71.5	50.4	24.5	6.2
2006[7]	50.3	35.5	20.1	60.3	79.1	75.4	55.3	26.8	6.5
2007[7]	51.8	36.5	20.4	61.9	79.8	76.9	58.0	28.7	6.8
2008[7]	51.8	35.9	20.1	59.7	78.1	75.7	58.8	30.2	7.5
2009[7]	49.9	34.0	18.8	56.3	74.4	73.0	57.1	29.7	7.8
2010[7]	47.5	31.1	16.8	52.0	70.0	69.2	56.3	29.6	8.0
2011[7]	46.0	28.4	14.9	48.2	66.7	67.8	56.2	29.9	8.2
2012[7]	45.3	26.7	13.7	45.8	64.7	67.2	56.3	30.9	8.5
2013[7]	44.3	20.0	11.9	42.1	63.1	66.7	56.6	31.8	8.3
2014[7]	43.4	22.0	9.6	39.4	61.6	67.6	58.1	33.4	8.5
2015[7]	43.9	20.2	10.6	36.5	59.7	66.9	60.3	34.1	9.0
White									
1980[6,7]	18.1	16.5	12.0	24.1	25.1	21.5	14.1	7.1	1.8
1981[6,7]	18.6	17.2	12.6	24.6	25.8	22.3	14.2	7.2	1.9
1982[6,7]	19.3	18.0	13.1	25.3	26.5	23.1	15.3	7.4	2.1
1983[6,7]	19.8	18.7	13.6	26.4	27.1	23.8	15.9	7.8	2.0
1984[6,7]	20.6	19.3	13.7	27.9	28.5	25.5	16.8	8.4	2.0
1985[7]	22.5	20.8	14.5	31.2	31.7	28.5	18.4	9.0	2.0
1986[7]	23.9	21.8	14.9	33.5	34.2	30.5	20.1	9.7	2.2
1987[7]	25.3	23.2	16.2	34.5	36.6	32.0	22.3	10.7	2.4
1988[7]	27.4	25.3	17.6	36.8	39.2	35.4	24.2	12.1	2.7
1989[7]	30.2	28.0	19.3	40.2	43.8	39.1	26.8	13.1	2.9
1990[7]	32.9	30.6	20.4	44.9	48.2	43.0	29.9	14.5	3.2
1991[7]	34.5	32.7	21.7	49.4	51.4	44.3	30.9	15.2	3.2
1992[7]	35.0	32.7	21.4	51.2	52.4	44.8	31.3	16.1	3.6
1993[7]	35.6	33.3	21.9	52.0	53.8	46.0	31.9	16.3	3.9
1994[7]	37.8	35.8	23.9	55.8	57.5	48.6	33.8	17.2	4.3
1995[7]	37.0	35.0	23.3	54.7	57.2	47.4	33.7	16.8	4.2
1996[7]	37.0	34.0	22.3	53.5	57.9	48.1	35.4	17.7	4.3
1997[7]	36.3	33.6	22.0	52.9	57.9	47.0	33.6	16.6	3.9
1998[7]	36.9	33.6	21.5	53.1	59.5	48.6	34.1	16.9	4.1
1999[7]	37.4	33.2	20.6	52.9	60.2	50.8	34.9	17.4	4.1

Note: Race and Hispanic origin are reported separately on birth certificates. Persons of Hispanic origin may be of any race. Race categories are consistent with 1977 Office of Management and Budget standards. Forty-nine states and the District of Columbia reported multiple-race data for 2015 that were bridged to single-race categories for comparability with other states. Multiple-race reporting areas vary for 2003–2015. Rates cannot be computed for unmarried non-Hispanic black women or for American Indian or Alaska Native women because the necessary populations are not available.

NA = Not available.

[1]Rates computed by relating total births to unmarried mothers, regardless of age of mother, to unmarried women age 15 to 44 years.

[2]Beginning in 1997, birth rates computed by relating births to unmarried mothers age 40 years and over to unmarried women age 40 to 44 years.

[3]Includes races other than White, Black, and Asian or Other Pacific Islander.

[4]Births to unmarried women are estimated for the United States from data for registration areas in which marital status of mother was reported.

[5]Based on a 50 percent sample of births.

[6]Based on 100 percent of births in selected states and on a 50 percent sample of births in all other states.

[7]Data for states in which marital status was not reported have been inferred and included with data from the remaining states.

Table 1-34. Birth Rates for Unmarried Women, by Age of Mother, Selected Years, 1970–2015, and by Age, Race, and Hispanic Origin of Mother, Selected Years, 1970–2015—*Continued*

(Births to unmarried women per 1,000 unmarried women.)

Characteristic	15 to 44 years[1]	15 to 19 years			20 to 24 years	25 to 29 years	30 to 34 years	35 to 39 years	40 to 44 years[2]
		Total	15 to 17 years	18 to 19 years					
2000[7]	38.2	32.7	19.7	53.1	61.7	52.9	35.9	17.9	4.5
2001[7]	38.4	31.2	18.1	51.9	61.5	54.9	37.2	18.6	4.9
2002[7]	39.0	30.3	17.5	50.8	61.6	57.5	38.8	19.5	5.1
2003[7]	40.5	29.9	17.1	50.0	63.2	61.7	42.3	21.3	5.5
2004[7]	41.8	29.9	17.0	49.9	64.5	65.0	46.2	22.8	5.6
2005[7]	43.2	29.7	16.7	50.3	67.0	67.7	49.8	23.9	5.9
2006[7]	46.4	31.1	17.3	53.3	71.7	72.4	55.5	26.6	6.3
2007[7]	48.3	32.3	17.9	55.1	72.6	74.3	59.5	29.1	6.5
2008[7]	48.4	31.9	17.8	53.3	70.9	73.1	60.0	31.1	7.3
2009[7]	46.6	30.4	16.7	50.5	67.3	69.7	57.7	30.6	7.8
2010[7]	44.5	27.9	15.1	46.9	63.4	65.8	56.8	30.7	8.1
2011[7]	42.7	25.5	13.4	43.4	60.1	63.8	56.2	30.6	8.3
2012[7]	45.3	26.7	13.7	45.8	64.7	67.2	56.3	30.9	8.5
2013[7]	44.3	24.0	11.9	42.1	63.1	66.7	56.6	31.8	8.3
2014[7]	43.9	22.0	10.6	39.4	61.6	67.6	58.1	33.4	8.5
2015[7]	40.4	18.8	8.8	34.3	54.6	63.3	59.8	34.8	8.2
Non-Hispanic White									
1990[7,8]	24.4	25.0	16.2	37.0	36.4	30.3	20.5	6.1	NA
1991[7]	NA	NA	NA	NA	NA	NA	NA	NA	NA
1992[7]	NA	NA	NA	NA	NA	NA	NA	NA	NA
1993[7]	NA	NA	NA	NA	NA	NA	NA	NA	NA
1994[7]	28.4	28.1	17.9	45.0	43.8	34.7	24.6	12.8	3.1
1995[7]	28.1	27.7	17.6	44.6	43.9	34.4	25.1	12.9	3.2
1996[7]	28.2	27.0	16.9	43.9	44.5	35.0	26.4	13.8	3.3
1997[7]	27.5	26.4	16.2	43.3	44.8	34.4	24.9	12.7	2.9
1998[7]	27.9	26.2	15.5	43.1	46.3	35.4	25.0	13.1	3.1
1999[7]	27.9	25.6	14.6	42.7	46.3	36.2	24.8	13.0	3.1
2000[7]	28.0	24.7	13.6	42.1	47.0	36.9	24.8	12.9	3.3
2001[7]	27.8	23.1	12.1	40.3	46.4	37.8	25.4	13.2	3.6
2002[7]	27.9	22.1	11.4	38.8	46.3	38.9	26.2	13.6	3.7
2003[7]	28.8	21.5	11.0	37.8	47.6	41.5	28.0	14.8	4.1
2004[7]	29.6	21.3	10.7	37.4	48.6	44.2	30.0	15.7	4.2
2005[7]	30.4	20.9	10.3	37.4	49.9	46.0	31.7	16.2	4.3
2006[7]	32.4	21.6	10.7	38.9	52.6	49.1	35.1	17.9	4.5
2007[7]	33.8	22.6	10.9	40.7	53.4	50.7	37.2	19.2	4.6
2008[7]	34.3	22.5	10.8	39.7	52.9	50.8	38.4	20.4	5.2
2009[7]	33.6	21.8	10.4	38.1	51.4	49.3	37.9	20.0	5.5
2010[7]	32.9	20.3	9.5	36.0	49.5	48.0	38.7	20.2	5.8
2011[7]	32.3	18.8	8.6	33.6	47.8	47.8	39.2	20.7	6.0
2012[7]	32.1	24.1	8.0	32.1	46.6	47.8	40.2	21.8	6.1
2013[7]	31.7	16.2	7.0	29.8	45.6	47.6	40.9	22.6	6.1
2014[7]	31.8	15.0	6.3	28.1	44.4	49.1	43.1	24.2	6.5
2015[7]	31.6	13.9	5.7	26.3	43.3	48.8	44.4	24.8	6.8
Black									
1980[6,7]	81.1	87.9	68.8	118.2	112.3	81.4	46.7	19.0	5.5
1981[6,7]	79.4	85.0	65.9	114.2	110.7	83.1	45.5	19.6	5.6
1982[6,7]	77.9	85.1	66.3	112.7	109.3	82.7	44.1	19.5	5.2
1983[6,7]	76.2	85.5	66.8	111.9	107.2	79.7	43.8	19.4	4.8
1984[6,7]	75.2	86.1	66.5	113.6	107.9	77.8	43.8	19.4	4.3
1985[7]	77.0	87.6	66.8	117.9	113.1	79.3	47.5	20.4	4.3
1986[7]	79.0	88.5	67.0	121.1	118.0	84.6	50.0	20.6	4.4
1987[7]	82.6	90.9	69.9	123.0	126.1	91.6	53.1	22.4	4.7
1988[7]	86.5	96.1	73.5	130.5	133.6	97.2	57.4	24.1	5.0
1989[7]	90.7	104.5	78.9	140.9	142.4	102.9	60.5	24.9	5.0
1990[7]	90.5	106.0	78.8	143.7	144.8	105.3	61.5	25.5	5.1
1991[7]	89.0	107.8	79.9	147.7	146.4	100.0	59.8	25.5	5.4
1992[7]	85.7	104.8	77.2	146.4	142.6	96.8	57.3	25.6	5.4
1993[7]	83.0	101.2	75.9	140.0	139.9	92.8	56.7	25.7	5.8
1994[7]	80.8	99.3	73.9	139.6	135.2	91.3	56.5	26.0	5.9
1995[7]	74.5	91.2	67.4	129.2	124.6	82.3	53.3	25.3	6.0
1996[7]	72.8	87.5	62.6	127.2	122.6	81.2	53.4	25.2	6.1
1997[7]	71.5	84.5	59.0	124.8	124.2	81.4	51.0	24.3	6.5
1998[7]	71.6	81.5	55.0	121.5	127.8	86.5	50.5	24.3	6.0
1999[7]	69.7	76.5	50.0	115.8	126.8	85.5	49.0	24.2	5.8

Note: Race and Hispanic origin are reported separately on birth certificates. Persons of Hispanic origin may be of any race. Race categories are consistent with 1977 Office of Management and Budget standards. Forty-nine states and the District of Columbia reported multiple-race data for 2015 that were bridged to single-race categories for comparability with other states. Multiple-race reporting areas vary for 2003–2015. Rates cannot be computed for unmarried non-Hispanic black women or for American Indian or Alaska Native women because the necessary populations are not available.

NA = Not available.

[1] Rates computed by relating total births to unmarried mothers, regardless of age of mother, to unmarried women age 15 to 44 years.
[2] Beginning in 1997, birth rates computed by relating births to unmarried mothers age 40 years and over to unmarried women age 40 to 44 years.
[6] Based on 100 percent of births in selected states and on a 50 percent sample of births in all other states.
[7] Data for states in which marital status was not reported have been inferred and included with data from the remaining states.
[8] Rates based on data for 48 states and the District of Columbia that reported Hispanic origin on the birth certificate. Rate for age group 35–39 years are based on births to unmarried women aged 35–44 years.

Table 1-34. Birth Rates for Unmarried Women, by Age of Mother, Selected Years, 1970–2015, and by Age, Race, and Hispanic Origin of Mother, Selected Years, 1970–2015—*Continued*

(Births to unmarried women per 1,000 unmarried women.)

| Characteristic | 15 to 44 years[1] | Age of mother | | | 20 to 24 years | 25 to 29 years | 30 to 34 years | 35 to 39 years | 40 to 44 years[2] |
| | | 15 to 19 years | | | | | | | |
		Total	15 to 17 years	18 to 19 years					
2000[7]	70.5	75.0	48.3	115.0	129.0	85.9	50.2	25.4	6.3
2001[7]	68.0	69.4	43.5	109.1	122.5	84.4	51.2	25.4	6.3
2002[7]	66.1	64.0	39.4	102.8	119.0	86.3	50.2	24.9	6.3
2003[7]	65.9	61.0	37.4	98.0	117.8	91.3	51.2	25.2	6.5
2004[7]	66.8	60.1	36.1	98.0	119.6	92.5	52.0	25.7	6.8
2005[7]	67.2	58.7	34.4	97.9	120.4	94.7	53.9	25.9	7.1
2006[7]	70.7	61.1	35.4	103.3	125.5	98.0	58.4	27.3	7.2
2007[7]	71.4	61.3	34.8	103.6	125.3	99.1	59.9	28.0	7.4
2008[7]	71.0	59.7	33.9	98.4	124.0	97.0	61.1	28.5	7.6
2009[7]	68.7	55.9	31.1	91.3	119.5	95.6	60.3	28.4	7.6
2010[7]	65.3	50.8	27.6	83.6	112.6	92.5	58.6	27.8	7.8
2011[7]	63.7	46.7	24.7	77.4	106.9	92.4	59.1	28.9	7.8
2012[7]	62.6	43.4	22.0	73.2	103.5	91.2	59.6	29.7	8.1
2013[7]	61.7	38.5	19.0	66.2	100.7	92.3	60.6	31.1	8.4
2014[7]	61.5	34.4	16.7	60.9	97.4	93.3	67.0	32.0	8.8
2015[7]	59.6	31.5	15.4	55.8	94.2	91.9	63.9	32.6	9.1
Asian or Pacific Islander									
2000[7]	20.9	15.2	9.6	23.2	24.2	25.4	29.7	18.4	6.9
2001[7]	20.5	14.2	8.5	22.4	23.9	25.7	28.7	19.5	6.3
2002[7]	20.6	13.0	7.3	21.0	24.4	26.7	29.4	19.1	6.9
2003[7]	21.1	12.3	7.1	19.6	24.2	29.0	31.8	19.8	7.9
2004[7]	22.1	12.3	7.3	19.4	24.8	30.7	35.8	20.7	8.6
2005[7]	22.8	11.9	6.8	19.3	25.8	31.4	36.8	24.6	9.3
2006[7]	23.4	12.0	7.3	18.9	26.8	30.5	37.6	29.7	9.4
2007[7]	23.9	11.9	6.7	19.2	27.1	32.3	36.9	28.8	9.9
2008[7]	23.9	11.4	6.3	18.4	26.4	33.5	37.9	30.3	10.8
2009[7]	23.6	10.6	5.9	17.1	25.3	36.2	39.2	27.3	9.9
2010[7]	22.3	9.2	4.8	15.4	23.2	35.0	40.0	26.6	9.9
2011[7]	22.4	8.6	4.4	14.8	22.3	35.1	42.3	27.0	9.9
2012[7]	22.9	8.1	3.9	14.2	22.0	35.2	43.6	30.1	12.1
2013[7]	21.8	7.2	3.5	12.6	20.7	31.5	44.1	31.5	12.6
2014[7]	21.7	6.2	3.0	10.6	19.4	31.4	47.0	36.0	12.6
2015[7]	20.4	5.5	2.5	9.7	17.9	28.8	47.3	33.6	11.2
Hispanic[9]									
1990[7,8]	89.6	65.9	45.9	98.9	129.8	131.7	88.1	50.8	13.7
1991[7]	92.5	71.0	49.5	107.5	134.2	135.1	88.2	47.6	14.1
1992[7]	92.8	70.3	49.2	106.6	138.2	133.4	89.9	47.8	14.6
1993[7]	91.4	71.1	49.6	108.8	134.3	130.4	87.8	47.1	14.1
1994[7]	95.8	77.7	55.7	115.4	144.5	131.7	91.2	47.4	13.9
1995[7]	88.8	73.2	52.8	108.6	135.8	122.3	84.1	42.2	12.1
1996[7]	86.2	69.3	49.7	102.3	131.6	122.0	84.6	41.2	12.3
1997[7]	83.2	69.2	50.7	100.6	122.8	114.8	78.8	40.5	12.1
1998[7]	82.8	69.3	49.8	101.2	120.6	115.9	78.2	38.8	12.0
1999[7]	84.9	68.6	48.7	99.9	126.1	119.6	84.2	42.4	11.2
2000[7]	87.2	68.5	47.0	102.2	130.5	121.6	89.4	46.1	12.2
2001[7]	86.8	65.5	43.4	101.1	129.8	121.0	91.4	49.6	12.2
2002[7]	87.0	63.9	41.9	100.7	127.2	125.1	91.0	52.4	12.8
2003[7]	89.9	63.5	41.1	101.2	130.2	135.6	98.7	54.0	13.2
2004[7]	92.7	64.2	41.2	102.9	133.4	142.5	108.8	56.0	13.7
2005[7]	96.2	63.7	40.3	103.9	142.5	151.2	116.7	58.1	14.1
2006[7]	101.5	65.9	40.5	110.2	155.1	160.7	122.9	61.3	14.8
2007[7]	102.1	65.4	40.6	109.2	153.8	161.1	127.0	64.9	14.9
2008[7]	97.3	62.4	39.4	101.1	141.0	151.1	121.6	66.9	16.2
2009[7]	89.4	56.7	35.3	90.9	125.4	139.4	112.4	63.7	17.1
2010[7]	80.6	50.0	30.8	79.8	110.5	123.9	105.8	61.7	16.3
2011[7]	75.1	44.7	27.0	71.7	100.6	116.2	106.0	58.0	16.2
2012[7]	72.6	41.8	24.5	68.5	96.5	113.2	103.9	57.6	16.5
2013[7]	69.9	37.6	21.1	63.0	93.1	112.0	100.1	56.8	16.8
2014[7]	68.5	34.4	18.6	59.5	92.3	111.2	97.3	58.2	16.8
2015[7]	67.4	31.6	16.6	55.7	87.9	109.1	101.4	60.3	18.1

Note: Race and Hispanic origin are reported separately on birth certificates. Persons of Hispanic origin may be of any race. Race categories are consistent with 1977 Office of Management and Budget standards. Forty-nine states and the District of Columbia reported multiple-race data for 2015 that were bridged to single-race categories for comparability with other states. Multiple-race reporting areas vary for 2003–2015. Rates cannot be computed for unmarried non-Hispanic black women or for American Indian or Alaska Native women because the necessary populations are not available.
NA = Not available.
[1]Rates computed by relating total births to unmarried mothers, regardless of age of mother, to unmarried women age 15 to 44 years.
[2]Beginning in 1997, birth rates computed by relating births to unmarried mothers age 40 years and over to unmarried women age 40 to 44 years.
[3]Includes races other than White, Black, and Asian or Other Pacific Islander.
[4]Births to unmarried women are estimated for the United States from data for registration areas in which marital status of mother was reported.
[5]Based on a 50 percent sample of births.
[6]Based on 100 percent of births in selected states and on a 50 percent sample of births in all other states.
[7]Data for states in which marital status was not reported have been inferred and included with data from the remaining states.
[8]Rates based on data for 48 states and the District of Columbia that reported Hispanic origin on the birth certificate. Rate for age group 35–39 years are based on births to unmarried women aged 35–44 years.
[9]Persons of Hispanic origin may be of any race.

Table 1-35. Births and Birth Rates for Unmarried Women, by Age, Race, and Hispanic Origin of Mother, 2015

(Number, rate, percent.)

Measure and age of mother	All races[1]	White Total[2]	White Non-Hispanic	Black Total[2]	Black Non-Hispanic	American Indian or Alaska Native[2]	Asian or Pacific Islander[2]	Hispanic[3]
Number								
All ages	1,601,527	1,077,618	621,314	448,531	415,554	29,130	46,248	489,358
Under 15 years	2,489	1,501	578	898	845	53	37	979
15 to 19 years	204,043	143,134	77,222	53,130	48,739	4,417	3,362	70,813
15 years	7,497	4,962	2,101	2,250	2,076	167	118	3,062
16 years	17,791	12,260	5,575	4,854	4,464	415	262	7,119
17 years	33,259	23,416	11,537	8,540	7,737	791	512	12,778
18 years	57,032	40,449	22,015	14,425	13,261	1,201	957	19,751
19 years	88,464	62,047	35,994	23,061	21,201	1,843	1,513	28,103
20 to 24 years	560,639	372,317	224,094	166,405	155,047	10,258	11,659	160,158
25 to 29 years	435,339	289,467	171,977	124,527	115,662	7,868	13,477	126,195
30 to 34 years	252,397	170,365	94,806	67,187	61,977	4,270	10,575	80,447
35 to 39 years	116,670	79,928	41,812	29,448	26,962	1,873	5,421	40,283
40 years and over	29,950	20,906	10,825	6,936	6,322	391	1,717	10,483
Rate per 1,000 Unmarried Women in Specified Group								
15 to 44 years[4]	43.4	40.4	31.6	59.6	NA	NA	20.4	67.4
15 to 19 years	20.2	18.8	13.9	31.5	NA	NA	5.5	31.6
15 to 17 years	9.6	8.8	5.7	15.4	NA	NA	2.5	16.6
18 to 19 years	36.5	34.3	26.3	55.8	NA	NA	9.7	55.7
20 to 24 years	59.7	54.6	43.3	94.2	NA	NA	17.9	87.9
25 to 29 years	66.9	63.3	48.8	91.9	NA	NA	28.8	109.1
30 to 34 years	60.3	59.8	44.4	63.9	NA	NA	47.3	101.4
35 to 39 years	34.1	34.8	24.8	32.6	NA	NA	33.6	60.3
40 to 44 years[5]	9.0	8.2	6.8	9.1	NA	NA	11.2	18.1
Percent of Births to Unmarried Women								
All ages	40.3	35.8	29.2	70.1	70.6	65.8	16.4	53.0
Under 15 years	99.6	99.3	99.3	100.0	100.0	100.0	100.0	99.3
15 to 19 years	88.8	86.3	85.0	97.1	97.4	93.2	78.2	88.1
15 years	98.8	98.4	98.4	99.8	99.9	99.4	95.9	98.5
16 years	96.5	95.5	95.2	99.4	99.5	98.8	92.3	95.8
17 years	94.6	93.2	92.9	99.0	99.2	96.1	88.0	93.7
18 years	89.8	87.4	86.6	97.5	97.9	93.3	82.2	88.8
19 years	84.2	81.0	80.0	95.3	95.9	90.3	70.6	82.8
20 to 24 years	65.9	60.0	56.1	87.6	88.3	76.2	44.5	67.8
25 to 29 years	37.8	32.7	26.8	69.1	69.7	61.3	18.4	49.3
30 to 34 years	23.1	20.0	14.7	51.4	51.7	50.2	10.0	38.4
35 to 39 years	22.1	20.0	14.4	44.3	44.3	49.0	9.4	36.0
40 years and over	24.8	23.7	18.1	40.3	39.9	44.5	11.9	36.6

Note: For 49 states, the District of Columbia, and New York City, marital status is reported in the birth registration process; for New York, mother's marital status is inferred. Rates cannot be computed for unmarried non-Hispanic black women or for American Indian or Alaska Native women because the neccessary populations are not available.

NA = Not available.

[1] Includes races other than White and Black and origin not stated.

[2] Race and Hispanic origin are reported separately on birth certificates. Persons of Hispanic origin may be of any race. Multiple-race data, when reported, were bridged to single-race categories in order to maintain comparability among all reported areas. Forty-nine states and the District of Columbia reported multiple-race data for 2015 that were bridged to single-race categories for comparability with other states

[3] Persons of Hispanic origin may be of any race.

[4] Birth rates computed by relating total births to unmarried mothers, regardless of age of mother, to unmarried women age 15 to 44 years.

[5] Birth rates computed by relating births to unmarried mothers age 40 years and over to unmarried women age 40 to 44 years.

Table 1-36. Selected Demographic Characteristics of Births, by Hispanic Origin of Mother and by Race for Mothers of Non-Hispanic Origin, 2015

(Birth rates are births per 1,000 population. Fertility rates are computed by relating total births, regardless of age of mother, to women aged 15 to 44. Total fertility rates are sums of birth rates for 5-year age groups multiplied by 5. Populations estimated as of July 1. Mean age at first birth is the arithmetic average of the age of mothers at the time of birth, computed directly from the frequency of first births by age of mother.)

Characteristic	All origins[1]	Hispanic (of any race)						Non-Hispanic		
		Total	Mexican	Puerto Rican	Cuban	Central and South American	Other and unknown Hispanic	Total[2]	White	Black
Number										
Births	3,978,497	924,048	546,169	70,987	21,107	142,249	143,536	3,021,999	2,130,279	589,047
Rate										
Birth rate[3]	12.4	16.3	NA	NA	NA	(3)	NA	11.5	10.7	14.2
Fertility rate[3]	62.5	71.7	NA	NA	NA	(3)	NA	60.2	59.3	64.1
Total fertility rate[3]	1,843.5	2,123.5	NA	NA	NA	(3)	NA	1,769.5	1,746.0	1,857.0
Sex ratio[4]	1,048	1,042	1,040	1,051	1,049	1,042	1,041	1,050	1,053	1,033
Percent										
Births to mothers under 20 years	5.8	8.8	9.3	9.8	3.7	5.9	10.0	5.0	4.3	8.6
4th and higher-order births[5]	12.4	16.1	18.3	12.9	5.6	13.9	13.3	11.2	10.2	16.5
Births to unmarried mothers	40.3	53.0	51.5	64.2	50.7	51.0	55.1	36.4	29.2	70.5
Mothers born in the 50 states and D.C.	77.4	50.8	51.4	74.8	47.4	17.0	70.7	85.5	93.4	84.7
Mean										
Age of mother at first birth	26.4	24.5	24.0	24.3	27.1	36.5	24.3	26.9	27.2	24.4

Note: Race and Hispanic origin are reported separately on birth certificates. Race categories are consistent with 1977 Office of Management and Budget standards. Forty-nine states and the District of Columbia reported multiple-race data for 2015 that were bridged to single-race categories for comparability with other states. Persons of Hispanic origin may be of any race. In this table, Hispanic women are classified only by place of origin; non-Hispanic women are classified by race.
NA = Not available.
[1]Includes origin not stated.
[2]Includes races other than White and Black.
[3]Rates for Central and South American include other and unknown Hispanic.
[4]Male births per 1,000 female births.
[5]Based on live-birth order.

Table 1-37. Percent of Births with Selected Medical or Health Characteristics, by Race of Mother, 2015

(Percent, rate.)

Characteristic	All races	White	Black	American or Alaska Indian Native	Asian or Pacific Islander
ALL BIRTHS					
Mother					
Diabetes during pregnancy	6.5	6.2	5.8	9.9	11.1
Weight gain of less than 11 lbs	9.1	8.3	13.1	13.1	7.1
Weight gain of more than 40 lbs	21.0	21.6	21.4	22.2	14.3
Induction of labor	23.8	24.5	22.9	24.2	18.5
CNM delivery[1]	8.5	8.7	7.4	17.8	7.2
Cesarean delivery	32.0	31.3	35.3	28.3	33.0
Infant					
Gestational age					
Preterm[2]	9.6	9.0	13.2	10.5	8.6
Early preterm[3]	2.8	2.4	4.7	2.8	2.2
Late preterm[4]	6.9	6.6	8.4	7.7	6.4
Birthweight					
Very low birthweight[5]	1.4	1.1	2.8	1.3	1.1
Low birthweight[6]	8.1	7.0	13.0	7.5	8.4
4,000 grams or more	8.0	9.0	4.6	10.1	4.8
Twin birth[7] (rate)	33.5	32.8	38.7	25.1	29.9
Triplet or higher-order multiple birth[8] (rate)	103.6	107.1	101.7	38.4	81.4

Note: Race and Hispanic origin are reported separately on birth certificates. Race categories are consistent with 1977 Office of Management and Budget standards. Forty-nine states and the District of Columbia reported multiple-race data for 2015 that were bridged to single-race categories for comparability with other states. In this table, all women, including Hispanic women, are classified only according to their race.
[1]Births delivered by certified nurse midwives.
[2]Born prior to 37 completed weeks of gestation based on the obstetric estimate.
[3]Born prior to 34 completed weeks of gestation based on the obstetric estimate.
[4]Born between 34 and 36 completed weeks of gestatio based on the obstetric estimaten.
[5]Birthweight of less than 1,500 grams (3 lb 4 oz).
[6]Birthweight of less than 2,500 grams (5 lb 8 oz).
[7]Live births in twin deliveries per 1,000 live births.
[8]Live births in triplet and other higher-order multiple deliveries per 100,000 live births.

Table 1-38. Percent of Births with Selected Medical or Health Characteristics, by Hispanic Origin of Mother and by Race for Mothers of Non-Hispanic Origin, 2015

(Percent, rate.)

Characteristic	All origins[1]	Origin of mother								
		Hispanic (may be of any race)						Non-Hispanic		
		Total	Mexican	Puerto Rican	Cuban	Central and South American	Other and unknown Hispanic	Total[2]	White	Black
ALL BIRTHS										
Mother										
Diabetes during pregnancy	6.5	7.1	7.7	6.8	5.3	6.4	6.1	6.3	5.8	5.7
Weight gain of less than 11 lbs	9.1	10.5	11.1	9.8	6.1	9.9	9.9	8.6	7.5	13.3
Weight gain of more than 40 lbs	21.0	16.5	15.3	22.2	25.2	14.8	18.6	22.5	23.7	21.5
Induction of labor	23.8	19.3	18.8	21.7	18.9	18.0	21.3	25.3	26.8	23.0
CNM delivery[3]	8.5	8.1	7.6	10.5	5.0	10.0	7.2	8.6	9.0	7.2
Cesarean delivery	32.0	31.7	30.4	34.2	47.4	31.5	33.2	32.1	31.1	35.5
Infant										
Gestational age										
Preterm[4]	9.6	9.1	8.9	11.0	9.3	8.7	9.6	9.8	8.9	13.4
Early preterm[5]	2.8	2.5	2.4	3.5	2.8	2.3	2.8	2.8	2.3	4.8
Late preterm[6]	6.9	6.6	6.5	7.5	6.5	6.4	6.8	6.9	6.5	8.6
Birthweight										
Very low birthweight[7]	1.4	1.2	1.1	1.7	1.4	1.1	1.4	1.4	1.1	2.9
Low birthweight[8]	8.1	7.2	6.8	9.4	7.2	6.7	8.1	8.3	6.9	13.3
4,000 grams or more	8.0	7.1	7.4	6.2	7.8	6.8	6.3	8.3	9.7	4.5
Twin birth[9] (rate)	33.5	24.5	23.0	31.9	31.6	24.0	25.9	36.0	36.1	39.4
Triplet or higher-order multiple birth[10] (rate)	103.6	66.1	59.7	67.6	94.8	78.0	73.8	114.4	122.8	104.4

[1]Includes origin not stated.
[2]Includes races other than White and Black.
[3]Births delivered by certified nurse midwives.
[4]Born prior to 37 completed weeks of gestation based on the obstetric estimate.
[5]Born prior to 34 completed weeks of gestation based on the obstetric estimate.
[6]Born between 34 and 36 completed weeks of gestation based on the obstetric estimate.
[7]Birthweight of less than 1,500 grams (3 lb 4 oz).
[8]Birthweight of less than 2,500 grams (5 lb 8 oz).
[9]Live births in twin deliveries per 1,000 live births.
[10]Live births in triplet and other higher-order multiple deliveries per 100,000 live births.

Table 1-39. Births to Unmarried Women, by Race and Hispanic Origin of Mother, by State and Territory of Residence, 2015

(Number, percent.)

| State and territory | Births to unmarried women | | | | Percent unmarried | | | |
| | | Non-Hispanic | | | | Non-Hispanic | | |
	All races[1]	White[2]	Black[2]	Hispanic[3]	All races[1]	White[2]	Black[2]	Hispanic[3]
United States[4]	1,601,527	621,314	415,554	489,358	40.3	29.2	70.5	53.0
Alabama	26,162	10,563	13,928	1,456	43.9	29.5	76.3	33.9
Alaska	4,071	1,593	164	256	36.1	24.3	38.8	31.6
Arizona	38,862	11,590	2,875	19,967	45.5	31.3	62.7	56.6
Arkansas	17,502	8,864	6,038	2,013	45.0	34.5	79.6	50.2
California	190,990	33,458	17,755	123,767	38.8	23.6	65.7	52.8
Colorado	15,136	7,033	1,330	6,024	22.7	17.2	38.5	33.2
Connecticut	13,410	4,982	2,890	5,267	37.5	24.4	65.1	63.6
Delaware	5,171	2,047	2,114	969	46.3	34.4	70.8	63.3
District of Columbia	4,721	179	3,720	764	49.3	6.0	77.5	57.6
Florida	107,125	38,372	34,287	32,940	47.8	37.4	69.1	51.4
Georgia	59,387	17,166	31,895	9,000	45.2	28.5	70.2	50.5
Hawaii	6,838	1,135	137	1,318	37.1	23.6	23.7	47.5
Idaho	6,332	4,320	76	1,641	27.7	23.9	31.7	45.0
Illinois	63,947	23,053	21,494	17,859	40.4	27.0	79.1	52.7
Indiana	36,349	23,723	8,080	4,207	43.3	37.4	78.1	55.1
Iowa	13,951	10,058	1,749	1,744	35.3	31.4	69.9	51.0
Kansas	14,115	8,504	1,980	3,270	36.0	30.1	68.0	51.9
Kentucky	23,295	17,559	3,877	1,638	41.6	37.9	73.6	54.6
Louisiana	34,209	11,850	19,134	2,756	52.9	34.8	79.5	57.1
Maine	5,104	4,671	161	127	40.5	40.4	34.8	50.6
Maryland	29,522	8,013	14,468	6,439	40.1	24.7	61.2	54.8
Massachusetts	23,900	10,960	3,766	7,861	33.4	25.1	53.7	60.4
Michigan	47,532	25,300	17,472	3,913	41.9	32.0	80.1	52.7
Minnesota	22,482	12,218	4,381	2,578	32.2	24.6	54.6	53.1
Mississippi	20,543	6,272	13,139	875	53.5	31.9	80.0	54.2
Missouri	30,345	18,979	8,663	2,052	40.4	33.2	76.6	50.8
Montana	4,573	3,061	47	278	36.3	29.8	52.8	48.5
Nebraska	8,777	4,888	1,282	2,170	32.9	25.5	68.5	51.1
Nevada	16,934	5,176	3,269	7,219	46.7	34.7	73.4	54.6
New Hampshire	4,233	3,735	89	315	34.0	34.2	37.6	49.4
New Jersey	36,215	8,852	9,990	16,332	35.1	18.7	67.1	58.5
New Mexico	13,453	2,195	258	8,427	52.1	30.7	54.7	58.4
New York	93,734	29,302	24,320	35,234	39.5	25.6	66.8	63.1
North Carolina	49,548	17,959	20,744	9,141	41.0	26.8	71.9	50.5
North Dakota	3,573	2,261	259	252	31.6	25.7	45.2	43.4
Ohio	60,325	36,913	18,395	4,097	43.3	35.6	77.5	58.7
Oklahoma	22,202	11,577	3,627	3,631	41.8	34.8	72.6	49.0
Oregon	16,452	10,472	758	4,237	36.0	32.6	56.8	49.7
Pennsylvania	58,081	31,079	15,590	9,779	41.2	31.8	77.3	65.4
Rhode Island	4,957	2,439	612	1,654	45.1	36.4	64.3	63.1
South Carolina	27,043	10,419	13,698	2,532	46.5	30.7	77.0	51.2
South Dakota	4,584	2,352	147	322	37.2	26.0	44.8	57.6
Tennessee	35,843	18,677	13,071	3,718	43.9	33.7	77.8	51.2
Texas	167,516	37,473	30,813	96,805	41.5	26.7	62.0	50.6
Utah	9,556	5,136	278	3,235	18.8	13.3	43.2	41.1
Vermont	2,375	2,199	53	59	40.2	40.9	40.5	42.4
Virginia	35,564	13,895	13,991	6,971	34.4	23.5	64.2	50.0
Washington	28,576	15,053	2,207	7,960	32.1	27.2	47.8	49.5
West Virginia	8,669	7,928	514	133	43.8	43.0	73.6	40.2
Wisconsin	25,113	13,950	5,929	3,691	37.5	28.5	83.5	55.9
Wyoming	2,630	1,861	40	465	33.9	30.0	46.0	48.3
Puerto Rico	21,298	932	89	20,218	68.4	64.1	66.4	68.6
Virgin Islands	895	40	659	176	67.5	38.5	69.7	74.3
Guam	2,004	20	7	4	59.5	10.2	*	*
American Samoa	398	NA	NA	NA	36.9	NA	NA	NA
Northern Marianas	347	1	–	-	81.3	*	*	*

NA = Not available.
- = Quantity zero.
* = Figure does not meet standards of reliability or precision; based on fewer than 20 births in the numerator.
[1]Includes races other than White and Black and origin not stated.
[2]Race and Hispanic origin are reported separately on birth certificates. Persons of Hispanic origin may be of any race. Multiple-race data, when reported, were bridged to single-race categories in order to maintain comparability among all reported areas. Forty-nine states and the District of Columbia reported multiple-race data for 2015 that were bridged to single-race categories for comparability with other states.
[3]Includes all persons of Hispanic origin of any race.
[4]Excludes data for the territories.

Table 1-40. Births, by Weight Gain of Mother During Pregnancy, by Plurality, Gestational Age, and Race and Hispanic Origin of Mother, 2014

(Number, percent distribution.)

Period of gestation,[1] race, and Hispanic origin of mother	All births	Less than 11 pounds	11 to 20 pounds	21 to 30 pounds	31 to 40 pounds	41 to 98 pounds	Not stated
NUMBER							
All Pluralities							
All Gestational Ages[2]							
All races[3]	3,978,497	346,111	643,532	1,079,464	945,854	803,256	160,280
Non-Hispanic White[4]	2,130,279	153,740	288,970	568,770	555,327	487,863	75,609
Non-Hispanic Black[4]	589,047	74,035	106,238	141,069	114,145	119,264	34,296
Hispanic[5]	924,048	93,446	189,262	265,317	195,290	146,609	34,124
Under 37 Weeks							
All races[3]	382,786	51,270	79,171	96,275	69,134	64,406	22,530
Non-Hispanic White[4]	189,146	20,849	34,502	48,132	38,105	37,659	9,899
Non-Hispanic Black[4]	78,911	13,909	17,155	17,569	11,779	12,189	6,310
Hispanic[5]	84,418	12,710	20,622	22,124	13,897	10,823	4,242
37 Weeks and Over							
All races[3]	3,592,785	294,438	564,072	982,820	876,496	738,658	136,301
Non-Hispanic White[4]	1,939,937	132,714	254,332	520,476	517,100	450,094	65,221
Non-Hispanic Black[4]	509,685	60,021	89,036	123,437	102,346	107,052	27,793
Hispanic[5]	839,029	80,651	168,558	243,087	181,327	135,737	29,669
Live Births in Singleton Deliveries							
All Gestational Ages[2]							
All races[3]	3,841,219	337,132	628,460	1,054,118	914,233	753,413	153,863
Non-Hispanic White[4]	2,050,814	149,606	281,726	555,202	536,414	455,570	72,296
Non-Hispanic Black[4]	565,228	71,455	102,855	136,584	109,798	111,914	32,622
Hispanic[5]	900,844	91,794	186,058	260,288	189,720	139,691	33,293
Under 37 Weeks							
All races[3]	300,063	44,660	68,497	79,757	50,531	38,344	18,274
Non-Hispanic White[4]	141,607	17,869	29,314	39,098	26,858	20,799	7,669
Non-Hispanic Black[4]	63,918	11,978	14,752	14,655	9,161	8,204	5,168
Hispanic[5]	70,514	11,476	18,448	18,967	10,699	7,213	3,711
37 Weeks and Over							
All races[3]	3,538,319	292,096	559,682	974,001	863,485	714,882	134,173
Non-Hispanic White[4]	1,908,048	131,570	252,281	515,944	509,438	434,662	64,153
Non-Hispanic Black[4]	500,886	59,384	88,058	121,870	100,620	103,687	27,267
Hispanic[5]	829,737	80,234	167,529	241,215	178,955	132,433	29,371
PERCENT DISTRIBUTION							
All Pluralities							
All Gestational Ages[2]							
All races[3]	100.0	9.1	16.9	28.3	24.8	21.0	X
Non-Hispanic White[4]	100.0	7.5	14.1	27.7	27.0	23.7	X
Non-Hispanic Black[4]	100.0	13.3	19.2	25.4	20.6	21.5	X
Hispanic[5]	100.0	10.5	21.3	29.8	21.9	16.5	X
Under 37 Weeks							
All races[3]	100.0	14.2	22.0	26.7	19.2	17.9	X
Non-Hispanic White[4]	100.0	11.6	19.2	26.9	21.3	21.0	X
Non-Hispanic Black[4]	100.0	19.2	23.6	24.2	16.2	16.8	X
Hispanic[5]	100.0	15.9	25.7	27.6	17.3	13.5	X
37 Weeks and Over							
All races[3]	100.0	8.5	16.3	28.4	25.4	21.4	X
Non-Hispanic White[4]	100.0	7.1	13.6	27.8	27.6	24.0	X
Non-Hispanic Black[4]	100.0	12.5	18.5	25.6	21.2	22.2	X
Hispanic[5]	100.0	10.0	20.8	30.0	22.4	16.8	X
Live Births in Singleton Deliveries							
All Gestational Ages[2]							
All races[3]	100.0	9.1	17.0	28.6	24.8	20.4	X
Non-Hispanic White[4]	100.0	7.6	14.2	28.1	27.1	23.0	X
Non-Hispanic Black[4]	100.0	13.4	19.3	25.6	20.6	21.0	X
Hispanic[5]	100.0	10.6	21.4	30.0	21.9	16.1	X
Under 37 Weeks							
All races[3]	100.0	15.8	24.3	28.3	17.9	13.6	X
Non-Hispanic White[4]	100.0	13.3	21.9	29.2	20.1	15.5	X
Non-Hispanic Black[4]	100.0	20.4	25.1	24.9	15.6	14.0	X
Hispanic[5]	100.0	17.2	27.6	28.4	16.0	10.8	X
37 Weeks and Over							
All races[3]	100.0	8.6	16.4	28.6	25.4	21.0	X
Non-Hispanic White[4]	100.0	7.1	13.7	28.0	27.6	23.6	X
Non-Hispanic Black[4]	100.0	12.5	18.6	25.7	21.2	21.9	X
Hispanic[5]	100.0	10.0	20.9	30.1	22.4	16.5	X

X = Not applicable.
[1]Expressed in completed weeks.
[2]Includes births with period of gestation not stated.
[3]Includes races other than White and Black and origin not stated.
[4]Race and Hispanic origin are reported separately on birth certificates. Persons of Hispanic origin may be of any race. Multiple-race data, when reported, were bridged to single-race categories in order to maintain comparability among all reported areas. Forty-nine states and the District of Columbia reported multiple-race data for 2015 that were bridged to single-race categories for comparability with other states.
[5]Includes all persons of Hispanic origin of any race.

Table 1-41. Births Delivered by Forceps or Vacuum Extraction, Selected Years, 1990–2015

(Percent.)

Year and type of birth	Forceps	Vacuum extraction	Forceps or vacuum
All Births			
1990[1]	5.1	3.9	9.0
1995	3.5	5.9	9.4
2000	2.1	4.9	7.0
1005	0.9	3.9	4.8
2007	0.8	3.5	4.2
2008	0.7	3.2	3.9
2009	0.7	3.0	3.7
2010	0.7	3.0	3.6
2011	0.7	2.9	3.5
2012	0.6	2.8	3.4
2013	0.6	2.7	3.2
2014	0.6	2.6	3.2
2015	0.6	2.6	3.1

[1]Excludes data for Oklahoma, which did not require reporting method of delivery.

Table 1-42. Births, by Method of Delivery and Race and Hispanic Origin of Mother, 1989–2015

(Number, rate.)

		Vaginal				Cesarean							
		Number				Number				Percentage of all live births by cesarean delivery			
Year	All births	Total[1]	Non-Hispanic White[2]	Non-Hispanic Black[2]	Hispanic[3]	Total[1]	Non-Hispanic White[2]	Non-Hispanic Black[2]	Hispanic[3]	Total[1]	Non-Hispanic White[2]	Non-Hispanic Black[2]	Hispanic[3]
1989[4]	3,798,734	2,793,463	1,806,753	440,310	385,462	826,955	556,585	125,290	105,268	22.8	23.6	22.2	21.5
1990[5]	4,110,563	3,111,421	1,972,754	503,720	458,242	914,096	603,467	142,838	122,969	22.7	23.4	22.1	21.2
1991[6]	4,110,907	3,100,891	1,941,726	507,522	472,126	905,077	587,802	142,417	129,752	22.6	23.2	21.9	21.6
1992[6]	4,065,014	3,100,710	1,916,414	502,669	494,338	888,622	566,788	143,153	133,369	22.3	22.8	22.2	21.2
1993	4,000,240	3,098,796	1,902,433	496,333	514,493	861,987	542,013	139,702	136,279	21.8	22.2	22.0	20.9
1994	3,952,767	3,087,576	1,896,609	480,551	525,928	830,517	518,021	134,526	135,569	21.2	21.5	21.9	20.5
1995	3,899,589	3,063,724	1,867,024	457,104	539,731	806,722	496,103	127,171	136,640	20.8	21.0	21.8	20.2
1996	3,891,494	3,061,092	1,851,058	449,544	558,105	797,119	485,530	124,836	139,554	20.7	20.8	21.7	20.0
1997	3,880,894	3,046,621	1,829,213	451,744	563,114	799,033	481,982	126,138	142,907	20.8	20.9	21.8	20.2
1998	3,941,553	3,078,537	1,842,420	457,186	580,143	825,870	495,550	131,999	150,317	21.2	21.2	22.4	20.6
1999	3,959,417	3,063,870	1,810,682	449,580	599,118	862,086	514,051	135,508	161,035	22.0	22.1	23.2	21.2
2000	4,058,814	3,108,188	1,804,550	454,736	633,220	923,991	540,794	146,042	179,583	22.9	23.1	24.3	22.1
2001	4,025,933	3,027,993	1,746,551	435,455	648,821	978,411	567,488	151,908	199,874	24.4	24.5	25.9	23.6
2002	4,021,726	2,958,423	1,687,144	416,516	653,516	1,043,846	598,682	159,297	219,777	26.1	26.2	27.7	25.2
2003	4,089,950	2,949,853	1,671,414	405,671	667,656	1,119,388	637,482	167,506	241,159	27.5	27.6	29.2	26.5
2004	4,112,052	2,903,341	1,617,994	397,877	679,118	1,190,210	667,836	178,461	263,454	29.1	29.2	31.0	28.0
2005	4,138,349	2,873,918	1,579,613	392,064	698,089	1,248,815	690,260	189,287	285,376	30.3	30.4	32.6	29.0
2006	4,265,555	2,929,590	1,580,794	411,097	728,854	1,321,054	718,960	203,723	307,981	31.1	31.3	33.1	29.7
2007	4,316,233	2,933,056	1,565,555	413,088	737,478	1,367,340	735,744	211,615	322,554	31.8	32.0	33.9	30.4
2008	4,247,694	2,864,343	1,527,340	406,379	716,811	1,369,273	732,641	214,416	321,859	32.3	32.4	34.5	31.0
2009	4,130,665	2,764,285	1,481,660	392,715	682,512	1,353,572	723,687	214,810	315,025	32.9	32.8	35.4	31.6
2010	3,999,386	2,680,947	1,454,861	379,617	643,682	1,309,182	702,548	208,520	300,138	32.8	32.6	35.5	31.8
2011	3,953,590	2,651,428	1,447,969	374,978	623,010	1,293,267	693,591	206,009	293,816	32.8	32.4	35.5	32.0
2012	3,952,841	2,650,744	1,441,894	374,035	615,095	1,296,070	688,932	208,562	291,637	32.8	32.3	35.8	32.2
2013	3,932,181	2,642,892	1,446,270	374,054	610,196	1,284,339	680,521	209,015	290,016	32.7	32.0	35.8	32.2
2014	3,988,076	2,699,951	1,473,298	379,055	622,033	1,284,551	674,254	209,361	291,520	32.2	31.4	35.6	31.9
2015	3,978,497	2,703,504	1,466,495	379,730	631,111	1,272,503	662,593	208,976	292,596	32.0	31.1	35.3	31.7

[1]Includes races other than White and Black and origin not stated.
[2]Race and Hispanic origin are reported separately on birth certificates. Persons of Hispanic origin may be of any race. Multiple-race data, when reported, were bridged to single-race categories in order to maintain comparability among all reported areas. Forty-nine states and the District of Columbia reported multiple-race data for 2015 that were bridged to single-race categories for comparability with other states. Multiple-race reporting areas vary for 2003–2015.
[3]Includes all persons of Hispanic origin of any race.
[4]Excludes data for Louisiana, Maryland, Nebraska, Nevada, and Oklahoma, which did not report method of delivery on the birth certificate; data by Hispanic origin also excludes New Hampshire, which did not report Hispanic origin.
[5]Excludes data for New Hampshire and Oklahoma, which did not report data by Hispanic origin. Oklahoma did not report method of delivery.
[6]Excludes data for New Hampshire, which did not report Hispanic origin.

Table 1-43. Cesarean Deliveries, by Race and Hispanic Origin of Mother, by State and Territory of Residence, 2015

(Percent.)

State and territory	Total cesarean delivery rate[1]				Low-risk cesarean delivery rate[2]			
	All races[3]	Non-Hispanic		Hispanic[5]	All races[3]	Non-Hispanic		Hispanic[5]
		White[4]	Black[4]			White[4]	Black[4]	
United States[6]............................	32.0	31.1	35.5	31.7	25.8	24.8	29.7	25.2
Alabama..................................	35.2	35.4	37.3	26.0	28.5	27.8	30.8	23.4
Alaska.....................................	22.9	24.8	32.9	28.1	20.2	21.2	34.3	21.1
Arizona....................................	27.6	28.2	32.4	26.4	22.5	22.7	28.3	21.5
Arkansas..................................	32.3	32.4	32.8	30.3	24.8	24.9	25.0	23.5
California..................................	32.3	31.1	37.3	32.1	25.3	24.6	29.5	25.1
Colorado	25.9	26.4	29.8	23.6	20.6	21.1	25.2	18.0
Connecticut..............................	34.0	33.5	36.6	33.1	28.3	27.6	31.9	26.9
Delaware..................................	31.9	31.8	33.3	29.4	25.3	25.0	27.7	21.9
District of Columbia	31.9	30.2	34.3	26.1	27.1	25.0	29.5	23.9
Florida.....................................	37.3	34.4	38.6	41.2	31.0	27.9	31.8	36.1
Georgia	33.6	33.5	35.5	29.1	27.7	26.9	30.0	23.3
Hawaii	25.9	24.5	28.3	25.6	20.3	16.6	20.4	21.1
Idaho.......................................	24.4	23.9	25.9	26.3	19.5	19.2	*	20.1
Illinois.....................................	31.0	31.0	31.7	29.2	24.2	24.0	25.0	22.8
Indiana....................................	29.6	29.5	32.2	27.3	22.9	22.6	26.0	19.0
Iowa..	29.8	29.7	30.4	29.8	23.8	23.7	26.0	22.8
Kansas.....................................	29.6	30.2	31.7	26.2	23.8	23.8	25.0	21.6
Kentucky	34.4	34.4	36.6	31.3	27.4	27.0	29.9	27.2
Louisiana..................................	37.5	38.5	37.2	32.9	30.8	31.0	30.8	29.2
Maine......................................	29.4	29.4	29.6	29.5	22.9	22.7	25.0	24.1
Maryland..................................	34.9	32.7	39.6	30.7	29.9	26.9	35.2	25.8
Massachusetts..........................	31.4	31.5	35.3	30.4	24.0	24.1	29.2	22.1
Michigan..................................	31.9	31.9	32.1	30.6	26.3	25.8	27.8	26.0
Minnesota................................	26.5	27.0	28.3	25.0	21.6	21.3	25.9	19.5
Mississippi...............................	38.0	38.1	38.7	32.0	31.2	30.7	31.8	31.3
Missouri...................................	30.3	30.0	31.8	28.5	23.6	22.9	27.0	20.6
Montana...................................	29.7	29.0	33.7	30.5	23.7	23.5	*	21.8
Nebraska..................................	31.1	31.6	32.8	28.2	24.4	24.7	29.1	21.7
Nevada....................................	34.6	33.9	41.3	32.0	29.7	28.0	34.0	29.0
New Hampshire.........................	30.8	30.6	32.1	33.9	24.6	24.7	*	24.5
New Jersey	36.8	35.5	39.2	36.8	30.9	30.1	32.3	30.5
New Mexico..............................	24.3	24.7	25.6	24.6	18.0	17.6	20.8	18.2
New York..................................	33.8	32.0	38.3	34.6	28.5	27.1	32.7	28.5
North Carolina...........................	29.3	29.7	32.2	23.3	22.7	22.2	26.2	18.6
North Dakota.............................	27.5	26.7	27.9	30.0	20.6	19.5	31.8	18.7
Ohio..	30.4	30.2	31.9	27.5	24.2	23.7	27.3	20.7
Oklahoma.................................	32.4	32.6	35.8	30.1	24.4	24.2	29.4	22.9
Oregon	27.1	26.9	30.6	26.4	21.7	21.5	26.5	20.7
Pennsylvania.............................	30.1	29.9	30.4	29.7	24.7	24.5	25.9	23.0
Rhode Island.............................	30.6	31.6	30.1	29.3	23.5	25.1	22.6	19.4
South Carolina	33.7	33.0	36.9	28.1	26.9	25.6	30.6	23.4
South Dakota	25.7	25.0	25.3	25.9	18.5	18.4	24.1	21.6
Tennessee................................	33.2	33.0	35.2	29.2	27.6	27.1	30.4	24.2
Texas......................................	34.4	34.3	38.4	33.2	27.0	27.5	32.3	24.7
Utah..	22.8	22.1	27.2	24.0	18.0	17.2	23.9	18.8
Vermont...................................	25.5	24.9	27.5	37.4	20.2	19.7	*	*
Virginia....................................	32.9	31.6	36.3	30.1	25.1	23.4	28.6	22.8
Washington...............................	27.5	26.4	34.4	26.3	22.8	21.6	30.2	21.1
West Virginia.............................	34.9	34.9	36.0	31.1	27.2	27.1	26.8	32.0
Wisconsin.................................	26.2	26.4	26.7	25.6	21.3	21.0	23.1	20.1
Wyoming	27.3	26.4	29.9	31.8	17.8	17.5	*	18.0
Puerto Rico...............................	46.7	45.9	49.3	46.8	41.4	39.3	*	41.5
Virgin Islands............................	31.5	26.7	31.8	31.6	25.5	*	25.0	*
Guam	26.4	21.3	*	*	11.6	*	*	*
American Samoa	NA	NA	NA	NA	NA	NA	NA	NA
Northern Marianas......................	28.8	*	*	*	27.9	*	*	*

NA = Not available.
* = Figure does not meet standards of reliability or precision; based on fewer than 20 births in the numerator.
[1]Percent of all live births by cesarean delivery.
[2]Low-risk cesarean is defined as singleton, term (37 or more weeks of gestation), vertex (not breech) cesarean deliveries to women having a first birth per 100 women delivering singleton, term, vertex first births.
[3]Includes races other than White and Black and origin not stated.
[4]Race and Hispanic origin are reported separately on birth certificates. Persons of Hispanic origin may be of any race. Multiple-race data, when reported, were bridged to single-race categories in order to maintain comparability among all reported areas. Forty-nine states and the District of Columbia reported multiple-race data for 2015 that were bridged to single-race categories for comparability with other states.
[5]Includes all persons of Hispanic origin of any race.
[6]Excludes data for the territories.

Table 1-44. Births, by Birthweight, Gestational Age, and Race and Hispanic Origin of Mother, 2015

(Number, percent.)

Birthweight,[1] race, and Hispanic origin of mother	All births	Period of gestation[2] Preterm Total under 37 weeks	Under 28 weeks	28 to 31 weeks	32 to 33 weeks	34 to 36 weeks	Term Total, 37 to 41 weeks	37 to 38 weeks	39 weeks	40 to 41 weeks	Postterm 42 weeks and over	Not stated
ALL RACES[3]												
Total............................	3,978,497	382,786	26,996	36,149	46,515	273,126	3,577,072	993,599	2,324,474	258,999	15,713	2,926
Less than 500 grams	5,863	5,808	5,721	80	3	4	3	3	–	–	–	52
500 to 999 grams	20,689	20,559	16,359	3,870	244	86	91	30	57	4	2	37
1,000 to 1,499 grams	29,040	28,348	3,594	17,764	4,918	2,072	663	310	331	22	4	25
1,500 to 1,999 grams	62,862	56,994	130	11,758	21,680	23,426	5,792	4,744	980	68	17	59
2,000 to 2,499 grams	202,415	109,747	97	1,523	15,946	92,181	92,402	70,369	21,273	760	94	172
2,500 to 2,999 grams	729,673	106,245	100	423	2,651	103,071	622,022	310,156	297,329	14,537	873	533
3,000 to 3,499 grams	1,544,024	41,871	–	387	701	40,783	1,496,975	409,077	1,000,978	86,920	4,389	789
3,500 to 3,999 grams	1,062,456	9,249	–	185	225	8,839	1,046,430	162,412	775,079	108,939	6,347	430
4,000 to 4,499 grams	274,404	1,896	–	–	37	1,859	269,270	30,096	198,589	40,585	3,116	122
4,500 to 4,999 grams	38,796	474	–	–	6	468	37,559	4,947	26,130	6,482	735	28
5,000 grams or more	4,654	118	–	–	4	114	4,419	1,080	2,796	543	114	3
Not stated	3,621	1,477	995	159	100	223	1,446	375	932	139	22	676
Percent												
Very low birthweight[4]..............	14	14.3	98.7	60.3	11.1	0.8	0.0	0.0	0.0	0.0	0.0	5.1
Low birthweight[5].....................	81	58.1	99.6	97.2	92.2	43.2	2.8	7.6	1.0	0.3	0.7	15.3
NON-HISPANIC WHITE												
Total............................	2,130,279	189,146	10,162	16,905	22,750	139,329	1,929,852	494,807	1,278,326	156,719	10,085	1,196
Less than 500 grams	2,009	1,990	1,948	37	1	4	1	1	–	–	–	18
500 to 999 grams	8,051	7,980	6,138	1,670	124	48	57	16	39	2	1	13
1,000 to 1,499 grams	13,058	12,735	1,582	8,029	2,154	970	308	137	156	15	2	13
1,500 to 1,999 grams	29,702	27,006	46	5,886	10,323	10,751	2,658	2,184	445	29	7	31
2,000 to 2,499 grams	94,659	53,830	46	735	8,305	44,744	40,702	31,264	9,089	349	48	79
2,500 to 2,999 grams	336,316	55,524	48	189	1,332	53,955	280,124	140,514	132,674	6,936	431	237
3,000 to 3,499 grams	801,773	23,086	–	173	313	22,600	775,855	207,776	520,195	47,884	2,484	348
3,500 to 3,999 grams	635,412	5,021	–	93	108	4,820	626,012	92,125	465,605	68,282	4,175	204
4,000 to 4,499 grams	179,165	1,003	–	–	21	982	175,833	17,449	130,391	27,993	2,265	64
4,500 to 4,999 grams	25,572	249	–	–	2	247	24,735	2,579	17,439	4,717	571	17
5,000 grams or more	2,734	67	–	–	2	65	2,581	512	1,665	404	85	1
Not stated	1,828	655	354	93	65	143	986	250	628	108	16	171
Percent												
Very low birthweight[4]..............	11	12.0	98.6	57.9	10.0	0.7	0.0	0.0	0.0	0.0	0.0	4.3
Low birthweight[5].....................	69	54.9	99.5	97.3	92.2	40.6	2.3	6.8	0.8	0.3	0.6	15.0
NON-HISPANIC BLACK												
Total............................	589,047	78,911	9,118	9,060	10,260	50,473	507,737	162,705	314,185	30,847	1,948	451
Less than 500 grams	2,238	2,223	2,197	26	–	–	2	2	–	–	–	13
500 to 999 grams	6,886	6,862	5,580	1,216	51	15	15	7	6	2	1	8
1,000 to 1,499 grams	7,889	7,750	909	4,863	1,466	512	133	66	64	3	2	4
1,500 to 1,999 grams	15,357	13,839	41	2,426	5,298	6,074	1,496	1,230	242	24	5	17
2,000 to 2,499 grams	46,144	22,999	25	286	2,807	19,881	23,089	17,592	5,341	156	19	37
2,500 to 2,999 grams	146,538	17,764	21	114	457	17,172	128,502	62,986	62,609	2,907	163	109
3,000 to 3,499 grams	226,291	5,551	–	69	116	5,366	219,908	59,274	147,967	12,667	701	131
3,500 to 3,999 grams	110,694	1,167	–	29	36	1,102	108,758	17,610	79,697	11,451	728	41
4,000 to 4,499 grams	22,668	234	–	–	3	231	22,157	3,138	15,867	3,152	270	7
4,500 to 4,999 grams	3,136	61	–	–	–	61	3,024	601	1,985	438	49	2
5,000 grams or more..............	478	11	–	–	1	10	458	142	279	37	8	1
Not stated	728	450	345	31	25	49	195	57	128	10	2	81
Percent												
Very low birthweight[4]..............	2.9	21.5	99.0	67.6	14.8	1.0	0.0	0.0	0.0	0.0	0.2	6.8
Low birthweight[5].....................	13.3	68.4	99.8	97.7	94.0	52.5	4.9	11.6	1.8	0.6	1.4	21.4
HISPANIC[6]												
Total............................	924,048	84,418	5,732	7,560	9,974	61,152	836,310	245,306	539,124	51,880	2,719	601
Less than 500 grams	1,175	1,162	1,149	12	1	–	–	–	–	–	–	13
500 to 999 grams	4,263	4,239	3,474	701	44	20	13	6	7	–	–	11
1,000 to 1,499 grams	5,923	5,750	849	3,583	908	410	170	84	83	3	–	3
1,500 to 1,999 grams	12,731	11,620	33	2,619	4,431	4,537	1,102	882	211	9	4	5
2,000 to 2,499 grams	42,531	23,537	19	387	3,628	19,503	18,948	14,134	4,640	174	24	22
2,500 to 2,999 grams	171,413	24,533	22	91	672	23,748	146,541	74,169	69,267	3,105	214	125

– = Quantity zero.
[0].0 = Quantity more than zero but less than 0.05.
[1]Equivalents of the gram weights in pounds and ounces.
[2]Expressed in completed weeks based on the obstetric estimate of gestation.
[4]Birthweight of less than 1,500 grams (3 lb 4 oz).
[5]Birthweight of less than 2,500 grams (5 lb 8 oz).
[6]Includes all persons of Hispanic origin of any race.

Table 1-44. Births, by Birthweight, Gestational Age, and Race and Hispanic Origin of Mother, 2015—*Continued*

(Number, percent.)

Birthweight,[1] race, and Hispanic origin of mother	All births	Period of gestation[2]										Not stated
		Preterm					Term				Postterm	
		Total under 37 weeks	Under 28 weeks	28 to 31 weeks	32 to 33 weeks	34 to 36 weeks	Total, 37 to 41 weeks	37 to 38 weeks	39 weeks	40 to 41 weeks	42 weeks and over	
3,000 to 3,499 grams	378,193	10,245	–	105	206	9,934	366,836	105,646	242,391	18,799	902	210
3,500 to 3,999 grams	242,028	2,413	–	46	63	2,304	238,439	41,057	175,695	21,687	1,062	114
4,000 to 4,499 grams	56,317	522	–	–	10	512	55,344	7,526	40,787	7,031	416	35
4,500 to 4,999 grams	7,933	136	–	–	4	132	7,708	1,423	5,295	990	82	7
5,000 grams or more..............	1,114	36	–	–	1	35	1,062	338	652	72	15	1
Not stated	427	225	186	16	6	17	147	41	96	10	–	55
Percent												
Very low birthweight[4]	1.2	13.2	98.7	56.9	9.6	0.7	0.0	0.0	0.0	0.0	0.0	4.9
Low birthweight[5]	7.2	55.0	99.6	96.8	90.4	40.0	2.4	6.2	0.9	0.4	1.0	9.9

– = Quantity zero.
0.0 = Quantity more than zero but less than 0.05.
[1]Equivalents of the gram weights in pounds and ounces.
[2]Expressed in completed weeks based on the obstetric estimate of gestation.
[4]Birthweight of less than 1,500 grams (3 lb 4 oz).
[5]Birthweight of less than 2,500 grams (5 lb 8 oz).

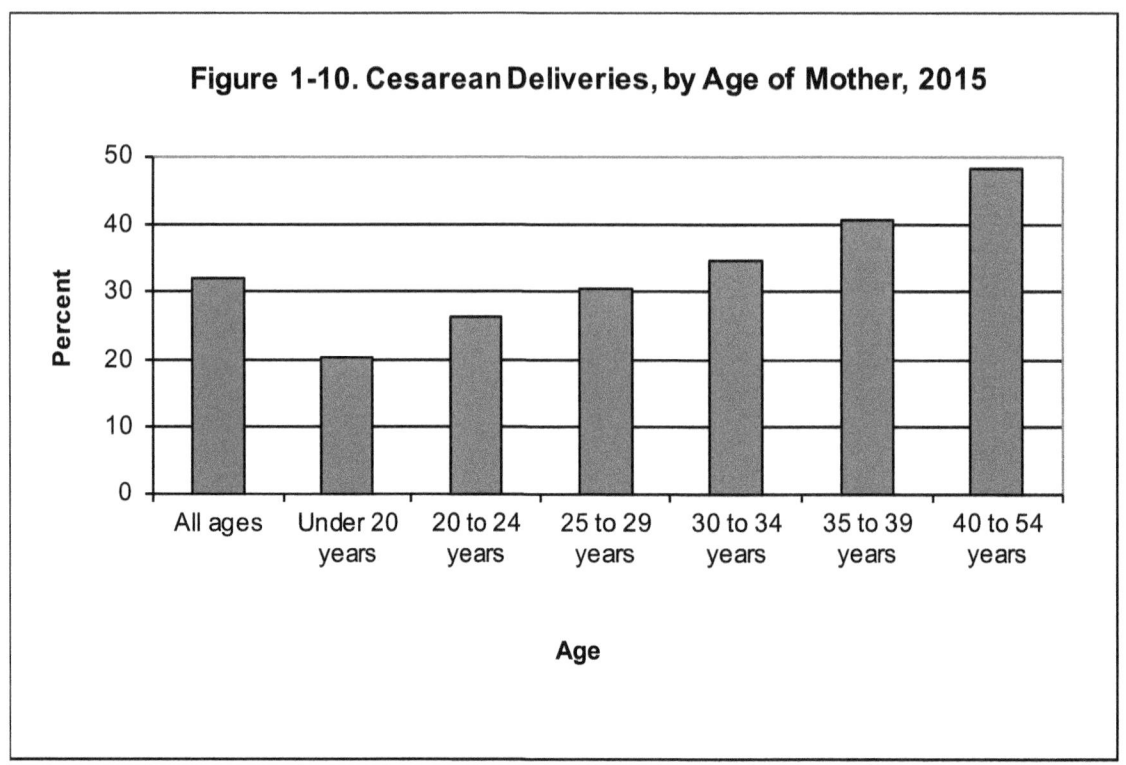

Figure 1-10. Cesarean Deliveries, by Age of Mother, 2015

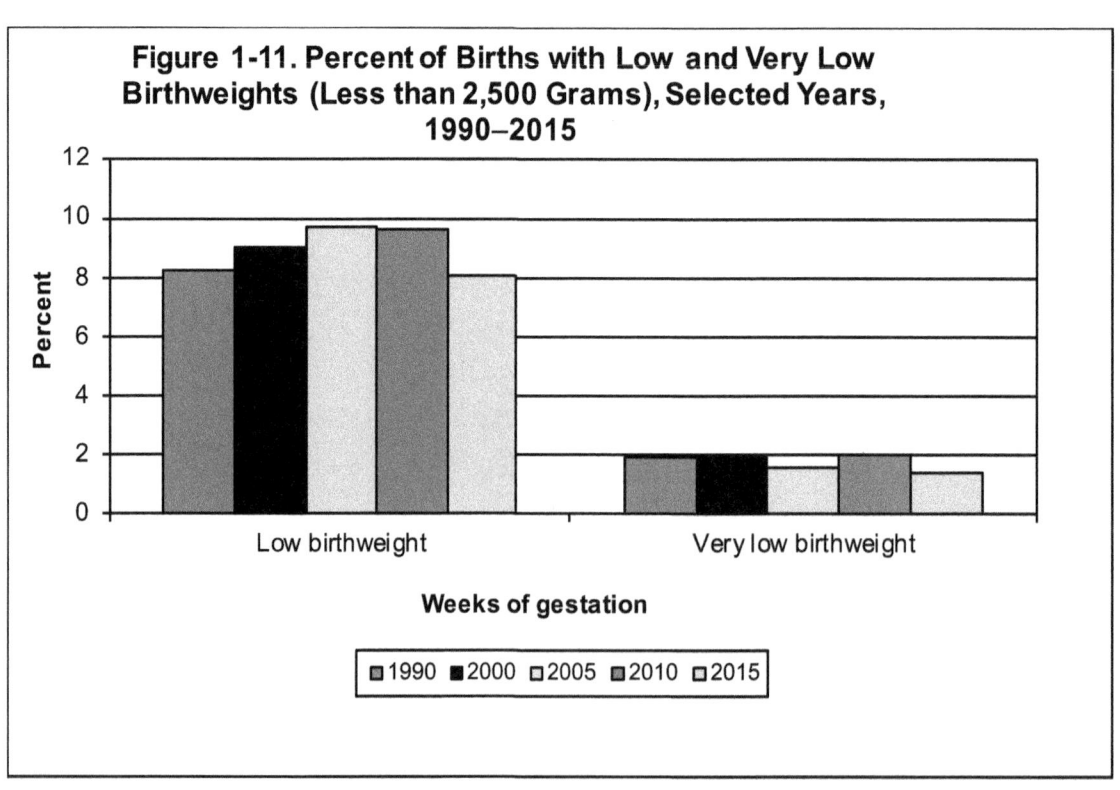

Figure 1-11. Percent of Births with Low and Very Low Birthweights (Less than 2,500 Grams), Selected Years, 1990–2015

Table 1-45. Very Preterm and Preterm Births and Very Low Birthweight and Low Birthweight Births, by Race and Hispanic Origin of Mother, 1989–2015

(Percent.)

Year	Very preterm[1]				Preterm[2]			
	All races[3]	Non-Hispanic		Hispanic[5]	All races[3]	Non-Hispanic		Hispanic[5]
		White[4]	Black[4]			White[4]	Black[4]	
2007	1.71	1.39	3.48	1.46	10.44	9.90	14.71	9.35
2008	1.67	1.37	3.26	1.43	10.36	9.81	14.38	9.38
2009	1.65	1.35	3.28	1.41	10.07	9.50	14.05	9.12
2010	1.65	1.36	3.20	1.41	9.98	9.41	13.81	9.09
2011	1.64	1.33	3.20	1.42	9.81	9.21	13.54	9.02
2012	1.63	1.32	3.19	1.45	9.76	9.13	13.48	9.09
2013	1.62	1.31	3.16	1.44	9.62	8.94	13.25	9.08
2014	1.60	1.29	3.08	1.45	9.57	8.91	13.21	9.03
2015	1.59	1.27	3.09	1.44	9.63	8.88	13.41	9.14

Year	Very low birthweight[6]				Low birthweight[7]			
	All races[3]	Non-Hispanic		Hispanic[5]	All races[3]	Non-Hispanic		Hispanic[5]
		White[4]	Black[4]			White[4]	Black[4]	
1989[8]	1.28	0.93	2.97	1.05	7.05	5.62	13.61	6.18
1990[9]	1.27	0.93	2.93	1.03	6.97	5.61	13.32	6.06
1991[10]	1.29	0.94	2.97	1.02	7.12	5.72	13.62	6.15
1992[10]	1.29	0.94	2.97	1.04	7.08	5.73	13.40	6.10
1993	1.33	1.00	2.99	1.06	7.22	5.92	13.43	6.24
1994	1.33	1.01	2.99	1.08	7.28	6.06	13.34	6.25
1995	1.35	1.04	2.98	1.11	7.32	6.20	13.21	6.29
1996	1.37	1.08	3.02	1.12	7.39	6.36	13.12	6.28
1997	1.42	1.12	3.05	1.13	7.51	6.47	13.11	6.42
1998	1.45	1.15	3.11	1.15	7.57	6.55	13.17	6.44
1999	1.45	1.15	3.18	1.14	7.62	6.64	13.23	6.38
2000	1.43	1.14	3.10	1.14	7.57	6.60	13.13	6.41
2001	1.44	1.17	3.08	1.14	7.68	6.76	13.07	6.47
2002	1.46	1.17	3.15	1.17	7.82	6.91	13.39	6.55
2003	1.45	1.18	3.12	1.16	7.93	7.04	13.55	6.69
2004	1.48	1.20	3.15	1.20	8.08	7.20	13.74	6.79
2005	1.49	1.21	3.27	1.20	8.19	7.29	14.02	6.88
2006	1.49	1.20	3.15	1.19	8.26	7.32	13.97	6.99
2007	1.49	1.19	3.20	1.21	8.22	7.28	13.90	6.93
2008	1.46	1.18	3.01	1.20	8.18	7.22	13.71	6.96
2009	1.45	1.16	3.06	1.19	8.16	7.19	13.61	6.94
2010	1.45	1.16	2.98	1.20	8.15	7.14	13.53	6.97
2011	1.44	1.14	2.99	1.20	8.10	7.09	13.33	7.02
2012	1.42	1.13	2.94	1.22	7.99	6.97	13.18	6.97
2013	1.41	1.11	2.90	1.21	8.02	6.98	13.08	7.09
2014	1.40	1.10	2.86	1.23	8.00	6.96	13.15	7.05
2015	1.40	1.09	2.89	1.23	8.07	6.93	13.35	7.21

[1]Births of less than 32 completed weeks of gestation.
[2]Births of less than 37 completed weeks of gestation.
[3]Includes races other than White and Black and origin not stated.
[4]Race and Hispanic origin are reported separately on birth certificates. Persons of Hispanic origin may be of any race. Multiple-race data, when reported, were bridged to single-race categories in order to maintain comparability among all reported areas. Forty-nine states and the District of Columbia reported multiple-race data for 2015 that were bridged to single-race categories for comparability with other states. Multiple-race reporting areas vary for 2003–2015.
[5]Includes all persons of Hispanic origin of any race.
[6]Less than 1,500 grams (3 lb. 4 oz.).
[7]Less than 2,500 grams (5 lb. 8 oz.).
[8]Data by Hispanic origin exclude New Hampshire, Oklahoma, and Louisiana, which did not report Hispanic origin.
[9]Data by Hispanic origin exclude New Hampshire and Oklahoma, which did not report Hispanic origin.
[10]Data by Hispanic origin exclude New Hampshire, which did not report Hispanic origin.

Table 1-46. Birthweight Distribution in 500-Gram Intervals, Selected Years, 1990–2014

(Percent.)

Weight	All births					Percent change		
	1990	2006	2008	2009	2014	1990–2009	1990–2014	2009–2014
Less than 1,000 grams	0.63	0.72	0.70	0.70	0.67	11.1	6.1	-4.5
1,000–1,499 grams.................................	0.65	0.76	0.75	0.75	0.73	15.4	13.0	-2.1
1,500–1,999 grams.................................	1.33	1.63	1.58	1.59	1.55	19.5	16.9	-2.2
2,000–2,499 grams.................................	4.37	5.15	5.14	5.12	5.04	17.2	15.3	-1.6
2,500–2,999 grams.................................	16.03	18.44	18.57	18.59	18.25	16.0	13.9	-1.8
3,000–3,499 grams.................................	36.71	38.87	39.20	39.22	38.77	6.8	5.6	-1.1
3,500–3,999 grams.................................	29.40	26.61	26.41	26.43	26.86	-10.1	-8.7	1.6
4,000–4,499 grams.................................	9.10	6.75	6.60	6.57	6.94	-27.8	-23.8	5.6
4,500–4,999 grams.................................	1.59	0.96	0.92	0.92	0.99	-42.1	-37.9	7.3
5,000 grams or more................................	0.19	0.11	0.10	0.10	0.12	-47.4	-37.4	19.0

Note: Totals do not sum to 100 due to rounding.

Table 1-47. Preterm and Low Birthweight Births, by Age and Race and Hispanic Origin of Mother, 2015

(Percent, number.)

Age, race, and Hispanic origin of mother	Preterm[1]							Low birthweight[2]						
	Percent			Number				Percent			Number			
	Total	Early[3]	Late[4]	Total	Early[3]	Late[4]	Unknown	Total	Very[5]	Moderately[6]	Total	Very[5]	Moderately[6]	Unknown
All Races[7]														
All ages	9.63	2.76	6.87	382,786	109,660	273,126	2,926	8.07	1.40	6.67	320,869	55,592	265,277	3,621
Under 15 years........................	13.78	5.75	8.04	343	143	200	11	12.57	3.32	9.25	314	83	231	2
15 to 19 years........................	9.91	3.05	6.86	22,735	6,989	15,746	243	9.48	1.64	7.84	21,756	3,765	17,991	163
15 years..........................	10.58	3.32	7.27	801	251	550	20	9.84	2.03	7.81	746	154	592	8
16 years..........................	10.53	3.45	7.08	1,938	635	1,303	33	10.20	1.89	8.30	1,878	349	1,529	10
17 years..........................	9.94	3.06	6.89	3,493	1,074	2,419	37	9.58	1.66	7.92	3,368	583	2,785	19
18 years..........................	9.95	3.12	6.82	6,310	1,982	4,328	60	9.62	1.74	7.88	6,103	1,104	4,999	47
19 years..........................	9.71	2.90	6.81	10,193	3,047	7,146	93	9.21	1.50	7.71	9,661	1,575	8,086	79
20 to 24 years........................	9.28	2.68	6.59	78,833	22,812	56,021	710	8.38	1.42	6.96	71,177	12,039	59,138	711
25 to 29 years........................	8.92	2.51	6.41	102,751	28,932	73,819	901	7.45	1.28	6.17	85,776	14,754	71,022	1,090
30 to 34 years........................	9.35	2.63	6.72	102,345	28,785	73,560	637	7.49	1.30	6.19	81,925	14,184	67,741	1,017
35 to 39 years........................	11.07	3.18	7.89	58,419	16,801	41,618	328	8.74	1.57	7.17	46,092	8,273	37,819	507
40 to 44 years........................	13.68	4.05	9.63	15,288	4,530	10,758	91	10.80	1.97	8.83	12,068	2,203	9,865	122
45 to 54 years........................	23.23	7.49	15.74	2,072	668	1,404	5	19.75	3.26	16.49	1,761	291	1,470	9
Non-Hispanic White[8]														
All ages	8.88	2.34	6.54	189,146	49,817	139,329	1,196	6.93	1.09	5.84	147,479	23,118	124,361	1,828
Under 15 years........................	13.25	4.99	8.26	77	29	48	1	10.15	3.61	6.54	59	21	38	1
15 to 19 years........................	9.56	2.85	6.72	8,677	2,583	6,094	83	8.45	1.42	7.02	7,668	1,292	6,376	59
15 years..........................	10.63	3.48	7.15	226	74	152	8	7.97	2.48	5.48	170	53	117	1
16 years..........................	10.22	3.30	6.91	597	193	404	11	9.06	1.62	7.43	530	95	435	3
17 years..........................	9.79	3.06	6.72	1,214	380	834	12	8.72	1.60	7.12	1,082	198	884	7
18 years..........................	9.86	2.96	6.90	2,504	752	1,752	18	8.82	1.50	7.32	2,241	381	1,860	14
19 years..........................	9.20	2.63	6.56	4,136	1,184	2,952	34	8.11	1.26	6.85	3,645	565	3,080	34
20 to 24 years........................	8.66	2.28	6.38	34,551	9,094	25,457	281	7.17	1.11	6.06	28,612	4,437	24,175	301
25 to 29 years........................	8.28	2.14	6.14	53,155	13,723	39,432	361	6.44	1.00	5.44	41,317	6,387	34,930	575
30 to 34 years........................	8.58	2.24	6.35	55,480	14,453	41,027	289	6.48	1.01	5.47	41,862	6,504	35,538	571
35 to 39 years........................	10.03	2.65	7.39	29,173	7,694	21,479	147	7.51	1.20	6.31	21,833	3,492	18,341	262
40 to 44 years........................	12.75	3.50	9.25	7,012	1,924	5,088	32	9.62	1.55	8.07	5,290	855	4,435	54
45 to 54 years........................	21.93	6.81	15.12	1,021	317	704	2	18.01	2.79	15.22	838	130	708	5
Non-Hispanic Black[8]														
All ages	13.41	4.83	8.58	78,911	28,438	50,473	451	13.35	2.89	10.45	78,514	17,013	61,501	728
Under 15 years........................	15.26	6.44	8.82	128	54	74	6	16.59	3.79	12.80	140	32	108	1
15 to 19 years........................	12.05	4.30	7.75	6,020	2,147	3,873	71	13.63	2.58	11.05	6,813	1,289	5,524	64
15 years..........................	12.46	4.20	8.26	258	87	171	8	12.92	2.51	10.41	268	52	216	5
16 years..........................	12.22	4.71	7.51	547	211	336	9	14.08	2.77	11.32	631	124	507	6
17 years..........................	12.13	3.82	8.30	945	298	647	10	13.60	2.13	11.47	1,060	166	894	9
18 years..........................	11.77	4.50	7.27	1,593	609	984	16	13.71	2.73	10.99	1,856	369	1,487	19
19 years..........................	12.12	4.26	7.85	2,677	942	1,735	28	13.57	2.62	10.95	2,998	578	2,420	25
20 to 24 years........................	12.38	4.36	8.02	21,722	7,653	14,069	135	13.20	2.63	10.57	23,144	4,614	18,530	217
25 to 29 years........................	12.91	4.66	8.25	21,396	7,726	13,670	111	12.77	2.80	9.97	21,162	4,645	16,517	193
30 to 34 years........................	14.08	5.11	8.97	16,880	6,122	10,758	78	13.09	3.08	10.01	15,683	3,690	11,993	151
35 to 39 years........................	16.17	6.01	10.16	9,835	3,653	6,182	32	14.59	3.53	11.06	8,870	2,145	6,725	83
40 to 44 years........................	17.99	6.64	11.35	2,622	968	1,654	18	16.47	3.70	12.78	2,401	539	1,862	17
45 to 54 years........................	24.84	9.27	15.56	308	115	193	–	24.31	4.77	19.55	301	59	242	2
Hispanic[9]														
All ages	9.14	2.52	6.62	84,418	23,266	61,152	601	7.21	1.23	5.98	66,623	11,361	55,262	427
Under 15 years........................	12.82	5.39	7.43	126	53	73	3	10.65	1.48	7.33	105	24	81	–
15 to 19 years........................	8.89	2.47	6.42	7,137	1,986	5,151	74	8.07	1.29	6.78	6,484	1,037	5,447	25
15 years..........................	9.17	2.64	6.53	285	82	203	3	8.81	1.48	7.33	274	46	228	1
16 years..........................	9.88	2.87	7.01	733	213	520	13	9.04	1.57	7.47	672	117	555	–
17 years..........................	8.71	2.55	6.16	1,187	347	840	11	8.06	1.39	6.67	1,099	189	910	2
18 years..........................	8.91	2.42	6.50	1,981	537	1,444	25	8.05	1.39	6.66	1,790	309	1,481	11
19 years..........................	8.7	2.38	6.32	2,951	807	2,144	22	7.81	1.11	6.70	2,649	376	2,273	11
20 to 24 years........................	8.07	2.17	5.91	19,062	5,118	13,944	165	6.86	1.06	5.79	16,191	2,505	13,686	94
25 to 29 years........................	8.35	2.22	6.13	21,370	5,693	15,677	165	6.54	1.10	5.44	16,740	2,807	13,933	118
30 to 34 years........................	9.49	2.65	6.84	19,887	5,551	14,336	121	7.02	1.27	5.75	14,719	2,666	12,053	106
35 to 39 years........................	11.41	3.28	8.13	12,775	3,670	9,105	60	8.42	1.55	6.87	9,427	1,736	7,691	66
40 to 44 years........................	13.65	4.00	9.65	3,699	1,083	2,616	13	9.85	1.97	7.88	2,670	534	2,136	18
45 to 54 years........................	23.83	7.37	16.46	362	112	250	–	18.89	3.42	15.47	287	52	235	–

- = Quantity zero.
[1]Less than 37 completed weeks of gestation based on the obstetric estimate.
[2]Less than 2,500 grams.
[3]Less than 34 completed weeks of gestatio based on the obstetric estimate.
[4]Includes 34 to 36 completed weeks of gestation based on the obstetric estimate.
[5]Less than 1,500 grams.
[6]Includes 1,500–2,499 grams.
[7]Includes races other than White and Black and origin not stated.
[8]Race and Hispanic origin are reported separately on birth certificates. Persons of Hispanic origin may be of any race. Race categories are consistent with 1977 Office of Management and Budget standards. Forty-nine states and the District of Columbia reported multiple-race data for 2015 that were bridged to single-race categories for comparability with other states.
[9]Includes all persons of Hispanic origin of any race.

Table 1-48. Births of Very Low Birthweight, by Race and Hispanic Origin of Mother and by State and Territory of Residence, 2015

(Number, percent.)

State and territory	Number				Percent			
	All races[1]	Non-Hispanic White[2]	Non-Hispanic Black[2]	Hispanic[3]	All races[1]	Non-Hispanic White[2]	Non-Hispanic Black[2]	Hispanic[3]
United States[4]	55,592	23,118	17,013	11,361	1.4	1.1	2.9	1.2
Alabama	1,176	478	640	46	2.0	1.3	3.5	1.1
Alaska	105	45	6	9	0.9	0.7	*	*
Arizona	961	363	100	395	1.1	1.0	2.2	1.1
Arkansas	609	327	232	35	1.6	1.3	3.1	0.9
California	5,527	1,276	612	2,655	1.1	0.9	2.3	1.1
Colorado	761	406	74	214	1.1	1.0	2.1	1.2
Connecticut	557	219	142	160	1.6	1.1	3.2	1.9
Delaware	208	86	92	24	1.9	1.4	3.1	1.6
District of Columbia	206	27	162	14	2.2	0.9	3.4	*
Florida	3,433	1,111	1,422	778	1.5	1.1	2.9	1.2
Georgia	2,354	685	1,371	213	1.8	1.1	3.0	1.2
Hawaii	245	37	15	41	1.3	0.8	*	1.5
Idaho	238	187	5	34	1.0	1.0	*	0.9
Illinois	2,319	917	826	448	1.5	1.1	3.0	1.3
Indiana	1,209	808	273	96	1.4	1.3	2.6	1.3
Iowa	486	368	49	55	1.2	1.1	2.0	1.6
Kansas	476	306	85	67	1.2	1.1	2.9	1.1
Kentucky	784	612	115	41	1.4	1.3	2.2	1.4
Louisiana	1,261	426	750	58	2.0	1.3	3.1	1.2
Maine	154	124	17	4	1.2	1.1	*	*
Maryland	1,202	333	650	155	1.6	1.0	2.8	1.3
Massachusetts	851	389	159	211	1.2	0.9	2.3	1.6
Michigan	1,707	866	678	92	1.5	1.1	3.1	1.2
Minnesota	799	503	163	44	1.1	1.0	2.0	0.9
Mississippi	817	230	559	16	2.1	1.2	3.4	*
Missouri	1,114	676	348	56	1.5	1.2	3.1	1.4
Montana	104	76	4	7	0.8	0.7	*	*
Nebraska	293	177	56	46	1.1	0.9	3.0	1.1
Nevada	478	149	133	141	1.3	1.0	3.0	1.1
New Hampshire	114	91	9	8	0.9	0.8	*	*
New Jersey	1,468	466	436	394	1.4	1.0	2.9	1.4
New Mexico	302	73	9	177	1.2	1.0	*	1.2
New York	3,188	1,139	968	767	1.3	1.0	2.7	1.4
North Carolina	2,106	795	992	232	1.7	1.2	3.4	1.3
North Dakota	138	100	6	7	1.2	1.1	*	*
Ohio	2,032	1,189	683	90	1.5	1.1	2.9	1.3
Oklahoma	726	391	132	93	1.4	1.2	2.6	1.3
Oregon	453	292	29	90	1.0	0.9	2.2	1.1
Pennsylvania	1,997	1,065	556	228	1.4	1.1	2.8	1.5
Rhode Island	155	74	29	44	1.4	1.1	3.0	1.7
South Carolina	1,029	396	557	50	1.8	1.2	3.1	1.0
South Dakota	127	83	7	2	1.0	0.9	*	*
Tennessee	1,318	710	501	75	1.6	1.3	3.0	1.0
Texas	5,683	1,612	1,401	2,414	1.4	1.1	2.8	1.3
Utah	515	350	14	104	1.0	0.9	*	1.3
Vermont	55	44	2	6	0.9	0.8	*	*
Virginia	1,545	682	597	169	1.5	1.2	2.7	1.2
Washington	973	524	108	169	1.1	0.9	2.3	1.1
West Virginia	284	260	15	1	1.4	1.4	*	*
Wisconsin	868	512	223	75	1.3	1.0	3.1	1.1
Wyoming	82	63	1	11	1.1	1.0	*	*
Puerto Rico	448	22	3	422	1.4	1.5	*	1.4
Virgin Islands	18	4	10	3	*	*	*	*
Guam	40	1	-	-	1.2	*	*	*
American Samoa	5	NA	NA	NA	*	NA	NA	NA
Northern Marianas	7	—	—	—	*	*	*	*

NA = Not available.
– = Quantity zero.
* = Figure does not meet standards of reliability or precision; based on fewer than 20 births in the numerator.
[1]Includes races other than White and Black and origin not stated.
[2]Race and Hispanic origin are reported separately on birth certificates. Persons of Hispanic origin may be of any race. Multiple-race data, when reported, were bridged to single-race categories in order to maintain comparability among all reported areas. Forty-nine states and the District of Columbia reported multiple-race data for 2015 that were bridged to single-race categories for comparability with other states.
[3]Includes all persons of Hispanic origin of any race.
[4]Excludes data for the territories.

Table 1-49. Preterm Births (Less Than 37 Completed Weeks of Gestation), by Race and Hispanic Origin of Mother, by State and Territory of Residence, 2015

(Number, percent.)

State and territory	Number All races[1]	Number Non-Hispanic White[2]	Number Non-Hispanic Black[2]	Number Hispanic[3]	Percent All races[1]	Percent Non-Hispanic White[2]	Percent Non-Hispanic Black[2]	Percent Hispanic[3]
United States[4]	382,786	189,146	78,911	84,418	9.63	8.88	13.41	9.14
Alabama	6,999	3,666	2,818	395	11.74	10.23	15.44	9.20
Alaska	1,008	505	40	59	8.95	7.73	9.48	7.28
Arizona	7,724	3,132	573	3,208	9.06	8.48	12.51	9.11
Arkansas	4,207	2,554	1,147	355	10.82	9.94	15.14	8.86
California	41,600	10,835	3,180	20,075	8.47	7.66	11.77	8.58
Colorado	5,770	3,348	389	1,613	8.67	8.19	11.27	8.89
Connecticut	3,340	1,674	555	869	9.35	8.21	12.51	10.50
Delaware	1,101	565	348	140	9.87	9.49	11.69	9.14
District of Columbia	984	227	605	108	10.28	7.63	12.61	8.14
Florida	22,407	9,175	6,696	5,764	10.00	8.95	13.51	9.00
Georgia	14,133	5,708	6,189	1,579	10.76	9.46	13.62	8.86
Hawaii	1,861	363	75	297	10.11	7.56	12.95	10.71
Idaho	1,859	1,436	25	319	8.15	7.94	10.42	8.75
Illinois	16,048	7,880	3,822	3,243	10.16	9.23	14.08	9.57
Indiana	8,061	5,828	1,326	707	9.59	9.18	12.82	9.26
Iowa	3,565	2,853	257	305	9.03	8.91	10.27	8.93
Kansas	3,426	2,410	332	522	8.75	8.54	11.40	8.29
Kentucky	6,026	4,950	700	266	10.77	10.68	13.30	8.87
Louisiana	7,964	3,575	3,735	466	12.32	10.50	15.53	9.67
Maine	1,065	977	44	21	8.45	8.45	9.52	8.37
Maryland	7,380	2,831	2,964	1,076	10.03	8.74	12.56	9.16
Massachusetts	6,002	3,394	734	1,199	8.40	7.78	10.46	9.22
Michigan	11,200	7,039	3,033	669	9.89	8.92	13.91	9.01
Minnesota	5,906	4,096	756	392	8.46	8.25	9.42	8.08
Mississippi	5,008	2,146	2,642	144	13.05	10.93	16.10	8.93
Missouri	7,504	5,353	1,572	358	10.01	9.39	13.93	8.87
Montana	1,059	799	7	54	8.42	7.78	*	9.42
Nebraska	2,629	1,830	242	430	9.86	9.53	12.96	10.12
Nevada	3,609	1,396	591	1,218	9.95	9.35	13.27	9.21
New Hampshire	981	851	22	58	7.90	7.80	9.36	9.09
New Jersey	10,064	4,151	1,977	2,729	9.76	8.76	13.30	9.78
New Mexico	2,462	685	55	1,358	9.54	9.57	11.65	9.42
New York	20,531	8,658	4,365	5,040	8.66	7.55	12.00	9.03
North Carolina	12,297	6,086	4,023	1,566	10.18	9.07	13.94	8.66
North Dakota	955	707	37	54	8.44	8.04	6.46	9.31
Ohio	14,300	9,758	3,341	730	10.28	9.43	14.09	10.47
Oklahoma	5,485	3,355	704	675	10.33	10.08	14.11	9.12
Oregon	3,459	2,363	120	688	7.58	7.35	9.00	8.08
Pennsylvania	13,224	8,470	2,544	1,465	9.39	8.67	12.64	9.81
Rhode Island	947	548	103	237	8.62	8.19	10.82	9.04
South Carolina	6,429	3,197	2,604	460	11.06	9.43	14.64	9.31
South Dakota	1,053	707	23	50	8.54	7.81	7.01	8.94
Tennessee	8,959	5,617	2,485	668	10.99	10.15	14.83	9.22
Texas	41,019	13,494	6,717	18,797	10.17	9.60	13.53	9.84
Utah	4,722	3,451	58	822	9.30	8.97	9.01	10.44
Vermont	429	386	10	12	7.28	7.20	*	*
Virginia	9,549	4,913	2,750	1,174	9.25	8.29	12.64	8.43
Washington	7,216	4,247	475	1,270	8.11	7.68	10.29	7.91
West Virginia	2,227	2,058	101	26	11.25	11.17	14.47	7.85
Wisconsin	6,271	4,314	996	585	9.38	8.81	14.11	8.93
Wyoming	762	585	4	103	9.81	9.44	*	10.70
Puerto Rico	3,547	163	14	3,360	11.39	11.22	*	11.41
Virgin Islands	110	10	81	16	10.59	*	10.84	*
Guam	335	10	-	1	10.01	*	*	*
American Samoa	NA	NA	NA	NA	NA	NA	NA	NA
Northern Marianas	41	–	–	–	9.67	*	*	*

NA = Not available.
– = Quantity zero.
* = Figure does not meet standards of reliability or precision; based on fewer than 20 births in the numerator.
[1]Includes races other than White and Black and origin not stated.
[2]Race and Hispanic origin are reported separately on birth certificates. Persons of Hispanic origin may be of any race. Race categories are consistent with 1977 Office of Management and Budget standards. Forty-nine states and the District of Columbia reported multilple-race data for 2015 that were bridged to single-race categories for comparability with other states.
[3]Includes all persons of Hispanic origin of any race.
[4]Excludes data for the territories.

Table 1-50. Low Birthweight Births (Less Than 2,500 Grams or 5 Lbs 8 Oz), by Race and Hispanic Origin of Mother, by State and Territory of Residence, 2015

(Number, percent.)

State and territory	Number				Percent			
	All races[1]	Non-Hispanic		Hispanic[3]	All races[1]	Non-Hispanic		Hispanic[3]
		White[2]	Black[2]			White[2]	Black[2]	
United States[4]	320,869	147,479	78,514	66,623	8.1	6.9	13.3	7.2
Alabama	6,218	2,892	2,898	305	10.4	8.1	15.9	7.1
Alaska	653	341	37	52	5.8	5.2	8.7	6.4
Arizona	6,128	2,442	557	2,454	7.2	6.6	12.2	7.0
Arkansas	3,564	1,990	1,169	267	9.2	7.7	15.4	6.7
California	33,666	8,369	3,112	15,246	6.8	5.9	11.5	6.5
Colorado	6,001	3,459	456	1,611	9.0	8.5	13.2	8.9
Connecticut	2,836	1,332	563	702	7.9	6.5	12.7	8.5
Delaware	1,036	457	394	133	9.3	7.7	13.2	8.7
District of Columbia	959	207	635	87	10.0	7.0	13.2	6.6
Florida	19,306	7,328	6,547	4,666	8.6	7.1	13.2	7.3
Georgia	12,464	4,278	6,270	1,235	9.5	7.1	13.8	6.9
Hawaii	1,531	276	64	232	8.3	5.8	11.1	8.4
Idaho	1,501	1,157	27	252	6.6	6.4	11.3	6.9
Illinois	13,069	5,834	3,727	2,407	8.3	6.8	13.7	7.1
Indiana	6,725	4,709	1,283	538	8.0	7.4	12.4	7.1
Iowa	2,663	2,073	252	219	6.7	6.5	10.1	6.4
Kansas	2,672	1,844	337	369	6.8	6.5	11.6	5.9
Kentucky	4,846	3,813	730	195	8.7	8.2	13.9	6.5
Louisiana	6,839	2,708	3,618	346	10.6	8.0	15.0	7.2
Maine	871	782	47	17	6.9	6.8	10.2	*
Maryland	6,297	2,164	2,796	841	8.6	6.7	11.8	7.2
Massachusetts	5,312	2,816	743	1,071	7.5	6.5	10.6	8.3
Michigan	9,612	5,486	3,119	555	8.5	7.0	14.3	7.5
Minnesota	4,494	2,881	754	293	6.4	5.8	9.4	6.0
Mississippi	4,387	1,533	2,704	91	11.4	7.8	16.5	5.6
Missouri	6,248	4,114	1,628	290	8.3	7.2	14.4	7.2
Montana	887	702	11	42	7.1	6.8	*	7.3
Nebraska	1,893	1,242	255	290	7.1	6.5	13.6	6.8
Nevada	3,093	1,168	605	970	8.5	7.8	13.6	7.3
New Hampshire	852	732	23	44	6.9	6.7	9.7	6.9
New Jersey	8,345	3,220	1,817	2,141	8.1	6.8	12.2	7.7
New Mexico	2,244	605	66	1,275	8.7	8.5	14.0	8.9
New York	18,507	7,277	4,359	4,335	7.8	6.4	12.0	7.8
North Carolina	11,023	4,998	4,142	1,252	9.1	7.5	14.4	6.9
North Dakota	700	531	41	42	6.2	6.0	7.2	7.2
Ohio	11,807	7,514	3,296	535	8.5	7.3	13.9	7.7
Oklahoma	4,172	2,429	675	540	7.9	7.3	13.5	7.3
Oregon	2,919	1,935	125	571	6.4	6.0	9.4	6.7
Pennsylvania	11,453	6,751	2,631	1,300	8.2	6.9	13.2	8.7
Rhode Island	833	460	104	205	7.6	6.9	10.9	7.8
South Carolina	5,535	2,485	2,579	315	9.5	7.3	14.5	6.4
South Dakota	754	525	19	31	6.1	5.8	*	5.5
Tennessee	7,460	4,312	2,452	490	9.2	7.8	14.7	6.8
Texas	33,275	10,016	6,526	14,676	8.2	7.1	13.1	7.7
Utah	3,561	2,547	60	652	7.0	6.6	9.3	8.3
Vermont	390	340	14	13	6.6	6.3	*	*
Virginia	8,111	3,881	2,654	891	7.9	6.6	12.2	6.4
Washington	5,730	3,228	453	980	6.4	5.8	9.8	6.1
West Virginia	1,891	1,735	95	26	9.6	9.4	13.6	7.9
Wisconsin	4,870	3,059	1,037	442	7.3	6.2	14.6	6.7
Wyoming	666	502	8	91	8.6	8.1	*	9.5
Puerto Rico	3,282	176	13	3,082	10.5	12.1	*	10.5
Virgin Islands	114	12	82	16	9.2	*	9.4	*
Guam	307	5	-	1	9.2	*	*	*
American Samoa	34	NA	NA	NA	3.2	NA	NA	NA
Northern Marianas	33	-	-	-	7.8	*	*	NA

NA = Not available.
– = Quantity zero.
* = Figure does not meet standards of reliability or precision; based on fewer than 20 births in the numerator.
[1]Includes races other than White and Black and origin not stated.
[2]Race and Hispanic origin are reported separately on birth certificates. Persons of Hispanic origin may be of any race. Race categories are consistent with 1977 Office of Management and Budget standards. Forty-nine states and the District of Columbia reported multiple-race data for 2015 that were bridged to single-race categories for comparability with other states.
[3]Includes all persons of Hispanic origin of any race.
[4]Excludes data for the territories.

Table 1-51. Births, by Plurality, Age, and Race and Hispanic Origin of Mother, 2015

(Number, rate as stated.)

Plurality, race, and Hispanic origin of mother	All ages	Under 15 years	Age of mother			20 to 24 years	25 to 29 years	30 to 34 years	35 to 39 years	40 to 44 years	45 to 54 years
			15 to 19 years								
			Total	15 to 17 years	18 to 19 years						
					Number						
All Live Births											
All races[1]	3,978,497	2,500	229,715	61,184	168,531	850,509	1,152,311	1,094,693	527,996	111,848	8,925
Non-Hispanic White[2]	2,130,279	582	90,833	20,406	70,427	399,373	642,150	646,767	290,877	55,040	4,657
Non-Hispanic Black[2]	589,047	845	50,039	14,366	35,673	175,597	165,895	119,976	60,863	14,592	1,240
Hispanic[3]	924,048	986	80,364	24,187	56,177	236,264	256,106	209,647	112,045	27,117	1,519
Live Births in Single Deliveries											
All races[1]	3,841,219	2,467	226,061	60,362	165,699	830,329	1,116,679	1,050,568	502,380	105,502	7,233
Non-Hispanic White[2]	2,050,814	571	89,448	20,138	69,310	390,268	621,557	618,646	275,304	51,284	3,736
Non-Hispanic Black[2]	565,228	833	48,972	14,105	34,867	169,638	158,894	114,216	57,723	13,892	1,060
Hispanic[3]	900,844	976	79,292	23,926	55,366	231,915	250,013	203,243	108,018	26,099	1,288
Live Births in Twin Deliveries											
All races[1]	133,155	33	3,613	807	2,806	19,797	34,634	42,617	24,748	6,079	1,634
Non-Hispanic White[2]	76,848	11	1,380	268	1,112	8,914	19,909	27,088	15,046	3,605	895
Non-Hispanic Black[2]	23,204	12	1,052	258	794	5,844	6,859	5,606	3,004	656	171
Hispanic[3]	22,593	10	1,057	249	808	4,285	5,964	6,200	3,887	970	220
Live Births in Triplet and Higher-Order Multiple Births[4]											
All races[1]	4,123	–	41	15	26	383	998	1,508	868	267	58
Non-Hispanic White[2]	2,617	–	5	–	5	191	684	1,033	527	151	26
Non-Hispanic Black[2]	615	–	15	3	12	115	142	154	136	44	9
Hispanic[3]	611	–	15	12	3	64	129	204	140	48	11
					Rate per 1,000 live births						
All Multiple Births											
All races[1]	34.5	13.2	15.9	13.4	16.8	23.7	30.9	40.3	48.5	56.7	189.6
Non-Hispanic White[2]	37.3	*	15.2	13.1	15.9	22.8	32.1	43.5	53.5	68.2	197.8
Non-Hispanic Black[2]	40.4	*	21.3	18.2	22.6	33.9	42.2	48.0	51.6	48.0	145.2
Hispanic[3]	25.1	*	13.3	10.8	14.4	18.4	23.8	30.5	35.9	37.5	152.1
Twin Births											
All races[1]	33.5	13.2	15.7	13.2	16.6	23.3	30.1	38.9	46.9	54.4	183.1
Non-Hispanic White[2]	36.1	*	15.2	13.1	15.8	22.3	31.0	41.9	51.7	65.5	192.2
Non-Hispanic Black[2]	39.4	*	21.0	18.0	22.3	33.3	41.3	46.7	49.4	45.0	137.9
Hispanic[3]	24.5	*	13.2	10.3	14.4	18.1	23.3	29.6	34.7	35.8	144.8
Triplet and Higher-Order Multiple Births[4]											
All races[1]	103.6	*	17.8	*	15.4	45.0	86.6	137.8	164.4	238.7	649.9
Non-Hispanic White[2]	122.8	*	*	*	*	47.8	106.5	159.7	181.2	274.3	558.3
Non-Hispanic Black[2]	104.4	*	*	*	*	65.5	85.6	128.4	223.5	301.5	*
Hispanic[3]	66.12	*	*	*	*	27.1	50.4	97.3	124.9	177.0	*

– = Quantity zero.
* = Figure does not meet standards of reliability or precision; based on fewer than 20 births in the numerator.
[1]Includes races other than White and Black and origin not stated.
[2]Race and Hispanic origin are reported separately on birth certificates. Persons of Hispanic origin may be of any race. Race categories are consistent with 1977 Office of Management and Budget standards. Forty-nine states and the District of Columbia reported multiple-race data for 2015 that were bridged to single-race categories for comparability with other states.
[3]Includes all persons of Hispanic origin of any race.
[4]Triplet, quadruplet, quintuplet, and higher-order multiple deliveries.

Table 1-52. Numbers and Rates of Twin and Triplet and Higher-Order Multiple Births, by Race and Hispanic Origin of Mother, 1980–2015

(Number, rate per 1,000 live births; rate per 100,000 live births, as stated.)

Year, race, and Hispanic origin of mother	Total births	Twin births	Triplet and higher-order births	Multiple birth rate[1]	Twin birth rate[2]	Triplet or higher-order birth rate[3]
All Races[4]						
1980	3,612,258	68,339	1,337	19.3	18.9	37.0
1981	3,629,238	70,049	1,385	19.7	19.3	38.2
1982	3,680,537	71,631	1,484	19.9	19.5	40.3
1983	3,638,933	72,287	1,575	20.3	19.9	43.3
1984	3,669,141	72,949	1,653	20.3	19.9	45.1
1985	3,760,561	77,102	1,925	21.0	20.5	51.2
1986	3,756,547	79,485	1,814	21.6	21.2	48.3
1987	3,809,394	81,778	2,139	22.0	21.5	56.2
1988	3,909,510	85,315	2,385	22.4	21.8	61.0
1989	4,040,958	90,118	2,798	23.0	22.3	69.2
1990	4,158,212	93,865	3,028	23.3	22.6	72.8
1991	4,110,907	94,779	3,346	23.9	23.1	81.4
1992	4,065,014	95,372	3,883	24.4	23.5	95.5
1993	4,000,240	96,445	4,168	25.2	24.1	104.2
1994	3,952,767	97,064	4,594	25.7	24.6	116.2
1995	3,899,589	96,736	4,973	26.1	24.8	127.5
1996	3,891,494	100,750	5,939	27.4	25.9	152.6
1997	3,880,894	104,137	6,737	28.6	26.8	173.6
1998	3,941,553	110,670	7,625	30.0	28.1	193.5
1999	3,959,417	114,307	7,321	30.7	28.9	184.9
2000	4,058,814	118,916	7,325	31.1	29.3	180.5
2001	4,025,933	121,246	7,471	32.0	30.1	185.6
2002	4,021,726	125,134	7,401	33.0	31.1	184.0
2003	4,089,950	128,665	7,663	33.3	31.5	187.4
2004	4,112,052	132,219	7,275	33.9	32.2	176.9
2005	4,138,349	133,122	6,694	33.8	32.2	161.8
2006	4,265,555	137,085	6,540	33.7	32.1	153.3
2007	4,316,233	138,961	6,427	33.7	32.2	148.9
2008	4,247,694	138,660	6,268	34.1	32.6	147.6
2009	4,130,665	137,217	6,340	34.8	33.2	153.5
2010	3,999,386	132,562	5,503	34.5	33.1	137.6
2011	3,953,590	131,269	5,417	34.6	33.2	137.0
2012	3,952,841	131,024	4,919	34.4	33.1	124.4
2013	3,932,181	135,336	4,700	34.8	33.7	119.5
2014	3,988,076		4,526	35.1	33.9	113.5
2015	3,978,497	133,155	4,123	34.5	33.5	103.6
Non-Hispanic White[5]						
1990[6]	2,626,500	60,210	2,358	23.8	22.9	89.8
1991[7]	2,589,878	60,904	2,612	24.5	23.5	100.9
1992[7]	2,527,207	60,640	3,115	25.2	24.0	123.3
1993	2,472,031	61,525	3,360	26.2	24.9	135.9
1994	2,438,855	62,476	3,721	27.1	25.6	152.6
1995	2,382,638	62,370	4,050	27.9	26.2	170.0
1996	2,358,989	65,523	4,885	29.8	27.8	207.1
1997	2,333,363	67,191	5,386	31.1	28.8	230.8
1998	2,283,986	71,270	6,206	32.8	30.2	262.8
1999	2,346,450	73,964	5,909	34.0	31.5	251.8
2000	2,362,968	76,018	5,821	34.6	32.2	246.3
2001	2,326,578	77,882	5,894	36.0	33.5	253.3
2002	2,298,156	79,949	5,754	37.3	34.8	250.4
2003	2,321,904	81,691	5,922	37.7	35.2	255.0
2004	2,296,683	83,346	5,590	38.7	36.3	243.4
2005	2,279,768	82,223	4,966	38.2	36.1	217.8
2006	2,308,640	83,108	4,805	38.1	36.0	208.1
2007	2,310,333	83,632	4,559	38.2	36.2	197.3
2008	2,267,817	82,903	4,493	38.5	36.6	198.1
2009	2,212,552	81,954	4,457	39.1	37.0	201.4
2010	2,162,406	79,728	3,842	38.6	36.9	177.7
2011	2,146,566	78,638	3,670	38.3	36.6	171.0
2012	2,134,196	78,449	3,264	38.3	36.8	152.9
2013	2,129,196	78,072	3,134	38.1	36.7	147.2
2014	2,149,302	78,788	3,028	38.1	36.7	140.9
2015	2,130,279	76,848	2,617	37.3	36.1	122.8

[1]The number of live births in all multiple deliveries per 1,000 live births.
[2]The number of live births in twin deliveries per 1,000 live births.
[3]The number of live births in triplet and other higher-order deliveries per 100,000 live births.
[4]Includes races other than White and Black and origin not stated.
[5]Race and Hispanic origin are reported separately on birth certificates. Persons of Hispanic origin may be of any race. Race categories are consistent with 1977 Office of Management and Budget standards. Forty-nine states and the District of Columbia reported multiple-race data for 2015 that were bridged to single-race categories for comparability with other statess. Multiple-race reporting areas vary for 2003–2015.
[6]Excludes data for New Hampshire and Oklahoma, which did not report Hispanic origin.
[7]Excludes data for New Hampshire, which did not report Hispanic origin.
[8]Includes all persons of Hispanic origin of any race.

Table 1-52. Numbers and Rates of Twin and Triplet and Higher-Order Multiple Births, by Race and Hispanic Origin of Mother, 1980–2015—*Continued*

(Number, rate per 1,000 live births; rate per 100,000 live births, as stated.)

Year, race, and Hispanic origin of mother	Total births	Twin births	Triplet and higher-order births	Multiple birth rate[1]	Twin birth rate[2]	Triplet or higher-order birth rate[3]
Non-Hispanic Black[5]						
1990[6]	661,701	17,646	306	27.1	26.7	46.2
1991[7]	666,758	18,243	367	27.9	27.4	55.0
1992[7]	657,450	18,294	346	28.4	27.8	52.6
1993	641,273	18,115	314	28.7	28.2	49.0
1994	619,198	17,934	357	29.5	29.0	57.7
1995	587,781	16,622	340	28.9	28.3	57.8
1996	578,099	16,873	425	29.9	29.2	73.5
1997	581,431	17,472	523	30.9	30.0	90.0
1998	593,127	18,589	518	32.2	31.3	87.3
1999	588,981	18,920	561	33.1	32.1	95.2
2000	604,346	20,173	506	34.2	33.4	83.7
2001	589,917	19,974	531	34.8	33.9	90.0
2002	578,335	20,064	591	35.7	34.7	102.2
2003	576,033	20,010	631	35.8	34.7	109.5
2004	578,772	20,605	577	36.6	35.6	99.7
2005	583,759	21,254	616	37.5	36.4	105.5
2006	617,247	22,702	580	37.7	36.8	94.0
2007	627,191	23,101	612	37.8	36.8	97.6
2008	623,029	22,924	569	37.7	36.8	91.3
2009	609,584	23,159	644	39.0	38.0	105.6
2010	589,808	21,804	574	37.9	37.0	97.3
2011	582,345	21,681	634	38.3	37.2	108.9
2012	583,489	21,545	629	38.0	36.9	107.8
2013	583,834	22,346	623	39.3	38.3	106.7
2014	588,891	23,546	528	40.9	40.0	89.7
2015	589,047	23,204	615	40.4	39.4	104.4
Hispanic[8]						
1990[6]	595,073	10,713	235	18.4	18.0	39.5
1991[7]	623,085	11,356	235	18.6	18.2	37.7
1992[7]	643,271	11,932	239	18.9	18.5	37.2
1993	654,418	12,294	321	19.3	18.8	49.1
1994	665,026	12,206	348	18.9	18.4	52.3
1995	679,768	12,685	355	19.2	18.7	52.2
1996	701,339	13,014	409	19.1	18.6	58.3
1997	709,767	13,821	516	20.2	19.5	72.7
1998	734,661	15,015	553	21.2	20.4	75.3
1999	764,339	15,388	583	20.9	20.1	76.3
2000	815,868	16,470	659	21.0	20.2	80.8
2001	851,851	17,257	710	21.1	20.3	83.3
2002	876,642	18,128	737	21.5	20.7	84.1
2003	912,329	19,472	784	22.2	21.3	85.9
2004	946,349	20,351	723	22.3	21.5	76.4
2005	985,505	21,723	761	22.8	22.0	77.2
2006	1,039,077	22,698	787	22.6	21.8	75.7
2007	1,062,779	23,405	857	22.8	22.0	80.6
2008	1,041,239	23,266	834	23.1	22.3	80.1
2009	999,548	22,481	835	23.3	22.5	83.5
2010	945,180	21,359	721	23.4	22.6	76.3
2011	918,129	21,236	723	23.9	23.1	78.7
2012	907,677	20,505	636	23.3	22.6	46.2
2013	901,033	21,511	643	24.6	23.9	64.3
2014	914,065	22,051	588	24.8	24.1	70.1
2015	924,048	22,593	611	25.1	24.5	66.1

[1]The number of live births in all multiple deliveries per 1,000 live births.
[2]The number of live births in twin deliveries per 1,000 live births.
[3]The number of live births in triplet and other higher-order deliveries per 100,000 live births.
[4]Includes races other than White and Black and origin not stated.
[5]Race and Hispanic origin are reported separately on birth certificates. Persons of Hispanic origin may be of any race. Race categories are consistent with 1977 Office of Management and Budget standards. Forty-nine states and the District of Columbia reported multiple-race data for 2015 that were bridged to single-race categories for comparability with other statess. Multiple-race reporting areas vary for 2003–2015.
[6]Excludes data for New Hampshire and Oklahoma, which did not report Hispanic origin.
[7]Excludes data for New Hampshire, which did not report Hispanic origin.
[8]Includes all persons of Hispanic origin of any race.

Table 1-53. Gestational Age and Birthweight Characteristics, by Plurality, 2015

(Number, percent.)

Characteristic	All births	Singletons	Twins	Triplets	Quadruplets	Quintuplets and higher-order multiples[1]
Number of Births	3,978,497	3,841,219	133,155	3,871	228	24
Percent, very preterm[2]	1.6	1.2	10.7	37.1	81.1	95.8
Percent, preterm[3]	9.6	7.8	59.1	98.6	98.3	100.0
Percent, very low birthweight[4]	1.4	1.1	9.6	36.4	79.1	100.0
Percent, low birthweight[5]	8.1	6.3	55.4	95.7	98.6	100.0

[1]Quintuplets, sextuplets, and higher-order multiple births are not differentiated in the national data set.
[2]Very preterm is less than 32 completed weeks of gestation.
[3]Preterm is less than 37 completed weeks of gestation.
[4]Very low birthweight is less than 1,500 grams.
[5]Low birthweight is less than 2,500 grams.

Table 1-54. Distribution of Births, by Selected Gestational Age, Selected Years, 1990–2015

(Percent; number.)

Gestational age	Obstetric estimate						
	1990	2000	2005	2006	2010	2014	2015
Under 28 weeks	0.7	0.7	0.8	0.8	0.7	0.7	0.7
28 to 31 weeks	1.2	1.2	1.3	1.3	1.2	0.9	0.9
32 to 33 weeks	1.4	1.5	1.6	1.6	1.5	1.2	1.2
Total under 34 weeks	3.3	3.4	3.6	3.7	3.5	2.7	2.8
34 to 36 weeks	7.3	8.2	9.1	9.2	8.5	6.8	6.9
Total under 37 weeks	10.6	11.6	12.7	12.8	12.0	9.6	9.6
37 to 38 weeks	19.7	24.5	28.3	28.9	26.9	24.8	25.0
39 to 40 weeks	NA	NA	NA	NA	NA	58.7	58.5
39 weeks	21.7	24.3	25.3	25.4	28.3	NA	NA
40 weeks	22.6	21.3	19.2	18.9	19.1	NA	NA
41 weeks	14.1	11.0	8.7	8.3	8.2	6.5	6.5
42 weeks or more	11.3	7.3	5.8	5.7	5.5	0.4	0.4
Not states	NA	NA	NA	6	10,538	3,246	2,926

NA = Not available.

Table 1-55. Quitting Smoking Prior to Pregnancy, by Race, Hispanic Origin, Age of Mother, and Reporting Area, 2011

(Percent.)

Reporting area	Race and Hispanic origin				Age of mother in years					
	Total	Non-Hispanic White	Non-Hispanic Black	Hispanic	Under 20 years	20 to 24 years	25 to 29 years	30 to 35 years	35 to 39 years	40 to 54 years
Total	23.8	22.4	23.1	39.2	22.6	22.3	24.6	26.7	24.3	20.0
California	34.6	31.2	25.2	45.4	33.4	34.7	34.3	36.4	35.3	24.3
Colorado	21.3	20.3	17.7	25.6	22.7	21.1	20.9	23.5	19.0	*
Delaware	14.3	13.5	13.5	*	*	15.0	13.4	17.6	*	*
District of Columbia	36.8	*	35.4	*	*	41.3	40.7	23.0	*	*
Florida	17.5	15.6	16.9	33.6	19.6	16.7	17.7	17.7	17.9	15.1
Georgia	12.8	12.1	12.5	28.3	10.5	12.9	12.7	14.4	12.9	*
Idaho	26.2	24.9	*	35.3	22.5	25.1	29.7	25.4	24.1	*
Illinois	16.1	16.1	12.0	29.1	17.3	14.4	17.2	18.1	13.9	12.3
Indiana	19.6	18.8	23.0	34.2	20.8	18.7	19.8	20.8	18.8	17.4
Iowa	25.8	25.5	22.4	38.9	25.3	23.8	28.5	27.5	23.3	*
Kansas	15.7	15.8	6.4	26.4	16.7	15.1	16.3	15.3	18.2	*
Kentucky	12.9	12.3	18.2	31.8	12.5	11.7	13.7	15.1	13.1	14.5
Louisiana	18.0	18.3	16.0	30.9	17.0	17.0	18.5	19.5	20.1	*
Maryland	35.8	34.3	35.1	58.2	30.3	33.8	37.4	39.5	36.5	30.8
Missouri	26.8	26.8	25.3	35.8	25.6	24.0	27.9	33.2	25.2	16.4
Montana	15.2	15.9	*	*	16.7	12.9	15.5	17.3	19.7	*
Nebraska	28.4	28.1	18.7	39.1	25.4	28.0	29.3	30.0	25.9	*
Nevada	15.4	13.4	15.1	22.7	14.0	18.4	15.5	14.1	11.3	*
New Hampshire	14.2	14.2	*	*	11.8	12.3	14.9	17.1	16.7	*
New Mexico	39.9	31.8	*	44.7	45.7	41.8	39.6	35.5	32.6	*
New York	28.1	26.0	28.0	41.8	23.8	24.1	28.7	34.4	31.7	28.0
North Carolina	25.2	23.5	28.0	43.1	25.9	25.6	24.5	26.1	23.1	18.6
North Dakota	26.0	27.2	*	45.3	22.7	22.6	30.4	28.3	27.4	*
Ohio	23.9	23.3	26.0	32.7	20.9	21.9	24.9	28.4	26.4	22.1
Oklahoma	18.5	18.2	15.3	31.4	19.3	18.3	18.8	19.1	15.3	*
Oregon	16.3	15.6	*	26.3	16.8	15.0	16.6	17.6	18.5	*
Pennsylvania	26.5	26.4	22.9	33.7	22.5	23.5	28.2	30.7	28.4	25.2
South Carolina	25.1	23.2	29.4	45.7	22.7	25.2	25.3	26.7	26.4	*
South Dakota	32.6	30.9	*	29.8	36.9	31.0	33.1	35.0	23.1	*
Tennessee	22.5	21.8	23.5	43.8	22.4	20.7	23.1	26.6	21.3	22.4
Texas	32.4	28.4	30.3	49.6	31.7	31.2	33.2	34.5	32.5	24.9
Utah	26.2	25.5	*	32.3	29.1	27.5	26.2	22.7	23.9	*
Vermont	17.7	17.4	*	*	21.7	13.7	16.8	28.4	*	*
Washington	19.6	18.9	15.0	28.7	18.3	19.8	20.0	19.4	19.9	19.4
Wisconsin	24.9	25.7	16.4	32.4	22.1	23.0	25.9	28.3	25.6	18.9
Wyoming	25.3	24.2	*	33.6	24.3	25.5	26.1	26.3	*	*

* = Figure does not meet standards of reliability or precision.

Table 1-56. Maternal Prepregnancy Body Mass Index, by Reporting Area, and Prepregnancy Obesity, by Race, Hispanic Origin, and Age of Mother, 36 States, the District of Columbia, and Puerto Rico, 2011

(Percent.)

Reporting area	BMI[1]					Race and Hispanic origin of mother	
	Total	Underweight (BMI less than 18.5)	Normal (BMI 18.5 to 24.9)	Overweight (BMI 25.0 to 29.9)	Obese (BMI greater than 30.0)	Total	Non-Hispanic White[2]
Total[4]	100.0	3.9	47.3	25.3	23.4	23.4	21.8
California..	100.0	3.8	48.5	26.2	21.6	21.6	17.1
Colorado...	100.0	4.1	52.3	24.8	18.8	18.8	16.6
Delaware...	100.0	4.5	45.1	25.7	24.7	24.7	21.8
District of Columbia	100.0	4.3	52.7	22.7	20.3	20.3	4.8
Florida..	100.0	4.8	48.3	25.1	21.8	21.8	19.3
Georgia	100.0	3.7	42.6	26.4	27.3	27.3	23.5
Idaho	100.0	3.3	50.1	24.8	21.7	21.7	20.7
Illinois	100.0	3.5	46.0	26.4	24.1	24.1	21.9
Indiana	100.0	4.2	45.0	25.2	25.7	25.7	24.9
Iowa	100.0	3.2	46.5	25.6	24.8	24.8	25.0
Kansas	100.0	3.5	46.8	26.0	23.7	23.7	23.4
Kentucky	100.0	4.6	43.7	24.3	27.4	27.4	27.1
Louisiana	100.0	4.4	43.8	24.6	27.2	27.2	23.2
Maryland...	100.0	3.5	46.5	26.3	23.7	23.7	19.8
Michigan	100.0	3.5	45.1	25.5	25.9	25.9	24.4
Missouri..	100.0	4.2	47.3	24.1	24.4	24.4	23.5
Montana..	100.0	3.1	49.0	25.0	22.9	22.9	21.3
Nebraska	100.0	3.3	48.4	24.9	23.5	23.5	22.7
Nevada..	100.0	4.7	48.8	25.4	21.1	21.1	19.5
New Hampshire..	100.0	3.5	50.1	23.8	22.6	22.6	23.2
New Mexico	100.0	4.0	43.2	28.1	24.8	24.8	19.1
New York...	100.0	4.2	50.0	25.4	20.4	20.4	19.5
North Carolina	100.0	4.2	46.4	25.0	24.4	24.4	21.1
North Dakota	100.0	2.6	41.0	27.9	28.5	28.5	27.2
Ohio	100.0	4.2	46.9	24.1	24.8	24.8	23.7
Oklahoma..	100.0	4.5	45.2	24.8	25.4	25.4	24.3
Oregon..	100.0	3.2	48.5	24.9	23.4	23.4	22.6
Pennsylvania...	100.0	3.9	49.2	24.1	22.9	22.9	21.8
South Carolina	100.0	4.1	42.5	24.8	28.6	28.6	23.2
South Dakota	100.0	3.6	47.8	25.5	23.2	23.2	22.2
Tennessee	100.0	4.8	46.5	24.3	24.3	24.3	22.6
Texas..	100.0	4.0	47.4	25.3	23.3	23.3	20.5
Utah	100.0	4.3	54.9	22.7	18.0	18.0	17.0
Vermont..	100.0	3.1	49.4	24.3	23.2	23.2	23.7
Washington...	100.0	2.9	46.4	25.9	24.7	24.7	24.1
Wisconsin	100.0	2.6	43.1	26.5	27.8	27.8	26.7
Wyoming	100.0	3.6	50.1	24.3	22.1	22.1	21.8
Puerto Rico...	100.0	7.4	46.9	25.2	20.5	20.5	NA

NA = Not available.
* = Figure does not meet standards of reliability or precision.
[1]BMI is Body Mass Index.
[2]Race and Hispanic origin are reported separately on birth certificates. Persons of Hispanic origin may be of any race. Multiple-race data, when reported, were bridged to single-race categories in order to maintain comparability among all reported areas.
[3]Includes all persons of Hispanic origin of any race.
[4]Excludes data for Puerto Rico.

Table 1-56. Maternal Prepregnancy Body Mass Index, by Reporting Area, and Prepregnancy Obesity, by Race, Hispanic Origin, and Age of Mother, 36 States, the District of Columbia, and Puerto Rico, 2011—Continued

(Percent.)

Reporting area	Race and Hispanic origin of mother		Age of mother in years					
	Non-Hispanic Black[2]	Hispanic[3]	Under 20 years	20 to 24 years	25 to 29 years	30 to 34 years	35 to 39 years	40 to 54 years
Total[4]	32.6	25.2	15.0	23.9	24.8	23.6	24.7	25.1
California..	29.4	26.8	13.6	22.7	23.5	21.4	21.2	22.2
Colorado..	24.2	24.5	11.6	19.9	20.3	18.1	19.3	19.4
Delaware..	33.3	25.4	15.3	23.4	24.8	26.6	29.0	26.0
District of Columbia	30.0	20.6	17.0	26.7	27.9	16.2	14.2	13.7
Florida...	30.5	20.2	13.7	21.8	23.0	22.1	23.1	23.8
Georgia..	35.9	24.6	18.6	28.2	28.8	27.1	29.1	30.3
Idaho...	19.2	27.2	13.9	20.4	22.2	23.0	26.0	28.0
Illinois...	34.1	26.4	15.9	25.1	25.4	23.7	25.6	25.6
Indiana..	33.9	26.0	15.9	25.6	26.4	27.4	28.3	30.9
Iowa...	29.5	25.5	16.0	25.3	25.3	24.6	29.1	23.7
Kansas...	28.8	25.8	14.2	24.2	24.8	24.5	25.7	28.2
Kentucky..	36.1	23.8	18.3	28.0	28.4	28.4	31.1	31.8
Louisiana...	34.7	22.0	17.2	26.2	29.3	29.4	31.3	33.7
Maryland..	33.6	22.0	17.1	25.0	24.6	23.0	23.8	26.8
Michigan..	34.5	27.7	17.1	26.2	26.7	26.1	29.1	28.9
Missouri...	31.5	24.1	14.6	24.2	25.5	25.6	27.1	29.8
Montana...	*	26.6	12.9	22.4	23.9	23.3	27.7	26.7
Nebraska..	30.4	25.7	14.6	23.2	23.5	23.5	28.3	31.9
Nevada..	24.2	23.7	11.0	20.8	22.5	22.4	22.7	24.4
New Hampshire....................................	22.0	22.6	16.1	23.1	23.9	22.0	23.1	20.4
New Mexico..	23.6	26.1	13.0	23.8	27.0	28.2	29.8	27.6
New York..	30.3	21.9	15.4	20.6	21.7	19.8	20.5	21.1
North Carolina.....................................	35.4	22.6	16.1	25.2	25.5	24.0	26.6	28.0
North Dakota..	22.9	31.9	16.6	27.6	27.7	30.2	39.6	29.0
Ohio...	32.5	26.3	15.7	25.1	26.1	24.8	27.9	28.6
Oklahoma...	30.8	26.0	15.1	25.1	26.7	27.9	30.6	30.8
Oregon...	27.7	27.4	15.3	24.6	24.8	22.6	24.1	23.1
Pennsylvania..	31.8	23.7	15.1	22.9	24.2	22.5	24.6	25.1
South Carolina.....................................	40.5	25.0	18.6	29.3	30.2	29.1	31.1	30.9
South Dakota.......................................	13.9	24.6	10.2	22.4	24.2	24.6	29.1	28.8
Tennessee..	33.0	21.3	15.2	24.4	26.0	24.9	27.9	27.7
Texas...	29.4	25.4	13.3	23.2	25.1	24.8	26.0	26.3
Utah...	25.0	21.7	12.7	15.5	17.5	19.4	24.0	25.5
Vermont...	*	*	20.9	25.8	25.1	21.8	20.6	15.6
Washington..	30.9	29.8	16.6	26.5	25.5	24.0	25.1	27.0
Wisconsin..	37.0	29.9	19.7	27.3	28.3	27.8	31.5	30.8
Wyoming..	*	22.2	13.8	21.4	22.2	24.9	26.1	20.6
Puerto Rico..	NA	20.4	10.3	18.8	24.1	25.0	27.3	32.4

NA = Not available.
* = Figure does not meet standards of reliability or precision.
[1]BMI is Body Mass Index.
[2]Race and Hispanic origin are reported separately on birth certificates. Persons of Hispanic origin may be of any race. Multiple-race data, when reported, were bridged to single-race categories in order to maintain comparability among all reported areas.
[3]Includes all persons of Hispanic origin of any race.
[4]Excludes data for Puerto Rico.

Table 1-57. Number of Live Births by Attendant, Place of Delivery, Race, and Hispanic Origin of Mother, 2014

(Number.)

Place of delivery and race and Hispanic origin of mother	All births	Physician			Midwife			Other	Unspecified
		Total	Doctor of medicine	Doctor of osteopathy	Total	Certified nurse midwife	Other midwife		
ALL RACES[1]									
Total...	3,988,076	3,594,759	3,331,630	263,129	363,808	332,107	31,701	27,542	1,967
In hospital[2].....................................	3,928,272	3,592,121	3,329,379	262,742	320,148	312,777	7,371	15,099	904
Not in hospital.................................	59,674	2,584	2,203	381	43,647	19,324	24,323	12,402	1,041
Freestanding birthing center	18,219	561	432	129	16,848	9,825	7,023	779	31
Clinic or doctor's office	404	192	148	44	189	172	17	19	4
Residence	38,094	1,365	1,197	168	25,892	9,102	16,790	10,023	814
Other..	2,957	466	426	40	718	225	493	1,581	192
Not specified	130	54	48	6	13	6	7	41	22
NON-HISPANIC WHITE[3]									
Total...	2,149,302	1,917,811	1,751,589	166,222	214,908	189,583	25,325	15,580	1,003
In hospital[2].....................................	2,100,900	1,916,178	1,750,278	165,900	177,684	173,269	4,415	6,593	445
Not in hospital.................................	48,333	1,606	1,287	319	37,213	16,308	20,905	8,962	552
Freestanding birthing center	14,986	506	378	128	13,794	8,068	5,726	666	20
Clinic or doctor's office	322	131	93	38	179	163	16	10	2
Residence	31,299	722	596	126	22,610	7,893	14,717	7,512	455
Other..	1,726	247	220	27	630	184	446	774	75
Not specified	69	27	24	3	11	6	5	25	6
NON-HISPANIC BLACK[3]									
Total...	588,891	541,062	512,921	28,141	43,537	41,802	1,735	3,992	300
In hospital[2].....................................	585,699	540,529	512,412	28,117	42,312	41,172	1,140	2,729	129
Not in hospital.................................	3,166	519	495	24	1,225	630	595	1,254	168
Freestanding birthing center	745	25	25	–	684	391	293	27	9
Clinic or doctor's office	25	21	19	2	–	–	–	4	–
Residence	2,033	371	355	16	518	226	292	1,011	133
Other..	363	102	96	6	23	13	10	212	26
Not specified	26	14	14	–	–	–	–	9	3
HISPANIC[4]									
Total...	914,065	831,250	777,780	53,470	76,725	73,446	3,279	5,762	328
In hospital[2].....................................	909,040	830,957	777,515	53,442	73,383	71,981	1,402	4,557	143
Not in hospital.................................	5,016	287	259	28	3,341	1,465	1,876	1,203	185
Freestanding birthing center	1,758	25	24	1	1,671	915	756	60	2
Clinic or doctor's office	22	13	13	–	7	6	1	1	1
Residence	2,810	188	166	22	1,620	526	1,094	869	133
Other..	426	61	56	5	43	18	25	273	49
Not specified	9	6	6	–	1	–	1	2	–

– = Quantity zero.
[1]Includes races other than White and Black and origin not stated.
[2]Includes births occurring en route to or on arrival at hospital.
[3]Race and Hispanic origin are reported separately on birth certificates. Persons of Hispanic origin may be of any race. Multiple-race data, when reported, were bridged to single-race categories in order to maintain comparability among all reported areas.
[4]Includes all persons of Hispanic origin of any race.

Table 1-58. Mother Received WIC Food During This Pregnancy, by Race and Hispanic Origin, and Age of Mother, 36 States, the District of Columbia, and Puerto Rico, 2011

(Percent.)

Reporting area		Race and Hispanic origin of mother			Age of mother in years					
	Total	Non-Hispanic White[1]	Non-Hispanic Black[1]	Hispanic[2]	Under 20 years	20 to 24 years	25 to 29 years	30 to 34 years	35 to 39 years	40 to 54 years
Total[3]	47.8	33.0	67.9	71.4	81.2	68.8	43.9	31.1	29.7	29.7
California	54.3	26.1	69.6	76.2	87.7	77.7	55.0	38.9	35.6	34.3
Colorado	33.0	19.8	53.1	60.2	71.7	53.8	30.3	18.9	17.4	16.9
Delaware	35.7	25.4	45.5	67.6	61.6	52.7	33.8	22.4	20.2	19.5
District of Columbia	44.5	2.4	59.2	77.5	76.9	67.4	54.3	27.9	21.3	14.5
Florida	54.0	39.9	73.0	64.5	83.7	73.8	50.9	38.3	37.0	36.8
Georgia	51.5	38.1	66.4	64.9	81.9	71.1	47.4	33.6	30.4	28.1
Idaho	44.2	38.0	69.5	73.1	80.6	60.4	39.7	27.1	28.8	28.3
Illinois	41.6	26.6	66.4	66.3	77.7	68.0	39.0	24.9	23.5	23.4
Indiana	46.9	40.0	73.0	75.1	81.3	67.6	38.6	28.0	28.2	28.8
Iowa	37.6	31.5	72.2	75.7	80.5	60.4	29.9	20.9	22.9	23.3
Kansas	39.0	29.8	63.3	70.0	71.8	57.8	31.6	22.8	22.3	22.6
Kentucky	49.5	46.9	65.4	69.5	81.0	68.1	41.1	28.3	28.1	28.0
Louisiana	55.2	42.5	72.6	61.8	81.8	70.4	47.8	36.5	35.0	34.2
Maryland	41.9	24.1	59.5	69.6	83.2	69.3	41.1	26.5	22.7	22.3
Michigan	46.7	38.9	70.3	69.7	80.6	70.7	42.3	26.7	27.0	26.2
Missouri	46.6	40.0	71.6	70.3	84.6	69.1	38.4	25.9	25.7	24.9
Montana	35.8	30.8	48.0	47.5	67.5	54.2	30.1	19.8	20.3	19.8
Nebraska	36.3	25.5	70.9	72.1	75.1	58.3	29.6	20.9	23.4	26.1
Nevada	40.7	23.0	53.5	61.3	68.8	53.7	35.7	30.2	30.1	28.5
New Hampshire	28.1	26.4	51.0	57.1	73.6	54.3	26.6	13.5	11.5	11.3
New Mexico	55.9	34.2	54.9	66.1	77.8	66.7	48.8	43.0	43.0	42.6
New York	48.0	30.1	69.7	68.9	81.0	72.4	51.2	33.8	30.4	30.2
North Carolina	49.1	34.8	69.3	73.5	83.0	69.9	43.9	31.1	27.1	29.1
North Dakota	31.6	23.8	74.2	46.8	73.1	50.5	24.6	15.1	21.4	20.9
Ohio	42.8	35.9	69.5	64.9	79.7	65.6	36.4	23.3	21.2	21.7
Oklahoma	53.9	45.2	69.6	75.5	83.1	69.6	44.0	35.5	34.8	35.6
Oregon	45.7	37.2	61.2	77.3	82.0	67.9	43.3	30.1	28.8	28.8
Pennsylvania	39.9	29.2	68.0	73.4	78.4	64.3	36.3	22.6	20.9	22.6
South Carolina	53.9	39.9	76.7	68.4	84.7	73.3	47.3	33.5	32.0	30.7
South Dakota	40.0	28.5	60.1	62.5	78.2	62.1	31.5	23.1	23.2	26.1
Tennessee	49.2	43.3	62.0	68.7	79.7	66.3	42.3	30.1	28.1	28.5
Texas	53.5	29.5	62.8	71.8	80.8	69.6	48.2	37.5	36.5	36.5
Utah	28.3	21.5	57.0	58.2	65.2	40.2	24.1	19.4	19.8	20.4
Vermont	42.9	42.7	73.2	38.0	82.6	71.9	42.7	24.5	18.3	19.7
Washington	41.5	32.2	56.8	73.8	79.5	63.9	39.3	26.8	24.5	23.9
Wisconsin	37.2	26.6	75.2	71.2	79.9	62.8	31.9	20.8	20.7	21.2
Wyoming	34.4	30.0	52.5	55.1	69.4	47.8	27.1	20.8	17.7	19.1
Puerto Rico	87.1	NA	NA	87.5	95.1	93.3	87.3	75.6	68.9	69.0

NA = Not available.
[1] Race and Hispanic origin are reported separately on birth certificates. Persons of Hispanic origin may be of any race. Multiple-race data, when reported, were bridged to single-race categories in order to maintain comparability among all reported areas.
[2] Includes all persons of Hispanic origin of any race.
[3] Excludes data for Puerto Rico.

Table 1-59. Pregnancy Resulted from Infertility Therapy, by Race and Hispanic Origin, and Age of Mother, 36 States, the District of Columbia, and Puerto Rico, 2011

(Percent.)

Reporting area	Race and Hispanic origin of mother				Age of mother in years					
	Total	Non-Hispanic White[1]	Non-Hispanic Black[1]	Hispanic[2]	Under 20 years	20 to 24 years	25 to 29 years	30 to 34 years	35 to 39 years	40 to 54 years
Total[3]	1.4	2.0	0.4	0.4	0.0	0.2	0.9	1.9	3.2	6.8
California	1.0	1.9	0.4	0.3	*	0.1	0.4	1.1	2.2	6.4
Colorado	1.8	2.4	*	0.5	*	0.2	1.0	2.3	3.9	10.9
Delaware	2.2	3.1	*	*	*	0.1	1.5	3.8	4.7	9.3
District of Columbia	2.7	7.9	*	*	*	*	*	2.4	6.6	17.1
Florida	0.6	1.0	0.2	0.4	*	0.1	0.3	1.0	1.6	3.3
Georgia	1.0	1.7	0.3	0.4	*	0.1	0.6	1.6	2.9	6.0
Idaho	1.2	1.4	*	*	*	0.3	1.1	1.8	2.7	7.5
Illinois	2.5	3.7	0.5	0.7	*	0.2	1.5	3.4	5.7	11.5
Indiana	0.9	1.1	0.2	*	*	0.2	0.8	1.6	2.1	2.9
Iowa	2.5	2.8	*	0.7	*	0.3	2.3	4.0	5.0	9.7
Kansas	1.2	1.5	*	0.3	*	*	1.1	2.1	3.0	3.9
Kentucky	0.8	0.9	*	*	*	0.1	0.8	1.3	1.9	4.5
Louisiana	0.5	0.9	0.2	*	*	*	0.5	1.2	1.3	3.5
Maryland	3.7	5.4	1.8	1.3	*	0.6	2.2	4.7	8.0	13.8
Michigan	1.1	1.3	0.2	0.5	*	0.1	0.9	1.6	2.5	4.4
Missouri	1.1	1.3	0.2	*	*	0.2	0.9	1.9	2.8	4.2
Montana	1.1	1.2	*	*	*	*	0.6	2.0	2.6	*
Nebraska	1.2	1.6	*	*	*	*	1.1	1.9	2.7	*
Nevada	1.5	2.4	*	0.6	*	0.3	1.0	2.0	3.8	*
New Hampshire	2.2	2.2	*	*	*	*	1.1	2.9	4.9	*
New Mexico	0.3	0.6	*	*	*	*	0.2	0.6	*	*
New York	1.6	3.3	0.8	0.6	*	0.3	1.1	2.6	4.2	8.8
North Carolina	0.9	1.3	0.3	0.3	*	0.1	0.6	1.4	2.1	4.6
North Dakota	1.5	1.8	*	*	*	*	1.1	2.7	3.4	*
Ohio	1.7	2.0	0.4	0.7	*	0.2	1.4	2.8	4.2	7.6
Oklahoma	0.8	1.1	*	*	*	*	0.8	1.4	2.2	4.3
Oregon	1.9	2.3	*	0.6	*	*	1.2	2.6	4.5	9.5
Pennsylvania	1.8	2.3	0.4	0.6	*	0.2	1.2	2.6	4.3	8.0
South Carolina	0.7	1.1	0.2	*	*	*	0.5	1.3	2.2	3.7
South Dakota	1.4	1.8	*	*	*	0.5	1.4	2.1	2.6	*
Tennessee	0.8	1.1	0.1	*	*	0.1	0.7	1.5	2.2	4.3
Texas	0.8	1.5	0.3	0.3	*	0.1	0.5	1.3	2.0	4.9
Utah	4.9	5.6	*	2.1	*	2.5	5.4	6.0	7.4	10.4
Vermont	2.0	2.1	*	*	*	*	1.0	2.3	5.4	*
Washington	1.2	1.4	0.4	0.5	*	0.1	0.7	1.6	2.8	7.4
Wisconsin	2.0	2.4	0.4	0.7	*	0.2	1.6	3.0	4.3	6.9
Wyoming	1.0	1.2	*	*	*	*	0.9	1.7	*	*
Puerto Rico	0.4	NA	NA	*	*	*	0.2	0.7	2.1	*

NA = Not available.
* = Figure does not meet standards of reliability or precision.
0.0 = Quantity more than zero but less than 0.05.
[1]Race and Hispanic origin are reported separately on birth certificates. Persons of Hispanic origin may be of any race. Multiple-race data, when reported, were bridged to single-race categories in order to maintain comparability among all reported areas.
[2]Includes all persons of Hispanic origin of any race.
[3]Excludes data for Puerto Rico.

Table 1-60. Principal Source of Payment for the Delivery, 36 States, the District of Columbia, and Puerto Rico, 2011

(Percent.)

Reporting area	All births	Medicaid	Private insurance	Self-pay[1]	Other
Total[2]	100.0	44.9	46.1	4.2	4.8
California...	100.0	46.9	46.5	2.1	4.5
Colorado	100.0	35.9	52.8	3.5	7.8
Delaware	100.0	49.2	46.5	1.4	2.9
District of Columbia	100.0	46.1	41.8	0.6	11.6
Florida..	100.0	49.8	38.9	8.6	2.6
Georgia	100.0	47.3	35.1	5.1	12.6
Idaho..	100.0	39.3	48.0	8.2	4.5
Illinois..	100.0	49.0	48.8	1.0	1.2
Indiana...	100.0	46.0	48.0	4.5	1.5
Iowa...	100.0	38.6	57.2	3.0	1.2
Kansas	100.0	33.8	50.8	7.2	8.2
Kentucky	100.0	43.7	43.9	2.8	9.5
Louisiana	100.0	64.2	32.3	0.9	2.7
Maryland	100.0	30.6	59.6	3.7	6.0
Michigan	100.0	45.0	53.1	1.3	0.5
Missouri..	100.0	45.0	49.8	3.1	2.1
Montana..	100.0	35.4	46.6	7.1	10.9
Nebraska	100.0	30.7	58.9	6.8	3.6
Nevada	100.0	32.7	47.6	14.5	5.2
New Hampshire..	100.0	31.1	63.7	2.1	3.0
New Mexico	100.0	58.2	23.9	6.9	11.1
New York...	100.0	45.6	48.8	1.6	4.0
North Carolina..	100.0	45.8	44.7	6.9	2.6
North Dakota..	100.0	28.8	56.6	3.1	11.6
Ohio..	100.0	40.5	49.8	4.9	4.7
Oklahoma...	100.0	54.8	33.9	2.2	9.1
Oregon	100.0	45.5	50.8	2.2	1.5
Pennsylvania..	100.0	32.7	59.5	5.1	2.8
South Carolina	100.0	51.0	38.6	5.1	5.3
South Dakota	100.0	35.4	56.0	2.2	6.4
Tennessee	100.0	53.8	41.8	1.8	2.6
Texas..	100.0	47.9	36.6	7.8	7.7
Utah..	100.0	29.4	60.8	6.0	3.8
Vermont..	100.0	45.9	49.4	1.7	3.0
Washington...	100.0	39.7	49.2	1.2	9.9
Wisconsin	100.0	38.9	54.1	2.9	4.1
Wyoming	100.0	37.6	51.9	5.8	4.7
Puerto Rico...	100.0	73.4	25.5	1.1	*

* = Figure does not meet standards of reliability or precision; based on fewer than 20 births in the numerator.
[1] No third-party payer listed; uninsured.
[2] Excludes data for Puerto Rico.

NOTES AND DEFINITIONS

Sources of Data

The tables in Part 1 are from the National Center for Health Statistics (NCHS), a component of the Centers for Disease Control and Prevention (CDC). Several different publications were used to obtain the data.

Most of the tables found in Part 1 were obtained from Martin JA, Hamilton BE, Osterman MJK, et al. *Births: Final Data for 2015*. National vital statistics report; vol 66, no 1. Hyattsville, MD: National Center for Health Statistics. 2017.

Some data for the year 2014 was derived from Hamilton BE, Martin JA, Osterman MJK, et al. *Births: Final Data for 2014*. National vital statistics reports; vol 64 no 12. Hyattsville, MD: National Center for Health Statistics. 2015.

Data for Tables 1-55 through 1-60 were obtained from Osterman MJK, Martin JA, Curtin, SC, et al. *Newly Released Data from the Revised U.S. Birth Certificate, 2011*. National Vital Statistics Reports: Volume 62, No 4. Hyattsville, MD: National Center for Health Statistics, 2013. Some data was also derived from Osterman MJK, Martin JA, Mathews TJ, Hamilton BE. *Expanded Data From The New Birth Certificate, 2008*. National Vital Statistics Reports: Volume 59, No 7. Hyattsville, MD: National Center for Health Statistics. July 2011.

Some data for tables relating to teenagers were derived from Abma JC, Martinez GM. *Sexual Activity and Contraceptive Use Among Teenagers in the United States, 2011–2015*. National Health Statistics Reports; no 104. Hyattsville, MD: National Center for Health Statistics. 2017. Data were also collected from Martinez G, Copen, CE, Abma, JC. *Teenagers in the United States: Sexual Activity, Contraceptive Use, and Childbearing, 2006–2010 National Survey of Family Growth*. National Center for Health Statistics. Vital Health Stat 23 (31). 2011.

Notes on the Data

Race and Hispanic origin are noted separately on birth certificates. Some rates for 2001 through 2009 have been revised using new population estimates that are based on the 2010 census; thus, these rates may differ from those previously published. Population estimates are generally for July 1 of the year shown.

Concepts and Definitions

Anencephaly—A congenital anomaly that consists of a partial or complete absence of the brain and skull.

Apgar score—This has been employed for over 50 years to assess the physical condition and short term prognosis of newborns. Historically, the score has been measured at 1 minute, 5 minutes, and if needed, at additional 5-minute intervals after delivery. Information on the 5 minute score is included in national birth certificate data. The Apgar score measures five easily identifiable characteristics of newborns. A 5-minute score of 0 to 3 indicates an infant in immediate need of resuscitation; 4 to 6 is considered intermediate, and 7 to 10 is considered normal. The Apgar score is a useful clinical indicator for reporting overall status of the neonate and need for, and response to resuscitation efforts.

Birth cohort—Consists of all persons born within a given period of time, such as a calendar year.

Birthweight—The first weight of the newborn obtained after birth. Low birthweight is defined as less than 2,500 grams or 5 pounds 8 ounces. Very low birthweight is defined as less than 1,500 grams or 3 pounds 4 ounces. Before 1979, low birthweight was defined as weighing 2,500 grams or less, and very low birthweight was defined as 1,500 grams or less. Equivalents of the gram weights in terms of pounds and ounces are as follows:

Less than 500 grams = 1 oz or less
500–999 grams = 2 oz–2 lb 3 oz
3 oz1,000–1,499 grams = 4 oz–3 lb 4 oz
1,500–1,999 grams = 5 oz–4 lb 6 oz
2,000–2,499 grams = 7 oz–5 lb 8 oz
2,500–2,999 grams = 9 oz–6 lb 9 oz
3,000–3,499 grams = 10 oz–7 lb 11 oz
3,500–3,999 grams = 12 oz–8 lb 13 oz
4,000–4,499 grams = 14 oz–9 lb 14 oz
4,500–4,999 grams = 15 oz–11 lb 0 oz
5,000 grams or more = 11lb 1oz or more

Birth rate—Calculated by dividing the number of live births in a population in a year by the midyear resident population. Birth rates are expressed as the number of live births per 1,000 population. The rate may be restricted to births to women of specific age, race, marital status, or geographic location (specific rate), or it may be related to the entire population (crude rate).

Breech/malpresentation—Presenting part of the fetus listed as breech, complete breech, frank breech, footling breech.

Cervical cerclage—Circumferential banding or suture of the cervix to prevent or treat early dilation of the cervix (e.g., incompetent cervix) in an attempt to avoid premature delivery.

Cleft lip/palate—Incomplete closure of the lip. May be unilateral, bilateral, or median. Cleft palate is incomplete fusion of the palatal shelves. May be limited to the soft palate, or may extend into the hard palate.

Contraception—The National Survey of Family Growth collects information on contraceptive use reported by women 15–44 years old. For current contraceptive use, women were asked about contraceptive use during the month of interview. Women were classified by whether they reported using any of the 19 methods of contraception at any time in the month of interview.

Cyanotic heart disease—Congenital heart defects resulting in lack of oxygen that cause cyanosis.

Down syndrome—The most common chromosomal defect (trisomy 21).

Fertility rate—Total number of live births per 1,000 women of reproductive age (defined as women age 15 to 44 years).

Gestation—The time period between the first day of the last normal menstrual period and the day of birth or day of termination of pregnancy according to the National Vital Statistics System and the CDC's Abortion Surveillance.

Hispanic origin—Includes persons of Mexican, Puerto Rican, Cuban, Central and South American, and other or unknown Latin American or Spanish origins. Persons of Hispanic origin may be of any race.

Hypertension, chronic—Diagnosis prior to the onset of this pregnancy of elevated blood pressure above normal for age, gender, and physiological condition.

Hypertension, pregnancy-associated—Diagnosis in pregnancy of elevated blood pressure above normal for age, gender, and physiological condition.

Induction of labor—Initiation of uterine contractions by medical and/or surgical means for the purpose of delivery before the spontaneous onset of labor.

Maternal morbidities—Information on six maternal morbidities is collected on the 2003 revised birth certificate: maternal transfusion, third-or fourth-degree perineal laceration, ruptured uterus, unplanned hysterectomy, admission to intensive care unit, and unplanned operating room procedure. More than one morbidity may be reported. Maternal morbidity data are not available for Delaware for 2011 because of concerns with data quality.

Meconium, moderate/heavy—Staining of the amniotic fluid caused by passage of fetal bowel contents during labor and/or at delivery that is more than enough to cause a greenish color change of an otherwise clear fluid.

Meningomyecele/Spina bifida—Meningomyelocele is herniation of meninges and spinal cord tissue. Meningocele (herniation of meninges without spinal cord tissue) should also be included in this category. Both open and closed (covered with skin) lesions should be included. Spina bifida is herniation of the meninges and/or spinal cord tissue through a bony defect of spine closure.

Nonvertex presentation—Includes any nonvertex fetal presentation, that is, presentation of a part of the infant's body other than the upper and back part of the infant's head.

Omphalocele/Gastroschisis—Omphalocele is a defect in the anterior abdominal wall, accompanied by herniation of some abdominal organs through a widened umbilical ring into the umbilical stalk. Gastroschisis is an abnormality of the anterior abdominal wall, lateral to the umbilicus, resulting in herniation of the abdominal contents directly into the amniotic cavity.

Precipitous labor—Labor lasting less than 3 hours.

Prenatal care—Medical care provided to a pregnant woman to prevent complications and decrease the incidence of maternal and prenatal mortality. Information on when pregnancy care began is recorded on the birth certificate. Between 1970 and 1980, the reporting area for prenatal care expanded. In 1970, 39 states and the District of Columbia (D.C.) reported prenatal care on the birth certificate. Data were not available from Alabama, Alaska, Arkansas, Connecticut, Delaware, Georgia, Idaho, Massachusetts, New Mexico, Pennsylvania, and Virginia. In 1975, these data were available from three additional states—Connecticut, Delaware, and Georgia—increasing the number of states reporting prenatal care to 42 and D.C. During 1980–2002, prenatal care information was available for the entire United States.

Prepregnancy BMI—The 2003 Standard Certificate of Live Birth includes the components needed to compute both prepregnancy BMI and maternal weight gain (i.e., maternal height, prepregnancy weight, and weight at delivery). BMI is calculated as weight in kilograms divided by height in meters squared (kg/m^2).

Suspected chromosomal disorder—Includes any constellation of congenital malformations resulting from, or compatible with, known syndromes caused by detectable defects in chromosome structure.

Tocolysis—Administration of any agent with the intent to inhibit preterm uterine contractions to extend the length of the pregnancy.

WIC Program—The WIC program is run by the U.S. Department of Agriculture. It is intended to help low-income pregnant women, infants, and children through age 5 years receive proper nutrition by providing vouchers for food, nutrition counseling, health care screenings, and referrals.

PART II: MORTALITY

PART II: MORTALITY

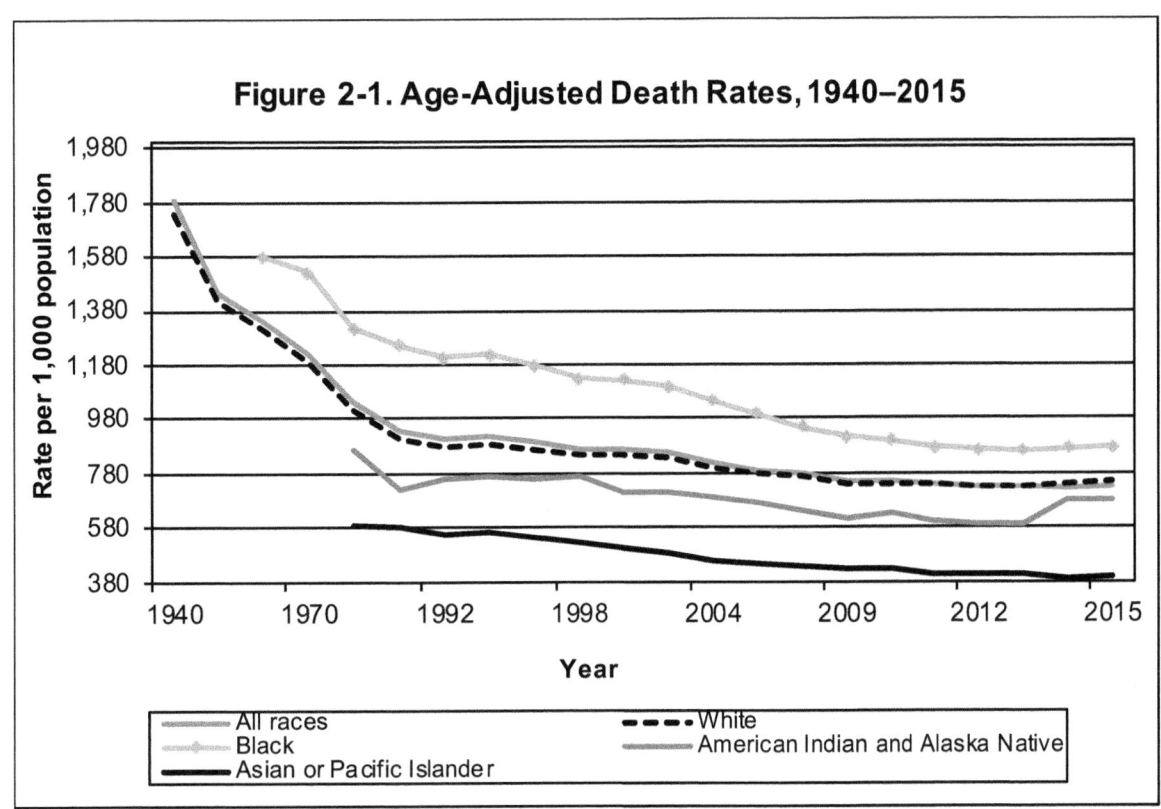

Figure 2-1. Age-Adjusted Death Rates, 1940–2015

HIGHLIGHTS

- In 2015, 2,712,630 deaths were registered in the United States. The age-adjusted death rate rose for the first time from one year to the next, increasing from 724.6 per 100,000 standard population in 2014 to 733.1 in 2015. Among all states, Mississippi had the highest age-adjusted death rate at 963.7, while Hawaii had the lowest age-adjusted death rate at 588.2. (Tables 2-1 and 2-31)

- Hispanics had the highest life expectancy of all races and ethnic origins at 82.0 years in 2015. Life expectancy remained at 78.8 years for the population as a whole. (Table 2-5)

- The infant mortality rate declined to 5.9 deaths per 1,000 live births in 2015, down from rates of 6.6 in 2008 and 6.4 in 2009. The neonatal mortality rate also declined, falling from 4.3 in 2008 to 3.9 in 3015). The postneonatal mortality rate declined from 2.3 in 2008 to 2.0 in 2015. (Table 2-39)

Table 2-1. Number of Deaths, Death Rates, and Age-Adjusted Death Rates, by Race, Hispanic Origin, and Sex, Selected Years, 1940–2015

(Number, rate per 100,000 population.)

Year	Total[1] Both sexes	Male	Female	Non-Hispanic White[2] Both sexes	Male	Female	Non-Hispanic Black[2] Both sexes	Male	Female
Number									
1940..................................	1,417,269	781,003	626,266	NA	NA	NA	NA	NA	NA
1950..................................	1,452,454	827,749	624,705	NA	NA	NA	NA	NA	NA
1960..................................	1,711,982	975,648	736,334	NA	NA	NA	NA	NA	NA
1970..................................	1,921,031	1,078,478	842,553	NA	NA	NA	NA	NA	NA
1980..................................	1,989,841	1,075,078	914,763	NA	NA	NA	NA	NA	NA
1990..................................	2,148,463	1,113,417	1,035,046	NA	NA	NA	NA	NA	NA
2000..................................	2,403,351	177,578	1,225,773	1,959,919	944,781	1,015,138	282,676	143,297	139,379
2010..................................	2,468,435	1,232,432	1,236,003	1,969,916	971,604	998,312	283,438	143,824	139,614
2011..................................	2,515,458	1,254,978	1,260,480	2,006,319	989,835	1,016,484	286,797	145,052	141,745
2012..................................	2,543,279	1,273,722	1,269,557	2,016,896	998,832	1,018,064	291,179	148,344	142,835
2013..................................	2,596,993	1,306,034	1,290,959	2,052,660	1,021,135	1,031,525	299,227	152,661	146,566
2014..................................	2,626,418	1,328,241	1,298,177	2,066,949	1,035,345	1,031,604	303,844	154,836	149,008
2015..................................	2,712,630	1,373,404	1,339,226	2,123,631	1,063,705	1,059,926	315,254	161,850	153,404
Crude Death Rate[5]									
1940..................................	1,076.4	1,197.4	954.6	NA	NA	NA	NA	NA	NA
1950..................................	963.8	1,106.1	823.5	NA	NA	NA	NA	NA	NA
1960..................................	954.7	1,104.5	809.2	NA	NA	NA	NA	NA	NA
1970..................................	945.3	1,090.3	807.8	NA	NA	NA	NA	NA	NA
1980..................................	878.3	976.9	785.3	NA	NA	NA	NA	NA	NA
1990..................................	863.8	918.4	812.0	NA	NA	NA	NA	NA	NA
2000..................................	854.0	853.0	855.0	993.2	978.5	1,007.3	805.5	859.5	756.7
2010..................................	799.5	812.0	787.4	984.3	987.5	981.2	718.7	764.5	676.9
2011..................................	807.3	818.7	796.3	1,001.0	1,004.1	998.1	718.0	760.4	679.2
2012..................................	810.2	824.5	796.4	1,004.9	1,011.2	998.8	720.9	768.5	677.3
2013..................................	821.5	839.1	804.4	1,021.6	1,032.1	1,011.5	733.4	782.5	688.4
2014..................................	823.7	846.4	801.7	1,028.1	1,045.4	1,011.3	735.4	783.3	691.4
2015..................................	844.0	868.0	820.7	1,055.3	1,072.5	1,038.5	754.6	809.4	704.3
Age-Adjusted Death Rate[6]									
1940..................................	1,785.0	1,976.0	1,599.4	NA	NA	NA	NA	NA	NA
1950..................................	1,446.0	1,674.2	1,236.0	NA	NA	NA	NA	NA	NA
1960..................................	1,339.2	1,609.0	1,105.3	NA	NA	NA	NA	NA	NA
1970..................................	1,222.6	1,542.1	971.4	NA	NA	NA	NA	NA	NA
1980..................................	1,039.1	1,348.1	817.9	NA	NA	NA	NA	NA	NA
1990..................................	938.7	1,202.8	750.9	NA	NA	NA	NA	NA	NA
2000..................................	869.0	1,053.8	731.4	855.5	1,035.4	721.5	1,137.0	1,422.0	941.2
2010..................................	747.0	887.1	634.9	755.0	892.5	643.3	920.4	1,131.7	770.8
2011..................................	741.3	875.3	632.4	754.3	887.2	644.6	901.6	1,098.3	759.8
2012..................................	732.8	865.1	624.7	745.8	876.2	637.6	887.1	1,086.4	742.1
2013..................................	731.9	863.6	623.5	747.1	876.8	638.4	885.2	1,083.3	740.6
2014..................................	724.6	855.1	616.7	742.8	872.3	633.8	870.7	1,060.3	731.2
2015..................................	733.1	863.2	624.2	753.2	881.3	644.1	876.1	1,070.1	731.0

Note: Beginning in 1970, excludes deaths of nonresidents of the United States. Data for specified race or Hispanic-origin groups other than non-Hispanic white and non-Hispanic black should be interpreted with caution because of inconsistencies in reporting these items on death certificates and surveys, although misclassification is very minor for the Hispanic and non-Hispanic Asian or Pacific Islander populations.
NA= Not available.
[1]Includes data for origin not stated.
[2]Multiple-race data reported according to 1997 OMB standards were bridged to the single-race categories of 1977 OMB standards.
[5]Per 100,000 population based on populations enumerated as of April 1 for census years and estimated as of July 1 for all other years.
[6]Per 100,000 U.S. standard population.

Table 2-1. Number of Deaths, Death Rates, and Age-Adjusted Death Rates, by Race, Hispanic Origin, and Sex, Selected Years, 1940–2015—*Continued*

(Number, rate per 100,000 population.)

Year	Non-Hispanic American Indian or Alaska Native[2,3]			Non-Hispanic Asian or Pacific Islander[2,4]			Hispanic		
	Both sexes	Male	Female	Both sexes	Male	Female	Both sexes	Male	Female
Number									
1940	NA	NA	NA	NA	NA	NA	NA	NA	NA
1950	NA	NA	NA	NA	NA	NA	NA	NA	NA
1960	NA	NA	NA	NA	NA	NA	NA	NA	NA
1970	NA	NA	NA	NA	NA	NA	NA	NA	NA
1980	NA	NA	NA	NA	NA	NA	NA	NA	NA
1990	NA	NA	NA	NA	NA	NA	NA	NA	NA
2000	11,025	5,973	5,052	34,226	18,653	15,573	107,254	60,172	47,082
2010	14,846	8,072	6,774	50,018	25,938	24,080	144,490	79,622	64,868
2011	15,181	8,175	7,006	52,346	26,909	25,437	149,635	81,887	67,748
2012	15,705	8,598	7,107	55,298	28,214	27,084	156,419	85,238	71,181
2013	16,219	8,840	7,379	58,702	30,343	28,359	163,241	88,880	74,361
2014	17,138	9,338	7,800	60,424	31,039	29,385	169,387	92,474	76,913
2015	18,039	9,869	8,170	65,277	33,306	31,971	179,457	98,170	81,287
Crude Death Rate[5]									
1940	NA	NA	NA	NA	NA	NA	NA	NA	NA
1950	NA	NA	NA	NA	NA	NA	NA	NA	NA
1960	NA	NA	NA	NA	NA	NA	NA	NA	NA
1970	NA	NA	NA	NA	NA	NA	NA	NA	NA
1980	NA	NA	NA	NA	NA	NA	NA	NA	NA
1990	NA	NA	NA	NA	NA	NA	NA	NA	NA
2000	470.3	517.0	425.0	301.4	338.3	266.5	303.8	331.3	274.6
2010	577.8	640.1	517.7	310.0	336.7	285.6	286.2	310.8	260.9
2011	584.2	640.9	529.5	315.7	339.9	293.7	287.5	309.7	264.6
2012	599.3	668.7	532.5	322.0	344.1	301.7	295.0	316.5	272.7
2013	613.7	681.4	548.3	331.8	359.2	306.7	301.9	323.7	279.4
2014	642.5	713.4	574.2	327.7	352.7	305.0	305.8	330.1	281.0
2015	670.7	747.4	596.7	341.5	364.9	320.1	317.1	343.2	290.4
Age-Adjusted Death Rate[6]									
1940	NA	NA	NA	NA	NA	NA	NA	NA	NA
1950	NA	NA	NA	NA	NA	NA	NA	NA	NA
1960	NA	NA	NA	NA	NA	NA	NA	NA	NA
1970	NA	NA	NA	NA	NA	NA	NA	NA	NA
1980	NA	NA	NA	NA	NA	NA	NA	NA	NA
1990	NA	NA	NA	NA	NA	NA	NA	NA	NA
2000	800.5	955.6	679.1	507.0	624.9	417.3	665.7	818.1	546.0
2010	818.8	965.8	696.8	425.6	513.0	360.6	558.6	677.7	463.4
2011	798.1	933.8	684.7	413.2	493.4	352.8	540.7	647.3	452.8
2012	787.8	929.9	666.3	409.6	486.3	351.4	539.1	643.9	452.5
2013	787.5	930.6	666.4	407.5	490.2	344.8	535.4	639.8	448.6
2014	796.9	935.0	677.4	390.5	464.2	333.3	523.3	626.8	437.5
2015	805.7	950.2	679.5	396.2	468.9	339.6	525.3	628.9	438.3

Note: Beginning in 1970, excludes deaths of nonresidents of the United States. Data for specified race or Hispanic-origin groups other than non-Hispanic white and non-Hispanic black should be interpreted with caution because of inconsistencies in reporting these items on death certificates and surveys, although misclassification is very minor for the Hispanic and non-Hispanic Asian or Pacific Islander populations.
NA= Not available.
[2]Multiple-race data reported according to 1997 OMB standards were bridged to the single-race categories of 1977 OMB standards.
[3]Includes Aleuts and Eskimos.
[4]Includes Chinese, Filipinos, Hawaiians, Japanese, and other Asian or Pacific Islander persons.
[5]Per 100,000 population based on populations enumerated as of April 1 for census years and estimated as of July 1 for all other years.
[6]Per 100,000 U.S. standard population.

Table 2-2. Number of Deaths and Death Rates, by Age, Race, and Sex, 2015

(Number, rate per 100,000 population in specified group.)

Year	Total[1]			Non-Hispanic White[2]			Non-Hispanic Black[2]		
	Both sexes	Male	Female	Both sexes	Male	Female	Both sexes	Male	Female
Number									
All ages	2,712,630	1,373,404	1,339,226	2,123,631	1,063,705	1,059,926	315,254	161,850	153,404
Under 1 year	23,455	13,008	10,447	10,277	5,758	4,519	6,907	3,815	3,092
1 to 4 years	3,965	2,281	1,684	1,895	1,083	812	1,016	608	408
5 to 9 years	2,402	1,377	1,025	1,192	669	523	553	317	236
10 to 14 years	3,009	1,776	1,233	1,643	965	678	634	386	248
15 to 19 years	10,186	7,187	2,999	5,456	3,692	1,764	2,336	1,795	541
20 to 24 years	20,308	15,159	5,149	11,080	8,061	3,019	4,760	3,691	1,069
25 to 29 years	23,898	17,173	6,725	14,349	10,097	4,252	5,006	3,680	1,326
30 to 34 years	27,619	18,608	9,011	17,143	11,499	5,644	5,310	3,549	1,761
35 to 39 years	31,417	20,190	11,227	19,392	12,398	6,994	6,273	3,942	2,331
40 to 44 years	41,671	25,480	16,191	26,245	16,039	10,206	8,029	4,668	3,361
45 to 49 years	64,377	38,807	25,570	42,315	25,542	16,773	11,774	6,686	5,088
50 to 54 years	110,117	66,740	43,377	76,263	46,369	29,894	19,398	11,126	8,272
55 to 59 years	159,589	97,172	62,417	113,442	69,459	43,983	28,015	16,180	11,835
60 to 64 years	198,196	120,454	77,742	144,070	88,164	55,906	32,871	19,263	13,608
65 to 69 years	235,482	137,630	97,852	179,608	105,474	74,134	32,541	18,438	14,103
70 to 74 years	259,534	144,717	114,817	204,486	114,786	89,700	30,777	16,429	14,348
75 to 79 years	290,405	153,719	136,686	232,080	123,883	108,197	30,976	15,455	15,521
80 to 84 years	347,161	170,127	177,034	285,606	141,645	143,961	30,485	13,485	17,000
85 years and over	859,701	321,704	537,997	737,032	278,085	458,947	57,576	18,325	39,251
Not stated	138	95	43	57	37	20	17	12	5
Rate									
All ages	844.0	868.0	820.7	1,055.3	1,072.5	1,038.5	754.6	809.4	704.3
Under 1 year[6]	589.6	639.2	537.7	494.6	541.1	445.7	1,123.1	1,215.0	1,027.3
1 to 4 years	24.9	38.0	21.6	22.9	25.5	20.1	41.6	48.9	34.0
5 to 9 years	11.7	13.2	10.2	11.1	12.1	10.0	17.7	20.0	15.4
10 to 14 years	14.6	16.9	12.2	14.6	16.7	12.4	20.7	24.9	16.4
15 to 19 years	48.3	66.6	29.1	46.2	61.0	30.7	72.8	110.1	34.2
20 to 24 years	89.3	129.9	46.5	87.2	123.6	48.8	133.0	203.3	60.7
25 to 29 years	106.4	150.5	60.8	111.6	154.7	67.2	154.6	230.1	80.9
30 to 34 years	127.4	170.9	83.5	136.7	181.9	90.8	185.5	258.2	118.4
35 to 39 years	154.2	198.5	110.1	165.0	209.4	119.9	233.6	310.1	164.9
40 to 44 years	206.1	254.0	159.0	218.8	266.3	170.9	307.2	380.5	242.4
45 to 49 years	308.7	375.5	243.1	320.2	386.4	253.9	446.6	539.0	364.5
50 to 54 years	493.0	608.7	381.5	504.2	619.1	391.5	703.1	861.7	563.6
55 to 59 years	731.8	916.9	556.8	733.0	913.5	558.7	1,078.9	1,347.6	847.8
60 to 64 years	1,039.3	1,321.2	781.1	1,025.1	1,293.8	772.2	1,571.1	2,052.3	1,179.6
65 to 69 years	1,465.6	1,811.8	1,155.1	1,464.5	1,790.6	1,163.1	2,069.7	2,684.5	1,592.8
70 to 74 years	2,260.1	2,732.5	1,855.8	2,286.1	2,736.6	1,888.3	2,964.9	3,780.6	2,377.6
75 to 79 years	3,754.7	4,257.1	3,028.8	3,655.3	4,316.7	3,109.8	4,311.4	5,424.0	3,580.2
80 to 84 years	5,986.2	7,051.4	5,227.4	6,176.9	7,236.0	5,399.3	6,427.4	7,879.9	5,607.5
85 years and over	13,673.9	14,795.8	13,080.8	14,324.3	15,526.0	13,682.6	12,364.4	13,344.0	11,954.7

Note: Beginning in 1970, excludes deaths of nonresidents of the United States. Data for specified race or Hispanic-origin groups other than non-Hispanic white and non-Hispanic black should be interpreted with caution because of inconsistencies in reporting these items on death certificates and surveys, although misclassification is very minor for the Hispanic and non-Hispanic Asian or Pacific Islander populations.
[1]Includes data for origin not stated.
[2]Multiple-race data reported according to 1997 OMB standards were bridged to the single-race categories of 1977 OMB standards.
[6]Death rates for "Under 1 year" (based on population estimates) differ from infant mortality rates (based on live births).

Table 2-2. Number of Deaths and Death Rates, by Age, Race, and Sex, 2015—*Continued*

(Number, rate per 100,000 population in specified group.)

Year	Non-Hispanic American Indian or Alaska Native[2,3]			Non-Hispanic Asian or Pacific Islander[2,4]			Hispanic		
	Both sexes	Male	Female	Both sexes	Male	Female	Both sexes	Male	Female
Number									
All ages	18,039	9,869	8,170	65,277	33,306	31,971	179,457	98,170	81,287
Under 1 year	300	161	139	892	501	391	4,805	2,619	2,186
1 to 4 years...............................	82	45	37	141	72	69	815	461	354
5 to 9 years...............................	47	28	19	108	58	50	495	301	194
10 to 14 years............................	52	23	29	104	66	38	568	332	236
15 to 19 years............................	174	112	62	321	225	96	1,868	1,341	527
20 to 24 years............................	351	250	101	552	405	147	3,485	2,698	787
25 to 29 years............................	454	317	137	610	435	175	3,396	2,592	804
30 to 34 years............................	543	345	198	722	452	270	3,786	2,676	1,110
35 to 39 years............................	589	370	219	824	503	321	4,202	2,890	1,312
40 to 44 years............................	688	439	249	1,223	709	514	5,288	3,495	1,793
45 to 49 years............................	997	609	388	1,763	1,032	731	7,159	4,672	2,487
50 to 54 years............................	1,368	812	556	2,449	1,429	1,020	10,030	6,558	3,472
55 to 59 years............................	1,628	995	633	3,462	2,067	1,395	12,128	7,826	4,302
60 to 64 years............................	1,700	987	713	4,547	2,679	1,868	13,859	8,540	5,319
65 to 69 years............................	1,727	946	781	5,463	3,152	2,311	14,920	8,776	6,144
70 to 74 years............................	1,771	962	809	6,033	3,347	2,686	15,355	8,477	6,878
75 to 79 years............................	1,692	888	804	7,323	3,934	3,389	17,242	8,926	8,316
80 to 84 years............................	1,532	705	827	8,592	4,171	4,421	19,847	9,557	10,290
85 years and over	2,344	875	1,469	20,147	8,069	12,078	40,203	15,428	24,775
Not stated	–	–	–	1	–	1	6	5	1
Rate									
All ages	670.7	747.4	596.7	341.5	364.9	320.1	317.1	343.2	290.4
Under 1 year[5]	732.6	771.9	691.8	405.5	444.1	364.9	469.2	500.4	436.6
1 to 4 years...............................	51.2	55.2	47.0	15.3	15.3	15.4	19.8	22.0	17.5
5 to 9 years...............................	22.8	26.9	*	9.2	9.8	8.7	9.5	11.3	7.6
10 to 14 years............................	25.4	22.2	28.7	8.8	11.2	6.5	11.5	13.3	9.7
15 to 19 years............................	82.4	104.5	59.6	27.4	38.0	16.6	39.6	55.6	22.9
20 to 24 years............................	153.8	214.8	90.3	39.2	56.7	21.2	72.4	108.0	34.0
25 to 29 years............................	219.7	303.7	133.9	37.5	54.7	21.0	74.9	108.7	37.5
30 to 34 years............................	296.0	380.3	213.4	44.1	58.3	31.4	85.0	115.1	52.2
35 to 39 years............................	354.2	450.8	260.0	54.0	70.5	39.5	99.0	132.2	63.8
40 to 44 years............................	430.0	560.3	305.0	80.8	99.9	63.9	134.5	175.4	92.4
45 to 49 years............................	609.4	766.2	461.3	131.4	164.3	102.5	204.8	262.9	144.7
50 to 54 years............................	760.1	940.7	593.7	199.7	249.6	156.0	329.5	430.3	228.4
55 to 59 years............................	956.6	1,242.4	702.6	311.0	404.0	231.9	494.7	651.1	344.2
60 to 64 years............................	1,235.8	1,532.5	974.6	479.7	629.6	357.6	753.9	976.4	551.9
65 to 69 years............................	1,627.1	1,891.8	1,391.2	712.2	920.3	544.3	1,099.0	1,401.2	840.2
70 to 74 years............................	2,578.8	3,032.6	2,189.2	1,166.9	1,446.7	940.3	1,678.8	2,097.7	1,347.2
75 to 79 years............................	3,794.0	4,501.4	3,232.8	2,001.1	2,414.7	1,669.3	2,670.2	3,264.0	2,234.0
80 to 84 years............................	5,770.0	6,503.1	5,264.2	3,592.7	4,221.3	3,150.2	4,556.7	5,480.7	3,939.8
85 years and over	9,792.4	10,272.4	9,527.2	8,653.4	9,459.6	8,187.2	9,585.2	10,145.7	9,266.4

Note: Beginning in 1970, excludes deaths of nonresidents of the United States. Data for specified race or Hispanic-origin groups other than non-Hispanic white and non-Hispanic black should be interpreted with caution because of inconsistencies in reporting these items on death certificates and surveys, although misclassification is very minor for the Hispanic and non-Hispanic Asian or Pacific Islander populations.

– = Quantity zero.

* = Figure does not meet standards of reliability or precision.

[2] Multiple-race data reported according to 1997 OMB standards were bridged to the single-race categories of 1977 OMB standards.

[3] Includes Aleuts and Eskimos.

[4] Includes Chinese, Filipinos, Hawaiians, Japanese, and other Asian or Pacific Islander persons.

[5] Death rates for "Under 1 year" (based on population estimates) differ from infant mortality rates (based on live births).

Table 2-3. Number of Deaths and Death Rates, by Age, and Age-Adjusted Death Rates, by Specified Hispanic Origin and Sex, 2015

(Number, rate per 100,000 population in specified group.)

Origin, race, and sex	All ages	Under 1 year[1]	1 to 4 years	5 to 14 years	15 to 24 years	25 to 34 years	35 to 44 years	45 to 54 years	55 to 64 years	65 to 74 years	75 to 84 years	85 years and over	Age not stated	Age-adjusted rate[2]
NUMBER														
Hispanic	179,457	4,805	815	1,063	5,353	7,182	9,490	17,189	25,987	30,275	37,089	40,203	6	X
Male	98,170	2,619	461	633	4,039	5,268	6,385	11,230	16,366	17,253	18,483	15,428	5	X
Female	81,287	2,186	354	430	1,314	1,914	3,105	5,959	9,621	13,022	18,606	24,775	1	X
Mexican	101,288	3,196	555	722	3,547	4,521	5,939	10,463	15,462	17,171	19,599	20,110	3	X
Male	56,952	1,749	329	431	2,687	3,314	3,994	6,862	9,831	9,816	9,854	8,082	3	X
Female	44,336	1,447	226	291	860	1,207	1,945	3,601	5,631	7,355	9,745	12,028	-	X
Puerto Rican	23,115	481	77	104	560	807	1,175	2,307	3,621	4,369	4,909	4,704	1	X
Male	12,449	265	39	61	414	565	789	1,515	2,237	2,494	2,385	1,685	-	X
Female	10,666	216	38	43	146	242	386	792	1,384	1,875	2,524	3,019	1	X
Cuban	15,826	94	9	19	134	177	239	756	1,393	2,198	4,486	6,319	2	X
Male	8,163	43	5	13	100	134	171	513	943	1,350	2,378	2,511	2	X
Female	7,663	51	4	6	34	43	68	243	450	848	2,108	3,808	-	X
Central and South American	16,840	438	68	112	545	803	1,024	1,662	2,270	2,827	3,331	3,760	-	X
Male	8,671	236	39	63	422	620	717	1,056	1,356	1,467	1,503	1,192	-	X
Female	8,169	202	29	49	123	183	307	606	914	1,360	1,828	2,568	-	X
Dominican	4,288	104	14	20	123	159	193	357	602	721	991	1,004	-	X
Male	2,119	54	7	13	92	119	111	201	339	406	462	315	-	X
Female	2,169	50	7	7	31	40	82	156	263	315	529	689	-	X
Other and unknown Hispanic	18,100	492	92	86	444	715	920	1,644	2,639	2,989	3,773	4,306	-	X
Male	9,816	272	42	52	324	516	603	1,083	1,660	1,720	1,901	1,643	-	X
Female	8,284	220	50	34	120	199	317	561	979	1,269	1,872	2,663	-	X
RATE[3]														
Hispanic	317.1	469.2	19.8	10.5	56.2	79.9	116.1	262.8	605.7	1,332.4	3,430.1	9,585.2	X	525.3
Male	343.2	500.4	22.0	12.2	82.2	111.8	152.8	340.2	788.2	1,674.3	4,127.1	10,145.7	X	628.9
Female	290.4	436.6	17.5	8.6	28.5	44.8	77.7	184.0	434.6	1,048.7	2,937.3	9,266.4	X	438.3
Mexican	283.0	502.2	19.9	10.3	56.2	80.3	115.4	271.4	637.3	1,401.6	3,641.0	9,912.8	X	548.7
Male	312.2	533.9	23.3	12.1	82.9	112.0	150.5	345.3	813.8	1,706.8	4,266.2	10,767.4	X	650.1
Female	252.5	468.6	16.4	8.4	28.0	45.2	78.1	192.7	462.3	1,131.6	3,171.1	9,410.8	X	460.5
Puerto Rican	430.2	533.2	20.1	11.3	61.9	98.8	158.4	365.4	807.5	1,635.0	3,943.0	11,647.9	X	643.0
Male	469.0	579.0	19.3	13.1	88.9	140.2	215.6	489.9	1,057.8	2,141.1	4,419.5	11,443.1	X	752.7
Female	392.3	486.1	21.0	9.4	33.2	58.4	102.6	245.9	584.2	1,243.9	3,578.4	11,765.4	X	547.6
Cuban	751.3	418.9	*	*	52.2	61.5	84.0	230.7	575.1	1,284.3	3,579.6	10,848.1	X	531.6
Male	764.0	332.9	*	*	74.3	88.3	113.5	296.5	779.2	1,722.7	4,625.1	11,574.1	X	656.0
Female	738.2	535.4	*	*	27.9	31.6	50.8	157.2	371.3	914.0	2,852.3	10,417.2	X	428.5
Central and South American	195.5	323.3	12.2	8.7	41.6	54.2	71.0	147.6	318.0	782.3	2,155.2	7,847.2	X	348.7
Male	200.6	352.7	13.7	9.5	61.6	78.0	97.2	192.3	419.1	988.2	2,817.0	8,996.2	X	435.5
Female	190.3	294.6	10.6	8.0	19.7	26.6	43.5	105.0	234.2	638.8	1,806.2	7,408.0	X	291.9
Dominican	228.9	321.5	*	7.2	37.5	52.4	75.8	152.1	355.0	856.2	2,480.3	7,626.3	X	368.2
Male	244.1	354.1	*	*	55.7	83.2	99.0	201.1	467.7	1,104.5	3,252.4	*	X	457.5
Female	215.8	292.4	*	*	19.0	25.0	57.5	115.8	270.8	663.9	2,054.4	7,349.3	X	309.9
Other and unknown Hispanic	662.5	1,203.1	53.9	20.1	96.2	186.0	267.4	500.0	967.9	1,729.7	4,283.6	10,702.1	X	728.7
Male	715.5	1,265.1	47.5	23.1	131.8	256.9	343.7	666.3	1,300.6	2,276.7	5,501.4	11,041.7	X	904.1
Female	609.0	1,134.3	60.8	16.7	55.7	108.4	188.0	337.5	675.1	1,304.8	3,497.4	10,502.9	X	584.7

Note: Rates are per 100,000 population in specifed group; age-adjusted rates are per 100,000 U.S. standard population. Data for Hispanic origin should be interpreted with caution because of inconsistencies between reporting Hispanic origin on death certifcates and on censuses and surveys.
X = Not applicable.
- = Quantity zero.
* = Figure does not meet standards of reliability or precision.
[1]Death rates for "Under 1 year" (based on population estimates) differ from infant mortality rates (based on live births); see chapter notes for more information.
[2]For method of computation, see chapter notes.
[3]Figures for age not stated are included in "All ages" but not distributed among age groups.

Table 2-4. Abridged Life Table for the Total Population, 2015

(Number.)

Age	Probability of dying between ages x to $x+n$ $_nq_x$	Number surviving to age x l_x	Number dying between ages x to $x+n$ $_nd_x$	Person-years lived between ages x to $x+n$ $_nL_x$	Total number of person-years lived above age x T_x	Expectancy of life at age x e_x
0 to 1 years	0.006	100,000	589	99,483	7,876,057	78.8
1 to 5 years	0.001	99,411	99	397,404	7,776,574	78.2
5 to 10 years	0.001	99,312	58	496,402	7,379,170	74.3
10 to 15 years	0.001	99,254	72	496,125	6,882,769	69.3
15 to 20 years	0.002	99,181	238	495,398	6,386,644	64.4
20 to 25 years	0.004	98,943	440	493,671	5,891,247	59.5
25 to 30 years	0.005	98,503	523	491,239	5,397,576	54.8
30 to 35 years	0.006	97,980	623	488,385	4,906,337	50.1
35 to 40 years	0.008	97,357	748	484,982	4,417,952	45.4
40 to 45 years	0.010	96,609	990	480,702	3,932,970	40.7
45 to 50 years	0.015	95,619	1,461	474,713	3,452,268	36.1
50 to 55 years	0.024	94,158	2,290	465,433	2,977,555	31.6
55 to 60 years	0.036	91,867	3,309	451,496	2,512,122	27.3
60 to 65 years	0.051	88,559	4,503	432,063	2,060,626	23.3
65 to 70 years	0.071	84,055	5,993	406,029	1,628,563	19.4
70 to 75 years	0.109	78,062	8,507	370,224	1,222,534	15.7
75 to 80 years	0.169	69,555	11,733	319,951	852,311	12.3
80 to 85 years	0.269	57,822	15,555	251,625	532,359	9.2
85 to 90 years	0.421	42,266	17,782	167,034	280,735	6.6
90 to 95 years	0.609	24,484	14,901	82,735	113,701	4.6
95 to 100 years	0.781	9,583	7,487	26,135	30,966	3.2
100 years and over	1.000	2,096	2,096	4,831	4,831	2.3

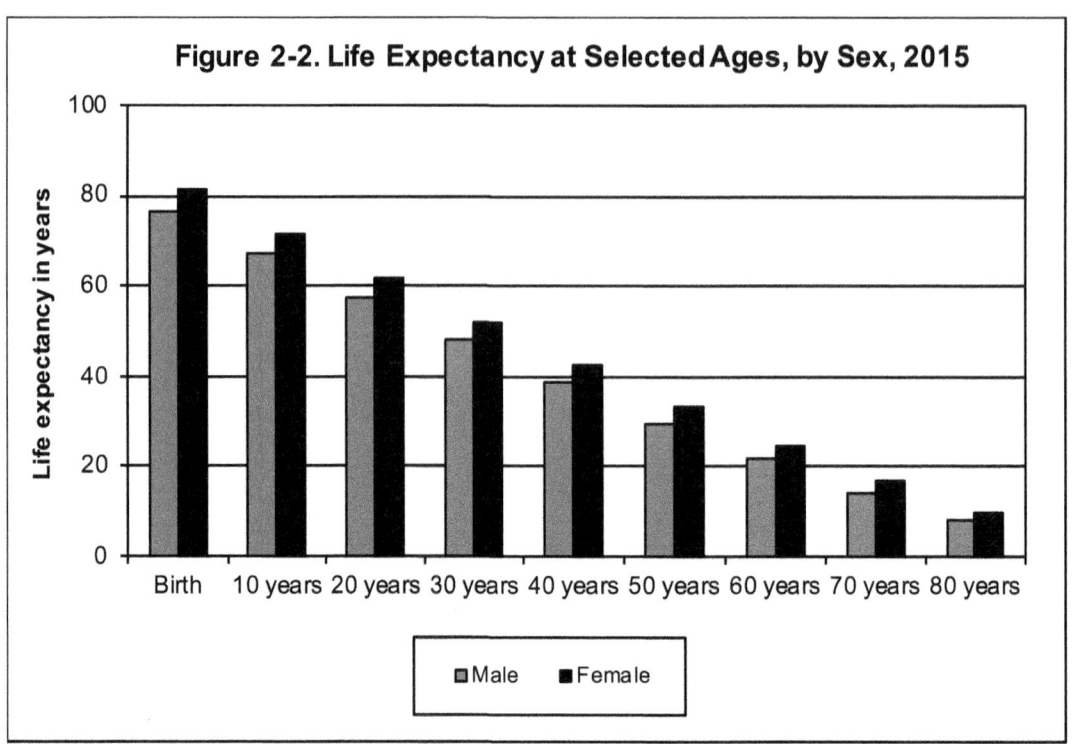

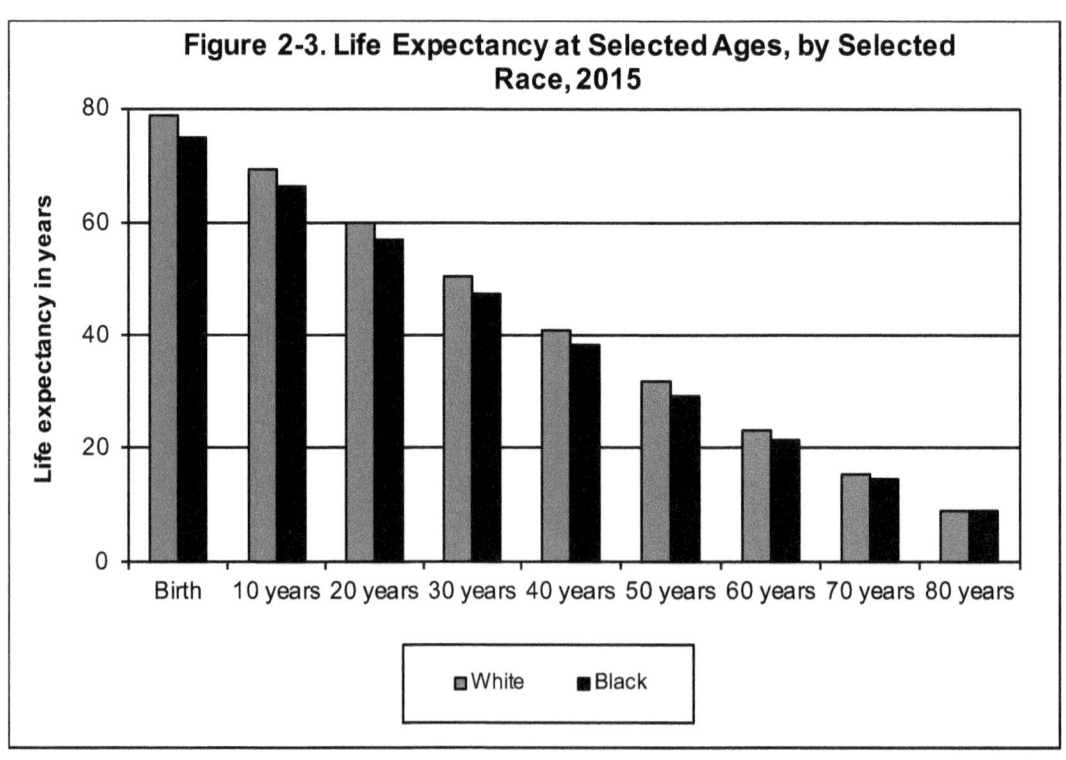

Table 2-5. Life Expectancy at Birth by Race and Sex, Selected Years, 1940–2015

(Number.)

Year	All races and origins[1]			Non-Hispanic White[2]			Non-Hispanic Black[2]			Hispanic[3]		
	Both sexes	Male	Female	Both sexes	Male	Female	Both sexes	Male	Female	Both sexes	Male	Female
1940	62.9	60.8	65.2	NA	NA	NA	NA	NA	NA	NA	NA	NA
1950	68.2	65.6	71.1	NA	NA	NA	NA	NA	NA	NA	NA	NA
1960	69.7	66.6	73.1	NA	NA	NA	NA	NA	NA	NA	NA	NA
1970	70.8	67.1	74.7	NA	NA	NA	NA	NA	NA	NA	NA	NA
1980	73.7	70.0	77.4	NA	NA	NA	NA	NA	NA	NA	NA	NA
1990	75.4	71.8	78.8	NA	NA	NA	NA	NA	NA	NA	NA	NA
2000	76.8	74.1	79.3	NA	NA	NA	NA	NA	NA	NA	NA	NA
2001[4]	77.0	74.3	79.5	NA	NA	NA	NA	NA	NA	NA	NA	NA
2002[4]	77.0	74.4	79.6	NA	NA	NA	NA	NA	NA	NA	NA	NA
2003[4,5]	77.2	74.5	79.7	NA	NA	NA	NA	NA	NA	NA	NA	NA
2004[4,5]	77.6	75.0	80.1	NA	NA	NA	NA	NA	NA	NA	NA	NA
2005[4,5]	77.6	75.0	80.1	NA	NA	NA	NA	NA	NA	NA	NA	NA
2006[4,5]	77.8	75.2	80.3	78.2	75.7	80.6	73.1	69.5	76.4	80.3	77.5	82.9
2007[4,5]	78.1	75.5	80.6	78.4	75.9	80.8	73.5	69.9	76.7	80.7	77.8	83.2
2008[4,5]	78.2	75.6	80.6	78.4	76.0	80.7	73.9	70.5	77.0	80.8	78.0	83.3
2009[4,5]	78.5	76.0	80.9	78.7	76.3	81.0	74.4	71.0	77.4	81.1	78.4	83.5
2010[4,5]	78.7	76.2	81.0	78.8	76.4	81.1	74.7	71.5	77.7	81.7	78.8	84.3
2011[4,5]	78.7	76.3	81.1	78.7	76.4	81.1	75.0	71.8	77.8	81.8	79.2	84.2
2012[4,5]	78.8	76.4	81.2	78.9	76.5	81.2	75.1	71.9	78.1	81.9	79.3	84.3
2013[4,5]	78.8	76.4	81.2	78.8	76.5	81.2	75.1	71.9	78.1	81.9	79.2	84.2
2014[4,5]	78.9	76.5	81.3	78.8	76.5	81.2	75.3	72.2	78.2	82.1	79.4	84.5
2015[4,5]	78.8	76.3	81.2	78.7	76.3	81.1	75.1	71.8	78.1	82.0	79.3	84.3

NA = Not available.

[1]Includes races other than White and Black.

[2]Includes Hispanic and non-Hispanic persons.

[3]Life expectancies for the Hispanic population are based on death rates adjusted for misclassification; please see chapter notes.

[4]Life table data for 2001–2013 are based on revised life table methodology.

[5]Race categories are consistent with the 1977 Office of Management and Budget (OMB) standards. Multiple-race data were reported by 42 states and the District of Columbia in 2012 and 2013, by 38 states and the District of Columbia in 2011, by 37 states and the District of Columbia in 2010, by 34 states and the District of Columbia in 2009 and 2008, by 27 states and the District of Columbia in 2007, by 25 states and the District of Columbia in 2006, by 21 states and the District of Columbia in 2005, by 15 states in 2004, and by 7 states in 2003. The multiple-race data for these reporting areas were bridged to the single-race categories of the 1977 OMB standards for comparability with other reporting areas.

Table 2-6. Life Expectancy at Selected Ages by Race, Hispanic Origin, Race for Non-Hispanic Population, and Sex, 2015

(Years.)

Exact age in years	All races and origins[1]			Non-Hispanic White[2]			Non-Hispanic Black[2]			Hispanic[3]		
	Both sexes	Male	Female	Both sexes	Male	Female	Both sexes	Male	Female	Both sexes	Male	Female
0 years	78.8	76.3	81.2	78.7	76.3	81.1	75.1	71.8	78.1	82.0	79.3	84.3
1 year	78.2	75.8	80.6	78.1	75.7	80.4	75.0	71.8	78.0	81.4	78.8	83.7
5 years	74.3	71.9	76.7	74.2	71.8	76.5	71.1	67.9	74.1	77.5	74.8	79.8
10 years	69.3	66.9	71.7	69.2	66.9	71.5	66.2	63.0	69.1	72.5	69.9	74.8
15 years	64.4	62.0	66.8	64.3	61.9	66.6	61.2	58.0	64.2	67.5	64.9	69.9
20 years	59.5	57.2	61.8	59.4	57.1	61.7	56.5	53.3	59.3	62.7	60.1	65.0
25 years	54.8	52.5	57.0	54.6	52.4	56.8	51.8	48.9	54.5	57.9	55.4	60.1
30 years	50.1	47.9	52.1	49.9	47.8	52.0	47.2	44.4	49.7	53.1	50.7	55.2
35 years	45.4	43.3	47.4	45.3	43.3	47.2	42.6	39.9	45.0	48.3	45.9	50.3
40 years	40.7	38.7	42.6	40.6	38.7	42.5	38.1	35.5	40.3	43.5	41.2	45.5
45 years	36.1	34.2	37.9	36.0	34.2	37.8	33.6	31.1	35.8	38.8	36.6	40.7
50 years	31.6	29.8	33.4	31.6	29.8	33.3	29.3	26.9	31.4	34.2	32.1	36.0
55 years	27.3	25.6	28.9	27.3	25.6	28.9	25.3	23.0	27.2	29.8	27.7	31.4
60 years	23.3	21.7	24.7	23.2	21.7	24.6	21.6	19.4	23.3	25.5	23.6	26.9
65 years	19.4	18.0	20.6	19.3	18.0	20.5	18.1	16.2	19.6	21.4	19.7	22.7
70 years	15.7	14.5	16.6	15.6	14.4	16.6	14.8	13.2	16.0	17.6	16.1	18.5
75 years	12.3	11.2	13.0	12.2	11.2	12.9	11.8	10.5	12.7	13.9	12.7	14.7
80 years	9.2	8.4	9.8	9.1	8.3	9.7	9.2	8.1	9.8	10.6	9.5	11.1
85 years	6.6	6.0	7.0	6.6	5.9	7.0	6.9	6.1	7.3	7.8	6.9	8.1
90 years	4.6	4.1	4.9	4.6	4.1	4.8	5.1	4.5	5.4	5.5	4.8	5.6
95 years	3.2	2.9	3.4	3.2	2.8	3.3	3.8	3.3	3.9	3.8	3.3	3.9
100 years	2.3	2.1	2.4	2.2	2.0	2.3	2.9	2.5	2.9	2.7	2.4	2.7

[1]Includes races and origins not shown separately.

[2]Multiple-race data reported according to 1997 OMB standards were bridged to the single-race categories of 1977 OMB standards.

[3]Life expectancies by Hispanic origin are based on death rates adjusted for misclassification.

Table 2-7. Life Expectancy at Birth, at 65 Years of Age, and at 75 Years of Age, by Race, Hispanic Origin and Sex, Selected Years, 1900–2013

(Number.)

Specified age and year	All races Both sexes	All races Male	All races Female	White Both sexes	White Male	White Female	Black or African American[1] Both sexes	Black or African American[1] Male	Black or African American[1] Female
	Remaining life expectancy in years								
At Birth									
1900[2,3]	47.3	46.3	48.3	47.6	46.6	48.7	33.0	32.5	33.5
1950[3]	68.2	65.6	71.1	69.1	66.5	72.2	60.8	59.1	62.9
1960[3]	69.7	66.6	73.1	70.6	67.4	74.1	63.6	61.1	66.3
1970	70.8	67.1	74.7	71.7	68.0	75.6	64.1	60.0	68.3
1975	72.6	68.8	76.6	73.4	69.5	77.3	66.8	62.4	71.3
1980	73.7	70.0	77.4	74.4	70.7	78.1	68.1	63.8	72.5
1981	74.1	70.4	77.8	74.8	71.1	78.4	68.9	64.5	73.2
1982	74.5	70.8	78.1	75.1	71.5	78.7	69.4	65.1	73.6
1983	74.6	71.0	78.1	75.2	71.6	78.7	69.4	65.2	73.5
1984	74.7	71.1	78.2	75.3	71.8	78.7	69.5	65.3	73.6
1985	74.7	71.1	78.2	75.3	71.8	78.7	69.3	65.0	73.4
1986	74.7	71.2	78.2	75.4	71.9	78.8	69.1	64.8	73.4
1987	74.9	71.4	78.3	75.6	72.1	78.9	69.1	64.7	73.4
1988	74.9	71.4	78.3	75.6	72.2	78.9	68.9	64.4	73.2
1989	75.1	71.7	78.5	75.9	72.5	79.2	68.8	64.3	73.3
1990	75.4	71.8	78.8	76.1	72.7	79.4	69.1	64.5	73.6
1991	75.5	72.0	78.9	76.3	72.9	79.6	69.3	64.6	73.8
1992	75.8	72.3	79.1	76.5	73.2	79.8	69.6	65.0	73.9
1993	75.5	72.2	78.8	76.3	73.1	79.5	69.2	64.6	73.7
1994	75.7	72.4	79.0	76.5	73.3	79.6	69.5	64.9	73.9
1995	75.8	72.5	78.9	76.5	73.4	79.6	69.6	65.2	73.9
1996	76.1	73.1	79.1	76.8	73.9	79.7	70.2	66.1	74.2
1997	76.5	73.6	79.4	77.1	74.3	79.9	71.1	67.2	74.7
1998	76.7	73.8	79.5	77.3	74.5	80.0	71.3	67.6	74.8
1999	76.7	73.9	79.4	77.3	74.6	79.9	71.4	67.8	74.7
2000	76.8	74.1	79.3	77.3	74.7	79.9	71.8	68.2	75.1
2001	76.9	74.2	79.4	77.4	74.8	79.9	72.0	68.4	75.2
2002	76.9	74.3	79.5	77.4	74.9	79.9	72.1	68.6	75.4
2003	77.1	74.5	79.6	77.6	75.0	80.0	72.3	68.8	75.6
2004	77.5	74.9	79.9	77.9	75.4	80.4	72.8	69.3	76.0
2005	77.4	74.9	79.9	77.9	75.4	80.4	72.8	69.3	76.1
2006	77.7	75.1	80.2	78.2	75.7	80.6	73.2	69.7	76.5
2007	77.9	75.4	80.4	78.4	75.9	80.8	73.6	70.0	76.8
2008	78.1	75.6	80.6	78.5	76.1	80.9	74.0	70.6	77.2
2009	78.5	76.0	80.9	78.8	76.4	81.2	74.5	71.1	77.6
2010	78.7	76.2	81.0	78.9	76.5	81.3	75.1	71.8	78.0
2011	78.7	76.3	81.1	79.0	76.6	81.3	75.3	72.2	78.2
2012	78.8	76.4	81.2	79.1	76.7	81.4	75.5	72.3	78.4
2013	78.8	76.4	81.2	79.1	76.7	81.4	75.5	72.3	78.4
At 65 Years									
1950[3]	13.9	12.8	15.0	14.1	12.8	15.1	13.9	12.9	14.9
1960[3]	14.3	12.8	15.8	14.4	12.9	15.9	13.9	12.7	15.1
1970	15.2	13.1	17.0	15.2	13.1	17.1	14.2	12.5	15.7
1975	16.1	13.8	18.1	16.1	13.8	18.2	15.0	13.1	16.7
1980	16.4	14.1	18.3	16.5	14.2	18.4	15.1	13.0	16.8
1981	16.6	14.3	18.6	16.7	14.4	18.7	15.5	13.4	17.2
1982	16.8	14.5	18.7	16.9	14.5	18.8	15.7	13.5	17.5
1983	16.7	14.4	18.6	16.8	14.5	18.7	15.4	13.2	17.2
1984	16.8	14.5	18.6	16.8	14.6	18.7	15.4	13.2	17.2
1985	16.7	14.5	18.5	16.8	14.5	18.7	15.2	13.0	16.9
1986	16.8	14.6	18.6	16.9	14.7	18.7	15.2	13.0	17.0
1987	16.9	14.7	18.7	17.0	14.8	18.8	15.2	13.0	17.0
1988	16.9	14.7	18.6	17.0	14.8	18.7	15.1	12.9	16.9
1989	17.1	15.0	18.8	17.2	15.1	18.9	15.2	13.0	16.9
1990	17.2	15.1	18.9	17.3	15.2	19.1	15.4	13.2	17.2
1991	17.4	15.3	19.1	17.5	15.4	19.2	15.5	13.4	17.2
1992	17.5	15.4	19.2	17.6	15.5	19.3	15.7	13.5	17.4
1993	17.3	15.3	18.9	17.4	15.4	19.0	15.5	13.4	17.1
1994	17.4	15.5	19.0	17.5	15.6	19.1	15.7	13.6	17.2
1995	17.4	15.6	18.9	17.6	15.7	19.1	15.6	13.6	17.1
1996	17.5	15.7	19.0	17.6	15.8	19.1	15.8	13.9	17.2
1997	17.7	15.9	19.2	17.8	16.0	19.3	16.1	14.2	17.6
1998	17.8	16.0	19.2	17.8	16.1	19.3	16.1	14.3	17.4
1999	17.7	16.1	19.1	17.8	16.1	19.2	16.0	14.3	17.3
2000	17.6	16.0	19.0	17.7	16.1	19.1	16.1	14.1	17.5
2001	17.7	16.2	19.0	17.8	16.3	19.1	16.2	14.2	17.6

[1]Data shown for 1900-1960 are for the Non-White population.
[2]Death registration area only. The death registration area increased from 10 states and the District of Columbia (D.C.) in 1900 to the coterminous United States in 1933.
[3]Includes deaths of persons who were not residents of the 50 states and D.C.

Table 2-7. Life Expectancy at Birth, at 65 Years of Age, and at 75 Years of Age, by Race, Hispanic Origin and Sex, Selected Years, 1900–2013—Continued

(Number.)

Specified age and year	All races			White			Black or African American[1]		
	Both sexes	Male	Female	Both sexes	Male	Female	Both sexes	Male	Female
	Remaining life expectancy in years								
2002	17.8	16.2	19.1	17.9	16.3	19.2	16.3	14.4	17.7
2003	17.9	16.4	19.2	18.0	16.5	19.3	16.4	14.5	17.9
2004	18.2	16.7	19.5	18.3	16.8	19.5	16.7	14.8	18.2
2005	18.2	16.8	19.5	18.3	16.9	19.5	16.8	14.9	18.2
2006	18.5	17.0	19.7	18.6	17.1	19.8	17.1	15.1	18.6
2007	18.6	17.2	19.9	18.7	17.3	19.9	17.2	15.2	18.7
2008	18.8	17.3	20.0	18.8	17.4	20.0	17.4	15.4	18.9
2009	19.2	17.6	20.3	19.1	17.7	20.4	17.8	15.8	19.3
2010	19.1	17.7	20.3	19.2	17.8	20.3	17.8	15.9	19.3
2011	19.2	17.8	20.3	19.2	17.8	20.4	18.0	16.2	19.4
2012	19.3	17.9	20.5	19.3	18.0	20.4	18.1	16.2	19.5
2013	19.3	17.9	20.5	19.3	18.0	20.5	18.1	16.3	19.5
At 75 years									
1980	10.4	8.8	11.5	10.4	8.8	11.5	9.7	8.3	10.7
1981	10.6	9.0	11.7	10.6	9.0	11.7	10.4	9.0	11.4
1982	10.7	9.1	11.9	10.7	9.0	11.9	10.6	9.1	11.6
1983	10.6	9.0	11.7	10.6	8.9	11.7	10.3	8.9	11.4
1984	10.7	9.0	11.8	10.7	9.0	11.8	10.3	8.9	11.4
1985	10.6	9.0	11.7	10.6	9.0	11.7	10.1	8.7	11.1
1986	10.7	9.1	11.7	10.7	9.1	11.8	10.1	8.6	11.1
1987	10.7	9.1	11.8	10.7	9.1	11.8	10.1	8.6	11.1
1988	10.6	9.1	11.7	10.7	9.1	11.7	10.0	8.5	11.0
1989	10.9	9.3	11.9	10.9	9.3	11.9	10.1	8.6	11.0
1990	10.9	9.4	12.0	11.0	9.4	12.0	10.2	8.6	11.2
1991	11.1	9.5	12.1	11.1	9.5	12.1	10.2	8.7	11.2
1992	11.2	9.6	12.2	11.2	9.6	12.2	10.4	8.9	11.4
1993	10.9	9.5	11.9	11.0	9.5	12.0	10.2	8.7	11.1
1994	11.0	9.6	12.0	11.1	9.6	12.0	10.3	8.9	11.2
1995	11.0	9.7	11.9	11.1	9.7	12.0	10.2	8.8	11.1
1996	11.1	9.8	12.0	11.1	9.8	12.0	10.3	9.0	11.2
1997	11.2	9.9	12.1	11.2	9.9	12.1	10.7	9.3	11.5
1998	11.3	10.0	12.2	11.3	10.0	12.2	10.5	9.2	11.3
1999	11.2	10.0	12.1	11.2	10.0	12.1	10.4	9.2	11.1
2000	11.0	9.8	11.8	11.0	9.8	11.9	10.4	9.0	11.3
2001	11.1	9.9	11.9	11.1	9.9	11.9	10.5	9.1	11.4
2002	11.0	9.9	11.9	11.1	9.9	11.9	10.5	9.2	11.4
2003	11.1	10.0	11.9	11.1	10.0	11.9	10.6	9.3	11.5
2004	11.4	10.3	12.2	11.4	10.3	12.2	10.8	9.5	11.7
2005	11.3	10.2	12.1	11.4	10.3	12.1	10.8	9.5	11.7
2006	11.6	10.5	12.3	11.5	10.5	12.3	11.1	9.8	12.0
2007	11.7	10.6	12.5	11.7	10.6	12.4	11.2	9.9	12.1
2008	11.8	10.7	12.6	11.8	10.7	12.6	11.3	9.9	12.3
2009	12.2	11.0	12.9	12.1	11.0	12.9	11.7	10.3	12.6
2010	12.1	11.0	12.9	12.1	11.0	12.8	11.6	10.2	12.5
2011	12.1	11.1	12.9	12.1	11.0	12.8	11.7	10.4	12.5
2012	12.2	11.2	12.9	12.1	11.1	12.9	11.8	10.4	12.7
2013	12.2	11.2	12.9	12.1	11.1	12.9	11.8	10.4	12.7

[1]Data shown for 1900-1960 are for the Non-White population.

Table 2-7. Life Expectancy at Birth, at 65 Years of Age, and at 75 Years of Age, by Race, Hispanic Origin and Sex, Selected Years, 1900–2013—*Continued*

(Number.)

Specified age and year	Hispanic[4]			Non-Hispanic White			Non-Hispanic Black		
	Both sexes	Male	Female	Both sexes	Male	Female	Both sexes	Male	Female
	Remaining life expectancy in years								
At birth									
2006	80.3	77.5	82.9	78.2	75.7	80.6	73.1	69.5	76.4
2007	80.7	77.8	83.2	78.4	75.9	80.8	73.5	69.9	76.7
2008	80.8	78.0	83.3	78.4	76.0	80.7	73.9	70.5	77.0
2009	81.1	78.4	83.5	78.7	76.3	81.1	74.3	70.9	77.4
2010	81.2	78.5	83.8	78.8	76.4	81.1	74.7	71.4	77.7
2011	81.4	78.8	83.7	78.8	76.4	81.1	74.9	71.7	77.8
2012	81.6	79.1	83.9	78.9	76.6	81.2	75.1	71.8	78.1
2013	81.6	79.1	83.8	78.9	76.5	81.2	75.1	71.8	78.1
At 65 Years									
2006	20.2	18.5	21.5	18.7	17.2	19.9	17.1	15.1	18.5
2007	20.5	18.7	21.7	18.8	17.4	20.0	17.2	15.3	18.7
2008	20.4	18.7	21.6	18.8	17.4	20.0	17.4	15.4	18.8
2009	20.7	19.0	21.9	19.1	17.7	19.5	17.7	15.8	19.1
2010	20.6	18.8	22.0	19.1	17.7	20.3	17.7	15.8	19.1
2011	20.7	19.1	21.8	19.1	17.8	20.3	17.9	16.1	19.2
2012	21.0	19.5	22.1	19.3	17.9	20.4	18.0	16.1	19.4
2013	20.9	19.3	22.0	19.3	17.9	20.4	18.0	16.1	19.4
At 75 Years									
2006	13.0	11.7	13.7	11.7	10.6	12.5	11.1	9.6	12.0
2007	13.1	11.8	13.8	11.8	10.7	12.6	11.2	9.7	12.1
2008	13.0	11.7	13.8	11.8	10.7	12.6	11.3	9.8	12.2
2009	13.3	12.0	13.8	12.0	11.0	12.9	11.6	10.1	12.4
2010	13.2	11.7	14.1	12.0	11.0	12.8	11.6	10.1	12.5
2011	13.2	12.0	13.9	12.0	11.0	12.8	11.7	10.4	12.5
2012	13.5	12.3	14.2	12.1	11.1	12.9	11.7	10.4	12.6
2013	13.4	12.3	14.1	12.1	11.1	12.9	11.7	10.4	12.6

[4]Hispanic origin was added to the U.S. standard death certificate in 1989 and was adopted by every state in 1997. To estimate life expectancy, age-specific death rates were corrected to address racial and ethnic misclassification, which underestimates deaths in the Hispanic population. To address the effects of age misstatement at the oldest ages, the probability of death for Hispanic persons older than 80 years is estimated as a function of non-Hispanic white mortality with the use of the Brass relational logit model.

Table 2-8. Death Rates by Age and Age-Adjusted Death Rates for the 10 Leading Causes of Death in 2015 and Drug-Induced Deaths, Alcohol-Induced Deaths, and Injury by Firearm, 1999–2015

(Rate per 100,000 population in specified group; age-adjusted rates per 100,000 U.S. standard population.)

Cause of death (based on ICD–10) and year	All ages[1]	Under 1 year[2]	1 to 4 years	5 to 14 years	15 to 24 years	25 to 34 years	35 to 44 years	45 to 54 years	55 to 64 years	65 to 74 years	75 to 84 years	85 years and over	Age-adjusted rate[3]
All Causes													
1999	857.0	736.0	34.2	18.6	79.3	102.2	198.0	418.2	1,005.0	2,457.3	5,714.5	15,554.6	875.6
2000	854.0	736.7	32.4	18.0	79.9	101.4	198.9	425.6	992.2	2,399.1	5,666.5	15,524.4	869.0
2001	848.0	687.0	33.4	17.2	80.2	105.6	203.5	426.7	972.5	2,344.2	5,573.7	15,432.6	858.8
2002	849.5	709.5	31.4	17.4	80.9	105.1	204.2	431.0	948.7	2,300.3	5,543.8	15,589.5	855.9
2003	843.9	704.9	31.8	16.9	81.1	105.2	202.6	433.1	937.3	2,235.0	5,451.3	15,401.4	843.5
2004	818.8	695.9	30.3	16.7	79.7	104.1	194.9	426.8	903.2	2,141.0	5,267.4	14,777.6	813.7
2005	828.4	710.2	29.9	16.3	80.7	106.8	194.9	431.9	898.5	2,109.7	5,251.8	14,982.4	815.0
2006	813.1	705.8	29.1	15.2	81.4	109.0	192.0	427.5	881.3	2,031.4	5,096.1	14,426.7	791.8
2007	804.6	702.5	29.4	15.2	78.8	107.2	186.0	420.3	866.7	1,976.0	4,987.1	14,160.9	775.3
2008	812.9	678.9	29.3	13.9	74.2	105.1	181.0	419.6	867.1	1,958.4	4,998.1	14,332.4	774.9
2009	794.5	659.7	27.4	13.8	69.8	104.4	180.0	418.1	856.7	1,888.7	4,820.2	13,660.1	749.6
2010	799.5	623.4	26.5	12.9	67.7	102.9	170.5	407.1	851.9	1,875.1	4,790.2	13,934.3	747.0
2011	807.3	600.1	26.3	13.2	67.7	104.7	172.0	409.8	849.4	1,846.2	4,753.0	13,779.3	741.3
2012	810.2	599.3	26.3	12.6	66.4	105.4	170.7	405.4	854.2	1,802.5	4,674.5	13,678.6	732.8
2013	821.5	594.7	25.5	13.0	64.8	106.1	172.0	406.1	860.0	1,802.1	4,648.1	13,660.4	731.9
2014	823.7	588.0	24.0	12.7	65.5	108.4	175.2	404.8	870.3	1,786.3	4,564.2	13,407.9	724.6
2015	844.0	589.6	24.9	13.2	69.5	116.7	180.1	404.0	875.3	1,796.8	4,579.2	13,673.9	733.1
Diseases of Heart (I00–I09, I11, I13, I20–I51)													
1999	259.9	13.8	1.2	0.7	2.8	7.6	30.2	95.7	269.9	701.7	1,849.9	6,063.0	266.5
2000	252.6	13.0	1.2	0.7	2.6	7.4	29.2	94.2	261.2	665.6	1,780.3	5,926.1	257.6
2001	245.7	11.9	1.5	0.7	2.5	8.0	29.6	92.4	248.9	632.6	1,723.0	5,784.1	249.5
2002	242.3	12.7	1.1	0.6	2.5	8.0	30.7	93.9	240.5	612.0	1,673.2	5,726.3	244.6
2003	236.1	11.0	1.2	0.6	2.7	8.3	30.8	92.4	232.3	579.8	1,607.7	5,570.7	236.3
2004	222.8	10.5	1.2	0.6	2.5	8.1	29.5	90.2	217.1	535.7	1,504.1	5,233.8	221.6
2005	220.7	8.9	0.9	0.6	2.6	8.3	29.2	89.7	212.8	512.3	1,458.5	5,188.3	216.8
2006	211.7	8.6	1.0	0.6	2.5	8.4	28.5	88.0	205.1	483.0	1,378.0	4,877.6	205.5
2007	204.5	10.2	1.1	0.6	2.5	8.1	27.7	85.2	197.8	454.8	1,308.6	4,668.1	196.1
2008	202.8	9.6	1.2	0.6	2.5	8.1	26.9	85.2	195.3	441.4	1,271.7	4,598.4	192.1
2009	195.4	9.6	0.9	0.5	2.4	7.8	26.7	82.3	190.0	422.8	1,210.8	4,316.9	182.8
2010	193.6	8.3	1.0	0.5	2.4	7.8	25.8	81.6	186.6	409.2	1,172.0	4,285.2	179.1
2011	191.5	7.7	1.0	0.5	2.3	7.9	26.2	80.7	183.2	399.0	1,134.7	4,111.6	173.7
2012	191.0	8.5	1.0	0.4	2.2	7.6	25.9	79.7	184.6	388.3	1,103.7	4,046.1	170.5
2013	193.3	7.8	1.1	0.4	2.1	7.6	25.6	80.3	184.6	390.3	1,095.1	4,013.9	169.8
2014	192.7	8.0	0.9	0.5	2.2	7.7	25.6	80.1	185.8	385.2	1,070.2	3,920.9	167.0
2015	197.2	7.3	0.9	0.5	2.3	8.0	25.6	79.3	188.1	389.5	1,071.6	3,986.5	168.5
Malignant Neoplasms (C00-C97)													
1999	197.0	1.8	2.7	2.5	4.5	10.0	37.1	127.6	374.6	827.1	1,331.5	1,805.8	200.8
2000	196.5	2.4	2.7	2.5	4.4	9.8	36.6	127.5	366.7	816.3	1,335.6	1,819.4	199.6
2001	194.3	1.6	2.7	2.4	4.2	10.1	36.8	125.8	359.4	799.7	1,313.7	1,802.9	196.5
2002	193.7	1.9	2.6	2.6	4.2	9.8	36.0	124.1	349.7	787.2	1,308.8	1,812.4	194.3
2003	192.0	1.9	2.5	2.6	4.0	9.5	35.1	122.1	341.6	763.5	1,299.7	1,792.3	190.9
2004	189.2	1.8	2.5	2.5	4.1	9.3	33.6	119.0	330.8	746.8	1,278.6	1,767.4	186.8
2005	189.3	1.9	2.4	2.5	4.0	9.2	33.5	118.6	323.9	733.2	1,272.8	1,778.2	185.1
2006	187.6	1.9	2.4	2.2	3.8	9.3	32.2	116.3	317.7	716.3	1,259.2	1,748.3	181.8
2007	186.9	1.7	2.3	2.4	3.8	8.7	31.0	114.2	311.4	702.9	1,250.1	1,739.4	179.3
2008	186.0	1.7	2.4	2.2	3.8	8.8	30.1	113.4	304.7	688.4	1,230.9	1,724.6	176.4
2009	185.0	1.8	2.2	2.2	3.8	9.0	30.2	112.8	301.7	668.2	1,213.0	1,699.3	173.5
2010	186.2	1.6	2.1	2.2	3.7	8.8	28.8	111.6	300.1	666.1	1,202.2	1,729.5	172.8
2011	185.1	1.8	2.2	2.1	3.7	8.4	28.8	109.3	295.8	647.6	1,179.1	1,676.2	169.0
2012	185.6	1.6	2.4	2.2	3.6	8.7	28.0	108.5	293.2	632.2	1,161.7	1,658.9	166.5
2013	185.0	1.6	2.1	2.2	3.4	8.6	28.1	105.5	288.2	616.9	1,139.4	1,635.4	163.2
2014	185.6	1.3	2.0	2.1	3.6	8.3	27.8	103.2	287.6	603.1	1,125.9	1,632.9	161.2
2015	185.4	1.3	2.2	2.1	3.4	8.4	26.9	99.7	284.1	594.3	1,100.8	1,628.6	158.5
Chronic Lower Respiratory Diseases (J40-J47)													
1999	44.5	0.9	0.4	0.3	0.5	0.8	2.0	8.5	47.5	177.2	397.8	646.0	45.4
2000	43.4	0.9	0.3	0.3	0.5	0.7	2.1	8.6	44.2	169.4	386.1	648.6	44.2
2001	43.2	1.0	0.3	0.3	0.4	0.7	2.2	8.4	44.5	167.3	379.3	658.3	43.9
2002	43.4	1.0	0.4	0.3	0.5	0.8	2.3	8.7	42.2	162.0	385.8	670.3	43.9
2003	43.6	0.8	0.4	0.3	0.5	0.7	2.2	8.7	43.1	161.7	382.2	670.2	43.7
2004	41.7	0.9	0.3	0.3	0.4	0.6	2.0	8.4	40.1	152.1	366.2	643.2	41.6
2005	44.3	0.8	0.4	0.3	0.3	0.7	2.0	9.4	41.6	158.4	385.0	691.9	43.9
2006	41.8	0.7	0.3	0.3	0.4	0.6	1.9	9.1	38.8	147.0	362.0	641.3	41.0
2007	42.5	1.0	0.4	0.3	0.3	0.7	1.9	9.5	38.6	145.5	367.1	652.0	41.4
2008	46.4	0.8	0.3	0.3	0.4	0.6	1.9	9.9	41.1	155.9	395.4	722.7	44.7
2009	44.8	0.7	0.4	0.3	0.4	0.7	1.8	10.4	40.0	147.5	376.4	684.9	42.7
2010	44.7	0.9	0.3	0.3	0.3	0.7	1.7	9.9	39.0	146.3	369.9	690.7	42.2
2011	45.9	0.8	0.3	0.3	0.4	0.6	1.8	10.4	39.5	144.3	374.9	697.9	42.5

[1] Figures for age not stated included in "All ages" but not distributed among age groups.
[2] Death rates for "Under 1 year" (based on population estimates) differ from infant mortality rates (based on live births); please see chapter notes for more information.
[3] For method of computation, please see chapter notes.

Table 2-8. Death Rates by Age and Age-Adjusted Death Rates for the 10 Leading Causes of Death in 2015 and Drug-Induced Deaths, Alcohol-Induced Deaths, and Injury by Firearm, 1999–2015—*Continued*

(Rate per 100,000 population in specified group; age-adjusted rates per 100,000 U.S. standard population.)

Cause of death (based on ICD–10) and year	All ages[1]	Under 1 year[2]	1 to 4 years	5 to 14 years	15 to 24 years	25 to 34 years	35 to 44 years	45 to 54 years	55 to 64 years	65 to 74 years	75 to 84 years	85 years and over	Age-adjusted rate[3]
2012	45.7	0.5	0.3	0.3	0.3	0.7	1.8	10.2	39.4	140.0	364.0	687.8	41.5
2013	47.2	0.6	0.4	0.4	0.4	0.7	1.9	10.6	40.5	141.2	367.0	699.3	42.1
2014	46.1	*	0.3	0.3	0.4	0.8	1.9	10.1	41.2	134.9	349.0	670.5	40.5
2015	48.2	0.7	0.3	0.4	0.5	0.7	1.7	10.1	42.7	136.6	357.9	705.1	41.6
Accidents (unintentional injuries) (V01–X59,Y85–Y86)													
1999	35.1	22.3	12.4	7.6	35.3	29.6	33.8	31.8	30.6	44.6	100.5	282.4	35.3
2000	34.8	23.1	11.9	7.3	36.0	29.5	34.1	32.6	30.9	41.9	95.1	273.5	34.9
2001	35.6	24.3	11.2	6.9	35.8	30.0	35.4	33.9	30.5	42.6	100.7	282.2	35.7
2002	37.1	23.9	10.6	6.6	37.7	31.9	37.4	36.7	31.3	44.0	101.1	289.6	37.1
2003	37.7	23.8	11.0	6.4	36.9	32.0	38.0	38.8	32.7	43.7	101.6	294.3	37.6
2004	38.3	26.2	10.4	6.5	36.8	33.2	37.6	40.7	32.9	43.5	103.6	295.8	38.1
2005	39.9	27.0	10.5	5.9	37.1	35.7	38.9	43.2	35.4	45.7	106.0	303.5	39.5
2006	40.8	28.4	10.1	5.6	37.9	38.0	40.5	45.5	35.8	43.8	104.7	299.2	40.2
2007	41.1	31.0	9.9	5.4	36.8	37.7	39.6	46.2	36.8	44.4	105.0	313.6	40.4
2008	40.1	31.8	9.1	4.6	32.5	36.3	38.1	45.8	37.4	43.9	105.7	318.3	39.2
2009	38.5	29.5	9.0	4.1	28.6	34.5	36.4	44.5	36.5	42.1	103.5	310.9	37.5
2010	39.1	28.1	8.6	4.0	28.3	35.5	36.0	43.7	38.4	43.3	106.1	328.4	38.0
2011	40.6	29.1	8.5	4.0	28.2	37.1	37.5	46.4	39.8	44.5	107.0	333.8	39.1
2012	40.7	29.6	8.4	3.8	27.1	37.5	37.1	46.1	41.0	44.0	107.8	336.9	39.1
2013	41.3	29.3	8.3	3.7	26.4	37.8	38.0	46.5	43.4	43.5	107.4	340.0	39.4
2014	42.6	29.4	7.6	3.6	26.8	39.8	39.6	47.4	44.9	45.1	108.7	349.1	40.5
2015	45.6	32.5	7.8	3.7	28.5	44.8	43.9	49.8	47.7	47.0	111.5	364.5	43.2
Cerebrovascular Diseases (I60–I69)													
1999	60.0	2.7	0.3	0.2	0.5	1.4	5.7	15.2	40.6	130.8	469.8	1,614.8	61.6
2000	59.6	3.3	0.3	0.2	0.5	1.5	5.8	16.0	41.0	128.6	461.3	1,589.2	60.9
2001	57.4	2.7	0.4	0.2	0.5	1.5	5.5	15.0	38.3	122.9	443.3	1,532.0	58.4
2002	56.6	3.0	0.3	0.2	0.4	1.4	5.4	15.1	37.1	119.6	430.0	1,520.1	57.2
2003	54.4	2.5	0.3	0.2	0.5	1.5	5.6	15.0	35.5	111.9	409.8	1,446.0	54.6
2004	51.3	3.2	0.3	0.2	0.5	1.4	5.4	14.8	34.0	106.6	385.6	1,331.9	51.2
2005	48.6	3.1	0.4	0.2	0.5	1.4	5.2	15.0	32.7	99.8	358.4	1,239.7	48.0
2006	46.0	3.5	0.3	0.2	0.5	1.3	5.1	14.6	32.9	94.9	333.9	1,131.7	44.8
2007	45.1	3.2	0.3	0.2	0.5	1.3	5.0	14.5	31.7	91.4	320.8	1,110.7	43.5
2008	44.1	3.4	0.4	0.2	0.4	1.3	4.8	13.7	30.6	87.3	313.3	1,071.0	42.1
2009	42.0	3.7	0.3	0.2	0.4	1.3	4.6	13.7	29.7	82.8	294.9	992.2	39.6
2010	41.9	3.3	0.3	0.2	0.4	1.3	4.6	13.1	29.3	81.7	288.3	993.8	39.1
2011	41.4	3.4	0.3	0.2	0.4	1.3	4.2	12.8	29.4	78.2	285.4	943.7	37.9
2012	40.9	2.6	0.3	0.2	0.4	1.3	4.3	12.8	28.7	75.7	272.2	931.2	36.9
2013	40.8	2.7	0.2	0.2	0.3	1.2	4.2	12.4	28.9	74.2	268.9	906.0	36.2
2014	41.7	2.4	0.2	0.2	0.4	1.3	4.3	12.3	29.3	74.5	265.7	929.7	36.5
2015	43.7	2.2	0.3	0.2	0.4	1.3	4.4	12.3	29.6	75.5	273.0	975.8	37.6
Alzheimer's Disease (G30)													
1999	16.0	*	*	*	*	*	*	0.2	1.9	17.4	129.5	601.3	16.5
2000	17.6	*	*	*	*	*	*	0.2	2.0	18.7	139.6	667.7	18.1
2001	18.9	*	*	*	*	*	*	0.2	2.1	18.6	147.2	725.4	19.3
2002	20.5	*	*	*	*	*	*	0.1	1.9	19.6	157.7	790.9	20.8
2003	21.9	*	*	*	*	*	*	0.2	2.0	20.7	164.1	846.8	22.1
2004	22.5	*	*	*	*	*	*	0.2	1.8	19.5	168.5	875.3	22.6
2005	24.2	*	*	*	*	*	*	0.2	2.1	20.2	177.0	935.5	24.0
2006	24.3	*	*	*	*	*	*	0.2	2.1	19.9	175.0	923.4	23.7
2007	24.8	*	*	*	*	*	*	0.2	2.2	20.2	175.8	928.7	23.8
2008	27.1	*	*	*	*	*	*	0.2	2.2	21.1	192.5	1,002.2	25.8
2009	25.8	*	*	*	*	*	*	0.2	2.0	19.4	179.1	945.3	24.2
2010	27.0	*	*	*	*	*	*	0.3	2.1	19.8	184.5	987.1	25.1
2011	27.3	*	*	*	*	*	*	0.2	2.2	19.2	183.9	967.1	24.7
2012	26.6	*	*	*	*	*	*	0.2	2.2	17.9	175.4	936.1	23.8
2013	26.8	*	*	*	*	*	*	0.2	2.2	18.1	171.6	929.5	23.5
2014	29.3	*	*	*	*	*	*	0.2	2.1	19.6	185.6	1,006.8	25.4
2015	34.4	*	*	*	*	*	*	0.2	2.4	22.4	211.9	1,174.2	29.4
Diabetes Mellitus (E10–E14)													
1999	24.5	*	*	0.1	0.4	1.4	4.3	12.9	38.3	91.8	178.0	317.2	25.0
2000	24.6	*	*	0.1	0.4	1.6	4.3	13.1	37.8	90.7	179.5	319.7	25.0
2001	25.0	*	*	0.1	0.4	1.5	4.3	13.6	38.1	91.0	181.1	328.6	25.4
2002	25.5	*	*	0.1	0.4	1.6	4.8	13.7	37.5	90.9	182.4	337.0	25.6
2003	25.6	*	*	0.1	0.4	1.7	4.6	13.9	38.3	90.0	180.7	335.1	25.5
2004	25.0	*	*	0.1	0.4	1.5	4.6	13.4	36.8	86.2	176.6	328.2	24.7
2005	25.4	*	*	0.1	0.5	1.6	4.7	13.4	36.9	85.7	177.0	338.8	24.9

* = Figure does not meet standards of reliability or precision.
[1] Figures for age not stated included in "All ages" but not distributed among age groups.
[2] Death rates for "Under 1 year" (based on population estimates) differ from infant mortality rates (based on live births); please see chapter notes for more information.
[3] For method of computation, please see chapter notes.

Table 2-8. Death Rates by Age and Age-Adjusted Death Rates for the 10 Leading Causes of Death in 2015 and Drug-Induced Deaths, Alcohol-Induced Deaths, and Injury by Firearm, 1999–2015—Continued

(Rate per 100,000 population in specified group; age-adjusted rates per 100,000 U.S. standard population.)

Cause of death (based on ICD–10) and year	All ages[1]	Under 1 year[2]	1 to 4 years	5 to 14 years	15 to 24 years	25 to 34 years	35 to 44 years	45 to 54 years	55 to 64 years	65 to 74 years	75 to 84 years	85 years and over	Age-adjusted rate[3]
2006	24.3	*	*	0.1	0.4	1.7	4.8	13.1	35.8	80.6	166.2	310.4	23.6
2007	23.7	*	*	0.1	0.4	1.5	4.6	13.1	34.1	76.7	161.9	302.2	22.8
2008	23.2	*	*	0.1	0.5	1.4	4.4	12.6	33.3	74.7	153.2	298.9	22.0
2009	22.4	*	*	0.1	0.4	1.5	4.5	12.8	32.1	69.6	145.8	282.6	21.0
2010	22.4	*	*	0.1	0.4	1.5	4.4	12.5	32.0	67.6	144.1	285.5	20.8
2011	23.7	*	*	0.1	0.4	1.6	4.5	13.4	33.3	72.0	148.8	289.5	21.6
2012	23.6	*	*	0.1	0.4	1.5	4.6	13.0	32.5	69.7	145.8	285.7	21.2
2013	23.9	*	*	0.1	0.4	1.6	4.8	13.5	33.2	68.5	145.7	279.5	21.2
2014	24.0	*	*	0.1	0.4	1.6	4.9	13.9	33.3	69.0	141.8	268.6	20.9
2015	24.7	*	*	0.1	0.4	1.8	4.9	14.4	34.7	70.6	143.0	267.0	21.3
Influenza and Pneumonia (J09–J18)													
1999	22.8	8.4	0.8	0.2	0.5	0.8	2.4	4.6	11.0	37.2	157.0	751.8	23.5
2000	23.2	7.6	0.7	0.2	0.5	0.9	2.4	4.7	11.9	39.1	160.3	744.1	23.7
2001	21.8	7.5	0.7	0.2	0.5	0.9	2.2	4.6	10.8	36.2	148.3	700.1	22.2
2002	22.8	6.7	0.7	0.2	0.4	0.9	2.2	4.8	11.2	37.2	156.6	732.4	23.2
2003	22.5	8.1	1.0	0.4	0.5	1.0	2.2	5.2	11.2	36.9	150.8	703.0	22.6
2004	20.4	6.8	0.8	0.2	0.4	0.8	2.0	4.6	10.8	34.2	139.1	622.8	20.4
2005	21.3	6.6	0.7	0.3	0.4	0.9	2.1	5.1	11.2	35.1	142.0	644.9	21.0
2006	18.9	6.5	0.8	0.2	0.4	0.9	1.9	4.6	9.9	31.6	127.3	547.0	18.4
2007	17.5	5.4	0.7	0.3	0.4	0.8	1.8	4.3	9.5	28.2	113.5	506.7	16.8
2008	18.5	5.5	0.9	0.2	0.5	0.9	2.1	5.1	10.9	30.5	118.6	512.3	17.6
2009	17.5	6.3	0.9	0.6	1.0	2.0	3.2	6.5	11.7	29.5	107.0	433.8	16.5
2010	16.2	4.9	0.6	0.2	0.4	0.9	1.9	4.3	9.9	27.9	102.4	426.2	15.1
2011	17.3	5.2	0.7	0.3	0.5	1.2	2.1	5.0	11.0	28.9	104.0	439.2	15.7
2012	16.1	4.0	0.6	0.2	0.3	0.8	1.7	4.1	10.2	26.1	98.2	408.4	14.4
2013	18.0	4.5	0.6	0.3	0.4	1.0	2.2	5.1	12.2	29.5	103.7	441.0	15.9
2014	17.3	4.7	0.7	0.2	0.5	1.3	2.8	6.3	13.4	29.8	96.4	385.9	15.1
2015	17.8	4.4	0.6	0.2	0.4	0.9	1.7	4.7	11.3	29.5	101.6	421.4	15.2
Nephritis, Nephrotic Syndrome and Nephrosis (N00–N07, N17–N19, N25–N27)													
1999	12.7	4.4	*	0.1	0.2	0.6	1.6	4.0	12.0	37.1	97.6	268.8	13.0
2000	13.2	4.3	*	0.1	0.2	0.6	1.6	4.4	12.8	38.0	100.8	277.8	13.5
2001	13.9	3.3	*	*	0.2	0.6	1.7	4.6	13.1	40.0	104.0	293.8	14.1
2002	14.2	4.4	*	0.1	0.2	0.7	1.7	4.7	12.9	39.0	108.9	303.4	14.4
2003	14.6	4.6	*	0.1	0.2	0.7	1.8	4.9	13.6	39.7	109.3	309.3	14.7
2004	14.5	4.3	*	0.1	0.2	0.6	1.8	5.0	13.5	38.1	108.2	306.4	14.5
2005	14.9	4.0	*	0.1	0.2	0.7	1.7	4.8	13.5	38.8	110.2	313.1	14.7
2006	15.2	4.0	*	*	0.2	0.7	1.8	5.2	13.7	38.8	111.0	316.2	14.8
2007	15.4	3.5	0.1	0.1	0.2	0.7	1.8	5.1	13.4	39.4	112.4	317.9	14.9
2008	15.9	3.5	*	*	0.2	0.6	1.8	5.0	14.1	39.9	113.3	325.6	15.1
2009	16.0	2.8	*	*	0.2	0.7	2.0	5.2	13.5	38.7	115.1	321.4	15.1
2010	16.3	2.7	*	0.1	0.2	0.6	1.8	4.9	13.9	39.3	115.7	333.8	15.3
2011	14.6	1.9	*	*	0.2	0.5	1.6	4.4	12.5	34.2	101.4	292.1	13.4
2012	14.5	2.1	*	*	0.2	0.5	1.6	4.7	12.3	33.3	99.9	280.0	13.1
2013	14.9	2.2	*	*	0.1	0.6	1.5	4.6	12.6	33.8	99.0	285.4	13.2
2014	15.1	2.3	*	*	0.2	0.5	1.7	4.7	12.6	34.3	98.6	282.4	13.2
2015	15.5	2,1	*	*	0.1	0.6	1.7	4.9	13.3	35.1	99.7	281.8	13.4
Intentional Self–Harm (Suicide) (*U03, X60–X84, Y87.0)[4]													
1999	10.5	NA	NA	0.6	10.1	12.7	14.3	13.9	12.2	13.4	18.1	19.3	10.5
2000	10.4	NA	NA	0.7	10.2	12.0	14.5	14.4	12.1	12.5	17.6	19.6	10.4
2001[5]	10.7	NA	NA	0.7	9.9	12.8	14.7	15.1	13.2	13.2	17.4	17.8	10.7
2002	11.0	NA	NA	0.6	9.8	12.8	15.3	15.8	13.5	13.4	17.7	18.9	10.9
2003	10.9	NA	NA	0.6	9.6	12.9	15.0	15.9	13.7	12.6	16.4	17.9	10.8
2004	11.1	NA	NA	0.7	10.3	12.9	15.2	16.6	13.7	12.2	16.3	17.6	11.0
2005	11.0	NA	NA	0.7	9.9	12.7	15.1	16.5	13.7	12.4	16.8	18.3	10.9
2006	11.2	NA	NA	0.5	9.8	12.7	15.2	17.2	14.4	12.4	15.8	17.3	11.0
2007	11.5	NA	NA	0.5	9.6	13.3	15.7	17.7	15.3	12.4	16.2	17.0	11.3
2008	11.8	NA	NA	0.5	9.9	13.2	15.9	18.6	16.0	13.6	16.1	16.4	11.6
2009	12.0	NA	NA	0.6	10.0	13.1	16.1	19.2	16.4	13.7	15.8	16.4	11.8
2010	12.4	NA	NA	0.7	10.5	14.0	16.0	19.6	17.5	13.7	15.7	17.6	12.1
2011	12.7	NA	NA	0.7	11.0	14.6	16.2	19.8	17.1	14.1	16.5	16.9	12.3

NA = Not applicable.

* = Figure does not meet standards of reliability or precision.

[1] Figures for age not stated included in "All ages" but not distributed among age groups.

[2] Death rates for "Under 1 year" (based on population estimates) differ from infant mortality rates (based on live births); please see chapter notes for more information.

[3] For method of computation, please see chapter notes.

[4] Asterisks (*) preceding cause-of-death codes indicate they are not part of the International Classification of Diseases, Tenth Revision (ICD–10).

[5] Data include September 11, 2001-related deaths for which death certificates were filed as of October 24, 2002; see Technical Notes for National Vital Statistics Reports vol 52 no 3, "Deaths: Final Data for 2001."

Table 2-8. Death Rates by Age and Age-Adjusted Death Rates for the 10 Leading Causes of Death in 2015 and Drug-Induced Deaths, Alcohol-Induced Deaths, and Injury by Firearm, 1999–2015—*Continued*

(Rate per 100,000 population in specified group; age-adjusted rates per 100,000 U.S. standard population.)

Cause of death (based on ICD–10) and year	All ages[1]	Under 1 year[2]	1 to 4 years	5 to 14 years	15 to 24 years	25 to 34 years	35 to 44 years	45 to 54 years	55 to 64 years	65 to 74 years	75 to 84 years	85 years and over	Age-adjusted rate[3]
2012	12.9	NA	NA	0.8	11.1	14.7	16.7	20.0	18.0	14.0	16.8	17.8	12.6
2013	13.0	NA	NA	1.0	11.1	14.8	16.2	19.7	18.1	15.0	17.1	18.6	12.6
2014	13.4	NA	NA	1.0	11.6	15.1	16.6	20.2	18.8	15.6	17.5	19.3	13.0
2015	13.7	NA	NA	1.0	12.5	15.7	17.1	20.3	18.9	15.2	17.9	19.4	13.2
Drug-Induced Causes[6]													
1999	6.9	0.6	0.2	0.1	3.5	8.9	15.7	12.6	4.9	3.0	3.8	4.8	6.8
2000	7.0	*	*	0.1	4.0	8.8	16.0	13.2	4.9	2.6	3.5	5.7	7.0
2001	7.6	0.5	0.2	0.1	4.5	9.5	17.0	14.7	5.4	3.0	3.5	5.2	7.6
2002	9.1	0.7	0.2	0.1	5.4	11.3	19.8	18.0	6.8	3.6	3.8	6.0	9.1
2003	9.9	0.6	0.2	0.1	6.3	12.3	20.7	20.0	8.0	4.1	4.2	6.3	9.9
2004	10.5	0.7	0.2	0.2	6.8	12.9	21.1	21.7	9.0	4.2	4.8	6.7	10.5
2005	11.3	0.9	0.2	0.1	7.3	14.6	21.5	23.6	10.6	4.7	5.4	8.3	11.3
2006	12.9	1.1	0.1	0.1	8.5	17.2	23.5	26.7	12.1	5.2	6.0	8.8	12.8
2007	12.7	0.8	0.3	0.2	8.5	17.5	22.6	26.8	13.4	4.6	3.9	5.2	12.6
2008	12.7	0.5	0.3	0.1	8.3	17.4	22.2	26.8	14.0	5.2	4.0	5.0	12.6
2009	12.8	0.8	0.2	0.1	8.0	17.8	21.5	26.9	14.9	5.4	4.5	5.1	12.6
2010	13.1	0.6	0.3	0.2	8.4	19.2	21.7	26.5	16.2	5.2	4.0	5.5	12.9
2011	14.0	0.6	0.2	0.1	8.9	20.9	23.4	28.2	17.1	6.0	4.0	4.9	13.9
2012	14.0	0.8	0.2	0.1	8.3	20.9	23.1	28.3	17.9	6.5	4.0	5.1	13.8
2013	14.7	0.8	0.3	0.1	8.6	21.7	24.1	29.0	20.6	7.1	4.4	5.3	14.6
2014	15.6	0.6	0.3	0.1	8.9	24.0	26.2	29.8	21.7	7.6	4.4	5.0	15.5
2015	17.2	0.7	0.4	0.1	10.0	28.0	29.6	31.9	23.3	8.1	4.4	5.6	17.2
Alcohol-Induced Causes[6]													
1999	7.0	*	*	*	0.3	1.6	8.5	16.4	18.7	15.9	10.6	5.5	7.1
2000	7.0	*	*	*	0.2	1.6	8.5	16.3	18.7	15.8	9.9	5.4	7.0
2001	7.1	*	*	*	0.3	1.6	8.3	17.1	18.3	15.5	9.6	5.1	7.0
2002	7.0	*	*	*	0.3	1.5	8.1	16.9	18.3	15.4	9.3	4.6	6.9
2003	7.1	*	*	*	0.3	1.5	8.1	17.3	18.5	15.0	9.2	4.3	7.0
2004	7.2	*	*	*	0.3	1.6	7.7	17.3	18.6	15.5	9.2	4.6	7.0
2005	7.3	*	*	*	0.4	1.4	7.5	17.6	19.4	14.9	9.2	5.0	7.0
2006	7.4	*	*	*	0.3	1.6	7.5	17.5	19.2	14.5	9.7	5.3	7.0
2007	7.7	*	*	*	0.4	1.9	7.3	18.2	19.9	15.2	9.6	5.0	7.2
2008	8.0	*	*	*	0.4	2.0	7.6	18.6	20.7	15.3	9.4	5.2	7.4
2009	8.0	*	*	*	0.4	1.8	7.6	18.7	20.8	15.1	9.2	4.8	7.4
2010	8.3	*	*	*	0.3	2.2	7.5	19.1	21.9	15.8	9.6	5.3	7.6
2011	8.6	*	*	*	0.4	2.1	7.6	19.8	22.7	15.2	9.6	5.1	7.7
2012	8.8	*	*	*	0.4	2.4	7.4	20.0	24.1	15.8	10.3	5.0	8.0
2013	9.2	*	*	*	0.3	2.5	7.7	20.1	25.3	16.6	10.3	4.9	8.2
2014	9.6	*	*	*	0.3	2.8	8.0	20.4	26.8	10.5	10.5	5.6	8.5
2015	10.3	*	*	*	0.4	3.2	8.7	21.6	28.2	11.2	11.2	5.8	9.1
Injury by Firearm[6]													
1999	10.3	*	0.4	1.0	17.6	14.9	11.6	10.2	9.7	11.0	14.2	13.5	10.3
2000	10.2	*	0.3	0.9	16.8	14.5	11.9	10.5	9.4	10.6	13.9	14.2	10.2
2001	10.4	*	0.5	0.8	16.6	15.5	11.7	10.5	10.1	10.9	14.3	13.1	10.3
2002	10.5	*	0.4	0.8	16.6	15.6	12.2	10.8	10.2	10.8	14.4	13.2	10.5
2003	10.4	*	0.3	0.8	16.5	15.8	11.6	11.1	10.0	10.3	13.4	13.2	10.3
2004	10.1	*	0.3	0.7	15.6	15.3	11.4	11.0	9.8	10.1	13.3	12.7	10.0
2005	10.4	*	0.4	0.8	16.1	16.1	11.7	11.2	9.7	10.2	13.6	13.0	10.3
2006	10.4	*	0.4	0.9	15.7	16.7	11.6	11.2	9.7	9.9	12.9	12.5	10.3
2007	10.4	*	0.4	0.8	15.9	16.0	12.0	11.1	10.1	9.8	13.1	12.7	10.3
2008	10.4	*	0.5	0.7	15.4	15.4	11.8	11.5	10.8	10.7	13.2	12.5	10.3
2009	10.2	*	0.4	0.7	14.4	14.5	11.9	11.8	10.8	10.9	13.3	12.5	10.1
2010	10.3	*	0.4	0.7	14.2	15.0	11.7	12.0	11.1	10.7	12.7	13.2	10.1
2011	10.4	*	0.5	0.8	14.4	15.0	11.7	12.2	11.0	10.9	13.7	13.1	10.2
2012	10.7	*	0.4	0.8	14.7	15.3	12.4	12.4	11.6	10.8	14.1	13.6	10.5
2013	10.8	*	0.4	0.8	14.1	15.3	12.3	12.3	11.5	11.3	14.1	13.9	10.4
2014	10.5	*	0.4	0.9	14.0	14.7	12.1	12.1	11.4	11.5	13.9	15.0	10.3
2015	11.3	*	0.5	0.9	15.7	16.8	13.1	13.1	11.7	11.3	14.5	14.5	11.1

NA = Not applicable.
* = Figure does not meet standards of reliability or precision.
[1] Figures for age not stated included in "All ages" but not distributed among age groups.
[2] Death rates for "Under 1 year" (based on population estimates) differ from infant mortality rates (based on live births); please see chapter notes for more information.
[3] For method of computation, please see chapter notes.
[6] For the list of ICD–10 codes included, see chapter notes.

Table 2-9. Number of Deaths from Selected Causes, by Age, 2015

(Number.)

Cause of death (based on ICD-10, 2004)	All ages	Under 1 year	1 to 4 years	5 to 14 years	15 to 24 years	25 to 34 years	35 to 44 years	45 to 54 years	55 to 64 years	65 to 74 years	75 to 84 years	85 years and over	Not stated
All causes	2,712,630	23,455	3,965	5,411	30,494	51,517	73,088	174,494	357,785	495,016	637,566	859,701	138
Enterocolitis due to Clostridium difficile (A047)	7,410	2	2	3	8	22	67	214	650	1,272	2,256	2,913	1
Septicemia (A40–A41)	40,773	180	54	64	130	379	829	2,542	5,774	8,655	10,481	11,681	4
Viral hepatitis (B15–B19)	7,461	1	–	1	4	47	248	1,496	3,559	1,464	478	163	–
Human immunodeficiency virus (HIV) disease (B20–B24)	6,465	2	2	1	100	529	1,055	2,027	1,824	710	184	31	–
Malignant neoplasms(C00–C97)	595,930	53	354	865	1,469	3,704	10,909	43,054	116,122	163,728	153,268	102,393	11
Malignant neoplasms of lip, oral cavity and pharynx (C00–C14)	9,754	–	–	1	19	66	174	1,009	2,662	2,657	1,869	1,297	–
Malignant neoplasm of esophagus (C15)	15,212	–	–	–	4	32	230	1,239	3,813	4,734	3,475	1,684	1
Malignant neoplasm of stomach (C16)	11,331	–	–	–	26	129	439	1,086	2,148	2,754	2,851	1,897	1
Malignant neoplasms of colon, rectum and anus (C18–C21)	53,176	–	–	–	41	368	1,407	4,972	10,225	12,586	12,572	11,004	1
Malignant neoplasms of liver and intrahepatic bile ducts (C22)	25,761	2	14	19	31	100	335	2,090	7,979	7,289	5,265	2,636	1
Malignant neoplasm of pancreas (C25)	41,615	–	–	–	14	62	446	2,704	8,307	12,438	11,030	6,614	–
Malignant neoplasms of trachea, bronchus and lung (C33–C34)	153,819	–	2	5	26	133	1,015	8,837	31,413	49,855	42,655	19,874	4
Malignant melanoma of skin (C43)	8,885	–	3	1	18	129	390	837	1,678	2,181	2,105	1,543	–
Malignant neoplasm of breast (C50)	41,987	–	–	–	9	390	1,842	5,220	9,255	9,931	8,156	7,183	1
Malignant neoplasm of cervix uteri (C53)	4,175	–	–	–	10	210	561	906	1,014	779	456	239	–
Malignant neoplasm of ovary (C56)	13,920	–	–	4	29	89	302	1,272	2,959	3,902	3,385	1,978	–
Malignant neoplasm of prostate (C61)	28,848	–	–	–	–	4	18	394	2,715	6,487	9,611	9,619	–
Malignant neoplasm of kidney and renal pelvis (C64–C65)	14,448	5	11	20	28	65	227	1,068	3,077	4,072	3,537	2,338	–
Malignant neoplasm of bladder (C67)	16,254	–	–	–	2	15	68	497	1,817	3,620	5,147	5,088	–
Malignant neoplasms of meninges, brain and other parts of central nervous system (C70–C72)	16,268	9	94	327	230	405	839	1,966	3,748	4,355	2,963	1,332	–
Non-Hodgkin's lymphoma (C82–C85)	20,154	–	3	32	86	186	340	1,032	2,795	4,899	6,189	4,592	–
Multiple myeloma and immunoproliferative neoplasms (C88,C90)	12,696	–	–	–	1	10	116	640	1,912	3,577	4,056	2,384	–
Leukemia (C91–C95)	22,665	22	115	206	335	419	495	1,180	2,795	5,338	6,724	5,036	–
In situ neoplasms, benign neoplasms and neoplasms of uncertain or unknown behavior (D00–D48)	16,277	47	34	72	83	147	261	675	1,619	3,156	4,837	5,346	–
Anemias (D50–D64)	5,250	17	25	33	84	146	176	257	476	793	1,132	2,111	–
Diabetes mellitus (E10–E14)	79,535	3	5	23	196	798	1,986	6,212	14,166	19,453	19,904	16,785	4
Nutritional deficiencies (E40–E64)	5,222	9	4	1	10	25	44	137	355	697	1,211	2,729	–
Obesity (E66)	7,430	–	1	4	75	397	887	1,586	1,951	1,568	742	219	–
Parkinson's disease (G20–G21)	27,972	–	–	–	3	–	6	66	628	3,813	11,473	11,983	–
Alzheimer's disease (G30)	110,561	–	–	–	–	–	11	87	968	6,167	29,503	73,825	–
Major cardiovascular diseases (I00–I78)	832,024	404	196	300	1,226	4,383	13,104	42,106	95,347	137,805	201,515	335,601	37
Diseases of heart (I00–I09,I11,I13,I20–I51)	633,842	292	147	210	997	3,522	10,387	34,248	76,872	107,303	149,199	250,636	29
Essential hypertension and hypertensive renal disease (I10,I12,I15)	32,200	3	4	–	15	121	470	1,477	3,595	4,979	7,533	14,003	–
Cerebrovascular diseases (I60–I69)	140,323	89	42	84	166	567	1,788	5,307	12,116	20,793	38,012	61,351	8
Atherosclerosis (I70)	6,088	5	–	–	1	7	22	96	364	741	1,506	3,346	–
Aortic aneurysm and dissection (I71)	9,988	1	–	4	33	124	322	620	1,322	2,122	2,769	2,671	–
Influenza and pneumonia (J09–J18)	57,062	174	88	83	184	397	708	2,050	4,601	8,131	14,149	26,494	3
Chronic lower respiratory diseases (J40–J47)	155,041	26	40	173	202	288	702	4,345	17,457	37,642	49,832	44,330	4
Pneumonitis due to solids and liquids (J69)	19,803	8	10	6	43	87	171	536	1,468	2,586	5,152	9,736	–
Chronic liver disease and cirrhosis (K70,K73–K74)	40,326	3	2	1	28	844	2,861	8,874	13,278	8,409	4,446	1,577	3
Alcoholic liver disease (K70)	21,028	–	–	–	19	681	2,147	5,997	7,574	3,413	1,012	183	2
Cholelithiasis and other disorders of gallbladder (K80–K82)	3,766	–	–	–	5	21	49	141	311	661	1,046	1,532	–
Nephritis, nephrotic syndrome and nephrosis (N00–N07,N17–N19,N25–N27)	49,959	85	16	17	57	262	686	2,124	5,452	9,662	13,881	17,715	2
Pregnancy, childbirth and the puerperium (O00–O99)	1,140	...	...	2	161	424	310	240	1	1	–	–	1
Certain conditions originating in the perinatal period (P00–P96)	11,715	11,613	50	21	11	3	2	8	5	1	–	1	–
Congenital malformations, deformations and chromosomal abnormalities (Q00–Q99)	10,017	4,825	435	337	386	443	483	781	1,085	542	341	358	1
Symptoms, signs and abnormal clinical and laboratory findings, not elsewhere classified (R00–R99)	32,042	2,819	252	115	552	1,125	1,299	2,152	2,957	3,518	4,924	12,301	28
Accidents (unintentional injuries) (V01–X59,Y85–Y86)	146,571	1,291	1,235	1,518	12,514	19,795	17,818	21,499	19,488	12,961	15,518	22,916	18
Motor vehicle accidents (V02–V04,V09 0,V09 2,V12–V14, V19 0–V19 2,V19 4–V19 6,V20–V79,V80 3–V80 5, V81 0–V81 1,V82 0–V82 1,V83–V86,V87 0–V87 8, V88 0–V88 8,V89 0,V89 2)	37,757	70	416	860	6,977	6,504	4,849	5,539	5,209	3,524	2,437	1,367	5
Falls (W00–W19)	33,381	4	30	25	217	324	492	1,298	2,504	4,091	8,668	15,727	1
Accidental discharge of firearms (W32–W34)	489	1	25	22	121	79	59	57	55	45	18	7	–
Accidental drowning and submersion (W65–W74)	3,602	30	390	216	504	445	374	450	491	343	267	89	3
Accidental hanging, strangulation, and suffocation (W75–W84)	6,914	1,125	131	57	97	181	240	469	777	923	1,231	1,683	–
Accidental exposure to smoke, fire and flames (X00–X09)	2,646	22	96	113	78	137	148	364	558	494	411	224	1
Accidental poisoning and exposure to noxious substances (X40–X49)	47,478	9	29	53	3,920	11,231	10,580	11,670	7,782	1,596	386	216	6
Intentional self-harm (suicide) (*U03,X60–X84,Y87 0)[1]	44,193	X	X	413	5,491	6,947	6,936	8,751	7,739	4,201	2,489	1,222	4
Intentional self-harm (suicide) by poisoning (X60–X69)	6,816	X	X	23	409	769	1,181	1,835	1,593	603	250	152	1
Intentional self-harm (suicide) by hanging, strangulation and suffocation (X70)	11,855	X	X	237	2,119	2,504	2,219	2,333	1,535	541	232	135	–
Intentional self-harm (suicide) by discharge of firearms (X72–X74)	22,018	X	X	140	2,461	3,118	2,952	3,882	3,951	2,779	1,872	860	3
Assault (homicide) (*U01–*U02,X85–Y09,Y87.1)[1]	17,793	253	369	298	4,733	4,863	2,895	2,106	1,309	550	294	109	4
Assault (homicide) by discharge of firearms (*U01.4,X93–X95)	12,979	8	50	190	4,140	3,996	2,197	1,299	681	258	119	40	1
Legal intervention (Y35,Y89.0)	530	-	-	-	88	163	109	101	53	10	4	2	-
Complications of medical and surgical care (Y40-Y84,Y88)	2,686	12	18	17	40	65	113	240	460	652	607	462	-
Drug-induced deaths[2]	56,403	29	56	60	4,401	12,379	12,013	13,760	9,511	2,230	606	353	5
Alcohol-induced deaths[2]	33,171	-	-	3	157	1,418	3,543	9,320	11,545	5,255	1,557	366	7
Injury by firearms[2]	36,252	9	78	356	6,883	7,406	5,337	5,361	4,766	3,114	2,024	914	4

X = Not applicable.
- = Quantity zero.
[1] Asterisks (*) preceding cause-of-death codes indicate they are not part of the International Classification of Diseases, Tenth Revision (ICD–10)
[2] Included in selected categories above.

Table 2-10. Death Rates for Selected Causes, by Age, 2015

(Number.)

Cause of death (based on ICD-10, 2004)	All ages[1]	Under 1 year[2]	1 to 4 years	5 to 14 years	15 to 24 years	25 to 34 years	35 to 44 years	45 to 54 years	55 to 64 years	65 to 74 years	75 to 84 years	85 years and over
All causes	844.0	589.6	24.9	13.2	69.5	116.7	180.1	404.0	875.3	1,796.8	4,579.2	13,673.9
Enterocolitis due to Clostridium difficile (A047)	2.3	*	*	*	*	0.0	0.2	0.5	1.6	4.6	16.2	46.3
Septicemia (A40–A41)	12.7	4.5	0.3	0.2	0.3	0.9	2.0	5.9	14.1	31.4	75.3	185.8
Viral hepatitis (B15–B19)	2.3	*	*	*	*	0.1	0.6	3.5	8.7	5.3	3.4	2.6
Human immunodeficiency virus (HIV) disease (B20–B24)	2.0	*	*	*	0.2	1.2	2.6	4.7	4.5	2.6	1.3	0.5
Malignant neoplasms (C00–C97)	185.4	1.3	2.2	2.1	3.4	8.4	26.9	99.7	284.1	594.3	1,100.8	1,628.6
Malignant neoplasms of lip, oral cavity and pharynx (C00–C14)	3.0	*	*	*	*	0.1	0.4	2.3	6.5	9.6	13.4	20.6
Malignant neoplasm of esophagus (C15)	4.7	*	*	*	*	0.1	0.6	2.9	9.3	17.2	25.0	26.8
Malignant neoplasm of stomach (C16)	3.5	*	*	*	0.1	0.3	1.1	2.5	5.3	10.0	20.5	30.2
Malignant neoplasms of colon, rectum and anus (C18–C21)	16.5	*	*	*	0.1	0.8	3.5	11.5	25.0	45.7	90.3	175.0
Malignant neoplasm of liver and intrahepatic bile ducts (C22)	8.0	*	*	*	0.1	0.2	0.8	4.8	19.5	26.5	37.8	41.9
Malignant neoplasm of pancreas (C25)	12.9	*	*	*	*	0.1	1.1	6.3	20.3	45.1	79.2	105.2
Malignant neoplasms of trachea, bronchus and lung (C33–C34)	47.9	*	*	*	0.1	0.3	2.5	20.5	76.8	181.0	306.4	316.1
Malignant melanoma of skin (C43)	2.8	*	*	*	*	0.3	1.0	1.9	4.1	7.9	15.1	24.5
Malignant neoplasm of breast (C50)	13.1	*	*	*	*	0.9	4.5	12.1	22.6	36.0	58.6	114.2
Malignant neoplasm of cervix uteri (C53)	1.3	*	*	*	*	0.5	1.4	2.1	2.5	2.8	3.3	3.8
Malignant neoplasm of ovary (C56)	4.3	*	*	*	0.1	0.2	0.7	2.9	7.2	14.2	24.3	31.5
Malignant neoplasm of prostate (C61)	9.0	*	*	*	*	*	*	0.9	6.6	23.5	69.0	153.0
Malignant neoplasms of kidney and renal pelvis (C64–C65)	4.5	*	*	0.0	0.1	0.1	0.6	2.5	7.5	14.8	25.4	37.2
Malignant neoplasm of bladder (C67)	5.1	*	*	*	*	*	0.2	1.2	4.4	13.1	37.0	80.9
Malignant neoplasms of meninges, brain and other parts of central nervous system (C70–C72)	5.1	*	0.6	0.8	0.5	0.9	2.1	4.6	9.2	15.8	21.3	21.2
Non-Hodgkin's lymphoma (C82–C85)	6.3	*	*	0.1	0.2	0.4	0.8	2.4	6.8	17.8	44.5	73.0
Multiple myeloma and immunoproliferative neoplasms (C88,C90)	3.9	*	*	*	*	*	0.3	1.5	4.7	13.0	29.1	37.9
Leukemia (C91–C95)	7.1	0.6	0.7	0.5	0.8	0.9	1.2	2.7	6.8	19.4	48.3	80.1
In situ neoplasms, benign neoplasms and neoplasms of uncertain or unknown behavior (D00–D48)	5.1	1.2	0.2	0.2	0.2	0.3	0.6	1.6	4.0	11.5	34.7	85.0
Anemias (D50–D64)	1.6	*	0.2	0.1	0.2	0.3	0.4	0.6	1.2	2.9	8.1	33.6
Diabetes mellitus (E10–E14)	24.7	*	*	0.1	0.4	1.8	4.9	14.4	34.7	70.6	143.0	267.0
Nutritional deficiencies (E40–E64)	1.6	*	*	*	*	0.1	0.1	0.3	0.9	2.5	8.7	43.4
Obesity (E66)	2.3	*	*	*	0.2	0.9	2.2	3.7	4.8	5.7	5.3	3.5
Parkinson's disease (G20–G21)	8.7	*	*	*	*	*	*	0.2	1.5	13.8	82.4	190.6
Alzheimer's disease (G30)	34.4	*	*	*	*	*	*	0.2	2.4	22.4	211.9	1,174.2
Major cardiovascular diseases (I00–I78)	258.9	10.2	1.2	0.7	2.8	9.9	32.3	97.5	233.2	500.2	1,447.3	5,337.9
Diseases of heart (I00–I09,I11,I13,I20–I51)	197.2	7.3	0.9	0.5	2.3	8.0	25.6	79.3	188.1	389.5	1,071.6	3,986.5
Essential hypertension and hypertensive renal disease (I10,I12,I15)	10.0	*	*	*	*	0.3	1.2	3.4	8.8	18.1	54.1	222.7
Cerebrovascular diseases (I60–I69)	43.7	2.2	0.3	0.2	0.4	1.3	4.4	12.3	29.6	75.5	273.0	975.8
Atherosclerosis (I70)	1.9	*	*	*	*	*	0.1	0.2	0.9	2.7	10.8	53.2
Aortic aneurysm and dissection (I71)	3.1	*	*	*	0.1	0.3	0.8	1.4	3.2	7.7	19.9	42.5
Influenza and pneumonia (J09–J18)	17.8	4.4	0.6	0.2	0.4	0.9	1.7	4.7	11.3	29.5	101.6	421.4
Chronic lower respiratory diseases (J40–J47)	48.2	0.7	0.3	0.4	0.5	0.7	1.7	10.1	42.7	136.6	357.9	705.1
Pneumonitis due to solids and liquids (J69)	6.2	*	*	*	0.1	0.2	0.4	1.2	3.6	9.4	37.0	154.9
Chronic liver disease and cirrhosis (K70,K73–K74)	12.5	*	*	*	0.1	1.9	7.0	20.5	32.5	30.5	31.9	25.1
Alcoholic liver disease (K70)	6.5	*	*	*	*	1.5	5.3	13.9	18.5	12.4	7.3	2.9
Cholelithiasis and other disorders of gallbladder (K80–K82)	1.2	*	*	*	*	0.0	0.1	0.3	0.8	2.4	7.5	24.4
Nephritis, nephrotic syndrome and nephrosis (N00–N07,N17–N19,N25–N27)	15.5	2.1	*	*	0.1	0.6	1.7	4.9	13.3	35.1	99.7	281.8
Pregnancy, childbirth and the puerperium O00–O99)	0.4	X	X	*	0.4	1.0	0.8	0.6	*	*	*	*
Certain conditions originating in the perinatal period (P00–P96)	3.6	291.9	0.3	0.1	*	*	*	*	*	*	*	*
Congenital malformations, deformations and chromosomal abnormalities (Q00–Q99)	3.1	121.3	2.7	0.8	0.9	1.0	1.2	1.8	2.7	2.0	2.4	5.7
Symptoms, signs and abnormal clinical and laboratory findings, not elsewhere classified (R00–R99)	10.0	70.9	1.6	0.3	1.3	2.5	3.2	5.0	7.2	12.8	35.4	195.7
Accidents (unintentional injuries) (V01–X59,Y85–Y86)	45.6	32.5	7.8	3.7	28.5	44.8	43.9	49.8	47.7	47.0	111.5	364.5
Motor vehicle accidents (V02–V04,V090,V092,V12–V14, V190–V192,V194–V196,V20–V79,V803–V805 V810–V811,V820–V821,V83–V86,V870–V878, V880–V888,V890,V892)	11.7	1.8	2.6	2.1	15.9	14.7	11.9	12.8	12.7	12.8	17.5	21.7
Falls (W00–W19)	10.4	*	0.2	0.1	0.5	0.7	1.2	3.0	6.1	14.8	62.3	250.1
Accidental discharge of firearms (W32–W34)	0.2	*	0.2	0.1	0.3	0.2	0.1	0.1	0.1	0.2	*	*
Accidental drowning and submersion (W65–W74)	1.1	0.8	2.4	0.5	1.1	1.0	0.9	1.0	1.2	1.2	1.9	1.4
Accidental hanging, strangulation, and suffocation (W75–W84)	2.2	28.3	0.8	0.1	0.2	0.4	0.6	1.1	1.9	3.4	8.8	26.8
Accidental exposure to smoke, fire and flames (X00–X09)	0.8	0.6	0.6	0.3	0.2	0.3	0.4	0.8	1.4	1.8	3.0	3.6
Accidental poisoning and exposure to noxious substances (X40–X49)	14.8	*	0.2	0.1	8.9	25.4	26.1	27.0	19.0	5.8	2.8	3.4
Intentional self-harm (suicide) (*U03,X60–X84,Y870)[3]	13.7	X	X	1.0	12.5	15.7	17.1	20.3	18.9	15.2	17.9	19.4
Intentional self-harm (suicide) by poisoning (X60–X69)	2.1	X	X	0.1	0.9	1.7	2.9	4.2	3.9	2.2	1.8	2.4
Intentional self-harm (suicide) by hanging, strangulation and suffocation (X70)	3.7	X	X	0.6	4.8	5.7	5.5	5.4	3.8	2.0	1.7	2.1
Intentional self-harm (suicide) by discharge of firearms (X72–X74)	6.9	X	X	0.3	5.6	7.1	7.3	9.0	9.7	10.1	13.4	13.7
Assault (homicide) (*U01–*U02,X85–Y09,Y871)[3]	5.5	6.6	2.3	0.7	10.8	11.0	7.1	4.9	3.2	2.0	2.1	1.7
Assault (homicide) by discharge of firearms (*U014,X93–X95)[3]	4.0	*	0.3	0.5	9.4	9.1	5.4	3.0	1.7	0.9	0.9	0.6
Legal intervention (Y35,Y890)	0.2	*	*	*	0.2	0.4	0.3	0.2	0.1	*	*	*
Complications of medical and surgical care (Y40–Y84,Y88)	0.8	*	*	*	0.1	0.1	0.3	0.6	1.1	2.4	4.4	7.3
Drug-induced deaths[4]	17.2	0.7	0.4	0.1	10.0	28.0	29.6	31.9	23.3	8.1	4.4	5.6
Alcohol-induced deaths[4]	10.3	*	*	*	0.4	3.2	8.7	21.6	28.2	19.1	11.2	5.8
Injury by firearms[4]	11.3	*	0.5	0.9	15.7	16.8	13.1	12.4	11.7	11.3	14.5	14.5

X = Not applicable.
* = Figure does not meet standards of reliability or precision.
0.0 = Quantity more than zero but less than 0.05.
[1]Figures for age not stated included in "All ages" but not distributed among age groups.
[2]Death rates for "Under 1 year" (based on population estimates) differ from infant mortality rates (based on live births); for more information, see chapter notes.
[3]Asterisks (*) preceding cause-of-death codes indicate they are not part of the International Classification of Diseases, Tenth Revision (ICD–10)
[4]Included in selected categories above.

Table 2-11. Number of Deaths from Selected Causes, by Race, Hispanic Origin, and Sex, 2015

(Number.)

Cause of death (based on ICD–10, 2004)	All races[1] Both sexes	Male	Female	Non-Hispanic White[2] Both sexes	Male	Female	Non-Hispanic Black[2] Both sexes	Male	Female
All causes	2,712,630	1,373,404	1,339,226	2,123,631	1,063,705	1,059,926	315,254	161,850	153,404
Enterocolitis due to Clostridium difficile (A04 7)	7,410	3,003	4,407	6,104	2,443	3,661	609	246	363
Septicemia (A40–A41)	40,773	19,385	21,388	30,240	14,309	15,931	6,576	3,061	3,515
Viral hepatitis (B15–B19)	7,461	4,977	2,484	4,797	3,203	1,594	1,124	747	377
Human immunodeficiency virus (HIV) disease (B20–B24)	6,465	4,796	1,669	1,984	1,660	324	3,379	2,230	1,149
Malignant neoplasms (C00–C97)	595,930	313,818	282,112	467,208	247,645	219,563	68,523	34,787	33,736
Malignant neoplasms of lip, oral cavity and pharynx (C00–C14)	9,754	6,882	2,872	7,631	5,386	2,245	1,065	748	317
Malignant neoplasm of esophagus (C15)	15,212	12,187	3,025	12,915	10,463	2,452	1,212	853	359
Malignant neoplasm of stomach (C16)	11,331	6,754	4,577	6,589	4,016	2,573	1,994	1,215	779
Malignant neoplasms of colon, rectum and anus (C18–C21)	53,176	27,805	25,371	40,045	20,838	19,207	7,123	3,675	3,448
Malignant neoplasm of liver and intrahepatic bile ducts (C22)	25,761	17,414	8,347	17,107	11,530	5,577	3,519	2,487	1,032
Malignant neoplasm of pancreas (C25)	41,615	21,392	20,223	32,138	16,842	15,296	5,022	2,355	2,667
Malignant neoplasms of trachea, bronchus and lung (C33–C34)	153,819	83,700	70,119	126,835	68,088	58,747	16,115	9,306	6,809
Malignant melanoma of skin (C43)	8,885	5,811	3,074	8,426	5,541	2,885	125	77	48
Malignant neoplasm of breast (C50)	41,987	463	41,524	31,339	340	30,999	6,314	85	6,229
Malignant neoplasm of cervix uteri (C53)	4,175	X	4,175	2,627	X	2,627	750	X	750
Malignant neoplasm of ovary (C56)	13,920	X	13,920	11,024	X	11,024	1,335	X	1,335
Malignant neoplasm of prostate (C61)	28,848	28,848	X	21,513	21,513	X	4,678	4,678	X
Malignant neoplasms of kidney and renal pelvis (C64–C65)	14,448	9,502	4,946	11,364	7,521	3,843	1,411	891	520
Malignant neoplasm of bladder (C67)	16,254	11,587	4,667	14,016	10,160	3,856	1,176	704	472
Malignant neoplasms of meninges,brain and other parts of central nervous system (C70–C72)	16,268	9,119	7,149	13,508	7,621	5,887	1,055	570	485
Non-Hodgkin's lymphoma (C82–C85)	20,154	11,381	8,773	16,396	9,290	7,106	1,511	824	687
Multiple myeloma and immunoproliferative neoplasms (C88,C90)	12,696	6,988	5,708	9,194	5,224	3,970	2,216	1,074	1,142
Leukemia (C91–C95)	22,665	13,251	9,414	18,447	10,874	7,573	1,863	1,009	854
In situ neoplasms, benign neoplasms and neoplasms of uncertain or unknown behavior (D00–D48)	16,277	8,647	7,630	13,404	7,253	6,151	1,466	695	771
Anemias (D50–D64)	5,250	2,253	2,997	3,754	1,594	2,160	1,039	451	588
Diabetes mellitus (E10–E14)	79,535	43,123	36,412	53,590	29,813	23,777	13,693	6,806	6,887
Nutritional deficiencies (E40–E64)	5,222	1,952	3,270	4,130	1,500	2,630	626	257	369
Obesity (E66)	7,430	3,788	3,642	5,344	2,802	2,542	1,386	599	787
Parkinson's disease (G20–G21)	27,972	16,867	11,105	24,339	14,778	9,561	1,181	684	497
Alzheimer's disease (G30)	110,561	33,690	76,871	93,325	28,631	64,694	8,072	2,154	5,918
Major cardiovascular diseases (I00–I78)	832,024	420,111	411,913	653,378	327,784	325,594	100,448	50,624	49,824
Diseases of heart (I00–I09,I11,I13,I20–I51)	633,842	335,002	298,840	503,172	264,784	238,388	74,093	38,638	35,455
Essential hypertension and hypertensive renal disease (I10,I12,I15)	32,200	13,934	18,266	22,628	9,526	13,102	5,740	2,599	3,141
Cerebrovascular diseases (I60–I69)	140,323	58,288	82,035	106,830	43,100	63,730	17,760	7,962	9,798
Atherosclerosis (I70)	6,088	2,549	3,539	5,105	2,106	2,999	530	225	305
Aortic aneurysm and dissection (I71)	9,988	5,870	4,118	8,084	4,755	3,329	1,026	580	446
Influenza and pneumonia (J09–J18)	57,062	26,903	30,159	45,242	20,995	24,247	5,554	2,729	2,825
Chronic lower respiratory diseases (J40–J47)	155,041	72,498	82,543	136,228	62,857	73,371	10,327	5,236	5,091
Pneumonitis due to solids and liquids (J69)	19,803	10,911	8,892	16,430	9,085	7,345	1,689	883	806
Chronic liver disease and cirrhosis (K70,K73–K74)	40,326	25,666	14,660	29,343	18,546	10,797	3,185	1,933	1,252
Alcoholic liver disease (K70)	21,028	14,715	6,313	14,978	10,327	4,651	1,571	986	585
Cholelithiasis and other disorders of gallbladder (K80–K82)	3,766	1,797	1,969	2,976	1,432	1,544	328	140	188
Nephritis, nephrotic syndrome and nephrosis (N00–N07,N17–N19, N25–N27)	49,959	25,441	24,518	35,481	18,351	17,130	9,083	4,351	4,732
Pregnancy, childbirth and the puerperium (O00–O99)	1,140	X	1,140	541	X	541	373	X	373
Certain conditions originating in the perinatal period (P00–P96)	11,715	6,494	5,221	4,670	2,573	2,097	3,827	2,130	1,697
Congenital malformations, deformations and chromosomal abnormalities (Q00–Q99)	10,017	5,316	4,701	6,139	3,235	2,904	1,590	876	714
Symptoms, signs and abnormal clinical and laboratory findings, not elsewhere classified (R00–R99)	32,042	14,912	17,130	24,688	11,046	13,642	4,232	2,152	2,080
Accidents (unintentional injuries) (V01–X59,Y85–Y86)	146,571	92,919	53,652	111,827	68,715	43,112	15,366	10,516	4,850
Motor vehicle accidents (V02–V04, V09 0,V09 2,V12–V14,V19 0–V19 2, V19 4–V19 6,V20–V79,V80 3–V80 5, V81 0–V81 1,V82 0–V82 1,V83–V86, V87 0–87 8,V88 0–V88 8,V89 0,V89 2)	37,757	26,895	10,862	25,156	17,709	7,447	5,323	3,934	1,389
Falls (W00–W19)	33,381	16,881	16,500	28,913	14,277	14,636	1,458	851	607
Accidental discharge of firearms (W32–W34)	489	418	71	333	286	47	95	81	14
Accidental drowning and submersion (W65–W74)	3,602	2,716	886	2,310	1,687	623	553	442	111
Accidental hanging, strangulation, and suffocation (W75–W84)	6,914	3,942	2,972	5,175	2,943	2,232	988	555	433
Accidental exposure to smoke, fire and flames (X00–X09)	2,646	1,586	1,060	1,833	1,095	738	570	343	227
Accidental poisoning and exposure to noxious substances (X40–X49)	47,478	31,436	16,042	37,024	23,963	13,061	4,799	3,254	1,545
Intentional self-harm (suicide) (*U03,X60–X84,Y87 0)[5]	44,193	33,994	10,199	36,465	28,045	8,420	2,415	1,951	464
Intentional self-harm (suicide) by poisoning (X60–X69)	6,816	3,407	3,409	5,922	2,952	2,970	279	152	127
Intentional self-harm (suicide) by hanging, strangulation and suffocation (X70)	11,855	9,134	2,721	8,826	6,848	1,978	664	519	145
Intentional self-harm (suicide) by discharge of firearms (X72–X74)	22,018	18,910	3,108	19,161	16,397	2,764	1,132	1,017	115
Assault (homicide) (*U01–*U02, X85–Y09,Y87 1)[5]	17,793	14,274	3,519	5,222	3,487	1,735	9,038	7,909	1,129
Assault (homicide) by discharge of firearms (*U01 4,X93–X95)[5]	12,979	11,029	1,950	3,075	2,134	941	7,515	6,821	694
Legal intervention (Y35, Y89.0)	530	508	22	283	271	12	120	113	7
Complications of medical and surgical care (Y40–Y84, Y88)	2,686	1,364	1,322	2,021	1,019	1,002	416	215	201
Drug-induced deaths[6]	55,403	34,815	20,588	43,917	26,902	17,015	5,505	3,664	1,841
Alcohol-induced deaths[6]	33,171	23,996	9,175	24,017	17,096	6,921	2,858	1,970	888
Injury by firearms[6]	36,252	31,032	5,220	23,026	19,208	3,818	8,904	8,068	836

X = Not applicable.
- = Quantity zero.
[1]Includes deaths for origin not stated.
[2]Multiple-race data reported according to 1997 OMB standards were bridged to the single-race categories of 1977 OMB standards.
[4]Includes Chinese, Filipinos, Hawaiians, Japanese, and other Asian and Pacific Islander persons.
[5]Asterisks (*) preceding cause-of-death codes indicate they are not part of the ICD-10.
[6]Included in selected categories above.

Table 2-11. Number of Deaths from Selected Causes, by Race, Hispanic Origin, and Sex, 2015—*Continued*

(Number.)

Cause of death (based on ICD–10, 2004)	Non-Hispanic American Indian and Alaskan Native[2,3]			Non-Hispanic Asian or Pacific Islander[2,4]			Hispanic		
	Both sexes	Male	Female	Both sexes	Male	Female	Both sexes	Male	Female
All causes	18,039	9,869	8,170	65,277	33,306	31,971	179,457	98,170	81,287
Enterocolitis due to Clostridium difficile (A04 7)	38	18	20	149	75	74	477	203	274
Septicemia (A40–A41)	296	130	166	798	418	380	2,692	1,370	1,322
Viral hepatitis (B15–B19)	102	70	32	224	121	103	1,144	785	359
Human immunodeficiency virus (HIV) disease (B20–B24)	53	34	19	73	64	9	889	734	155
Malignant neoplasms (C00–C97)	3,192	1,699	1,493	17,306	8,774	8,532	37,804	19,847	17,957
Malignant neoplasms of lip, oral cavity and pharynx (C00–C14)	54	37	17	396	270	126	564	407	157
Malignant neoplasm of esophagus (C15)	90	76	14	260	208	52	683	545	138
Malignant neoplasm of stomach (C16)	81	55	26	874	472	402	1,753	977	776
Malignant neoplasms of colon, rectum and anus (C18–C21)	325	184	141	1,718	866	852	3,787	2,140	1,647
Malignant neoplasms of liver and intrahepatic bile ducts (C22)	240	162	78	1,618	1,086	532	3,187	2,080	1,107
Malignant neoplasm of pancreas (C25)	207	101	106	1,309	623	686	2,821	1,402	1,419
Malignant neoplasms of trachea, bronchus and lung (C33–C34)	796	425	371	3,831	2,195	1,636	5,701	3,360	2,341
Malignant melanoma of skin (C43)	10	3	7	58	32	26	238	141	97
Malignant neoplasm of breast (C50)	210	1	209	1,218	7	1,211	2,767	28	2,739
Malignant neoplasm of cervix uteri (C53)	32	X	32	191	X	191	563	X	563
Malignant neoplasm of ovary (C56)	91	X	91	442	X	442	999	X	999
Malignant neoplasm of prostate (C61)	143	143	X	574	574	X	1,867	1,867	X
Malignant neoplasms of kidney and renal pelvis (C64–C65)	108	72	36	301	199	102	1,232	804	428
Malignant neoplasm of bladder (C67)	48	30	18	262	183	79	688	463	225
Malignant neoplasms of meninges, brain and other parts of central nervous system (C70–C72)	60	39	21	436	225	211	1,181	645	536
Non-Hodgkin's lymphoma (C82–C85)	93	53	40	657	359	298	1,442	826	616
Multiple myeloma and immunoproliferative neoplasms (C88,C90)	60	33	27	298	152	146	891	483	408
Leukemia (C91–C95)	93	61	32	583	349	234	1,611	914	697
In situ neoplasms, benign neoplasms and neoplasms of uncertain or unknown behavior (D00–D48)	72	38	34	426	204	222	860	429	431
Anemias (D50–D64)	36	17	19	111	47	64	293	137	156
Diabetes mellitus (E10–E14)	1,034	537	497	2,599	1,322	1,277	8,278	4,426	3,852
Nutritional deficiencies (E40–E64)	35	18	17	112	55	57	299	117	182
Obesity (E66)	74	40	34	79	49	30	505	275	230
Parkinson's disease (G20–G21)	93	56	37	747	448	299	1,546	860	686
Alzheimer's disease (G30)	307	100	207	2,180	675	1,505	6,444	2,035	4,409
Major cardiovascular diseases (I00–I78)	4,274	2,359	1,915	20,497	10,557	9,940	49,806	26,587	23,219
Diseases of heart (I00–I09,I11,I13,I20–I51)	3,303	1,916	1,387	13,974	7,612	6,362	36,401	20,225	16,176
Essential hypertension and hypertensive renal disease (I10,I12,I15)	192	87	105	1,136	515	621	2,384	1,139	1,245
Cerebrovascular diseases (I60–I69)	646	291	355	4,798	2,153	2,645	9,795	4,544	5,251
Atherosclerosis (I70)	31	14	17	112	52	60	280	131	149
Aortic aneurysm and dissection (I71)	46	30	16	317	167	150	477	312	165
Influenza and pneumonia (J09–J18)	330	181	149	2,161	1,109	1,052	3,497	1,735	1,762
Chronic lower respiratory diseases (J40–J47)	859	398	461	1,874	1,061	813	5,159	2,606	2,553
Pneumonitis due to solids and liquids (J69)	97	58	39	500	285	215	1,006	546	460
Chronic liver disease and cirrhosis (K70,K73–K74)	1,006	563	443	598	384	214	6,018	4,109	1,909
Alcoholic liver disease (K70)	769	451	318	262	208	54	3,334	2,653	681
Cholelithiasis and other disorders of gallbladder (K80–K82)	30	17	13	114	55	59	308	145	163
Nephritis, nephrotic syndrome and nephrosis (N00–N07,N17–N19, N25–N27)	340	159	181	1,318	651	667	3,581	1,837	1,744
Pregnancy, childbirth and the puerperium (O00–O99)	19	X	19	47	X	47	158	X	158
Certain conditions originating in the perinatal period (P00–P96)	104	55	49	478	265	213	2,454	1,368	1,086
Congenital malformations, deformations and chromosomal abnormalities (Q00–Q99)	109	57	52	347	179	168	1,768	931	837
Symptoms, signs and abnormal clinical and laboratory findings, not elsewhere classified (R00–R99)	241	120	121	527	250	277	2,164	1,233	931
Accidents (unintentional injuries) (V01–X59,Y85–Y86)	1,953	1,282	671	2,839	1,788	1,051	13,806	10,067	3,739
Motor vehicle accidents (V02–V04, V09 0,V09 2,V12–V14,V19 0–V19 2, V19 4–V19 6,V20–V79,V80 3–V80 5, V81 0–V81 1,V82 0–V82 1,V83–V86, V87 0–87 8,V88 0–V88 8,V89 0,V89 2)	715	472	243	919	559	360	5,510	4,118	1,392
Falls (W00–W19)	183	102	81	821	450	371	1,894	1,133	761
Accidental discharge of firearms (W32–W34)	12	10	2	8	8	–	37	30	7
Accidental drowning and submersion (W65–W74)	67	49	18	187	136	51	467	388	79
Accidental hanging, strangulation, and suffocation (W75–W84)	73	41	32	131	78	53	513	305	208
Accidental exposure to smoke, fire and flames (X00–X09)	38	28	10	48	29	19	137	78	59
Accidental poisoning and exposure to noxious substances (X40–X49)	654	427	227	469	361	108	4,150	3,153	997
Intentional self-harm (suicide) (*U03,X60–X84,Y87 0)[5]	535	395	140	1,273	855	418	3,303	2,587	716
Intentional self-harm (suicide) by poisoning (X60–X69)	54	23	31	153	76	77	373	184	189
Intentional self-harm (suicide) by hanging, strangulation and suffocation (X70)	249	183	66	613	390	223	1,441	1,143	298
Intentional self-harm (suicide) by discharge of firearms (X72–X74)	197	165	32	289	246	43	1,162	1,017	145
Assault (homicide) (*U01–*U02, X85–Y09,Y87 1)[5]	262	209	53	304	212	92	2,886	2,391	495
Assault (homicide) by discharge of firearms (*U01 4,X93–X95)[5]	129	114	15	192	158	34	2,021	1,761	260
Legal intervention (Y35, Y89.0)	8	8	–	15	13	2	99	98	1
Complications of medical and surgical care (Y40–Y84, Y88)	16	7	9	59	30	29	163	87	76
Drug-induced deaths[6]	593	353	240	577	416	161	4,387	3,175	1,212
Alcohol-induced deaths[6]	1,179	762	417	391	313	78	4,474	3,643	831
Injury by firearms[6]	353	301	52	504	426	78	3,332	2,912	420

X = Not applicable.
- = Quantity zero.
[1]Includes deaths for origin not stated.
[2]Multiple-race data reported according to 1997 OMB standards were bridged to the single-race categories of 1977 OMB standards.
[3]Includes Aleuts and Eskimos.
[4]Includes Chinese, Filipinos, Hawaiians, Japanese, and other Asian and Pacific Islander persons.
[5]Asterisks (*) preceding cause-of-death codes indicate they are not part of the ICD-10.
[6]Included in selected categories above.

Table 2-12. Death Rates for Selected Causes, by Race, Hispanic Origin, and Sex, 2015

(Number.)

Cause of death (based on ICD–10, 2004)	All races[1]			Non-Hispanic White[2]			Non-Hispanic Black[2]		
	Both sexes	Male	Female	Both sexes	Male	Female	Both sexes	Male	Female
All causes	844.0	868.0	820.7	1,055.3	1,072.5	1,038.5	754.6	809.4	704.3
Enterocolitis due to Clostridium difficile (A04 7)	2.3	1.9	2.7	3.0	2.5	3.6	1.5	1.2	1.7
Septicemia (A40–A41)	12.7	12.3	13.1	15.0	14.4	15.6	15.7	15.3	16.1
Viral hepatitis (B15–B19)	2.3	3.1	1.5	2.4	3.2	1.6	2.7	3.7	1.7
Human immunodeficiency virus (HIV) disease (B20–B24)	2.0	3.0	1.0	1.0	1.7	0.3	8.1	11.2	5.3
Malignant neoplasms (C00–C97)	185.4	198.3	172.9	232.2	249.7	215.1	164.0	174.0	154.9
Malignant neoplasms of lip, oral cavity and pharynx (C00–C14)	3.0	4.3	1.8	3.8	5.4	2.2	2.5	3.7	1.5
Malignant neoplasm of esophagus (C15)	4.7	7.7	1.9	6.4	10.5	2.4	2.9	4.3	1.6
Malignant neoplasm of stomach (C16)	3.5	4.3	2.8	3.3	4.0	2.5	4.8	6.1	3.6
Malignant neoplasms of colon, rectum and anus (C18–C21)	16.5	17.6	15.5	19.9	21.0	18.8	17.0	18.4	15.8
Malignant neoplasms of liver and intrahepatic bile ducts (C22)	8.0	11.0	5.1	8.5	11.6	5.5	8.4	12.4	4.7
Malignant neoplasms of pancreas (C25)	12.9	13.5	12.4	16.0	17.0	15.0	12.0	11.8	12.2
Malignant neoplasms of trachea, bronchus and lung (C33–C34)	47.9	52.9	43.0	63.0	68.6	57.6	38.6	46.5	31.3
Malignant melanoma of skin (C43)	2.8	3.7	1.9	4.2	5.6	2.8	0.3	0.4	0.2
Malignant neoplasm of breast (C50)	13.1	0.3	25.4	15.6	0.3	30.4	15.1	0.4	28.6
Malignant neoplasm of cervix uteri (C53)	1.3	...	2.6	1.3	...	2.6	1.8	...	3.4
Malignant neoplasm of ovary (C56)	4.3	...	8.5	5.5	...	10.8	3.2	...	6.1
Malignant neoplasm of prostate (C61)	9.0	18.2	...	10.7	21.7	...	11.2	23.4	...
Malignant neoplasms of kidney and renal pelvis (C64–C65)	4.5	6.0	3.0	5.6	7.6	3.8	3.4	4.5	2.4
Malignant neoplasm of bladder (C67)	5.1	7.3	2.9	7.0	10.2	3.8	2.8	3.5	2.2
Malignant neoplasms of meninges, brain and other parts of central nervous system (C70–C72)	5.1	5.8	4.4	6.7	7.7	5.8	2.5	2.9	2.2
Non-Hodgkin's lymphoma (C82–C85)	6.3	7.2	5.4	8.1	9.4	7.0	3.6	4.1	3.2
Multiple myeloma and immunoproliferative neoplasms (C88,C90)	3.9	4.4	3.5	4.6	5.3	3.9	5.3	5.4	5.2
Leukemia (C91–C95)	7.1	8.4	5.8	9.2	11.0	7.4	4.5	5.0	3.9
In situ neoplasms, benign neoplasms and neoplasms of uncertain or unknown behavior (D00–D48)	5.1	5.5	4.7	6.7	7.3	6.0	3.5	3.5	3.5
Anemias (D50–D64)	1.6	1.4	1.8	1.9	1.6	2.1	2.5	2.3	2.7
Diabetes mellitus (E10–E14)	24.7	27.3	22.3	26.6	30.1	23.3	32.8	34.0	31.6
Nutritional deficiencies (E40–E64)	1.6	1.2	2.0	2.1	1.5	2.6	1.5	1.3	1.7
Obesity (E66)	2.3	2.4	2.2	2.7	2.8	2.5	3.3	3.0	3.6
Parkinson's disease (G20–G21)	8.7	10.7	6.8	12.1	14.9	9.4	2.8	3.4	2.3
Alzheimer's disease (G30)	34.4	21.3	47.1	46.4	28.9	63.4	19.3	10.8	27.2
Major cardiovascular diseases (I00–I78)	258.9	265.5	252.4	324.7	330.5	319.0	240.4	253.2	228.7
Diseases of heart (I00–I09,I11,I13,I20–I51)	197.2	211.7	183.1	250.0	267.0	233.6	177.4	193.2	162.8
Essential hypertension and hypertensive renal disease (I10,I12,I15)	10.0	8.8	11.2	11.2	9.6	12.8	13.7	13.0	14.4
Cerebrovascular diseases (I60–I69)	43.7	36.8	50.3	53.1	43.5	62.4	42.5	39.8	45.0
Atherosclerosis (I70)	1.9	1.6	2.2	2.5	2.1	2.9	1.3	1.1	1.4
Aortic aneurysm and dissection (I71)	3.1	3.7	2.5	4.0	4.8	3.3	2.5	2.9	2.0
Influenza and pneumonia (J09–J18)	17.8	17.0	18.5	22.5	21.2	23.8	13.3	13.6	13.0
Chronic lower respiratory diseases (J40–J47)	48.2	45.8	50.6	67.7	63.4	71.9	24.7	26.2	23.4
Pneumonitis due to solids and liquids (J69)	6.2	6.9	5.4	8.2	9.2	7.2	4.0	4.4	3.7
Chronic liver disease and cirrhosis (K70,K73–K74)	12.5	16.2	9.0	14.6	18.7	10.6	7.6	9.7	5.7
Alcoholic liver disease (K70)	6.5	9.3	3.9	7.4	10.4	4.6	3.8	4.9	2.7
Cholelithiasis and other disorders of gallbladder (K80–K82)	1.2	1.1	1.2	1.5	1.4	1.5	0.8	0.7	0.9
Nephritis, nephrotic syndrome and nephrosis (N00–N07,N17–N19, N25–N27)	15.5	16.1	15.0	17.6	18.5	16.8	21.7	21.8	21.7
Pregnancy, childbirth and the puerperium (O00–O99)	0.4	X	0.7	0.3	X	0.5	0.9	X	1.7
Certain conditions originating in the perinatal period (P00–P96)	3.6	4.1	3.2	2.3	2.6	2.1	9.2	10.7	7.8
Congenital malformations, deformations and chromosomal abnormalities (Q00–Q99)	3.1	3.4	2.9	3.1	3.3	2.8	3.8	4.4	3.3
Symptoms, signs and abnormal clinical and laboratory findings, not elsewhere classified (R00–R99)	10.0	9.4	10.5	12.3	11.1	13.4	10.1	10.8	9.5
Accidents (unintentional injuries) (V01–X59,Y85–Y86)	45.6	58.7	32.9	55.6	69.3	42.2	36.8	52.6	22.3
Motor vehicle accidents (V02–V04, V09 0,V09 2,V12–V14,V19 0–V19 2, V19 4–V19 6,V20–V79,V80 3–V80 5, V81 0–V81 1,V82 0–V82 1,V83–V86, V87 0–87 8,V88 0–V88 8,V89 0,V89 2)	11.7	17.0	6.7	12.5	17.9	7.3	12.7	19.7	6.4
Falls (W00–W19)	10.4	10.7	10.1	14.4	14.4	14.3	3.5	4.3	2.8
Accidental discharge of firearms (W32–W34)	0.2	0.3	0.0	0.2	0.3	0.0	0.2	0.4	*
Accidental drowning and submersion (W65–W74)	1.1	1.7	0.5	1.1	1.7	0.6	1.3	2.2	0.5
Accidental hanging, strangulation, and suffocation (W75–W84)	2.2	2.5	1.8	2.6	3.0	2.2	2.4	2.8	2.0
Accidental exposure to smoke, fire and flames (X00–X09)	0.8	1.0	0.6	0.9	1.1	0.7	1.4	1.7	1.0
Accidental poisoning and exposure to noxious substances (X40–X49)	14.8	19.9	9.8	18.4	24.2	12.8	11.5	16.3	7.1
Intentional self-harm (suicide) (*U03,X60–X84,Y87 0)[3]	13.7	21.5	6.2	18.1	28.3	8.3	5.8	9.8	2.1
Intentional self-harm (suicide) by poisoning (X60–X69)	2.1	2.2	2.1	2.9	3.0	2.9	0.7	0.8	0.6
Intentional self-harm (suicide) by hanging, strangulation and suffocation (X70)	3.7	5.8	1.7	4.4	6.9	1.9	1.6	2.6	0.7
Intentional self-harm (suicide) by discharge of firearms (X72–X74)	6.9	12.0	1.9	9.5	16.5	2.7	2.7	5.1	0.5
Assault (homicide) (*U01–*U02, X85–Y09,Y87 1)[3]	5.5	9.0	2.2	2.6	3.5	1.7	21.6	39.6	5.2
Assault (homicide) by discharge of firearms (*U01 4,X93–X95)[3]	4.0	7.0	1.2	1.5	2.2	0.9	18.0	34.1	3.2
Legal intervention (Y35, Y89.0)	0.2	0.3	0.0	0.1	0.3	*	0.3	0.6	*
Complications of medical and surgical care (Y40-Y84, Y88)	0.8	0.9	0.8	1.0	1.0	1.0	1.0	1.1	0.9
Drug-induced deaths[6]	17.2	22.0	12.6	21.8	27.1	16.7	13.2	18.3	8.5
Alcohol-induced deaths[6]	10.3	15.2	5.6	11.9	17.2	6.8	6.8	9.9	4.1
Injury by firearms[6]	11.3	19.6	3.2	11.4	19.4	3.7	21.3	40.3	3.8

X = Not applicable.
- = Quantity zero.
[1]Includes deaths for origin not stated.
[2]Multiple-race data reported according to 1997 OMB standards were bridged to the single-race categories of 1977 OMB standards.
[3]Asterisks (*) preceding cause-of-death codes indicate they are not part of the ICD-10.
[6]Included in selected categories above.

Table 2-12. Death Rates for Selected Causes, by Race, Hispanic Origin, and Sex, 2015—Continued

(Number.)

Cause of death (based on ICD–10, 2004)	Non-Hispanic American Indian and Alaskan Native[2,3]			Non-Hispanic Asian or Pacific Islander[2,4]			Hispanic		
	Both sexes	Male	Female	Both sexes	Male	Female	Both sexes	Male	Female
All causes	670.7	747.4	596.7	341.5	364.9	320.1	317.1	343.2	290.4
Enterocolitis due to Clostridium difficile (A04 7)	1.4	*	1.5	0.8	0.8	0.7	0.8	0.7	1.0
Septicemia (A40–A41)	11.0	9.8	12.1	4.2	4.6	3.8	4.8	4.8	4.7
Viral hepatitis (B15–B19)	3.8	5.3	2.3	1.2	1.3	1.0	2.0	2.7	1.3
Human immunodeficiency virus (HIV) disease (B20–B24)	2.0	2.6	*	0.4	0.7	*	1.6	2.6	0.6
Malignant neoplasms (C00–C97)	118.7	128.7	109.0	90.5	96.1	85.4	66.8	69.4	64.2
Malignant neoplasm of lip, oral cavity and pharynx (C00–C14)	2.0	2.8	*	2.1	3.0	1.3	1.0	1.4	0.6
Malignant neoplasm of esophagus (C15)	3.3	5.8	*	1.4	2.3	0.5	1.2	1.9	0.5
Malignant neoplasm of stomach (C16)	3.0	4.2	1.9	4.6	5.2	4.0	3.1	3.4	2.8
Malignant neoplasms of colon, rectum and anus (C18–C21)	12.1	13.9	10.3	9.0	9.5	8.5	6.7	7.5	5.9
Malignant neoplasms of liver and intrahepatic bile ducts (C22)	8.9	12.3	5.7	8.5	11.9	5.3	5.6	7.3	4.0
Malignant neoplasm of pancreas (C25)	7.7	7.6	7.7	6.8	6.8	6.9	5.0	4.9	5.1
Malignant neoplasms of trachea, bronchus and lung (C33–C34)	29.6	32.2	27.1	20.0	24.0	16.4	10.1	11.7	8.4
Malignant melanoma of skin (C43)	*	*	*	0.3	0.4	0.3	0.4	0.5	0.3
Malignant neoplasm of breast (C50)	7.8	*	15.3	6.4	*	12.1	4.9	0.1	9.8
Malignant neoplasm of cervix uteri (C53)	1.2	...	2.3	1.0	...	1.9	1.0	...	2.0
Malignant neoplasm of ovary (C56)	3.4	...	6.6	2.3	...	4.4	1.8	...	3.6
Malignant neoplasm of prostate (C61)	5.3	10.8	...	3.0	6.3	...	3.3	6.5	...
Malignant neoplasms of kidney and renal pelvis (C64–C65)	4.0	5.5	2.6	1.6	2.2	1.0	2.2	2.8	1.5
Malignant neoplasm of bladder (C67)	1.8	2.3	*	1.4	2.0	0.8	1.2	1.6	0.8
Malignant neoplasms of meninges, brain and other parts of central nervous system (C70–C72)	2.2	3.0	1.5	2.3	2.5	2.1	2.1	2.3	1.9
Non-Hodgkin's lymphoma (C82–C85)	3.5	4.0	2.9	3.4	3.9	3.0	2.5	2.9	2.2
Multiple myeloma and immunoproliferative neoplasms (C88,C90)	2.2	2.5	2.0	1.6	1.7	1.5	1.6	1.7	1.5
Leukemia (C91–C95)	3.5	4.6	2.3	3.0	3.8	2.3	2.8	3.2	2.5
In situ neoplasms, benign neoplasms and neoplasms of uncertain or unknown behavior (D00–D48)	2.7	2.9	2.5	2.2	2.2	2.2	1.5	1.5	1.5
Anemias (D50–D64)	1.3	*	*	0.6	0.5	0.6	0.5	0.5	0.6
Diabetes mellitus (E10–E14)	38.4	40.7	36.3	13.6	14.5	12.8	14.6	15.5	13.8
Nutritional deficiencies (E40–E64)	1.3	*	*	0.6	0.6	0.6	0.5	0.4	0.7
Obesity (E66)	2.8	3.0	2.5	0.4	0.5	0.3	0.9	1.0	0.8
Parkinson's disease (G20–G21)	3.5	4.2	2.7	3.9	4.9	3.0	2.7	3.0	2.5
Alzheimer's disease (G30)	11.4	7.6	15.1	11.4	7.4	15.1	11.4	7.1	15.8
Major cardiovascular diseases (I00–I78)	158.9	178.7	139.9	107.2	115.7	99.5	88.0	93.0	83.0
Diseases of heart (I00–I09,I11,I13,I20–I51)	122.8	145.1	101.3	73.1	83.4	63.7	64.3	70.7	57.8
Essential hypertension and hypertensive renal disease (I10,I12,I15)	7.1	6.6	7.7	5.9	5.6	6.2	4.2	4.0	4.4
Cerebrovascular diseases (I60–I69)	24.0	22.0	25.9	25.1	23.6	26.5	17.3	15.9	18.8
Atherosclerosis (I70)	1.2	*	*	0.6	0.6	0.6	0.5	0.5	0.5
Aortic aneurysm and dissection (I71)	1.7	2.3	*	1.7	1.8	1.5	0.8	1.1	0.6
Influenza and pneumonia (J09–J18)	12.3	13.7	10.9	11.3	12.2	10.5	6.2	6.1	6.3
Chronic lower respiratory diseases (J40–J47)	31.9	30.1	33.7	9.8	11.6	8.1	9.1	9.1	9.1
Pneumonitis due to solids and liquids (J69)	3.6	4.4	2.8	2.6	3.1	2.2	1.8	1.9	1.6
Chronic liver disease and cirrhosis (K70,K73–K74)	37.4	42.6	32.4	3.1	4.2	2.1	10.6	14.4	6.8
Alcoholic liver disease (K70)	28.6	34.2	23.2	1.4	2.3	0.5	5.9	9.3	2.4
Cholelithiasis and other disorders of gallbladder (K80–K82)	1.1	*	*	0.6	0.6	0.6	0.5	0.5	0.6
Nephritis, nephrotic syndrome and nephrosis (N00–N07,N17–N19, N25–N27)	12.6	12.0	13.2	6.9	7.1	6.7	6.3	6.4	6.2
Pregnancy, childbirth and the puerperium (O00–O99)	*	X	*	0.2	X	0.5	0.3	X	0.6
Certain conditions originating in the perinatal period (P00–P96)	3.9	4.2	3.6	2.5	2.9	2.1	4.3	4.8	3.9
Congenital malformations, deformations and chromosomal abnormalities (Q00–Q99)	4.1	4.3	3.8	1.8	2.0	1.7	3.1	3.3	3.0
Symptoms, signs and abnormal clinical and laboratory findings, not elsewhere classified (R00–R99)	9.0	9.1	8.8	2.8	2.7	2.8	3.8	4.3	3.3
Accidents (unintentional injuries) (V01–X59,Y85–Y86)	72.6	97.1	49.0	14.9	19.6	10.5	24.4	35.2	13.4
Motor vehicle accidents (V02–V04, V09 0,V09 2,V12–V14,V19 0–V19 2, V19 4–V19 6,V20–V79,V80 3–V80 5, V81 0–V81 1,V82 0–V82 1,V83–V86, V87 0–87 8,V88 0–V88 8,V89 0,V89 2)	26.6	35.7	17.7	4.8	6.1	3.6	9.7	14.4	5.0
Falls (W00–W19)	6.8	7.7	5.9	4.3	4.9	3.7	3.3	4.0	2.7
Accidental discharge of firearms (W32–W34)	*	*	*	*	*	*	0.1	0.1	*
Accidental drowning and submersion (W65–W74)	2.5	3.7	*	1.0	1.5	0.5	0.8	1.4	0.3
Accidental hanging, strangulation, and suffocation (W75–W84)	2.7	3.1	2.3	0.7	0.9	0.5	0.9	1.1	0.7
Accidental exposure to smoke, fire and flames (X00–X09)	1.4	2.1	*	0.3	0.3	*	0.2	0.3	0.2
Accidental poisoning and exposure to noxious substances (X40–X49)	24.3	32.3	16.6	2.5	4.0	1.1	7.3	11.0	3.6
Intentional self-harm (suicide) (*U03,X60–X84,Y87 0)[5]	19.9	29.9	10.2	6.7	9.4	4.2	5.8	9.0	2.6
Intentional self-harm (suicide) by poisoning (X60–X69)	2.0	1.7	2.3	0.8	0.8	0.8	0.7	0.6	0.7
Intentional self-harm (suicide) by hanging, strangulation and suffocation (X70)	9.3	13.9	4.8	3.2	4.3	2.2	2.5	4.0	1.1
Intentional self-harm (suicide) by discharge of firearms (X72–X74)	7.3	12.5	2.3	1.5	2.7	0.4	2.1	3.6	0.5
Assault (homicide) (*U01–*U02, X85–Y09,Y87 1)[5]	9.7	15.8	3.9	1.6	2.3	0.9	5.1	8.4	1.8
Assault (homicide) by discharge of firearms (*U01 4,X93–X95)[5]	4.8	8.6	*	1.0	1.7	0.3	3.6	6.2	0.9
Legal intervention (Y35, Y89.0)	*	*	*	*	*	*	0.2	0.3	*
Complications of medical and surgical care (Y40-Y84, Y88)	*	*	*	0.3	0.3	0.3	0.3	0.3	0.3
Drug-induced deaths[6]	22.0	26.7	17.5	3.0	4.6	1.6	7.8	11.1	4.3
Alcohol-induced deaths[6]	43.8	57.7	30.5	2.0	3.4	0.8	7.9	12.7	3.0
Injury by firearms[6]	13.1	22.8	3.8	2.6	4.7	0.8	5.9	10.2	1.5

X = Not applicable.
- = Quantity zero.
[2]Multiple-race data reported according to 1997 OMB standards were bridged to the single-race categories of 1977 OMB standards.
[3]Includes Aleuts and Eskimos.
[4]Includes Chinese, Filipinos, Hawaiians, Japanese, and other Asian and Pacific Islander persons.
[5]Asterisks (*) preceding cause-of-death codes indicate they are not part of the ICD-10.
[6]Included in selected categories above.

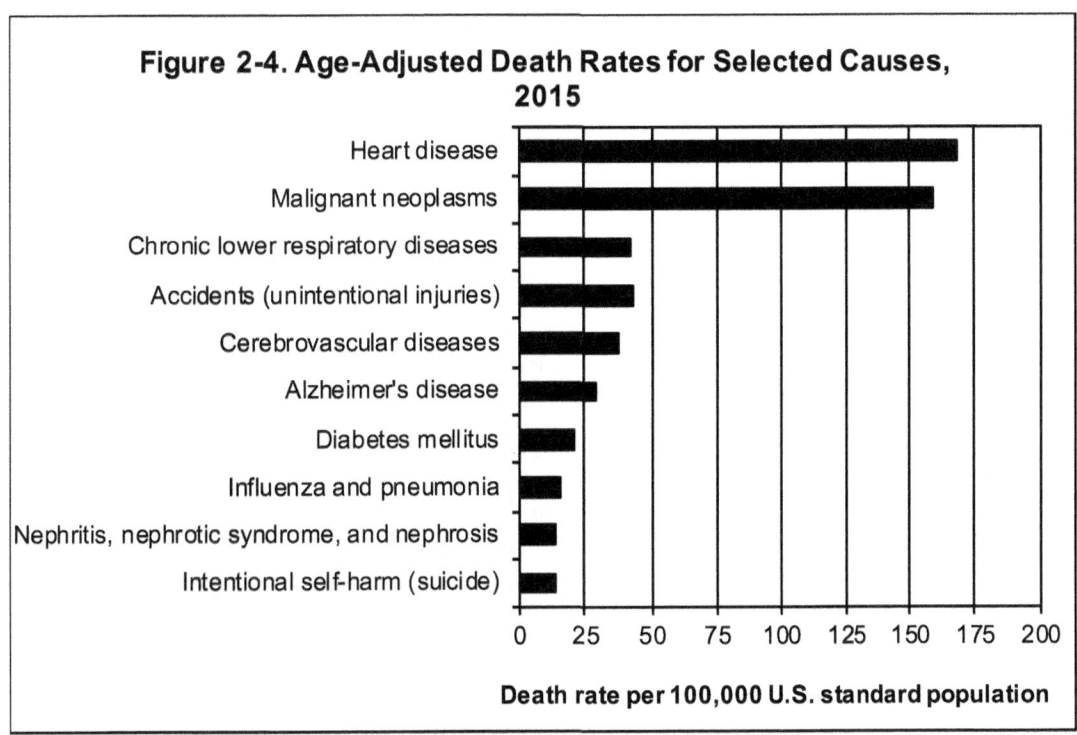

Figure 2-4. Age-Adjusted Death Rates for Selected Causes, 2015

Table 2-13. Age-Adjusted Death Rates from Selected Causes, by Race and Sex, 2015

(Age-adjusted rates per 100,000 U.S. standard population.)

Cause of death (based on ICD–10, 2004)	All races[1] Both sexes	All races[1] Male	All races[1] Female	Non-Hispanic White[2] Both sexes	Non-Hispanic White[2] Male	Non-Hispanic White[2] Female	Non-Hispanic Black[2] Both sexes	Non-Hispanic Black[2] Male	Non-Hispanic Black[2] Female
All causes	733.1	863.2	624.2	753.2	881.3	644.1	876.1	1,070.1	731.0
Enterocolitis due to Clostridium difficile (A04 7)	2.0	2.0	2.0	2.1	2.0	2.1	1.8	1.8	1.8
Septicemia (A40–A41)	11.0	12.1	10.1	10.6	11.6	9.8	18.6	21.4	16.8
Viral hepatitis (B15–B19)	1.9	2.6	1.2	1.7	2.3	1.1	2.5	3.7	1.6
Human immunodeficiency virus (HIV) disease (B20–B24)	1.9	2.8	1.0	0.9	1.4	0.3	8.2	11.6	5.3
Malignant neoplasms (C00–C97)	158.5	189.2	135.9	163.7	194.3	140.6	185.1	231.0	156.6
Malignant neoplasms of lip, oral cavity and pharynx (C00–C14)	2.5	3.9	1.4	2.6	4.1	1.4	2.7	4.2	1.4
Malignant neoplasm of esophagus (C15)	4.0	7.0	1.4	4.5	7.9	1.5	3.1	5.2	1.6
Malignant neoplasm of stomach (C16)	3.1	4.1	2.3	2.3	3.2	1.6	5.6	8.2	3.8
Malignant neoplasms of colon, rectum and anus (C18–C21)	14.2	16.8	12.1	14.1	16.6	12.1	19.3	23.9	16.2
Malignant neoplasms of liver and intrahepatic bile ducts (C22)	6.6	9.7	4.0	5.9	8.5	3.6	8.6	13.8	4.7
Malignant neoplasm of pancreas (C25)	11.0	12.6	9.6	11.1	12.9	9.6	13.7	15.2	12.5
Malignant neoplasms of trachea, bronchus and lung (C33–C34)	40.5	49.5	33.5	43.8	52.2	37.3	43.1	60.3	31.5
Malignant melanoma of skin C43)	2.4	3.6	1.5	3.1	4.5	1.9	0.3	0.5	0.2
Malignant neoplasm of breast (C50)	11.2	0.3	20.3	11.2	0.3	20.4	16.7	0.6	28.5
Malignant neoplasm of cervix uteri (C53)	1.2	X	2.3	1.1	X	2.1	1.9	X	3.4
Malignant neoplasm of ovary (C56)	3.7	X	6.7	3.9	X	7.2	3.6	X	6.2
Malignant neoplasm of prostate (C61)	7.7	18.8	X	7.3	17.7	X	14.1	37.8	X
Malignant neoplasms of kidney and renal pelvis (C64–C65)	3.8	5.6	2.4	3.9	5.8	2.4	3.8	5.6	2.5
Malignant neoplasm of bladder (C67)	4.4	7.4	2.2	4.8	8.2	2.3	3.4	5.4	2.3
Malignant neoplasms of meninges, brain and other parts of central nervous system (C70–C72)	4.4	5.4	3.6	5.1	6.1	4.1	2.7	3.2	2.2
Non-Hodgkin's lymphoma (C82–C85)	5.4	7.1	4.2	5.8	7.5	4.4	4.2	5.3	3.3
Multiple myeloma and immunoproliferative neoplasms (C88,C90)	3.4	4.3	2.7	3.2	4.2	2.5	6.3	7.6	5.5
Leukemia (C91–C95)	6.2	8.3	4.6	6.6	8.9	4.8	5.2	6.9	4.1
In situ neoplasms, benign neoplasms and neoplasms of uncertain or unknown behavior (D00–D48)	4.4	5.6	3.6	4.7	6.0	3.8	4.3	5.1	3.8
Anemias (D50–D64)	1.4	1.4	1.4	1.3	1.3	1.3	2.8	2.8	2.8
Diabetes mellitus E10–E14)	21.3	26.2	17.3	18.9	23.8	14.9	38.0	45.1	32.8
Nutritional deficiencies (E40–E64)	1.4	1.3	1.5	1.4	1.2	1.5	1.9	2.1	1.9
Obesity (E66)	2.1	2.2	1.9	2.1	2.3	1.9	3.5	3.3	3.6
Parkinson's disease (G20–G21)	7.7	11.6	5.1	8.4	12.6	5.5	3.9	6.2	2.6
Alzheimer's disease (G30)	29.4	23.7	32.8	30.8	24.9	34.4	27.3	21.3	30.0
Major cardiovascular diseases (I00–I78)	221.5	266.6	184.4	223.0	268.4	185.1	287.2	350.3	239.9
Diseases of heart (I00–I09,I11,I13,I20–I51)	168.5	211.8	133.6	171.9	216.3	135.6	210.1	264.9	169.9
Essential hypertension and hypertensive renal disease (I10,I12,I15)	8.5	8.8	8.1	7.6	7.8	7.3	16.7	18.4	15.2
Cerebrovascular diseases (I60–I69)	37.6	37.8	36.9	36.4	35.8	36.2	52.2	57.0	47.9
Atherosclerosis (I70)	1.6	1.7	1.5	1.7	1.7	1.6	1.6	1.8	1.5
Aortic aneurysm and dissection (I71)	2.7	3.7	1.9	2.9	3.8	2.0	2.9	3.7	2.2
Influenza and pneumonia (J09–J18)	15.2	17.7	13.5	15.4	17.6	13.9	16.3	20.3	13.7
Chronic lower respiratory diseases (J40–J47)	41.6	46.0	38.6	46.9	50.5	44.4	29.7	38.5	24.3
Pneumonitis due to solids and liquids (J69)	5.3	7.3	4.0	5.6	7.7	4.2	5.1	7.2	3.9
Chronic liver disease and cirrhosis (K70,K73–K74)	10.8	14.5	7.6	11.1	14.6	7.9	7.6	10.2	5.5
Alcoholic liver disease (K70)	5.7	8.3	3.4	5.9	8.2	3.8	3.7	5.1	2.5
Cholelithiasis and other disorders of gallbladder (K80–K82)	1.0	1.1	0.9	1.0	1.2	0.9	1.0	1.0	0.9
Nephritis, nephrotic syndrome and nephrosis (N00–N07,N17–N19,N25–N27)	13.4	16.3	11.3	12.2	15.2	10.1	26.2	31.4	22.9
Pregnancy, childbirth and the puerperium (O00–O99)	0.4	X	0.8	0.3	X	0.6	0.9	X	1.8
Certain conditions originating in the perinatal period (P00–P96)	4.1	4.4	3.7	3.1	3.3	2.8	8.6	9.4	7.8
Congenital malformations, deformations and chromosomal abnormalities (Q00–Q99)	3.2	3.4	3.0	3.2	3.4	3.0	3.7	4.1	3.3
Symptoms, signs and abnormal clinical and laboratory findings, not elsewhere classified (R00–R99)	8.9	9.6	8.1	9.3	9.9	8.5	11.3	12.7	9.9
Accidents (unintentional injuries) (V01–X59, Y85–Y86)	43.2	58.7	28.7	49.0	65.2	33.6	38.2	56.8	22.6
Motor vehicle accidents (V02–V04,V090, V092,V12–V14,V190–V192, V194–V196,V20–V79,V803–V805, V810–V811,V820–V821,V83–V86, V870–V878,V880–V888,V890,V892)	11.4	16.7	6.4	11.8	17.0	6.8	12.7	19.9	6.3
Falls (W00–W19)	9.0	11.1	7.3	9.9	12.1	8.2	4.2	6.1	3.0
Accidental discharge of firearms (W32–W34)	0.2	0.3	0.0	0.2	0.3	0.0	0.2	0.4	*
Accidental drowning and submersion (W65–W74)	1.1	1.7	0.5	1.1	1.6	0.6	1.3	2.2	0.5
Accidental hanging, strangulation, and suffocation (W75–W84)	2.0	2.5	1.5	2.1	2.7	1.6	2.6	3.3	2.0
Accidental exposure to smoke, fire and flames (X00–X09)	0.8	0.9	0.6	0.7	1.0	0.6	1.5	2.1	1.0
Accidental poisoning and exposure to noxious substances (X40–X49)	14.8	19.8	9.8	18.8	24.6	13.0	11.5	16.7	7.0
Intentional self-harm (suicide) (*U03,X60–X84,Y87 0)[3]	13.3	21.1	6.0	17.0	26.6	7.8	5.8	10.0	2.1
Intentional self-harm (suicide) by poisoning (X60–X69)	2.0	2.1	2.0	2.7	2.7	2.6	0.7	0.8	0.6
Intentional self-harm (suicide) by hanging, strangulation and suffocation (X70)	3.7	5.8	1.7	4.5	7.0	2.0	1.6	2.5	0.7
Intentional self-harm (suicide) by discharge of firearms (X72–X74)	6.5	11.6	1.8	8.6	15.1	2.6	2.7	5.3	0.5
Assault (homicide) (*U01–*U02, X85–Y09,Y87 1)[3]	5.7	9.1	2.2	2.6	3.6	1.7	20.9	37.6	5.1
Assault (homicide) by discharge of firearms (*U01 4,X93–X95)[3]	4.2	7.1	1.2	1.6	2.2	0.9	17.3	32.2	3.1
Legal intervention (Y35, Y89.0)	0.2	0.3	0.0	0.1	0.3	*	0.3	0.5	*
Complications of medical and surgical care (Y40–Y84, Y88)	0.7	0.8	0.7	0.7	0.8	0.7	1.1	1.3	0.9
Drug-induced deaths[4]	17.2	21.9	12.5	22.1	27.5	16.7	13.2	18.7	8.4
Alcohol-induced deaths[4]	9.1	13.6	5.0	9.6	13.8	5.6	6.7	10.3	3.9
Injury by firearms[4]	11.1	19.4	3.2	10.6	18.0	3.6	20.7	38.6	3.8

X = Not applicable.
0.0 = Quantity more than zero but less than 0.05.
* = Figure does not meet standards of reliability or precision.
[1]Includes deaths for origin not stated.
[2]Multiple-race data reported according to 1997 OMB standards were bridged to the single-race categories of 1977 OMB standards.
[3]Asterisks (*) preceding cause-of-death codes indicate they are not part of the ICD-10.
[4]Included in selected categories above.

Table 2-13. Age-Adjusted Death Rates from Selected Causes, by Race and Sex, 2015—Continued

(Age-adjusted rates per 100,000 U.S. standard population.)

Cause of death (based on ICD–10, 2004)	Non-Hispanic American Indian and Alaskan Native[2,3]			Non-Hispanic Asian or Pacific Islander[2,4]			Hispanic		
	Both sexes	Male	Female	Both sexes	Male	Female	Both sexes	Male	Female
All causes	805.7	950.2	679.5	396.2	468.9	339.6	525.3	628.9	438.3
Enterocolitis due to Clostridium difficile (A04 7)	1.9	*	1.7	0.9	1.1	0.8	1.6	1.6	1.5
Septicemia (A40–A41)	13.0	12.3	13.5	4.9	6.0	4.0	8.1	9.3	7.2
Viral hepatitis (B15–B19)	3.7	5.6	2.1	1.2	1.5	1.1	2.7	3.8	1.7
Human immunodeficiency virus (HIV) disease (B20–B24)	2.0	2.8	*	0.4	0.7	*	1.8	3.1	0.6
Malignant neoplasms (C00–C97)	140.9	167.5	120.1	99.8	117.7	86.9	110.3	133.8	93.6
Malignant neoplasms of lip, oral cavity and pharynx (C00–C14)	2.3	3.2	*	2.2	3.3	1.2	1.6	2.6	0.9
Malignant neoplasm of esophagus (C15)	3.7	6.7	*	1.5	2.6	0.5	2.0	3.5	0.7
Malignant neoplasm of stomach (C16)	3.4	4.9	2.1	5.1	6.4	4.2	4.9	6.2	3.9
Malignant neoplasms of colon, rectum and anus (C18–C21)	14.8	19.3	11.5	9.9	11.4	8.7	10.9	13.9	8.6
Malignant neoplasms of liver and intrahepatic bile ducts (C22)	9.7	13.6	6.3	9.1	13.6	5.6	9.0	12.7	6.0
Malignant neoplasm of pancreas (C25)	8.9	9.0	8.6	7.7	8.4	7.2	8.4	9.2	7.8
Malignant neoplasms of trachea, bronchus and lung (C33–C34)	34.8	42.2	29.0	22.4	29.8	16.9	17.8	24.3	12.9
Malignant melanoma of skin C43)	*	*	*	0.3	0.4	0.3	0.7	0.9	0.5
Malignant neoplasm of breast (C50)	9.3	*	16.7	6.6	*	11.8	7.4	0.2	13.5
Malignant neoplasm of cervix uteri (C53)	1.3	X	2.4	1.0	X	1.8	1.3	X	2.5
Malignant neoplasm of ovary (C56)	3.8	X	6.9	2.4	X	4.3	2.8	X	5.1
Malignant neoplasm of prostate (C61)	7.4	17.7	X	3.6	8.9	X	6.4	15.6	X
Malignant neoplasms of kidney and renal pelvis (C64–C65)	4.8	7.2	3.1	1.7	2.6	1.1	3.5	5.2	2.3
Malignant neoplasm of bladder (C67)	2.3	3.4	*	1.7	2.8	0.9	2.3	3.8	1.3
Malignant neoplasms of meninges, brain and other parts of central nervous system (C70–C72)	2.6	3.4	1.8	2.4	2.7	2.1	3.0	3.5	2.5
Non-Hodgkin's lymphoma (C82–C85)	4.5	5.3	3.7	3.9	5.0	3.1	4.3	5.5	3.4
Multiple myeloma and immunoproliferative neoplasms (C88,C90)	2.9	3.8	2.2	1.7	2.0	1.5	2.8	3.4	2.3
Leukemia (C91–C95)	4.3	6.3	2.7	3.4	4.7	2.4	4.3	5.4	3.4
In situ neoplasms, benign neoplasms and neoplasms of uncertain or unknown behavior (D00–D48)	3.6	4.4	3.0	2.6	2.9	2.4	2.7	3.1	2.4
Anemias (D50–D64)	1.7	*	*	0.7	0.7	0.7	0.9	1.0	0.8
Diabetes mellitus E10–E14)	45.0	50.6	40.2	15.8	18.5	13.8	25.2	29.8	21.4
Nutritional deficiencies (E40–E64)	1.9	*	*	0.7	0.9	0.6	1.0	1.0	1.0
Obesity (E66)	2.8	3.2	2.3	0.4	0.6	0.3	1.1	1.2	1.1
Parkinson's disease (G20–G21)	5.3	7.9	3.7	5.0	7.4	3.3	5.7	7.9	4.2
Alzheimer's disease (G30)	18.9	15.2	21.0	14.7	11.7	16.5	24.2	19.7	26.9
Major cardiovascular diseases (I00–I78)	202.9	243.4	168.2	127.4	153.0	107.3	160.9	194.0	133.8
Diseases of heart (I00–I09,I11,I13,I20–I51)	154.9	195.8	121.1	86.6	109.8	68.6	116.9	146.4	93.0
Essential hypertension and hypertensive renal disease (I10,I12,I15)	9.4	8.7	9.5	7.3	7.8	6.8	7.9	8.5	7.2
Cerebrovascular diseases (I60–I69)	32.0	31.9	31.6	30.0	31.4	28.6	32.3	34.2	30.4
Atherosclerosis (I70)	1.7	*	*	0.7	0.8	0.7	1.0	1.1	0.9
Aortic aneurysm and dissection (I71)	2.2	3.0	*	1.9	2.3	1.6	1.4	2.0	0.9
Influenza and pneumonia (J09–J18)	16.2	20.5	13.0	14.1	17.8	11.4	11.4	13.4	10.0
Chronic lower respiratory diseases (J40–J47)	40.4	44.0	38.2	12.1	16.8	9.0	17.7	21.7	14.9
Pneumonitis due to solids and liquids (J69)	4.8	6.7	3.5	3.3	4.7	2.4	3.4	4.5	2.7
Chronic liver disease and cirrhosis (K70,K73–K74)	39.2	45.3	33.5	3.2	4.5	2.2	14.9	20.8	9.4
Alcoholic liver disease (K70)	29.7	36.0	24.0	1.3	2.3	0.5	7.5	12.7	2.9
Cholelithiasis and other disorders of gallbladder (K80–K82)	1.5	*	*	0.7	0.9	0.6	1.0	1.1	0.9
Nephritis, nephrotic syndrome and nephrosis (N00–N07,N17–N19,N25–N27)	16.0	17.2	15.2	8.3	9.8	7.2	11.4	13.4	9.9
Pregnancy, childbirth and the puerperium (O00–O99)	*	X	*	0.2	X	0.4	0.3	X	0.6
Certain conditions originating in the perinatal period (P00–P96)	3.5	3.6	3.4	3.0	3.2	2.7	3.3	3.6	3.0
Congenital malformations, deformations and chromosomal abnormalities (Q00–Q99)	3.8	4.0	3.7	2.1	2.2	2.0	2.7	2.8	2.6
Symptoms, signs and abnormal clinical and laboratory findings, not elsewhere classified (R00–R99)	10.4	11.2	9.8	3.2	3.4	3.0	5.2	6.2	4.3
Accidents (unintentional injuries) (V01–X59, Y85–Y86)	77.1	104.3	51.7	16.0	21.9	11.0	28.6	41.5	16.1
Motor vehicle accidents (V02–V04,V090, V092,V12–V14,V190–V192, V194–V196,V20–V79,V803–V805, V810–V811,V820–V821,V83–V86, V870–V878,V880–V888,V890,V892)	26.7	36.2	17.7	4.9	6.3	3.6	10.2	15.2	5.2
Falls (W00-W19)	8.9	11.0	7.2	5.2	6.8	4.1	5.8	7.5	4.4
Accidental discharge of firearms (W32–W34)	*	*	*	*	*	*	0.0	0.1	*
Accidental drowning and submersion (W65–W74)	2.5	3.7	*	1.0	1.5	0.5	0.8	1.4	0.3
Accidental hanging, strangulation, and suffocation (W75–W84)	3.0	3.4	2.6	0.8	1.1	0.6	1.2	1.5	0.9
Accidental exposure to smoke, fire and flames (X00–X09)	1.5	2.3	*	0.3	0.4	*	0.4	0.4	0.3
Accidental poisoning and exposure to noxious substances (X40–X49)	25.1	33.4	17.1	2.3	3.7	1.0	7.7	11.5	3.8
Intentional self-harm (suicide) (*U03,X60–X84,Y87 0)[5]	20.0	30.3	10.2	6.5	9.2	4.0	6.2	9.9	2.6
Intentional self-harm (suicide) by poisoning (X60–X69)	2.1	1.9	2.3	0.7	0.8	0.8	0.7	0.7	0.7
Intentional self-harm (suicide) by hanging, strangulation and suffocation (X70)	9.0	13.6	4.5	3.1	4.3	2.1	2.6	4.2	1.0
Intentional self-harm (suicide) by discharge of firearms (X72–X74)	7.5	12.9	2.5	1.4	2.6	0.4	2.2	4.0	0.5
Assault (homicide) (*U01–*U02, X85–Y09,Y87 1)[5]	9.8	16.0	3.9	1.5	2.2	0.9	4.9	7.9	1.8
Assault (homicide) by discharge of firearms (*U01 4,X93–X95)[5]	4.8	8.6	*	1.0	1.6	0.3	3.3	5.6	0.9
Legal intervention (Y35, Y89.0)	*	*	*	*	*	*	0.2	0.3	*
Complications of medical and surgical care (Y40-Y84, Y88)	*	*	*	0.4	0.4	0.3	0.5	0.5	0.4
Drug-induced deaths[6]	22.8	27.6	18.1	2.8	4.3	1.6	8.2	11.7	4.7
Alcohol-induced deaths[6]	45.6	60.9	31.5	1.9	3.4	0.7	9.9	16.9	3.5
Injury by firearms[6]	13.3	23.0	4.0	2.5	4.4	0.8	5.8	10.1	1.5

X = Not applicable.
0.0 = Quantity more than zero but less than 0.05.
* = Figure does not meet standards of reliability or precision.
[2]Multiple-race data reported according to 1997 OMB standards were bridged to the single-race categories of 1977 OMB standards.
[3]Includes Aleuts and Eskimos.
[4]Includes Chinese, Filipinos, Hawaiians, Japanese, and other Asian and Pacific Islander persons.
[5]Asterisks (*) preceding cause-of-death codes indicate they are not part of the ICD-10.
[6]Included in selected categories above.

Table 2-14. Age-Adjusted Death Rates, by Race, Hispanic Origin, Average Annual 1979–1981, 1989–1991, 2009–2011, and 2013–2015

(Age-adjusted death rate per 100,000 population.[1])

State	All persons				White		Black or African American		American Indian or Alaska Native[1]		Asian or Pacific Islander[1]		Hispanic or Latino[1]		White, not Hispanic or Latino[1]	
	1979–1981	1989–1991	2009–2011	2013–2015	2009–2011	2013–2015	2009–2011	2013–2015	2009–2011	2013–2015	2009–2011	2013–2015	2009–2011	2013–2015	2009–2011	2013–2015
United States[2]	1,022.8	942.2	745.9	729.9	741.1	730.5	895.8	853.9	614.7	594.1	419.4	395.9	552.6	527.8	754.8	747.7
Alabama	1,091.2	1,037.9	937.8	919.5	913.7	906.1	1,045.7	994.8	315.3	326.9	411.2	219.6	366.0	346.2	920.5	914.8
Alaska	1,087.4	944.6	760.8	736.2	709.0	680.9	675.1	657.1	1,162.6	1,169.7	475.9	479.3	454.8	356.7	714.2	690.3
Arizona	951.5	873.5	691.9	669.2	685.8	663.9	785.2	763.4	867.9	843.4	413.1	376.0	616.4	590.1	694.9	672.1
Arkansas	1,017.0	996.3	894.9	893.1	877.1	885.0	1,059.1	992.6	364.2	250.2	554.7	519.6	386.8	303.2	888.7	894.6
California	975.5	911.0	647.7	619.1	674.3	651.4	853.2	807.6	363.2	380.2	422.6	394.5	540.5	514.4	704.5	686.4
Colorado	941.1	856.1	683.3	661.7	687.7	667.6	785.5	741.6	450.5	462.4	404.7	389.0	671.8	652.5	682.5	663.1
Connecticut	961.5	857.5	657.6	649.6	656.8	655.2	725.3	683.2	213.2	194.9	357.9	311.7	532.3	519.8	656.5	657.0
Delaware	1,069.7	1,001.9	767.3	734.2	761.4	733.2	845.6	790.5	Y	Y	288.3	329.3	446.9	403.9	764.2	739.9
District of Columbia	1,243.1	1,255.3	793.4	748.1	495.9	463.6	1,010.3	969.7	Y	Y	340.2	345.4	396.3	362.8	492.7	458.7
Florida	960.8	870.9	692.5	662.7	684.1	657.8	798.3	741.2	300.7	285.2	347.0	331.9	540.7	507.4	715.7	694.7
Georgia	1,094.3	1,037.4	834.2	805.4	815.7	795.0	920.6	869.3	185.1	205.7	424.0	394.4	313.9	316.2	831.9	816.0
Hawaii	801.2	752.2	598.4	589.2	645.3	652.8	536.6	532.6	Y	Y	582.6	568.5	776.3	828.2	651.5	638.3
Idaho	936.7	856.6	734.1	727.4	735.5	731.7	577.9	413.7	798.5	716.4	476.7	411.6	508.7	486.7	742.9	741.0
Illinois	1,063.7	973.8	740.4	726.1	721.6	712.9	943.3	915.0	177.1	127.1	392.5	370.6	470.4	451.2	735.7	730.9
Indiana	1,048.3	962.0	822.2	829.5	815.1	824.6	964.3	951.2	162.8	192.3	391.8	384.2	447.9	461.3	820.0	833.2
Iowa	919.9	848.2	722.5	723.8	720.6	722.7	926.5	877.9	719.7	540.7	444.5	447.3	410.4	382.9	723.5	727.3
Kansas	940.1	867.2	762.4	763.8	754.1	756.2	953.6	936.0	1,157.0	1,127.3	437.6	445.5	557.3	528.0	759.4	763.2
Kentucky	1,088.9	1,024.5	912.5	910.3	912.3	915.8	986.3	914.6	290.8	161.2	399.8	390.9	330.7	319.9	917.6	921.2
Louisiana	1,132.6	1,074.6	899.3	888.5	854.7	844.7	1,033.9	1,019.3	439.3	367.4	431.6	423.5	349.7	393.5	869.0	859.9
Maine	1,002.9	918.7	751.6	758.9	753.4	762.4	451.6	464.6	1,070.5	793.4	334.2	292.6	363.1	243.3	752.5	762.2
Maryland	1,063.3	985.2	731.4	705.1	706.7	692.6	849.5	799.8	180.0	253.5	373.0	338.3	315.2	312.2	718.3	708.3
Massachusetts	982.6	884.8	677.6	670.5	689.4	689.5	640.6	583.9	240.4	289.7	360.1	353.1	453.1	446.0	690.2	684.3
Michigan	1,050.2	966.0	784.5	783.5	761.0	763.8	975.9	961.9	851.5	819.5	348.4	341.1	641.0	623.9	761.4	763.8
Minnesota	892.9	825.2	657.6	650.6	652.2	643.3	681.2	736.0	1,074.5	1,066.6	512.1	480.1	400.8	402.4	653.9	645.5
Mississippi	1,108.7	1,071.4	956.2	953.6	911.9	919.5	1,061.5	1,029.8	783.2	740.6	476.1	494.2	296.1	243.4	917.7	929.7
Missouri	1,033.7	952.4	815.6	810.6	805.5	799.6	948.6	956.7	409.8	376.2	376.7	399.9	333.9	417.0	811.9	804.9
Montana	1,013.6	890.2	757.7	751.9	738.1	726.0	Y	Y	1,172.2	1,268.9	Y	413.6	487.9	511.8	732.5	721.6
Nebraska	930.6	867.9	716.3	724.1	708.6	719.5	961.3	892.9	881.5	823.8	410.6	365.9	434.5	450.7	713.8	726.7
Nevada	1,077.4	1,017.4	793.2	758.5	820.3	788.5	840.8	815.1	570.4	525.1	434.7	429.9	492.7	462.1	866.9	845.3
New Hampshire	982.3	891.7	697.6	702.1	703.1	711.2	532.4	374.2	Y	Y	301.8	331.4	349.3	243.6	705.0	715.3
New Jersey	1,047.5	956.0	690.4	669.3	688.3	677.4	843.9	791.2	206.4	148.2	347.1	317.1	483.2	460.0	702.5	697.3
New Mexico	967.1	891.9	749.2	740.8	747.4	736.5	726.2	707.7	789.7	826.1	370.4	339.0	721.9	709.4	738.9	729.0
New York	1,051.8	973.7	668.5	643.2	681.9	663.9	696.7	654.8	192.1	180.0	361.6	354.6	530.6	492.2	678.0	663.4
North Carolina	1,050.4	986.0	799.9	781.2	778.3	761.8	913.9	884.9	781.0	759.9	349.6	374.2	295.8	321.2	788.0	774.4
North Dakota	922.4	818.4	704.6	699.7	681.0	677.8	Y	397.1	1,364.4	1,278.2	Y	504.2	545.9	527.9	679.8	677.3
Ohio	1,070.6	967.4	817.4	816.6	804.5	808.3	962.0	932.6	268.5	249.8	401.9	368.1	481.4	468.6	806.6	811.4
Oklahoma	1,025.6	961.4	910.2	904.2	896.8	890.9	1,051.6	1,014.5	987.6	1,015.8	525.4	478.2	518.7	522.3	909.3	903.6
Oregon	953.9	893.0	725.2	715.5	732.4	724.5	797.8	761.3	679.5	674.7	433.0	424.7	456.2	450.3	740.5	734.3
Pennsylvania	1,076.4	963.4	772.5	760.0	759.6	751.9	960.3	908.1	236.7	280.3	380.1	390.2	507.8	563.2	760.8	748.5
Rhode Island	990.8	889.6	713.4	710.8	720.5	726.9	596.8	474.7	549.3	560.3	475.1	402.8	419.0	404.2	724.8	733.9
South Carolina	1,104.6	1,030.0	847.0	835.6	811.6	808.2	972.3	942.6	457.4	351.4	430.3	365.6	404.9	368.2	813.6	818.9
South Dakota	941.9	846.4	714.1	701.7	679.1	664.1	364.8	273.7	1,278.9	1,283.2	Y	375.5	349.5	254.1	680.3	667.9
Tennessee	1,045.5	1,011.8	885.1	882.5	870.2	875.4	1,021.0	967.1	253.7	229.2	448.1	394.1	295.3	338.4	877.6	882.4
Texas	1,014.9	947.6	765.2	747.2	761.5	748.5	934.7	889.8	156.7	150.7	382.3	383.6	643.4	626.6	793.4	787.0
Utah	924.9	823.2	696.4	710.7	698.6	714.5	760.2	600.7	752.6	713.0	529.0	543.3	540.1	538.9	705.4	724.0
Vermont	990.2	908.6	704.2	706.7	708.0	711.1	Y	497.0	Y	Y	Y	375.3	Y	329.3	707.2	713.2
Virginia	1,054.0	963.1	744.6	721.3	729.1	714.6	892.7	847.4	387.3	283.7	390.2	364.3	387.1	350.1	736.1	725.5
Washington	947.7	869.4	696.9	679.9	706.1	694.1	776.6	734.4	901.6	856.5	458.2	418.6	479.0	454.0	713.1	702.5
West Virginia	1,100.3	1,031.5	944.7	932.0	946.0	935.3	1,027.5	981.0	Y	Y	338.2	276.2	239.3	226.6	949.4	940.2
Wisconsin	956.4	879.1	714.5	716.0	701.5	702.9	977.9	948.6	985.9	958.6	430.4	499.8	449.0	449.4	704.9	706.6
Wyoming	1,016.1	897.4	767.4	740.8	762.7	742.9	Y	333.2	1,093.8	1,042.5	Y	Y	661.8	533.9	764.5	752.0
American Samoa[3]	NA	NA	1,063.0	1,042.0	NA	NA	NA	NA	NA	NA	NA	NA	NA	NA	NA	NA
Guam[3]	NA	NA	729.9	793.4	NA	NA	NA	NA	NA	NA	NA	NA	NA	NA	NA	NA
Northern Marianas[3]	NA	NA	816.2	861.3	NA	NA	NA	NA	NA	NA	NA	NA	NA	NA	NA	NA
Puerto Rico[3]	NA	NA	708.8	656.4	NA	NA	NA	NA	NA	NA	NA	NA	NA	NA	NA	NA
Virgin Islands[3]	NA	NA	628.1	†644.0	NA	NA	NA	NA	NA	NA	NA	NA	NA	NA	NA	NA

Note: Data are based on death certificates. Age-adjusted average annual death rates are calculated using the year 2000. Prior to 2001, age-adjusted rates were calculated using standard million proportions based on rounded population numbers. Starting with 2001 data, unrounded population numbers are used to calculate age-adjusted rates. Age-adjusted rates for Puerto Rico, Virgin Islands, Guam, American Samoa, and Northern Marianas were computed by applying the age-specific death rates to the U.S. standard population combining the age groups for age 75 and over. For the territories, age groups were not available for those age 75 and over by age. Prior to 2009–2011, denominators for rates are resident population estimates for the middle year of each 3-year period, multiplied by 3. Starting with 2009–2011 estimates, denominators for rates are the 3-year average population. The race groups, White, Black, American Indian or Alaska Native, and Asian or Pacific Islander, include persons of Hispanic and non-Hispanic origin. Persons of Hispanic origin may be of any race. United States, state, and territory rates for 2011 and beyond were calculated using 2010-based postcensal population estimates. Starting with 2003 data, some states began to collect information on more than one race on the death certificate, according to 1997 Office of Management and Budget (OMB) standards. The multiple-race data for these states were bridged to the single-race categories of the 1977 OMB standards, for comparability with other states. Rates are rounded at the end of the calculation process. They may differ from rates based on the same data presented elsewhere if rounding is done earlier in the calculation process. Data for additional years are available.

NA = Not available.

Y = Prior to 2009–2011, data for states with populations under 10,000 in the middle year of a 3-year period, or fewer than 50 deaths for the 3-year period, are considered unreliable and are not shown. Starting with 2009–2011 estimates (shown in spreadsheet file), data for states with an average population for the 3-year period of under 10,000, or fewer than 50 deaths for the 3-year period, are considered unreliable and are not shown.

† = Rate shown is for 2010-2012 because death data were not available for the Virgin Islands for 2013.

[1]Death rates for Hispanic, American Indian or Alaska Native, and Asian or Pacific Islander persons should be interpreted with caution because of inconsistencies in reporting Hispanic origin or race on the death certificate (death rate numerators) compared with population figures (death rate denominators). The net effect of misclassification is an underestimation of deaths and death rates for races other than White and Black.

[2]Excludes data for American Samoa, Guam, Northern Marianas, Puerto Rico, and Virgin Islands.

[3]Comparable population data were not available for all time periods and for all racial and ethnicity groups. Therefore, only selected rates are presented for the territories.

Table 2-15. Age-Adjusted Death Rates for Selected Causes of Death, by Sex, Race, and Hispanic Origin, Selected Years, 1950–2015

(Age-adjusted rate per 100,000 population.)

Sex, race, Hispanic origin, and cause of death[1]	1950[2,3]	1960[2,3]	1970[3]	1980[3]	1985[3]	1990[3]	1995[3]	2000[4]	2005[4]	2006[4]	2007[4]	2008[4]	2009[4]	2010[4]	2011[4]	2012[4]	2013[4]	2014[4]	2015[4]
	Age-adjusted death rate per 100,000 population[5]																		
All Persons																			
All causes	1,446.0	1,339.2	1,222.6	1,039.1	988.1	938.7	909.8	869.0	815.0	791.8	775.3	774.9	749.6	747.0	741.3	732.8	731.9	724.6	733.1
Diseases of heart	588.8	559.0	492.7	412.1	375.0	321.8	293.4	257.6	216.8	205.5	196.1	192.1	182.8	179.1	173.7	170.5	169.8	167.0	168.5
Ischemic heart disease	NA	NA	NA	345.2	296.2	249.6	219.7	186.8	148.2	138.3	129.2	126.1	117.7	113.6	109.2	105.4	102.6	98.8	97.2
Cerebrovascular diseases	180.7	177.9	147.7	96.2	76.4	65.3	63.1	60.9	48.0	44.8	43.5	42.1	39.6	39.1	37.9	36.9	36.2	36.5	37.6
Malignant neoplasms	193.9	193.9	198.6	207.9	211.3	216.0	209.9	199.6	185.1	181.8	179.3	176.4	173.5	172.8	169.0	166.5	163.2	161.2	158.5
Trachea, bronchus, and lung	15.0	24.1	37.1	49.9	54.6	59.3	58.4	56.1	52.7	51.5	50.6	49.5	48.4	47.6	46.0	44.9	43.4	42.1	40.5
Colon, rectum, and anus	NA	30.3	28.9	27.4	26.3	24.5	22.5	20.8	17.7	17.4	17.0	16.6	16.0	15.8	15.3	14.9	14.6	14.3	14.2
Chronic lower respiratory diseases[6]	NA	NA	NA	28.3	34.5	37.2	40.1	44.2	43.9	41.0	41.4	44.7	42.7	42.2	42.5	41.5	42.1	40.5	41.6
Influenza and pneumonia[7]	48.1	53.7	41.7	31.4	34.5	36.8	33.4	23.7	21.0	18.4	16.8	17.6	16.5	15.1	15.7	14.4	15.9	15.1	15.2
Chronic liver disease and cirrhosis	11.3	13.3	17.8	15.1	12.3	11.1	9.9	9.5	8.9	8.8	9.1	9.2	9.1	9.4	9.7	9.9	10.2	10.4	10.8
Diabetes mellitus[8]	23.1	22.5	24.3	18.1	17.4	20.7	23.2	25.0	24.9	23.6	22.8	22.0	21.0	20.8	21.6	21.2	21.2	20.9	21.3
Alzheimer's disease	NA	NA	NA	V	V	V	V	18.1	24.0	23.7	23.8	25.8	24.2	25.1	24.7	23.8	23.5	25.4	29.4
Human immunodeficiency virus (HIV) disease	X	X	X	X	NA	10.2	16.2	5.2	4.2	4.0	3.7	3.3	3.0	2.6	2.4	2.2	2.1	2.0	1.9
Unintentional injuries	78.0	62.3	60.1	46.4	38.5	36.3	34.4	34.9	39.5	40.2	40.4	39.2	37.5	38.0	39.1	39.1	39.4	40.5	43.2
Motor vehicle-related injuries	24.6	23.1	27.6	22.3	18.6	18.5	16.3	15.4	15.2	15.0	14.4	12.9	11.6	11.3	11.1	11.4	10.9	10.8	11.4
Poisoning	2.5	1.7	2.8	1.9	2.2	2.3	3.4	4.5	8.0	9.2	9.9	10.2	10.3	10.6	11.6	11.5	12.2	13.1	14.8
Nephritis, nephrotic syndrome, and nephrosis[8]	NA	NA	NA	9.1	10.4	9.3	9.4	13.5	14.7	14.8	14.9	15.1	15.1	15.3	13.4	13.1	13.2	13.2	13.4
Suicide[9]	13.2	12.5	13.1	12.2	12.5	12.5	11.8	10.4	10.9	11.0	11.3	11.6	11.8	12.1	12.3	12.6	12.6	13.0	13.3
Homicide[9]	5.1	5.0	8.8	10.4	7.9	9.4	8.3	5.9	6.1	6.2	6.1	5.9	5.5	5.3	5.3	5.4	5.2	5.1	5.7
Male																			
All causes	1,674.2	1,609.0	1,542.1	1,348.1	1,278.1	1,202.8	1,143.9	1,053.8	971.9	943.5	922.9	918.8	890.9	887.1	875.3	865.1	863.6	855.1	863.2
Diseases of heart	699.0	687.6	634.0	538.9	488.0	412.4	371.0	320.0	268.2	254.9	243.7	238.5	229.4	225.1	218.1	214.7	214.5	210.9	211.8
Ischemic heart disease	NA	NA	NA	459.7	393.7	328.2	286.5	241.4	192.3	180.7	169.2	165.1	156.2	151.3	145.6	141.1	138.2	133.5	131.2
Cerebrovascular diseases	186.4	186.1	157.4	102.2	79.9	68.5	65.9	62.4	48.4	45.2	43.7	42.2	39.9	39.3	37.9	37.1	36.7	36.9	37.8
Malignant neoplasms	208.1	225.1	247.6	271.2	274.4	280.4	267.5	248.9	227.2	221.7	218.8	214.9	210.9	209.9	204.0	200.3	196.0	192.9	189.2
Trachea, bronchus, and lung	24.6	43.6	67.5	85.2	88.6	91.1	84.2	76.7	69.1	67.0	64.9	63.5	61.4	60.3	57.7	56.1	53.7	51.7	49.5
Colon, rectum, and anus	NA	31.8	32.3	32.8	31.8	30.4	27.4	25.1	21.2	20.7	20.3	19.7	19.1	19.0	18.1	17.7	17.4	16.9	16.8
Prostate	28.6	28.7	28.8	32.8	33.4	38.4	37.0	30.4	25.3	24.2	24.2	23.0	22.1	21.9	20.7	19.5	19.2	19.0	18.8
Chronic lower respiratory diseases[6]	NA	NA	NA	49.9	56.2	55.4	54.8	55.8	52.2	48.4	48.8	52.3	49.5	48.7	48.6	47.2	47.5	45.4	46.0
Influenza and pneumonia[7]	55.0	65.8	54.0	42.1	46.8	47.8	42.8	28.9	24.9	22.1	20.2	20.7	19.6	18.2	18.8	17.3	18.6	17.8	17.7
Chronic liver disease and cirrhosis	15.0	18.5	24.8	21.3	17.4	15.9	14.2	13.4	12.4	12.1	12.7	12.7	12.5	12.9	13.1	13.4	13.8	14.1	14.5
Diabetes mellitus[8]	18.8	19.9	23.0	18.1	17.7	21.7	25.0	27.8	28.8	27.7	26.6	25.9	25.0	24.9	26.0	25.5	25.6	25.6	26.2
Alzheimer's disease	NA	NA	NA	V	V	V	V	15.2	19.5	19.4	19.5	21.3	20.2	21.0	20.4	19.8	19.3	20.6	23.7
Human immunodeficiency virus (HIV) disease	X	X	X	X	NA	18.5	27.3	7.9	6.3	5.9	5.4	4.8	4.4	3.8	3.4	3.2	3.1	3.0	2.8
Unintentional injuries	101.8	85.5	87.4	69.0	57.1	52.9	49.6	49.3	55.0	56.0	55.9	54.3	51.4	51.5	52.8	52.6	53.1	54.6	58.7
Motor vehicle-related injuries	38.5	35.4	41.5	33.6	27.2	26.5	22.8	21.7	21.9	21.5	21.0	18.9	16.8	16.2	16.1	16.5	16.5	15.9	16.7
Poisoning	3.3	2.3	3.9	2.7	3.2	3.5	5.3	6.6	10.8	12.6	13.1	13.6	13.5	13.8	15.1	15.0	16.0	17.3	19.8
Nephritis, nephrotic syndrome, and nephrosis[8]	NA	NA	NA	12.2	13.8	12.1	12.2	16.9	18.1	18.3	18.3	18.5	18.4	18.7	16.5	16.0	16.1	16.2	16.3
Suicide[9]	21.2	20.0	19.8	19.9	21.1	21.5	20.3	17.7	18.1	18.1	18.5	19.0	19.2	19.8	20.0	20.4	20.3	20.7	21.1
Homicide[9]	7.9	7.5	14.3	16.6	12.2	14.8	12.8	9.0	9.7	9.8	9.7	9.3	8.6	8.4	8.3	8.5	8.2	8.0	9.1
Female																			
All causes	1,236.0	1,105.3	971.4	817.9	784.5	750.9	739.4	731.4	692.3	672.2	658.1	659.9	636.8	634.9	632.4	624.7	623.5	616.7	624.2
Diseases of heart	486.6	447.0	381.6	320.8	294.5	257.0	236.6	210.9	177.5	167.2	159.0	155.9	146.6	143.3	138.7	135.5	134.3	131.8	133.6
Ischemic heart disease	NA	NA	NA	263.1	227.0	193.9	171.3	146.5	115.0	106.3	98.8	96.3	88.4	84.9	81.0	77.8	74.9	71.6	70.5
Cerebrovascular diseases	175.8	170.7	140.0	91.7	73.3	62.6	60.5	59.1	47.0	43.9	42.7	41.4	38.8	38.3	37.2	36.1	35.2	35.6	36.9
Malignant neoplasms	182.3	168.7	163.2	166.7	171.2	175.7	173.6	167.6	156.7	154.7	152.3	149.6	147.4	146.7	144.0	142.1	139.5	138.1	135.9
Trachea, bronchus, and lung	5.8	7.5	13.1	24.4	30.6	37.1	40.4	41.3	40.6	40.1	40.1	39.1	38.6	38.1	37.1	36.4	35.5	34.7	33.5
Colon, rectum, and anus	NA	29.1	26.5	23.8	22.7	20.6	19.1	17.7	15.0	14.9	14.6	14.2	13.5	13.3	13.0	12.6	12.3	12.1	12.1
Breast	31.9	31.7	32.1	31.9	33.0	33.3	30.5	26.8	24.2	23.6	23.0	22.6	22.3	22.1	21.6	21.3	20.8	20.6	20.3
Chronic lower respiratory diseases[6]	NA	NA	NA	14.9	21.7	26.6	31.8	37.4	38.7	36.4	36.6	39.8	38.3	38.0	38.5	37.8	38.5	37.1	38.6
Influenza and pneumonia[7]	41.9	43.8	32.7	25.1	27.6	30.5	28.1	20.7	18.6	16.1	14.7	15.6	14.5	13.1	13.7	12.5	14.0	13.2	13.5
Chronic liver disease and cirrhosis	7.8	8.7	11.9	9.9	7.9	7.1	6.2	6.2	5.8	5.8	5.9	6.0	6.1	6.2	6.6	6.7	6.8	7.1	7.6
Diabetes mellitus[8]	27.0	24.7	25.1	18.0	17.0	19.9	21.8	23.0	21.9	20.4	19.8	19.1	17.9	17.6	18.2	17.7	17.6	17.2	17.3
Alzheimer's disease	NA	NA	NA	V	V	V	V	19.3	26.2	25.9	26.2	28.2	26.3	27.3	27.1	26.1	25.9	28.3	32.8
Human immunodeficiency virus (HIV) disease	X	X	X	X	NA	2.2	5.3	2.5	2.3	2.2	2.1	1.9	1.7	1.4	1.3	1.2	1.1	1.1	1.0

NA = Not available.
V = Data for Alzheimer's disease are only presented for data years 1999 and beyond due to large differences in death rates caused by changes in the coding of the causes of death between ICD-9 and ICD-10.
X = Not applicable.
[1] Underlying cause of death code numbers are based on the applicable revision of the International Classification of Diseases (ICD) for data years shown.
[2] Includes deaths of persons who were not residents of the 50 states and the District of Columbia.
[3] Underlying cause of death was coded according to the 6th Revision of the ICD in 1950, 7th Revision in 1960, 8th Revision in 1970, and 9th Revision in 1980-1998.
[4] Starting with 1999 data, cause of death is coded according to ICD-10.
[5] Age-adjusted rates are calculated using the year 2000 standard population. Prior to 2001, age-adjusted rates were calculated using standard million proportions based on rounded population numbers. Starting with 2001 data, unrounded population numbers are used to calculate age-adjusted rates.
[6] Between 1998 and 1999, the cause of death title for Chronic obstructive pulmonary diseases in the ICD–9 was renamed to Chronic lower respiratory diseases (CLRD) in ICD–10.
[7] Starting with 1999 data, the rules for selecting CLRD and Pneumonia as the underlying cause of death changed, resulting in an increase in the number of deaths for CLRD and a decrease in the number of deaths for pneumonia. Therefore, trend data for these two causes of death should be interpreted with caution.
[8] Starting with 2011 data, the rules for selecting Renal failure as the underlying cause of death were changed, affecting the number of deaths in the Nephritis, nephrotic syndrome and nephrosis and Diabetes categories. These changes directly affect deaths with mention of Renal failure and other associated conditions, such as Diabetes mellitus with renal complications. The result is a decrease in the number of deaths for Nephritis, nephrotic syndrome and nephrosis and an increase in the number of deaths for Diabetes mellitus. Therefore, trend data for these two causes of death should be interpreted with caution.
[9] Figures for 2001 include September 11-related deaths, for which death certificates were filed as of October 24, 2002.

Table 2-15. Age-Adjusted Death Rates for Selected Causes of Death, by Sex, Race, and Hispanic Origin, Selected Years, 1950–2015—*Continued*

(Age-adjusted rate per 100,000 population.)

Sex, race, Hispanic origin, and cause of death[1]	1950[2,3]	1960[2,3]	1970[3]	1980[3]	1985[3]	1990[3]	1995[3]	2000[4]	2005[4]	2006[4]	2007[4]	2008[4]	2009[4]	2010[4]	2011[4]	2012[4]	2013[4]	2014[4]	2015[4]
	Age-adjusted death rate per 100,000 population[5]																		
Unintentional injuries	54.0	40.0	35.1	26.1	22.2	21.5	21.0	22.0	25.3	25.8	26.1	25.4	24.8	25.6	26.5	26.4	26.6	27.3	28.7
Motor vehicle-related injuries	11.5	11.7	14.9	11.8	10.7	11.0	10.3	9.5	8.9	8.8	8.2	7.2	6.7	6.5	6.3	6.5	6.2	6.1	6.4
Poisoning	1.7	1.1	1.8	1.3	1.2	1.2	1.6	2.5	5.1	5.9	6.6	6.8	7.1	7.5	8.2	8.1	8.5	9.1	9.8
Nephritis, nephrotic syndrome, and nephrosis[8]	NA	NA	NA	7.3	8.5	7.7	7.8	11.5	12.6	12.6	12.8	13.0	13.0	13.0	11.4	11.1	11.3	11.1	11.3
Suicide[9]	5.6	5.6	7.4	5.7	5.2	4.8	4.3	4.0	4.4	4.5	4.6	4.8	4.9	5.0	5.2	5.4	5.5	5.8	6.0
Homicide[9]	2.4	2.6	3.7	4.4	3.8	4.0	3.7	2.8	2.5	2.6	2.5	2.4	2.4	2.3	2.2	2.2	2.1	2.1	2.2
White[10]																			
All causes	1,410.8	1,311.3	1,193.3	1,012.7	963.6	909.8	882.3	849.8	801.1	779.3	764.3	767.2	742.8	741.8	738.8	730.9	731.0	725.4	735.0
Diseases of heart	586.0	559.0	492.2	409.4	371.4	317.0	288.6	253.4	213.2	202.0	192.8	189.3	180.1	176.9	172.2	168.9	168.2	165.9	167.9
Ischemic heart disease	NA	NA	NA	347.6	298.0	249.7	219.1	185.6	147.3	137.4	128.5	125.8	117.4	113.5	109.3	105.6	102.9	99.3	98.0
Cerebrovascular diseases	175.5	172.7	143.5	93.2	73.7	62.8	60.7	58.8	46.0	42.9	41.6	40.4	38.1	37.7	36.5	35.6	34.9	35.2	36.4
Malignant neoplasms	194.6	193.1	196.7	204.2	207.3	211.6	206.2	197.2	183.9	181.0	178.5	175.9	173.3	172.4	168.8	166.6	163.7	161.9	159.4
Trachea, bronchus, and lung	15.2	24.0	36.7	49.2	53.9	58.6	58.1	56.2	53.2	52.1	51.2	50.2	49.1	48.3	46.7	45.6	44.1	42.9	41.4
Colon, rectum, and anus	NA	30.9	29.2	27.4	26.1	24.1	22.0	20.3	17.1	16.9	16.6	16.1	15.6	15.3	14.8	14.5	14.3	14.0	13.9
Chronic lower respiratory diseases[6]	NA	NA	NA	29.3	35.6	38.3	41.5	46.0	46.0	43.1	43.5	47.1	45.1	44.6	45.1	44.1	44.8	43.1	44.5
Influenza and pneumonia[7]	44.8	50.4	39.8	30.9	34.3	36.4	33.0	23.5	20.9	18.2	16.6	17.4	16.3	14.9	15.6	14.3	15.8	15.1	15.2
Chronic liver disease and cirrhosis	11.5	13.2	16.6	13.9	11.4	10.5	9.7	9.6	9.2	9.1	9.5	9.6	9.6	9.9	10.2	10.5	10.7	11.2	11.7
Diabetes mellitus[8]	22.9	21.7	22.9	16.7	15.9	18.8	20.9	22.8	22.8	21.4	20.7	20.2	19.2	19.0	19.8	19.4	19.4	19.3	19.6
Alzheimer's disease	NA	NA	NA	V	V	V	V	18.8	24.7	24.5	24.6	26.7	25.0	26.0	25.7	24.7	24.4	26.4	30.5
Human immunodeficiency virus (HIV) disease	X	X	X	X	NA	8.3	11.4	2.8	2.2	2.1	1.9	1.7	1.5	1.4	1.3	1.2	1.2	1.1	1.1
Unintentional injuries	77.0	60.4	57.8	45.3	37.7	35.5	33.9	35.1	40.7	41.7	42.1	41.4	39.5	40.3	41.6	41.5	41.9	43.1	46.0
Motor vehicle-related injuries	24.4	22.9	27.1	22.6	18.8	18.5	16.3	15.6	15.7	15.5	14.9	13.4	12.0	11.7	11.5	11.8	11.3	11.1	11.7
Poisoning	2.4	1.6	2.4	1.8	2.0	2.1	3.1	4.5	8.5	9.8	10.7	11.3	11.4	11.9	13.0	12.9	13.7	14.8	16.7
Nephritis, nephrotic syndrome, and nephrosis[8]	NA	NA	NA	8.0	9.3	8.3	8.5	12.1	13.2	13.3	13.5	13.8	13.7	14.0	12.2	12.0	12.1	12.1	12.2
Suicide[9]	13.9	13.1	13.8	13.0	13.4	13.4	12.6	11.3	12.1	12.2	12.6	13.0	13.2	13.6	13.9	14.1	14.2	14.7	15.1
Homicide[9]	2.6	2.7	4.7	6.7	5.3	5.5	5.0	3.6	3.7	3.7	3.7	3.7	3.4	3.3	3.2	3.2	3.1	3.0	3.3
Black or African American[10]																			
All causes	1,722.1	1,577.5	1,518.1	1,314.8	1,261.2	1,250.3	1,213.9	1,121.4	1,035.1	997.9	972.0	947.7	912.8	898.2	877.1	864.8	860.8	849.3	851.9
Diseases of heart	588.7	548.3	512.0	455.3	430.6	391.5	363.8	324.8	278.0	263.5	252.5	243.4	231.8	224.9	214.1	211.7	210.4	206.3	205.1
Ischemic heart disease	NA	NA	NA	334.5	293.4	267.0	244.9	218.3	175.7	165.4	154.0	146.8	137.4	131.2	125.3	121.3	117.5	112.8	108.9
Cerebrovascular diseases	233.6	235.2	197.1	129.1	105.2	91.6	86.9	81.9	67.0	63.1	61.7	58.8	54.0	53.0	50.9	49.3	49.0	49.7	50.8
Malignant neoplasms	176.4	199.1	225.3	256.4	266.5	279.5	267.7	248.5	223.5	217.6	215.1	208.5	204.5	203.8	198.8	193.8	189.2	185.6	180.1
Trachea, bronchus, and lung	11.1	23.7	41.3	59.7	65.8	72.4	69.0	64.0	58.1	56.3	55.1	52.9	51.3	51.4	49.2	48.3	46.8	44.5	42.0
Colon, rectum, and anus	NA	22.8	26.1	28.3	30.0	30.6	29.3	28.2	25.1	24.4	23.6	22.9	22.0	21.8	21.2	20.0	19.4	18.6	18.8
Chronic lower respiratory diseases[6]	NA	NA	NA	19.2	24.6	28.1	30.1	31.6	31.1	28.5	28.5	30.8	28.9	29.0	29.2	29.0	29.5	28.4	28.9
Influenza and pneumonia[7]	76.7	81.1	57.2	34.4	35.8	39.4	36.4	25.6	22.6	20.4	19.2	19.5	18.0	16.8	16.8	15.7	16.7	16.1	15.9
Chronic liver disease and cirrhosis	9.0	13.6	28.1	25.0	19.3	16.5	12.0	9.4	7.6	6.8	7.2	6.8	6.8	6.7	7.0	6.9	7.3	7.2	7.4
Diabetes mellitus[8]	23.5	30.9	38.8	32.7	33.0	40.5	46.7	49.5	47.5	45.5	43.1	40.8	39.1	38.7	39.6	38.7	38.4	37.3	37.0
Alzheimer's disease	NA	NA	NA	V	V	V	V	13.0	20.8	19.7	20.5	21.2	20.6	20.6	20.8	19.9	20.1	22.3	26.6
Human immunodeficiency virus (HIV) disease	X	X	X	X	NA	26.7	54.2	23.3	19.2	18.3	17.0	14.9	13.7	11.6	10.3	9.5	8.9	8.3	7.9
Unintentional injuries	79.9	74.0	78.3	57.6	47.1	43.8	41.0	37.7	38.8	38.2	36.5	33.1	31.6	31.3	31.6	31.4	32.6	33.7	36.8
Motor vehicle-related injuries	26.0	24.2	31.1	20.2	17.8	18.8	16.7	15.7	14.4	14.5	14.0	12.1	11.5	10.9	10.7	11.3	10.9	11.1	12.2
Poisoning	2.8	2.9	5.8	3.1	3.6	4.1	6.2	6.0	8.1	9.3	8.4	7.7	7.4	7.3	8.0	8.1	8.9	9.6	11.1
Nephritis, nephrotic syndrome, and nephrosis[8]	NA	NA	NA	20.9	22.7	19.8	19.3	28.7	30.3	30.8	29.9	29.9	29.9	29.3	25.9	25.2	25.0	24.6	25.4
Suicide[9]	4.5	5.0	6.2	6.5	6.6	7.1	6.8	5.5	5.2	5.0	4.9	5.2	5.1	5.2	5.4	5.6	5.4	5.5	5.6
Homicide[9]	28.3	26.0	44.0	39.0	28.1	36.3	29.7	20.5	21.1	21.5	20.9	19.3	18.1	17.7	17.6	18.4	17.8	17.2	19.8
American Indian or Alaska Native[10]																			
All causes	NA	NA	NA	867.0	731.7	716.3	771.2	709.3	701.1	676.6	661.3	644.0	616.0	628.3	600.9	595.3	591.7	594.1	596.9
Diseases of heart	NA	NA	NA	240.6	219.0	200.6	204.6	178.2	156.6	153.2	140.5	132.6	130.7	128.6	124.2	119.6	120.6	119.1	118.5
Ischemic heart disease	NA	NA	NA	173.6	158.3	139.1	141.4	129.1	106.1	107.2	95.9	88.0	86.5	84.9	81.4	79.2	78.2	76.4	73.4
Cerebrovascular diseases	NA	NA	NA	57.8	46.2	40.7	48.6	45.0	38.8	33.4	34.2	27.7	29.2	28.1	27.1	25.2	24.6	25.4	24.7
Malignant neoplasms	NA	NA	NA	113.7	113.5	121.8	138.2	127.8	128.8	125.4	124.1	125.0	114.9	122.4	109.4	111.4	110.2	106.7	107.9

NA = Not available.
V = Data for Alzheimer's disease are only presented for data years 1999 and beyond due to large differences in death rates caused by changes in the coding of the causes of death between ICD-9 and ICD-10.
X = Not applicable.
[1]Underlying cause of death code numbers are based on the applicable revision of the International Classification of Diseases (ICD) for data years shown.
[2]Includes deaths of persons who were not residents of the 50 states and the District of Columbia.
[3]Underlying cause of death was coded according to the 6th Revision of the ICD in 1950, 7th Revision in 1960, 8th Revision in 1970, and 9th Revision in 1980-1998.
[4]Starting with 1999 data, cause of death is coded according to ICD-10.
[5]Age-adjusted rates are calculated using the year 2000 standard population. Prior to 2001, age-adjusted rates were calculated using standard million proportions based on rounded population numbers. Starting with 2001 data, unrounded population numbers are used to calculate age-adjusted rates.
[6]Between 1998 and 1999, the cause of death title for Chronic obstructive pulmonary diseases in the ICD–9 was renamed to Chronic lower respiratory diseases (CLRD) in ICD–10.
[7]Starting with 1999 data, the rules for selecting CLRD and Pneumonia as the underlying cause of death changed, resulting in an increase in the number of deaths for CLRD and a decrease in the number of deaths for pneumonia. Therefore, trend data for these two causes of death should be interpreted with caution.
[8]Starting with 2011 data, the rules for selecting Renal failure as the underlying cause of death were changed, affecting the number of deaths in the Nephritis, nephrotic syndrome and nephrosis and Diabetes categories. These changes directly affect deaths with mention of Renal failure and other associated conditions, such as Diabetes mellitus with renal complications. The result is a decrease in the number of deaths for Nephritis, nephrotic syndrome and nephrosis and an increase in the number of deaths for Diabetes mellitus. Therefore, trend data for these two causes of death should be interpreted with caution.
[9]Figures for 2001 include September 11-related deaths, for which death certificates were filed as of October 24, 2002.
[10]The race groups White, Black, Asian or Pacific Islander, and American Indian or Alaska Native, include persons of Hispanic and non-Hispanic origin. Persons of Hispanic origin may be of any race. Death rates for the American Indian or Alaska Native, Asian or Pacific Islander, and Hispanic populations are known to be underestimated.

Table 2-15. Age-Adjusted Death Rates for Selected Causes of Death, by Sex, Race, and Hispanic Origin, Selected Years, 1950–2015—*Continued*

(Age-adjusted rate per 100,000 population.)

Sex, race, Hispanic origin, and cause of death[1]	1950[2,3]	1960[2,3]	1970[3]	1980[3]	1985[3]	1990[3]	1995[3]	2000[4]	2005[4]	2006[4]	2007[4]	2008[4]	2009[4]	2010[4]	2011[4]	2012[4]	2013[4]	2014[4]	2015[4]
	Age-adjusted death rate per 100,000 population[5]																		
Trachea, bronchus, and lung	NA	NA	NA	20.7	25.8	30.9	37.4	32.3	35.3	32.3	34.1	34.8	29.5	33.1	30.0	30.1	27.7	27.8	26.7
Colon, rectum, and anus	NA	NA	NA	9.5	10.5	12.0	14.9	13.4	12.6	11.7	12.1	14.6	13.0	11.7	12.3	11.1	12.6	10.9	11.1
Chronic lower respiratory diseases[6]	NA	NA	NA	14.2	17.6	25.4	27.6	32.8	31.6	29.8	33.9	31.9	30.7	33.8	28.7	29.8	30.8	29.9	30.9
Influenza and pneumonia[7]	NA	NA	NA	44.4	33.6	36.1	36.1	22.3	23.6	16.3	15.9	19.6	17.9	15.9	15.5	13.1	15.0	15.1	12.5
Chronic liver disease and cirrhosis	NA	NA	NA	45.3	27.9	24.1	27.4	24.3	21.6	20.9	23.1	23.6	21.3	22.8	22.9	25.3	24.8	24.2	26.4
Diabetes mellitus[8]	NA	NA	NA	29.6	29.0	34.1	45.9	41.5	44.1	42.2	40.0	36.3	34.9	36.4	36.5	36.9	34.1	31.3	34.2
Alzheimer's disease	NA	NA	NA	V	V	V	V	9.1	15.0	13.6	14.3	15.1	13.1	17.2	13.4	12.3	12.7	15.2	15.4
Human immunodeficiency virus (HIV) disease	X	X	X	X	NA	1.8	6.5	2.2	2.5	2.1	2.3	1.8	1.7	1.6	1.2	1.0	1.3	1.2	1.4
Unintentional injuries	NA	NA	NA	99.0	67.4	62.6	55.3	51.3	51.3	52.6	50.8	49.0	48.7	46.9	48.3	49.5	47.1	49.5	50.7
Motor vehicle-related injuries	NA	NA	NA	54.5	34.8	32.5	29.1	27.3	22.6	24.1	20.8	18.4	17.2	15.7	16.6	16.3	15.4	16.6	16.9
Poisoning	NA	NA	NA	2.3	3.1	3.2	4.6	4.7	8.6	9.4	10.3	12.4	13.8	13.0	14.0	15.1	14.2	15.5	16.1
Nephritis, nephrotic syndrome, and nephrosis[8]	NA	NA	NA	12.2	10.7	11.6	10.6	15.0	15.6	15.1	15.9	17.2	14.4	16.4	12.5	12.6	11.4	12.4	12.2
Suicide[9]	NA	NA	NA	11.9	10.9	11.7	10.6	9.8	10.7	10.4	10.1	10.1	10.0	10.8	10.6	10.8	11.7	10.9	12.6
Homicide[9]	NA	NA	NA	15.5	11.7	10.4	9.9	6.8	6.8	6.6	5.6	6.2	5.9	5.7	5.9	5.8	5.3	5.8	6.2
Asian or Pacific Islander[10]																			
All causes	NA	NA	NA	589.9	586.5	582.0	554.8	506.4	459.6	450.7	436.2	435.1	424.6	424.3	410.3	407.1	405.4	388.3	394.8
Diseases of heart	NA	NA	NA	202.1	196.7	181.7	171.3	146.0	119.7	115.8	108.3	107.7	103.8	100.9	93.2	92.2	92.8	86.1	86.5
Ischemic heart disease	NA	NA	NA	168.2	153.3	139.6	128.0	109.6	85.6	82.2	75.9	75.9	70.7	68.7	62.7	60.5	59.9	55.1	54.9
Cerebrovascular diseases	NA	NA	NA	66.1	58.7	56.9	55.2	52.9	40.8	39.3	36.6	35.2	33.0	33.2	31.6	30.8	29.4	28.3	29.8
Malignant neoplasms	NA	NA	NA	126.1	132.3	134.2	131.8	121.9	113.2	109.6	109.5	108.8	106.8	108.9	105.6	104.2	100.5	98.9	99.0
Trachea, bronchus, and lung	NA	NA	NA	28.4	27.2	30.2	29.9	28.1	26.3	25.9	26.0	25.6	25.2	24.8	24.6	24.0	23.3	22.7	22.2
Colon, rectum, and anus	NA	NA	NA	16.4	16.6	14.4	14.0	12.7	11.5	11.3	11.2	11.6	10.5	11.4	10.8	10.8	9.8	9.5	9.8
Chronic lower respiratory diseases[6]	NA	NA	NA	12.9	17.6	19.4	19.3	18.6	15.9	15.4	14.3	15.2	14.3	13.9	14.5	12.8	13.6	12.5	12.2
Influenza and pneumonia[7]	NA	NA	NA	24.0	26.1	31.4	29.1	19.7	16.8	16.1	14.9	15.7	15.0	14.4	14.2	14.0	15.0	12.9	14.0
Chronic liver disease and cirrhosis	NA	NA	NA	6.1	5.9	5.2	3.9	3.5	3.6	3.5	3.3	3.4	3.3	3.2	3.3	3.3	3.3	3.5	3.3
Diabetes mellitus[8]	NA	NA	NA	12.6	12.1	14.6	16.8	16.4	17.3	16.6	17.0	16.8	16.2	15.5	15.9	15.7	15.8	15.0	15.7
Alzheimer's disease	NA	NA	NA	V	V	V	V	5.5	8.5	9.4	9.1	10.1	10.9	10.9	11.1	11.7	11.1	12.1	14.7
Human immunodeficiency virus (HIV) disease	X	X	X	X	NA	2.2	3.2	0.6	0.6	0.6	0.5	0.6	0.4	0.4	0.4	0.4	0.4	0.3	0.4
Unintentional injuries	NA	NA	NA	27.0	24.8	23.9	20.2	17.9	18.1	17.1	16.9	15.3	14.9	15.0	15.7	15.1	15.2	15.1	16.1
Motor vehicle-related injuries	NA	NA	NA	13.9	12.9	14.0	11.4	8.6	7.5	7.3	6.9	6.0	4.9	5.1	4.8	4.6	4.8	4.6	4.9
Poisoning	NA	NA	NA	0.5	0.6	0.7	0.8	0.7	1.3	1.4	1.4	1.3	1.5	1.4	1.7	1.8	2.0	2.0	2.4
Nephritis, nephrotic syndrome, and nephrosis[8]	NA	NA	NA	7.2	7.2	7.1	6.5	8.4	8.7	9.4	9.2	8.9	9.8	9.6	7.7	8.0	8.1	8.2	8.3
Suicide[9]	NA	NA	NA	7.8	7.1	6.7	6.7	5.5	5.1	5.4	5.9	5.5	5.9	6.2	5.9	6.3	5.9	6.0	6.4
Homicide[9]	NA	NA	NA	5.9	4.1	5.0	4.7	3.0	2.8	2.7	2.2	2.1	2.0	1.8	2.0	1.9	1.5	1.5	1.6
Hispanic or Latino[10,11]																			
All causes	NA	NA	NA	NA	698.8	692.0	700.2	665.7	627.6	604.0	586.1	579.8	559.7	558.6	540.7	539.1	535.4	523.3	525.3
Diseases of heart	NA	NA	NA	NA	239.8	217.1	211.0	196.0	170.4	157.8	149.5	141.4	135.8	132.8	123.9	122.0	121.2	116.0	116.9
Ischemic heart disease	NA	NA	NA	NA	187.9	173.3	166.4	153.2	127.9	116.4	107.5	100.8	94.7	92.3	84.2	81.1	80.3	75.3	74.5
Cerebrovascular diseases	NA	NA	NA	NA	51.9	45.2	46.3	46.4	38.6	37.2	35.8	34.4	32.2	32.1	30.7	30.0	29.6	30.2	32.3
Malignant neoplasms	NA	NA	NA	NA	125.9	136.8	138.5	134.9	127.9	123.7	121.8	121.0	119.7	119.7	117.0	116.9	114.5	112.4	110.3
Trachea, bronchus, and lung	NA	NA	NA	NA	22.9	26.5	25.9	24.8	23.3	21.6	21.9	21.6	20.4	20.4	19.8	19.2	18.7	18.3	17.8
Colon, rectum, and anus	NA	NA	NA	NA	13.0	14.7	14.1	14.1	13.1	13.4	12.8	12.7	12.7	12.3	11.9	11.7	11.7	11.1	10.9
Chronic lower respiratory diseases[6]	NA	NA	NA	NA	17.4	19.3	22.6	21.1	20.9	19.0	19.3	20.5	19.8	19.6	19.1	18.5	18.7	17.5	17.7
Influenza and pneumonia[7]	NA	NA	NA	NA	30.2	29.7	26.2	20.6	18.5	16.7	14.7	15.9	15.6	13.7	13.6	12.0	13.2	12.8	11.4
Chronic liver disease and cirrhosis	NA	NA	NA	NA	20.3	18.3	17.4	16.5	14.1	13.6	14.0	14.0	14.0	13.7	14.1	14.1	14.0	14.5	14.9
Diabetes mellitus[8]	NA	NA	NA	NA	23.0	28.2	35.7	36.9	35.4	31.7	30.6	29.8	27.0	27.1	27.2	26.9	26.3	25.1	25.2
Alzheimer's disease	NA	NA	NA	NA	V	V	V	10.4	15.6	16.1	15.6	18.0	16.9	18.5	17.7	17.4	17.7	19.8	24.2
Human immunodeficiency virus (HIV) disease	X	X	X	X	NA	16.3	24.9	6.7	4.8	4.5	4.1	3.6	3.2	2.8	2.7	2.2	2.1	2.0	1.8
Unintentional injuries	NA	NA	NA	NA	34.3	34.6	32.2	30.1	31.8	32.0	30.5	28.4	26.3	25.8	26.3	26.5	26.9	26.8	28.6
Motor vehicle-related injuries	NA	NA	NA	NA	17.1	19.5	16.4	14.7	14.6	14.6	13.1	11.2	10.1	9.6	9.3	9.6	9.7	9.6	10.2
Poisoning	NA	NA	NA	NA	3.2	3.2	4.9	4.1	5.2	5.7	5.8	5.9	5.8	5.6	6.2	6.2	6.7	6.8	7.7
Nephritis, nephrotic syndrome, and nephrosis[8]	NA	NA	NA	NA	10.3	8.4	6.9	11.8	12.8	13.5	13.3	13.6	13.8	14.1	11.2	11.3	11.1	11.1	11.4
Suicide[9]	NA	NA	NA	NA	6.3	7.8	7.2	5.9	5.6	5.3	6.0	5.5	5.8	5.9	5.7	5.8	5.7	6.3	6.2
Homicide[9]	NA	NA	NA	NA	14.6	16.2	12.5	7.5	7.4	7.2	6.8	6.4	6.0	5.3	5.0	4.9	4.5	4.5	4.9

NA = Not available.
V = Data for Alzheimer's disease are only presented for data years 1999 and beyond due to large differences in death rates caused by changes in the coding of the causes of death between ICD-9 and ICD-10.
X = Not applicable.
[1]Underlying cause of death code numbers are based on the applicable revision of the International Classification of Diseases (ICD) for data years shown.
[2]Includes deaths of persons who were not residents of the 50 states and the District of Columbia.
[3]Underlying cause of death was coded according to the 6th Revision of the ICD in 1950, 7th Revision in 1960, 8th Revision in 1970, and 9th Revision in 1980-1998.
[4]Starting with 1999 data, cause of death is coded according to ICD-10.
[5]Age-adjusted rates are calculated using the year 2000 standard population. Prior to 2001, age-adjusted rates were calculated using standard million proportions based on rounded population numbers. Starting with 2001 data, unrounded population numbers are used to calculate age-adjusted rates.
[6]Between 1998 and 1999, the cause of death title for Chronic obstructive pulmonary diseases in the ICD–9 was renamed to Chronic lower respiratory diseases (CLRD) in ICD–10.
[7]Starting with 1999 data, the rules for selecting CLRD and Pneumonia as the underlying cause of death changed, resulting in an increase in the number of deaths for CLRD and a decrease in the number of deaths for pneumonia. Therefore, trend data for these two causes of death should be interpreted with caution.
[8]Starting with 2011 data, the rules for selecting Renal failure as the underlying cause of death were changed, affecting the number of deaths in the Nephritis, nephrotic syndrome and nephrosis and Diabetes categories. These changes directly affect deaths with mention of Renal failure and other associated conditions, such as Diabetes mellitus with renal complications. The result is a decrease in the number of deaths for Nephritis, nephrotic syndrome and nephrosis and an increase in the number of deaths for Diabetes mellitus. Therefore, trend data for these two causes of death should be interpreted with caution.
[9]Figures for 2001 include September 11-related deaths, for which death certificates were filed as of October 24, 2002.
[10]The race groups White, Black, Asian or Pacific Islander, and American Indian or Alaska Native, include persons of Hispanic and non-Hispanic origin. Persons of Hispanic origin may be of any race. Death rates for the American Indian or Alaska Native, Asian or Pacific Islander, and Hispanic populations are known to be underestimated.
[11]Prior to 1997, data from states that did not report Hispanic origin on the death certificate were excluded.

Table 2-15. Age-Adjusted Death Rates for Selected Causes of Death, by Sex, Race, and Hispanic Origin, Selected Years, 1950–2015—*Continued*

(Age-adjusted rate per 100,000 population.)

Sex, race, Hispanic origin, and cause of death[1]	1950[2,3]	1960[2,3]	1970[3]	1980[3]	1985[3]	1990[3]	1995[3]	2000[4]	2005[4]	2006[4]	2007[4]	2008[4]	2009[4]	2010[4]	2011[4]	2012[4]	2013[4]	2014[4]	2015[4]
								Age-adjusted death rate per 100,000 population[5]											
White, not Hispanic or Latino[9]																			
All causes	NA	NA	NA	NA	942.1	914.5	882.3	855.5	810.1	789.1	775.3	779.4	755.1	755.0	754.3	745.8	747.1	742.8	753.2
Diseases of heart	NA	NA	NA	NA	366.7	319.7	289.9	255.5	215.5	204.5	195.5	192.4	182.9	179.9	175.6	172.3	171.8	169.9	171.9
Ischemic heart disease	NA	NA	NA	NA	296.0	251.9	219.9	186.6	148.3	138.6	129.9	127.4	118.9	115.0	111.1	107.4	104.6	101.2	99.7
Cerebrovascular diseases	NA	NA	NA	NA	72.2	63.5	60.8	59.0	46.2	42.9	41.7	40.5	38.3	37.8	36.7	35.8	35.0	35.4	36.4
Malignant neoplasms	NA	NA	NA	NA	202.1	215.4	208.9	200.6	187.8	185.1	182.6	179.9	177.4	176.5	173.0	170.6	167.7	166.2	163.7
Trachea, bronchus, and lung	NA	NA	NA	NA	53.2	60.3	59.6	58.2	55.5	54.5	53.7	52.6	51.6	50.8	49.2	48.0	46.6	45.4	43.8
Colon, rectum, and anus	NA	NA	NA	NA	25.7	24.6	22.3	20.5	17.4	17.1	16.9	16.4	15.8	15.5	15.0	14.7	14.5	14.3	14.1
Chronic lower respiratory diseases[6]	NA	NA	NA	NA	36.3	39.2	42.1	47.2	47.7	44.8	45.3	49.1	47.1	46.6	47.2	46.3	47.0	45.4	46.9
Influenza and pneumonia[7]	NA	NA	NA	NA	35.2	36.5	33.0	23.5	21.0	18.3	16.7	17.4	16.2	14.9	15.7	14.4	15.9	15.1	15.4
Chronic liver disease and cirrhosis	NA	NA	NA	NA	10.9	9.9	9.0	9.0	8.7	8.6	8.9	9.1	9.1	9.4	9.7	10.0	10.3	10.6	11.1
Diabetes mellitus[8]	NA	NA	NA	NA	14.8	18.3	20.1	21.8	21.8	20.6	19.9	19.3	18.5	18.2	19.1	18.5	18.6	18.6	18.9
Alzheimer's disease	NA	NA	NA	NA	V	V	V	19.1	25.1	24.9	25.1	27.2	25.4	26.4	26.1	25.1	24.8	26.8	30.8
Human immunodeficiency virus (HIV) disease	X	X	X	X	NA	7.4	9.8	2.2	1.8	1.7	1.5	1.4	1.2	1.1	1.0	1.0	0.9	0.9	0.9
Unintentional injuries	NA	NA	NA	NA	35.2	35.0	33.4	35.3	41.5	42.7	43.6	43.2	41.3	42.4	44.0	43.9	44.2	45.8	49.0
Motor vehicle-related injuries	NA	NA	NA	NA	17.4	18.2	16.1	15.6	15.7	15.4	15.1	13.7	12.2	11.9	11.9	12.1	11.5	11.3	11.8
Poisoning	NA	NA	NA	NA	2.2	2.0	2.9	4.6	9.1	10.6	11.8	12.4	12.6	13.3	14.6	14.4	15.3	16.7	18.8
Nephritis, nephrotic syndrome, and nephrosis[8]	NA	NA	NA	NA	8.8	8.1	8.4	12.0	13.1	13.2	13.4	13.6	13.5	13.8	12.2	11.9	12.1	12.1	12.2
Suicide[9]	NA	NA	NA	NA	13.8	13.8	13.1	12.0	13.0	13.3	13.7	14.3	14.5	15.0	15.5	15.7	15.9	16.4	17.0
Homicide[9]	NA	NA	NA	NA	4.4	4.0	3.6	2.8	2.7	2.7	2.8	2.9	2.6	2.5	2.6	2.6	2.5	2.5	2.6

NA = Not available.
V = Data for Alzheimer's disease are only presented for data years 1999 and beyond due to large differences in death rates caused by changes in the coding of the causes of death between ICD-9 and ICD-10.
X = Not applicable.
[1]Underlying cause of death code numbers are based on the applicable revision of the International Classification of Diseases (ICD) for data years shown.
[2]Includes deaths of persons who were not residents of the 50 states and the District of Columbia.
[3]Underlying cause of death was coded according to the 6th Revision of the ICD in 1950, 7th Revision in 1960, 8th Revision in 1970, and 9th Revision in 1980-1998.
[4]Starting with 1999 data, cause of death is coded according to ICD-10.
[5]Age-adjusted rates are calculated using the year 2000 standard population. Prior to 2001, age-adjusted rates were calculated using standard million proportions based on rounded population numbers. Starting with 2001 data, unrounded population numbers are used to calculate age-adjusted rates.
[6]Between 1998 and 1999, the cause of death title for Chronic obstructive pulmonary diseases in the ICD–9 was renamed to Chronic lower respiratory diseases (CLRD) in ICD–10.
[7]Starting with 1999 data, the rules for selecting CLRD and Pneumonia as the underlying cause of death changed, resulting in an increase in the number of deaths for CLRD and a decrease in the number of deaths for pneumonia. Therefore, trend data for these two causes of death should be interpreted with caution.
[8]Starting with 2011 data, the rules for selecting Renal failure as the underlying cause of death were changed, affecting the number of deaths in the Nephritis, nephrotic syndrome and nephrosis and Diabetes categories. These changes directly affect deaths with mention of Renal failure and other associated conditions, such as Diabetes mellitus with renal complications. The result is a decrease in the number of deaths for Nephritis, nephrotic syndrome and nephrosis and an increase in the number of deaths for Diabetes mellitus. Therefore, trend data for these two causes of death should be interpreted with caution.
[9]Figures for 2001 include September 11-related deaths, for which death certificates were filed as of October 24, 2002.

Table 2-16. Number of Deaths, Death Rates, and Age-Adjusted Death Rates for Injury Deaths, by Mechanism and Intent of Death, 2015

(Number; rates per 100,000 population; age-adjusted rates per 100,000 U.S. standard population.)

Mechanism and intent of death (based on the ICD, Tenth Revision)	Number	Rate	Age-adjusted rate[1]
All Injury (*U01'-*U03, V01'-Y36, Y85'-Y87, Y89)	214,008	66.6	63.9
Unintentional (V01'-X59, Y85'-Y86)	146,571	45.6	43.2
Suicide (*U03,X60'-X84, Y87.0)	44,193	13.7	13.3
Homicide (*U01'-*U02, X85'-Y09, Y87.1)	17,793	5.5	5.7
Undetermined (Y10'-Y34, Y87.2, Y89.9)	4,915	1.5	1.5
Legal intervention/war (Y35'-Y36, Y89[.0,.1])	536	0.2	0.2
Poisoning (*U01[.6–.7],X40–X49,X60–X69,X85–X90,Y10–Y19,Y35.2)	57,567	17.9	17.8
Unintentional (W25'-W29, W45)	47,478	14.8	14.8
Suicide (X78)	6,816	2.1	2.0
Homicide (X99)	111	0.0	0.0
Undetermined (Y28)	3,162	1.0	1.0
Legal intervention/war (Y35.4)	–	*	*
Firearm (*U01.4, W32'-W34, X72'-X74, X93'-X95, Y22'-Y24, Y35.0)	36,252	11.3	11.1
Unintentional (W65'-W74)	489	0.2	0.2
Suicide (X71)	22,018	6.9	6.5
Homicide (X92)	12,979	4.0	4.2
Undetermined (Y21)	282	0.1	0.1
Legal intervention/war (Y35.4)	484	0.2	0.1
Motor vehicle traffic (V02'-V04[.1,.9], V09.2, V12'-V14[.3'-.9], V19[.4'-.6], V20'-V28[.3'-.9], V29'-V79[.4'-.9], V80[.3'- .5],V81.1, V82.1,V83'-V86[.0'-.3], V87[.0'-.8],V89.2)[2]	36,161	11.3	10.9
Occupant (V30'-V79[.4'-.9], V83'-V86[.0'-.3])[2]	8,313	2.6	2.5
Motorcyclist (V20'-V28[.3'-.9], V29[.4'-.9])[2]	4,431	1.4	1.3
Pedal cyclist (V12'-V14[.3'-.9], V19[.4'-.6])[2]	675	0.2	0.2
Pedestrian (V02'-V04[.1,.9], V09.2)[2]	5,719	1.8	1.7
Other (V80[.3'-.5], V81.1, V82.1)[2]	15	*	*
Unspecified (V87[.0'-.8], V89.2)[2]	17,008	5.3	5.2
Fall (W00'-W19, X80, Y01, Y30)	34,488	10.7	9.3
Unintentional (W00'-W19)	33,381	10.4	9.0
Suicide (X80)	1,008	0.3	0.3
Homicide (Y01)	7	*	*
Undetermined (Y30)	92	0.0	0.0

– = Quantity zero.
* = Figure does not meet standard of reliability or precision.
0.0 = Quantity more than zero but less than 0.05.
[1]For method of computation, see chapter notes.
[2]Intent of death is unintentional.

Table 2-17. Leading Causes of Death and Numbers of Death, by Sex, Race, and Hispanic Origin, 1980 and 2015

(Number.)

Sex, race, Hispanic origin, and rank order	1980		Sex, race, Hispanic origin, and rank order	2015	
	Cause of death	Deaths		Cause of death	Deaths
All Persons			**All Persons**		
Rank..........	All causes....................	1,989,841	Rank..........	All causes....................	2,712,630
1..........	Diseases of heart	761,085	1..........	Diseases of heart	633,842
2..........	Malignant neoplasms....................	416,509	2..........	Malignant neoplasms....................	595,930
3..........	Cerebrovascular diseases....................	170,225	3..........	Chronic lower respiratory diseases[1,2]....................	155,041
4..........	Unintentional injuries....................	105,718	4..........	Unintentional injuries....................	146,571
5..........	Chronic obstructive pulmonary diseases[1]....................	56,050	5..........	Cerebrovascular diseases....................	140,323
6..........	Pneumonia and influenza[2]....................	54,619	6..........	Alzheimer's disease....................	110,561
7..........	Diabetes mellitus....................	34,851	7..........	Diabetes mellitus[3]....................	79,535
8..........	Chronic liver disease and cirrhosis....................	30,583	8..........	Influenza and pneumonia[2]....................	57,062
9..........	Atherosclerosis....................	29,449	9..........	Nephritis, nephrotic syndrome, and nephrosis[3] ..	49,959
10..........	Suicide....................	26,869	10..........	Suicide....................	44,193
Male			**Male**		
Rank..........	All causes....................	1,075,078	Rank..........	All causes....................	1,373,404
1..........	Diseases of heart	405,661	1..........	Diseases of heart	335,002
2..........	Malignant neoplasms....................	225,948	2..........	Malignant neoplasms....................	313,818
3..........	Unintentional injuries....................	74,180	3..........	Unintentional injuries....................	92,919
4..........	Cerebrovascular diseases....................	69,973	4..........	Chronic lower respiratory diseases[1,2]....................	72,498
5..........	Chronic obstructive pulmonary diseases[1]....................	38,625	5..........	Cerebrovascular diseases....................	58,288
6..........	Pneumonia and influenza[2]....................	27,574	6..........	Diabetes mellitus[3]....................	43,123
7..........	Suicide....................	20,505	7..........	Suicide....................	33,994
8..........	Chronic liver disease and cirrhosis....................	19,768	8..........	Alzheimer's disease....................	33,690
9..........	Homicide....................	18,779	9..........	Influenza and pneumonia[2]....................	26,903
10..........	Diabetes mellitus....................	14,325	10..........	Chronic liver disease and cirrhosis....................	25,666
Female			**Female**		
Rank..........	All causes....................	914,763	Rank..........	All causes....................	1,339,226
1..........	Diseases of heart	355,424	1..........	Diseases of heart	298,840
2..........	Malignant neoplasms....................	190,561	2..........	Malignant neoplasms....................	282,112
3..........	Cerebrovascular diseases....................	100,252	3..........	Chronic lower respiratory diseases[1,2]....................	82,543
4..........	Unintentional injuries....................	31,538	4..........	Cerebrovascular diseases....................	82,035
5..........	Pneumonia and influenza[2]....................	27,045	5..........	Alzheimer's disease....................	76,871
6..........	Diabetes mellitus....................	20,526	6..........	Unintentional injuries....................	53,652
7..........	Atherosclerosis....................	17,848	7..........	Diabetes mellitus[3]....................	36,412
8..........	Chronic obstructive pulmonary diseases[1]....................	17,425	8..........	Influenza and pneumonia[2]....................	30,159
9..........	Chronic liver disease and cirrhosis....................	10,815	9..........	Nephritis, nephrotic syndrome, and nephrosis[3] ..	24,518
10..........	Certain conditions originating in the perinatal period....................	9,815	10..........	Septicemia....................	21,388
White			**White**		
Rank..........	All causes....................	1,738,607	Rank..........	All causes....................	2,306,861
1..........	Diseases of heart	683,347	1..........	Diseases of heart	540,857
2..........	Malignant neoplasms....................	368,162	2..........	Malignant neoplasms....................	505,613
3..........	Cerebrovascular diseases....................	148,734	3..........	Chronic lower respiratory diseases[1,2]....................	141,766
4..........	Unintentional injuries....................	90,122	4..........	Unintentional injuries....................	125,773
5..........	Chronic obstructive pulmonary diseases[1]....................	52,375	5..........	Cerebrovascular diseases....................	116,788
6..........	Pneumonia and influenza[2]....................	48,369	6..........	Alzheimer's disease....................	99,866
7..........	Diabetes mellitus....................	28,868	7..........	Diabetes mellitus[3]....................	61,938
8..........	Atherosclerosis....................	27,069	8..........	Influenza and pneumonia[2]....................	48,877
9..........	Chronic liver disease and cirrhosis....................	25,240	9..........	Suicide....................	39,796
10..........	Suicide....................	24,829	10..........	Nephritis, nephrotic syndrome, and nephrosis[3] ..	39,078
Black			**Black**		
Rank..........	All causes....................	233,135	Rank..........	All causes....................	320,072
1..........	Diseases of heart	72,956	1..........	Diseases of heart	75,249
2..........	Malignant neoplasms....................	45,037	2..........	Malignant neoplasms....................	69,389
3..........	Cerebrovascular diseases....................	20,135	3..........	Cerebrovascular diseases....................	17,988
4..........	Unintentional injuries....................	13,480	4..........	Unintentional injuries....................	15,745
5..........	Homicide....................	10,172	5..........	Diabetes mellitus[3]....................	13,869
6..........	Certain conditions originating in the perinatal period....................	6,961	6..........	Chronic lower respiratory diseases[1,2]....................	10,475
7..........	Pneumonia and influenza[2]....................	5,648	7..........	Homicide....................	9,173
8..........	Diabetes mellitus....................	5,544	8..........	Nephritis, nephrotic syndrome, and nephrosis[3] ..	9,170
9..........	Chronic liver disease and cirrhosis....................	4,790	9..........	Alzheimer's disease....................	8,156
10..........	Nephritis, nephrotic syndrome, and nephrosis	3,416	10..........	Septicemia....................	6,647

NA = Not available. Complete coverage of all states for the Hispanic origin variable began in 1997.

[1]Between 1998 and 1999, the cause of death title for Chronic obstructive pulmonary diseases in the International Classification of Diseases, 9th Revision (ICD–9) was renamed to Chronic lower respiratory diseases (CLRD) in ICD–10.

[2]Starting with 1999 data, the rules for selecting CLRD and Pneumonia as the underlying cause of death changed, resulting in an increase in the number of deaths for CLRD and a decrease in the number of deaths for pneumonia. Therefore, trend data for these two causes of death should be interpreted with caution.

[3]Starting with 2011 data, the rules for selecting Renal failure as the underlying cause of death were changed, affecting the number of deaths in the Nephritis, nephrotic syndrome, and nephrosis and Diabetes categories. These changes directly affect deaths with mention of Renal failure and other associated conditions, such as Diabetes mellitus with renal complications. The result is a decrease in the number of deaths for Nephritis, nephrotic syndrome, and nephrosis and an increase in the number of deaths for Diabetes mellitus. Therefore, trend data for these two causes of death should be interpreted with caution.

Table 2-17. Leading Causes of Death and Numbers of Death, by Sex, Race, and Hispanic Origin, 1980 and 2015—*Continued*

(Number.)

Sex, race, Hispanic origin, and rank order	1980 Cause of death	Deaths	Sex, race, Hispanic origin, and rank order	2015 Cause of death	Deaths
American Indian or Alaska Native			**American Indian or Alaska Native**		
Rank	All causes	6,923	Rank	All causes	19,016
1	Diseases of heart	1,494	1	Diseases of heart	3,463
2	Unintentional injuries	1,290	2	Malignant neoplasms	3,358
3	Malignant neoplasms	770	3	Unintentional injuries	2,078
4	Chronic liver disease and cirrhosis	410	4	Diabetes mellitus[3]	1,087
5	Cerebrovascular diseases	322	5	Chronic liver disease and cirrhosis	1,061
6	Pneumonia and influenza[2]	257	6	Chronic lower respiratory diseases[1,2]	883
7	Homicide	217	7	Cerebrovascular diseases	676
8	Diabetes mellitus	210	8	Suicide	577
9	Certain conditions originating in the perinatal period	199	9	Nephritis, nephrotic syndrome, and nephrosis[3]	352
10	Suicide	181	10	Influenza and pneumonia[2]	342
Asian or Pacific Islander			**Asian or Pacific Islander**		
Rank	All causes	11,071	Rank	All causes	66,681
1	Diseases of heart	3,265	1	Malignant neoplasms	17,570
2	Malignant neoplasms	2,522	2	Diseases of heart	14,273
3	Cerebrovascular diseases	1,028	3	Cerebrovascular diseases	4,871
4	Unintentional injuries	810	4	Unintentional injuries	2,975
5	Pneumonia and influenza[2]	342	5	Diabetes mellitus[3]	2,641
6	Suicide	249	6	Alzheimer's disease	2,212
7	Certain conditions originating in the perinatal period	246	7	Influenza and pneumonia[2]	2,202
8	Diabetes mellitus	227	8	Chronic lower respiratory diseases[1,2]	1,917
9	Homicide	211	9	Nephritis, nephrotic syndrome, and nephrosis[3]	1,359
10	Chronic obstructive pulmonary diseases[1]	207	10	Suicide	1,316
Hispanic or Latino[1]			**Hispanic or Latino[1]**		
Rank	NA	NA	Rank	All causes	179,457
1	NA	NA	1	Malignant neoplasms	37,804
2	NA	NA	2	Diseases of heart	36,401
3	NA	NA	3	Unintentional injuries	13,806
4	NA	NA	4	Cerebrovascular diseases	9,795
5	NA	NA	5	Diabetes mellitus[3]	8,278
6	NA	NA	6	Alzheimer's disease	6,444
7	NA	NA	7	Chronic liver disease and cirrhosis	6,018
8	NA	NA	8	Chronic lower respiratory diseases[1,2]	5,159
9	NA	NA	9	Nephritis, nephrotic syndrome, and nephrosis[3]	3,581
10	NA	NA	10	Influenza and pneumonia[2]	3,497
White Male			**White Male**		
Rank	All causes	933,878	Rank	All causes	1,164,176
1	Diseases of heart	364,679	1	Diseases of heart	285,884
2	Malignant neoplasms	198,188	2	Malignant neoplasms	267,885
3	Unintentional injuries	62,963	3	Unintentional injuries	78,887
4	Cerebrovascular diseases	60,095	4	Chronic lower respiratory diseases[1,2]	65,680
5	Chronic obstructive pulmonary diseases[1]	35,977	5	Cerebrovascular diseases	47,713
6	Pneumonia and influenza[2]	23,810	6	Diabetes mellitus[3]	34,299
7	Suicide	18,901	7	Alzheimer's disease	30,710
8	Chronic liver disease and cirrhosis	16,407	8	Suicide	30,658
9	Diabetes mellitus	12,125	9	Influenza and pneumonia[2]	22,794
10	Atherosclerosis	10,543	10	Chronic liver disease and cirrhosis	22,681
Black or African American Male			**Black or African American male**		
Rank	All causes	130,138	Rank	All causes	164,670
1	Diseases of heart	37,877	1	Diseases of heart	39,325
2	Malignant neoplasms	25,861	2	Malignant neoplasms	35,250
3	Unintentional injuries	9,701	3	Unintentional injuries	10,779
4	Cerebrovascular diseases	9,194	4	Cerebrovascular diseases	8,073
5	Homicide	8,274	5	Homicide	8,021
6	Certain conditions originating in the perinatal period	3,869	6	Diabetes mellitus[3]	6,909
7	Pneumonia and influenza[2]	3,386	7	Chronic lower respiratory diseases[1,2]	5,328
8	Chronic liver disease and cirrhosis	3,020	8	Nephritis, nephrotic syndrome, and nephrosis[3]	4,401
9	Chronic obstructive pulmonary diseases[1]	2,429	9	Septicemia	3,098
10	Diabetes mellitus	2,010	10	Influenza and pneumonia[2]	2,787

NA = Not available. Complete coverage of all states for the Hispanic origin variable began in 1997.
[1]Between 1998 and 1999, the cause of death title for Chronic obstructive pulmonary diseases in the International Classification of Diseases, 9th Revision (ICD–9) was renamed to Chronic lower respiratory diseases (CLRD) in ICD–10.
[2]Starting with 1999 data, the rules for selecting CLRD and Pneumonia as the underlying cause of death changed, resulting in an increase in the number of deaths for CLRD and a decrease in the number of deaths for pneumonia. Therefore, trend data for these two causes of death should be interpreted with caution.
[3]Starting with 2011 data, the rules for selecting Renal failure as the underlying cause of death were changed, affecting the number of deaths in the Nephritis, nephrotic syndrome, and nephrosis and Diabetes categories. These changes directly affect deaths with mention of Renal failure and other associated conditions, such as Diabetes mellitus with renal complications. The result is a decrease in the number of deaths for Nephritis, nephrotic syndrome, and nephrosis and an increase in the number of deaths for Diabetes mellitus. Therefore, trend data for these two causes of death should be interpreted with caution.

Table 2-17. Leading Causes of Death and Numbers of Death, by Sex, Race, and Hispanic Origin, 1980 and 2015—Continued

(Number.)

Sex, race, Hispanic origin, and rank order	1980		Sex, race, Hispanic origin, and rank order	2015	
	Cause of death	Deaths		Cause of death	Deaths
American Indian or Alaska Native Male			**American Indian or Alaska Native Male**		
Rank...........	All causes...................	4,193	Rank...........	All causes...................	10,451
1...............	Unintentional injuries	946	1...............	Diseases of heart	2,009
2...............	Diseases of heart	917	2...............	Malignant neoplasms	1,781
3...............	Malignant neoplasms	408	3...............	Unintentional injuries	1,364
4...............	Chronic liver disease and cirrhosis	239	4...............	Chronic liver disease and cirrhosis	598
5...............	Cerebrovascular diseases	163	5...............	Diabetes mellitus[3]	573
6...............	Homicide	162	6...............	Suicide	426
7[1]...............	Pneumonia and influenza[2]	148	7[1]...............	Chronic lower respiratory diseases[1,2]	408
8...............	Suicide	147	8...............	Cerebrovascular diseases	308
9...............	Certain conditions originating in the perinatal period	107	9...............	Homicide	228
10...............	Diabetes mellitus	86	10...............	Influenza and pneumonia[2]	189
Asian or Pacific Islander Male			**Asian or Pacific Islander Male**		
Rank...........	All causes...................	6,809	Rank...........	All causes...................	34,107
1...............	Diseases of heart	2,174	1...............	Malignant neoplasms	8,902
2...............	Malignant neoplasms	1,485	2...............	Diseases of heart	7,784
3...............	Unintentional injuries	556	3...............	Cerebrovascular diseases	2,194
4...............	Cerebrovascular diseases	521	4...............	Unintentional injuries	1,889
5...............	Pneumonia and influenza[2]	227	5...............	Diabetes mellitus[3]	1,342
6...............	Suicide	159	6...............	Influenza and pneumonia[2]	1,133
7...............	Chronic obstructive pulmonary diseases[1]	158	7...............	Chronic lower respiratory diseases[1,2]	1,082
8...............	Homicide	151	8...............	Suicide	887
9...............	Certain conditions originating in the perinatal period	128	9...............	Alzheimer's disease	688
10...............	Diabetes mellitus	103	10...............	Nephritis, nephrotic syndrome, and nephrosis[3] ..	672
Hispanic or Latino Male[1]			**Hispanic or Latino Male[1]**		
Rank...........	NA...................	NA	Rank...........	All causes...................	98,170
1...............	NA	NA	1...............	Diseases of heart	20,225
2...............	NA	NA	2...............	Malignant neoplasms	19,847
3...............	NA	NA	3...............	Unintentional injuries	10,067
4...............	NA	NA	4...............	Cerebrovascular diseases	4,544
5...............	NA	NA	5...............	Diabetes mellitus[3]	4,426
6...............	NA	NA	6...............	Chronic liver disease and cirrhosis	4,109
7...............	NA	NA	7...............	Chronic lower respiratory diseases[1,2]	2,606
8...............	NA	NA	8...............	Suicide	2,587
9...............	NA	NA	9...............	Homicide	2,391
10...............	NA	NA	10...............	Alzheimer's disease	2,035
White Female			**White Female**		
Rank...........	All causes...................	804,729	Rank...........	All causes...................	1,142,685
1...............	Diseases of heart	318,668	1...............	Diseases of heart	254,973
2...............	Malignant neoplasms	169,974	2...............	Malignant neoplasms	237,728
3...............	Cerebrovascular diseases	88,639	3...............	Chronic lower respiratory diseases[1,2]	76,086
4...............	Unintentional injuries	27,159	4...............	Alzheimer's disease	69,156
5...............	Pneumonia and influenza[2]	24,559	5...............	Cerebrovascular diseases	69,075
6...............	Diabetes mellitus	16,743	6...............	Unintentional injuries	46,886
7...............	Atherosclerosis	16,526	7...............	Diabetes mellitus[3]	27,639
8...............	Chronic obstructive pulmonary diseases[1]	16,398	8...............	Influenza and pneumonia[2]	26,083
9...............	Chronic liver disease and cirrhosis	8,833	9...............	Nephritis, nephrotic syndrome, and nephrosis[3] ..	18,876
10...............	Certain conditions originating in the perinatal period	6,512	10...............	Septicemia	17,282
Black or African American Female			**Black or African American Female**		
Rank...........	All causes...................	102,997	Rank...........	All causes...................	155,402
1...............	Diseases of heart	35,079	1...............	Diseases of heart	35,924
2...............	Malignant neoplasms	19,176	2...............	Malignant neoplasms	34,139
3...............	Cerebrovascular diseases	10,941	3...............	Cerebrovascular diseases	9,915
4...............	Unintentional injuries	3,779	4...............	Diabetes mellitus[3]	6,960
5...............	Diabetes mellitus	3,534	5...............	Alzheimer's disease	5,973
6...............	Certain conditions originating in the perinatal period	3,092	6...............	Chronic lower respiratory diseases[1,2]	5,147
7...............	Pneumonia and influenza[2]	2,262	7...............	Unintentional injuries	4,966
8...............	Homicide	1,898	8...............	Nephritis, nephrotic syndrome, and nephrosis[3] ..	4,769
9...............	Chronic liver disease and cirrhosis	1,770	9...............	Septicemia	3,549
10...............	Nephritis, nephrotic syndrome, and nephrosis	1,722	10...............	Essential hypertension and hypertensive renal disease	3,175

NA = Not available. Complete coverage of all states for the Hispanic origin variable began in 1997.

[1]Between 1998 and 1999, the cause of death title for Chronic obstructive pulmonary diseases in the International Classification of Diseases, 9th Revision (ICD–9) was renamed to Chronic lower respiratory diseases (CLRD) in ICD–10.

[2]Starting with 1999 data, the rules for selecting CLRD and Pneumonia as the underlying cause of death changed, resulting in an increase in the number of deaths for CLRD and a decrease in the number of deaths for pneumonia. Therefore, trend data for these two causes of death should be interpreted with caution.

[3]Starting with 2011 data, the rules for selecting Renal failure as the underlying cause of death were changed, affecting the number of deaths in the Nephritis, nephrotic syndrome, and nephrosis and Diabetes categories. These changes directly affect deaths with mention of Renal failure and other associated conditions, such as Diabetes mellitus with renal complications. The result is a decrease in the number of deaths for Nephritis, nephrotic syndrome, and nephrosis and an increase in the number of deaths for Diabetes mellitus. Therefore, trend data for these two causes of death should be interpreted with caution.

Table 2-17. Leading Causes of Death and Numbers of Death, by Sex, Race, and Hispanic Origin, 1980 and 2015—*Continued*

(Number.)

Sex, race, Hispanic origin, and rank order	1980		Sex, race, Hispanic origin, and rank order	2015	
	Cause of death	Deaths		Cause of death	Deaths
American Indian or Alaska Native Female			**American Indian or Alaska Native Female**		
Rank................................	All causes................................	2,730	Rank................................	All causes................................	8,565
1................................	Diseases of heart	577	1................................	Malignant neoplasms................................	1,577
2................................	Malignant neoplasms	362	2................................	Diseases of heart	1,454
3................................	Unintentional injuries	344	3................................	Unintentional injuries	714
4................................	Chronic liver disease and cirrhosis	171	4................................	Diabetes mellitus[3]	514
5................................	Cerebrovascular diseases	159	5................................	Chronic lower respiratory diseases[1,2]	475
6................................	Diabetes mellitus................................	124	6................................	Chronic liver disease and cirrhosis	463
7................................	Pneumonia and influenza[2]................................	109	7................................	Cerebrovascular diseases	368
8................................	Certain conditions originating in the perinatal period................................	92	8................................	Alzheimer's disease................................	218
9................................	Nephritis, nephrotic syndrome, and nephrosis	56	9................................	Nephritis, nephrotic syndrome, and nephrosis[3]..	186
10................................	Homicide................................	55	10................................	Septicemia................................	167
Asian or Pacific Islander Female			**Asian or Pacific Islander Female**		
Rank................................	All causes................................	4,262	Rank................................	All causes................................	32,574
1................................	Diseases of heart	1,091	1................................	Malignant neoplasms................................	8,668
2................................	Malignant neoplasms	1,037	2................................	Diseases of heart	6,489
3................................	Cerebrovascular diseases	507	3................................	Cerebrovascular diseases	2,677
4................................	Unintentional injuries	254	4................................	Alzheimer's disease................................	1,524
5................................	Diabetes mellitus................................	124	5................................	Diabetes mellitus[3]	1,299
6................................	Certain conditions originating in the perinatal period................................	118	6................................	Unintentional injuries	1,086
7................................	Pneumonia and influenza[2]................................	115	7................................	Influenza and pneumonia[2]................................	1,069
8................................	Congenital anomalies	104	8................................	Chronic lower respiratory diseases[1,2]................................	835
9................................	Suicide	90	9................................	Nephritis, nephrotic syndrome, and nephrosis[3]..	687
10................................	Homicide................................	60	10................................	Essential hypertension and hypertensive renal disease................................	635
Hispanic or Latina Female			**Hispanic or Latina Female**		
Rank................................	NA................................	NA	Rank................................	All causes................................	81,287
1................................	NA................................	NA	1................................	Malignant neoplasms................................	17,957
2................................	NA................................	NA	2................................	Diseases of heart	16,176
3................................	NA................................	NA	3................................	Cerebrovascular diseases	5,251
4................................	NA................................	NA	4................................	Alzheimer's disease................................	4,409
5................................	NA................................	NA	5................................	Diabetes mellitus[3]	3,852
6................................	NA................................	NA	6................................	Unintentional injuries	3,739
7................................	NA................................	NA	7................................	Chronic lower respiratory diseases[1,2]................................	2,553
8................................	NA................................	NA	8................................	Chronic liver disease and cirrhosis	1,909
9................................	NA................................	NA	9................................	Influenza and pneumonia[2]................................	1,762
10................................	NA................................	NA	10................................	Nephritis, nephrotic syndrome, and nephrosis[3]..	1,744

NA = Not available. Complete coverage of all states for the Hispanic origin variable began in 1997.

[1]Between 1998 and 1999, the cause of death title for Chronic obstructive pulmonary diseases in the International Classification of Diseases, 9th Revision (ICD–9) was renamed to Chronic lower respiratory diseases (CLRD) in ICD–10.

[2]Starting with 1999 data, the rules for selecting CLRD and Pneumonia as the underlying cause of death changed, resulting in an increase in the number of deaths for CLRD and a decrease in the number of deaths for pneumonia. Therefore, trend data for these two causes of death should be interpreted with caution.

[3]Starting with 2011 data, the rules for selecting Renal failure as the underlying cause of death were changed, affecting the number of deaths in the Nephritis, nephrotic syndrome, and nephrosis and Diabetes categories. These changes directly affect deaths with mention of Renal failure and other associated conditions, such as Diabetes mellitus with renal complications. The result is a decrease in the number of deaths for Nephritis, nephrotic syndrome, and nephrosis and an increase in the number of deaths for Diabetes mellitus. Therefore, trend data for these two causes of death should be interpreted with caution.

Table 2-18. Leading Causes of Death and Numbers of Deaths, by Age, 1980 and 2015

(Number.)

	1980			2015	
Age and rank order	Cause of death	Deaths	Age and rank order	Cause of death	Deaths
Under 1 Year			**Under 1 Year**		
Rank..................................	All causes..................	45,526	Rank..................................	All causes..................	23,455
				Congenital malformations/deformations/chromo-somal abnormalities..................	
1............................	Congenital anomalies..................	9,220	1............................		4,825
				Disorders related to short gestation and low birth weight..................	
2............................	Sudden infant death syndrome..................	5,510	2............................		4,084
3............................	Respiratory distress syndrome..................	4,989	3............................	Sudden infant death syndrome..................	1,568
	Disorders relating to short gestation and unspecified low birthweight..................			Newborn affected by maternal complications of pregnancy..................	
4............................		3,648	4............................		1,522
	Newborn affected by maternal complications of pregnancy..................				
5............................		1,572	5............................	Unintentional injuries..................	1,291
				Newborn affected by complications of placenta, cord and membranes..................	
6............................	Intrauterine hypoxia and birth asphyxia..................	1,497	6............................		910
7............................	Unintentional injuries..................	1,166	7............................	Bacterial sepsis of newborn..................	599
8............................	Birth trauma..................	1,058	8............................	Respiratory distress of newborn..................	462
9............................	Pneumonia and influenza[1]..................	1,012	9............................	Diseases of circulatory system..................	428
	Newborn affected by complications of placenta, cord, and membranes..................				
10............................		985	10............................	Neonatal hemorrhage..................	406
1 to 4 Years			**1 to 4 Years**		
Rank..................................	All causes..................	8,187	Rank..................................	All causes..................	3,965
1............................	Unintentional injuries..................	3,313	1............................	Unintentional injuries..................	1,235
				Congenital malformations/deformations/chromo-somal abnormalities..................	
2............................	Congenital anomalies..................	1,026	2............................		435
3............................	Malignant neoplasms..................	573	3............................	Homicide..................	369
4............................	Diseases of heart..................	338	4............................	Malignant neoplasms..................	354
5............................	Homicide..................	319	5............................	Diseases of heart..................	147
6............................	Pneumonia and influenza[1]..................	267	6............................	Influenza and pneumonia[1]..................	88
7............................	Meningitis..................	223	7............................	Septicemia..................	54
8............................	Meningococcal infection..................	110	8............................	Conditions originating in perinatal period..................	50
9............................	Certain conditions originating in the perinatal period..................	84	9............................	Cerebrovascular diseases..................	42
10............................	Septicemia..................	71	10............................	Chronic lower respiratory diseases[1,2]..................	40
5 to 14 Years			**5 to 14 Years**		
Rank..................................	All causes..................	10,689	Rank..................................	All causes..................	5,411
1............................	Unintentional injuries..................	5,224	1............................	Unintentional injuries..................	1,518
2............................	Malignant neoplasms..................	1,497	2............................	Malignant neoplasms..................	865
3............................	Congenital anomalies..................	561	3............................	Suicide..................	413
				Congenital malformations/deformations/chromo-somal abnormalities..................	
4............................	Homicide..................	415	4............................		337
5............................	Diseases of heart..................	330	5............................	Homicide..................	298
6............................	Pneumonia and influenza[1]..................	194	6............................	Diseases of heart..................	210
7............................	Suicide..................	142	7............................	Chronic lower respiratory diseases[1,2]..................	173
8............................	Benign neoplasms..................	104	8............................	Cerebrovascular diseases..................	84
9............................	Cerebrovascular diseases..................	95	9............................	Influenza and pneumonia[1]..................	83
				In situ neoplasms/benign neoplasms/neoplasms of uncertain/unknown behavior..................	
10............................	Chronic obstructive pulmonary diseases[2]..................	85	10............................		72
15 to 24 Years			**15 to 24 Years**		
Rank..................................	All causes..................	49,027	Rank..................................	All causes..................	30,494
1............................	Unintentional injuries..................	26,206	1............................	Unintentional injuries..................	12,514
2............................	Homicide..................	6,537	2............................	Suicide..................	5,491
3............................	Suicide..................	5,239	3............................	Homicide..................	4,733
4............................	Malignant neoplasms..................	2,683	4............................	Malignant neoplasms..................	1,469
5............................	Diseases of heart..................	1,223	5............................	Diseases of heart..................	997
				Congenital malformations/deformations/chromo-somal abnormalities..................	
6............................	Congenital anomalies..................	600	6............................		386
7............................	Cerebrovascular diseases..................	418	7............................	Chronic lower respiratory diseases[1,2]..................	202
8............................	Pneumonia and influenza[1]..................	348	8............................	Diabetes mellitus[3]..................	196
9............................	Chronic obstructive pulmonary diseases[2]..................	141	9............................	Influenza and pneumonia[1]..................	184
10............................	Anemias..................	133	10............................	Cerebrovascular diseases..................	166
25 to 44 Years			**25 to 44 Years**		
Rank..................................	All causes..................	108,658	Rank..................................	All causes..................	124,605
1............................	Unintentional injuries..................	26,722	1............................	Unintentional injuries..................	37,613
2............................	Malignant neoplasms..................	17,551	2............................	Malignant neoplasms..................	14,613
3............................	Diseases of heart..................	14,513	3............................	Diseases of heart..................	13,909
4............................	Homicide..................	10,983	4............................	Suicide..................	13,883
5............................	Suicide..................	9,855	5............................	Homicide..................	7,758
6............................	Chronic liver disease and cirrhosis..................	4,782	6............................	Chronic liver disease and cirrhosis..................	3,705
7............................	Cerebrovascular diseases..................	3,154	7............................	Diabetes mellitus[3]..................	2,784
8............................	Diabetes mellitus..................	1,472	8............................	Cerebrovascular diseases..................	2,355
9............................	Pneumonia and influenza[1]..................	1,467	9............................	Human immunodeficiency virus (HIV) disease..................	1,584
10............................	Congenital anomalies..................	817	10............................	Septicemia..................	1,208

[1]Starting with 1999 data, the rules for selecting CLRD and Pneumonia as the underlying cause of death changed, resulting in an increase in the number of deaths for CLRD and a decrease in the number of deaths for pneumonia. Therefore, trend data for these two causes of death should be interpreted with caution.

[2]Between 1998 and 1999, the cause of death title for Chronic obstructive pulmonary diseases in the ICD–9 was renamed to Chronic lower respiratory diseases (CLRD) in ICD–10.

[3]Starting with 2011 data, the rules for selecting Renal failure as the underlying cause of death were changed, affecting the number of deaths in the Nephritis, nephrotic syndrome and nephrosis and Diabetes categories. These changes directly affect deaths with mention of Renal failure and other associated conditions, such as Diabetes mellitus with renal complications. The result is a decrease in the number of deaths for Nephritis, nephrotic syndrome and nephrosis and an increase in the number of deaths for Diabetes mellitus. Therefore, trend data for these two causes of death should be interpreted with caution.

Table 2-18. Leading Causes of Death and Numbers of Deaths, by Age, 1980 and 2015—*Continued*

(Number.)

	1980			2015	
Age and rank order	Cause of death	Deaths	Age and rank order	Cause of death	Deaths
45 to 64 Years			**45 to 64 Years**		
Rank..........	All causes..........	425,338	Rank..........	All causes..........	532,279
1..........	Diseases of heart	148,322	1..........	Malignant neoplasms..........	159,176
2..........	Malignant neoplasms..........	135,675	2..........	Diseases of heart..........	111,120
3..........	Cerebrovascular diseases	19,909	3..........	Unintentional injuries..........	40,987
4..........	Unintentional injuries..........	18,140	4..........	Chronic liver disease and cirrhosis..........	22,152
5..........	Chronic liver disease and cirrhosis	16,089	5..........	Chronic lower respiratory diseases[1,2]..........	21,802
6..........	Chronic obstructive pulmonary diseases[2]..........	11,514	6..........	Diabetes mellitus[3]..........	20,378
7..........	Diabetes mellitus..........	7,977	7..........	Cerebrovascular diseases	17,423
8..........	Suicide..........	7,079	8..........	Suicide..........	16,490
9..........	Pneumonia and influenza[1]..........	5,804	9..........	Septicemia	8,316
10..........	Homicide..........	4,019	10..........	Nephritis, nephrotic syndrome, and nephrosis[3]..........	7,576
65 Years and Over			**65 Years and Over**		
Rank..........	All causes..........	1,341,848	Rank..........	All causes..........	1,992,283
1..........	Diseases of heart	595,406	1..........	Diseases of heart	507,138
2..........	Malignant neoplasms..........	258,389	2..........	Malignant neoplasms..........	419,389
3..........	Cerebrovascular diseases	146,417	3..........	Chronic lower respiratory diseases[1,2]..........	131,804
4..........	Pneumonia and influenza[1]..........	45,512	4..........	Cerebrovascular diseases	120,156
5..........	Chronic obstructive pulmonary diseases[2]..........	43,587	5..........	Alzheimer's disease..........	109,495
6..........	Atherosclerosis	28,081	6..........	Diabetes mellitus[3]..........	56,142
7..........	Diabetes mellitus..........	25,216	7..........	Unintentional injuries..........	51,395
8..........	Unintentional injuries..........	24,844	8..........	Influenza and pneumonia..........	48,774
9..........	Nephritis, nephrotic syndrome, and nephrosis	12,968	9..........	Nephritis, nephrotic syndrome, and nephrosis[3]........	41,258
10..........	Chronic liver disease and cirrhosis	9,519	10..........	Septicemia	30,817

[1]Starting with 1999 data, the rules for selecting CLRD and Pneumonia as the underlying cause of death changed, resulting in an increase in the number of deaths for CLRD and a decrease in the number of deaths for pneumonia. Therefore, trend data for these two causes of death should be interpreted with caution.
[2]Between 1998 and 1999, the cause of death title for Chronic obstructive pulmonary diseases in the ICD–9 was renamed to Chronic lower respiratory diseases (CLRD) in ICD-10.
[3]Starting with 2011 data, the rules for selecting Renal failure as the underlying cause of death were changed, affecting the number of deaths in the Nephritis, nephrotic syndrome and nephrosis and Diabetes categories. These changes directly affect deaths with mention of Renal failure and other associated conditions, such as Diabetes mellitus with renal complications. The result is a decrease in the number of deaths for Nephritis, nephrotic syndrome and nephrosis and an increase in the number of deaths for Diabetes mellitus. Therefore, trend data for these two causes of death should be interpreted with caution.

Table 2-19. Deaths from Selected Occupational Diseases Among Persons 15 Years of Age and Over, Selected Years, 1980–2013

(Number of deaths.)

Cause of death	1980[1]	1985[1]	1990[1]	1995[1]	2000[2]	2005[2]	2006[2]	2007[2]	2008[2]	2009[2]	2010[2]	2011[2]	2012[2]	2013[2]
Multiple Cause of Death (Number of Death Certificates with Cause of Death Code(s) Mentioned)														
Angiosarcoma of liver[3]..........	NA	NA	NA	NA	16	26	23	22	17	27	29	22	29	22
Malignant mesothelioma[4]..........	699	715	874	897	2,531	2,704	2,588	2,606	2,709	2,753	2,744	2,832	2,874	2,686
Pneumoconiosis[5]..........	4,151	3,783	3,644	3,151	2,859	2,425	2,308	2,189	2,155	1,993	2,028	1,890	1,850	1,859
Coal workers' pneumoconiosis..........	2,576	2,615	1,990	1,413	949	652	654	524	470	480	486	409	399	361
Asbestosis	339	534	948	1,169	1,486	1,416	1,340	1,393	1,341	1,255	1,308	1,243	1,208	1,229
Silicosis	448	334	308	242	151	160	126	122	146	121	101	88	103	111
Other (including unspecified)..........	814	321	413	343	290	222	206	163	215	158	146	166	153	170
Underlying Cause of Death														
Angiosarcoma of liver[3]..........	NA	NA	NA	NA	15	23	21	20	16	25	28	20	27	19
Malignant mesothelioma[4]..........	531	573	725	780	2,384	2,553	2,452	2,432	2,538	2,606	2,573	2,651	2,686	2,497
Pneumoconiosis..........	1,581	1,355	1,335	1,117	1,142	983	907	898	891	830	820	752	755	781
Coal workers' pneumoconiosis..........	982	958	734	533	389	270	266	209	183	206	213	160	158	151
Asbestosis	101	139	302	355	558	532	485	538	520	485	486	460	466	475
Silicosis	207	143	150	114	71	74	67	72	85	66	52	56	58	70
Other (including unspecified)..........	291	115	149	115	124	107	89	79	103	73	69	76	73	85

NA = Not available.
Note: Multiple cause of death includes underlying and nonunderlying causes of death. Cause-of-death titles for selected occupational diseases and corresponding code numbers according to the International Classification of Diseases, 9th and 10th Revisions.
[1]For the period 1980-1998, underlying cause of death was coded according to the 9th Revision of the International Classification of Diseases (ICD).
[2]Starting with 1999 data, ICD-10 was introduced for coding cause of death. Discontinuities exist between 1998 and 1999 due to ICD-10 coding and classification changes.
[3]Prior to 1999, there was no discrete code for this condition.
[4]Prior to 1999, the combined ICD-9 categories of malignant neoplasm of peritoneum and malignant neoplasm of pleura served as a crude surrogate for malignant mesothelioma category under ICD-10.
[5]For multiple cause of death, counts for pneumoconiosis subgroups may sum to slightly more than total pneumoconiosis due to the reporting of more than one type of pneumoconiosis on some death certificates. Multiple cause of death includes underlying and nonunderlying causes of death.

Table 2-20. Death Rates for Motor Vehicle–Related Injuries, by Sex and Age, Selected Years, 1950–2015

(Rate per 100,000 population.)

Sex, race, Hispanic origin, and age	1950[1,2]	1960[1,2]	1970[2]	1980[2]	1985[2]	1990[2]	1995[2]	2000[3]	2005[3]	2006[3]	2007[3]	2008[3]	2009[3]	2010[3]	2011[3]	2012[3]	2013[3]	2014[3]	2015[3]
	Deaths per 100,000 resident population																		
All Persons																			
All ages, age-adjusted[4]	24.6	23.1	27.6	22.3	18.6	18.5	16.3	15.4	15.2	15.0	14.4	12.9	11.6	11.3	11.1	11.4	10.9	10.8	11.4
All ages, crude	23.1	21.3	26.9	23.5	19.3	18.8	16.3	15.4	15.3	15.2	14.6	13.1	11.8	11.4	11.3	11.6	11.2	11.1	11.7
Under 1 year	8.4	8.1	9.8	7.0	4.9	4.9	4.7	4.4	3.6	3.5	3.0	2.5	2.4	2.0	2.4	1.8	1.7	1.7	1.8
1-14 years	9.8	8.6	10.5	8.2	7.0	6.0	5.3	4.3	3.7	3.4	3.2	2.6	2.5	2.3	2.3	2.2	2.2	2.2	2.2
1-4 years	11.5	10.0	11.5	9.2	7.2	6.3	5.2	4.2	3.9	3.7	3.4	2.9	2.9	2.8	2.6	2.9	2.7	2.5	2.6
5-14 years	8.8	7.9	10.2	7.9	6.9	5.9	5.3	4.3	3.6	3.3	3.2	2.5	2.4	2.2	2.1	2.0	2.1	2.0	2.1
15-24 years	34.4	38.0	47.2	44.8	35.7	34.1	28.9	26.9	25.7	25.7	24.5	20.6	17.6	16.6	16.2	16.1	15.2	15.3	15.9
15-19 years	29.6	33.9	43.6	43.0	33.5	33.1	28.1	26.0	23.1	22.6	21.4	17.4	15.2	13.6	13.2	12.6	11.4	11.9	12.4
20-24 years	38.8	42.9	51.3	46.6	37.6	35.0	29.7	28.0	28.3	28.9	27.7	24.0	20.2	19.7	19.1	19.3	18.8	18.3	19.2
25-34 years	24.6	24.3	30.9	29.1	23.0	23.6	19.2	17.3	18.4	18.7	17.8	16.3	14.5	14.0	13.7	14.5	13.9	13.9	14.7
35-44 years	20.3	19.3	24.9	20.9	17.2	16.9	15.3	15.3	15.5	15.4	14.9	13.4	12.2	11.6	11.3	11.8	11.4	11.1	11.9
45-64 years	25.2	23.0	26.5	18.0	15.4	15.7	14.1	14.3	14.8	14.8	14.1	13.3	12.2	11.9	11.9	12.4	12.1	12.0	12.8
45-54 years	22.2	21.4	25.5	18.6	15.2	15.6	13.8	14.2	15.1	15.3	14.9	13.7	12.7	12.0	12.3	12.6	12.2	12.1	12.8
55-64 years	29.0	25.1	27.9	17.4	15.6	15.9	14.5	14.4	14.5	14.1	13.2	12.8	11.5	11.9	11.5	12.2	11.9	11.9	12.7
65 years and over	43.1	34.7	36.2	22.5	21.7	23.1	22.6	21.4	20.1	19.0	18.7	16.9	15.8	16.0	15.9	15.7	15.1	14.8	15.3
65-74 years	39.1	31.4	32.8	19.2	17.9	18.6	17.5	16.5	16.5	15.2	14.9	13.8	12.7	12.3	13.0	13.0	12.2	11.9	12.8
75-84 years	52.7	41.8	43.5	28.1	27.4	29.1	28.4	25.7	22.9	22.2	21.7	19.2	18.6	18.8	18.3	17.9	17.8	17.5	17.5
85 years and over	45.1	37.9	34.2	27.6	26.5	31.2	31.0	30.4	27.3	25.5	25.3	23.2	20.9	23.8	21.8	22.1	21.0	20.9	21.7
Male																			
All ages, age-adjusted[4]	38.5	35.4	41.5	33.6	27.2	26.5	22.8	21.7	21.9	21.5	21.0	18.9	16.8	16.2	16.1	16.5	15.9	15.8	16.7
All ages, crude	35.4	31.8	39.7	35.3	28.0	26.7	22.4	21.3	21.8	21.6	21.0	18.9	16.9	16.3	16.3	16.6	16.1	16.0	17.0
Under 1 year	9.1	8.6	9.3	7.3	5.0	5.0	4.9	4.6	3.6	3.4	2.7	2.9	2.6	2.2	2.8	1.9	1.7	1.9	2.2
1-14 years	12.3	10.7	13.0	10.0	8.5	7.0	6.1	4.9	4.1	3.7	3.7	3.1	2.9	2.7	2.5	2.5	2.5	2.5	2.5
1-4 years	13.0	11.5	12.9	10.2	8.3	6.9	5.6	4.7	4.3	3.9	3.8	3.2	3.4	3.0	2.7	3.1	3.0	2.8	2.9
5-14 years	11.9	10.4	13.1	9.9	8.6	7.0	6.3	5.0	4.1	3.7	3.7	3.0	2.7	2.5	2.5	2.3	2.4	2.4	2.4
15-24 years	56.7	61.2	73.2	68.4	52.7	49.5	40.5	37.4	36.3	36.3	34.6	29.3	24.5	23.1	22.8	22.5	21.2	21.5	22.2
15-19 years	46.3	51.7	64.1	62.6	46.5	45.5	36.1	33.9	29.9	29.5	27.7	22.6	19.2	17.8	17.2	16.2	14.7	16.1	16.3
20-24 years	66.7	73.2	84.4	74.3	58.2	53.3	45.0	41.2	42.8	43.4	41.9	36.3	30.0	28.5	28.2	28.4	27.3	26.5	27.7
25-34 years	40.8	40.1	49.4	46.3	35.9	35.7	28.1	25.5	27.9	28.5	27.2	25.2	21.7	21.0	20.4	21.5	20.8	20.8	21.8
35-44 years	32.5	29.9	37.7	31.7	25.2	24.7	21.7	22.0	22.5	22.1	22.1	19.9	18.2	16.9	16.7	17.6	16.9	16.4	17.9
45-64 years	37.7	33.3	38.9	26.5	22.0	21.9	19.5	20.2	21.6	21.6	20.9	19.7	18.2	17.9	18.2	18.6	18.2	18.1	19.4
45-54 years	33.6	31.6	37.2	27.6	21.9	22.0	19.3	20.4	22.2	22.6	22.2	20.2	19.0	17.9	18.6	18.8	18.3	18.2	19.1
55-64 years	43.1	35.6	40.9	25.4	22.1	21.7	19.6	19.8	20.7	20.3	19.2	19.0	17.2	17.8	17.7	18.5	18.1	18.1	19.8
65 years and over	66.6	52.1	54.4	33.9	30.4	32.1	30.7	29.5	28.4	26.4	26.9	24.1	22.0	22.2	22.3	22.1	21.5	21.0	22.1
65-74 years	59.1	45.8	47.3	27.3	23.0	24.2	22.2	21.7	22.8	20.7	21.1	19.4	17.5	17.1	18.2	18.5	17.5	17.0	18.5
75-84 years	85.0	66.0	68.2	44.3	41.3	41.2	39.9	35.6	32.1	30.4	31.4	27.3	25.8	25.9	25.7	24.8	24.9	24.8	24.9
85 years and over	78.1	62.7	63.1	56.1	55.3	64.5	61.5	57.5	49.0	45.6	44.4	40.2	35.3	40.2	35.4	35.3	35.3	34.0	35.6
Female																			
All ages, age-adjusted[4]	11.5	11.7	14.9	11.8	10.7	11.0	10.3	9.5	8.9	8.8	8.2	7.2	6.7	6.5	6.3	6.5	6.2	6.1	6.4
All ages, crude	10.9	11.0	14.7	12.3	11.0	11.3	10.4	9.7	9.1	9.0	8.4	7.4	6.9	6.8	6.5	6.7	6.4	6.3	6.7
Under 1 year	7.6	7.5	10.4	6.7	4.7	4.9	4.5	4.2	3.7	3.5	3.3	2.0	2.1	1.8	1.9	1.8	1.8	1.5	1.3
1-14 years	7.2	6.3	7.9	6.3	5.4	4.9	4.4	3.7	3.1	3.1	2.8	2.2	2.2	2.0	2.0	1.9	1.9	1.8	1.9
1-4 years	10.0	8.4	10.0	8.1	6.0	5.6	4.8	3.8	3.4	3.5	3.1	2.5	2.5	2.5	2.6	2.6	2.3	2.3	2.3
5-14 years	5.7	5.4	7.2	5.7	5.1	4.7	4.2	3.6	3.0	2.9	2.6	2.0	2.0	1.8	1.8	1.7	1.8	1.6	1.8
15-24 years	12.6	15.1	21.6	20.8	18.2	17.9	16.8	15.9	14.5	14.5	13.8	11.5	10.5	9.9	9.4	9.3	8.9	8.7	9.3
15-19 years	12.9	16.0	22.7	22.8	20.1	20.0	19.7	17.5	15.9	15.4	14.8	11.8	10.9	9.2	9.0	8.9	7.9	7.6	8.4
20-24 years	12.2	14.0	20.4	18.9	16.7	16.0	13.8	14.2	13.2	13.6	12.8	11.2	10.0	10.5	9.7	9.8	9.9	9.7	10.2
25-34 years	9.3	9.2	13.0	12.2	10.1	11.5	10.2	8.8	8.9	8.8	8.5	7.4	7.2	6.9	7.0	7.4	6.9	6.8	7.5
35-44 years	8.5	9.1	12.9	10.4	9.4	9.2	9.0	8.8	8.6	8.8	7.8	7.0	6.2	6.2	6.0	6.2	5.9	5.8	6.1
45-64 years	12.6	13.1	15.3	10.3	9.5	10.1	9.0	8.7	8.4	8.3	7.7	7.2	6.5	6.3	5.9	6.4	6.3	6.2	6.4
45-54 years	10.9	11.6	14.5	10.2	9.0	9.6	8.4	8.2	8.2	8.2	7.8	7.4	6.6	6.3	6.1	6.5	6.3	6.2	6.7
55-64 years	14.9	15.2	16.2	10.5	9.9	10.8	9.9	9.5	8.8	8.5	7.5	6.9	6.3	6.3	5.7	6.4	6.2	6.1	6.1
65 years and over	21.9	20.3	23.1	15.0	15.8	17.2	17.0	15.8	14.1	13.6	12.6	11.5	11.1	11.3	10.9	10.8	10.0	9.9	10.0
65-74 years	20.6	19.0	21.6	13.0	14.0	14.1	13.7	12.3	11.1	10.5	9.6	8.9	8.5	8.2	8.4	8.2	7.5	7.5	7.8
75-84 years	25.2	23.0	27.2	18.5	19.2	21.9	21.2	19.2	16.5	16.5	15.0	13.5	13.5	13.7	12.8	12.9	12.5	12.0	11.9
85 years and over	22.1	22.0	18.0	15.2	15.0	18.3	19.3	19.3	17.6	16.4	16.5	15.3	14.0	15.9	15.1	15.5	13.7	14.1	14.4
White Male[5]																			
All ages, age-adjusted[4]	37.9	34.8	40.4	33.8	27.2	26.3	22.6	21.8	22.4	22.1	21.6	19.6	17.3	16.7	16.6	17.0	16.3	16.1	17.0
All ages, crude	35.1	31.5	39.1	35.9	28.3	26.7	22.4	21.6	22.5	22.2	21.7	19.7	17.5	17.0	16.9	17.3	16.7	16.5	17.4
Under 1 year	9.1	8.8	9.1	7.0	4.6	4.8	4.3	4.2	3.4	3.3	2.9	2.9	2.5	2.0	2.5	1.9	1.7	1.8	1.9
1-14 years	12.4	10.6	12.5	9.8	8.3	6.6	5.9	4.8	4.1	3.6	3.8	3.1	2.8	2.7	2.6	2.4	2.4	2.4	2.5

Note: Data are based on death certificates.
NA = Not available.
*Rates based on fewer than 20 deaths are considered unreliable and are not shown.
[1]Includes deaths of persons who were not residents of the 50 states and the District of Columbia.
[2]Underlying cause of death was coded according to the 6th Revision of the International Classification of Diseases (ICD) in 1950, 7th Revision in 1960, 8th Revision in 1970, and 9th Revision in 1980-1998.
[3]Starting with 1999 data, cause of death is coded according to ICD-10.
[4]Age-adjusted rates are calculated using the year 2000 standard population. Prior to 2001, age-adjusted rates were calculated using standard million proportions based on rounded population numbers. Starting with 2001 data, unrounded population numbers are used to calculate age-adjusted rates.
[5]The race groups, white, black, Asian or Pacific Islander, and American Indian or Alaska Native, include persons of Hispanic and non-Hispanic origin. Persons of Hispanic origin may be of any race. Death rates for Hispanic, American Indian or Alaska Native, and Asian or Pacific Islander persons should be interpreted with caution because of inconsistencies in reporting Hispanic origin or race on the death certificate (death rate numerators) compared with population figures (death rate denominators). The net effect of misclassification is an underestimation of deaths and death rates for races other than White and Black.

Table 2-20. Death Rates for Motor Vehicle–Related Injuries, by Sex and Age, Selected Years, 1950–2015—*Continued*

(Rate per 100,000 population.)

Sex, race, Hispanic origin, and age	1950[1,2]	1960[1,2]	1970[2]	1980[2]	1985[2]	1990[2]	1995[2]	2000[3]	2005[3]	2006[3]	2007[3]	2008[3]	2009[3]	2010[3]	2011[3]	2012[3]	2013[3]	2014[3]	2015[3]
	Deaths per 100,000 resident population																		
15-24 years	58.3	62.7	75.2	73.8	56.5	52.5	42.4	39.6	39.2	39.3	37.4	31.7	26.6	24.6	24.6	24.5	22.9	23.0	23.3
25-34 years	39.1	38.6	47.0	46.6	35.8	35.4	27.9	25.1	28.4	28.8	27.8	26.2	21.8	21.4	20.9	22.0	21.1	20.8	22.1
35-44 years	30.9	28.4	35.2	30.7	24.3	23.7	21.1	21.8	22.8	22.6	22.2	20.3	18.5	17.4	17.0	18.0	17.3	16.6	18.0
45-64 years	36.2	31.7	36.5	25.2	20.8	20.6	18.7	19.7	21.7	21.6	21.1	20.1	18.7	18.3	18.5	19.0	18.5	18.3	19.5
65 years and over	67.1	52.1	54.2	32.7	29.9	31.4	30.1	29.4	28.7	26.6	27.0	24.5	22.3	22.7	22.8	22.6	22.1	21.5	22.7
Black or African American Male[5]																			
All ages, age-adjusted[4]	34.8	39.6	51.0	34.2	29.0	29.9	26.1	24.4	22.5	22.6	22.3	18.9	17.8	16.7	16.7	17.4	17.0	17.4	19.1
All ages, crude	37.2	33.1	44.3	31.1	27.1	28.1	24.1	22.5	21.1	21.4	21.0	18.0	16.7	15.9	15.8	16.6	16.4	16.8	18.7
Under 1 year	NA	*	10.6	7.8	*	*	8.7	6.7	*	*	*	*	*	*	*	*	*	*	*
1-14 years[6]	10.4	11.2	16.3	11.4	9.7	8.9	7.5	5.5	4.4	4.8	4.0	3.1	3.5	3.0	2.7	3.2	3.3	2.9	3.2
15-24 years	42.5	46.4	58.1	34.9	32.0	36.1	33.9	30.2	27.8	26.9	26.9	22.4	18.5	19.4	17.7	17.5	17.6	18.7	21.8
25-34 years	54.4	51.0	70.4	44.9	37.7	39.5	32.2	32.6	32.1	34.4	32.0	27.0	26.9	24.9	22.4	25.6	25.1	25.7	26.7
35-44 years	46.7	43.6	59.5	41.2	34.7	33.5	28.7	27.2	25.8	25.1	27.2	23.0	21.9	19.4	20.8	20.8	20.5	21.2	23.7
45-64 years	54.6	47.8	61.7	39.5	32.9	33.3	26.2	27.1	24.1	25.2	24.0	21.5	19.3	19.1	20.2	20.8	21.1	21.1	24.5
65 years and over	52.6	48.2	53.4	42.4	35.2	36.3	36.9	32.1	29.1	26.1	27.4	22.9	22.8	20.0	21.3	21.8	18.5	19.8	19.6
American Indian or Alaska Native Male[5]																			
All ages, age-adjusted[4]	NA	NA	NA	78.9	50.9	48.3	40.7	35.8	31.5	33.5	28.6	24.1	22.7	21.1	22.5	22.2	20.0	23.4	22.8
All ages, crude	NA	NA	NA	74.6	51.7	47.6	40.1	33.6	31.3	32.2	27.3	23.5	22.0	19.8	21.8	22.2	19.0	22.2	22.1
1-14 years	NA	NA	NA	15.1	16.2	11.6	7.6	7.8	9.6	4.6	4.4	4.6	4.8	*	*	6.8	3.9	4.2	4.4
15-24 years	NA	NA	NA	126.1	77.3	75.2	69.0	56.8	44.1	47.9	40.0	37.5	35.2	31.9	30.9	27.3	26.8	27.3	24.9
25-34 years	NA	NA	NA	107.0	84.0	78.2	67.8	49.8	49.0	45.2	42.7	30.5	29.3	23.8	34.8	32.0	30.3	31.8	32.4
35-44 years	NA	NA	NA	82.8	55.8	57.0	45.2	36.3	36.9	34.3	32.0	29.3	28.5	24.5	21.9	30.4	19.8	24.2	30.3
45-64 years	NA	NA	NA	77.4	52.2	45.9	38.8	32.0	31.9	41.4	27.9	25.8	22.8	23.2	27.4	27.0	20.4	30.5	26.6
65 years and over	NA	NA	NA	97.0	*	43.0	*	48.5	27.8	37.4	38.5	24.5	22.2	26.6	23.7	*	25.8	26.8	26.3
Asian or Pacific Islander Male[5]																			
All ages, age-adjusted[4]	NA	NA	NA	19.0	17.3	17.9	14.5	10.6	9.5	9.3	9.1	7.9	6.2	6.5	6.6	5.9	6.4	6.2	6.3
All ages, crude	NA	NA	NA	17.1	16.0	15.8	12.6	9.8	8.7	8.6	8.3	7.5	5.8	6.2	6.2	5.6	5.9	6.0	6.1
1-14 years	NA	NA	NA	8.2	5.2	6.3	4.5	2.5	1.7	2.6	1.8	1.6	1.5	*	*	*	1.5	1.2	*
15-24 years	NA	NA	NA	27.2	28.1	25.7	18.5	17.0	14.5	14.9	15.7	11.6	8.8	9.6	9.3	8.9	8.1	8.6	9.7
25-34 years	NA	NA	NA	18.8	18.4	17.0	12.4	10.4	8.9	8.4	7.0	8.5	7.3	7.8	6.6	5.8	5.9	8.0	6.7
35-44 years	NA	NA	NA	13.1	12.0	12.2	9.9	6.9	6.6	6.0	6.1	6.4	4.5	4.1	4.8	3.5	5.3	4.1	3.8
45-64 years	NA	NA	NA	13.7	13.4	15.1	14.3	10.1	9.0	8.6	7.7	7.4	5.6	6.0	6.5	6.3	5.9	5.7	6.4
65 years and over	NA	NA	NA	37.3	37.3	33.6	32.1	21.1	20.8	19.7	20.9	16.1	11.9	14.6	14.9	12.5	14.3	13.1	13.5
Hispanic or Latino Male[5,7]																			
All ages, age-adjusted[4]	NA	NA	NA	NA	25.4	29.5	24.4	21.3	21.4	21.4	19.4	16.7	14.7	14.0	13.7	13.9	14.2	14.3	15.2
All ages, crude	NA	NA	NA	NA	25.6	29.2	22.4	20.1	20.8	20.9	18.6	16.1	14.2	12.8	12.9	13.1	13.3	13.5	14.4
1-14 years	NA	NA	NA	NA	7.7	7.2	5.7	4.4	4.6	4.4	4.1	2.9	3.0	2.5	2.3	2.5	2.5	2.5	2.6
15-24 years	NA	NA	NA	NA	44.9	48.2	37.1	34.7	37.6	38.1	32.8	26.9	24.1	20.2	20.7	20.3	20.5	22.0	22.8
25-34 years	NA	NA	NA	NA	31.2	41.0	28.8	24.9	28.0	27.6	25.9	24.7	20.1	18.0	17.4	19.9	18.2	19.6	21.2
35-44 years	NA	NA	NA	NA	26.3	28.0	23.2	21.6	20.9	21.6	18.6	16.4	15.5	13.9	13.9	13.9	14.5	13.4	14.8
45-64 years	NA	NA	NA	NA	25.9	28.9	23.0	21.7	20.2	21.6	18.8	16.9	14.4	14.3	15.2	14.7	15.9	14.9	15.9
65 years and over	NA	NA	NA	NA	22.9	35.3	37.0	28.9	27.6	24.8	25.6	19.7	16.9	20.7	18.0	17.5	18.8	19.5	20.1
White, not Hispanic or Latino Male[7]																			
All ages, age-adjusted[4]	NA	NA	NA	NA	24.9	25.7	22.1	21.7	22.2	21.8	21.6	19.8	17.4	17.1	17.0	17.3	16.5	16.2	17.0
All ages, crude	NA	NA	NA	NA	25.9	26.0	21.9	21.5	22.5	22.1	22.0	20.2	17.9	17.6	17.6	18.0	17.2	16.9	17.9
1-14 years	NA	NA	NA	NA	7.8	6.4	5.8	4.9	3.9	3.2	3.5	3.1	2.6	2.7	2.7	2.2	2.3	2.3	2.4
15-24 years	NA	NA	NA	NA	53.3	52.3	42.7	40.3	38.8	38.8	37.9	32.5	26.6	25.4	25.3	25.3	23.0	22.6	22.8
25-34 years	NA	NA	NA	NA	33.2	34.0	27.1	24.7	27.8	28.5	27.6	26.1	21.8	21.9	21.5	22.0	21.4	20.7	21.7
35-44 years	NA	NA	NA	NA	21.6	23.1	20.3	21.6	22.9	22.4	22.7	20.9	18.9	18.0	17.5	18.9	17.8	17.2	18.6
45-64 years	NA	NA	NA	NA	18.0	19.8	18.1	19.3	21.7	21.4	21.1	20.2	19.0	18.6	18.7	19.3	18.6	18.6	19.8
65 years and over	NA	NA	NA	NA	27.6	31.1	29.4	29.3	28.6	26.6	27.0	24.7	22.6	22.7	23.0	22.9	22.3	21.5	22.8
White Female[5]																			
All ages, age-adjusted[4]	11.4	11.7	14.9	12.2	10.9	11.2	10.4	9.8	9.3	9.2	8.6	7.5	6.9	6.8	6.6	6.8	6.4	6.3	6.6
All ages, crude	10.9	11.2	14.8	12.8	11.4	11.6	10.7	10.0	9.6	9.4	8.8	7.8	7.2	7.1	6.9	7.1	6.7	6.6	6.9
Under 1 year	7.8	7.5	10.2	7.1	3.9	4.7	4.5	3.5	3.0	3.1	2.9	1.8	1.5	1.9	1.4	1.6	1.7	1.5	*
1-14 years	7.2	6.2	7.5	6.2	5.4	4.8	4.3	3.7	3.2	3.1	2.7	2.1	2.1	2.1	2.0	1.9	1.8	1.8	1.8

Note: Data are based on death certificates.
NA = Not available.
*Rates based on fewer than 20 deaths are considered unreliable and are not shown.
[1]Includes deaths of persons who were not residents of the 50 states and the District of Columbia.
[2]Underlying cause of death was coded according to the 6th Revision of the International Classification of Diseases (ICD) in 1950, 7th Revision in 1960, 8th Revision in 1970, and 9th Revision in 1980-1998.
[3]Starting with 1999 data, cause of death is coded according to ICD-10.
[4]Age-adjusted rates are calculated using the year 2000 standard population. Prior to 2001, age-adjusted rates were calculated using standard million proportions based on rounded population numbers. Starting with 2001 data, unrounded population numbers are used to calculate age-adjusted rates.
[5]The race groups, white, black, Asian or Pacific Islander, and American Indian or Alaska Native, include persons of Hispanic and non-Hispanic origin. Persons of Hispanic origin may be of any race. Death rates for Hispanic, American Indian or Alaska Native, and Asian or Pacific Islander persons should be interpreted with caution because of inconsistencies in reporting Hispanic origin or race on the death certificate (death rate numerators) compared with population figures (death rate denominators). The net effect of misclassification is an underestimation of deaths and death rates for races other than White and Black.
[6]In 1950, rate is for the age group under 15 years.
[7]Prior to 1997, data from states that did not report Hispanic origin on the death certificate were excluded.

Table 2-20. Death Rates for Motor Vehicle–Related Injuries, by Sex and Age, Selected Years, 1950–2015—Continued

(Rate per 100,000 population.)

Sex, race, Hispanic origin, and age	1950[1,2]	1960[1,2]	1970[2]	1980[2]	1985[2]	1990[2]	1995[2]	2000[3]	2005[3]	2006[3]	2007[3]	2008[3]	2009[3]	2010[3]	2011[3]	2012[3]	2013[3]	2014[3]	2015[3]
	Deaths per 100,000 resident population																		
15-24 years	12.6	15.6	22.7	23.0	20.0	19.5	18.1	17.1	15.7	15.9	15.1	12.6	11.3	10.8	10.1	10.0	9.5	9.2	9.8
25-34 years	9.0	9.0	12.7	12.2	10.1	11.6	10.2	8.9	9.4	9.1	9.0	7.6	7.4	7.1	7.3	7.6	7.1	7.1	7.7
35-44 years	8.1	8.9	12.3	10.6	9.4	9.2	8.9	8.9	9.0	9.2	8.1	7.4	6.5	6.5	6.4	6.6	6.1	6.1	6.4
45-64 years	12.7	13.1	15.1	10.4	9.5	9.9	8.9	8.7	8.6	8.3	7.8	7.3	6.6	6.4	6.1	6.5	6.4	6.3	6.6
65 years and over	22.2	20.8	23.7	15.3	16.2	17.4	17.5	16.2	14.5	14.0	13.0	11.8	11.4	11.5	11.3	11.3	10.4	10.3	10.3
Black or African American Female[5]																			
All ages, age-adjusted[4]	9.3	10.4	14.1	8.5	8.5	9.6	9.0	8.4	7.6	7.7	7.0	6.4	6.2	5.9	5.7	5.9	5.7	5.6	6.1
All ages, crude	10.2	9.7	13.4	8.3	8.3	9.4	8.8	8.2	7.5	7.6	6.9	6.3	6.1	5.8	5.7	5.9	5.7	5.6	6.1
Under 1 year	NA	8.1	11.9	*	8.1	7.0	*	*	6.9	*	*	*	*	*	*	*	*	*	*
1-14 years[6]	7.2	6.9	10.2	6.3	5.1	5.3	4.9	3.9	3.4	3.4	3.3	2.5	2.6	2.0	2.3	2.4	2.3	2.3	2.6
15-24 years	11.6	9.9	13.4	8.0	9.1	9.9	10.5	11.7	10.5	9.8	9.5	8.4	8.1	7.8	7.6	7.7	7.7	7.7	8.9
25-34 years	10.8	9.8	13.3	10.6	9.3	11.1	10.3	9.4	7.6	8.7	7.5	7.1	7.6	6.8	7.1	7.4	7.2	6.9	7.8
35-44 years	11.1	11.0	16.1	8.3	9.1	9.4	9.7	8.2	7.7	8.0	7.0	6.7	6.0	5.8	5.4	5.7	6.4	5.7	6.1
45-64 years	11.8	12.7	16.7	9.2	9.0	10.7	9.3	9.0	8.2	8.8	7.4	7.0	6.5	6.3	5.9	6.5	6.2	6.2	6.3
65 years and over	14.3	13.2	15.7	9.5	11.2	13.5	11.4	10.4	9.9	9.5	8.7	8.4	7.9	8.6	7.6	7.7	5.9	6.4	6.8
American Indian or Alaska Native Female[5]																			
All ages, age-adjusted[4]	NA	NA	NA	32.0	19.8	17.5	18.2	19.5	14.0	15.1	13.5	12.8	11.8	10.6	10.8	10.2	11.0	10.1	11.2
All ages, crude	NA	NA	NA	32.0	20.6	17.3	18.8	18.6	13.8	14.9	13.5	12.4	11.7	10.0	10.5	10.1	10.7	10.0	11.2
1-14 years	NA	NA	NA	15.0	9.2	8.1	8.1	6.5	*	*	*	*	*	*	*	*	4.9	*	*
15-24 years	NA	NA	NA	42.3	29.5	31.4	30.4	30.3	22.0	24.5	21.4	17.4	19.8	13.4	14.7	16.2	13.6	16.5	13.8
25-34 years	NA	NA	NA	52.5	30.2	18.8	33.7	22.3	22.1	19.1	19.4	19.2	13.8	17.7	18.0	15.1	17.0	13.4	21.2
35-44 years	NA	NA	NA	38.1	27.0	18.2	17.2	22.0	15.7	17.7	18.8	15.3	16.9	13.1	11.3	11.6	14.2	12.0	12.6
45-64 years	NA	NA	NA	32.6	19.5	17.6	15.7	17.8	10.6	13.5	10.8	10.3	11.7	8.4	8.7	10.5	8.7	9.7	11.9
65 years and over	NA	NA	NA	*	*	*	*	24.0	*	17.1	*	17.8	*	14.8	14.4	*	*	*	*
Asian or Pacific Islander Female[5]																			
All ages, age-adjusted[4]	NA	NA	NA	9.3	8.8	10.4	8.6	6.7	5.7	5.4	5.0	4.2	3.8	3.9	3.3	3.3	3.4	3.2	3.6
All ages, crude	NA	NA	NA	8.2	7.9	9.0	7.7	5.9	5.3	5.1	4.6	3.9	3.5	3.6	3.1	3.3	3.4	3.2	3.6
1-14 years	NA	NA	NA	7.4	5.0	3.6	3.2	2.3	1.5	1.7	*	1.4	1.5	*	*	*	*	*	*
15-24 years	NA	NA	NA	7.4	7.4	11.4	11.5	6.0	7.0	6.3	6.7	4.5	4.3	3.3	3.7	3.0	3.0	3.0	3.4
25-34 years	NA	NA	NA	7.3	8.4	7.3	4.8	4.5	3.4	3.2	2.9	3.1	2.9	3.1	1.9	2.8	2.5	2.5	2.6
35-44 years	NA	NA	NA	8.6	7.0	7.5	5.9	4.9	4.3	4.1	2.7	2.2	2.1	2.0	2.3	1.7	*	2.0	1.7
45-64 years	NA	NA	NA	8.5	8.6	11.8	10.4	6.4	6.4	6.0	5.4	4.4	3.0	4.3	3.0	4.2	4.1	3.3	4.0
65 years and over	NA	NA	NA	18.6	20.5	24.3	18.9	18.5	13.9	13.6	13.4	12.1	11.4	12.2	10.2	8.7	10.8	9.4	11.2
Hispanic or Latina Female[5,7]																			
All ages, age-adjusted[4]	NA	NA	NA	NA	8.8	9.6	8.8	7.9	7.8	7.6	6.8	5.5	5.5	5.3	4.8	5.3	5.2	5.0	5.2
All ages, crude	NA	NA	NA	NA	7.9	8.9	8.0	7.2	7.3	7.0	6.3	5.0	5.1	4.9	4.5	4.9	4.8	4.7	5.0
1-14 years	NA	NA	NA	NA	4.8	4.8	4.3	3.9	3.3	3.1	2.7	2.1	2.3	2.0	1.7	1.9	1.7	1.9	1.8
15-24 years	NA	NA	NA	NA	10.1	11.6	11.8	10.6	12.7	10.9	10.1	7.8	7.8	7.7	6.3	7.2	7.4	7.5	7.7
25-34 years	NA	NA	NA	NA	7.5	9.4	7.2	6.5	7.1	6.8	6.6	5.4	5.5	5.0	5.1	5.4	5.1	5.3	6.1
35-44 years	NA	NA	NA	NA	8.8	8.0	7.9	7.3	7.3	7.1	6.7	4.8	4.6	4.5	4.6	4.5	4.7	4.1	4.6
45-64 years	NA	NA	NA	NA	9.4	11.4	9.3	8.3	7.4	8.0	6.7	5.1	5.5	5.6	4.8	5.6	5.3	5.3	5.2
65 years and over	NA	NA	NA	NA	14.8	14.9	14.6	13.4	11.4	12.0	10.5	10.7	9.5	9.4	8.6	9.2	9.0	8.1	8.3
White, not Hispanic or Latina Female[7]																			
All ages, age-adjusted[4]	NA	NA	NA	NA	10.4	11.3	10.5	10.0	9.5	9.4	8.8	7.9	7.1	7.0	6.9	7.0	6.6	6.5	6.8
All ages, crude	NA	NA	NA	NA	10.9	11.7	10.9	10.3	9.9	9.8	9.2	8.3	7.5	7.5	7.3	7.5	7.1	7.0	7.3
1-14 years	NA	NA	NA	NA	4.9	4.7	4.2	3.5	3.0	3.0	2.6	2.1	1.9	2.0	2.1	1.8	1.8	1.7	1.8
15-24 years	NA	NA	NA	NA	20.2	20.4	19.0	18.4	16.3	16.9	16.2	13.7	12.0	11.4	11.0	10.7	10.0	9.6	10.3
25-34 years	NA	NA	NA	NA	9.8	11.7	10.5	9.3	9.9	9.6	9.5	8.1	7.7	7.6	7.7	8.2	7.5	7.5	8.0
35-44 years	NA	NA	NA	NA	8.6	9.3	8.9	9.0	9.2	9.4	8.3	7.9	6.8	6.9	6.7	7.0	6.4	6.6	6.8
45-64 years	NA	NA	NA	NA	8.6	9.7	8.6	8.7	8.6	8.3	7.9	7.6	6.7	6.4	6.2	6.6	6.5	6.4	6.7
65 years and over	NA	NA	NA	NA	15.3	17.5	17.5	16.3	14.7	14.1	13.1	11.8	11.5	11.6	11.5	11.4	10.5	10.4	10.5

Note: Data are based on death certificates.

NA = Not available.

* Rates based on fewer than 20 deaths are considered unreliable and are not shown.

[1] Includes deaths of persons who were not residents of the 50 states and the District of Columbia.

[2] Underlying cause of death was coded according to the 6th Revision of the International Classification of Diseases (ICD) in 1950, 7th Revision in 1960, 8th Revision in 1970, and 9th Revision in 1980-1998.

[3] Starting with 1999 data, cause of death is coded according to ICD-10.

[4] Age-adjusted rates are calculated using the year 2000 standard population. Prior to 2001, age-adjusted rates were calculated using standard million proportions based on rounded population numbers. Starting with 2001 data, unrounded population numbers are used to calculate age-adjusted rates.

[5] The race groups, white, black, Asian or Pacific Islander, and American Indian or Alaska Native, include persons of Hispanic and non-Hispanic origin. Persons of Hispanic origin may be of any race. Death rates for Hispanic, American Indian or Alaska Native, and Asian or Pacific Islander persons should be interpreted with caution because of inconsistencies in reporting Hispanic origin or race on the death certificate (death rate numerators) compared with population figures (death rate denominators). The net effect of misclassification is an underestimation of deaths and death rates for races other than White and Black.

[6] In 1950, rate is for the age group under 15 years.

[7] Prior to 1997, data from states that did not report Hispanic origin on the death certificate were excluded.

Table 2-21. Occupational Fatal Injuries, by Industry, Sex, Age, Race, and Hispanic Origin, 2003–2015

(Number.)

Characteristic	2003	2004	2005	2006	2007	2008	2009	2010	2011	2012	2013	2014	2015
Rate													
Total workforce	5,575	5,764	5,734	5,840	5,657	5,214	4,551	4,690	4,693	4,628	4,585	4,821	4,836
Sex													
Male	5,129	5,349	5,328	5,396	5,228	4,827	4,216	4,322	4,308	4,277	4,265	4,454	4,492
Female	446	415	406	444	429	387	335	368	385	351	319	367	344
Unspecified	NA	NA	NA	NA	NA	NA	NA	NA	NA	NA	1	0	0
Age													
Under 16 years	25	13	23	11	18	11	13	16	10	19	5	8	12
16-17 years	28	25	31	21	20	23	14	18	13	10	9	14	12
18-19 years	84	103	111	106	97	66	57	56	61	59	57	42	50
20-24 years	462	421	403	390	424	353	275	245	292	287	279	292	329
25-34 years	1,018	996	1,017	1,041	991	850	704	785	714	736	777	753	758
35-44 years	1,329	1,342	1,243	1,288	1,168	1,113	908	868	875	829	853	860	864
45-54 years	1,301	1,384	1,389	1,417	1,425	1,292	1,173	1,169	1,222	1,161	1,115	1,161	1,130
55-64 years	802	907	933	963	934	920	853	948	936	936	933	1,007	1,031
65 years and over	523	569	578	599	574	580	551	582	569	588	557	684	650
Unspecified	3	4	6	4	6	6	3	3	1	3	0	0	0
Race and Hispanic origin													
Hispanic or Latino (may be of any race)	794	902	923	990	937	804	713	707	749	748	817	804	903
Not Hispanic or Latino	4,781	4,862	4,811	4,850	4,720	4,410	3,838	3,983	3,944	3,880	3,768	4,017	3,933
White	3,988	4,066	3,977	4,019	3,867	3,663	3,204	3,363	3,323	3,177	3,125	3,332	3,241
Black or African American	543	546	584	565	609	533	421	412	440	486	439	475	495
American Indian or Alaska Native	42	28	50	46	29	32	33	32	30	37	35	34	36
Asian	147	168	154	148	166	145	141	143	121	147	125	137	114
Native Hawaiian or Other Pacific Islander	11	12	9	11	6	7	7	6	3	7	7	5	9
Multiple races	3	4	*	11	10	6	7	8	15	5	12	20	12
Other races or not reported	47	38	35	50	33	24	25	19	12	21	25	14	26
Industry[1]													
Private sector	5,043	5,229	5,214	5,320	5,112	4,670	4,090	4,206	4,188	4,175	4,101	4,386	4,379
Agriculture, forestry, fishing, and hunting	709	669	715	655	585	672	575	621	566	509	500	584	570
Mining[2]	141	152	159	192	183	176	99	172	155	181	155	183	120
Utilities	32	51	30	53	34	37	16	26	39	23	24	17	22
Construction	1,131	1,234	1,192	1,239	1,204	975	834	774	738	806	828	899	937
Manufacturing	420	463	393	456	400	411	319	329	327	327	312	349	353
Wholesale trade	191	205	209	222	207	180	190	191	190	204	201	191	175
Retail trade	344	377	400	359	348	301	307	311	268	273	263	272	269
Transportation and warehousing	808	840	885	860	890	796	633	661	749	741	733	766	765
Information	64	55	65	66	79	47	33	43	56	42	40	35	42
Finance and insurance	45	46	42	44	46	24	33	24	36	21	21	29	19
Real estate and rental and leasing	84	70	57	82	73	82	75	89	62	64	66	88	64
Professional and technical services	97	77	83	78	77	69	85	76	74	57	87	80	76
Management, administrative, and waste services[3]	NA	NA	NA	NA	NA	NA	NA	NA	359	352	343	345	401
Educational services	41	44	46	49	34	28	27	30	37	34	32	40	30
Health care and social assistance	102	113	104	129	115	113	123	141	117	107	103	106	109
Arts, entertainment, and recreation	88	99	77	80	96	92	80	84	93	80	69	81	82
Accommodation and food services	187	148	136	185	164	146	151	154	138	152	138	135	143
Other services (except public administration)	194	207	210	183	175	178	173	192	183	199	186	186	202
Government[4]	532	535	520	520	545	544	461	484	505	453	484	435	457

Note: Fatal work injuries are based on revised data and may differ from originally published data from the Census of Fatal Occupational Injuries (CFOI). NA = Not available.
* = Estimates are unreliable or data do not meet publication criteria.
[1]Industry data from 2003 to 2008 are based on the North American Industry Classification System (NAICS), 2002. Industry data from 2009 to the present are based on NAICS 2007. NAICS replaces the Standard Industrial Classification (SIC) system. Because of substantial differences between these systems, industry data classified by these two systems are not comparable.
[2]Includes fatal injuries at all establishments categorized as Mining (Sector 21) in the NAICS, including establishments not governed by the Mine Safety and Health Administration (MSHA) rules and reporting, such as those in Oil and Gas Extraction.
[3]Starting with 2011 data, CFOI combined the categories "Management of companies and enterprises" and "Administrative and support and waste management and remediation services" into one category entitled "Management, administrative, and waste services."
[4]Includes fatal work injuries to workers employed by governmental organizations, regardless of industry.

Table 2-22. Number of Fatal Work Injuries, by Most Frequent Type, 1992–2016

(Number.)

Year	Total	Roadway incidents	Homicides	Falls, slips, trips	Struck by object
1992	6,217	1,158	1,044	600	557
1993	6,331	1,242	1,074	618	565
1994	6,632	1,343	1,080	665	591
1995	6,275	1,346	1,036	651	547
1996	6,202	1,346	927	691	582
1997	6,238	1,393	860	716	579
1998	6,055	1,442	714	706	520
1999	6,054	1,496	651	721	585
2000	5,920	1,365	677	734	571
2001	5,915	1,409	643	810	553
2002	5,534	1,373	609	719	505
2003	5,575	1,353	632	696	531
2004	5,764	1,398	559	822	602
2005	5,734	1,437	567	770	607
2006	5,840	1,356	540	827	589
2007	5,657	1,414	628	847	504
2008	5,214	1,215	526	700	520
2009	4,551	985	542	645	420
2010	4,690	1,044	518	646	404
2011	4,693	1,103	468	681	476
2012	4,383	1,044	463	668	519
2013	4,585	1,099	404	724	509
2014	4,821	1,157	409	818	503
2015	4,836	1,264	417	800	519
2016	5,190	1,252	500	849	533

Table 2-23. Number of Fatal Occupational Injuries, by Selected Industry Sector and Occupation, and Percentage of Fatal Incidents, 2016

(Number, percent.)

Characteristic	Count	Percent
Total	5,190	100.0
Industry		
Private industry..	4,693	90.4
Government	497	9.6
Construction	991	19.1
Transportation and warehousing...	825	15.9
Agriculture, forestry, fishing and hunting...	593	11.4
Government	497	9.6
Professional and business services	540	10.4
Manufacturing..	318	6.1
Retail trade...	282	5.4
Leisure and hospitality	NA	NA
Other services (exc. public administration)...	223	4.3
Public administration	1	0.0
Wholesale trade...	179	3.4
Real estate and rental and leasing..	91	1.8
Mining[1]..	89	1.7
Educational and health services	159	3.1
Health care and social assistance...	117	2.3
Arts, entertainment, and recreation...	96	1.8
Financial activities...	117	2.3
Information...	46	0.9
Utilities...	30	0.6
Administrative and waste services	439	8.5
Occupation..		
Fishers and related fishing workers	24	0.5
Logging workers...	95	2.0
Aircraft pilots and flight engineers	75	1.6
Farmers, ranchers, and other agricultural managers.............................	260	5.6
Extraction workers	87	1.9
Roofers	101	2.2
Refuse and recyclable material collectors	31	0.7
Driver/sales workers and truck drivers..	918	19.6
Industrial machinery installation, repair, and maintenance workers........	35	0.7
Police and sheriff's patrol officers...	108	2.3

NA = Not available.

[1]CFOI has used several versions of the Standard Occupation Classification (SOC) system since 2003 to define occupation. For more information on the version of SOC used in this year, see the definitions page at http://www.bls.gov/iif/oshcfdef.htm.

Table 2-24. Number of Fatal Work Injuries, by State, 2015 and 2016

(Number.)

State	2015	2016	Net change
Total	4,585	4,383	202
Alabama	70	100	30
Alaska	14	35	21
Arizona	69	77	8
Arkansas	74	68	6
California	388	376	12
Colorado	75	81	6
Connecticut	44	28	16
Delaware	8	12	4
District of Columbia	8	5	3
Florida	272	309	37
Georgia	180	171	9
Hawaii	18	29	11
Idaho	36	30	6
Illinois	172	171	1
Indiana	115	137	22
Iowa	60	76	16
Kansas	60	74	14
Kentucky	99	92	7
Louisiana	112	95	17
Maine	15	18	3
Maryland	69	92	23
Massachusetts	69	109	40
Michigan	134	162	28
Minnesota	74	92	18
Mississippi	77	71	6
Missouri	117	124	7
Montana	36	38	2
Nebraska	50	60	10
Nevada	44	54	10
New Hampshire	18	22	4
New Jersey	97	101	4
New Mexico	35	41	6
New York	256	272	16
North Carolina	150	174	24
North Dakota	47	28	19
Ohio	202	164	38
Oklahoma	91	92	1
Oregon	44	72	28
Pennsylvania	173	163	10
Rhode Island	6	9	3
South Carolina	117	96	21
South Dakota	21	31	10
Tennessee	112	122	10
Texas	527	545	18
Utah	42	44	2
Vermont	9	10	1
Virginia	106	153	47
Washington	70	78	8
West Virginia	35	47	12
Wisconsin	104	105	1
Wyoming	34	34	0

Table 2-25. Years of Potential Life Lost Before Age 75 for Selected Causes of Death, by Sex, Race, and Hispanic Origin, Selected Years, 1980–2015

(Years lost before 75 per 100,000 population.)

	Crude	Age-adjusted[2]														
Sex, race, Hispanic origin, and cause of death[1]	2015[3]	1980[2]	1990[2]	1995[2]	2000[3]	2005[3]	2006[3]	2007[3]	2008[3]	2009[3]	2010[3]	2011[3]	2012[3]	2013[3]	2014[3]	2015[3]
ALL PERSONS																
All causes	7,214.0	10,448.4	9,085.5	8,626.2	7,578.1	7,315.7	7,228.7	7,087.0	6,957.7	6,833.1	6,642.9	6,635.2	6,588.0	6,593.1	6,622.1	6,757.7
Diseases of heart	1,090.7	2,238.7	1,617.7	1,475.4	1,253.0	1,107.5	1,074.8	1,037.8	1,022.9	992.6	972.4	962.4	951.9	952.3	952.0	956.6
Ischemic heart disease	622.5	1,729.3	1,153.6	1,013.2	841.8	698.9	672.5	638.2	624.4	591.5	577.3	567.0	558.4	546.1	537.1	530.3
Cerebrovascular diseases	183.0	357.5	259.6	246.5	223.3	192.9	189.7	183.7	177.9	172.8	169.3	164.0	161.6	158.1	160.1	161.0
Malignant neoplasms	1,501.2	2,108.8	2,003.8	1,841.6	1,674.1	1,519.8	1,484.6	1,452.7	1,427.8	1,413.9	1,395.8	1,370.9	1,356.2	1,328.6	1,310.4	1,283.3
Trachea, bronchus, and lung	342.1	548.5	561.4	497.3	443.1	390.5	376.1	363.5	350.5	341.7	331.3	318.7	309.9	298.2	287.7	273.4
Colorectal	140.6	190.0	164.7	152.0	141.9	124.3	125.6	126.0	126.8	124.3	125.0	124.1	123.0	123.5	122.2	123.3
Prostate[4]	59.1	84.9	96.8	83.5	63.6	54.4	54.1	52.7	52.2	50.1	52.2	48.5	48.1	47.5	47.6	46.7
Breast[5]	272.0	463.2	451.6	398.6	332.6	295.4	285.9	274.0	269.2	269.6	262.4	259.4	256.0	250.0	245.9	241.9
Chronic lower respiratory diseases	217.1	169.1	187.4	190.4	188.1	180.1	169.7	170.5	179.8	177.2	172.4	174.7	171.6	176.6	174.1	175.9
Influenza and pneumonia	81.7	160.2	141.5	126.9	87.1	83.6	76.5	71.6	80.7	108.7	71.4	81.8	67.4	82.3	93.3	74.2
Chronic liver disease and cirrhosis	205.9	300.3	196.9	173.7	164.1	152.5	149.8	157.3	158.7	160.1	163.9	169.1	173.3	176.9	180.7	190.3
Diabetes mellitus[6]	200.8	134.4	155.9	174.7	178.4	179.4	176.0	169.3	164.4	161.2	158.2	167.6	164.3	168.3	170.8	176.2
Alzheimer's disease	17.1	V	V	V	10.9	11.7	11.7	11.9	12.3	11.4	11.7	11.5	11.0	11.1	11.4	13.0
Human immunodeficiency virus (HIV) disease	50.2														55.0	50.4
Unintentional injuries	1,139.2	1,543.5	1,162.1	1,057.2	1,026.5	1,137.2	1,173.3	1,162.1	1,095.8	1,028.2	1,025.2	1,056.8	1,046.1	1,051.2	1,080.1	1,172.0
Motor vehicle-related injuries	394.4	912.9	716.4	616.3	574.3	565.9	563.0	538.4	473.2	421.7	400.6	394.8	402.4	386.6	383.0	404.9
Poisoning	510.4	68.0	81.2	123.1	163.6	289.1	335.1	356.1	364.0	365.7	379.7	414.8	408.8	430.9	465.8	531.2
Nephritis, nephrotic syndrome and nephrosis[6]	79.6	NA	50.4	47.5	70.7	74.2	76.5	74.8	75.5	75.7	73.1	65.0	65.2	65.7	66.7	69.3
Suicide[7]	418.7	392.0	393.1	384.7	334.5	348.9	350.6	358.6	367.4	372.5	385.2	395.6	402.1	401.6	413.6	428.6
Homicide[7]	241.8	425.5	417.4	378.6	266.5	278.2	283.4	279.0	267.6	248.0	239.0	236.2	240.9	229.8	224.5	251.9
MALE																
All causes	8,960.1	13,777.2	11,973.5	11,289.2	9,572.2	9,244.2	9,130.1	8,945.0	8,764.7	8,560.7	8,329.5	8,304.1	8,249.1	8,249.5	8,276.4	8,474.7
Diseases of heart	1,482.8	3,352.1	2,356.0	2,117.4	1,766.0	1,559.0	1,514.5	1,463.3	1,433.5	1,399.2	1,370.8	1,351.1	1,336.6	1,338.2	1,326.9	1,327.6
Ischemic heart disease	895.4	2,715.1	1,766.3	1,531.5	1,255.4	1,040.6	1,005.2	956.9	927.8	886.5	864.8	848.6	831.8	816.2	797.6	784.1
Cerebrovascular diseases	204.3	396.7	286.6	276.9	244.6	213.3	211.5	205.4	197.7	195.7	190.7	185.3	183.7	182.1	184.9	183.1
Malignant neoplasms	1,583.8	2,360.8	2,214.6	2,008.5	1,810.8	1,632.9	1,587.4	1,554.7	1,540.7	1,515.6	1,500.8	1,467.6	1,450.9	1,415.9	1,396.9	1,365.3
Trachea, bronchus, and lung	385.2	821.1	764.8	645.6	554.9	472.8	450.6	429.5	418.8	403.4	390.5	374.0	361.1	345.1	331.8	315.8
Colorectal	161.7	214.9	194.3	179.4	167.3	145.7	144.7	147.6	148.8	145.6	148.0	146.0	144.4	146.8	144.3	144.2
Prostate	59.1	84.9	96.8	83.5	63.6	54.4	54.1	52.7	52.2	50.1	52.2	48.5	48.1	47.5	47.6	46.7
Chronic lower respiratory diseases	221.5	235.1	224.8	213.1	206.0	194.3	180.8	185.6	192.2	186.9	182.8	185.5	179.7	185.2	182.8	184.5
Influenza and pneumonia	92.9	202.5	180.0	155.7	102.8	98.0	89.0	83.6	91.7	119.5	82.6	93.5	77.5	94.1	103.7	85.6
Chronic liver disease and cirrhosis	270.8	415.0	283.9	254.8	236.9	216.4	211.1	222.4	223.2	222.8	226.9	228.9	237.2	242.1	242.6	252.5
Diabetes mellitus[6]	245.9	140.4	170.4	194.6	203.8	216.1	212.8	206.3	200.7	201.2	194.8	206.4	203.5	208.6	214.0	220.7
Alzheimer's disease	14.7	V	V	V	10.6	10.8	11.4	11.0	11.5	11.0	10.7	10.6	10.2	10.2	10.3	11.7
Human immunodeficiency virus (HIV) disease	72.8	X	686.2	991.2	258.9	194.0	180.3	162.6	141.0	126.7	109.5	94.8	87.0	84.3	79.0	72.7
Unintentional injuries	1,608.3	2,342.7	1,715.1	1,531.6	1,475.6	1,622.6	1,675.9	1,652.0	1,562.6	1,449.8	1,432.1	1,472.5	1,459.7	1,463.5	1,509.6	1,642.4
Motor vehicle-related injuries	571.5	1,359.7	1,018.4	851.1	796.4	802.0	797.8	771.0	683.8	600.5	569.2	563.5	574.3	552.2	550.4	579.7
Poisoning	697.2	96.4	123.6	193.1	242.1	400.4	468.1	486.4	499.6	493.0	503.8	550.6	541.5	573.1	623.8	722.2
Nephritis, nephrotic syndrome and nephrosis[6]	90.7	NA	58.9	55.6	81.1	85.8	89.7	84.6	86.9	86.5	82.3	75.6	75.3	75.3	78.6	80.3
Suicide[7]	643.4	605.6	634.8	628.4	539.1	553.4	555.0	566.6	578.6	585.6	607.0	618.4	625.9	619.8	635.1	654.2
Homicide[7]	397.5	675.0	658.0	589.6	410.5	443.6	452.0	443.2	426.6	390.3	380.3	373.7	383.6	365.9	357.3	407.0
FEMALE																
All causes	5,481.1	7,350.3	6,333.1	6,057.5	5,644.6	5,429.0	5,365.9	5,267.2	5,188.6	5,143.7	4,994.0	5,000.3	4,959.6	4,967.9	4,999.8	5,070.7
Diseases of heart	701.5	1,246.0	948.5	883.9	774.6	680.2	658.1	634.2	633.2	606.5	593.6	592.5	585.4	584.5	595.2	603.4
Ischemic heart disease	351.6	852.1	600.3	537.8	457.6	377.2	358.7	337.3	338.0	312.7	305.2	300.2	299.3	290.0	290.2	289.7
Cerebrovascular diseases	161.8	324.0	235.9	218.7	203.9	173.9	169.2	163.5	159.4	151.1	149.1	143.9	140.7	135.4	136.5	140.1
Malignant neoplasms	1,419.2	1,896.8	1,826.6	1,698.9	1,555.3	1,419.0	1,393.1	1,361.9	1,325.8	1,322.6	1,301.0	1,284.0	1,271.0	1,250.3	1,232.6	1,209.8
Trachea, bronchus, and lung	299.3	310.4	382.2	365.2	342.1	315.2	307.8	303.1	287.7	285.0	276.9	267.9	262.8	255.1	247.1	234.4
Colorectal	119.6	168.7	138.7	127.5	118.7	104.5	107.9	105.9	106.2	104.5	103.4	103.5	102.8	101.5	101.4	103.6
Breast	272.0	463.2	451.6	398.6	332.6	295.4	285.9	274.0	269.2	269.6	262.4	259.4	256.0	250.0	245.9	241.9
Chronic lower respiratory diseases	212.8	114.0	155.9	171.0	172.3	167.2	159.5	156.7	168.5	168.3	162.8	164.7	164.1	168.7	166.1	167.9
Influenza and pneumonia	70.7	122.0	106.2	100.2	72.3	69.9	64.7	60.1	70.3	98.4	60.7	70.7	57.8	70.9	83.4	63.1
Chronic liver disease and cirrhosis	141.6	194.5	115.1	96.6	94.5	91.4	91.1	95.0	96.9	99.9	103.5	111.9	111.9	114.4	121.5	130.6
Diabetes mellitus[6]	156.0	128.5	142.3	155.9	154.4	144.5	141.1	134.1	129.9	123.2	123.5	130.8	127.0	129.8	129.6	133.8
Alzheimer's disease	19.5	V	V	V	11.1	12.5	11.9	12.7	13.0	11.8	12.6	12.4	11.8	12.0	12.5	14.1
Human immunodeficiency virus (HIV) disease	27.8	X	87.8	205.7	92.0	76.4	74.7	70.1	60.5	52.7	44.4	41.9	37.2	32.5	31.6	28.7
Unintentional injuries	673.6	755.3	607.4	580.1	573.2	647.9	666.3	668.5	625.8	604.6	616.4	638.5	629.6	635.7	647.5	698.3
Motor vehicle-related injuries	218.7	470.4	411.6	378.4	348.5	326.4	324.9	302.8	260.1	241.3	230.5	224.4	228.7	219.0	213.6	228.1
Poisoning	325.0	40.2	39.1	53.6	85.0	177.3	201.4	225.0	227.6	237.8	255.1	278.0	275.1	287.7	306.6	338.9
Nephritis, nephrotic syndrome and nephrosis[6]	68.7	NA	42.4	40.0	60.8	63.3	64.0	65.7	64.8	65.5	64.6	55.0	55.6	56.6	55.3	58.8
Suicide[7]	195.7	184.2	153.3	140.8	129.1	144.1	145.8	150.4	156.2	159.6	163.7	172.3	177.6	182.5	191.2	201.7
Homicide[7]	87.3	181.3	174.3	163.2	118.9	108.8	110.5	111.0	105.1	102.8	94.9	95.5	94.9	90.4	88.7	93.1
WHITE[8]																
All causes	7,090.6	9,554.1	8,159.5	7,744.9	6,949.5	6,823.2	6,763.4	6,664.3	6,590.9	6,486.5	6,342.8	6,365.7	6,321.6	6,338.2	6,390.1	6,514.8
Diseases of heart	1,056.0	2,100.8	1,490.3	1,353.0	1,149.4	1,012.4	987.0	952.8	941.9	912.2	900.9	895.3	882.5	881.8	883.0	889.0
Ischemic heart disease	635.4	1,682.7	1,113.4	975.2	805.3	671.4	647.8	616.4	606.6	573.7	563.7	553.3	544.8	532.0	524.8	519.2

NA = Not available.
V = Data for Alzheimer's disease are only presented for data years 1999 and beyond due to large differences in death rates caused by changes in the coding of the causes of death between ICD-9 and ICD-10.
X = Not applicable.
* = Figure does not meet standards of reliability or precision.
[1]Underlying cause of death code was coded according to the 9th Revision of the International Classification of Diseases (ICD) in 1980-1998.
[2]Age-adjusted rates are calculated using the year 2000 standard population. Prior to 2001, age-adjusted rates were calculated using standard million proportions based on rounded population numbers. Starting with 2001 data, unrounded population numbers are used to calculate age-adjusted rates.
[3]Starting with 1999 data, cause of death is coded according to ICD-10.
[4]Rate for male population only.
[5]Rate for female population only.
[6]Starting with 2011 data, the rules for selecting Renal failure as the underlying cause of death were changed, affecting the number of deaths in the Nephritis, nephrotic syndrome and nephrosis and Diabetes categories. These changes directly affect deaths with mention of Renal failure and other associated conditions, such as Diabetes mellitus with renal complications. The result is a decrease in the number of deaths for Nephritis, nephrotic syndrome and nephrosis and an increase in the number of deaths for Diabetes mellitus. Therefore, trend data for these two causes of death should be interpreted with caution.
[7]Figures for 2001 include September 11th-related deaths for which death certificates were filed as of October 24, 2002.
[8]The race groups, White, Black, Asian or Pacific Islander, and American Indian or Alaska Native, include persons of Hispanic and non-Hispanic origin. Persons of Hispanic origin may be of any race. Death rates for the American Indian or Alaska Native, Asian or Pacific Islander, and Hispanic populations are known to be Indian or Alaska Native, Asian or Pacific Islander, and Hispanic populations are known to be underestimated.

Table 2-25. Years of Potential Life Lost Before Age 75 for Selected Causes of Death, by Sex, Race, and Hispanic Origin, Selected Years, 1980–2015—*Continued*

(Years lost before 75 per 100,000 population.)

Sex, race, Hispanic origin, and cause of death[1]	Crude	Age-adjusted[2]														
	2015[3]	1980[2]	1990[2]	1995[2]	2000[3]	2005[3]	2006[3]	2007[3]	2008[3]	2009[3]	2010[3]	2011[3]	2012[3]	2013[3]	2014[3]	2015[3]
Cerebrovascular diseases	163.3	300.7	213.1	205.2	187.1	160.5	158.3	154.1	149.5	147.2	142.7	139.5	138.7	135.1	138.1	137.9
Malignant neoplasms	1,549.3	2,035.9	1,929.3	1,780.5	1,627.8	1,485.8	1,456.8	1,427.3	1,404.5	1,396.1	1,375.8	1,351.9	1,340.7	1,317.7	1,301.5	1,274.9
Trachea, bronchus, and lung	365.1	529.9	544.2	487.1	436.3	388.1	373.4	363.1	351.9	343.7	332.8	320.5	311.4	300.4	291.0	277.8
Colorectal	140.7	186.8	157.8	145.0	134.1	117.3	118.9	119.6	120.0	118.6	118.4	117.9	117.9	118.6	117.6	119.3
Prostate[4]	55.2	74.8	86.6	73.0	54.3	46.6	46.8	45.6	45.6	42.6	45.3	41.7	42.1	41.9	41.8	40.9
Breast5	263.7	460.2	441.7	381.5	315.6	275.2	269.3	256.9	253.5	255.7	245.0	241.6	239.3	236.0	230.3	226.7
Chronic lower respiratory diseases	236.7	165.4	182.3	185.7	185.3	181.5	171.2	173.1	182.9	180.4	176.1	178.3	175.3	180.1	178.7	180.1
Influenza and pneumonia	79.6	130.8	116.9	108.3	77.7	76.7	70.8	65.6	74.6	103.4	66.7	77.1	63.2	78.4	90.1	70.2
Chronic liver disease and cirrhosis	228.2	257.3	175.8	164.6	162.7	157.2	156.0	164.3	166.8	169.0	173.5	179.6	185.9	189.3	195.1	206.3
Diabetes mellitus[6]	186.5	115.7	133.7	149.4	155.6	156.3	153.0	147.7	145.6	142.7	139.0	148.7	145.4	149.2	152.6	157.5
Alzheimer's disease	19.2	V	V	V	11.4	12.3	12.4	12.6	13.0	12.1	12.4	12.3	11.7	11.8	12.0	13.6
Human immunodeficiency virus (HIV) disease	27.6	X	309.0	422.6	94.7	70.5	65.4	58.8	51.8	44.5	39.9	36.1	32.8	31.5	30.2	27.3
Unintentional injuries	1,208.7	1,520.4	1,139.7	1,040.9	1,031.8	1,183.1	1,225.2	1,223.0	1,167.6	1,092.1	1,098.6	1,134.9	1,119.7	1,125.2	1,156.4	1,258.9
Motor vehicle-related injuries	398.5	939.9	726.7	623.6	586.1	591.1	587.2	563.4	497.3	438.5	419.0	413.1	420.1	401.2	395.9	415.4
Poisoning	578.7	64.9	74.4	115.4	167.2	314.4	366.0	397.4	412.4	415.7	435.4	475.3	467.6	493.0	534.7	610.6
Nephritis, nephrotic syndrome and nephrosis[6]	66.5	NA	37.0	36.1	52.5	56.5	58.8	57.7	58.8	59.4	57.4	50.9	51.1	52.7	53.6	55.2
Suicide[7]	469.3	414.5	417.7	411.6	362.0	385.1	388.3	398.5	409.4	417.1	430.8	444.8	450.8	451.2	468.3	484.7
Homicide[7]	127.3	271.7	234.9	220.2	156.6	161.7	162.4	164.7	160.9	147.6	138.7	135.5	135.9	127.7	125.7	135.9
BLACK OR AFRICAN AMERICAN[8]																
All causes	9,764.6	17,873.4	16,593.0	15,809.7	12,897.1	11,788.4	11,515.2	11,098.2	10,611.2	10,319.6	9,832.5	9,659.5	9,555.7	9,528.5	9,490.6	9,702.3
Diseases of heart	1,613.8	3,619.9	2,891.8	2,681.8	2,275.2	2,011.1	1,929.1	1,859.8	1,813.4	1,766.6	1,691.1	1,647.8	1,645.0	1,647.0	1,638.9	1,637.9
Ischemic heart disease	737.4	2,305.1	1,676.1	1,510.2	1,300.1	1,058.3	1,009.8	945.0	905.2	859.5	818.8	803.3	792.0	776.7	756.5	740.4
Cerebrovascular diseases	318.0	883.2	656.4	583.6	507.0	434.1	422.8	406.0	386.6	362.3	358.1	338.0	326.5	319.2	322.3	322.9
Malignant neoplasms	1,610.4	2,946.1	2,894.8	2,597.1	2,294.7	2,030.4	1,957.5	1,913.4	1,864.2	1,823.3	1,796.7	1,770.5	1,724.1	1,666.7	1,651.6	1,598.8
Trachea, bronchus, and lung	328.8	776.0	811.3	683.0	593.0	500.4	483.4	456.3	426.7	417.6	405.6	387.2	377.5	362.4	340.8	318.3
Colorectal	171.3	232.3	241.8	226.9	222.4	195.7	194.4	193.9	192.8	185.3	188.6	185.3	177.0	174.2	176.5	172.9
Prostate[4]	102.4	200.3	223.5	210.0	171.0	139.6	134.2	132.1	125.6	129.6	127.3	120.1	113.6	109.9	109.0	106.9
Breast[5]	378.6	524.2	592.9	577.4	500.0	480.1	444.0	437.7	421.6	415.1	420.8	420.2	406.2	389.8	386.7	379.2
Chronic lower respiratory diseases	201.7	203.7	240.6	244.0	232.7	207.4	193.6	188.0	197.9	195.9	187.7	192.7	192.8	200.1	193.6	198.3
Influenza and pneumonia	114.9	384.9	330.8	269.8	161.2	143.7	125.8	121.6	129.4	152.2	109.8	123.4	106.2	122.9	130.9	114.5
Chronic liver disease and cirrhosis	121.6	644.0	371.8	250.3	185.6	136.0	124.3	126.9	122.1	119.7	120.2	123.1	116.2	122.4	120.4	122.5
Diabetes mellitus[6]	325.5	305.3	361.5	400.8	383.4	373.1	367.6	349.6	323.2	317.0	316.4	324.1	316.6	323.8	321.4	329.6
Alzheimer's disease	12.6	V	V	V	8.3	10.9	10.2	9.6	10.8	10.4	10.0	10.0	9.3	9.8	11.2	13.0
Human immunodeficiency virus (HIV) disease	192.4	X	1,014.7	1,945.4	763.3	590.3	561.1	514.8	435.4	397.3	329.5	287.8	259.0	238.4	222.9	203.5
Unintentional injuries	1,081.0	1,751.5	1,392.7	1,272.1	1,152.8	1,129.7	1,163.6	1,106.2	979.2	934.0	896.7	918.4	925.8	953.0	986.8	1,082.6
Motor vehicle-related injuries	457.4	750.2	699.5	621.8	580.8	530.4	538.7	516.7	443.6	420.0	393.4	386.6	404.0	402.6	404.6	450.7
Poisoning	326.8	99.4	144.3	209.6	196.6	252.2	293.3	259.8	230.0	221.3	218.9	240.8	242.1	265.6	289.7	342.1
Nephritis, nephrotic syndrome and nephrosis[6]	172.9	NA	160.9	140.0	216.9	214.8	214.5	210.5	206.5	201.5	193.2	174.3	172.4	165.7	167.1	174.6
Suicide[7]	218.5	238.0	261.4	254.2	208.7	193.6	186.5	185.9	195.3	189.1	196.4	202.3	210.4	207.0	209.0	216.1
Homicide[7]	942.0	1,580.8	1,612.9	1,352.8	941.6	967.5	996.2	961.8	897.2	834.8	821.2	813.0	842.9	813.5	785.1	907.4
AMERICAN INDIAN OR ALASKA NATIVE[8]																
All causes	6,895.3	13,390.9	9,506.2	9,332.5	7,758.2	7,705.7	7,449.2	7,233.7	7,121.7	7,000.8	6,771.3	6,712.5	6,842.6	6,698.8	6,954.0	7,176.2
Diseases of heart	770.5	1,819.9	1,391.0	1,296.3	1,030.1	945.6	927.9	887.0	853.9	839.3	820.6	796.0	797.4	807.4	822.2	850.0
Ischemic heart disease	437.5	1,208.2	901.8	877.3	709.3	591.1	572.7	536.8	510.2	502.3	487.6	484.2	486.4	484.4	492.0	487.5
Cerebrovascular diseases	124.3	269.3	223.3	255.3	198.1	195.8	161.9	153.5	137.3	130.6	129.7	144.3	121.5	124.1	123.2	138.6
Malignant neoplasms	776.0	1,101.3	1,141.1	1,099.5	995.7	1,021.4	913.5	909.3	940.2	925.5	929.5	836.0	856.9	852.4	809.9	848.8
Trachea, bronchus, and lung	148.5	181.1	268.1	267.7	227.8	255.5	213.3	212.8	207.3	196.8	211.0	185.1	188.5	166.0	168.4	166.0
Colorectal	84.1	78.8	82.4	103.5	93.8	102.9	82.5	92.2	107.2	102.5	95.8	104.5	90.0	103.3	90.2	94.5
Prostate[4]	28.3	66.7	42.0	51.1	44.5	36.3	37.6	31.9	41.5	36.2	36.8	30.8	36.7	32.6	39.0	32.6
Breast[5]	119.1	205.5	213.4	195.9	174.1	139.2	158.2	149.0	142.7	135.4	145.0	121.7	120.0	108.5	110.9	129.7
Chronic lower respiratory diseases	147.0	89.3	129.0	145.3	151.8	146.8	134.3	157.6	156.1	138.4	154.5	137.6	133.2	135.6	140.5	158.2
Influenza and pneumonia	69.5	307.9	206.3	199.7	124.0	102.5	89.4	94.1	141.5	174.5	99.3	100.5	80.8	109.0	129.0	75.5
Chronic liver disease and cirrhosis	543.8	1,190.3	535.1	604.8	519.4	459.3	433.2	509.7	504.0	477.1	510.8	518.8	553.3	562.2	549.9	605.3
Diabetes mellitus[6]	269.5	305.5	292.3	360.6	305.6	327.7	301.7	268.3	264.5	260.4	267.6	297.1	286.4	281.7	279.4	300.7
Alzheimer's disease	4.3	V	V	V	*	*	*	9.9	5.8	6.7	8.8	7.7	6.2	5.7	6.7	5.3
Human immunodeficiency virus (HIV) disease	33.2	X	70.1	246.9	68.4	81.4	67.4	69.3	57.3	49.5	46.1	32.1	32.1	33.8	29.5	36.2
Unintentional injuries	1,512.5	3,541.0	2,183.9	1,980.9	1,700.1	1,670.0	1,637.4	1,581.6	1,482.0	1,481.4	1,377.7	1,437.1	1,505.2	1,388.2	1,509.3	1,523.6
Motor vehicle-related injuries	652.8	2,102.4	1,301.5	1,210.3	1,032.2	894.0	891.4	790.8	698.6	667.4	570.6	614.2	637.0	575.7	605.4	638.0
Poisoning	516.1	92.9	119.5	161.5	180.1	302.0	317.6	359.3	433.5	479.0	449.6	479.1	514.1	487.3	537.8	543.5
Nephritis, nephrotic syndrome and nephrosis[6]	67.2	NA	88.5	70.3	102.0	94.6	112.2	85.9	94.9	92.3	81.7	68.3	67.5	73.7	80.5	74.1
Suicide[7]	513.0	515.0	495.9	445.2	403.1	446.5	427.4	403.5	411.9	415.3	437.9	423.4	437.6	463.0	437.1	497.7
Homicide[7]	263.2	628.9	434.2	432.7	278.5	298.4	284.7	237.4	264.2	253.3	256.4	234.4	244.5	227.8	239.0	256.2
ASIAN OR PACIFIC ISLANDER[8]																
All causes	3,073.6	5,378.4	4,705.2	4,333.2	3,811.1	3,433.5	3,361.3	3,262.2	3,154.7	3,114.2	3,061.2	3,014.4	3,049.4	3,050.9	2,954.4	3,049.7
Diseases of heart	414.8	952.8	702.2	664.9	567.9	505.8	465.0	443.0	431.6	433.2	400.1	403.8	404.0	413.1	402.1	400.6
Ischemic heart disease	249.9	697.7	486.6	440.6	381.1	322.5	302.2	289.2	275.4	270.5	250.6	255.7	248.3	250.4	239.8	240.1
Cerebrovascular diseases	133.8	266.9	233.5	220.0	199.4	160.5	161.9	149.6	152.5	141.7	148.3	136.5	136.0	134.3	121.8	129.5

NA = Not available.
V = Data for Alzheimer's disease are only presented for data years 1999 and beyond due to large differences in death rates caused by changes in the coding of the causes of death between ICD-9 and ICD-10.
X = Not applicable.
* = Figure does not meet standards of reliability or precision.
[1]Underlying cause of death code was coded according to the 9th Revision of the International Classification of Diseases (ICD) in 1980-1998.
[2]Age-adjusted rates are calculated using the year 2000 standard population. Prior to 2001, age-adjusted rates were calculated using standard million proportions based on rounded population numbers. Starting with 2001 data, unrounded population numbers are used to calculate age-adjusted rates.
[3]Starting with 1999 data, cause of death is coded according to ICD-10.
[4]Rate for male population only.
[5]Rate for female population only.
[6]Starting with 2011 data, the rules for selecting Renal failure as the underlying cause of death were changed, affecting the number of deaths in the Nephritis, nephrotic syndrome and nephrosis and Diabetes categories. These changes directly affect deaths with mention of Renal failure and other associated conditions, such as Diabetes mellitus with renal complications. The result is a decrease in the number of deaths for Nephritis, nephrotic syndrome and nephrosis and an increase in the number of deaths for Diabetes mellitus. Therefore, trend data for these two causes of death should be interpreted with caution.
[7]Figures for 2001 include September 11th-related deaths for which death certificates were filed as of October 24, 2002.
[8]The race groups, White, Black, Asian or Pacific Islander, and American Indian or Alaska Native, include persons of Hispanic and non-Hispanic origin. Persons of Hispanic origin may be of any race. Death rates for the American Indian or Alaska Native, Asian or Pacific Islander, and Hispanic populations are known to be Indian or Alaska Native, Asian or Pacific Islander, and Hispanic populations are known to be underestimated.

Table 2-25. Years of Potential Life Lost Before Age 75 for Selected Causes of Death, by Sex, Race, and Hispanic Origin, Selected Years, 1980–2015—*Continued*

(Years lost before 75 per 100,000 population.)

Sex, race, Hispanic origin, and cause of death[1]	Crude 2015[3]	Age-adjusted[2]														
		1980[2]	1990[2]	1995[2]	2000[3]	2005[3]	2006[3]	2007[3]	2008[3]	2009[3]	2010[3]	2011[3]	2012[3]	2013[3]	2014[3]	2015[3]
Malignant neoplasms	839.1	1,218.6	1,166.4	1,122.1	1,033.8	931.0	899.0	871.2	854.5	834.4	874.7	853.6	855.5	830.7	799.4	809.9
Trachea, bronchus, and lung	137.1	238.2	204.7	197.0	185.8	167.1	169.3	158.9	156.2	144.6	148.2	146.6	145.2	136.7	136.5	130.5
Colorectal	84.0	115.9	105.1	99.5	91.6	77.7	80.3	80.2	83.7	78.3	87.6	84.5	85.6	87.0	79.1	80.8
Prostate[4]	18.6	17.0	32.4	25.3	18.8	20.3	18.1	16.3	16.1	16.3	17.0	18.2	14.7	14.4	16.8	18.6
Breast[5]	165.6	222.2	216.5	237.8	200.8	175.0	169.7	151.0	155.2	149.7	156.9	156.5	161.7	146.5	160.6	155.1
Chronic lower respiratory diseases	29.1	56.4	72.8	65.8	56.5	35.4	36.6	34.8	33.8	34.3	33.2	34.2	30.6	35.0	32.7	28.0
Influenza and pneumonia	36.5	79.3	74.0	64.3	48.6	39.3	36.0	35.5	39.9	61.5	38.4	43.3	33.5	36.4	42.8	36.1
Chronic liver disease and cirrhosis	45.5	85.6	72.4	48.4	44.8	43.2	44.0	40.5	40.6	45.2	41.7	40.9	37.8	42.9	41.6	44.0
Diabetes mellitus[6]	78.9	83.1	74.0	83.5	77.0	77.1	79.7	77.5	74.9	72.8	69.5	72.3	77.0	74.0	73.8	75.4
Alzheimer's disease	4.4	V	V	V	3.5	3.1	2.0	2.8	3.4	2.3	3.2	2.7	3.8	3.6	2.6	4.3
Human immunodeficiency virus (HIV) disease	11.2	X	77.0	110.4	19.9	16.6	15.4	14.6	18.0	11.6	10.7	10.0	9.9	11.2	9.8	11.0
Unintentional injuries	336.8	742.7	636.6	525.7	425.7	393.5	389.4	385.3	332.3	308.0	303.0	306.6	311.8	308.5	307.0	328.6
Motor vehicle-related injuries	144.3	472.6	445.5	351.9	263.4	228.9	229.0	210.7	184.2	154.0	147.9	138.5	135.9	136.5	141.2	140.4
Poisoning	89.6	*	17.6	24.5	25.9	40.6	45.1	49.8	43.7	50.5	46.5	62.9	64.9	71.5	67.6	84.3
Nephritis, nephrotic syndrome and nephrosis[6]	33.6	NA	26.7	23.8	33.6	31.5	36.2	31.8	33.9	35.5	38.1	26.7	29.9	31.1	29.1	32.3
Suicide[7]	229.9	217.1	200.6	211.1	168.6	158.0	175.8	190.3	170.4	182.0	199.7	190.2	207.6	206.0	203.1	222.0
Homicide[7]	61.5	201.1	205.8	202.3	113.1	123.3	113.8	89.4	85.6	80.0	68.8	78.0	68.3	64.4	59.7	60.6

HISPANIC OR LATINO[8,9]

All causes	4,452.8	NA	7,963.3	7,426.7	6,037.6	5,701.3	5,556.2	5,377.7	5,153.6	5,055.4	4,795.1	4,681.7	4,678.4	4,668.1	4,676.8	4,750.4
Diseases of heart	474.5	NA	1,082.0	962.0	821.3	726.9	687.8	664.6	629.0	630.2	598.1	585.0	570.7	571.0	567.9	578.0
Ischemic heart disease	268.9	NA	756.6	665.8	564.6	483.5	447.0	417.0	396.6	381.9	366.6	351.7	341.7	340.0	334.1	339.9
Cerebrovascular diseases	116.9	NA	238.0	232.0	207.8	184.8	184.6	175.4	162.5	155.8	150.4	149.0	144.3	145.5	140.2	141.1
Malignant neoplasms	752.0	NA	1,232.2	1,172.0	1,098.2	1,016.7	988.5	986.6	971.7	955.1	951.2	925.6	947.3	927.9	909.3	900.6
Trachea, bronchus, and lung	74.6	NA	193.7	173.9	152.1	138.2	125.1	125.7	122.9	117.4	115.0	108.6	107.3	102.9	96.8	96.9
Colorectal	75.5	NA	100.2	97.9	101.4	86.5	91.7	92.6	92.8	92.3	94.0	88.7	86.7	92.8	87.4	92.4
Prostate[4]	26.0	NA	47.7	60.8	42.9	42.1	44.3	43.9	41.5	37.3	38.2	38.1	37.0	35.9	36.5	37.8
Breast[5]	143.0	NA	299.3	257.7	230.7	194.9	200.6	190.7	184.0	186.0	180.0	176.2	192.5	181.2	183.4	169.0
Chronic lower respiratory diseases	44.3	NA	78.8	82.1	68.5	62.2	56.9	56.2	59.1	58.6	59.6	54.3	53.2	56.2	52.7	54.3
Influenza and pneumonia	47.9	NA	130.1	108.5	76.0	69.1	64.8	54.7	65.8	114.1	57.5	59.3	53.1	64.3	79.1	54.3
Chronic liver disease and cirrhosis	182.7	NA	329.1	281.4	252.1	210.7	202.2	210.2	208.4	207.5	201.6	209.3	209.5	206.1	216.4	219.2
Diabetes mellitus[6]	130.9	NA	177.8	228.8	215.6	202.4	181.4	178.1	171.8	161.6	158.5	160.2	160.0	161.6	160.9	163.1
Alzheimer's disease	6.8	NA	V	V	6.9	7.8	8.9	7.7	8.5	7.2	8.4	8.2	7.7	8.5	8.9	10.2
Human immunodeficiency virus (HIV) disease	41.6	X	600.1	865.0	209.4	140.2	130.2	115.9	98.5	86.5	74.9	69.5	55.2	52.5	49.5	47.0
Unintentional injuries	827.8	NA	1,190.6	1,017.9	920.1	966.1	980.6	907.4	812.0	755.5	708.7	727.9	719.5	735.9	740.1	808.7
Motor vehicle-related injuries	392.1	NA	740.8	593.0	540.2	558.0	553.9	493.3	414.2	379.5	340.3	334.3	346.0	344.8	348.3	370.7
Poisoning	263.2	NA	121.9	173.9	145.9	179.5	196.4	200.4	200.5	194.7	191.2	213.1	207.7	224.3	234.1	269.1
Nephritis, nephrotic syndrome and nephrosis[6]	49.0	NA	54.4	35.3	62.0	65.9	69.6	68.9	69.2	73.5	67.7	56.3	57.1	57.5	56.3	60.1
Suicide[7]	221.6	NA	256.2	245.1	188.5	190.9	183.2	196.5	179.9	191.9	193.6	195.0	198.1	195.6	214.3	215.4
Homicide[7]	229.1	NA	720.8	575.4	335.1	336.2	328.1	311.5	289.7	267.9	238.0	221.5	215.4	199.3	197.6	213.5

WHITE, NOT HISPANIC OR LATINO[9]

All causes	7,661.5	NA	8,022.5	7,607.5	6,960.5	6,903.8	6,863.2	6,791.1	6,753.3	6,643.9	6,545.3	6,614.9	6,560.4	6,593.2	6,659.4	6,799.9
Diseases of heart	1,193.0	NA	1,504.0	1,368.2	1,175.1	1,045.9	1,023.4	988.3	982.9	948.9	943.2	939.9	929.3	930.5	932.4	939.2
Ischemic heart disease	721.6	NA	1,127.2	988.7	824.7	692.9	671.9	641.7	633.6	598.9	590.8	582.3	574.7	560.9	553.6	546.4
Cerebrovascular diseases	172.0	NA	210.1	199.6	183.0	155.5	154.2	149.2	145.0	143.3	139.1	135.5	135.2	130.3	134.9	134.1
Malignant neoplasms	1,737.4	NA	1,974.1	1,814.2	1,668.4	1,532.2	1,503.3	1,471.1	1,447.7	1,443.8	1,421.5	1,400.2	1,383.3	1,362.2	1,349.1	1,320.0
Trachea, bronchus, and lung	439.1	NA	566.8	507.0	460.3	414.5	400.3	389.8	378.3	370.5	359.1	347.4	337.7	327.2	318.6	304.0
Colorectal	155.7	NA	162.1	147.8	136.2	120.6	121.6	122.6	123.2	121.7	121.2	122.2	124.4	122.1	122.3	123.0
Prostate[4]	62.4	NA	89.2	73.6	54.9	46.8	47.0	45.6	45.9	43.0	45.9	41.9	42.4	42.3	42.2	41.0
Breast[5]	291.1	NA	451.5	389.3	322.3	283.8	275.8	263.4	260.5	264.0	252.6	249.0	243.5	242.3	235.4	234.1
Chronic lower respiratory diseases	285.4	NA	188.1	190.6	193.8	192.9	182.2	185.2	195.8	193.3	189.1	193.4	190.0	195.9	195.9	197.1
Influenza and pneumonia	86.3	NA	112.3	105.8	76.4	77.1	70.7	66.9	75.7	98.0	67.8	79.8	64.5	80.5	91.1	72.3
Chronic liver disease and cirrhosis	234.4	NA	162.4	151.4	150.9	148.0	147.6	155.8	158.7	160.6	166.9	172.6	179.6	183.9	188.6	200.7
Diabetes mellitus[6]	197.1	NA	131.2	142.8	150.2	151.4	150.0	144.3	142.5	139.8	136.7	147.4	143.0	147.0	150.6	156.2
Alzheimer's disease	22.2	NA	V	V	11.7	12.6	12.6	13.1	13.4	12.5	12.7	12.6	12.1	12.1	12.3	13.8
Human immunodeficiency virus (HIV) disease	22.4	X	271.2	362.1	76.0	57.0	52.0	46.2	41.3	34.7	31.3	27.8	26.9	25.7	24.7	21.1
Unintentional injuries	1,285.9	NA	1,114.7	1,026.1	1,041.4	1,214.1	1,263.4	1,282.1	1,240.1	1,157.4	1,183.0	1,227.3	1,210.5	1,214.6	1,253.8	1,365.1
Motor vehicle-related injuries	390.8	NA	715.7	618.0	588.8	586.9	583.4	569.7	508.9	441.9	430.6	426.3	431.0	407.4	398.9	417.6
Poisoning	652.3	NA	68.3	105.4	169.4	342.2	403.3	442.2	461.2	467.6	494.0	540.8	533.1	561.8	613.2	700.8
Nephritis, nephrotic syndrome and nephrosis[6]	69.8	NA	34.5	35.7	51.1	54.9	57.1	56.0	57.0	56.6	55.3	49.5	49.8	51.2	52.7	53.7
Suicide[7]	529.2	NA	433.0	427.7	389.2	421.2	427.9	439.5	458.3	465.2	483.8	502.5	510.2	512.9	531.3	554.1
Homicide[7]	96.1	NA	162.0	148.6	113.2	110.7	111.6	117.4	118.5	105.1	103.4	103.4	106.6	100.6	98.4	106.2

NA = Not available.
V = Data for Alzheimer's disease are only presented for data years 1999 and beyond due to large differences in death rates caused by changes in the coding of the causes of death between ICD-9 and ICD-10.
X = Not applicable.
* = Figure does not meet standards of reliability or precision.
[1]Underlying cause of death code was coded according to the 9th Revision of the International Classification of Diseases (ICD) in 1980-1998.
[2]Age-adjusted rates are calculated using the year 2000 standard population. Prior to 2001, age-adjusted rates were calculated using standard million proportions based on rounded population numbers. Starting with 2001 data, unrounded population numbers are used to calculate age-adjusted rates.
[3]Starting with 1999 data, cause of death is coded according to ICD-10.
[4]Rate for male population only.
[5]Rate for female population only.
[6]Starting with 2011 data, the rules for selecting Renal failure as the underlying cause of death were changed, affecting the number of deaths in the Nephritis, nephrotic syndrome and nephrosis and Diabetes categories. These changes directly affect deaths with mention of Renal failure and other associated conditions, such as Diabetes mellitus with renal complications. The result is a decrease in the number of deaths for Nephritis, nephrotic syndrome and nephrosis and an increase in the number of deaths for Diabetes mellitus. Therefore, trend data for these two causes of death should be interpreted with caution.
[7]Figures for 2001 include September 11th-related deaths for which death certificates were filed as of October 24, 2002.
[8]The race groups, White, Black, Asian or Pacific Islander, and American Indian or Alaska Native, include persons of Hispanic and non-Hispanic origin. Persons of Hispanic origin may be of any race. Death rates for the American Indian or Alaska Native, Asian or Pacific Islander, and Hispanic populations are known to be Indian or Alaska Native, Asian or Pacific Islander, and Hispanic populations are known to be underestimated.
[9]Prior to 1997, excludes data from states lacking an Hispanic origin item on the death certificate.

Table 2-26. Number of Deaths, Death Rates, and Age-Adjusted Death Rates for Major Causes of Death, by State and Territory, 2015

(Number, rates per 100,000 population, age–adjusted rates per 100,000 U.S. standard population.)

State and territory	All causes			Human immunodeficiency virus (HIV) disease (B20–B24)			Malignant neoplasms (C00–C97)			Diabetes mellitus (E10–E14)		
	Number	Rate	Age-adjusted rate[1]	Number	Rate	Age-adjusted rate[1]	Number	Rate	Age-adjusted rate[1]	Number	Rate	Age-adjusted rate[1]
United States[2]	2,712,630	844.0	733.1	6,465	2.0	1.9	595,930	185.4	158.5	79,535	24.7	21.3
Alabama	51,909	1,068.3	924.5	126	2.6	2.5	10,354	213.1	175.6	1,255	25.8	21.7
Alaska	4,316	584.5	747.4	3	*	*	978	132.4	159.8	142	19.2	23.9
Arizona	54,299	795.2	671.8	110	1.6	1.5	11,776	172.5	141.3	2,081	30.5	25.3
Arkansas	31,617	1,061.6	901.8	54	1.8	1.8	6,727	225.9	185.4	886	29.7	24.7
California	259,206	662.2	621.6	710	1.8	1.7	59,629	152.3	142.8	8,845	22.6	21.2
Colorado	36,349	666.2	665.0	56	1.0	1.0	7,604	139.4	134.4	887	16.3	15.9
Connecticut	30,535	850.3	656.1	69	1.9	1.6	6,666	185.6	146.2	653	18.2	13.9
Delaware	8,582	907.3	741.5	31	3.3	2.8	2,010	212.5	165.6	215	22.7	18.1
District of Columbia	4,871	724.6	748.6	70	10.4	10.3	1,072	159.5	167.5	162	24.1	25.7
Florida	191,737	945.9	662.9	873	4.3	3.9	44,027	217.2	150.6	5,403	26.7	18.6
Georgia	79,942	782.6	808.1	377	3.7	3.6	16,945	165.9	163.0	2,210	21.6	21.4
Hawaii	11,053	772.1	588.2	13	*	*	2,462	172.0	135.3	263	18.4	14.5
Idaho	13,026	787.1	727.8	4	*	*	2,849	172.2	153.6	403	24.4	22.1
Illinois	106,872	831.0	728.3	224	1.7	1.6	24,713	192.2	167.6	2,817	21.9	19.2
Indiana	62,713	947.4	833.9	78	1.2	1.2	13,511	204.1	176.3	2,030	30.7	26.9
Iowa	29,600	947.5	724.6	17	*	*	6,513	208.5	164.1	1,077	34.5	26.7
Kansas	26,664	915.8	774.1	28	1.0	0.9	5,604	192.5	164.6	684	23.5	20.2
Kentucky	46,564	1,052.3	924.7	41	0.9	0.9	10,312	233.0	195.9	1,458	32.9	28.2
Louisiana	43,716	936.0	874.2	213	4.6	4.5	9,397	201.2	180.2	1,199	25.7	23.5
Maine	14,479	1,089.2	783.5	8	*	*	3,398	255.6	178.0	407	30.6	21.9
Maryland	47,247	786.6	705.7	193	3.2	2.9	10,568	175.9	155.0	1,243	20.7	18.3
Massachusetts	57,806	850.8	684.8	91	1.3	1.1	12,750	187.7	152.9	1,398	20.6	16.7
Michigan	95,140	958.8	784.4	109	1.1	1.0	20,732	208.9	168.0	2,751	27.7	22.5
Minnesota	42,800	779.7	653.8	30	0.5	0.5	9,925	180.8	153.0	1,221	22.2	18.6
Mississippi	31,783	1,062.1	963.7	107	3.6	3.5	6,485	216.7	188.4	1,092	36.5	32.4
Missouri	59,871	984.1	816.9	52	0.9	0.8	12,965	213.1	173.4	1,468	24.1	19.7
Montana	9,942	962.5	762.7	6	*	*	2,130	206.2	156.9	321	31.1	24.5
Nebraska	16,740	882.8	739.2	12	*	*	3,514	185.3	157.8	553	29.2	24.8
Nevada	22,879	791.4	757.2	53	1.8	1.8	5,015	173.5	157.2	420	14.5	13.4
New Hampshire	11,984	900.6	720.6	10	*	*	2,773	208.4	161.3	308	23.1	17.9
New Jersey	72,271	806.8	666.0	255	2.8	2.5	16,270	181.6	150.8	1,933	21.6	17.9
New Mexico	17,685	848.2	741.5	32	1.5	1.6	3,591	172.2	143.3	608	29.2	24.9
New York	153,628	776.1	644.0	581	2.9	2.6	35,089	177.3	148.4	4,045	20.4	17.1
North Carolina	89,133	887.5	789.9	234	2.3	2.2	19,322	192.4	164.7	2,746	27.3	23.6
North Dakota	6,223	822.1	696.8	4	*	*	1,320	174.4	152.9	195	25.8	22.6
Ohio	118,188	1,017.7	828.4	116	1.0	0.9	25,396	218.7	175.1	3,645	31.4	25.3
Oklahoma	39,422	1,007.9	904.3	66	1.7	1.7	8,280	211.7	184.3	1,442	36.9	32.4
Oregon	35,705	886.2	722.3	46	1.1	1.0	8,093	200.9	160.2	1,148	28.5	22.9
Pennsylvania	132,598	1,035.7	768.3	177	1.4	1.2	28,697	224.2	167.2	3,777	29.5	22.1
Rhode Island	10,163	962.1	721.9	12	*	*	2,226	210.7	163.1	276	26.1	20.2
South Carolina	47,198	964.0	840.0	138	2.8	2.7	9,950	203.2	166.6	1,347	27.5	23.4
South Dakota	7,731	900.6	715.4	2	*	*	1,640	191.0	154.0	282	32.8	26.3
Tennessee	66,570	1,008.6	886.4	158	2.4	2.3	14,214	215.4	180.5	1,798	27.2	23.4
Texas	189,654	690.4	745.0	637	2.3	2.3	39,121	142.4	149.2	5,521	20.1	21.2
Utah	17,334	578.6	712.1	13	*	*	3,091	103.2	125.2	604	20.2	24.6
Vermont	5,919	945.5	714.7	1	*	*	1,399	223.5	165.3	159	25.4	19.8
Virginia	65,577	782.3	721.6	118	1.4	1.3	14,947	178.3	159.5	2,044	24.4	21.9
Washington	54,595	761.4	687.4	61	0.9	0.8	12,687	176.9	156.4	1,811	25.3	22.4
West Virginia	22,752	1,233.8	943.4	15	*	*	4,839	262.4	190.4	784	42.5	31.7
Wisconsin	51,264	888.3	715.9	29	0.5	0.4	11,423	197.9	159.3	1,382	23.9	19.4
Wyoming	4,778	815.2	748.3	2	*	*	931	158.8	139.4	136	23.2	20.8
Puerto Rico	28,085	808.4	624.7	197	5.7	5.3	5,158	148.5	112.4	2,926	84.2	62.8
Virgin Islands	673	649.8	531.0	7	*	*	137	132.3	96.7	38	36.7	29.8
Guam	985	608.8	798.6	2	*	*	189	116.8	146.9	51	31.5	38.6
American Samoa	303	557.6	1,165.0	–	*	*	46	84.6	175.3	47	86.5	172.6
Northern Marianas	223	426.0	876.0	–	*	*	49	93.6	185.2	29	55.4	106.7

- = Quantity zero.
* = Figure does not meet standards of reliability or precision.
[1]Death rates are affected by the population composition of the area. Age-adjusted death rates should be used for comparisons between areas.
[2]Excludes data for Puerto Rico, Virgin Islands, Guam, American Samoa and Northern Marianas.

Table 2-26. Number of Deaths, Death Rates, and Age-Adjusted Death Rates for Major Causes of Death, by State and Territory, 2015—Continued

(Number, rates per 100,000 population, age–adjusted rates per 100,000 U.S. standard population.)

State and territory	Parkinson's disease (G20–G21)			Alzheimer's disease (G30)			Disease of the heart (I00–I09, I11, I13, I20–I51)			Essential hypertension and hypertensive renal disease (I10, I12, I15)		
	Number	Rate	Age-adjusted rate[1]	Number	Rate	Age-adjusted rate[1]	Number	Rate	Age-adjusted rate[1]	Number	Rate	Age-adjusted rate[1]
United States[2]	27,972	8.7	7.7	110,561	34.4	29.4	633,842	197.2	168.5	32,200	10.0	8.5
Alabama	461	9.5	8.4	2,282	47.0	41.8	12,981	267.2	229.7	519	10.7	9.2
Alaska	38	5.1	8.7	68	9.2	16.7	846	114.6	154.1	38	5.1	7.2
Arizona	720	10.5	8.8	2,943	43.1	35.8	11,458	167.8	138.8	963	14.1	11.6
Arkansas	248	8.3	7.0	1,457	48.9	41.5	7,938	266.5	223.2	329	11.0	9.4
California	2,896	7.4	7.2	15,065	38.5	35.7	61,289	156.6	145.6	5,118	13.1	12.1
Colorado	452	8.3	9.0	1,612	29.5	31.3	7,009	128.5	128.4	273	5.0	5.1
Connecticut	334	9.3	7.2	966	26.9	19.0	7,205	200.6	147.8	317	8.8	6.4
Delaware	84	8.9	7.3	264	27.9	22.6	1,940	205.1	165.2	64	6.8	5.4
District of Columbia	33	4.9	5.5	129	19.2	19.2	1,217	181.0	187.6	87	12.9	13.4
Florida	2,228	11.0	7.2	7,031	34.7	21.8	45,441	224.2	149.8	2,187	10.8	7.2
Georgia	733	7.2	8.2	3,714	36.4	42.4	17,769	174.0	180.2	1,076	10.5	10.9
Hawaii	141	9.8	7.3	422	29.5	19.5	2,605	182.0	135.6	86	6.0	4.2
Idaho	169	10.2	9.8	552	33.4	31.6	2,825	170.7	156.4	101	6.1	5.8
Illinois	1,079	8.4	7.6	3,686	28.7	24.4	25,652	199.5	171.5	1,137	8.8	7.6
Indiana	638	9.6	8.7	2,513	38.0	33.1	13,948	210.7	182.3	694	10.5	9.1
Iowa	341	10.9	8.1	1,339	42.9	29.9	6,813	218.1	160.9	390	12.5	8.9
Kansas	326	11.2	9.4	865	29.7	23.5	5,624	193.2	158.5	245	8.4	6.8
Kentucky	395	8.9	8.1	1,694	38.3	34.9	10,077	227.7	197.8	441	10.0	8.8
Louisiana	371	7.9	7.9	2,018	43.2	42.5	10,665	228.3	212.1	369	7.9	7.4
Maine	147	11.1	8.1	544	40.9	28.4	3,009	226.4	157.3	97	7.3	4.9
Maryland	461	7.7	7.2	1,095	18.2	16.4	11,481	191.1	169.3	521	8.7	7.7
Massachusetts	640	9.4	7.8	1,815	26.7	20.2	12,130	178.5	138.5	603	8.9	6.9
Michigan	960	9.7	8.1	3,771	38.0	30.1	24,794	249.9	198.9	922	9.3	7.3
Minnesota	620	11.3	9.6	1,789	32.6	26.0	7,844	142.9	116.6	518	9.4	7.6
Mississippi	247	8.3	7.8	1,402	46.9	44.1	7,969	266.3	240.5	508	17.0	15.3
Missouri	560	9.2	7.7	2,173	35.7	28.7	14,808	243.4	197.9	513	8.4	6.7
Montana	114	11.0	8.5	277	26.8	20.7	2,104	203.7	155.8	61	5.9	4.4
Nebraska	220	11.6	9.8	598	31.5	24.8	3,591	189.4	154.5	247	13.0	10.4
Nevada	213	7.4	7.5	874	30.2	32.9	6,114	211.5	200.9	194	6.7	6.6
New Hampshire	143	10.7	8.9	432	32.5	25.5	2,571	193.2	149.0	89	6.7	5.3
New Jersey	716	8.0	6.6	2,260	25.2	19.8	18,647	208.2	166.7	733	8.2	6.5
New Mexico	172	8.2	7.2	483	23.2	19.9	3,508	168.2	142.4	154	7.4	6.1
New York	1,247	6.3	5.3	3,174	16.0	12.6	44,450	224.5	181.6	2,287	11.6	9.3
North Carolina	897	8.9	8.3	3,803	37.9	34.8	18,474	184.0	162.4	944	9.4	8.3
North Dakota	65	8.6	7.1	376	49.7	36.7	1,323	174.8	142.4	79	10.4	8.3
Ohio	1,139	9.8	8.0	4,643	40.0	31.1	28,069	241.7	191.7	1,395	12.0	9.5
Oklahoma	334	8.5	7.8	1,498	38.3	34.7	10,310	263.6	234.0	502	12.8	11.4
Oregon	429	10.6	8.9	1,652	41.0	33.0	6,859	170.2	136.1	565	14.0	11.1
Pennsylvania	1,348	10.5	7.6	4,012	31.3	21.0	32,042	250.3	177.8	1,108	8.7	6.1
Rhode Island	117	11.1	8.4	453	42.9	28.8	2,371	224.5	160.4	108	10.2	7.1
South Carolina	420	8.6	7.8	2,453	50.1	46.2	10,092	206.1	177.8	482	9.8	8.7
South Dakota	80	9.3	7.2	421	49.0	34.8	1,711	199.3	150.9	104	12.1	8.8
Tennessee	604	9.2	8.4	3,122	47.3	43.4	15,730	238.3	207.3	649	9.8	8.6
Texas	1,983	7.2	8.5	8,903	32.4	38.2	43,298	157.6	171.6	2,089	7.6	8.3
Utah	229	7.6	10.2	906	30.2	40.7	3,598	120.1	152.9	136	4.5	5.7
Vermont	83	13.3	10.2	298	47.6	35.1	1,311	209.4	152.5	57	9.1	6.7
Virginia	638	7.6	7.4	2,248	26.8	25.6	14,077	167.9	154.2	684	8.2	7.5
Washington	654	9.1	8.7	3,490	48.7	44.4	11,025	153.8	137.6	594	8.3	7.4
West Virginia	163	8.8	6.7	738	40.0	30.0	4,727	256.3	191.3	297	16.1	11.9
Wisconsin	600	10.4	8.3	2,087	36.2	27.5	11,473	198.8	156.0	485	8.4	6.6
Wyoming	42	7.2	6.8	151	25.8	24.2	1,030	175.7	159.4	41	7.0	6.4
Puerto Rico	159	4.6	3.4	2,124	61.1	44.7	4,972	143.1	106.7	479	13.8	10.2
Virgin Islands	–	*	*	33	31.9	29.9	133	128.4	97.1	36	34.8	30.1
Guam	6	*	*	8	*	*	303	187.3	260.6	5	*	*
American Samoa	2	*	*	–	*	*	61	112.2	227.7	3	*	*
Northern Marianas	1	*	*	–	*	*	47	89.8	201.1	3	*	*

- = Quantity zero.
* = Figure does not meet standards of reliability or precision.
[1]Death rates are affected by the population composition of the area. Age-adjusted death rates should be used for comparisons between areas.
[2]Excludes data for Puerto Rico, Virgin Islands, Guam, American Samoa and Northern Marianas.

Table 2-26. Number of Deaths, Death Rates, and Age-Adjusted Death Rates for Major Causes of Death, by State and Territory, 2015—*Continued*

(Number, rates per 100,000 population, age–adjusted rates per 100,000 U.S. standard population.)

State and territory	Cerebrovascular disease (I60–I69) Number	Rate	Age-adjusted rate[1]	Influenza and pneumonia (J09–J18) Number	Rate	Age-adjusted rate[1]	Chronic lower respiratory disease (J40–J47) Number	Rate	Age-adjusted rate[1]	Chronic liver disease and cirrhosis (K70,K73–K74) Number	Rate	Age-adjusted rate[1]
United States[2]	140,323	43.7	37.6	57,062	17.8	15.2	155,041	48.2	41.6	40,326	12.5	10.8
Alabama	2,937	60.4	52.2	1,097	22.6	19.5	3,279	67.5	56.4	716	14.7	12.5
Alaska	182	24.6	36.8	41	5.6	8.4	204	27.6	37.8	114	15.4	15.4
Arizona	2,522	36.9	30.7	775	11.4	9.5	3,681	53.9	43.8	1,149	16.8	15.0
Arkansas	1,653	55.5	46.8	700	23.5	20.0	2,270	76.2	62.4	421	14.1	12.1
California	15,065	38.5	36.2	6,188	15.8	14.8	13,621	34.8	33.1	5,425	13.9	12.7
Colorado	1,856	34.0	34.9	659	12.1	12.3	2,577	47.2	47.8	735	13.5	12.2
Connecticut	1,388	38.7	28.5	667	18.6	13.6	1,369	38.1	29.7	365	10.2	8.4
Delaware	466	49.3	39.4	189	20.0	16.1	510	53.9	42.5	111	11.7	9.6
District of Columbia	242	36.0	38.3	104	15.5	16.2	147	21.9	23.4	61	9.1	8.8
Florida	11,433	56.4	37.1	2,676	13.2	8.9	11,705	57.7	38.4	3,084	15.2	11.7
Georgia	4,335	42.4	45.3	1,467	14.4	15.5	4,607	45.1	46.7	1,003	9.8	9.0
Hawaii	735	51.3	38.2	557	38.9	27.4	332	23.2	17.3	138	9.6	8.1
Idaho	641	38.7	36.3	218	13.2	12.4	843	50.9	46.3	218	13.2	12.2
Illinois	5,709	44.4	38.4	2,343	18.2	15.7	5,544	43.1	38.2	1,289	10.0	8.7
Indiana	2,959	44.7	39.1	1,044	15.8	13.9	4,212	63.6	55.4	859	13.0	11.4
Iowa	1,418	45.4	33.2	618	19.8	14.2	2,011	64.4	49.1	328	10.5	9.1
Kansas	1,364	46.8	38.6	682	23.4	18.9	1,704	58.5	49.7	313	10.7	9.7
Kentucky	2,050	46.3	40.8	967	21.9	19.3	3,331	75.3	64.3	657	14.8	12.6
Louisiana	2,280	48.8	46.0	753	16.1	15.3	2,178	46.6	43.2	553	11.8	10.5
Maine	616	46.3	32.6	333	25.1	17.6	1,025	77.1	53.6	195	14.7	11.1
Maryland	2,540	42.3	37.8	1,176	19.6	17.7	2,040	34.0	30.7	471	7.8	6.7
Massachusetts	2,475	36.4	28.4	1,512	22.3	17.1	2,784	41.0	33.0	661	9.7	8.2
Michigan	4,666	47.0	37.6	1,894	19.1	15.2	5,848	58.9	47.5	1,287	13.0	10.8
Minnesota	2,238	40.8	33.5	738	13.4	10.9	2,351	42.8	36.4	542	9.9	8.5
Mississippi	1,734	57.9	52.6	791	26.4	24.0	1,924	64.3	57.1	382	12.8	11.1
Missouri	3,037	49.9	40.8	1,337	22.0	17.9	3,935	64.7	52.8	678	11.1	9.6
Montana	458	44.3	33.8	183	17.7	13.7	679	65.7	50.2	179	17.3	15.7
Nebraska	776	40.9	33.4	397	20.9	16.9	1,174	61.9	52.2	165	8.7	7.8
Nevada	1,078	37.3	37.0	630	21.8	21.3	1,617	55.9	54.1	475	16.4	14.5
New Hampshire	457	34.3	26.9	275	20.7	16.1	705	53.0	41.9	161	12.1	9.3
New Jersey	3,413	38.1	31.1	1,402	15.7	12.5	3,202	35.7	29.6	782	8.7	7.3
New Mexico	786	37.7	32.5	322	15.4	13.6	1,109	53.2	44.7	566	27.1	24.8
New York	6,292	31.8	26.0	4,881	24.7	20.0	7,109	35.9	29.9	1,571	7.9	6.7
North Carolina	5,033	50.1	44.7	2,115	21.1	18.7	5,221	52.0	45.5	1,254	12.5	10.7
North Dakota	308	40.7	33.4	172	22.7	17.7	351	46.4	40.0	86	11.4	11.6
Ohio	5,945	51.2	40.7	2,445	21.1	16.6	7,211	62.1	49.6	1,506	13.0	10.7
Oklahoma	1,881	48.1	43.0	717	18.3	16.5	2,924	74.8	65.8	597	15.3	13.7
Oregon	1,873	46.5	37.5	453	11.2	9.0	2,119	52.6	42.4	667	16.6	13.7
Pennsylvania	6,987	54.6	38.8	2,899	22.6	15.9	6,664	52.1	38.1	1,438	11.2	8.9
Rhode Island	394	37.3	27.1	246	23.3	16.2	510	48.3	36.9	139	13.2	10.6
South Carolina	2,600	53.1	46.7	848	17.3	15.3	2,908	59.4	49.9	716	14.6	12.2
South Dakota	383	44.6	33.2	213	24.8	18.2	502	58.5	45.3	139	16.2	16.1
Tennessee	3,447	52.2	46.0	1,723	26.1	23.3	4,239	64.2	54.9	957	14.5	12.2
Texas	10,485	38.2	42.7	3,214	11.7	13.0	10,231	37.2	41.3	3,844	14.0	13.8
Utah	888	29.6	38.4	372	12.4	15.7	811	27.1	33.9	244	8.1	9.3
Vermont	307	49.0	36.4	85	13.6	10.0	357	57.0	42.3	71	11.3	8.6
Virginia	3,393	40.5	38.0	1,416	16.9	15.7	3,370	40.2	37.1	943	11.2	9.6
Washington	2,703	37.7	34.2	851	11.9	10.8	3,154	44.0	39.7	1,024	14.3	12.4
West Virginia	1,079	58.5	43.8	526	28.5	21.2	1,628	88.3	64.6	338	18.3	14.2
Wisconsin	2,618	45.4	35.6	1,052	18.2	14.2	2,846	49.3	39.3	591	10.2	8.5
Wyoming	198	33.8	31.4	99	16.9	16.0	368	62.8	57.1	118	20.1	18.9
Puerto Rico	1,298	37.4	27.8	632	18.2	13.6	1,014	29.2	21.8	246	7.1	5.4
Virgin Islands	44	42.5	31.7	6	*	*	10	*	*	6	*	*
Guam	70	43.3	62.9	20	12.4	14.7	34	21.0	29.6	16	*	*
American Samoa	29	53.4	134.5	7	*	*	14	*	*	3	*	*
Northern Marianas	13	*	*	7	*	*	5	*	*	2	*	*

- = Quantity zero.
* = Figure does not meet standards of reliability or precision.
[1]Death rates are affected by the population composition of the area. Age-adjusted death rates should be used for comparisons between areas.
[2]Excludes data for Puerto Rico, Virgin Islands, Guam, American Samoa and Northern Marianas.

Table 2-26. Number of Deaths, Death Rates, and Age-Adjusted Death Rates for Major Causes of Death, by State and Territory, 2015—*Continued*

(Number, rates per 100,000 population, age–adjusted rates per 100,000 U.S. standard population.)

State and territory	Nephritis, nephrotic syndrome, and nephrosis (N00–N07, N–17–N19, N–25–N27)			Accidents (V01–X59, Y85–Y86)			Motor vehicle accidents[3]			Intentional self–harm (suicide) (*U03, X60–X84, Y87.0)		
	Number	Rate	Age-adjusted rate[1]	Number	Rate	Age-adjusted rate[1]	Number	Rate	Age-adjusted rate[1]	Number	Rate	Age-adjusted rate[1]
United States[2]	49,959	15.5	13.4	146,571	45.6	43.2	37,757	11.7	11.4	44,193	13.7	13.3
Alabama	1,040	21.4	18.4	2,552	52.5	50.9	962	19.8	19.4	750	15.4	14.9
Alaska	50	6.8	10.0	388	52.5	57.9	74	10.0	10.6	201	27.2	26.9
Arizona	458	6.7	5.5	3,539	51.8	49.2	920	13.5	13.4	1,276	18.7	18.2
Arkansas	707	23.7	19.8	1,538	51.6	49.6	593	19.9	19.6	577	19.4	19.1
California	3,557	9.1	8.6	12,544	32.0	30.6	3,721	9.5	9.2	4,167	10.6	10.3
Colorado	458	8.4	8.5	2,725	49.9	49.7	587	10.8	10.4	1,093	20.0	19.5
Connecticut	584	16.3	12.1	1,799	50.1	44.8	286	8.0	7.6	384	10.7	9.9
Delaware	174	18.4	14.5	449	47.5	46.0	129	13.6	13.2	122	12.9	12.6
District of Columbia	65	9.7	9.9	265	39.4	40.2	43	6.4	6.6	34	5.1	4.9
Florida	3,203	15.8	10.8	10,578	52.2	46.2	2,983	14.7	14.3	3,205	15.8	14.4
Georgia	1,881	18.4	19.2	4,344	42.5	43.2	1,471	14.4	14.3	1,317	12.9	12.7
Hawaii	202	14.1	10.8	536	37.4	32.2	105	7.3	6.9	201	14.0	13.5
Idaho	154	9.3	8.7	746	45.1	44.7	243	14.7	14.9	359	21.7	22.1
Illinois	2,543	19.8	17.3	4,850	37.7	35.8	1,108	8.6	8.3	1,363	10.6	10.3
Indiana	1,450	21.9	18.9	3,258	49.2	47.7	854	12.9	12.6	960	14.5	14.4
Iowa	336	10.8	8.0	1,537	49.2	42.1	352	11.3	10.6	433	13.9	13.9
Kansas	582	20.0	16.8	1,475	50.7	47.2	398	13.7	13.4	477	16.4	16.3
Kentucky	998	22.6	19.7	2,962	66.9	66.0	831	18.8	18.6	776	17.5	17.1
Louisiana	1,160	24.8	23.2	2,578	55.2	54.7	805	17.2	17.0	722	15.5	15.2
Maine	211	15.9	11.4	802	60.3	53.8	151	11.4	11.3	235	17.7	16.0
Maryland	834	13.9	12.3	1,903	31.7	29.7	518	8.6	8.3	553	9.2	8.8
Massachusetts	1,228	18.1	14.3	3,229	47.5	44.0	393	5.8	5.4	642	9.4	8.9
Michigan	1,921	19.4	15.6	4,647	46.8	43.9	880	8.9	8.6	1,410	14.2	13.8
Minnesota	639	11.6	9.7	2,574	46.9	42.0	476	8.7	8.3	730	13.3	13.2
Mississippi	731	24.4	22.0	1,814	60.6	59.8	769	25.7	25.7	431	14.4	14.0
Missouri	1,483	24.4	19.9	3,309	54.4	50.9	932	15.3	14.8	1,052	17.3	17.1
Montana	121	11.7	9.3	637	61.7	56.3	220	21.3	21.1	272	26.3	25.3
Nebraska	264	13.9	11.2	799	42.1	38.9	268	14.1	13.9	223	11.8	11.7
Nevada	316	10.9	10.5	1,340	46.4	45.4	365	12.6	12.6	558	19.3	18.4
New Hampshire	194	14.6	11.4	815	61.3	59.0	106	8.0	7.5	228	17.1	16.5
New Jersey	1,582	17.7	14.4	3,218	35.9	33.7	591	6.6	6.3	789	8.8	8.3
New Mexico	316	15.2	12.9	1,430	68.6	67.3	342	16.4	16.5	500	24.0	23.7
New York	2,245	11.3	9.3	6,515	32.9	30.2	1,189	6.0	5.7	1,652	8.3	7.8
North Carolina	1,821	18.1	16.0	4,991	49.7	47.9	1,518	15.1	14.7	1,406	14.0	13.4
North Dakota	118	15.6	12.5	368	48.6	44.1	137	18.1	17.2	124	16.4	17.5
Ohio	2,100	18.1	14.5	6,756	58.2	55.9	1,257	10.8	10.5	1,650	14.2	13.9
Oklahoma	616	15.7	14.2	2,422	61.9	60.1	673	17.2	17.1	790	20.2	20.3
Oregon	409	10.2	8.2	1,999	49.6	44.5	501	12.4	11.9	762	18.9	17.8
Pennsylvania	3,021	23.6	16.9	7,324	57.2	52.0	1,296	10.1	9.6	1,894	14.8	14.0
Rhode Island	142	13.4	9.8	649	61.4	53.1	55	5.2	5.0	127	12.0	11.2
South Carolina	886	18.1	15.5	2,737	55.9	54.0	985	20.1	19.8	742	15.2	14.8
South Dakota	79	9.2	7.4	469	54.6	49.5	143	16.7	16.2	173	20.2	20.4
Tennessee	1,090	16.5	14.4	3,873	58.7	56.4	988	15.0	14.6	1,068	16.2	15.7
Texas	4,052	14.8	16.1	9,976	36.3	37.4	3,722	13.5	13.6	3,403	12.4	12.5
Utah	363	12.1	15.6	1,223	40.8	45.6	282	9.4	9.9	630	21.0	22.4
Vermont	39	6.2	4.5	346	55.3	48.4	54	8.6	8.0	103	16.5	14.8
Virginia	1,470	17.5	16.1	3,429	40.9	39.6	791	9.4	9.1	1,118	13.3	12.7
Washington	474	6.6	5.9	3,192	44.5	41.9	641	8.9	8.7	1,137	15.9	15.4
West Virginia	510	27.7	20.4	1,516	82.2	77.9	304	16.5	16.3	340	18.4	17.4
Wisconsin	996	17.3	13.7	3,206	55.6	49.3	611	10.6	10.1	877	15.2	14.7
Wyoming	86	14.7	13.3	400	68.2	65.8	134	22.9	23.1	157	26.8	28.0
Puerto Rico	795	22.9	17.2	911	26.2	22.7	328	9.4	8.9	226	6.5	6.0
Virgin Islands	13	*	*	28	27.0	23.8	12	*	*	3	*	*
Guam	21	13.0	19.2	31	19.2	21.0	9	*	*	33	20.4	19.4
American Samoa	3	*	*	9	*	*	2	*	*	2	*	*
Northern Marianas	5	*	*	10	*	*	1	*	*	10	*	*

- = Quantity zero.
* = Figure does not meet standards of reliability or precision.
[1]Death rates are affected by the population composition of the area. Age-adjusted death rates should be used for comparisons between areas.
[2]Excludes data for Puerto Rico, Virgin Islands, Guam, American Samoa and Northern Marianas.
[3]ICD–10 codes for Motor vehicle accidents are V02-V04,V09.0,V09.2,V12-V14,V19.0-V19.2,V19.4-V19.6,V20-V79,V80.3-V80.5,V81.0-V81.1,V82.0-V82.1,V83-V86,V87.0-V87.8,V88.0-V88.8,V89.0, and V89.

Table 2-26. Number of Deaths, Death Rates, and Age-Adjusted Death Rates for Major Causes of Death, by State and Territory, 2015—Continued

(Number, rates per 100,000 population, age-adjusted rates per 100,000 U.S. standard population.)

State and territory	Assault (homicide) (*U01–*U02,X85–Y09, Y87.1)			Alcohol–induced causes[4]			Drug–induced causes[5]			Injury by firearms[6]		
	Number	Rate	Age-adjusted rate[1]	Number	Rate	Age-adjusted rate[1]	Number	Rate	Age-adjusted rate[1]	Number	Rate	Age-adjusted rate[1]
United States[2]	17,793	5.5	5.7	33,171	10.3	9.1	55,403	17.2	17.2	36,252	11.3	11.1
Alabama	473	9.7	10.2	316	6.5	5.8	810	16.7	17.2	958	19.7	19.6
Alaska	62	8.4	8.0	161	21.8	21.1	127	17.2	16.8	177	24.0	23.4
Arizona	364	5.3	5.5	1,277	18.7	17.3	1,351	19.8	20.1	970	14.2	13.8
Arkansas	217	7.3	7.4	242	8.1	7.2	425	14.3	14.9	520	17.5	16.9
California	1,987	5.1	5.0	5,150	13.2	12.1	5,025	12.8	12.2	3,095	7.9	7.7
Colorado	206	3.8	3.7	857	15.7	14.5	893	16.4	15.8	701	12.8	12.6
Connecticut	124	3.5	3.6	341	9.5	8.0	827	23.0	22.8	189	5.3	5.3
Delaware	65	6.9	7.5	80	8.5	7.6	208	22.0	23.0	112	11.8	12.1
District of Columbia	136	20.2	17.5	80	11.9	11.6	130	19.3	19.2	120	17.9	15.2
Florida	1,208	6.0	6.3	2,489	12.3	9.9	3,377	16.7	16.9	2,559	12.6	12.0
Georgia	738	7.2	7.3	726	7.1	6.4	1,370	13.4	13.3	1,448	14.2	14.1
Hawaii	31	2.2	2.2	95	6.6	5.8	175	12.2	11.8	55	3.8	3.6
Idaho	33	2.0	2.0	240	14.5	13.5	224	13.5	14.6	247	14.9	14.7
Illinois	863	6.7	6.9	946	7.4	6.5	1,872	14.6	14.4	1,220	9.5	9.5
Indiana	389	5.9	6.0	689	10.4	9.4	1,310	19.8	20.5	846	12.8	12.7
Iowa	73	2.3	2.5	344	11.0	9.8	332	10.6	11.0	247	7.9	7.8
Kansas	132	4.5	4.7	278	9.5	8.9	349	12.0	12.5	330	11.3	11.4
Kentucky	250	5.6	5.8	466	10.5	9.1	1,332	30.1	31.3	694	15.7	15.2
Louisiana	569	12.2	12.4	388	8.3	7.6	901	19.3	19.9	952	20.4	20.4
Maine	22	1.7	1.7	194	14.6	11.6	278	20.9	22.0	144	10.8	9.8
Maryland	596	9.9	10.3	301	5.0	4.4	1,320	22.0	21.4	708	11.8	11.9
Massachusetts	144	2.1	2.1	633	9.3	7.9	1,851	27.2	27.5	213	3.1	3.0
Michigan	597	6.0	6.4	985	9.9	8.7	2,316	23.3	23.9	1,164	11.7	11.7
Minnesota	147	2.7	2.8	599	10.9	9.6	653	11.9	11.7	410	7.5	7.4
Mississippi	325	10.9	11.3	175	5.8	5.2	369	12.3	13.0	589	19.7	19.6
Missouri	547	9.0	9.6	512	8.4	7.5	1,098	18.0	18.4	1,094	18.0	18.1
Montana	38	3.7	4.0	194	18.8	17.1	152	14.7	15.2	205	19.8	19.2
Nebraska	75	4.0	4.0	199	10.5	9.8	139	7.3	7.6	169	8.9	8.9
Nevada	191	6.6	6.7	433	15.0	13.2	629	21.8	20.7	446	15.4	14.9
New Hampshire	18	*	*	173	13.0	10.0	433	32.5	35.3	121	9.1	8.9
New Jersey	388	4.3	4.5	527	5.9	5.1	1,506	16.8	16.9	475	5.3	5.4
New Mexico	157	7.5	8.0	656	31.5	30.8	516	24.7	26.0	390	18.7	18.6
New York	671	3.4	3.4	1,479	7.5	6.5	3,009	15.2	14.7	849	4.3	4.2
North Carolina	593	5.9	6.1	915	9.1	8.0	1,636	16.3	16.4	1,289	12.8	12.5
North Dakota	22	2.9	3.1	96	12.7	12.6	65	8.6	9.1	92	12.2	12.8
Ohio	669	5.8	6.0	1,027	8.8	7.6	3,418	29.4	30.9	1,397	12.0	11.9
Oklahoma	324	8.3	8.5	530	13.6	12.4	751	19.2	19.7	706	18.1	18.0
Oregon	138	3.4	3.4	896	22.2	18.6	609	15.1	14.2	486	12.1	11.4
Pennsylvania	673	5.3	5.6	879	6.9	5.6	3,376	26.4	27.1	1,485	11.6	11.4
Rhode Island	28	2.7	2.8	146	13.8	11.9	318	30.1	28.9	51	4.8	4.7
South Carolina	448	9.2	9.5	495	10.1	8.6	793	16.2	16.3	850	17.4	17.3
South Dakota	35	4.1	4.2	152	17.7	18.2	72	8.4	9.3	96	11.2	11.1
Tennessee	460	7.0	7.2	637	9.7	8.4	1,546	23.4	23.5	1,075	16.3	16.0
Texas	1,538	5.6	5.6	2,073	7.5	7.3	2,732	9.9	9.9	3,203	11.7	11.7
Utah	60	2.0	2.0	266	8.9	9.8	667	22.3	24.2	367	12.2	12.8
Vermont	16	*	*	96	15.3	11.9	111	17.7	18.5	70	11.2	9.6
Virginia	374	4.5	4.5	655	7.8	6.9	1,070	12.8	12.7	946	11.3	10.9
Washington	239	3.3	3.4	1,100	15.3	13.4	1,189	16.6	16.0	718	10.0	9.8
West Virginia	80	4.3	4.5	193	10.5	8.4	750	40.7	42.9	278	15.1	14.0
Wisconsin	243	4.2	4.5	638	11.1	9.3	894	15.5	15.7	613	10.6	10.4
Wyoming	17	*	*	152	25.9	24.4	99	16.9	16.8	113	19.3	19.6
Puerto Rico	588	16.9	17.9	189	5.4	4.4	52	1.5	1.3	587	16.9	17.9
Virgin Islands	43	41.5	48.3	9	*	*	2	*	*	36	34.8	43.2
Guam	7	*	*	2	*	*	-	*	*	7	*	*
American Samoa	2	*	*	1	*	*	1	*	*	-	*	*
Northern Marianas	2	*	*	3	*	*	-	*	*	1	*	*

- = Quantity zero.
* = Figure does not meet standards of reliability or precision.
[1]Death rates are affected by the population composition of the area. Age-adjusted death rates should be used for comparisons between areas.
[2]Excludes data for Puerto Rico, Virgin Islands, Guam, American Samoa and Northern Marianas.
[4]Causes of death attributable to alcohol-induced mortality include ICD–10 codes E24.4,F10,G31.2,G62.1,G72.1,I42.6,K29.2,K70,K85.2,K86.0,R78.0,X45,X65, and Y15.
[5]Causes of death attributable to drug-induced mortality include ICD–10 codes D52.1,D59.0,D59.2,D61.1,D64.2,E06.4,E16.0,E23.1,E24.2,E27.3,E66.1,F11.1-F11.5,F11.7-F11.9,F12.1-F12.5,F12.7-F12.9, F13.1-F13.5,F13.7-
F13.9,F14.1-F14.5,F14.7-F14.9,F15.1-F15.5,F15.7-F15.9,F16.1-F16.5,F16.7-F16.9,F17.3-F17.5,F17.7-F17.9,F18.1-F18.5,F18.7-F18.9,F19.1-F19.5,F19.7-F19.9,G21.1,G24.0,G25.1, G25.4,G25.6,G44.4,G62.0,G72.0,I95.
2,J70.2-J70.4,K85.3,L10.5,L27.0-L27.1,M10.2,M32.0,M80.4,M81.4,M83.5,M87.1,R50.2,R78.1-R78.5,X40-X44,X60-X64,X85, and Y10-Y14.
[6]ICD–10 codes for Injury by firearms are *U01.4,W32-W34,X72-X74,X93-X95,Y22-Y24, and Y35.0.

Table 2-27. Death Rates for All Causes, by Sex, Race, Hispanic Origin, and Age, Selected Years 1950–2015

(Deaths per 100,000 resident population.)

Sex, race, Hispanic origin, and age	1950[1]	1960[1]	1970	1980	1985	1990	1995	2000	2005	2006
All Persons										
All ages, age-adjusted[2]	1,446.0	1,339.2	1,222.6	1,039.1	988.1	938.7	909.8	869.0	815.0	791.8
All ages, crude	963.8	954.7	945.3	878.3	876.9	863.8	868.3	854.0	828.4	813.1
Under 1 year	3,299.2	2,696.4	2,142.4	1,288.3	1,088.1	971.9	780.3	736.7	710.2	705.8
1 to 4 years	139.4	109.1	84.5	63.9	51.8	46.8	40.4	32.4	29.9	29.1
5 to 14 years	60.1	46.6	41.3	30.6	26.5	24.0	22.2	18.0	16.3	15.2
15 to 24 years	128.1	106.3	127.7	115.4	94.9	99.2	93.4	79.9	80.7	81.4
25 to 34 years	178.7	146.4	157.4	135.5	124.4	139.2	137.3	101.4	106.8	109.0
35 to 44 years	358.7	299.4	314.5	227.9	207.7	223.2	239.4	198.9	194.9	192.0
45 to 54 years	853.9	756.0	730.0	584.0	519.3	473.4	454.3	425.6	431.9	427.5
55 to 64 years	1,901.0	1,735.1	1,658.8	1,346.3	1,294.2	1,196.9	1,104.7	992.2	898.5	881.3
65 to 74 years	4,104.3	3,822.1	3,582.7	2,994.9	2,862.8	2,648.6	2,549.0	2,399.1	2,109.7	2,031.4
75 to 84 years	9,331.1	8,745.2	8,004.4	6,692.6	6,398.7	6,007.2	5,811.3	5,666.5	5,251.8	5,096.1
85 years and over	20,196.9	19,857.5	16,344.9	15,980.3	15,712.4	15,327.4	15,248.6	15,524.4	14,982.4	14,426.7
Male										
All ages, age-adjusted[2]	1,674.2	1,609.0	1,542.1	1,348.1	1,278.1	1,202.8	1,143.9	1,053.8	971.9	943.5
All ages, crude	1,106.1	1,104.5	1,090.3	976.9	948.6	918.4	900.8	853.0	831.7	819.6
Under 1 year	3,728.0	3,059.3	2,410.0	1,428.5	1,219.9	1,082.8	856.3	806.5	782.2	773.5
1 to 4 years	151.7	119.5	93.2	72.6	58.5	52.4	44.5	35.9	34.0	31.3
5 to 14 years	70.9	55.7	50.5	36.7	31.8	28.5	26.4	20.9	18.5	17.5
15 to 24 years	167.9	152.1	188.5	172.3	138.9	147.4	137.4	114.9	117.1	118.5
25 to 34 years	216.5	187.9	215.3	196.1	179.6	204.3	198.0	138.6	148.6	152.7
35 to 44 years	428.8	372.8	402.6	299.2	278.9	310.4	331.0	255.2	246.3	242.4
45 to 54 years	1,067.1	992.2	958.5	767.3	671.6	610.3	589.9	542.8	548.2	541.4
55 to 64 years	2,395.3	2,309.5	2,282.7	1,815.1	1,711.4	1,553.4	1,400.7	1,230.7	1,119.8	1,097.5
65 to 74 years	4,931.4	4,914.4	4,873.8	4,105.2	3,856.3	3,491.5	3,263.8	2,979.6	2,566.0	2,464.5
75 to 84 years	10,426.0	10,178.4	10,010.2	8,816.7	8,501.6	7,888.6	7,399.6	6,972.6	6,300.3	6,103.8
85 years and over	21,636.0	21,186.3	17,821.5	18,801.1	18,614.1	18,056.6	17,861.0	17,501.4	16,538.9	15,910.1
Female										
All ages, age-adjusted[2]	1,236.0	1,105.3	971.4	817.9	784.5	750.9	739.4	731.4	692.3	672.2
All ages, crude	823.5	809.2	807.8	785.3	809.1	812.0	837.2	855.0	825.1	806.9
Under 1 year	2,854.6	2,321.3	1,863.7	1,141.7	950.6	855.7	700.5	663.4	634.9	635.0
1 to 4 years	126.7	98.4	75.4	54.7	44.8	41.0	36.0	28.7	25.6	26.9
5 to 14 years	48.9	37.3	31.8	24.2	21.0	19.3	17.9	15.0	13.9	12.7
15 to 24 years	89.1	61.3	68.1	57.5	49.6	49.0	47.3	43.1	42.2	42.3
25 to 34 years	142.7	106.6	101.6	75.9	69.4	74.2	76.1	63.5	64.7	65.0
35 to 44 years	290.3	229.4	231.1	159.3	138.7	137.9	149.3	143.2	144.0	142.2
45 to 54 years	641.5	526.7	517.2	412.9	375.2	342.7	324.1	312.5	319.5	317.4
55 to 64 years	1,404.8	1,196.4	1,098.9	934.3	925.6	878.8	835.2	772.2	692.4	680.0
65 to 74 years	3,333.2	2,871.8	2,579.7	2,144.7	2,096.9	1,991.2	1,975.8	1,921.2	1,721.3	1,661.0
75 to 84 years	8,399.6	7,633.1	6,677.6	5,440.1	5,162.1	4,883.1	4,818.6	4,814.7	4,532.3	4,397.2
85 years and over	19,194.7	19,008.4	15,518.0	14,746.9	14,553.9	14,274.3	14,242.3	14,719.2	14,290.8	13,753.8
White Male[3]										
All ages, age-adjusted[2]	1,642.5	1,586.0	1,513.7	1,317.6	1,249.8	1,165.9	1,107.5	1,029.4	952.9	925.8
All ages, crude	1,089.5	1,098.5	1,086.7	983.3	963.6	930.9	921.0	887.8	873.5	862.3
Under 1 year	3,400.5	2,694.1	2,113.2	1,230.3	1,056.5	896.1	720.7	667.6	664.5	653.2
1 to 4 years	135.5	104.9	83.6	66.1	52.8	45.9	39.0	32.6	31.7	28.4
5 to 14 years	67.2	52.7	48.0	35.0	30.1	26.4	24.3	19.8	17.1	16.5
15 to 24 years	152.4	143.7	170.8	167.0	134.2	131.3	120.1	105.8	110.6	112.2
25 to 34 years	185.3	163.2	176.6	171.3	158.8	176.1	171.9	124.1	136.2	141.7
35 to 44 years	380.9	332.6	343.5	257.4	243.1	268.2	286.8	233.6	232.4	228.8
45 to 54 years	984.5	932.2	882.9	698.9	611.7	548.7	528.3	496.9	512.1	508.6
55 to 64 years	2,304.4	2,225.2	2,202.6	1,728.5	1,625.8	1,467.2	1,319.3	1,163.3	1,061.3	1,043.2
65 to 74 years	4,864.9	4,848.4	4,810.1	4,035.7	3,770.7	3,397.7	3,173.3	2,905.7	2,511.6	2,409.6
75 to 84 years	10,526.3	10,299.6	10,098.8	8,829.8	8,486.1	7,844.9	7,347.3	6,933.1	6,277.9	6,089.7
85 years and over	22,116.3	21,750.0	18,551.7	19,097.3	18,980.1	18,268.3	18,050.7	17,716.4	16,693.3	16,059.2
Black or African American Male[3]										
All ages, age-adjusted[2]	1,909.1	1,811.1	1,873.9	1,697.8	1,634.5	1,644.5	1,585.7	1,403.5	1,281.3	1,239.5
All ages, crude	1,257.7	1,181.7	1,186.6	1,034.1	989.3	1,008.0	960.2	834.1	796.1	781.4
Under 1 year	NA	5,306.8	4,298.9	2,586.7	2,219.9	2,112.4	1,664.7	1,567.6	1,478.6	1,449.5
1 to 4 years[4]	1,412.6	208.5	150.5	110.5	90.1	85.8	73.1	54.5	48.7	49.3
5 to 14 years	95.1	75.1	67.1	47.4	42.3	41.2	38.5	28.2	26.4	24.2

NA = Not available.

[1] Includes deaths of persons who were not residents of the 50 states and the District of Columbia (DC).

[2] Age-adjusted rates are calculated using the year 2000 standard population. Prior to 2001, age-adjusted rates were calculated using standard million proportions based on rounded population numbers. Starting with 2001 data, unrounded population numbers are used to calculate age-adjusted rates.

[3] The race groups, White, Black, Asian or Pacific Islander, and American Indian and Alaska Native, include persons of Hispanic and non-Hispanic origin. Persons of Hispanic origin may be of any race. Death rates for the American Indian and Alaska Native, Asian or Pacific Islander, and Hispanic populations are known to be underestimated.

[4] In 1950, rate is for the age group under 5 years.

Table 2-27. Death Rates for All Causes, by Sex, Race, Hispanic Origin, and Age, Selected Years 1950–2015—Continued

(Deaths per 100,000 resident population.)

Sex, race, Hispanic origin, and age	2007	2008	2009	2010	2011	2012	2013	2014	2015
All Persons									
All ages, age-adjusted[2]	775.3	774.9	749.6	747.0	741.3	732.8	731.9	724.6	733.1
All ages, crude	804.6	812.9	794.5	799.5	807.3	810.2	821.5	823.7	844.0
Under 1 year	702.5	678.9	659.7	623.4	600.1	599.3	594.7	588.0	589.6
1 to 4 years	29.4	29.3	27.4	26.5	26.3	26.3	25.5	24.0	24.9
5 to 14 years	15.2	13.9	13.8	12.9	13.2	12.6	13.0	12.7	13.2
15 to 24 years	78.8	74.2	69.8	67.7	67.7	66.4	64.8	65.5	69.5
25 to 34 years	107.2	105.1	104.4	102.9	104.7	105.4	106.1	108.4	116.7
35 to 44 years	186.0	181.0	180.0	170.5	172.0	170.7	172.0	175.2	180.1
45 to 54 years	420.3	419.6	418.1	407.1	409.8	405.4	406.1	404.8	404.0
55 to 64 years	866.7	867.1	856.7	851.9	849.4	854.2	860.0	870.3	875.3
65 to 74 years	1,976.0	1,958.4	1,888.7	1,875.1	1,846.2	1,802.5	1,802.1	1,786.3	1,796.8
75 to 84 years	4,987.1	4,998.1	4,820.2	4,790.2	4,753.0	4,674.5	4,648.1	4,564.2	4,579.2
85 years and over	14,160.9	14,332.4	13,660.1	13,934.3	13,779.3	13,678.6	13,660.4	13,407.9	13,673.9
Male									
All ages, age-adjusted[2]	922.9	918.8	890.9	887.1	875.3	865.1	863.6	855.1	863.2
All ages, crude	813.1	820.3	807.2	812.0	818.7	824.5	839.1	846.4	868.0
Under 1 year	768.2	742.7	725.0	680.2	652.1	651.5	650.5	638.6	639.2
1 to 4 years	32.3	32.7	30.1	29.6	29.1	29.2	28.6	26.7	28.0
5 to 14 years	17.3	15.8	15.6	14.6	15.2	14.4	14.6	14.9	15.0
15 to 24 years	114.3	108.0	100.0	97.6	97.7	95.3	92.6	93.8	99.5
25 to 34 years	149.5	146.8	142.7	141.5	143.0	144.3	145.4	148.8	160.5
35 to 44 years	235.3	227.1	225.5	212.5	213.7	212.8	213.8	216.7	226.0
45 to 54 years	529.8	526.2	520.3	505.9	507.3	500.8	500.7	496.5	495.6
55 to 64 years	1,086.5	1,089.8	1,078.4	1,075.5	1,071.1	1,080.2	1,088.4	1,098.2	1,103.9
65 to 74 years	2,398.6	2,372.3	2,290.5	2,275.1	2,236.2	2,186.4	2,186.0	2,175.5	2,190.0
75 to 84 years	5,948.6	5,939.4	5,725.8	5,693.7	5,610.8	5,500.6	5,474.2	5,369.2	5,376.3
85 years and over	15,620.2	15,709.6	15,142.9	15,414.3	15,069.8	14,974.4	14,911.6	14,642.2	14,795.8
Female									
All ages, age-adjusted[2]	658.1	659.9	636.8	634.9	632.4	624.7	623.5	616.7	624.2
All ages, crude	796.4	805.8	782.1	787.4	796.3	796.4	804.4	801.7	820.7
Under 1 year	633.6	612.5	591.5	564.0	545.8	544.6	536.1	535.0	537.7
1 to 4 years	26.5	25.8	24.6	23.3	23.3	23.2	22.4	21.3	21.6
5 to 14 years	12.9	11.9	12.0	11.1	11.1	10.8	11.2	10.5	11.2
15 to 24 years	41.3	38.6	38.1	36.4	36.2	36.0	35.6	35.8	38.1
25 to 34 years	64.6	63.1	65.6	64.0	65.9	65.8	66.0	67.2	72.1
35 to 44 years	137.2	135.3	134.9	128.9	130.7	129.0	130.5	134.1	134.5
45 to 54 years	314.4	316.4	319.1	311.4	315.2	312.7	314.1	315.6	315.0
55 to 64 years	661.8	659.6	650.1	643.5	642.9	643.8	647.4	658.2	662.3
65 to 74 years	1,612.8	1,601.0	1,540.5	1,527.5	1,505.8	1,466.1	1,464.6	1,444.2	1,450.9
75 to 84 years	4,313.2	4,331.8	4,172.2	4,137.7	4,124.2	4,062.5	4,029.1	3,955.1	3,971.3
85 years and over	13,486.3	13,684.3	12,951.6	13,219.2	13,143.4	13,030.0	13,021.6	12,765.7	13,080.8
White Male[3]									
All ages, age-adjusted[2]	907.1	907.1	880.5	878.5	870.2	860.0	859.2	853.4	861.9
All ages, crude	857.8	870.6	858.2	866.1	876.4	882.8	899.1	909.4	932.9
Under 1 year	653.2	635.8	611.2	584.3	560.6	558.5	566.4	551.3	541.8
1 to 4 years	29.4	30.5	28.3	27.4	27.2	27.3	26.2	23.8	24.9
5 to 14 years	16.2	14.6	14.5	13.8	14.5	13.3	13.9	14.0	14.1
15 to 24 years	108.1	102.4	94.9	91.8	92.5	89.7	87.1	88.3	92.3
25 to 34 years	140.4	139.3	135.9	135.6	138.0	139.3	139.8	145.3	157.0
35 to 44 years	222.7	218.3	216.8	206.6	208.9	207.2	208.0	212.6	221.3
45 to 54 years	501.9	504.8	502.3	491.9	495.1	489.0	491.7	488.9	487.4
55 to 64 years	1,034.7	1,044.0	1,032.2	1,033.0	1,033.3	1,043.5	1,050.7	1,063.8	1,070.9
65 to 74 years	2,345.4	2,324.8	2,245.3	2,232.4	2,199.7	2,150.5	2,152.0	2,143.3	2,159.9
75 to 84 years	5,939.7	5,938.3	5,737.1	5,703.6	5,650.4	5,529.5	5,507.2	5,419.1	5,426.8
85 years and over	15,776.0	15,922.9	15,362.2	15,640.3	15,335.7	15,271.5	15,220.4	15,000.3	15,202.8
Black or African American Male[3]									
All ages, age-adjusted[2]	1,204.8	1,168.0	1,123.1	1,104.0	1,067.1	1,058.6	1,052.8	1,034.0	1,040.3
All ages, crude	768.1	750.6	735.3	725.4	719.4	728.0	739.3	742.6	765.3
Under 1 year	1,406.0	1,343.0	1,357.2	1,206.5	1,149.9	1,147.3	1,120.1	1,125.4	1,150.2
1 to 4 years[4]	47.6	48.2	41.9	42.9	42.7	41.6	40.6	42.2	45.7
5 to 14 years	23.9	22.6	22.2	19.6	20.5	21.3	19.6	21.0	21.0

[2]Age-adjusted rates are calculated using the year 2000 standard population. Prior to 2001, age-adjusted rates were calculated using standard million proportions based on rounded population numbers. Starting with 2001 data, unrounded population numbers are used to calculate age-adjusted rates.
[3]The race groups, White, Black, Asian or Pacific Islander, and American Indian and Alaska Native, include persons of Hispanic and non-Hispanic origin. Persons of Hispanic origin may be of any race. Death rates for the American Indian and Alaska Native, Asian or Pacific Islander, and Hispanic populations are known to be underestimated.
[4]In 1950, rate is for the age group under 5 years.

Table 2-27. Death Rates for All Causes, by Sex, Race, Hispanic Origin, and Age, Selected Years 1950–2015—*Continued*

(Deaths per 100,000 resident population.)

Sex, race, Hispanic origin, and age	1950¹	1960¹	1970	1980	1985	1990	1995	2000	2005	2006
15 to 24 years	289.7	212.0	320.6	209.1	173.6	252.2	246.6	181.4	170.8	169.5
25 to 34 years	503.5	402.5	559.5	407.3	351.9	430.8	407.4	261.0	264.8	265.0
35 to 44 years	878.1	762.0	956.6	689.8	630.2	699.6	716.8	453.0	394.1	389.1
45 to 54 years	1,905.0	1,624.8	1,777.5	1,479.9	1,292.9	1,261.0	1,238.9	1,017.7	923.1	891.5
55 to 64 years	3,773.2	3,316.4	3,256.9	2,873.0	2,779.8	2,618.4	2,382.0	2,080.1	1,877.9	1,805.8
65 to 74 years	5,310.3	5,798.7	5,803.2	5,131.1	5,172.4	4,946.1	4,707.8	4,253.5	3,606.8	3,511.6
75 to 84 years⁵	10,101.9	8,605.1	9,454.9	9,231.6	9,262.3	9,129.5	8,862.0	8,486.0	7,674.6	7,381.4
85 years and over	NA	14,844.8	12,222.3	16,098.8	15,774.2	16,954.9	17,016.0	16,791.0	16,769.2	16,110.0
American Indian or Alaska Native Male³										
All ages, age-adjusted²	NA	NA	NA	1,111.5	926.1	916.2	932.0	841.5	824.5	780.8
All ages, crude	NA	NA	NA	597.1	492.5	476.4	459.4	415.6	428.4	413.7
Under 1 year	NA	NA	NA	1,598.1	1,080.0	1,056.6	696.0	700.2	600.5	706.2
1 to 4 years	NA	NA	NA	82.7	105.3	77.4	73.3	44.9	49.8	39.5
5 to 14 years	NA	NA	NA	43.7	39.2	33.4	27.0	20.2	19.7	14.1
15 to 24 years	NA	NA	NA	311.1	214.4	219.8	182.1	136.2	126.7	133.1
25 to 34 years	NA	NA	NA	360.6	275.0	256.1	263.6	179.1	191.6	176.3
35 to 44 years	NA	NA	NA	556.8	363.5	365.4	377.4	295.2	304.7	298.7
45 to 54 years	NA	NA	NA	871.3	687.9	619.9	601.0	520.0	541.6	534.2
55 to 64 years	NA	NA	NA	1,547.5	1,319.1	1,211.3	1,276.0	1,090.4	1,076.8	974.9
65 to 74 years	NA	NA	NA	2,968.4	2,692.3	2,461.7	2,660.8	2,478.3	2,243.8	2,127.5
75 to 84 years	NA	NA	NA	5,607.0	5,572.7	5,389.2	5,787.7	5,351.2	4,877.8	4,722.6
85 years and over	NA	NA	NA	12,635.2	8,900.0	11,243.9	10,604.7	10,725.8	11,841.9	10,735.7
Asian or Pacific Islander Male³										
All ages, age-adjusted²	NA	NA	NA	786.5	755.4	716.4	693.4	624.2	560.6	544.9
All ages, crude	NA	NA	NA	375.3	344.6	334.3	341.4	332.9	326.6	323.4
Under 1 year	NA	NA	NA	816.5	750.0	605.3	468.3	529.4	439.3	457.8
1 to 4 years	NA	NA	NA	50.9	43.4	45.0	28.0	23.3	19.7	17.4
5 to 14 years	NA	NA	NA	23.4	22.5	20.7	19.6	12.9	13.5	10.7
15 to 24 years	NA	NA	NA	80.8	76.0	76.0	73.0	55.2	51.2	54.7
25 to 34 years	NA	NA	NA	83.5	77.3	79.6	75.4	55.0	54.9	53.5
35 to 44 years	NA	NA	NA	128.3	114.4	130.8	124.9	104.9	96.5	92.3
45 to 54 years	NA	NA	NA	342.3	284.8	287.1	273.0	249.7	242.4	232.9
55 to 64 years	NA	NA	NA	881.1	869.4	789.1	714.2	642.4	540.4	546.1
65 to 74 years	NA	NA	NA	2,236.1	2,102.0	2,041.4	1,894.8	1,661.0	1,388.9	1,315.0
75 to 84 years	NA	NA	NA	5,389.5	5,551.2	5,008.6	4,729.9	4,328.2	3,875.2	3,730.6
85 years and over	NA	NA	NA	13,753.6	12,750.0	12,446.3	13,252.0	12,125.3	11,343.4	11,154.9
Hispanic or Latino Male³,⁶										
All ages, age-adjusted²	NA	NA	NA	NA	889.2	886.4	897.6	818.1	771.2	732.3
All ages, crude	NA	NA	NA	NA	374.6	411.6	391.6	331.3	335.6	326.1
Under 1 year	NA	NA	NA	NA	1,044.6	921.8	684.6	637.1	637.6	613.6
1 to 4 years	NA	NA	NA	NA	53.8	53.8	39.3	31.5	33.0	28.9
5 to 14 years	NA	NA	NA	NA	23.0	26.0	24.6	17.9	15.1	16.0
15 to 24 years	NA	NA	NA	NA	147.5	159.3	147.3	107.7	112.3	111.8
25 to 34 years	NA	NA	NA	NA	202.1	234.0	196.7	120.2	123.0	121.7
35 to 44 years	NA	NA	NA	NA	290.1	341.8	333.6	211.0	188.8	184.6
45 to 54 years	NA	NA	NA	NA	495.7	533.9	528.5	439.0	421.7	409.6
55 to 64 years	NA	NA	NA	NA	1,129.4	1,123.7	1,076.9	965.7	880.2	849.4
65 to 74 years	NA	NA	NA	NA	2,484.9	2,368.2	2,429.3	2,287.9	2,052.2	1,936.1
75 to 84 years	NA	NA	NA	NA	5,696.1	5,369.1	5,557.4	5,395.3	5,096.5	4,739.5
85 years and over	NA	NA	NA	NA	12,156.2	12,272.1	13,295.9	13,086.2	12,746.1	12,135.6
White, not Hispanic or Latino Male⁶										
All ages, age-adjusted²	NA	NA	NA	NA	1,215.6	1,170.9	1,105.6	1,035.4	961.5	935.7
All ages, crude	NA	NA	NA	NA	956.3	985.9	984.8	978.5	978.1	969.4
Under 1 year	NA	NA	NA	NA	1,002.0	865.4	703.8	658.7	656.4	647.8
1 to 4 years	NA	NA	NA	NA	48.8	43.8	37.8	32.4	30.6	27.4
5 to 14 years	NA	NA	NA	NA	28.9	25.7	23.5	20.0	17.5	16.2
15 to 24 years	NA	NA	NA	NA	125.0	123.4	111.5	103.5	107.6	109.6
25 to 34 years	NA	NA	NA	NA	151.2	165.3	163.5	123.0	137.7	145.0
35 to 44 years	NA	NA	NA	NA	231.8	257.1	276.5	233.9	238.4	235.3
45 to 54 years	NA	NA	NA	NA	587.7	544.5	520.7	497.7	518.8	516.8
55 to 64 years	NA	NA	NA	NA	1,550.7	1,479.7	1,322.7	1,170.9	1,070.8	1,054.0
65 to 74 years	NA	NA	NA	NA	3,648.1	3,434.5	3,188.5	2,930.5	2,536.0	2,435.4

NA = Not available.

¹Includes deaths of persons who were not residents of the 50 states and the District of Columbia (DC).

²Age-adjusted rates are calculated using the year 2000 standard population. Prior to 2001, age-adjusted rates were calculated using standard million proportions based on rounded population numbers. Starting with 2001 data, unrounded population numbers are used to calculate age-adjusted rates.

³The race groups, White, Black, Asian or Pacific Islander, and American Indian and Alaska Native, include persons of Hispanic and non-Hispanic origin. Persons of Hispanic origin may be of any race. Death rates for the American Indian and Alaska Native, Asian or Pacific Islander, and Hispanic populations are known to be underestimated.

⁵In 1950, rate is for the age group 75 years and over.

⁶Prior to 1997, excludes data from states lacking an Hispanic-origin item on the death certificate.

Table 2-27. Death Rates for All Causes, by Sex, Race, Hispanic Origin, and Age, Selected Years 1950–2015—Continued

(Deaths per 100,000 resident population.)

Sex, race, Hispanic origin, and age	2007	2008	2009	2010	2011	2012	2013	2014	2015
15 to 24 years	165.5	156.2	142.5	142.8	140.3	138.7	135.5	135.4	150.9
25 to 34 years	251.0	235.7	226.1	216.7	212.2	212.8	218.6	212.1	229.0
35 to 44 years	374.3	342.0	336.8	307.5	304.8	306.1	312.4	308.5	325.8
45 to 54 years	842.5	790.7	760.4	716.3	706.3	696.3	678.8	671.8	678.1
55 to 64 years	1,774.9	1,723.4	1,707.1	1,662.1	1,623.4	1,615.8	1,628.0	1,611.5	1,612.9
65 to 74 years	3,428.7	3,347.9	3,250.1	3,205.6	3,127.2	3,077.9	3,064.4	3,047.4	3,041.8
75 to 84 years[5]	7,142.9	7,084.2	6,727.9	6,721.5	6,358.9	6,416.8	6,362.4	6,172.6	6,204.5
85 years and over	15,879.4	15,380.0	14,562.9	14,715.3	14,159.4	13,775.7	13,657.1	13,291.7	13,066.3
American Indian or Alaska Native Male[3]									
All ages, age-adjusted[2]	780.3	757.2	709.0	730.2	691.7	690.5	689.2	685.4	693.6
All ages, crude	411.1	408.7	389.9	397.5	395.1	410.2	416.5	433.2	454.7
Under 1 year	646.4	600.1	548.7	542.5	486.5	528.4	493.4	509.7	486.4
1 to 4 years	42.0	34.6	31.2	34.3	28.8	34.2	41.5	41.0	35.2
5 to 14 years	17.9	14.7	15.5	18.1	13.1	16.8	12.1	12.3	15.2
15 to 24 years	119.2	122.0	121.0	116.4	107.0	107.9	98.0	103.8	101.1
25 to 34 years	175.6	171.3	154.9	156.2	161.9	175.3	172.7	179.1	191.4
35 to 44 years	285.4	262.9	275.6	258.2	250.9	248.6	244.4	264.4	281.4
45 to 54 years	507.1	535.2	486.7	496.1	500.6	500.8	506.4	508.5	543.5
55 to 64 years	973.7	961.8	941.0	951.2	894.8	939.2	937.8	984.7	994.2
65 to 74 years	2,105.8	2,128.4	1,969.9	1,971.0	1,908.1	1,948.9	1,845.9	1,830.2	1,840.6
75 to 84 years	4,737.9	4,729.6	4,342.4	4,451.8	4,240.5	4,190.2	4,224.5	4,097.9	4,171.0
85 years and over	11,274.5	9,880.9	9,174.7	10,268.1	9,169.4	8,618.1	9,034.3	8,610.4	8,277.3
Asian or Pacific Islander Male[3]									
All ages, age-adjusted[2]	525.9	518.5	509.2	512.1	490.7	484.1	487.8	462.0	467.6
All ages, crude	318.7	320.0	321.2	327.0	328.6	332.8	347.4	341.3	354.5
Under 1 year	462.5	443.8	412.0	434.4	410.0	430.9	408.9	384.3	437.8
1 to 4 years	24.3	16.8	19.3	19.3	15.4	16.3	19.3	14.3	15.1
5 to 14 years	11.4	11.5	11.0	8.4	9.2	9.0	11.1	9.9	10.3
15 to 24 years	52.2	41.5	41.3	43.0	42.5	41.5	42.2	44.7	48.6
25 to 34 years	47.9	50.9	50.3	52.6	53.9	54.9	54.2	54.1	55.7
35 to 44 years	92.0	89.1	93.7	83.5	84.2	92.0	88.5	83.0	84.5
45 to 54 years	227.6	219.3	226.5	213.7	216.8	216.5	220.4	212.3	205.3
55 to 64 years	514.8	516.3	509.9	519.0	502.8	505.9	517.6	519.9	507.9
65 to 74 years	1,278.2	1,273.1	1,218.8	1,226.0	1,167.1	1,109.2	1,126.4	1,107.1	1,130.7
75 to 84 years	3,650.5	3,595.7	3,456.9	3,438.7	3,311.2	3,218.0	3,239.9	3,047.8	3,091.6
85 years and over	10,580.0	10,492.8	10,477.3	10,824.5	10,143.4	10,116.5	10,142.8	9,263.1	9,405.8
Hispanic or Latino Male[3,8]									
All ages, age-adjusted[2]	711.4	695.3	675.5	677.7	647.3	643.9	639.8	626.8	628.9
All ages, crude	321.6	316.0	311.8	310.8	309.7	316.5	323.7	330.1	343.2
Under 1 year	616.5	605.0	569.5	556.8	487.6	509.1	501.1	508.3	500.4
1 to 4 years	28.4	29.0	25.9	25.0	25.5	23.5	23.1	20.1	22.0
5 to 14 years	15.3	12.3	14.1	11.4	12.5	12.3	11.7	12.5	12.2
15 to 24 years	104.2	91.9	87.6	79.4	78.5	76.4	72.9	75.4	82.2
25 to 34 years	117.4	112.3	107.1	100.9	98.5	100.0	99.9	103.6	111.8
35 to 44 years	173.7	165.5	158.5	146.2	142.4	142.7	143.3	149.4	152.8
45 to 54 years	404.3	377.2	376.9	351.9	357.3	342.7	348.0	341.0	340.2
55 to 64 years	836.0	837.0	818.9	815.1	791.0	816.3	797.4	787.7	788.2
65 to 74 years	1,884.2	1,854.9	1,789.2	1,775.0	1,722.4	1,679.1	1,710.4	1,655.1	1,674.3
75 to 84 years	4,612.2	4,563.6	4,396.7	4,461.9	4,303.5	4,250.9	4,218.1	4,103.3	4,127.1
85 years and over	11,719.4	11,453.4	11,225.7	11,779.8	10,707.8	10,799.6	10,596.0	10,318.0	10,145.7
White, not Hispanic or Latino Male[6]									
All ages, age-adjusted[2]	918.4	920.2	893.7	892.5	887.2	876.2	876.8	872.3	881.3
All ages, crude	968.3	987.5	975.7	987.5	1,004.1	1,011.2	1,032.1	1,045.4	1,072.5
Under 1 year	647.5	627.9	604.4	575.9	572.6	558.2	571.5	549.9	541.1
1 to 4 years	29.1	30.3	28.3	27.5	27.0	27.9	26.9	24.9	25.5
5 to 14 years	16.1	15.1	14.2	14.3	14.8	13.3	14.4	14.2	14.5
15 to 24 years	106.8	103.2	94.4	93.4	94.8	92.0	89.6	90.6	93.4
25 to 34 years	145.0	145.1	142.1	143.6	147.9	149.0	149.9	155.8	168.1
35 to 44 years	230.7	227.9	227.9	219.1	223.8	221.7	223.1	227.4	238.1
45 to 54 years	510.5	518.2	515.4	508.1	512.3	508.0	511.5	511.2	510.0
55 to 64 years	1,046.7	1,056.2	1,045.1	1,046.2	1,050.0	1,058.0	1,069.0	1,085.3	1,093.3
65 to 74 years	2,372.1	2,350.7	2,269.9	2,256.9	2,227.4	2,175.8	2,174.3	2,170.0	2,184.0

[2]Age-adjusted rates are calculated using the year 2000 standard population. Prior to 2001, age-adjusted rates were calculated using standard million proportions based on rounded population numbers. Starting with 2001 data, unrounded population numbers are used to calculate age-adjusted rates.

[3]The race groups, White, Black, Asian or Pacific Islander, and American Indian and Alaska Native, include persons of Hispanic and non-Hispanic origin. Persons of Hispanic origin may be of any race. Death rates for the American Indian and Alaska Native, Asian or Pacific Islander, and Hispanic populations are known to be underestimated.

[5]In 1950, rate is for the age group 75 years and over.

[6]Prior to 1997, excludes data from states lacking an Hispanic-origin item on the death certificate.

Table 2-27. Death Rates for All Causes, by Sex, Race, Hispanic Origin, and Age, Selected Years 1950–2015—*Continued*

(Deaths per 100,000 resident population.)

Sex, race, Hispanic origin, and age	1950¹	1960¹	1970	1980	1985	1990	1995	2000	2005	2006
75 to 84 years	NA	NA	NA	NA	8,361.0	7,920.4	7,367.4	6,977.8	6,329.5	6,154.5
85 years and over	NA	NA	NA	NA	18,635.3	18,505.4	18,132.6	17,853.2	16,840.7	16,206.8
White Female³										
All ages, age-adjusted²	1,198.0	1,074.4	944.0	796.1	764.3	728.8	718.7	715.3	680.9	662.3
All ages, crude	803.3	800.9	812.6	806.1	840.1	846.9	883.2	912.3	888.1	870.3
Under 1 year	2,566.8	2,007.7	1,614.6	962.5	799.3	690.0	574.4	550.5	535.5	533.3
1 to 4 years	112.2	85.2	66.1	49.3	40.0	36.1	31.3	25.5	23.5	24.3
5 to 14 years	45.1	34.7	29.9	22.9	19.5	17.9	16.5	14.1	12.9	12.0
15 to 24 years	71.5	54.9	61.6	55.5	48.1	45.9	43.7	41.1	41.5	41.8
25 to 34 years	112.8	85.0	84.1	65.4	59.4	61.5	62.9	55.1	59.0	60.2
35 to 44 years	235.8	191.1	193.3	138.2	121.9	117.4	125.5	125.7	131.3	130.1
45 to 54 years	546.4	458.8	462.9	372.7	341.4	309.3	291.9	281.4	291.8	292.6
55 to 64 years	1,293.8	1,078.9	1,014.9	876.2	869.1	822.7	783.4	730.9	659.7	649.9
65 to 74 years	3,242.8	2,779.3	2,470.7	2,066.6	2,027.1	1,923.5	1,913.2	1,868.3	1,687.6	1,631.5
75 to 84 years	8,481.5	7,696.6	6,698.7	5,401.7	5,111.6	4,839.1	4,775.3	4,785.3	4,526.1	4,397.1
85 years and over	19,679.5	19,477.7	15,980.2	14,979.6	14,745.4	14,400.6	14,405.8	14,890.7	14,438.0	13,905.7
Black or African American Female³										
All ages, age-adjusted²	1,545.5	1,369.7	1,228.7	1,033.3	994.4	975.1	955.9	927.6	862.7	828.4
All ages, crude	1,002.0	905.0	829.2	733.3	734.2	747.9	743.2	733.0	699.2	678.3
Under 1 year	NA	4,162.2	3,368.8	2,123.7	1,821.4	1,735.5	1,399.9	1,279.8	1,203.3	1,215.9
1 to 4 years⁴	1,139.3	173.3	129.4	84.4	71.1	67.6	59.5	45.3	38.2	41.2
5 to 14 years	72.8	53.8	43.8	30.5	28.6	27.5	25.4	20.0	19.0	17.0
15 to 24 years	213.1	107.5	111.9	70.5	59.6	68.7	68.9	58.3	50.3	50.2
25 to 34 years	393.3	273.2	231.0	150.0	137.6	159.5	162.8	121.8	110.2	107.0
35 to 44 years	758.1	568.5	533.0	323.9	276.5	298.6	324.9	271.9	248.4	243.0
45 to 54 years	1,576.4	1,177.0	1,043.9	768.2	667.6	639.4	612.1	588.3	562.0	540.9
55 to 64 years	3,089.4	2,510.9	1,986.2	1,561.0	1,532.5	1,452.6	1,354.3	1,227.2	1,083.0	1,052.9
65 to 74 years	4,000.2	4,064.2	3,860.9	3,057.4	2,967.8	2,865.7	2,837.5	2,689.6	2,300.8	2,196.1
75 to 84 years⁵	8,347.0	6,730.0	6,691.5	6,212.1	6,078.0	5,688.3	5,671.9	5,696.5	5,278.5	5,042.4
85 years and over	NA	13,052.6	10,706.6	12,367.2	12,703.0	13,309.5	13,073.3	13,941.3	14,183.6	13,535.1
American Indian or Alaska Native Female³										
All ages, age-adjusted²	NA	NA	NA	662.4	577.2	561.8	643.9	604.5	601.8	589.0
All ages, crude	NA	NA	NA	380.1	342.5	330.4	360.1	346.1	354.8	347.6
Under 1 year	NA	NA	NA	1,352.6	910.5	688.7	780.6	492.2	500.1	453.5
1 to 4 years	NA	NA	NA	87.5	54.8	37.8	54.4	39.8	31.3	34.0
5 to 14 years	NA	NA	NA	33.5	23.0	25.5	20.0	17.7	14.5	13.6
15 to 24 years	NA	NA	NA	90.3	72.8	69.0	60.4	58.9	61.5	56.3
25 to 34 years	NA	NA	NA	178.5	121.5	102.3	106.3	84.8	80.8	80.7
35 to 44 years	NA	NA	NA	286.0	185.6	156.4	171.9	171.9	171.2	176.1
45 to 54 years	NA	NA	NA	491.4	415.5	380.9	349.1	284.9	338.9	311.6
55 to 64 years	NA	NA	NA	837.1	851.9	805.9	876.2	772.1	675.6	656.8
65 to 74 years	NA	NA	NA	1,765.5	1,630.3	1,679.4	1,935.6	1,899.8	1,770.0	1,639.8
75 to 84 years	NA	NA	NA	3,612.9	3,200.0	3,073.2	4,067.6	3,850.0	3,812.8	3,967.9
85 years and over	NA	NA	NA	8,567.4	7,740.0	8,201.1	9,201.8	9,118.2	9,752.1	9,413.5
Asian or Pacific Islander Female³										
All ages, age-adjusted²	NA	NA	NA	425.9	456.7	469.3	446.7	416.8	385.2	381.2
All ages, crude	NA	NA	NA	222.5	224.9	234.3	250.4	262.3	271.4	273.4
Under 1 year	NA	NA	NA	755.8	622.0	518.2	396.6	434.3	373.8	348.6
1 to 4 years	NA	NA	NA	35.4	36.8	32.0	24.9	20.0	16.2	19.8
5 to 14 years	NA	NA	NA	21.5	19.1	13.0	15.4	11.7	11.4	9.8
15 to 24 years	NA	NA	NA	32.3	30.7	28.8	31.1	22.4	23.1	22.2
25 to 34 years	NA	NA	NA	45.4	36.5	37.5	35.6	27.6	27.1	26.9
35 to 44 years	NA	NA	NA	89.7	77.8	69.9	66.2	65.6	57.9	56.8
45 to 54 years	NA	NA	NA	214.1	184.9	182.7	184.1	155.5	140.1	142.1
55 to 64 years	NA	NA	NA	440.8	468.0	483.4	457.7	390.9	342.8	321.9
65 to 74 years	NA	NA	NA	1,027.7	1,130.8	1,089.2	1,037.8	996.4	896.0	887.7
75 to 84 years	NA	NA	NA	2,833.6	2,873.9	3,127.9	3,089.9	2,882.4	2,613.2	2,623.3
85 years and over	NA	NA	NA	7,923.3	9,808.3	10,254.0	9,406.1	9,052.2	8,769.0	8,664.5
Hispanic or Latina Female³,⁶										
All ages, age-adjusted²	NA	NA	NA	NA	546.1	537.1	546.1	546.0	513.8	500.2
All ages, crude	NA	NA	NA	NA	251.9	285.4	281.9	274.6	272.7	269.0
Under 1 year	NA	NA	NA	NA	791.4	746.6	572.0	553.6	526.3	512.0
1 to 4 years	NA	NA	NA	NA	42.3	42.1	33.1	27.5	24.3	24.0
5 to 14 years	NA	NA	NA	NA	16.0	17.3	15.0	13.4	11.8	11.6

NA = Not available.

¹Includes deaths of persons who were not residents of the 50 states and the District of Columbia (DC).

²Age-adjusted rates are calculated using the year 2000 standard population. Prior to 2001, age-adjusted rates were calculated using standard million proportions based on rounded population numbers. Starting with 2001 data, unrounded population numbers are used to calculate age-adjusted rates.

³The race groups, White, Black, Asian or Pacific Islander, and American Indian and Alaska Native, include persons of Hispanic and non-Hispanic origin. Persons of Hispanic origin may be of any race. Death rates for the American Indian and Alaska Native, Asian or Pacific Islander, and Hispanic populations are known to be underestimated.

⁴In 1950, rate is for the age group under 5 years.

⁵In 1950, rate is for the age group 75 years and over.

⁶Prior to 1997, excludes data from states lacking an Hispanic-origin item on the death certificate.

Table 2-27. Death Rates for All Causes, by Sex, Race, Hispanic Origin, and Age, Selected Years 1950–2015—*Continued*

(Deaths per 100,000 resident population.)

Sex, race, Hispanic origin, and age	2007	2008	2009	2010	2011	2012	2013	2014	2015
75 to 84 years	6,008.4	6,009.9	5,810.0	5,770.3	5,727.3	5,599.2	5,582.7	5,499.0	5,500.5
85 years and over	15,946.0	16,114.4	15,552.9	15,816.6	15,568.2	15,504.4	15,485.9	15,286.4	15,526.0
White Female[3]									
All ages, age-adjusted[2]	649.4	653.7	631.3	630.8	630.3	623.8	623.6	617.6	627.0
All ages, crude	860.6	874.6	849.3	857.3	868.9	869.9	879.4	876.7	899.2
Under 1 year	537.1	525.0	502.3	488.0	469.8	471.5	456.8	457.6	455.1
1 to 4 years	24.1	23.8	22.6	21.6	21.7	21.7	20.1	19.6	19.7
5 to 14 years	12.5	11.4	11.1	10.6	10.5	10.4	10.6	10.0	10.6
15 to 24 years	41.1	37.6	37.1	36.2	36.0	35.5	35.5	35.5	37.8
25 to 34 years	60.7	59.2	62.9	61.4	63.6	64.6	64.6	66.9	72.0
35 to 44 years	127.2	126.8	128.2	122.8	124.9	124.1	126.8	130.7	131.7
45 to 54 years	291.4	296.1	301.6	295.1	301.8	300.1	303.4	305.8	306.6
55 to 64 years	632.5	633.2	624.8	617.8	619.2	620.5	623.4	635.1	640.4
65 to 74 years	1,584.0	1,577.5	1,517.9	1,504.9	1,491.2	1,450.9	1,453.2	1,433.1	1,443.8
75 to 84 years	4,319.4	4,352.9	4,190.9	4,165.4	4,158.2	4,110.6	4,072.0	4,001.3	4,028.0
85 years and over	13,636.6	13,868.7	13,132.7	13,419.3	13,380.8	13,281.9	13,316.1	13,079.1	13,442.5
Black or African American Female[3]									
All ages, age-adjusted[2]	808.1	792.0	763.3	752.5	739.8	723.9	720.6	713.3	710.8
All ages, crude	668.2	661.8	645.6	642.7	643.4	642.3	651.1	655.5	665.7
Under 1 year	1,160.8	1,105.1	1,070.0	994.4	962.3	944.4	980.7	956.3	970.0
1 to 4 years[4]	41.0	36.3	37.7	33.2	33.8	33.0	33.4	31.9	32.0
5 to 14 years	16.6	15.8	16.6	14.5	14.6	14.0	14.8	14.3	15.0
15 to 24 years	47.5	48.8	46.6	43.3	43.5	43.6	41.2	42.5	45.8
25 to 34 years	102.1	97.2	97.5	92.9	94.9	89.5	91.0	88.6	92.9
35 to 44 years	226.4	218.2	207.7	199.3	198.5	192.9	187.9	193.9	191.8
45 to 54 years	528.3	515.1	500.5	481.0	467.6	461.5	454.4	455.8	447.0
55 to 64 years	1,021.0	1,000.1	983.7	972.2	952.3	950.4	962.2	974.8	969.6
65 to 74 years	2,159.9	2,101.7	2,041.2	2,021.2	1,969.2	1,918.7	1,909.2	1,880.2	1,864.4
75 to 84 years[5]	4,918.6	4,843.3	4,694.0	4,580.9	4,535.3	4,396.0	4,418.0	4,356.8	4,310.0
85 years and over	13,323.3	13,177.9	12,378.5	12,589.9	12,364.2	12,149.6	11,929.2	11,656.8	11,741.3
American Indian or Alaska Native Female[3]									
All ages, age-adjusted[2]	565.2	548.7	536.4	541.7	522.5	512.3	508.3	514.1	511.3
All ages, crude	339.0	332.9	332.4	332.4	338.1	340.9	348.2	363.5	375.8
Under 1 year	528.3	437.3	444.2	366.4	411.6	425.9	305.9	412.5	431.0
1 to 4 years	30.3	35.8	23.5	24.4	25.1	22.7	25.5	20.4	26.5
5 to 14 years	9.9	13.1	16.2	10.5	12.3	9.6	10.9	10.8	13.7
15 to 24 years	53.1	49.4	56.3	43.6	45.4	47.7	42.8	46.8	47.1
25 to 34 years	77.8	83.6	81.9	85.6	88.0	98.8	93.5	88.0	104.7
35 to 44 years	164.3	177.6	171.8	146.6	164.9	162.2	172.4	179.0	170.5
45 to 54 years	309.8	300.0	346.5	326.2	336.6	329.6	334.5	354.3	354.2
55 to 64 years	659.0	626.3	603.9	623.8	611.5	587.2	616.6	606.2	622.2
65 to 74 years	1,589.6	1,528.3	1,472.4	1,481.7	1,376.1	1,390.3	1,314.7	1,368.6	1,360.3
75 to 84 years	3,656.9	3,472.8	3,332.7	3,391.9	3,300.8	3,256.9	3,221.9	3,226.6	3,192.5
85 years and over	9,155.0	9,024.2	8,619.3	9,277.9	8,448.2	7,987.3	8,008.4	7,893.5	7,636.6
Asian or Pacific Islander Female[3]									
All ages, age-adjusted[2]	369.2	372.4	361.1	359.0	349.8	348.8	343.0	331.1	338.0
All ages, crude	269.5	277.0	273.5	277.3	283.8	292.0	297.4	295.5	310.8
Under 1 year	380.0	360.7	373.7	341.8	342.5	349.0	329.3	338.6	358.1
1 to 4 years	16.8	19.3	12.7	16.3	11.8	14.8	18.4	12.5	15.0
5 to 14 years	9.0	7.9	10.0	7.9	7.9	7.2	8.8	6.5	7.3
15 to 24 years	20.5	19.1	21.1	17.0	15.9	18.4	17.7	17.8	19.1
25 to 34 years	25.4	30.4	26.0	27.1	24.6	24.4	25.7	24.8	26.2
35 to 44 years	54.3	48.0	50.8	49.0	52.5	50.4	51.5	49.1	51.1
45 to 54 years	131.7	129.9	122.0	127.9	130.2	130.3	128.0	122.3	127.6
55 to 64 years	315.0	310.2	294.8	298.8	303.7	301.5	287.2	283.2	288.0
65 to 74 years	813.6	835.8	776.8	788.7	719.4	731.9	703.9	700.5	704.8
75 to 84 years	2,566.2	2,531.2	2,472.3	2,445.5	2,446.0	2,330.6	2,346.7	2,237.5	2,263.5
85 years and over	8,546.0	8,859.2	8,685.4	8,590.1	8,251.9	8,469.0	8,240.4	7,945.3	8,142.0
Hispanic or Latina Female[3,6]									
All ages, age-adjusted[2]	484.4	484.7	466.1	463.4	452.8	452.5	448.6	437.5	438.3
All ages, crude	264.0	265.8	261.4	260.9	264.6	272.7	279.4	281.0	290.4
Under 1 year	522.8	499.2	480.1	462.9	430.2	428.9	433.7	432.1	436.6
1 to 4 years	24.1	22.8	23.4	20.2	21.3	20.0	18.4	17.2	17.5
5 to 14 years	11.9	11.0	11.8	8.9	9.5	10.0	9.9	9.7	8.6

NA = Not available.
[1]Includes deaths of persons who were not residents of the 50 states and the District of Columbia (DC).
[2]Age-adjusted rates are calculated using the year 2000 standard population. Prior to 2001, age-adjusted rates were calculated using standard million proportions based on rounded population numbers. Starting with 2001 data, unrounded population numbers are used to calculate age-adjusted rates.
[3]The race groups, White, Black, Asian or Pacific Islander, and American Indian and Alaska Native, include persons of Hispanic and non-Hispanic origin. Persons of Hispanic origin may be of any race. Death rates for the American Indian and Alaska Native, Asian or Pacific Islander, and Hispanic populations are known to be underestimated.
[4]In 1950, rate is for the age group under 5 years.
[5]In 1950, rate is for the age group 75 years and over.
[6]Prior to 1997, excludes data from states lacking an Hispanic-origin item on the death certificate.

Table 2-27. Death Rates for All Causes, by Sex, Race, Hispanic Origin, and Age, Selected Years 1950–2015—*Continued*

(Deaths per 100,000 resident population.)

Sex, race, Hispanic origin, and age	1950[1]	1960[1]	1970	1980	1985	1990	1995	2000	2005	2006
15 to 24 years	NA	NA	NA	NA	36.2	40.6	37.5	31.7	34.5	33.0
25 to 34 years	NA	NA	NA	NA	56.3	62.9	58.6	43.4	40.5	42.6
35 to 44 years	NA	NA	NA	NA	100.0	109.3	118.9	100.5	89.1	85.7
45 to 54 years	NA	NA	NA	NA	251.3	253.3	238.8	223.8	213.7	212.5
55 to 64 years	NA	NA	NA	NA	619.7	607.5	602.3	548.4	489.0	481.0
65 to 74 years	NA	NA	NA	NA	1,449.5	1,453.8	1,457.2	1,423.2	1,285.1	1,216.0
75 to 84 years	NA	NA	NA	NA	3,551.8	3,351.3	3,506.4	3,624.5	3,464.7	3,329.0
85 years and over	NA	NA	NA	NA	10,228.6	10,098.7	10,540.5	11,202.8	10,769.7	10,682.9
White, not Hispanic or Latina Female[6]										
All ages, age-adjusted[2]	NA	NA	NA	NA	754.3	734.6	721.1	721.5	690.7	672.4
All ages, crude	NA	NA	NA	NA	861.7	903.6	951.7	1,007.3	999.7	982.8
Under 1 year	NA	NA	NA	NA	763.0	655.3	553.9	530.9	522.3	526.7
1 to 4 years	NA	NA	NA	NA	36.5	34.0	30.3	24.4	22.7	23.8
5 to 14 years	NA	NA	NA	NA	19.0	17.6	16.4	13.9	13.0	11.8
15 to 24 years	NA	NA	NA	NA	47.9	46.0	44.0	42.6	42.6	43.3
25 to 34 years	NA	NA	NA	NA	59.0	60.6	62.2	56.8	63.3	64.0
35 to 44 years	NA	NA	NA	NA	122.8	116.8	124.1	128.1	138.1	137.7
45 to 54 years	NA	NA	NA	NA	335.7	312.1	293.0	285.0	299.4	300.8
55 to 64 years	NA	NA	NA	NA	853.3	834.5	789.8	742.1	672.7	662.8
65 to 74 years	NA	NA	NA	NA	1,998.1	1,940.2	1,925.9	1,891.0	1,715.2	1,660.9
75 to 84 years	NA	NA	NA	NA	5,059.1	4,887.3	4,794.9	4,819.3	4,577.1	4,451.4
85 years and over	NA	NA	NA	NA	14,560.4	14,533.1	14,450.9	14,971.7	14,560.9	14,014.9

NA = Not available.
[1]Includes deaths of persons who were not residents of the 50 states and the District of Columbia (DC).
[2]Age-adjusted rates are calculated using the year 2000 standard population. Prior to 2001, age-adjusted rates were calculated using standard million proportions based on rounded population numbers. Starting with 2001 data, unrounded population numbers are used to calculate age-adjusted rates.
[6]Prior to 1997, excludes data from states lacking an Hispanic-origin item on the death certificate.

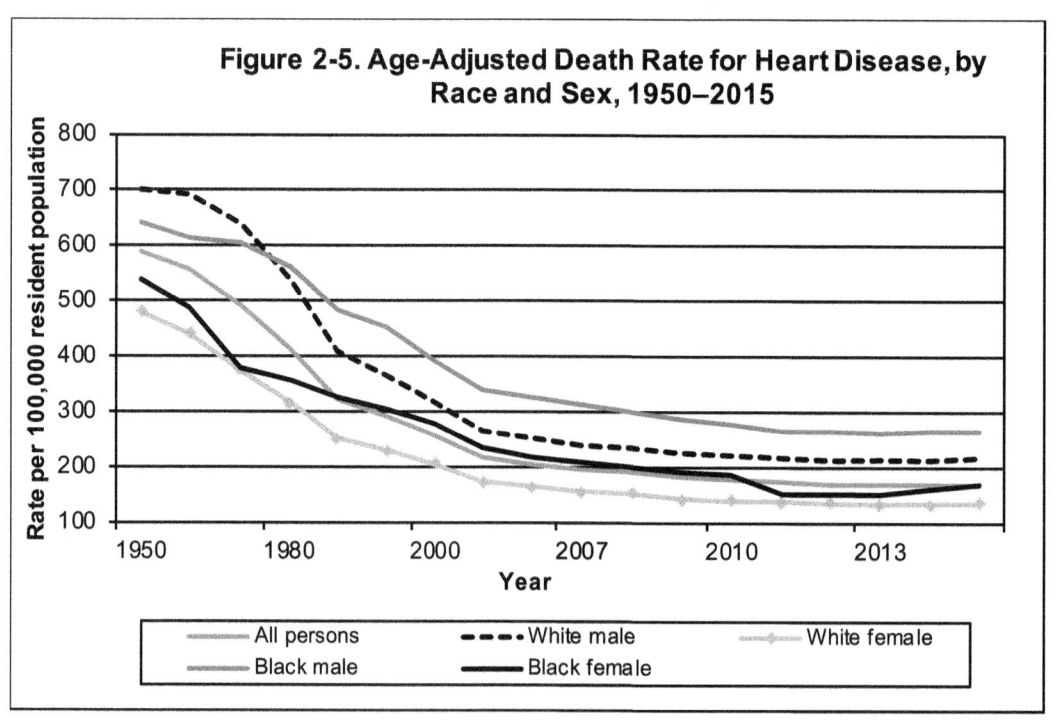

Figure 2-5. Age-Adjusted Death Rate for Heart Disease, by Race and Sex, 1950–2015

Table 2-27. Death Rates for All Causes, by Sex, Race, Hispanic Origin, and Age, Selected Years 1950–2015—_Continued_

(Deaths per 100,000 resident population.)

Sex, race, Hispanic origin, and age	2007	2008	2009	2010	2011	2012	2013	2014	2015
15 to 24 years	30.8	28.4	29.1	26.3	25.6	25.5	25.6	27.2	28.5
25 to 34 years	42.0	40.2	42.5	38.9	39.2	40.0	41.4	41.3	44.8
35 to 44 years	80.7	79.3	81.0	75.2	74.1	73.6	78.3	78.5	77.7
45 to 54 years	199.9	195.4	200.0	193.9	185.7	192.0	189.6	185.3	184.0
55 to 64 years	468.8	467.0	456.8	450.1	435.9	442.8	437.2	443.3	434.6
65 to 74 years	1,149.2	1,137.4	1,106.7	1,085.5	1,077.4	1,046.7	1,039.9	1,036.7	1,048.7
75 to 84 years	3,299.5	3,244.7	3,160.1	3,067.4	3,085.1	3,063.5	3,037.8	2,931.3	2,937.3
85 years and over	10,276.7	10,636.2	9,794.3	10,237.3	9,727.2	9,805.6	9,651.3	9,250.2	9,266.4
White, not Hispanic or Latina Female[6]									
All ages, age-adjusted[2]	660.6	665.4	643.1	643.3	644.6	637.6	638.4	633.8	644.1
All ages, crude	976.1	995.6	969.1	981.2	998.1	998.8	1,011.5	1,011.3	1,038.5
Under 1 year	525.3	516.0	494.2	480.4	468.6	469.2	448.5	451.0	445.7
1 to 4 years	23.5	23.5	21.6	21.8	21.1	21.7	20.4	20.2	20.1
5 to 14 years	12.4	11.1	10.5	10.9	10.6	10.1	10.6	9.8	11.2
15 to 24 years	43.2	39.6	38.6	38.4	38.4	37.8	38.0	37.5	40.1
25 to 34 years	65.0	63.8	67.5	66.8	69.6	70.7	70.2	73.2	78.8
35 to 44 years	135.8	136.1	137.7	133.1	136.6	136.0	138.6	143.8	145.7
45 to 54 years	301.6	308.0	313.5	307.7	317.8	315.2	320.5	325.5	327.7
55 to 64 years	645.5	646.2	638.5	631.5	635.2	635.9	640.5	653.5	661.0
65 to 74 years	1,616.4	1,609.8	1,548.1	1,535.9	1,522.8	1,480.2	1,483.9	1,462.9	1,472.8
75 to 84 years	4,375.2	4,416.1	4,252.4	4,232.6	4,227.0	4,178.1	4,142.2	4,078.9	4,103.1
85 years and over	13,761.8	13,984.1	13,264.8	13,543.5	13,544.3	13,437.0	13,502.5	13,290.4	13,682.6

[2]Age-adjusted rates are calculated using the year 2000 standard population. Prior to 2001, age-adjusted rates were calculated using standard million proportions based on rounded population numbers. Starting with 2001 data, unrounded population numbers are used to calculate age-adjusted rates.
[6]Prior to 1997, excludes data from states lacking an Hispanic-origin item on the death certificate.

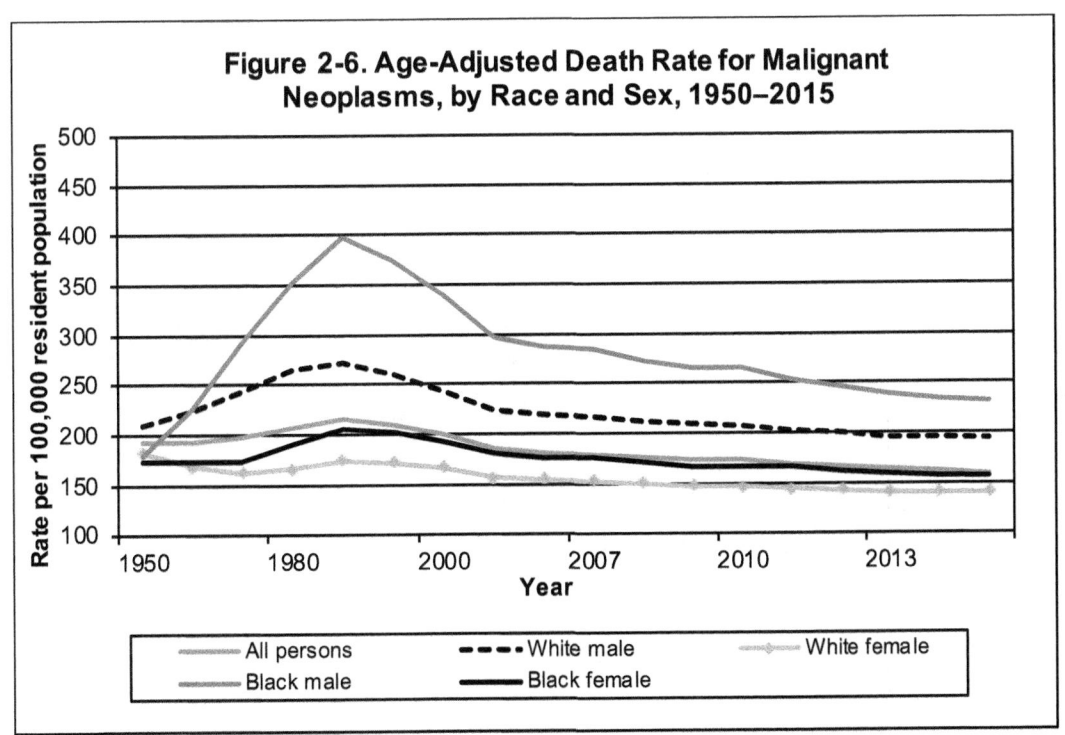

Figure 2-6. Age-Adjusted Death Rate for Malignant Neoplasms, by Race and Sex, 1950–2015

Table 2-28. Death Rates for Diseases of the Heart, by Sex, Race, Hispanic Origin, and Age, Selected Years, 1950–2015

(Deaths per 100,000 resident population.)

Sex, race, Hispanic origin, and age	1950[1,2]	1960[1,2]	1970[2]	1980[2]	1985[2]	1990[2]	1995[2]	2000[3]	2005[3]	2006[3]
All Persons										
All ages, age-adjusted[4]	588.8	559.0	492.7	412.1	375.0	321.8	293.4	257.6	216.8	205.5
All ages, crude	356.8	369.0	362.0	336.0	324.1	289.5	277.0	252.6	220.7	211.7
Under 1 year	4.1	6.6	13.1	22.8	25.0	20.1	17.4	13.0	8.9	8.6
1 to 4 years	1.6	1.3	1.7	2.6	2.2	1.9	1.6	1.2	0.9	1.0
5 to 14 years	3.9	1.3	0.8	0.9	1.0	0.9	0.8	0.7	0.6	0.6
15 to 24 years	8.2	4.0	3.0	2.9	2.8	2.5	2.8	2.6	2.6	2.5
25 to 34 years	20.9	15.6	11.4	8.3	8.3	7.6	8.2	7.4	8.3	8.4
35 to 44 years	88.3	74.6	66.7	44.6	38.1	31.4	31.8	29.2	29.2	28.5
45 to 54 years	309.2	271.8	238.4	180.2	153.8	120.5	109.6	94.2	89.7	88.0
55 to 64 years	804.3	737.9	652.3	494.1	443.0	367.3	320.1	261.2	212.8	205.1
65 to 74 years	1,857.2	1,740.5	1,558.2	1,218.6	1,089.8	894.3	795.4	665.6	512.3	483.0
75 to 84 years	4,311.0	4,089.4	3,683.8	2,993.1	2,693.1	2,295.7	2,050.5	1,780.3	1,458.5	1,378.0
85 years and over	9,152.5	9,317.8	7,891.3	7,777.1	7,384.1	6,739.9	6,391.5	5,926.1	5,188.3	4,877.6
Male										
All ages, age-adjusted[4]	699.0	687.6	634.0	538.9	488.0	412.4	371.0	320.0	268.2	254.9
All ages, crude	424.7	439.5	422.5	368.6	344.1	297.6	278.5	249.8	222.3	215.3
Under 1 year	4.7	7.8	15.1	25.5	27.8	21.9	17.7	13.3	9.6	9.1
1 to 4 years	1.7	1.4	1.9	2.8	2.2	1.9	1.7	1.4	1.0	1.1
5 to 14 years	3.5	1.4	0.9	1.0	0.9	0.9	0.8	0.8	0.6	0.7
15 to 24 years	8.3	4.2	3.7	3.7	3.5	3.1	3.5	3.2	3.5	3.2
25 to 34 years	24.4	20.1	15.2	11.4	11.6	10.3	11.0	9.6	11.2	11.6
35 to 44 years	120.4	112.7	103.2	68.7	58.6	48.1	46.9	41.4	41.3	40.1
45 to 54 years	441.2	420.4	376.4	282.6	237.8	183.0	166.1	140.2	131.6	128.9
55 to 64 years	1,100.5	1,066.9	987.2	746.8	659.1	537.3	460.1	371.7	303.9	293.4
65 to 74 years	2,310.2	2,291.3	2,170.3	1,728.0	1,535.8	1,250.0	1,095.3	898.3	680.1	646.9
75 to 84 years	4,825.8	4,742.4	4,534.8	3,834.3	3,496.9	2,968.2	2,622.9	2,248.1	1,815.1	1,722.7
85 years and over	9,661.4	9,788.9	8,426.2	8,752.7	8,251.8	7,418.4	6,993.5	6,430.0	5,713.2	5,359.2
Female										
All ages, age-adjusted[4]	486.6	447.0	381.6	320.8	294.5	257.0	236.6	210.9	177.5	167.2
All ages, crude	289.7	300.6	304.5	305.1	305.2	281.8	275.5	255.3	219.0	208.2
Under 1 year	3.4	5.4	10.9	20.0	22.0	18.3	17.0	12.5	8.2	8.0
1 to 4 years	1.6	1.1	1.6	2.5	2.2	1.9	1.5	1.0	0.9	0.9
5 to 14 years	4.3	1.2	0.8	0.9	1.0	0.8	0.7	0.5	0.6	0.6
15 to 24 years	8.2	3.7	2.3	2.1	2.1	1.8	2.1	2.1	1.7	1.8
25 to 34 years	17.6	11.3	7.7	5.3	5.0	5.0	5.4	5.2	5.3	5.1
35 to 44 years	57.0	38.2	32.2	21.4	18.3	15.1	17.0	17.2	17.2	17.1
45 to 54 years	177.8	127.5	109.9	84.5	74.4	61.0	55.4	49.8	49.1	48.4
55 to 64 years	507.0	429.4	351.6	272.1	252.1	215.7	192.6	159.3	128.0	122.8
65 to 74 years	1,434.9	1,261.3	1,082.7	828.6	746.1	616.8	554.9	474.0	369.5	342.8
75 to 84 years	3,873.0	3,582.7	3,120.8	2,497.0	2,220.4	1,893.8	1,692.7	1,475.1	1,213.8	1,139.0
85 years and over	8,798.1	9,016.8	7,591.8	7,350.5	7,037.6	6,478.1	6,159.6	5,720.9	4,955.1	4,659.1
White Male[5]										
All ages, age-adjusted[4]	701.4	694.5	640.2	539.6	487.3	409.2	367.0	316.7	264.8	251.1
All ages, crude	434.2	454.6	438.3	384.0	360.3	312.7	294.4	265.8	237.3	229.5
45 to 54 years	424.1	413.2	365.7	269.8	225.5	170.6	153.9	130.7	122.0	120.0
55 to 64 years	1,082.6	1,056.0	979.3	730.6	640.1	516.7	439.2	351.8	286.4	276.9
65 to 74 years	2,309.4	2,297.9	2,177.2	1,729.7	1,522.7	1,230.5	1,071.8	877.8	661.1	624.6
75 to 84 years	4,908.0	4,839.9	4,617.6	3,883.2	3,527.0	2,983.4	2,625.6	2,247.0	1,812.9	1,717.2
85 years and over	9,952.3	10,135.8	8,818.0	8,958.0	8,481.7	7,558.7	7,125.1	6,560.8	5,824.6	5,450.2
Black or African American Male[5]										
All ages, age-adjusted[4]	641.5	615.2	607.3	561.4	533.9	485.4	451.3	392.5	338.8	328.3
All ages, crude	348.4	330.6	330.3	301.0	288.6	256.8	239.1	211.1	194.0	190.5
45 to 54 years	624.1	514.0	512.8	433.4	385.2	328.9	308.6	247.2	231.1	222.2
55 to 64 years	1,434.0	1,236.8	1,135.4	987.2	935.3	824.0	740.5	631.2	527.6	502.5
65 to 74 years	2,140.1	2,281.4	2,237.8	1,847.2	1,839.2	1,632.9	1,514.1	1,268.8	1,002.5	999.7
75 to 84 years[6]	4,107.9	3,533.6	3,783.4	3,578.8	3,436.6	3,107.1	2,908.7	2,597.6	2,206.2	2,126.5
85 years and over	NA	6,037.9	5,367.6	6,819.5	6,393.5	6,479.6	6,088.5	5,633.5	5,137.1	4,968.8
American Indian or Alaska Native Male[5]										
All ages, age-adjusted[4]	NA	NA	NA	320.5	280.5	264.1	256.4	222.2	191.7	186.1
All ages, crude	NA	NA	NA	130.6	117.9	108.0	101.0	90.1	82.8	83.1
45 to 54 years	NA	NA	NA	238.1	209.1	173.8	136.2	108.5	103.2	107.8
55 to 64 years	NA	NA	NA	496.3	438.3	411.0	375.7	285.0	263.4	242.6

[1]Includes deaths of persons who were not residents of the 50 states and the District of Columbia.
[2]Underlying cause of death was coded according to the 6th Revision of the International Classification of Diseases (ICD) in 1950, 7th Revision in 1960, 8th Revision in 1970, and 9th Revision in 1980-1998.
[3]Starting with 1999 data, cause of death is coded according to ICD-10.
[4]Age-adjusted rates are calculated using the year 2000 standard population. Prior to 2001, age-adjusted rates were calculated using standard million proportions based on rounded population numbers. Starting with 2001 data, unrounded population numbers are used to calculate age-adjusted rates.
[5]The race groups, White, Black, Asian or Pacific Islander, and American Indian or Alaska Native, include persons of Hispanic and non-Hispanic origin. Persons of Hispanic origin may be of any race. Death rates for the American Indian or Alaska Native, Asian or Pacific Islander, and Hispanic populations are known to be underestimated.
[6]In 1950, rate is for the age group 75 years and over.

Table 2-28. Death Rates for Diseases of the Heart, by Sex, Race, Hispanic Origin, and Age, Selected Years, 1950–2015—*Continued*

(Deaths per 100,000 resident population.)

Sex, race, Hispanic origin, and age	2007[3]	2008[3]	2009[3]	2010[3]	2011[3]	2012[3]	2013[3]	2014[3]	2015[3]
All Persons									
All ages, age-adjusted[4]	196.1	192.1	182.8	179.1	173.7	170.5	169.8	167.0	168.5
All ages, crude	204.5	202.8	195.4	193.6	191.5	191.0	193.3	192.7	197.2
Under 1 year	10.2	9.6	9.6	8.3	7.7	8.5	7.8	8.0	7.3
1 to 4 years	1.1	1.2	0.9	1.0	1.0	1.0	1.1	0.9	0.9
5 to 14 years	0.6	0.6	0.5	0.5	0.5	0.4	0.4	0.5	0.5
15 to 24 years	2.5	2.5	2.4	2.4	2.3	2.2	2.1	2.2	2.3
25 to 34 years	8.1	8.1	7.8	7.8	7.9	7.6	7.6	7.7	8.0
35 to 44 years	27.7	26.9	26.7	25.8	26.2	25.9	25.6	25.6	25.6
45 to 54 years	85.2	85.2	82.3	81.6	80.7	79.7	80.3	80.1	79.3
55 to 64 years	197.8	195.3	190.0	186.6	183.2	184.6	184.6	185.8	188.1
65 to 74 years	454.8	441.4	422.8	409.2	399.0	388.3	390.3	385.2	389.5
75 to 84 years	1,308.6	1,271.7	1,210.8	1,172.0	1,134.7	1,103.7	1,095.1	1,070.2	1,071.6
85 years and over	4,668.1	4,598.4	4,316.9	4,285.2	4,111.6	4,046.1	4,013.9	3,920.9	3,986.5
Male									
All ages, age-adjusted[4]	243.7	238.5	229.4	225.1	218.1	214.7	214.5	210.9	211.8
All ages, crude	209.2	208.2	203.7	202.5	201.2	202.3	206.5	207.1	211.7
Under 1 year	11.2	10.3	10.5	9.8	7.9	9.6	8.7	8.6	7.5
1 to 4 years	1.0	1.2	0.9	1.1	1.0	1.0	1.2	0.9	1.0
5 to 14 years	0.6	0.6	0.5	0.5	0.5	0.5	0.4	0.5	0.5
15 to 24 years	3.2	3.3	3.1	3.2	3.0	2.9	2.8	2.7	3.0
25 to 34 years	10.9	10.8	10.6	10.7	10.5	10.4	10.2	10.3	10.3
35 to 44 years	39.2	37.4	37.5	36.0	36.6	35.8	35.5	34.8	35.1
45 to 54 years	124.6	122.9	119.8	117.8	116.7	114.3	115.1	113.5	112.1
55 to 64 years	285.1	280.8	274.1	269.5	263.6	266.4	267.3	268.1	269.4
65 to 74 years	610.0	594.0	571.1	553.0	540.4	527.7	530.9	525.7	529.7
75 to 84 years	1,631.9	1,584.3	1,514.8	1,475.7	1,426.6	1,388.1	1,382.4	1,354.8	1,354.4
85 years and over	5,154.3	5,083.6	4,862.8	4,833.6	4,622.7	4,582.7	4,564.2	4,453.4	4,495.1
Female									
All ages, age-adjusted[4]	159.0	155.9	146.6	143.3	138.7	135.5	134.3	131.8	133.6
All ages, crude	199.9	197.7	187.3	184.9	182.0	180.2	180.6	178.6	183.1
Under 1 year	9.2	8.8	8.8	6.8	7.5	7.3	6.9	7.4	7.2
1 to 4 years	1.2	1.1	1.0	0.9	1.0	0.9	0.9	0.9	0.9
5 to 14 years	0.5	0.5	0.5	0.4	0.5	0.4	0.4	0.4	0.5
15 to 24 years	1.8	1.6	1.6	1.5	1.5	1.5	1.5	1.6	1.5
25 to 34 years	5.3	5.4	5.0	4.9	5.3	4.8	4.9	5.0	5.6
35 to 44 years	16.2	16.4	16.0	15.6	15.9	16.0	15.7	16.4	16.2
45 to 54 years	47.1	48.8	46.0	46.5	45.9	46.0	46.6	47.5	47.4
55 to 64 years	116.4	115.6	111.6	109.3	108.4	108.4	107.5	109.3	112.3
65 to 74 years	321.4	309.7	294.2	284.2	275.7	266.2	266.8	261.7	266.2
75 to 84 years	1,082.0	1,050.4	993.3	952.7	920.7	893.0	879.8	854.8	855.9
85 years and over	4,443.3	4,370.0	4,056.0	4,020.3	3,859.7	3,777.5	3,732.9	3,643.8	3,717.6
White Male[5]									
All ages, age-adjusted[4]	240.3	235.8	226.6	222.9	216.9	213.1	213.1	210.0	211.2
All ages, crude	223.6	223.3	218.4	217.8	217.1	218.0	222.6	223.9	229.1
45 to 54 years	117.0	117.1	113.1	111.2	110.8	108.3	109.8	107.7	106.6
55 to 64 years	269.3	266.9	258.9	257.0	251.7	253.2	254.0	255.9	256.5
65 to 74 years	590.1	573.9	551.1	536.3	524.9	513.5	516.0	512.7	516.8
75 to 84 years	1,629.3	1,580.9	1,516.2	1,475.1	1,434.2	1,392.6	1,389.0	1,361.5	1,362.9
85 years and over	5,252.0	5,192.6	4,972.4	4,943.1	4,754.6	4,712.4	4,701.6	4,603.9	4,663.2
Black or African American Male[5]									
All ages, age-adjusted[4]	312.4	301.2	289.0	280.6	266.1	265.3	262.8	259.5	258.6
All ages, crude	184.7	180.5	178.1	174.6	171.0	174.7	177.2	178.7	182.8
45 to 54 years	207.9	192.4	194.1	190.9	184.1	182.4	178.3	179.5	177.3
55 to 64 years	489.8	465.5	463.2	437.8	425.2	435.9	430.0	425.5	430.9
65 to 74 years	941.0	925.0	893.3	847.8	825.5	805.5	807.5	794.6	801.5
75 to 84 years[6]	1,992.0	1,958.6	1,821.7	1,807.1	1,680.2	1,677.7	1,660.0	1,651.4	1,644.6
85 years and over	4,751.8	4,519.0	4,260.8	4,202.7	3,846.9	3,822.1	3,754.5	3,693.0	3,583.2
American Indian or Alaska Native Male[5]									
All ages, age-adjusted[4]	175.5	163.5	162.2	158.7	153.4	152.5	152.3	149.7	148.0
All ages, crude	79.3	76.5	76.5	75.0	76.9	78.3	82.3	84.4	87.4
45 to 54 years	99.5	106.1	86.4	98.0	91.8	87.4	101.6	95.9	102.2
55 to 64 years	221.4	219.4	230.2	217.2	210.6	198.5	206.2	217.2	231.7

[3]Starting with 1999 data, cause of death is coded according to ICD-10.
[4]Age-adjusted rates are calculated using the year 2000 standard population. Prior to 2001, age-adjusted rates were calculated using standard million proportions based on rounded population numbers. Starting with 2001 data, unrounded population numbers are used to calculate age-adjusted rates.
[5]The race groups, White, Black, Asian or Pacific Islander, and American Indian or Alaska Native, include persons of Hispanic and non-Hispanic origin. Persons of Hispanic origin may be of any race. Death rates for the American Indian or Alaska Native, Asian or Pacific Islander, and Hispanic populations are known to be underestimated.
[6]In 1950, rate is for the age group 75 years and over.

Table 2-28. Death Rates for Diseases of the Heart, by Sex, Race, Hispanic Origin, and Age, Selected Years, 1950–2015—Continued

(Deaths per 100,000 resident population.)

Sex, race, Hispanic origin, and age	1950[1,2]	1960[1,2]	1970[2]	1980[2]	1985[2]	1990[2]	1995[2]	2000[3]	2005[3]	2006[3]
65 to 74 years	NA	NA	NA	1,009.4	984.6	839.1	938.2	748.2	551.9	568.4
75 to 84 years	NA	NA	NA	2,062.2	2,118.2	1,788.8	1,858.5	1,655.7	1,253.6	1,323.6
85 years and over	NA	NA	NA	4,413.7	2,766.7	3,860.3	3,306.5	3,318.3	3,529.4	2,942.8
Asian or Pacific Islander Male[5]										
All ages, age-adjusted[4]	NA	NA	NA	286.9	258.9	220.7	214.5	185.5	149.4	145.4
All ages, crude	NA	NA	NA	119.8	103.5	88.7	93.2	90.6	81.7	80.6
45 to 54 years	NA	NA	NA	112.0	81.1	70.4	69.8	61.1	58.1	55.8
55 to 64 years	NA	NA	NA	306.7	291.2	226.1	205.4	182.6	143.9	144.1
65 to 74 years	NA	NA	NA	852.4	753.5	623.5	581.0	482.5	370.9	340.7
75 to 84 years	NA	NA	NA	2,010.9	2,025.6	1,642.2	1,533.8	1,354.7	1,014.6	996.4
85 years and over	NA	NA	NA	5,923.0	4,937.5	4,617.8	4,888.9	4,154.2	3,518.6	3,497.0
Hispanic or Latino Male[5,7]										
All ages, age-adjusted[4]	NA	NA	NA	NA	296.6	270.0	260.8	238.2	210.5	193.7
All ages, crude	NA	NA	NA	NA	92.1	91.0	83.1	74.7	72.3	68.2
45 to 54 years	NA	NA	NA	NA	128.1	116.4	102.0	84.3	78.7	76.7
55 to 64 years	NA	NA	NA	NA	398.8	363.0	311.2	264.8	220.4	203.7
65 to 74 years	NA	NA	NA	NA	971.1	829.9	784.6	684.8	567.9	512.3
75 to 84 years	NA	NA	NA	NA	2,150.0	1,971.3	1,854.0	1,733.2	1,541.7	1,380.2
85 years and over	NA	NA	NA	NA	4,912.5	4,711.9	5,104.0	4,897.5	4,442.3	4,190.2
White, Not Hispanic or Latino Male[7]										
All ages, age-adjusted[4]	NA	NA	NA	NA	480.4	413.6	369.1	319.9	267.9	254.6
All ages, crude	NA	NA	NA	NA	362.8	336.5	320.6	297.5	269.9	262.3
45 to 54 years	NA	NA	NA	NA	219.9	172.8	155.9	134.3	126.6	124.9
55 to 64 years	NA	NA	NA	NA	610.6	521.3	443.2	356.3	290.6	281.8
65 to 74 years	NA	NA	NA	NA	1,471.3	1,243.4	1,077.0	885.1	664.8	630.1
75 to 84 years	NA	NA	NA	NA	3,512.8	3,007.7	2,635.3	2,261.9	1,823.1	1,732.6
85 years and over	NA	NA	NA	NA	8,538.4	7,663.4	7,156.4	6,606.6	5,876.4	5,495.9
White Female[5]										
All ages, age-adjusted[4]	479.2	441.7	376.7	315.9	289.1	250.9	230.8	205.6	173.2	163.4
All ages, crude	290.5	306.5	313.8	319.2	321.8	298.4	294.7	274.5	236.9	225.9
45 to 54 years	142.4	103.4	91.4	71.2	62.5	50.2	45.5	40.9	40.9	40.9
55 to 64 years	460.7	383.0	317.7	248.1	227.1	192.4	172.0	141.3	113.8	110.6
65 to 74 years	1,401.6	1,229.8	1,044.0	796.7	713.3	583.6	523.2	445.2	349.2	323.0
75 to 84 years	3,926.2	3,629.7	3,143.5	2,493.6	2,207.5	1,874.3	1,670.3	1,452.4	1,195.1	1,124.4
85 years and over	9,086.9	9,280.8	7,839.9	7,501.6	7,170.0	6,563.4	6,251.3	5,801.4	5,017.5	4,721.8
Black or African American Female[5]										
All ages, age-adjusted[4]	538.9	488.9	435.6	378.6	357.7	327.5	304.0	277.6	234.5	218.1
All ages, crude	289.9	268.5	261.0	249.7	250.3	237.0	226.3	212.6	184.0	172.9
45 to 54 years	526.8	360.7	290.9	202.4	176.2	155.3	141.5	125.0	114.1	109.6
55 to 64 years	1,210.7	952.3	710.5	530.1	510.7	442.0	386.0	332.8	266.9	245.8
65 to 74 years	1,659.4	1,680.5	1,553.2	1,210.3	1,149.9	1,017.5	938.2	815.2	604.2	567.1
75 to 84 years[6]	3,499.3	2,926.9	2,964.1	2,707.2	2,533.4	2,250.9	2,100.7	1,913.1	1,599.6	1,465.7
85 years and over	NA	5,650.0	5,003.8	5,796.5	5,686.5	5,766.1	5,448.5	5,298.7	4,841.3	4,493.7
American Indian or Alaska Native Female[5]										
All ages, age-adjusted[4]	NA	NA	NA	175.4	170.0	153.1	164.8	143.6	129.3	126.1
All ages, crude	NA	NA	NA	80.3	84.3	77.5	80.2	71.9	66.8	65.3
45 to 54 years	NA	NA	NA	65.2	59.2	62.0	62.4	40.2	48.2	38.0
55 to 64 years	NA	NA	NA	193.5	230.8	197.0	200.7	149.4	118.0	119.8
65 to 74 years	NA	NA	NA	577.2	472.7	492.8	514.2	391.8	346.6	318.9
75 to 84 years	NA	NA	NA	1,364.3	1,258.8	1,050.3	1,184.3	1,044.1	896.3	993.4
85 years and over	NA	NA	NA	2,893.3	3,180.0	2,868.7	3,118.1	3,146.3	2,962.1	2,672.2
Asian or Pacific Islander Female[5]										
All ages, age-adjusted[4]	NA	NA	NA	132.3	149.4	149.2	137.6	115.7	97.5	93.7
All ages, crude	NA	NA	NA	57.0	60.3	62.0	66.3	65.0	63.6	62.1
45 to 54 years	NA	NA	NA	28.6	23.8	17.5	20.8	15.9	15.5	15.6
55 to 64 years	NA	NA	NA	92.9	103.0	99.0	89.5	68.8	55.2	46.8
65 to 74 years	NA	NA	NA	313.3	341.0	323.9	288.3	229.6	192.3	185.3

NA = Not available.
[1]Includes deaths of persons who were not residents of the 50 states and the District of Columbia.
[2]Underlying cause of death was coded according to the 6th Revision of the International Classification of Diseases (ICD) in 1950, 7th Revision in 1960, 8th Revision in 1970, and 9th Revision in 1980-1998.
[3]Starting with 1999 data, cause of death is coded according to ICD-10.
[4]Age-adjusted rates are calculated using the year 2000 standard population. Prior to 2001, age-adjusted rates were calculated using standard million proportions based on rounded population numbers. Starting with 2001 data, unrounded population numbers are used to calculate age-adjusted rates.
[5]The race groups, White, Black, Asian or Pacific Islander, and American Indian or Alaska Native, include persons of Hispanic and non-Hispanic origin. Persons of Hispanic origin may be of any race. Death rates for the American Indian or Alaska Native, Asian or Pacific Islander, and Hispanic populations are known to be underestimated.
[6]In 1950, rate is for the age group 75 years and over.
[7]Prior to 1997, excludes data from states lacking an Hispanic-origin item on the death certificate.

Table 2-28. Death Rates for Diseases of the Heart, by Sex, Race, Hispanic Origin, and Age, Selected Years, 1950–2015—Continued

(Deaths per 100,000 resident population.)

Sex, race, Hispanic origin, and age	2007[3]	2008[3]	2009[3]	2010[3]	2011[3]	2012[3]	2013[3]	2014[3]	2015[3]
65 to 74 years	515.2	520.5	518.1	425.1	470.4	451.5	465.2	444.0	408.5
75 to 84 years	1,276.2	1,058.5	1,097.2	1,042.6	1,068.8	1,138.9	1,071.8	978.2	1,042.1
85 years and over	2,805.9	2,684.7	2,560.7	2,833.1	2,395.7	2,278.2	2,269.1	2,415.9	2,184.3
Asian or Pacific Islander Male[5]									
All ages, age-adjusted[4]	134.4	133.0	130.2	127.2	115.1	116.1	118.4	109.1	109.7
All ages, crude	76.6	77.3	78.4	77.0	74.2	76.8	81.9	78.4	80.9
45 to 54 years	51.1	50.8	54.1	49.2	52.7	51.8	50.9	53.4	49.0
55 to 64 years	129.4	131.3	129.2	119.3	112.9	118.4	133.3	121.4	121.2
65 to 74 years	314.8	308.0	307.6	294.4	270.3	255.1	274.9	250.5	254.1
75 to 84 years	935.0	924.3	874.4	855.5	772.1	748.7	754.6	726.6	718.6
85 years and over	3,162.6	3,170.9	3,080.5	3,132.9	2,695.9	2,842.2	2,848.5	2,459.7	2,543.8
Hispanic or Latino Male[5,7]									
All ages, age-adjusted[4]	183.1	171.2	169.4	165.1	152.2	151.6	151.5	145.7	146.4
All ages, crude	66.5	63.7	65.0	64.1	62.5	64.3	66.9	67.4	70.7
45 to 54 years	74.3	68.4	71.0	66.1	66.0	61.7	63.5	64.0	64.8
55 to 64 years	203.0	196.6	195.5	185.9	172.3	177.5	178.0	169.5	176.4
65 to 74 years	482.5	459.1	452.0	424.5	412.9	406.1	416.6	391.6	395.6
75 to 84 years	1,303.4	1,219.9	1,211.9	1,160.9	1,092.7	1,069.1	1,057.5	1,019.7	1,046.6
85 years and over	3,875.4	3,569.9	3,486.6	3,577.9	3,076.1	3,147.0	3,106.2	2,987.5	2,883.7
White, Not Hispanic or Latino Male[7]									
All ages, age-adjusted[4]	244.0	240.0	230.4	226.9	221.6	217.7	217.9	215.2	216.3
All ages, crude	256.4	257.3	251.8	251.8	252.4	253.2	259.0	261.0	267.0
45 to 54 years	122.0	123.0	118.4	117.2	117.1	115.2	117.2	115.0	113.8
55 to 64 years	273.8	271.5	263.1	261.9	258.0	259.1	260.2	263.6	263.4
65 to 74 years	595.7	579.8	555.4	542.2	530.9	518.3	520.2	518.9	522.2
75 to 84 years	1,645.5	1,599.4	1,531.7	1,491.4	1,452.9	1,409.6	1,408.1	1,382.1	1,379.4
85 years and over	5,310.7	5,263.8	5,042.8	5,006.6	4,841.0	4,796.1	4,794.2	4,703.8	4,781.2
White Female[5]									
All ages, age-adjusted[4]	155.4	152.5	143.4	140.4	136.5	133.4	132.0	130.0	132.4
All ages, crude	216.9	215.0	203.7	201.5	198.8	196.7	196.8	195.1	200.6
45 to 54 years	40.2	41.3	39.5	40.7	40.5	40.7	41.0	42.2	42.4
55 to 64 years	104.4	103.4	99.7	98.2	98.0	97.8	95.9	98.8	101.6
65 to 74 years	301.1	292.6	276.8	268.4	261.3	251.7	252.5	247.6	253.8
75 to 84 years	1,069.4	1,038.5	982.3	941.6	912.8	888.1	871.8	849.0	855.3
85 years and over	4,496.0	4,437.7	4,119.8	4,086.7	3,938.3	3,855.8	3,821.0	3,746.8	3,835.1
Black or African American Female[5]									
All ages, age-adjusted[4]	209.8	202.5	191.0	185.3	176.2	172.7	172.1	167.7	165.7
All ages, crude	168.1	164.8	157.6	154.8	150.3	150.9	153.4	152.3	153.9
45 to 54 years	105.3	109.7	99.5	96.6	91.6	92.6	94.2	94.9	92.4
55 to 64 years	236.4	234.1	228.5	218.6	209.2	211.1	213.0	211.0	214.3
65 to 74 years	550.8	514.0	498.5	475.9	461.6	449.3	450.8	437.9	433.5
75 to 84 years[6]	1,388.4	1,342.1	1,272.0	1,227.2	1,158.4	1,114.8	1,122.2	1,085.7	1,050.5
85 years and over	4,399.9	4,153.1	3,833.3	3,783.8	3,559.7	3,513.5	3,425.3	3,269.8	3,282.5
American Indian or Alaska Native Female[5]									
All ages, age-adjusted[4]	112.2	106.8	104.6	103.5	99.4	92.9	93.9	94.0	94.0
All ages, crude	59.0	56.9	56.9	55.9	57.3	55.7	58.4	61.0	63.8
45 to 54 years	32.8	35.1	42.0	37.7	40.9	39.4	37.3	40.8	44.0
55 to 64 years	103.3	99.9	102.1	89.0	99.3	83.9	100.5	90.4	93.9
65 to 74 years	284.5	260.0	262.7	248.1	225.8	245.0	220.1	269.0	247.5
75 to 84 years	829.1	764.1	734.4	684.7	715.5	698.2	664.6	657.3	690.7
85 years and over	2,487.8	2,469.0	2,352.1	2,614.1	2,259.3	1,874.7	2,089.2	1,931.7	1,813.0
Asian or Pacific Islander Female[5]									
All ages, age-adjusted[4]	88.5	88.5	83.6	81.2	76.2	74.0	73.3	68.2	68.5
All ages, crude	60.0	61.7	59.4	59.0	59.1	59.6	61.8	59.2	61.9
45 to 54 years	11.7	12.7	11.4	10.6	12.0	10.5	12.5	11.9	12.3
55 to 64 years	44.8	48.5	38.6	40.6	42.1	40.9	41.7	34.9	40.6
65 to 74 years	164.6	158.0	150.2	141.6	125.4	126.8	124.7	124.8	122.1

[3]Starting with 1999 data, cause of death is coded according to ICD-10.
[4]Age-adjusted rates are calculated using the year 2000 standard population. Prior to 2001, age-adjusted rates were calculated using standard million proportions based on rounded population numbers. Starting with 2001 data, unrounded population numbers are used to calculate age-adjusted rates.
[5]The race groups, White, Black, Asian or Pacific Islander, and American Indian or Alaska Native, include persons of Hispanic and non-Hispanic origin. Persons of Hispanic origin may be of any race. Death rates for the American Indian or Alaska Native, Asian or Pacific Islander, and Hispanic populations are known to be underestimated.
[6]In 1950, rate is for the age group 75 years and over.
[7]Prior to 1997, excludes data from states lacking an Hispanic-origin item on the death certificate.

Table 2-28. Death Rates for Diseases of the Heart, by Sex, Race, Hispanic Origin, and Age, Selected Years, 1950–2015—*Continued*

(Deaths per 100,000 resident population.)

Sex, race, Hispanic origin, and age	1950[1,2]	1960[1,2]	1970[2]	1980[2]	1985[2]	1990[2]	1995[2]	2000[3]	2005[3]	2006[3]
75 to 84 years	NA	NA	NA	1,053.2	1,056.5	1,130.9	1,001.8	866.2	705.4	664.5
85 years and over	NA	NA	NA	3,211.0	4,208.3	4,161.2	3,942.4	3,367.2	2,881.1	2,856.6
Hispanic or Latina Female[5,7]										
All ages, age-adjusted[4]	NA	NA	NA	NA	195.9	177.2	173.8	163.7	139.9	130.1
All ages, crude	NA	NA	NA	NA	75.0	79.4	76.5	71.5	64.9	61.4
45 to 54 years	NA	NA	NA	NA	46.6	43.5	32.0	28.2	25.9	26.9
55 to 64 years	NA	NA	NA	NA	184.7	153.2	141.0	111.2	91.7	85.9
65 to 74 years	NA	NA	NA	NA	534.1	460.4	419.0	366.3	304.3	271.5
75 to 84 years	NA	NA	NA	NA	1,457.3	1,259.7	1,231.3	1,169.4	1,002.0	924.0
85 years and over	NA	NA	NA	NA	4,528.6	4,440.3	4,653.1	4,605.8	3,968.1	3,735.5
White, not Hispanic or Latina Female[7]										
All ages, age-adjusted[4]	NA	NA	NA	NA	287.2	252.6	231.5	206.8	174.8	165.2
All ages, crude	NA	NA	NA	NA	334.2	320.0	319.7	304.9	268.3	256.8
45 to 54 years	NA	NA	NA	NA	61.3	50.2	46.1	41.9	42.5	42.4
55 to 64 years	NA	NA	NA	NA	219.6	193.6	172.0	142.9	115.3	112.3
65 to 74 years	NA	NA	NA	NA	700.5	584.7	525.2	448.5	351.7	325.9
75 to 84 years	NA	NA	NA	NA	2,201.7	1,890.2	1,674.9	1,458.9	1,202.9	1,133.4
85 years and over	NA	NA	NA	NA	7,164.2	6,615.2	6,265.8	5,822.7	5,049.4	4,753.9

NA = Not available.

[1]Includes deaths of persons who were not residents of the 50 states and the District of Columbia.

[2]Underlying cause of death was coded according to the 6th Revision of the International Classification of Diseases (ICD) in 1950, 7th Revision in 1960, 8th Revision in 1970, and 9th Revision in 1980-1998.

[3]Starting with 1999 data, cause of death is coded according to ICD-10.

[4]Age-adjusted rates are calculated using the year 2000 standard population. Prior to 2001, age-adjusted rates were calculated using standard million proportions based on rounded population numbers. Starting with 2001 data, unrounded population numbers are used to calculate age-adjusted rates.

[5]The race groups, White, Black, Asian or Pacific Islander, and American Indian or Alaska Native, include persons of Hispanic and non-Hispanic origin. Persons of Hispanic origin may be of any race. Death rates for the American Indian or Alaska Native, Asian or Pacific Islander, and Hispanic populations are known to be underestimated.

[7]Prior to 1997, excludes data from states lacking an Hispanic-origin item on the death certificate.

Table 2-28. Death Rates for Diseases of the Heart, by Sex, Race, Hispanic Origin, and Age, Selected Years, 1950–2015—Continued

(Deaths per 100,000 resident population.)

Sex, race, Hispanic origin, and age	2007[3]	2008[3]	2009[3]	2010[3]	2011[3]	2012[3]	2013[3]	2014[3]	2015[3]
75 to 84 years	635.0	637.8	594.4	574.3	551.7	505.2	521.0	485.4	469.3
85 years and over	2,733.3	2,730.3	2,644.6	2,581.8	2,364.5	2,381.5	2,272.4	2,097.2	2,131.6
Hispanic or Latina Female[6,7]									
All ages, age-adjusted[4]	123.2	117.6	109.6	107.8	101.2	98.6	97.0	92.4	93.0
All ages, crude	59.0	57.3	54.9	54.6	54.1	54.7	55.9	55.3	57.8
45 to 54 years	22.9	23.7	23.8	24.5	22.3	21.9	22.2	21.3	21.8
55 to 64 years	80.0	77.9	74.0	72.3	71.3	71.9	63.1	70.2	64.7
65 to 74 years	246.9	242.4	224.5	212.2	202.2	192.3	195.8	190.0	196.6
75 to 84 years	884.3	799.9	793.7	756.0	720.3	711.9	702.3	657.5	654.8
85 years and over	3,568.0	3,486.5	3,080.0	3,140.3	2,868.0	2,781.3	2,738.8	2,558.9	2,599.1
White, not Hispanic or Latina Female[7]									
All ages, age-adjusted[4]	157.3	154.6	145.4	142.5	138.8	135.8	134.6	133.0	135.6
All ages, crude	247.7	246.5	234.3	232.2	230.0	227.5	228.0	226.9	233.6
45 to 54 years	42.2	43.5	41.5	42.9	43.1	43.5	44.0	45.8	46.3
55 to 64 years	106.2	105.3	101.7	100.3	100.2	99.9	99.0	101.4	105.5
65 to 74 years	304.6	295.6	279.9	271.9	265.3	255.5	256.3	251.3	257.3
75 to 84 years	1,078.5	1,052.0	992.3	951.5	923.8	898.1	881.3	862.1	867.6
85 years and over	4,528.6	4,470.5	4,161.5	4,122.8	3,985.5	3,903.8	3,876.5	3,813.8	3,907.6

[3]Starting with 1999 data, cause of death is coded according to ICD-10.
[4]Age-adjusted rates are calculated using the year 2000 standard population. Prior to 2001, age-adjusted rates were calculated using standard million proportions based on rounded population numbers. Starting with 2001 data, unrounded population numbers are used to calculate age-adjusted rates.
[6]The race groups, White, Black, Asian or Pacific Islander, and American Indian or Alaska Native, include persons of Hispanic and non-Hispanic origin. Persons of Hispanic origin may be of any race. Death rates for the American Indian or Alaska Native, Asian or Pacific Islander, and Hispanic populations are known to be underestimated.
[7]Prior to 1997, excludes data from states lacking an Hispanic-origin item on the death certificate.

Table 2-29. Death Rates for Cerebrovascular Diseases, by Sex, Race, Hispanic Origin, and Age, Selected Years, 1950–2015

(Deaths per 100,000 resident population.)

Sex, race, Hispanic origin, and age	1950[1,2]	1960[1,2]	1970[2]	1980[2]	1985[2]	1990[2]	1995[2]	2000[3]	2005[3]	2006[3]
All Persons										
All ages, age-adjusted[4]	180.7	177.9	147.7	96.2	76.4	65.3	63.1	60.9	48.0	44.8
All ages, crude	104.0	108.0	101.9	75.0	64.2	57.8	59.2	59.6	48.6	46.0
Under 1 year	5.1	4.1	5.0	4.4	3.6	3.8	5.9	3.3	3.1	3.5
1 to 4 years	0.9	0.8	1.0	0.5	0.3	0.3	0.4	0.3	0.4	0.3
5 to 14 years	0.5	0.7	0.7	0.3	0.2	0.2	0.2	0.2	0.2	0.2
15 to 24 years	1.6	1.8	1.6	1.0	0.8	0.6	0.5	0.5	0.5	0.5
25 to 34 years	4.2	4.7	4.5	2.6	2.2	2.2	1.7	1.5	1.4	1.3
35 to 44 years	18.7	14.7	15.6	8.5	7.2	6.4	6.5	5.8	5.2	5.1
45 to 54 years	70.4	49.2	41.6	25.2	21.2	18.7	17.4	16.0	15.0	14.6
55 to 64 years	194.2	147.3	115.8	65.1	54.7	47.9	45.6	41.0	32.7	32.9
65 to 74 years	554.7	469.2	384.1	219.0	172.4	144.2	136.2	128.6	99.8	94.9
75 to 84 years	1,499.6	1,491.3	1,254.2	786.9	600.1	498.0	477.1	461.3	358.4	333.9
85 years and over	2,990.1	3,680.5	3,014.3	2,283.7	1,858.5	1,628.9	1,607.2	1,589.2	1,239.7	1,131.7
Male										
All ages, age-adjusted[4]	186.4	186.1	157.4	102.2	79.9	68.5	65.9	62.4	48.4	45.2
All ages, crude	102.5	104.5	94.5	63.4	52.4	46.7	47.2	46.9	39.0	37.2
Under 1 year	6.4	5.0	5.8	5.0	4.6	4.4	6.4	3.8	3.6	4.0
1 to 4 years	1.1	0.9	1.2	0.4	0.4	0.3	0.4	*	0.5	0.3
5 to 14 years	0.5	0.7	0.8	0.3	0.2	0.2	0.2	0.2	0.3	0.3
15 to 24 years	1.8	1.9	1.8	1.1	0.7	0.7	0.5	0.5	0.4	0.5
25 to 34 years	4.2	4.5	4.4	2.6	2.2	2.1	1.8	1.5	1.5	1.5
35 to 44 years	17.5	14.6	15.7	8.7	7.4	6.8	7.0	5.8	5.3	5.4
45 to 54 years	67.9	52.2	44.4	27.2	23.1	20.5	19.5	17.5	16.5	16.4
55 to 64 years	205.2	163.8	138.7	74.6	63.4	54.3	52.7	47.2	38.2	38.3
65 to 74 years	589.6	530.7	449.5	258.6	201.0	166.6	154.7	145.0	111.6	105.8
75 to 84 years	1,543.6	1,555.9	1,361.6	866.3	659.4	551.1	517.7	490.8	370.0	341.4
85 years and over	3,048.6	3,643.1	2,895.2	2,193.6	1,723.8	1,528.5	1,522.1	1,484.3	1,136.7	1,036.8
Female										
All ages, age-adjusted[4]	175.8	170.7	140.0	91.7	73.3	62.6	60.5	59.1	47.0	43.9
All ages, crude	105.6	111.4	109.0	85.9	75.3	68.4	70.7	71.8	57.9	54.4
Under 1 year	3.7	3.2	4.0	3.8	2.7	3.1	5.3	2.7	2.7	3.0
1 to 4 years	0.7	0.7	0.7	0.5	0.3	0.3	0.3	0.4	0.3	0.4
5 to 14 years	0.4	0.6	0.6	0.3	0.3	0.2	0.1	0.2	0.2	0.2
15 to 24 years	1.5	1.6	1.4	0.8	0.8	0.6	0.4	0.5	0.5	0.5
25 to 34 years	4.3	4.9	4.7	2.6	2.1	2.2	1.6	1.5	1.3	1.2
35 to 44 years	19.9	14.8	15.6	8.4	6.9	6.1	6.0	5.7	5.1	4.9
45 to 54 years	72.9	46.3	39.0	23.3	19.4	17.0	15.3	14.5	13.6	13.0
55 to 64 years	183.1	131.8	95.3	56.8	47.1	42.2	39.1	35.3	27.7	28.0
65 to 74 years	522.1	415.7	333.3	188.7	150.4	126.7	121.4	115.1	89.7	85.6
75 to 84 years	1,462.2	1,441.1	1,183.1	740.1	565.1	466.2	451.8	442.1	350.4	328.6
85 years and over	2,949.4	3,704.4	3,081.0	2,323.1	1,912.3	1,667.6	1,640.0	1,632.0	1,285.5	1,174.8
White Male[5]										
All ages, age-adjusted[4]	182.1	181.6	153.7	98.7	77.1	65.5	62.9	59.8	46.0	42.8
All ages, crude	100.5	102.7	93.5	63.1	52.5	46.9	48.0	48.4	40.1	38.1
45 to 54 years	53.7	40.9	35.6	21.7	18.0	15.4	14.7	13.6	12.9	12.9
55 to 64 years	182.2	139.0	119.9	64.0	54.5	45.7	44.2	39.7	31.5	31.3
65 to 74 years	569.7	501.0	420.0	239.8	185.9	152.9	142.1	133.8	101.3	95.3
75 to 84 years	1,556.3	1,564.8	1,361.6	852.7	648.1	539.2	503.8	480.0	361.0	333.4
85 years and over	3,127.1	3,734.8	3,018.1	2,230.8	1,758.7	1,545.4	1,536.0	1,490.7	1,138.5	1,037.0
Black or African American Male[5]										
All ages, age-adjusted[4]	228.8	238.5	206.4	142.0	112.5	102.2	97.0	89.6	72.7	68.8
All ages, crude	122.0	122.9	108.8	73.0	59.2	53.0	49.8	46.1	40.1	39.0
45 to 54 years	211.9	166.1	136.1	82.1	71.1	68.4	62.3	49.5	43.6	42.1
55 to 64 years	522.8	439.9	343.4	189.7	160.5	141.7	130.8	115.4	99.6	101.7
65 to 74 years	783.6	899.2	780.1	472.3	379.4	326.9	297.0	268.5	215.9	209.3
75 to 84 years[6]	1,504.9	1,475.2	1,445.7	1,066.3	813.2	721.5	705.9	659.2	504.2	470.4
85 years and over	NA	2,700.0	1,963.1	1,873.2	1,427.4	1,421.5	1,410.1	1,458.8	1,194.3	1,076.0
American Indian or Alaska Native Male[5]										
All ages, age-adjusted[4]	NA	NA	NA	66.4	48.4	44.3	51.7	46.1	35.0	28.4
All ages, crude	NA	NA	NA	23.1	18.4	16.0	18.4	16.8	14.0	12.5
45 to 54 years	NA	NA	NA	*	*	*	25.5	13.3	12.6	14.7
55 to 64 years	NA	NA	NA	72.0	38.4	39.8	42.6	48.6	34.5	33.2

NA = Not available.
* = Rates based on fewer than 20 deaths are considered unreliable and are not shown.
[1]Includes deaths of persons who were not residents of the 50 states and the District of Columbia.
[2]Underlying cause of death was coded according to the 6th Revision of the International Classification of Diseases (ICD) in 1950, 7th Revision in 1960, 8th Revision in 1970, and 9th Revision in 1980-1998.
[3]Starting with 1999 data, cause of death is coded according to ICD-10.
[4]Age-adjusted rates are calculated using the year 2000 standard population. Prior to 2001, age-adjusted rates were calculated using standard million proportions based on rounded population numbers. Starting with 2001 data, unrounded population numbers are used to calculate age-adjusted rates.
[5]The race groups, White, Black, Asian or Pacific Islander, and American Indian or Alaska Native, include persons of Hispanic and non-Hispanic origin. Persons of Hispanic origin may be of any race. Death rates for the American Indian or Alaska Native, Asian or Pacific Islander, and Hispanic populations are known to be underestimated.
[6]In 1950, rate is for the age group 75 years and over.

Table 2-29. Death Rates for Cerebrovascular Diseases, by Sex, Race, Hispanic Origin, and Age, Selected Years, 1950–2015—Continued

(Deaths per 100,000 resident population.)

Sex, race, Hispanic origin, and age	2007[3]	2008[3]	2009[3]	2010[3]	2011[3]	2012[3]	2013[3]	2014[3]	2015[3]
All Persons									
All ages, age-adjusted[4]	43.5	42.1	39.6	39.1	37.9	36.9	36.2	36.5	37.6
All ages, crude	45.1	44.1	42.0	41.9	41.4	40.9	40.8	41.7	43.7
Under 1 year	3.2	3.4	3.7	3.3	3.4	2.6	2.7	2.4	2.2
1 to 4 years	0.3	0.4	0.3	0.3	0.3	0.3	0.2	0.2	0.3
5 to 14 years	0.2	0.2	0.2	0.2	0.2	0.2	0.2	0.2	0.2
15 to 24 years	0.5	0.4	0.4	0.4	0.4	0.4	0.3	0.4	0.4
25 to 34 years	1.3	1.3	1.3	1.3	1.3	1.3	1.2	1.3	1.3
35 to 44 years	5.0	4.8	4.6	4.6	4.2	4.3	4.2	4.3	4.4
45 to 54 years	14.5	13.7	13.7	13.1	12.8	12.8	12.4	12.3	12.3
55 to 64 years	31.7	30.6	29.7	29.3	29.4	28.7	28.9	29.3	29.6
65 to 74 years	91.4	87.3	82.8	81.7	78.2	75.7	74.2	74.5	75.5
75 to 84 years	320.8	313.3	294.9	288.3	285.4	272.2	268.9	265.7	273.0
85 years and over	1,110.7	1,071.0	992.2	993.8	943.7	931.2	906.0	929.7	975.8
Male									
All ages, age-adjusted[4]	43.7	42.2	39.9	39.3	37.9	37.1	36.7	36.9	37.8
All ages, crude	36.5	35.8	34.5	34.5	34.1	34.1	34.5	35.3	36.8
Under 1 year	3.6	3.3	4.4	3.2	3.6	2.6	3.0	2.6	2.6
1 to 4 years	0.2	0.4	0.3	0.3	0.4	0.4	0.3	*	0.3
5 to 14 years	0.2	0.2	0.2	0.3	0.2	0.2	0.2	0.2	0.2
15 to 24 years	0.5	0.5	0.5	0.5	0.5	0.5	0.4	0.5	0.4
25 to 34 years	1.3	1.5	1.5	1.3	1.3	1.4	1.3	1.5	1.4
35 to 44 years	5.4	5.2	5.1	5.0	4.5	4.8	4.7	5.0	4.9
45 to 54 years	16.2	15.3	15.3	14.9	14.5	14.2	14.2	14.0	13.6
55 to 64 years	37.5	35.5	35.0	34.7	34.9	34.5	35.1	35.2	35.4
65 to 74 years	102.7	97.6	94.2	92.0	88.1	85.7	85.0	85.1	86.3
75 to 84 years	328.2	320.4	300.9	295.2	289.7	277.7	277.9	272.8	282.2
85 years and over	998.9	965.2	891.6	892.0	840.0	832.1	808.4	832.0	863.3
Female									
All ages, age-adjusted[4]	42.7	41.4	38.8	38.3	37.2	36.1	35.2	35.6	36.9
All ages, crude	53.4	52.1	49.2	49.1	48.4	47.6	46.9	47.9	50.3
Under 1 year	2.7	3.6	3.0	3.4	3.1	2.6	2.5	2.1	1.9
1 to 4 years	0.4	0.4	0.3	0.3	*	0.3	*	*	*
5 to 14 years	0.2	0.2	0.1	0.2	0.2	0.2	0.2	0.2	0.2
15 to 24 years	0.4	0.4	0.4	0.4	0.4	0.3	0.3	0.3	0.4
25 to 34 years	1.3	1.2	1.2	1.2	1.2	1.1	1.1	1.2	1.1
35 to 44 years	4.6	4.5	4.2	4.2	4.0	3.8	3.7	3.7	3.9
45 to 54 years	12.9	12.2	12.2	11.4	11.0	11.4	10.6	10.7	11.0
55 to 64 years	26.3	26.1	24.8	24.3	24.4	23.3	23.1	23.8	24.3
65 to 74 years	81.7	78.4	72.9	72.8	69.6	67.0	64.8	65.2	66.0
75 to 84 years	315.5	308.2	290.6	283.4	282.1	268.2	262.1	260.3	266.0
85 years and over	1,162.4	1,120.8	1,040.2	1,043.0	994.9	980.9	955.8	980.6	1,035.3
White Male[5]									
All ages, age-adjusted[4]	41.3	40.2	38.0	37.6	36.2	35.4	35.0	35.2	36.1
All ages, crude	37.5	37.0	35.7	35.8	35.4	35.3	35.8	36.7	38.2
45 to 54 years	13.1	12.0	12.7	12.2	11.8	11.4	11.7	11.9	11.2
55 to 64 years	31.2	29.9	29.3	29.0	29.3	29.4	29.9	29.6	29.8
65 to 74 years	92.3	88.2	86.2	83.3	80.3	78.1	77.6	77.3	78.2
75 to 84 years	317.3	313.3	292.9	288.3	283.4	270.9	271.1	265.3	273.5
85 years and over	999.3	968.9	896.0	903.2	846.2	838.2	815.2	841.4	878.9
Black or African American Male[5]									
All ages, age-adjusted[4]	68.7	63.5	58.8	56.6	55.3	53.8	54.1	55.1	55.5
All ages, crude	39.1	36.8	35.0	34.5	34.5	34.1	35.1	36.5	37.5
45 to 54 years	39.4	39.4	34.5	33.6	33.9	33.4	30.7	29.6	30.4
55 to 64 years	94.7	85.1	84.5	83.2	81.4	76.0	78.1	79.4	78.4
65 to 74 years	212.4	195.0	182.8	182.6	172.0	164.9	165.0	169.8	169.9
75 to 84 years[6]	490.1	443.5	412.7	398.0	384.7	385.0	387.4	393.2	410.8
85 years and over	1,061.7	1,002.8	887.4	804.5	826.7	796.8	814.1	827.6	804.3
American Indian or Alaska Native Male[5]									
All ages, age-adjusted[4]	35.6	27.5	32.0	29.8	25.8	25.5	22.7	25.3	24.5
All ages, crude	13.9	11.7	12.7	12.0	11.8	12.0	11.3	13.0	13.4
45 to 54 years	12.3	13.0	14.4	11.7	10.4	10.7	9.2	8.4	10.9
55 to 64 years	34.8	28.1	25.2	22.1	29.0	26.9	23.8	29.8	23.8

NA = Not available.

* = Rates based on fewer than 20 deaths are considered unreliable and are not shown.

[3]Starting with 1999 data, cause of death is coded according to ICD-10.

[4]Age-adjusted rates are calculated using the year 2000 standard population. Prior to 2001, age-adjusted rates were calculated using standard million proportions based on rounded population numbers. Starting with 2001 data, unrounded population numbers are used to calculate age-adjusted rates.

[5]The race groups, White, Black, Asian or Pacific Islander, and American Indian or Alaska Native, include persons of Hispanic and non-Hispanic origin. Persons of Hispanic origin may be of any race. Death rates for the American Indian or Alaska Native, Asian or Pacific Islander, and Hispanic populations are known to be underestimated.

[6]In 1950, rate is for the age group 75 years and over.

Table 2-29. Death Rates for Cerebrovascular Diseases, by Sex, Race, Hispanic Origin, and Age, Selected Years, 1950–2015—Continued

(Deaths per 100,000 resident population.)

Sex, race, Hispanic origin, and age	1950[1,2]	1960[1,2]	1970[2]	1980[2]	1985[2]	1990[2]	1995[2]	2000[3]	2005[3]	2006[3]
65 to 74 years	NA	NA	NA	170.5	196.2	120.3	156.4	144.7	112.5	82.1
75 to 84 years	NA	NA	NA	523.9	372.7	325.9	351.2	373.3	255.8	196.1
85 years and over	NA	NA	NA	1,384.7	733.3	949.8	1,072.4	834.9	655.7	490.5
Asian or Pacific Islander Male[5]										
All ages, age-adjusted[4]	NA	NA	NA	71.4	65.2	59.1	64.0	58.0	43.9	42.5
All ages, crude	NA	NA	NA	28.7	24.0	23.3	27.5	27.2	23.3	23.1
45 to 54 years	NA	NA	NA	17.0	13.9	15.6	16.5	15.0	14.4	13.5
55 to 64 years	NA	NA	NA	59.9	48.8	51.8	59.6	49.3	33.1	36.0
65 to 74 years	NA	NA	NA	197.9	155.6	167.9	155.6	135.6	103.9	107.7
75 to 84 years	NA	NA	NA	619.5	583.7	483.9	521.9	438.7	347.8	305.1
85 years and over	NA	NA	NA	1,399.0	1,387.5	1,196.6	1,382.1	1,415.6	1,007.2	1,014.1
Hispanic or Latino Male[5,7]										
All ages, age-adjusted[4]	NA	NA	NA	NA	57.5	46.5	51.2	50.5	41.6	39.4
All ages, crude	NA	NA	NA	NA	17.2	15.6	16.2	15.8	14.5	14.4
45 to 54 years	NA	NA	NA	NA	23.6	20.0	20.3	18.1	18.0	17.3
55 to 64 years	NA	NA	NA	NA	64.0	49.2	46.9	48.8	40.5	41.4
65 to 74 years	NA	NA	NA	NA	163.3	126.4	138.1	136.1	107.4	101.4
75 to 84 years	NA	NA	NA	NA	394.7	356.6	373.3	392.9	308.5	308.9
85 years and over	NA	NA	NA	NA	1,181.2	866.3	1,079.5	1,029.9	870.3	748.4
White, Not Hispanic or Latino Male[7]										
All ages, age-adjusted[4]	NA	NA	NA	NA	74.8	66.3	62.8	59.9	46.0	42.7
All ages, crude	NA	NA	NA	NA	52.1	50.6	51.9	53.9	45.1	42.9
45 to 54 years	NA	NA	NA	NA	15.9	14.9	13.9	13.0	12.1	12.2
55 to 64 years	NA	NA	NA	NA	50.4	45.1	43.3	38.7	30.5	30.0
65 to 74 years	NA	NA	NA	NA	178.2	154.5	141.4	133.1	100.5	94.3
75 to 84 years	NA	NA	NA	NA	635.2	547.3	506.2	482.3	363.0	333.7
85 years and over	NA	NA	NA	NA	1,729.1	1,578.7	1,544.8	1,505.9	1,148.7	1,048.5
White Female[5]										
All ages, age-adjusted[4]	169.7	165.0	135.5	89.0	70.7	60.3	58.6	57.3	45.3	42.3
All ages, crude	103.3	110.1	109.8	88.6	78.2	71.6	75.1	76.9	62.0	58.3
45 to 54 years	55.0	33.8	30.5	18.6	15.5	13.5	12.6	11.2	10.5	10.4
55 to 64 years	156.9	103.0	78.1	48.6	39.9	35.8	33.3	30.2	23.7	23.9
65 to 74 years	498.1	383.3	303.2	172.5	137.6	116.1	111.7	107.3	82.6	78.6
75 to 84 years	1,471.3	1,444.7	1,176.8	728.8	551.7	456.5	443.4	434.2	343.4	321.6
85 years and over	3,017.9	3,795.7	3,167.6	2,362.7	1,938.0	1,685.9	1,656.7	1,646.7	1,292.6	1,182.1
Black or African American Female[5]										
All ages, age-adjusted[4]	238.4	232.5	189.3	119.6	99.2	84.0	79.4	76.2	62.4	58.4
All ages, crude	128.3	127.7	112.2	77.8	68.5	60.7	59.1	58.3	48.8	46.2
45 to 54 years	248.9	166.2	119.4	61.8	50.8	44.1	36.0	38.1	34.6	30.9
55 to 64 years	567.7	452.0	272.4	138.4	113.5	96.9	85.6	76.4	58.7	59.8
65 to 74 years	754.4	830.5	673.5	361.7	285.1	236.7	222.3	190.9	151.0	146.0
75 to 84 years[6]	1,496.7	1,413.1	1,338.3	917.5	752.4	595.0	565.1	549.2	451.5	416.8
85 years and over	NA	2,578.9	2,210.5	1,891.6	1,653.4	1,495.2	1,518.4	1,556.5	1,282.5	1,176.9
American Indian or Alaska Native Female[5]										
All ages, age-adjusted[4]	NA	NA	NA	51.2	44.3	38.4	46.3	43.7	41.1	35.4
All ages, crude	NA	NA	NA	22.0	21.5	19.3	22.0	21.5	21.3	17.2
45 to 54 years	NA	NA	NA	*	*	*	*	14.4	16.3	*
55 to 64 years	NA	NA	NA	*	40.4	40.7	41.5	37.9	34.6	15.5
65 to 74 years	NA	NA	NA	128.3	118.2	100.5	114.8	79.5	114.5	78.0
75 to 84 years	NA	NA	NA	404.2	317.6	282.0	364.4	391.1	304.7	283.4
85 years and over	NA	NA	NA	1,095.5	980.0	776.2	983.9	931.5	865.8	919.7
Asian or Pacific Islander Female[5]										
All ages, age-adjusted[4]	NA	NA	NA	60.8	54.8	54.9	48.3	49.1	38.3	37.0
All ages, crude	NA	NA	NA	26.4	23.3	24.3	24.2	28.7	25.6	25.5
45 to 54 years	NA	NA	NA	20.3	15.1	19.7	15.6	13.3	9.7	10.2
55 to 64 years	NA	NA	NA	43.7	49.0	42.1	37.6	33.3	26.4	27.8
65 to 74 years	NA	NA	NA	136.1	129.9	124.0	101.0	102.8	80.1	79.9

NA = Not available.
* = Rates based on fewer than 20 deaths are considered unreliable and are not shown.
[1]Includes deaths of persons who were not residents of the 50 states and the District of Columbia.
[2]Underlying cause of death was coded according to the 6th Revision of the International Classification of Diseases (ICD) in 1950, 7th Revision in 1960, 8th Revision in 1970, and 9th Revision in 1980-1998.
[3]Starting with 1999 data, cause of death is coded according to ICD-10.
[4]Age-adjusted rates are calculated using the year 2000 standard population. Prior to 2001, age-adjusted rates were calculated using standard million proportions based on rounded population numbers. Starting with 2001 data, unrounded population numbers are used to calculate age-adjusted rates.
[5]The race groups, White, Black, Asian or Pacific Islander, and American Indian or Alaska Native, include persons of Hispanic and non-Hispanic origin. Persons of Hispanic origin may be of any race. Death rates for the American Indian or Alaska Native, Asian or Pacific Islander, and Hispanic populations are known to be underestimated.
[6]In 1950, rate is for the age group 75 years and over.
[7]Prior to 1997, excludes data from states lacking an Hispanic-origin item on the death certificate.

Table 2-29. Death Rates for Cerebrovascular Diseases, by Sex, Race, Hispanic Origin, and Age, Selected Years, 1950–2015—Continued

(Deaths per 100,000 resident population.)

Sex, race, Hispanic origin, and age	2007[3]	2008[3]	2009[3]	2010[3]	2011[3]	2012[3]	2013[3]	2014[3]	2015[3]
65 to 74 years	82.2	94.5	68.4	68.0	66.8	84.4	72.5	74.7	76.5
75 to 84 years	300.5	193.8	288.5	267.5	226.3	172.2	191.0	193.0	183.3
85 years and over	709.9	492.5	629.2	580.4	425.6	506.3	348.3	463.9	424.5
Asian or Pacific Islander Male[5]									
All ages, age-adjusted[4]	37.9	36.2	35.4	35.2	33.5	33.2	31.2	29.4	31.3
All ages, crude	21.2	20.9	20.8	21.5	21.2	21.7	21.3	20.7	22.8
45 to 54 years	14.6	13.1	12.9	14.7	12.9	13.2	15.7	11.0	11.9
55 to 64 years	31.0	31.3	31.1	31.7	31.4	30.0	27.7	30.0	32.2
65 to 74 years	88.9	88.2	76.2	84.9	75.6	78.1	73.0	66.4	73.0
75 to 84 years	282.8	265.1	278.0	260.0	258.2	239.3	230.5	217.2	239.8
85 years and over	888.2	835.2	800.0	778.7	746.2	776.0	686.7	666.1	669.1
Hispanic or Latino Male[5,7]									
All ages, age-adjusted[4]	38.1	37.3	34.0	33.9	32.6	32.0	31.8	32.1	34.2
All ages, crude	14.1	13.9	13.1	13.2	13.3	13.5	14.0	14.6	15.9
45 to 54 years	16.7	15.4	14.7	14.3	13.9	13.5	13.8	13.3	11.5
55 to 64 years	43.2	35.3	33.7	31.9	35.2	33.3	33.9	33.2	32.7
65 to 74 years	95.6	90.6	92.6	84.4	80.4	75.5	82.1	77.0	86.4
75 to 84 years	278.6	292.2	253.0	266.5	245.4	248.1	242.1	245.8	265.9
85 years and over	778.3	758.4	678.8	679.1	665.4	644.9	620.6	656.6	706.9
White, Not Hispanic or Latino Male[7]									
All ages, age-adjusted[4]	41.1	40.0	37.9	37.5	36.1	35.3	34.9	35.1	35.8
All ages, crude	42.3	41.9	40.6	40.7	40.3	40.3	40.8	41.8	43.5
45 to 54 years	12.4	11.3	12.1	11.6	11.2	10.8	11.0	11.3	10.9
55 to 64 years	29.7	29.1	28.6	28.4	28.3	28.5	29.0	28.7	28.9
65 to 74 years	91.5	87.4	85.1	82.6	79.8	77.7	76.6	76.7	76.5
75 to 84 years	318.6	313.6	294.7	288.6	284.9	271.2	272.0	265.8	272.0
85 years and over	1,008.2	976.7	906.2	913.2	854.8	848.0	825.6	851.2	887.3
White Female[5]									
All ages, age-adjusted[4]	41.2	39.9	37.6	37.2	36.2	35.2	34.2	34.7	35.9
All ages, crude	57.3	56.0	53.1	53.0	52.3	51.5	50.6	51.8	54.4
45 to 54 years	10.0	9.5	9.6	9.1	9.0	9.3	9.0	8.8	9.5
55 to 64 years	22.3	21.9	21.1	20.6	21.1	19.8	19.8	20.4	21.1
65 to 74 years	75.0	72.8	67.5	66.8	64.6	62.3	60.0	60.2	61.4
75 to 84 years	310.6	302.0	286.4	280.2	278.0	265.4	257.7	257.1	260.1
85 years and over	1,168.7	1,129.7	1,052.0	1,052.8	1,008.1	994.7	970.4	995.7	1,055.0
Black or African American Female[5]									
All ages, age-adjusted[4]	56.4	54.8	50.0	49.6	47.0	45.4	44.7	45.2	46.7
All ages, crude	45.1	44.2	41.0	41.1	39.6	39.2	39.2	40.5	42.5
45 to 54 years	32.4	30.1	28.8	26.7	23.6	25.0	21.1	22.4	21.3
55 to 64 years	57.0	57.5	53.5	51.3	48.2	48.8	47.7	48.4	48.1
65 to 74 years	140.5	127.4	122.5	126.2	116.7	111.2	109.1	112.6	110.1
75 to 84 years[6]	389.1	399.3	360.1	347.2	342.0	321.6	333.0	322.6	345.3
85 years and over	1,166.7	1,106.4	989.6	1,001.5	948.1	927.2	894.1	934.0	977.5
American Indian or Alaska Native Female[5]									
All ages, age-adjusted[4]	32.8	27.2	27.0	26.5	27.9	24.8	25.5	25.0	24.4
All ages, crude	16.7	14.2	14.4	14.2	15.9	14.4	15.4	15.7	16.1
45 to 54 years	8.9	9.3	11.6	10.6	11.2	7.2	9.0	11.2	11.2
55 to 64 years	22.5	24.4	24.6	22.4	19.2	20.0	19.1	21.6	19.8
65 to 74 years	82.2	54.5	69.3	59.4	64.2	58.8	60.6	52.4	58.2
75 to 84 years	211.4	221.3	169.7	173.6	237.7	205.5	187.2	183.2	176.0
85 years and over	879.0	615.3	692.2	700.0	550.3	531.3	593.6	618.8	559.4
Asian or Pacific Islander Female[5]									
All ages, age-adjusted[4]	35.5	34.2	31.2	31.4	30.0	28.9	27.9	27.2	28.3
All ages, crude	24.8	24.7	22.9	23.5	23.7	23.7	23.8	23.8	25.5
45 to 54 years	9.6	10.2	9.4	7.9	9.1	9.2	8.6	8.6	7.6
55 to 64 years	24.1	24.6	20.6	22.1	22.5	20.0	18.2	18.4	18.3
65 to 74 years	70.9	74.9	61.4	65.6	55.8	56.3	54.0	52.3	51.3

NA = Not available.

* = Rates based on fewer than 20 deaths are considered unreliable and are not shown.

[1]Includes deaths of persons who were not residents of the 50 states and the District of Columbia.

[2]Underlying cause of death was coded according to the 6th Revision of the International Classification of Diseases (ICD) in 1950, 7th Revision in 1960, 8th Revision in 1970, and 9th Revision in 1980-1998.

[3]Starting with 1999 data, cause of death is coded according to ICD-10.

[4]Age-adjusted rates are calculated using the year 2000 standard population. Prior to 2001, age-adjusted rates were calculated using standard million proportions based on rounded population numbers. Starting with 2001 data, unrounded population numbers are used to calculate age-adjusted rates.

[5]The race groups, White, Black, Asian or Pacific Islander, and American Indian or Alaska Native, include persons of Hispanic and non-Hispanic origin. Persons of Hispanic origin may be of any race. Death rates for the American Indian or Alaska Native, Asian or Pacific Islander, and Hispanic populations are known to be underestimated.

[6]In 1950, rate is for the age group 75 years and over.

[7]Prior to 1997, excludes data from states lacking an Hispanic-origin item on the death certificate.

Table 2-29. Death Rates for Cerebrovascular Diseases, by Sex, Race, Hispanic Origin, and Age, Selected Years, 1950–2015—*Continued*

(Deaths per 100,000 resident population.)

Sex, race, Hispanic origin, and age	1950[1,2]	1960[1,2]	1970[2]	1980[2]	1985[2]	1990[2]	1995[2]	2000[3]	2005[3]	2006[3]
75 to 84 years	NA	NA	NA	446.6	387.0	396.6	381.8	386.0	278.1	295.2
85 years and over	NA	NA	NA	1,545.2	1,383.3	1,395.0	1,197.0	1,246.6	1,044.6	890.5
Hispanic or Latina Female[5,7]										
All ages, age-adjusted[4]	NA	NA	NA	NA	47.5	43.7	42.7	43.0	36.0	35.0
All ages, crude	NA	NA	NA	NA	18.2	20.1	19.4	19.4	17.3	17.1
45 to 54 years	NA	NA	NA	NA	15.8	15.2	15.1	12.4	11.9	11.6
55 to 64 years	NA	NA	NA	NA	35.3	38.5	36.5	31.9	26.9	27.5
65 to 74 years	NA	NA	NA	NA	108.6	102.6	102.3	95.2	75.4	76.5
75 to 84 years	NA	NA	NA	NA	340.0	308.5	307.3	311.3	270.3	248.5
85 years and over	NA	NA	NA	NA	1,185.7	1,055.3	1,021.0	1,108.9	905.5	901.5
White, not Hispanic or Latina Female[7]										
All ages, age-adjusted[4]	NA	NA	NA	NA	69.7	61.0	58.7	57.6	45.6	42.5
All ages, crude	NA	NA	NA	NA	80.8	77.2	81.5	85.5	70.1	66.0
45 to 54 years	NA	NA	NA	NA	14.3	13.2	12.3	10.9	10.2	10.1
55 to 64 years	NA	NA	NA	NA	37.8	35.7	32.6	29.9	23.2	23.4
65 to 74 years	NA	NA	NA	NA	133.2	116.9	111.4	107.6	82.9	78.3
75 to 84 years	NA	NA	NA	NA	550.8	461.9	445.9	438.3	347.0	325.2
85 years and over	NA	NA	NA	NA	1,920.7	1,714.7	1,666.8	1,661.6	1,306.0	1,192.2

NA = Not available.
* = Rates based on fewer than 20 deaths are considered unreliable and are not shown.
[1]Includes deaths of persons who were not residents of the 50 states and the District of Columbia.
[2]Underlying cause of death was coded according to the 6th Revision of the International Classification of Diseases (ICD) in 1950, 7th Revision in 1960, 8th Revision in 1970, and 9th Revision in 1980-1998.
[3]Starting with 1999 data, cause of death is coded according to ICD-10.
[4]Age-adjusted rates are calculated using the year 2000 standard population. Prior to 2001, age-adjusted rates were calculated using standard million proportions based on rounded population numbers. Starting with 2001 data, unrounded population numbers are used to calculate age-adjusted rates.
[5]The race groups, White, Black, Asian or Pacific Islander, and American Indian or Alaska Native, include persons of Hispanic and non-Hispanic origin. Persons of Hispanic origin may be of any race. Death rates for the American Indian or Alaska Native, Asian or Pacific Islander, and Hispanic populations are known to be underestimated.
[7]Prior to 1997, excludes data from states lacking an Hispanic-origin item on the death certificate.

Table 2-29. Death Rates for Cerebrovascular Diseases, by Sex, Race, Hispanic Origin, and Age, Selected Years, 1950–2015—*Continued*

(Deaths per 100,000 resident population.)

Sex, race, Hispanic origin, and age	2007[a]	2008[a]	2009[a]	2010[a]	2011[a]	2012[a]	2013[a]	2014[a]	2015[a]
75 to 84 years	269.8	247.2	237.1	218.4	237.2	213.4	203.0	197.9	219.2
85 years and over	935.0	898.2	814.3	872.8	758.7	770.1	754.6	747.4	757.6
Hispanic or Latina Female[5,7]									
All ages, age-adjusted[4]	33.5	32.0	30.4	30.2	29.0	28.2	27.6	28.3	30.4
All ages, crude	16.6	16.0	15.6	15.7	15.7	15.8	16.1	16.9	18.8
45 to 54 years	10.8	10.0	9.1	9.2	9.5	8.8	9.1	7.7	8.8
55 to 64 years	25.0	20.7	22.9	22.1	21.0	19.9	19.7	17.2	19.3
65 to 74 years	70.8	65.9	58.4	60.6	59.2	59.3	53.6	54.7	54.0
75 to 84 years	252.1	248.9	234.0	221.6	233.9	217.6	211.4	219.7	230.0
85 years and over	845.7	804.0	774.8	799.3	692.5	705.9	698.4	744.6	831.1
White, not Hispanic or Latina Female[7]									
All ages, age-adjusted[4]	41.5	40.2	37.8	37.4	36.5	35.5	34.5	35.0	36.2
All ages, crude	65.3	64.0	60.8	60.8	60.2	59.2	58.3	59.7	62.4
45 to 54 years	9.8	9.3	9.6	9.0	8.8	9.2	8.8	8.9	9.4
55 to 64 years	21.9	21.8	20.7	20.3	20.9	19.6	19.6	20.6	21.0
65 to 74 years	75.0	73.1	68.0	66.9	64.8	62.1	60.2	60.3	61.5
75 to 84 years	313.7	304.6	289.1	283.4	280.6	268.1	260.3	259.0	260.9
85 years and over	1,181.4	1,142.1	1,062.9	1,063.0	1,022.8	1,008.1	984.3	1,009.2	1,066.0

NA = Not available.

* = Rates based on fewer than 20 deaths are considered unreliable and are not shown.

[a]Starting with 1999 data, cause of death is coded according to ICD-10.

[4]Age-adjusted rates are calculated using the year 2000 standard population. Prior to 2001, age-adjusted rates were calculated using standard million proportions based on rounded population numbers. Starting with 2001 data, unrounded population numbers are used to calculate age-adjusted rates.

[5]The race groups, White, Black, Asian or Pacific Islander, and American Indian or Alaska Native, include persons of Hispanic and non-Hispanic origin. Persons of Hispanic origin may be of any race. Death rates for the American Indian or Alaska Native, Asian or Pacific Islander, and Hispanic populations are known to be underestimated.

[7]Prior to 1997, excludes data from states lacking an Hispanic-origin item on the death certificate.

Table 2-30. Death Rates for Malignant Neoplasms, by Sex, Race, Hispanic Origin, and Age, Selected Years, 1950–2015

(Deaths per 100,000 resident population.)

Sex, race, Hispanic origin, and age	1950[1,2]	1960[1,2]	1970[2]	1980[2]	1985[2]	1990[2]	1995[2]	2000[3]	2005[3]	2006[3]
All Persons										
All ages, age-adjusted[4]	193.9	193.9	198.6	207.9	211.3	216.0	209.9	199.6	185.1	181.8
All ages, crude	139.8	149.2	162.8	183.9	194.0	203.2	202.2	196.5	189.3	187.6
Under 1 year	8.7	7.2	4.7	3.2	3.1	2.3	1.8	2.4	1.9	1.9
1 to 4 years	11.7	10.9	7.5	4.5	3.8	3.5	3.1	2.7	2.4	2.4
5 to 14 years	6.7	6.8	6.0	4.3	3.5	3.1	2.7	2.5	2.5	2.2
15 to 24 years	8.6	8.3	8.3	6.3	5.4	4.9	4.5	4.4	4.0	3.8
25 to 34 years	20.0	19.5	16.5	13.7	13.2	12.6	11.6	9.8	9.2	9.3
35 to 44 years	62.7	59.7	59.5	48.6	45.9	43.3	40.1	36.6	33.5	32.2
45 to 54 years	175.1	177.0	182.5	180.0	170.1	158.9	140.4	127.5	118.6	116.3
55 to 64 years	390.7	396.8	423.0	436.1	454.6	449.6	412.3	366.7	323.9	317.7
65 to 74 years	698.8	713.9	754.2	817.9	845.5	872.3	863.3	816.3	733.2	716.3
75 to 84 years	1,153.3	1,127.4	1,169.2	1,232.3	1,271.8	1,348.5	1,355.4	1,335.6	1,272.8	1,259.2
85 years and over	1,451.0	1,450.0	1,320.7	1,594.6	1,615.4	1,752.9	1,797.7	1,819.4	1,778.2	1,748.3
Male										
All ages, age-adjusted[4]	208.1	225.1	247.6	271.2	274.4	280.4	267.5	248.9	227.2	221.7
All ages, crude	142.9	162.5	182.1	205.3	213.4	221.3	216.3	207.2	200.0	197.8
Under 1 year	9.7	7.7	4.4	3.7	3.0	2.4	1.9	2.6	2.2	1.9
1 to 4 years	12.5	12.4	8.3	5.2	4.3	3.7	3.6	3.0	2.7	2.5
5 to 14 years	7.4	7.6	6.7	4.9	3.9	3.5	3.0	2.7	2.7	2.4
15 to 24 years	9.7	10.2	10.4	7.8	6.4	5.7	5.4	5.1	4.8	4.6
25 to 34 years	17.7	18.8	16.3	13.4	13.2	12.6	11.3	9.2	9.2	9.0
35 to 44 years	45.6	48.9	53.0	44.0	42.4	38.5	36.3	32.7	29.3	27.8
45 to 54 years	156.2	170.8	183.5	188.7	175.2	162.5	141.5	130.9	121.7	119.1
55 to 64 years	413.1	459.9	511.8	520.8	536.9	532.9	475.1	415.8	365.8	359.4
65 to 74 years	791.5	890.5	1,006.8	1,093.2	1,105.2	1,122.2	1,083.0	1,001.9	883.1	852.5
75 to 84 years	1,332.6	1,389.4	1,588.3	1,790.5	1,839.7	1,914.4	1,847.9	1,760.6	1,636.8	1,611.8
85 years and over	1,668.3	1,741.2	1,720.8	2,369.5	2,451.8	2,739.9	2,818.7	2,710.7	2,576.2	2,500.3
Female										
All ages, age-adjusted[4]	182.3	168.7	163.2	166.7	171.2	175.7	173.6	167.6	156.7	154.7
All ages, crude	136.8	136.4	144.4	163.6	175.7	186.0	188.8	186.2	178.9	177.8
Under 1 year	7.6	6.8	5.0	2.7	3.2	2.2	1.8	2.3	1.5	1.9
1 to 4 years	10.8	9.3	6.7	3.7	3.4	3.2	2.6	2.5	2.1	2.2
5 to 14 years	6.0	6.0	5.2	3.6	3.1	2.8	2.3	2.2	2.2	2.0
15 to 24 years	7.6	6.5	6.2	4.8	4.3	4.1	3.5	3.6	3.3	3.1
25 to 34 years	22.2	20.1	16.7	14.0	13.2	12.6	11.9	10.4	9.2	9.6
35 to 44 years	79.3	70.0	65.6	53.1	49.2	48.1	43.8	40.4	37.6	36.5
45 to 54 years	194.0	183.0	181.5	171.8	165.3	155.5	139.3	124.2	115.7	113.5
55 to 64 years	368.2	337.7	343.2	361.7	381.8	375.2	355.1	321.3	284.8	278.9
65 to 74 years	612.3	560.2	557.9	607.1	645.3	677.4	687.1	663.6	605.6	599.8
75 to 84 years	1,000.7	924.1	891.9	903.1	937.8	1,010.3	1,047.5	1,058.5	1,023.0	1,014.6
85 years and over	1,299.7	1,263.9	1,096.7	1,255.7	1,281.4	1,372.1	1,404.4	1,456.4	1,423.6	1,407.2
White Male[5]										
All ages, age-adjusted[4]	210.0	224.7	244.8	265.1	267.1	272.2	260.6	243.9	224.3	219.3
All ages, crude	147.2	166.1	185.1	208.7	218.1	227.7	225.3	218.1	212.8	211.1
25 to 34 years	17.7	18.8	16.2	13.6	13.1	12.3	11.0	9.2	8.8	9.0
35 to 44 years	44.5	46.3	50.1	41.1	39.8	35.8	34.1	30.9	28.9	27.2
45 to 54 years	150.8	164.1	172.0	175.4	162.0	149.9	132.7	123.5	116.3	114.3
55 to 64 years	409.4	450.9	498.1	497.4	512.0	508.2	456.0	401.9	354.2	350.4
65 to 74 years	798.7	887.3	997.0	1,070.7	1,076.5	1,090.7	1,056.1	984.3	875.6	845.8
75 to 84 years	1,367.6	1,413.7	1,592.7	1,779.7	1,817.1	1,883.2	1,817.4	1,736.0	1,629.2	1,606.9
85 years and over	1,732.7	1,791.4	1,772.2	2,375.6	2,449.1	2,715.1	2,789.4	2,693.7	2,558.2	2,487.9
Black or African American Male[5]										
All ages, age-adjusted[4]	178.9	227.6	291.9	353.4	373.9	397.9	374.3	340.3	297.2	287.2
All ages, crude	106.6	136.7	171.6	205.5	214.9	221.9	204.8	188.5	174.7	171.2
25 to 34 years	18.0	18.4	18.8	14.1	14.9	15.7	14.8	10.1	12.4	10.4
35 to 44 years	55.7	72.9	81.3	73.8	69.9	64.3	57.2	48.4	36.1	36.2
45 to 54 years	211.7	244.7	311.2	333.0	315.9	302.6	243.9	214.2	181.1	176.1
55 to 64 years	490.8	579.7	689.2	812.5	859.2	859.2	738.1	626.4	546.0	518.2
65 to 74 years	636.5	938.5	1,168.9	1,417.2	1,532.8	1,613.9	1,541.4	1,363.8	1,139.4	1,106.8

[1] Includes deaths of persons who were not residents of the 50 states and the District of Columbia.
[2] Underlying cause of death was coded according to the 6th Revision of the International Classification of Diseases (ICD) in 1950, 7th Revision in 1960, 8th Revision in 1970, and 9th Revision in 1980-1998.
[3] Starting with 1999 data, cause of death is coded according to ICD-10.
[4] Age-adjusted rates are calculated using the year 2000 standard population. Prior to 2001, age-adjusted rates were calculated using standard million proportions based on rounded population numbers. Starting with 2001 data, unrounded population numbers are used to calculate age-adjusted rates.
[5] The race groups, White, Black, Asian or Pacific Islander, and American Indian or Alaska Native, include persons of Hispanic and non-Hispanic origin. Persons of Hispanic origin may be of any race. Death rates for the American Indian or Alaska Native, Asian or Pacific Islander, and Hispanic populations are known to be underestimated.

Table 2-30. Death Rates for Malignant Neoplasms, by Sex, Race, Hispanic Origin, and Age, Selected Years, 1950–2015—Continued

(Deaths per 100,000 resident population.)

Sex, race, Hispanic origin, and age	2007[3]	2008[3]	2009[3]	2010[3]	2011[3]	2012[3]	2013[3]	2014[3]	2015[3]
All Persons									
All ages, age-adjusted[4]	179.3	176.4	173.5	172.8	169.0	166.5	163.2	161.2	158.5
All ages, crude	186.9	186.0	185.0	186.2	185.1	185.6	185.0	185.6	185.4
Under 1 year	1.7	1.7	1.8	1.6	1.8	1.6	1.6	1.3	1.3
1 to 4 years	2.3	2.4	2.2	2.1	2.2	2.4	2.1	2.0	2.2
5 to 14 years	2.4	2.2	2.2	2.2	2.1	2.2	2.2	2.1	2.1
15 to 24 years	3.8	3.8	3.8	3.7	3.7	3.6	3.4	3.6	3.4
25 to 34 years	8.7	8.8	9.0	8.8	8.4	8.7	8.6	8.3	8.4
35 to 44 years	31.0	30.1	30.2	28.8	28.8	28.0	28.1	27.8	26.9
45 to 54 years	114.2	113.4	112.8	111.6	109.3	108.5	105.5	103.2	99.7
55 to 64 years	311.4	304.7	301.7	300.1	295.8	293.2	288.2	287.6	284.1
65 to 74 years	702.9	688.4	668.2	666.1	647.6	632.2	616.9	603.1	594.3
75 to 84 years	1,250.1	1,230.9	1,213.0	1,202.2	1,179.1	1,161.7	1,139.4	1,125.9	1,100.8
85 years and over	1,739.4	1,724.6	1,699.3	1,729.5	1,676.2	1,658.9	1,635.4	1,632.9	1,628.6
Male									
All ages, age-adjusted[4]	218.8	214.9	210.9	209.9	204.0	200.3	196.0	192.9	189.2
All ages, crude	197.8	197.5	196.8	198.3	197.2	197.9	197.6	198.4	198.3
Under 1 year	1.8	2.3	2.2	1.5	1.9	1.7	1.5	1.1	1.5
1 to 4 years	2.3	2.6	2.2	2.4	2.2	2.7	2.2	2.2	2.4
5 to 14 years	2.4	2.2	2.3	2.3	2.3	2.4	2.2	2.3	2.2
15 to 24 years	4.5	4.6	4.5	4.5	4.3	4.1	3.8	4.2	3.9
25 to 34 years	8.5	8.8	8.8	8.6	8.1	8.4	8.6	8.2	8.2
35 to 44 years	26.8	26.2	26.1	25.2	24.9	24.0	24.0	24.0	23.0
45 to 54 years	117.4	117.7	115.3	113.8	110.7	110.1	106.5	102.9	99.4
55 to 64 years	353.9	349.3	345.9	344.9	340.4	336.9	331.3	330.3	325.5
65 to 74 years	834.1	817.0	790.4	789.2	765.8	746.7	726.2	711.9	701.7
75 to 84 years	1,593.3	1,563.1	1,538.3	1,514.2	1,478.5	1,447.6	1,414.5	1,387.5	1,355.8
85 years and over	2,508.4	2,444.4	2,412.2	2,452.6	2,339.8	2,303.1	2,272.6	2,250.4	2,220.2
Female									
All ages, age-adjusted[4]	152.3	149.6	147.4	146.7	144.0	142.1	139.5	138.1	135.9
All ages, crude	176.3	174.8	173.7	174.4	173.4	173.7	172.8	173.2	172.9
Under 1 year	1.6	1.1	1.5	1.6	1.6	1.5	1.8	1.6	1.1
1 to 4 years	2.2	2.2	2.1	1.9	2.1	2.2	1.9	1.8	2.0
5 to 14 years	2.3	2.2	2.0	2.2	1.9	2.0	2.1	1.8	2.0
15 to 24 years	3.2	3.0	3.0	2.8	3.0	3.0	3.0	2.9	2.8
25 to 34 years	8.9	8.7	9.1	9.0	8.6	8.9	8.6	8.5	8.6
35 to 44 years	35.3	34.0	34.2	32.3	32.8	31.9	32.1	31.6	30.7
45 to 54 years	111.0	109.2	110.4	109.4	108.0	107.0	104.6	103.4	100.0
55 to 64 years	271.8	263.3	260.6	258.5	254.1	252.5	248.1	247.9	245.4
65 to 74 years	590.3	577.3	562.2	559.1	544.5	531.9	520.8	507.5	499.8
75 to 84 years	1,009.6	995.9	980.1	977.0	959.6	950.0	933.3	928.0	906.4
85 years and over	1,383.9	1,385.9	1,358.6	1,380.1	1,349.1	1,336.4	1,310.1	1,311.7	1,315.8
White Male[5]									
All ages, age-adjusted[4]	216.3	212.9	209.2	208.2	203.1	199.7	195.5	193.0	189.7
All ages, crude	211.2	211.5	211.0	212.7	212.0	213.1	213.0	214.4	214.7
25 to 34 years	8.5	8.8	8.9	8.8	8.1	8.5	8.5	8.4	8.4
35 to 44 years	26.4	25.6	25.9	25.2	25.2	24.2	23.9	24.0	23.1
45 to 54 years	112.8	113.9	112.5	111.6	108.6	108.2	105.7	102.3	98.8
55 to 64 years	344.1	340.4	335.8	334.9	332.4	329.4	323.1	323.5	320.5
65 to 74 years	827.3	811.1	784.2	782.8	759.5	742.8	723.3	707.6	698.7
75 to 84 years	1,588.2	1,560.4	1,538.3	1,511.6	1,485.2	1,453.0	1,421.7	1,400.4	1,369.4
85 years and over	2,488.1	2,437.8	2,412.5	2,453.5	2,347.1	2,318.7	2,290.7	2,279.7	2,251.6
Black or African American Male[5]									
All ages, age-adjusted[4]	284.2	273.1	266.7	264.8	252.6	246.1	238.7	231.9	224.8
All ages, crude	171.3	168.4	168.2	169.0	166.4	166.4	165.6	165.1	163.8
25 to 34 years	9.9	9.9	10.4	9.2	9.2	9.1	10.2	8.3	8.7
35 to 44 years	33.6	33.7	31.3	30.1	28.9	26.6	27.3	28.8	26.3
45 to 54 years	171.1	165.4	157.4	150.9	145.6	145.0	132.4	128.8	123.8
55 to 64 years	516.3	501.3	502.0	496.7	478.4	468.8	464.0	450.5	437.4
65 to 74 years	1,083.8	1,047.3	1,038.6	1,027.8	1,004.1	970.2	941.5	925.8	895.8

[3]Starting with 1999 data, cause of death is coded according to ICD-10.
[4]Age-adjusted rates are calculated using the year 2000 standard population. Prior to 2001, age-adjusted rates were calculated using standard million proportions based on rounded population numbers. Starting with 2001 data, unrounded population numbers are used to calculate age-adjusted rates.
[5]The race groups, White, Black, Asian or Pacific Islander, and American Indian or Alaska Native, include persons of Hispanic and non-Hispanic origin. Persons of Hispanic origin may be of any race. Death rates for the American Indian or Alaska Native, Asian or Pacific Islander, and Hispanic populations are known to be underestimated.

Table 2-30. Death Rates for Malignant Neoplasms, by Sex, Race, Hispanic Origin, and Age, Selected Years, 1950–2015—*Continued*

(Deaths per 100,000 resident population.)

Sex, race, Hispanic origin, and age	1950[1,2]	1960[1,2]	1970[2]	1980[2]	1985[2]	1990[2]	1995[2]	2000[3]	2005[3]	2006[3]
75 to 84 years[6]	853.5	1,053.3	1,624.8	2,029.6	2,229.6	2,478.3	2,449.8	2,351.8	2,019.5	1,976.0
85 years and over	NA	1,155.2	1,387.0	2,393.9	2,629.0	3,238.3	3,395.5	3,264.8	3,258.8	3,102.5
American Indian or Alaska Native Male[5]										
All ages, age-adjusted[4]	NA	NA	NA	140.5	142.1	145.8	169.0	155.8	158.5	146.0
All ages, crude	NA	NA	NA	58.1	62.8	61.4	67.8	67.0	73.0	66.0
25 to 34 years	NA	NA	NA	*	*	*	*	*	*	*
35 to 44 years	NA	NA	NA	*	28.8	22.8	14.3	21.4	24.3	13.3
45 to 54 years	NA	NA	NA	86.9	89.4	86.9	79.2	70.3	75.2	67.3
55 to 64 years	NA	NA	NA	213.4	276.6	246.2	279.8	255.6	257.7	211.0
65 to 74 years	NA	NA	NA	613.0	584.6	530.6	684.7	648.0	619.3	578.3
75 to 84 years	NA	NA	NA	936.4	963.6	1,038.4	1,346.3	1,152.5	1,138.4	1,143.9
85 years and over	NA	NA	NA	1,471.2	1,133.3	1,654.4	1,549.0	1,584.2	1,832.2	1,653.0
Asian or Pacific Islander Male[5]										
All ages, age-adjusted[4]	NA	NA	NA	165.2	173.4	172.5	164.3	150.8	137.4	131.6
All ages, crude	NA	NA	NA	81.9	82.6	82.7	83.7	85.2	84.8	82.6
25 to 34 years	NA	NA	NA	6.3	10.0	9.2	8.2	7.4	7.1	6.9
35 to 44 years	NA	NA	NA	29.4	25.7	27.7	26.1	26.1	20.6	20.4
45 to 54 years	NA	NA	NA	108.2	98.0	92.6	82.4	78.5	75.9	70.3
55 to 64 years	NA	NA	NA	298.5	315.0	274.6	244.8	229.2	197.5	195.6
65 to 74 years	NA	NA	NA	581.2	631.3	687.2	614.3	559.4	487.0	455.0
75 to 84 years	NA	NA	NA	1,147.6	1,251.2	1,229.9	1,167.2	1,086.1	1,022.0	974.7
85 years and over	NA	NA	NA	1,798.7	1,800.0	1,837.0	2,081.3	1,823.2	1,716.2	1,685.3
Hispanic or Latino Male[5,7]										
All ages, age-adjusted[4]	NA	NA	NA	NA	161.3	174.7	180.9	171.7	162.4	153.5
All ages, crude	NA	NA	NA	NA	56.1	65.5	65.4	61.3	63.2	60.9
25 to 34 years	NA	NA	NA	NA	9.7	8.0	8.4	6.9	6.9	6.5
35 to 44 years	NA	NA	NA	NA	22.9	22.5	24.7	20.1	18.5	16.8
45 to 54 years	NA	NA	NA	NA	83.5	96.6	85.0	79.4	76.7	72.4
55 to 64 years	NA	NA	NA	NA	259.0	294.0	281.6	253.1	238.1	226.4
65 to 74 years	NA	NA	NA	NA	598.2	655.5	697.9	651.2	610.3	582.5
75 to 84 years	NA	NA	NA	NA	1,210.5	1,233.4	1,359.8	1,306.4	1,219.2	1,158.8
85 years and over	NA	NA	NA	NA	1,743.8	2,019.4	2,018.6	2,049.7	2,013.0	1,852.2
White, Not Hispanic or Latino Male[7]										
All ages, age-adjusted[4]	NA	NA	NA	NA	259.0	276.7	263.5	247.7	228.4	223.7
All ages, crude	NA	NA	NA	NA	217.4	246.2	246.0	244.4	242.5	241.7
25 to 34 years	NA	NA	NA	NA	13.5	12.8	11.2	9.7	9.3	9.5
35 to 44 years	NA	NA	NA	NA	39.1	36.8	34.8	32.3	30.8	29.2
45 to 54 years	NA	NA	NA	NA	159.9	153.9	135.6	127.2	120.7	119.1
55 to 64 years	NA	NA	NA	NA	496.4	520.6	464.9	412.0	363.1	360.0
65 to 74 years	NA	NA	NA	NA	1,044.2	1,109.0	1,069.9	1,002.1	893.3	863.5
75 to 84 years	NA	NA	NA	NA	1,765.5	1,906.6	1,825.4	1,750.2	1,650.0	1,630.1
85 years and over	NA	NA	NA	NA	2,327.3	2,744.4	2,810.8	2,714.1	2,578.7	2,511.9
White Female[5]										
All ages, age-adjusted[4]	182.0	167.7	162.5	165.2	169.9	174.0	172.1	166.9	156.4	154.7
All ages, crude	139.9	139.8	149.4	170.3	184.4	196.1	200.6	199.4	192.3	191.5
25 to 34 years	20.9	18.8	16.3	13.5	12.7	11.9	11.2	10.1	8.8	9.3
35 to 44 years	74.5	66.6	62.4	50.9	47.3	46.2	41.9	38.2	36.2	35.2
45 to 54 years	185.8	175.7	177.3	166.4	161.6	150.9	135.0	120.1	110.9	109.9
55 to 64 years	362.5	329.0	338.6	355.5	376.3	368.5	350.3	319.7	282.2	277.1
65 to 74 years	616.5	562.1	554.7	605.2	644.9	675.1	685.6	665.6	611.5	606.1
75 to 84 years	1,026.6	939.3	903.5	905.4	938.2	1,011.8	1,047.9	1,063.4	1,032.0	1,023.5
85 years and over	1,348.3	1,304.9	1,126.6	1,266.8	1,285.4	1,372.3	1,405.4	1,459.1	1,426.4	1,413.0
Black or African American Female[5]										
All ages, age-adjusted[4]	174.1	174.3	173.4	189.5	195.5	205.9	203.8	193.8	180.3	176.6
All ages, crude	111.8	113.8	117.3	136.5	145.2	156.1	155.8	151.8	148.1	146.5
25 to 34 years	34.3	31.0	20.9	18.3	17.2	18.7	16.5	13.5	12.7	12.6
35 to 44 years	119.8	102.4	94.6	73.5	69.0	67.4	61.7	58.9	52.1	50.3
45 to 54 years	277.0	254.8	228.6	230.2	212.4	209.9	190.6	173.9	164.5	156.6
55 to 64 years	484.6	442.7	404.8	450.4	474.9	482.4	444.9	391.0	358.6	349.1
65 to 74 years	477.3	541.6	615.8	662.4	704.2	773.2	803.5	753.1	667.7	659.8

NA = Not available.

* = Rates based on fewer than 20 deaths are considered unreliable and are not shown.

[1]Includes deaths of persons who were not residents of the 50 states and the District of Columbia.

[2]Underlying cause of death was coded according to the 6th Revision of the International Classification of Diseases (ICD) in 1950, 7th Revision in 1960, 8th Revision in 1970, and 9th Revision in 1980-1998.

[3]Starting with 1999 data, cause of death is coded according to ICD-10.

[4]Age-adjusted rates are calculated using the year 2000 standard population. Prior to 2001, age-adjusted rates were calculated using standard million proportions based on rounded population numbers. Starting with 2001 data, unrounded population numbers are used to calculate age-adjusted rates.

[5]The race groups, White, Black, Asian or Pacific Islander, and American Indian or Alaska Native, include persons of Hispanic and non-Hispanic origin. Persons of Hispanic origin may be of any race. Death rates for the American Indian or Alaska Native, Asian or Pacific Islander, and Hispanic populations are known to be underestimated.

[6]In 1950, rate is for the age group 75 years and over.

[7]Prior to 1997, excludes data from states lacking an Hispanic-origin item on the death certificate.

Table 2-30. Death Rates for Malignant Neoplasms, by Sex, Race, Hispanic Origin, and Age, Selected Years, 1950–2015—*Continued*

(Deaths per 100,000 resident population.)

Sex, race, Hispanic origin, and age	2007[3]	2008[3]	2009[3]	2010[3]	2011[3]	2012[3]	2013[3]	2014[3]	2015[3]
75 to 84 years[6]	1,929.9	1,875.6	1,835.3	1,826.8	1,705.6	1,685.7	1,633.2	1,569.4	1,526.9
85 years and over	3,230.0	2,956.8	2,791.3	2,854.6	2,675.3	2,540.2	2,465.6	2,378.6	2,316.0
American Indian or Alaska Native Male[5]									
All ages, age-adjusted[4]	150.7	151.8	132.8	151.0	132.7	127.9	132.3	130.4	127.1
All ages, crude	70.1	72.7	66.4	74.1	68.0	70.5	73.6	76.1	77.5
25 to 34 years	*	*	6.5	7.4	*	*	6.2	*	5.4
35 to 44 years	13.7	17.7	12.3	13.4	11.3	14.2	13.1	15.2	14.7
45 to 54 years	69.3	82.5	73.2	70.0	70.6	65.9	61.9	58.7	70.0
55 to 64 years	248.4	225.4	229.6	249.5	197.2	216.2	233.5	221.2	202.7
65 to 74 years	558.7	620.8	541.3	597.7	523.8	558.4	477.8	520.7	505.3
75 to 84 years	1,112.3	1,144.2	936.9	1,104.4	1,018.5	885.2	1,009.1	1,015.8	971.8
85 years and over	1,876.3	1,588.6	1,390.1	1,741.3	1,459.3	1,288.7	1,488.1	1,256.3	1,229.2
Asian or Pacific Islander Male[5]									
All ages, age-adjusted[4]	134.8	132.8	131.0	131.0	125.7	123.1	120.9	116.4	116.7
All ages, crude	85.5	86.3	86.7	88.6	89.0	89.0	90.5	90.2	92.5
25 to 34 years	6.2	6.8	5.7	6.5	6.8	7.4	6.5	6.0	5.3
35 to 44 years	19.5	18.9	21.2	18.2	16.1	19.4	20.3	15.9	18.0
45 to 54 years	72.9	69.5	67.5	67.4	67.6	65.9	67.6	64.6	61.6
55 to 64 years	187.0	189.4	193.4	195.2	193.7	186.7	186.4	190.7	179.8
65 to 74 years	461.2	464.1	425.8	446.2	436.6	396.5	387.5	399.6	410.2
75 to 84 years	1,046.7	1,004.1	988.2	980.4	917.6	936.3	899.5	839.8	843.2
85 years and over	1,693.4	1,689.0	1,762.0	1,707.2	1,626.3	1,577.7	1,575.3	1,468.0	1,492.8
Hispanic or Latino Male[5,7]									
All ages, age-adjusted[4]	151.7	151.4	148.6	149.4	144.9	141.9	138.8	135.9	133.8
All ages, crude	61.6	62.8	62.9	64.2	65.0	66.3	66.9	68.0	69.4
25 to 34 years	6.7	8.0	7.7	7.2	6.7	7.6	7.8	7.1	7.7
35 to 44 years	18.2	18.2	18.0	16.5	16.4	17.3	16.4	17.2	17.0
45 to 54 years	75.2	71.7	70.7	69.7	69.2	67.6	66.4	65.1	63.3
55 to 64 years	223.1	228.8	222.9	225.4	224.3	224.8	217.4	207.8	208.8
65 to 74 years	566.8	565.5	545.9	552.0	528.2	524.3	515.6	497.9	487.9
75 to 84 years	1,133.4	1,137.6	1,128.7	1,118.7	1,104.5	1,068.1	1,051.3	1,026.5	1,016.4
85 years and over	1,855.9	1,820.3	1,794.7	1,861.2	1,728.5	1,652.6	1,606.6	1,624.9	1,573.7
White, Not Hispanic or Latino Male[7]									
All ages, age-adjusted[4]	220.8	217.2	213.6	212.6	207.6	204.0	200.0	197.7	194.3
All ages, crude	242.6	243.3	243.5	245.8	245.6	247.0	247.3	249.3	249.7
25 to 34 years	8.9	8.9	9.1	9.1	8.4	8.5	8.5	8.6	8.4
35 to 44 years	28.0	27.1	27.6	27.0	27.2	25.7	25.6	25.6	24.5
45 to 54 years	117.2	119.3	117.9	117.2	114.4	114.2	111.9	108.5	105.0
55 to 64 years	354.0	349.4	345.4	344.2	341.8	338.6	332.9	335.0	331.7
65 to 74 years	845.7	827.6	800.4	798.5	775.7	757.4	737.2	722.1	713.1
75 to 84 years	1,614.0	1,583.8	1,561.8	1,534.4	1,508.2	1,475.9	1,444.8	1,424.1	1,391.1
85 years and over	2,514.5	2,464.5	2,440.5	2,480.8	2,377.1	2,353.6	2,330.5	2,319.1	2,294.1
White Female[5]									
All ages, age-adjusted[4]	152.3	149.8	147.9	146.9	144.0	142.5	140.2	138.8	136.8
All ages, crude	190.0	188.7	187.8	188.2	186.8	187.5	186.8	187.2	187.1
25 to 34 years	8.8	8.6	9.1	8.8	8.3	8.7	8.5	8.3	8.6
35 to 44 years	34.2	32.8	33.6	31.3	31.4	31.0	31.8	31.2	29.9
45 to 54 years	107.4	106.0	108.4	106.5	105.0	104.5	103.0	101.8	98.7
55 to 64 years	269.5	261.7	258.9	255.3	250.6	249.7	245.4	244.9	242.1
65 to 74 years	595.9	581.9	567.1	563.7	549.2	535.5	526.4	512.4	505.9
75 to 84 years	1,018.1	1,008.3	991.2	988.6	970.1	962.1	945.4	943.2	922.7
85 years and over	1,392.7	1,393.2	1,370.0	1,389.8	1,359.9	1,351.4	1,326.5	1,329.0	1,338.3
Black or African American Female[5]									
All ages, age-adjusted[4]	174.9	170.1	167.0	167.1	166.1	161.7	158.5	156.8	152.2
All ages, crude	146.5	144.2	143.5	145.5	147.5	146.3	146.2	147.5	146.2
25 to 34 years	12.0	10.4	11.4	10.8	12.2	12.1	10.4	11.2	10.9
35 to 44 years	47.9	47.7	44.6	44.5	46.4	42.5	40.7	40.5	40.9
45 to 54 years	153.5	149.0	145.7	146.4	144.9	140.2	134.8	133.4	126.2
55 to 64 years	343.6	330.7	327.2	331.1	327.6	320.9	320.0	321.9	317.2
65 to 74 years	665.7	652.1	638.2	631.0	623.1	617.8	593.4	583.7	566.7

NA = Not available.

* = Rates based on fewer than 20 deaths are considered unreliable and are not shown.

[3]Starting with 1999 data, cause of death is coded according to ICD-10.

[4]Age-adjusted rates are calculated using the year 2000 standard population. Prior to 2001, age-adjusted rates were calculated using standard million proportions based on rounded population numbers. Starting with 2001 data, unrounded population numbers are used to calculate age-adjusted rates.

[5]The race groups, White, Black, Asian or Pacific Islander, and American Indian or Alaska Native, include persons of Hispanic and non-Hispanic origin. Persons of Hispanic origin may be of any race. Death rates for the American Indian or Alaska Native, Asian or Pacific Islander, and Hispanic populations are known to be underestimated.

[6]In 1950, rate is for the age group 75 years and over.

[7]Prior to 1997, excludes data from states lacking an Hispanic-origin item on the death certificate.

Table 2-30. Death Rates for Malignant Neoplasms, by Sex, Race, Hispanic Origin, and Age, Selected Years, 1950–2015—Continued

(Deaths per 100,000 resident population.)

Sex, race, Hispanic origin, and age	1950[1,2]	1960[1,2]	1970[2]	1980[2]	1985[2]	1990[2]	1995[2]	2000[3]	2005[3]	2006[3]
75 to 84 years[6]	605.3	696.3	763.3	923.9	986.3	1,059.9	1,120.8	1,124.0	1,074.9	1,068.2
85 years and over	NA	728.9	791.5	1,159.9	1,284.2	1,431.3	1,446.2	1,527.7	1,514.6	1,469.8
American Indian or Alaska Native Female[5]										
All ages, age-adjusted[4]	NA	NA	NA	94.0	93.0	106.9	117.7	108.3	108.9	111.9
All ages, crude	NA	NA	NA	50.4	52.5	62.1	64.5	61.3	65.7	66.7
25 to 34 years	NA	NA	NA	*	*	*	10.2	*	*	*
35 to 44 years	NA	NA	NA	36.9	23.4	31.0	29.7	23.7	20.7	21.8
45 to 54 years	NA	NA	NA	96.9	90.1	104.5	76.9	59.7	79.1	66.3
55 to 64 years	NA	NA	NA	198.4	192.3	213.3	213.2	200.9	194.6	185.3
65 to 74 years	NA	NA	NA	350.8	378.8	438.9	437.0	458.3	473.0	464.9
75 to 84 years	NA	NA	NA	446.4	505.9	554.3	819.9	714.0	742.4	801.6
85 years and over	NA	NA	NA	786.5	700.0	843.7	1,039.4	983.2	802.0	971.7
Asian or Pacific Islander Female[5]										
All ages, age-adjusted[4]	NA	NA	NA	93.0	99.6	103.0	107.4	100.7	96.2	94.2
All ages, crude	NA	NA	NA	54.1	57.5	60.5	69.5	72.1	75.0	74.5
25 to 34 years	NA	NA	NA	9.5	9.9	7.3	9.9	8.1	7.3	6.9
35 to 44 years	NA	NA	NA	38.7	33.1	29.8	27.6	28.9	25.0	24.7
45 to 54 years	NA	NA	NA	99.8	91.3	93.9	94.4	78.2	73.9	72.0
55 to 64 years	NA	NA	NA	174.7	195.5	196.2	203.5	176.5	166.2	155.0
65 to 74 years	NA	NA	NA	301.9	330.8	346.2	343.3	357.4	324.7	327.1
75 to 84 years	NA	NA	NA	522.1	589.1	641.4	681.0	650.1	626.8	625.7
85 years and over	NA	NA	NA	800.0	908.3	971.7	1,092.7	988.5	1,060.1	1,006.7
Hispanic or Latina Female[5,7]										
All ages, age-adjusted[4]	NA	NA	NA	NA	101.5	111.9	110.8	110.8	104.9	103.8
All ages, crude	NA	NA	NA	NA	49.8	60.7	58.7	58.5	58.3	58.5
25 to 34 years	NA	NA	NA	NA	9.7	9.7	8.5	7.8	7.0	8.4
35 to 44 years	NA	NA	NA	NA	30.9	34.8	30.7	30.7	26.6	27.5
45 to 54 years	NA	NA	NA	NA	90.1	100.5	89.7	84.7	78.9	77.1
55 to 64 years	NA	NA	NA	NA	199.2	205.4	203.0	192.5	170.8	172.5
65 to 74 years	NA	NA	NA	NA	356.4	404.8	398.0	410.0	380.6	368.2
75 to 84 years	NA	NA	NA	NA	600.0	663.0	706.2	716.5	708.7	687.8
85 years and over	NA	NA	NA	NA	907.1	1,022.7	1,028.6	1,056.5	1,045.6	1,073.8
White, not Hispanic or Latina Female[7]										
All ages, age-adjusted[4]	NA	NA	NA	NA	167.1	177.5	174.7	170.0	160.1	158.4
All ages, crude	NA	NA	NA	NA	187.1	210.6	217.3	220.6	216.6	216.5
25 to 34 years	NA	NA	NA	NA	12.2	11.9	11.5	10.5	9.1	9.4
35 to 44 years	NA	NA	NA	NA	47.2	47.0	42.7	38.9	37.8	36.3
45 to 54 years	NA	NA	NA	NA	158.8	154.9	137.8	123.0	114.2	113.4
55 to 64 years	NA	NA	NA	NA	372.7	379.5	359.3	328.9	291.7	286.3
65 to 74 years	NA	NA	NA	NA	638.4	688.5	697.9	681.0	629.1	625.1
75 to 84 years	NA	NA	NA	NA	917.8	1,027.2	1,056.1	1,075.3	1,048.9	1,042.3
85 years and over	NA	NA	NA	NA	1,241.5	1,385.7	1,411.6	1,468.7	1,440.0	1,424.6

NA = Not available.

* = Rates based on fewer than 20 deaths are considered unreliable and are not shown.

[1] Includes deaths of persons who were not residents of the 50 states and the District of Columbia.

[2] Underlying cause of death was coded according to the 6th Revision of the International Classification of Diseases (ICD) in 1950, 7th Revision in 1960, 8th Revision in 1970, and 9th Revision in 1980-1998.

[3] Starting with 1999 data, cause of death is coded according to ICD-10.

[4] Age-adjusted rates are calculated using the year 2000 standard population. Prior to 2001, age-adjusted rates were calculated using standard million proportions based on rounded population numbers. Starting with 2001 data, unrounded population numbers are used to calculate age-adjusted rates.

[5] The race groups, White, Black, Asian or Pacific Islander, and American Indian or Alaska Native, include persons of Hispanic and non-Hispanic origin. Persons of Hispanic origin may be of any race. Death rates for the American Indian or Alaska Native, Asian or Pacific Islander, and Hispanic populations are known to be underestimated.

[6] In 1950, rate is for the age group 75 years and over.

[7] Prior to 1997, excludes data from states lacking an Hispanic-origin item on the death certificate.

Table 2-30. Death Rates for Malignant Neoplasms, by Sex, Race, Hispanic Origin, and Age, Selected Years, 1950–2015—*Continued*

(Deaths per 100,000 resident population.)

Sex, race, Hispanic origin, and age	2007[3]	2008[3]	2009[3]	2010[3]	2011[3]	2012[3]	2013[3]	2014[3]	2015[3]
75 to 84 years[6]	1,075.1	1,021.3	1,026.7	1,008.2	1,010.4	985.6	984.3	960.8	925.2
85 years and over	1,405.0	1,427.8	1,345.7	1,418.6	1,390.9	1,318.4	1,306.5	1,297.5	1,267.9
American Indian or Alaska Native Female[5]									
All ages, age-adjusted[4]	105.8	105.6	102.2	102.0	92.6	99.1	94.3	88.5	93.0
All ages, crude	63.6	64.2	64.4	64.8	61.3	66.7	65.8	63.4	69.2
25 to 34 years	*	*	6.6	6.3	*	*	6.4	*	6.5
35 to 44 years	17.0	22.5	20.4	14.2	16.2	16.1	18.8	17.5	18.0
45 to 54 years	67.6	64.3	70.5	68.7	68.4	62.5	69.1	67.1	62.7
55 to 64 years	180.8	169.8	183.1	185.9	160.7	176.2	155.1	139.5	161.3
65 to 74 years	438.2	443.9	414.4	432.2	375.6	394.4	373.0	359.8	350.7
75 to 84 years	757.7	732.5	696.4	682.3	621.8	753.5	656.2	611.5	654.8
85 years and over	937.1	986.0	863.4	885.7	828.6	763.3	844.8	817.9	884.0
Asian or Pacific Islander Female[5]									
All ages, age-adjusted[4]	91.7	91.8	89.6	93.5	91.5	90.9	86.0	86.2	86.2
All ages, crude	73.4	74.4	73.7	78.5	79.8	80.9	78.6	80.6	82.7
25 to 34 years	5.4	7.8	5.8	7.1	5.1	5.6	6.4	6.2	5.3
35 to 44 years	23.7	20.5	21.3	21.7	23.3	23.2	22.1	21.7	21.7
45 to 54 years	67.7	67.1	60.2	69.5	69.9	71.2	63.6	64.1	67.1
55 to 64 years	155.2	145.6	144.9	152.6	155.9	149.9	139.7	143.8	146.6
65 to 74 years	301.7	316.1	300.8	314.4	299.6	290.3	280.7	278.8	279.5
75 to 84 years	624.4	633.4	618.7	654.5	640.9	626.5	601.5	597.1	589.1
85 years and over	1,019.8	1,027.2	1,053.5	994.4	957.6	1,012.6	925.7	963.7	941.5
Hispanic or Latina Female[5,7]									
All ages, age-adjusted[4]	101.7	100.1	99.8	99.4	97.5	99.3	97.3	95.7	93.6
All ages, crude	58.1	57.8	58.4	59.0	59.4	62.4	63.0	63.6	64.2
25 to 34 years	8.6	7.7	7.4	8.4	7.2	8.1	8.8	7.2	8.3
35 to 44 years	25.9	25.0	24.4	23.5	24.0	24.4	25.4	25.4	25.2
45 to 54 years	74.0	69.8	70.8	74.0	66.2	73.2	69.1	68.6	67.9
55 to 64 years	172.7	175.2	170.0	165.9	161.6	165.1	164.7	163.2	161.4
65 to 74 years	360.4	346.3	351.7	355.2	348.2	342.8	342.0	335.9	330.6
75 to 84 years	687.2	684.5	665.4	657.6	672.0	662.9	656.7	636.6	621.7
85 years and over	1,005.8	1,020.6	1,061.0	1,043.4	1,006.5	1,073.7	996.6	1,004.3	946.7
White, not Hispanic or Latina Female[7]									
All ages, age-adjusted[4]	156.1	153.6	151.8	150.6	147.9	146.0	143.9	142.7	140.6
All ages, crude	215.6	214.7	214.2	215.0	213.9	214.4	214.0	215.1	215.1
25 to 34 years	8.6	8.7	9.3	8.8	8.4	8.6	8.1	8.4	8.4
35 to 44 years	35.6	34.1	35.4	32.8	32.8	32.3	32.9	32.3	30.6
45 to 54 years	111.3	110.3	113.1	110.5	110.4	108.8	108.0	107.1	103.7
55 to 64 years	278.1	269.2	266.9	263.4	259.0	257.9	253.3	253.3	250.6
65 to 74 years	615.2	600.9	584.6	580.4	566.0	551.1	541.4	527.0	520.4
75 to 84 years	1,037.7	1,028.1	1,012.4	1,010.4	990.3	983.0	966.6	967.1	945.6
85 years and over	1,407.8	1,407.4	1,382.3	1,403.8	1,375.6	1,362.4	1,343.5	1,345.8	1,360.0

NA = Not available.

* = Rates based on fewer than 20 deaths are considered unreliable and are not shown.

[3]Starting with 1999 data, cause of death is coded according to ICD-10.

[4]Age-adjusted rates are calculated using the year 2000 standard population. Prior to 2001, age-adjusted rates were calculated using standard million proportions based on rounded population numbers. Starting with 2001 data, unrounded population numbers are used to calculate age-adjusted rates.

[5]The race groups, White, Black, Asian or Pacific Islander, and American Indian or Alaska Native, include persons of Hispanic and non-Hispanic origin. Persons of Hispanic origin may be of any race. Death rates for the American Indian or Alaska Native, Asian or Pacific Islander, and Hispanic populations are known to be underestimated.

[6]In 1950, rate is for the age group 75 years and over.

[7]Prior to 1997, excludes data from states lacking an Hispanic-origin item on the death certificate.

Table 2-31. Number of Infant Deaths and Infant Mortality Rates, by Selected Cause and Race, 2015

(Infant deaths [under 1 year] per 100,000 live births in specified group. Infant deaths based on race of decedent; live births based on race of mother.)

Cause of death (based on ICD–10, 2004)	Number[1] Total[2]	Non-Hispanic White[3]	Non-Hispanic Black[3]	Hispanic	Rate Total[2]	Non-Hispanic White[3]	Non-Hispanic Black[3]	Hispanic
All causes	23,455	10,277	6,907	4,805	589.5	482.4	1,172.6	520.0
Certain intestinal infectious diseases (A00-A08)	11	5	2	–	*	*	*	*
Diarrhea and gastroenteritis of infectious origin (A09)	210	73	80	42	5.3	3.4	13.6	4.5
Tuberculosis (A16-A19)	–	–	–	–	*	*	*	*
Tetanus (A33,A35)	–	–	–	–	*	*	*	*
Diphtheria (A36)	–	–	–	–	*	*	*	*
Whooping cough (A37)	6	–	1	5	*	*	*	*
Meningococcal infection (A39)	2	1	1	–	*	*	*	*
Septicemia (A40-A41)	180	71	58	41	4.5	3.3	9.8	4.4
Congenital syphilis (A50)	2	–	2	–	*	*	*	*
Gonococcal infection (A54)	–	–	–	–	*	*	*	*
Acute poliomyelitis (A80)	–	–	–	–	*	*	*	*
Varicella (chickenpox) (B01)	–	–	–	–	*	*	*	*
Measles (B05)	–	–	–	–	*	*	*	*
Human immunodeficiency virus (HIV) disease (B20-B24)	2	1	1	–	*	*	*	*
Mumps (B26)	–	–	–	–	*	*	*	*
Candidiasis (B37)	7	4	1	2	*	*	*	*
Malaria (B50-B54)	–	–	–	–	*	*	*	*
Pneumocystosis (B59)	–	–	–	–	*	*	*	*
Malignant neoplasms (C00-C97)	53	25	8	13	1.3	1.2	*	*
In situ neoplasms, benign neoplasms and neoplasms of uncertain or unknown behavior (D00-D48)	47	28	7	8	1.2	1.3	*	*
Diseases of the blood and blood-forming organs and certain disorders involving the immune mechanism (D50-D89)	95	40	28	16	2.4	1.9	4.8	*
Short stature, not elsewhere classified (E34.3)	4	2	–	1	*	*	*	*
Nutritional deficiencies (E40-E64)	9	5	1	3	*	*	*	*
Cystic fibrosis (E84)	7	5	–	1	*	*	*	*
Volume depletion, disorders of fluid, electrolyte and acid-base balance (E86-E87)	43	23	13	7	1.1	1.1	*	*
Meningitis (G00,G03)	51	22	15	12	1.3	1.0	*	*
Infantile spinal muscular atrophy, type I (Werdnig-Hoffman) (G12.0)	2	–	1	1	*	*	*	*
Infantile cerebral palsy (G80)	2	1	1	–	*	*	*	*
Anoxic brain damage, not elsewhere classified (G93.1)	50	32	–	6	1.3	1.5	*	*
Diseases of the ear and mastoid process (H60-H93)	2	–	1	–	*	*	*	*
Diseases of the circulatory system (I00-I99)	428	196	128	74	10.8	9.2	21.7	8.0
Acute upper respiratory infections (J00-J06)	15	7	6	2	*	*	*	*
Influenza and pneumonia (J09-J18)	174	77	56	30	4.4	3.6	9.5	3.2
Acute bronchitis and acute bronchiolitis (J20-J21)	50	21	18	6	1.3	1.0	*	*
Bronchitis, chronic and unspecified (J40-J42)	19	8	8	3	*	*	*	*
Asthma (J45-J46)	3	–	2	1	*	*	*	*
Pneumonitis due to solids and liquids (J69)	8	2	3	2	*	*	*	*
Gastritis, duodenitis, and noninfective enteritis and colitis (K29,K50-K55)	30	10	10	9	0.8	*	*	*
Hernia of abdominal cavity and intestinal obstruction without hernia (K40-K46,K56)	52	29	12	7	1.3	1.4	*	*
Renal failure and other disorders of kidney (N17-N19,N25,N27)	83	35	24	19	2.1	1.6	4.1	*
Newborn affected by maternal hypertensive disorders (P00.0)	87	26	39	17	2.2	1.2	6.6	*
Newborn affected by other maternal conditions which may be unrelated to present pregnancy (P00.1-P00.9)	85	40	22	17	2.1	1.9	3.7	*
Newborn affected by other maternal complications of pregnancy (P01.2-P01.4,P01.6-P01.9)	1,522	606	458	339	38.3	28.4	77.8	36.7
Newborn affected by complications of placenta, cord and membranes (P02)	910	379	270	194	22.9	17.8	45.8	21.0
Newborn affected by other complications of labor and delivery (P03)	127	46	34	28	3.2	2.2	5.8	3.0
Newborn affected by noxious influences transmitted via placenta or breast milk (P04)	51	28	11	10	1.3	1.3	*	*
Slow fetal growth and fetal malnutrition (P05)	112	54	38	12	2.8	2.5	6.5	*
Disorders related to short gestation and low birth weight, not elsewhere classified (P07)	4,084	1,485	1,513	824	102.7	69.7	256.9	89.2
Disorders related to long gestation and high birth weight (P08)	1	1	–	–	*	*	*	*
Birth trauma (P10-P15)	13	8	4	1	*	*	*	*
Intrauterine hypoxia and birth asphyxia (P20–P21)	314	150	93	56	7.9	7.0	15.8	6.1
Respiratory distress of newborn (P22)	462	184	168	87	11.6	8.6	28.5	9.4
Other respiratory conditions originating in the perinatal period (P23-P28)	790	345	252	156	19.9	16.2	42.8	16.9
Congenital pneumonia (P23)	49	18	11	16	1.2	*	*	*
Neonatal aspiration syndromes (P24)	46	31	4	8	1.2	1.5	*	*
Interstitial emphysema and related conditions originating in the perinatal period (P25)	93	37	37	15	2.3	1.7	6.3	*
Pulmonary hemorrhage originating in the perinatal period (P26)	152	58	55	28	3.8	2.7	9.3	3.0
Chronic respiratory disease originating in the perinatal period (P27)	115	46	46	20	2.9	2.2	7.8	2.2
Atelectasis (P28.0-P28.1)	273	118	84	62	6.9	5.5	14.3	6.7
Bacterial sepsis of newborn (P36)	599	230	208	127	15.1	10.8	35.3	13.7
Omphalitis of newborn with or without mild hemorrhage (P38)	1	1	–	–	*	*	*	*
Neonatal hemorrhage (P50-P52,P54)	406	177	99	99	10.2	8.3	16.8	10.7
Hemorrhagic disease of newborn (P53)	1	–	–	1	*	*	*	*
Hemolytic disease of newborn due to isoimmunization and other perinatal jaundice (P55-P59)	6	3	2	1	*	*	*	*
Hematological disorders (P60-P61)	102	48	22	23	2.6	2.3	3.7	2.5
Syndrome of infant of a diabetic mother and neonatal diabetes mellitus (P70.0-P70.2)	6	1	2	–	*	*	*	*
Necrotizing enterocolitis of newborn (P77)	363	133	126	82	9.1	6.2	21.4	8.9
Hydrops fetalis not due to hemolytic disease (P83.2)	177	95	21	47	4.4	4.5	3.6	5.1
Congenital malformations, deformations and chromosomal abnormalities (Q00-Q99)	4,825	2,373	930	1,216	121.3	111.4	157.9	131.6
Symptoms, signs and abnormal clinical and laboratory findings, not elsewhere classified (R00-R99)	2,819	1,328	928	423	70.9	62.3	157.5	45.8
Sudden infant death syndrome (R95)	1,568	771	513	202	39.4	36.2	87.1	21.9
Accidents (unintentional injuries) (V01-X59)	1,291	632	410	187	32.4	29.7	69.6	20.2
Assault (homicide) (*U01,X85-Y09)[4]	263	119	92	40	6.6	5.6	15.6	4.3
Complications of medical and surgical care (Y40-Y84)	12	7	4	1	*	*	*	*

- = Quantity zero.
* = Figure does not meet standards of reliability or precision.
[1] Only selected causes of deaths are shown; therefore, subcategories do not add to totals.
[2] Includes races and origins not shown separately.
[3] Multiple-race data reported according to 1997 OMB standards were bridged to the single-race categories of 1977 OMB standards.
[4] Asterisks (*) preceding cause-of-death codes indicate they are not part of the International Classification of Diseases, Tenth Revision.

This page is intentionally left blank

Table 2-32. Death Rates for Malignant Neoplasms of the Trachea, Bronchus, and Lung, by Sex, Race, Hispanic Origin, and Age, Selected Years, 1950–2015

(Deaths per 100,000 resident population.)

Sex, race, Hispanic origin, and age	1950[1,2]	1960[1,2]	1970[2]	1980[2]	1985[2]	1990[2]	1995[2]	2000[3]	2005[3]	2006[3]
All Persons										
All ages, age-adjusted[4]	15.0	24.1	37.1	49.9	54.6	59.3	58.4	56.1	52.7	51.5
All ages, crude	12.2	20.3	32.1	45.8	51.5	56.8	56.8	55.3	53.9	53.2
Under 25 years	0.1	0.0	0.1	0.0	0.0	0.0	0.0	0.0	0.0	0.0
25 to 34 years	0.8	1.0	0.9	0.6	0.6	0.7	0.6	0.5	0.3	0.4
35 to 44 years	4.5	6.8	11.0	9.2	7.8	6.8	6.0	6.1	5.3	4.7
45 to 54 years	20.4	29.6	43.4	54.1	50.9	46.8	37.5	31.6	29.7	29.1
55 to 64 years	48.7	75.3	109.1	138.2	153.8	160.6	141.6	122.4	102.4	98.1
65 to 74 years	59.7	108.1	164.5	233.3	261.2	288.4	295.4	284.2	256.3	249.3
75 to 84 years	55.8	91.5	163.2	240.5	282.0	333.3	358.9	370.8	375.0	372.1
85 years and over	42.3	65.6	101.7	176.0	195.2	242.5	279.9	302.1	328.2	327.1
Male										
All ages, age-adjusted[4]	24.6	43.6	67.5	85.2	88.6	91.1	84.2	76.7	69.1	67.0
All ages, crude	19.9	35.4	53.4	68.6	72.5	75.1	70.5	65.5	62.1	60.9
Under 25 years	0.0	0.0	0.1	0.1	*	0.0	0.1	*	*	*
25 to 34 years	1.1	1.4	1.3	0.8	0.7	0.9	0.7	0.5	0.4	0.4
35 to 44 years	7.1	10.5	16.1	11.9	10.0	8.5	7.0	6.9	5.5	4.8
45 to 54 years	35.0	50.6	67.5	76.0	67.5	59.7	46.3	38.5	35.1	33.8
55 to 64 years	83.8	139.3	189.7	213.6	223.5	222.9	185.3	154.0	126.3	120.2
65 to 74 years	98.7	204.3	320.8	403.9	416.2	430.4	414.3	377.9	324.8	312.9
75 to 84 years	82.6	167.1	330.8	488.8	537.6	572.9	553.8	532.2	511.1	503.8
85 years and over	62.5	107.7	194.0	368.1	433.2	513.2	540.3	521.2	519.9	508.9
Female										
All ages, age-adjusted[4]	5.8	7.5	13.1	24.4	30.6	37.1	40.4	41.3	40.6	40.1
All ages, crude	4.5	6.4	11.9	24.3	31.7	39.4	43.6	45.4	46.0	45.7
Under 25 years	0.1	0.0	0.0	*	*	*	*	*	*	*
25 to 34 years	0.5	0.5	0.5	0.5	0.6	0.5	0.6	0.5	0.3	0.4
35 to 44 years	1.9	3.2	6.1	6.5	5.6	5.2	5.0	5.3	5.1	4.6
45 to 54 years	5.8	9.2	21.0	33.7	35.2	34.5	29.1	25.0	24.5	24.6
55 to 64 years	13.6	15.4	36.8	72.0	92.1	105.0	101.9	93.3	80.0	77.4
65 to 74 years	23.3	24.4	43.1	102.7	141.8	177.6	200.0	206.9	197.9	195.0
75 to 84 years	32.9	32.8	52.4	94.1	131.7	190.1	237.2	265.6	281.6	280.8
85 years and over	28.2	38.8	50.0	91.9	100.2	138.1	179.6	212.8	243.1	244.6
White Male[5]										
All ages, age-adjusted[4]	25.1	43.6	67.1	83.8	86.8	89.0	82.6	75.7	68.8	66.7
All ages, crude	20.8	36.4	54.6	70.2	74.5	77.8	74.0	69.4	66.6	65.4
45 to 54 years	35.1	49.2	63.3	70.9	62.7	55.2	43.2	35.7	33.5	31.9
55 to 64 years	85.4	139.2	186.8	205.6	214.2	213.7	178.9	150.8	122.6	117.4
65 to 74 years	101.5	207.5	325.0	401.0	409.5	422.1	408.0	374.9	326.5	313.8
75 to 84 years	85.5	170.4	336.7	493.5	540.3	572.2	550.8	529.9	514.5	506.9
85 years and over	67.4	109.4	199.6	374.1	440.0	516.3	539.3	522.4	517.6	511.1
Black or African American Male[5]										
All ages, age-adjusted[4]	17.8	42.6	75.4	107.6	117.2	125.4	115.1	101.1	86.1	83.0
All ages, crude	12.1	28.1	47.7	66.6	71.2	73.7	65.6	58.3	52.8	51.7
45 to 54 years	34.4	68.4	115.4	133.8	122.5	114.9	85.2	70.7	55.4	55.0
55 to 64 years	68.3	146.8	234.3	321.1	351.5	358.6	288.5	223.5	191.3	175.9
65 to 74 years	53.8	168.3	300.5	472.3	539.6	585.4	559.5	488.8	393.5	385.4
75 to 84 years[6]	36.2	107.3	271.6	472.9	556.4	645.4	667.1	642.5	565.7	563.0
85 years and over	NA	82.8	137.0	311.3	382.3	499.5	583.0	562.8	601.6	539.6
American Indian or Alaska Native Male[5]										
All ages, age-adjusted[4]	NA	NA	NA	31.7	41.2	47.5	53.6	42.9	42.6	39.6
All ages, crude	NA	NA	NA	14.2	18.4	20.0	21.8	18.1	20.1	18.4
45 to 54 years	NA	NA	NA	*	*	26.6	23.8	14.5	18.2	16.5
55 to 64 years	NA	NA	NA	72.0	85.1	97.8	98.9	86.0	79.5	61.0
65 to 74 years	NA	NA	NA	202.8	223.1	194.3	261.5	184.8	190.3	200.4

NA = Not available.

* = Rates based on fewer than 20 deaths are considered unreliable and are not shown.

0.0 = Quantity more than zero but less than 0.05.

[1] Includes deaths of persons who were not residents of the 50 states and the District of Columbia.

[2] Underlying cause of death was coded according to the 6th Revision of the International Classification of Diseases (ICD) in 1950, 7th Revision in 1960, 8th Revision in 1970, and 9th Revision in 1980-1998.

[3] Starting with 1999 data, cause of death is coded according to ICD-10.

[4] Age-adjusted rates are calculated using the year 2000 standard population. Prior to 2001, age-adjusted rates were calculated using standard million proportions based on rounded population numbers. Starting with 2001 data, unrounded population numbers are used to calculate age-adjusted rates.

[5] The race groups, White, Black, Asian or Pacific Islander, and American Indian or Alaska Native, include persons of Hispanic and non-Hispanic origin. Persons of Hispanic origin may be of any race. Death rates for the American Indian or Alaska Native, Asian or Pacific Islander, and Hispanic populations are known to be underestimated.

[6] In 1950, rate is for the age group 75 years and over.

Table 2-32. Death Rates for Malignant Neoplasms of the Trachea, Bronchus, and Lung, by Sex, Race, Hispanic Origin, and Age, Selected Years, 1950–2015—*Continued*

(Deaths per 100,000 resident population.)

Sex, race, Hispanic origin, and age	2007[3]	2008[3]	2009[3]	2010[3]	2011[3]	2012[3]	2013[3]	2014[3]	2015[3]
All Persons									
All ages, age-adjusted[4]	50.6	49.5	48.4	47.6	46.0	44.9	43.4	42.1	40.5
All ages, crude	52.7	52.2	51.6	51.3	50.4	50.2	49.4	48.8	47.9
Under 25 years	0.0	0.0	0.0	0.0	0.0	0.0	0.0	0.0	0.0
25 to 34 years	0.3	0.4	0.4	0.4	0.3	0.4	0.3	0.3	0.3
35 to 44 years	4.3	3.8	3.7	3.7	3.3	3.1	2.9	2.8	2.7	2.5
45 to 54 years	28.4	28.2	27.8	26.9	25.7	25.1	23.9	22.4	20.5
55 to 64 years	94.2	90.2	87.5	85.4	83.5	81.5	79.9	78.5	76.8
65 to 74 years	244.5	235.5	228.6	223.9	214.3	206.1	196.6	189.4	181.0
75 to 84 years	369.5	366.7	359.8	357.2	345.9	339.6	328.5	321.2	306.4
85 years and over	328.0	332.9	328.0	332.4	323.7	323.7	320.0	311.7	316.1
Male									
All ages, age-adjusted[4]	64.9	63.5	61.4	60.3	57.7	56.1	53.7	51.7	49.5
All ages, crude	59.7	59.3	58.2	57.8	56.6	56.1	55.1	54.1	52.9
Under 25 years	0.0	0.1	0.0	*	0.0	0.0	*	*	*
25 to 34 years	0.4	0.4	0.4	0.4	0.3	0.5	0.3	0.3	0.3
35 to 44 years	4.3	4.0	3.7	3.2	3.1	2.9	2.8	2.9	2.6
45 to 54 years	32.1	32.3	31.0	30.0	28.1	27.7	25.9	23.8	22.1
55 to 64 years	114.7	111.1	107.9	104.9	102.5	98.3	96.9	93.8	92.1
65 to 74 years	302.8	291.2	279.4	274.9	262.8	250.0	236.0	229.5	217.1
75 to 84 years	490.9	482.0	470.5	461.9	442.4	432.0	413.4	395.7	378.3
85 years and over	505.2	511.0	489.1	492.3	467.3	473.4	463.0	442.8	434.4
Female									
All ages, age-adjusted[4]	40.1	39.1	38.6	38.1	37.1	36.4	35.5	34.7	33.5
All ages, crude	46.0	45.3	45.1	45.0	44.4	44.4	44.0	43.7	43.0
Under 25 years	*	*	*	0.0	*	*	*	*	0.0
25 to 34 years	0.3	0.3	0.3	0.4	0.3	0.3	0.3	0.3	0.3
35 to 44 years	4.4	3.6	3.6	3.3	3.1	2.9	2.9	2.6	2.4
45 to 54 years	24.8	24.3	24.7	23.8	23.3	22.6	21.9	21.0	18.8
55 to 64 years	75.2	70.7	68.4	67.2	65.7	65.9	64.2	64.2	62.7
65 to 74 years	194.3	187.4	184.5	179.5	171.9	167.5	161.9	154.2	149.1
75 to 84 years	284.4	285.1	280.6	281.7	275.3	271.1	264.9	264.8	251.5
85 years and over	246.0	249.1	251.0	255.2	252.9	248.7	246.9	243.5	253.6
White Male[5]									
All ages, age-adjusted[4]	64.6	63.4	61.3	60.1	57.7	56.0	53.7	51.8	49.7
All ages, crude	64.1	63.9	62.8	62.3	61.2	60.6	59.5	58.7	57.4
45 to 54 years	30.4	31.0	30.3	28.8	27.4	26.9	25.6	23.7	22.0
55 to 64 years	112.2	108.9	105.2	101.8	100.7	96.4	94.6	92.1	91.1
65 to 74 years	303.8	293.3	280.7	275.7	262.9	250.8	236.5	230.2	216.9
75 to 84 years	493.6	484.0	474.3	465.5	446.7	434.4	416.8	400.4	383.5
85 years and over	500.5	509.4	489.5	495.0	471.0	475.7	466.8	446.6	439.6
Black or African American Male[5]									
All ages, age-adjusted[4]	81.5	77.8	75.0	73.7	69.6	68.6	65.7	61.9	58.6
All ages, crude	51.0	49.2	48.7	48.7	47.2	47.3	46.8	45.0	43.7
45 to 54 years	52.0	48.7	45.1	45.2	40.4	40.6	35.2	31.0	28.8
55 to 64 years	168.6	159.0	158.1	155.4	145.4	138.4	141.0	131.4	124.4
65 to 74 years	376.3	345.5	348.8	341.3	333.1	312.8	302.6	287.7	275.3
75 to 84 years[6]	544.2	544.3	516.0	509.1	479.7	494.6	465.7	435.1	407.5
85 years and over	618.3	591.2	526.6	521.8	473.9	485.0	458.5	456.0	433.4
American Indian or Alaska Native Male[5]									
All ages, age-adjusted[4]	43.7	44.3	35.4	41.6	38.1	35.9	34.4	34.1	32.1
All ages, crude	20.0	20.8	17.7	20.8	18.9	19.4	18.2	19.8	19.0
45 to 54 years	12.8	16.7	14.4	19.7	16.4	13.0	10.7	8.8	13.1
55 to 64 years	77.4	66.2	65.4	67.6	52.9	59.7	55.8	53.2	42.0
65 to 74 years	200.2	221.0	183.2	213.2	164.1	185.8	131.3	177.8	160.5

NA = Not available.

* = Rates based on fewer than 20 deaths are considered unreliable and are not shown.

0.0 = Quantity more than zero but less than 0.05.

[3]Starting with 1999 data, cause of death is coded according to ICD-10.

[4]Age-adjusted rates are calculated using the year 2000 standard population. Prior to 2001, age-adjusted rates were calculated using standard million proportions based on rounded population numbers. Starting with 2001 data, unrounded population numbers are used to calculate age-adjusted rates.

[5]The race groups, White, Black, Asian or Pacific Islander, and American Indian or Alaska Native, include persons of Hispanic and non-Hispanic origin. Persons of Hispanic origin may be of any race. Death rates for the American Indian or Alaska Native, Asian or Pacific Islander, and Hispanic populations are known to be underestimated.

[6]In 1950, rate is for the age group 75 years and over.

Table 2-32. Death Rates for Malignant Neoplasms of the Trachea, Bronchus, and Lung, by Sex, Race, Hispanic Origin, and Age, Selected Years, 1950–2015—*Continued*

(Deaths per 100,000 resident population.)

Sex, race, Hispanic origin, and age	1950[1,2]	1960[1,2]	1970[2]	1980[2]	1985[2]	1990[2]	1995[2]	2000[3]	2005[3]	2006[3]
75 to 84 years	NA	NA	NA	*	263.6	356.2	409.7	367.9	341.1	330.9
85 years and over	NA	NA	NA	*	*	*	*	*	*	*
Asian or Pacific Islander Male[5]										
All ages, age-adjusted[4]	NA	NA	NA	43.3	42.7	44.2	41.0	40.9	37.1	36.6
All ages, crude	NA	NA	NA	22.1	20.4	20.7	20.7	22.7	22.4	22.7
45 to 54 years	NA	NA	NA	33.3	21.7	18.8	18.6	17.2	15.6	18.1
55 to 64 years	NA	NA	NA	94.4	98.1	74.4	64.4	61.4	56.7	55.7
65 to 74 years	NA	NA	NA	174.3	180.8	215.8	184.0	183.2	142.6	139.7
75 to 84 years	NA	NA	NA	301.3	295.3	307.5	296.6	323.2	295.0	295.5
85 years and over	NA	NA	NA	*	350.0	421.3	439.0	378.0	439.5	401.3
Hispanic or Latino Male[5,7]										
All ages, age-adjusted[4]	NA	NA	NA	NA	39.2	44.1	42.2	39.0	35.2	32.3
All ages, crude	NA	NA	NA	NA	12.9	16.2	14.8	13.3	13.1	12.1
45 to 54 years	NA	NA	NA	NA	16.7	21.5	17.5	14.8	12.1	10.6
55 to 64 years	NA	NA	NA	NA	68.6	80.7	69.9	58.6	52.5	45.1
65 to 74 years	NA	NA	NA	NA	169.9	195.5	192.0	167.3	153.1	142.0
75 to 84 years	NA	NA	NA	NA	292.1	313.4	324.4	327.5	295.5	268.2
85 years and over	NA	NA	NA	NA	393.8	420.7	382.8	368.8	338.1	339.4
White, Not Hispanic or Latino Male[7]										
All ages, age-adjusted[4]	NA	NA	NA	NA	84.2	91.1	84.1	77.9	71.3	69.3
All ages, crude	NA	NA	NA	NA	74.5	84.7	81.5	78.9	77.4	76.4
45 to 54 years	NA	NA	NA	NA	62.6	57.8	44.9	37.7	36.2	34.6
55 to 64 years	NA	NA	NA	NA	209.8	221.0	184.8	157.7	128.6	123.7
65 to 74 years	NA	NA	NA	NA	398.4	431.4	416.0	387.3	339.1	326.6
75 to 84 years	NA	NA	NA	NA	518.2	580.4	554.8	537.7	526.6	520.7
85 years and over	NA	NA	NA	NA	413.8	520.9	542.7	527.3	525.1	517.8
White Female[5]										
All ages, age-adjusted[4]	5.9	6.8	13.1	24.5	31.0	37.6	41.1	42.3	41.7	41.2
All ages, crude	4.7	5.9	12.3	25.6	33.9	42.4	47.5	49.9	50.7	50.6
45 to 54 years	5.7	9.0	20.9	33.0	35.4	34.6	29.3	24.8	24.1	24.1
55 to 64 years	13.7	15.1	37.2	71.9	92.4	105.7	104.0	96.1	82.2	79.9
65 to 74 years	23.7	24.8	42.9	104.6	145.5	181.3	203.8	213.2	205.6	203.3
75 to 84 years	34.0	32.7	52.6	95.2	134.8	194.6	243.3	272.7	288.9	288.9
85 years and over	29.3	39.1	50.6	92.4	99.3	138.3	181.0	215.9	245.9	248.8
Black or African American Female[5]										
All ages, age-adjusted[4]	4.5	6.8	13.7	24.8	29.7	36.8	38.8	39.8	39.9	38.8
All ages, crude	2.8	4.3	9.4	18.3	22.5	28.1	29.5	30.8	32.5	32.0
45 to 54 years	7.5	11.3	23.9	43.4	39.1	41.3	34.5	32.9	33.2	34.2
55 to 64 years	12.9	17.9	33.5	79.9	103.5	117.9	106.9	95.3	86.3	80.8
65 to 74 years	14.0	18.1	46.1	88.0	117.2	164.3	196.2	194.1	181.3	175.6
75 to 84 years[6]	*	31.3	49.1	79.4	101.2	148.1	183.2	224.3	254.2	252.0
85 years and over	NA	34.2	44.8	85.8	114.3	134.9	158.9	185.9	228.4	213.0
American Indian or Alaska Native Female[5]										
All ages, age-adjusted[4]	NA	NA	NA	11.7	14.2	19.3	25.9	24.8	30.0	26.9
All ages, crude	NA	NA	NA	6.0	8.2	11.2	13.8	14.0	17.8	16.1
45 to 54 years	NA	NA	NA	*	*	22.9	*	12.1	17.2	11.0
55 to 64 years	NA	NA	NA	*	38.5	53.7	45.7	52.6	54.9	57.1
65 to 74 years	NA	NA	NA	*	93.9	78.5	134.6	151.5	165.1	143.1
75 to 84 years	NA	NA	NA	*	*	111.8	209.5	136.3	204.1	183.2
85 years and over	NA	NA	NA	*	*	*	*	*	*	*
Asian or Pacific Islander Female[5]										
All ages, age-adjusted[4]	NA	NA	NA	15.4	14.4	18.9	21.4	18.4	18.5	18.1
All ages, crude	NA	NA	NA	8.4	7.9	10.5	13.0	12.6	13.9	13.9
45 to 54 years	NA	NA	NA	13.5	12.5	11.3	11.6	9.9	10.6	10.0
55 to 64 years	NA	NA	NA	24.6	26.0	38.3	37.6	30.4	27.3	26.6

NA = Not available.

* = Rates based on fewer than 20 deaths are considered unreliable and are not shown.

0.0 = Quantity more than zero but less than 0.05.

[1] Includes deaths of persons who were not residents of the 50 states and the District of Columbia.

[2] Underlying cause of death was coded according to the 6th Revision of the International Classification of Diseases (ICD) in 1950, 7th Revision in 1960, 8th Revision in 1970, and 9th Revision in 1980-1998.

[3] Starting with 1999 data, cause of death is coded according to ICD-10.

[4] Age-adjusted rates are calculated using the year 2000 standard population. Prior to 2001, age-adjusted rates were calculated using standard million proportions based on rounded population numbers. Starting with 2001 data, unrounded population numbers are used to calculate age-adjusted rates.

[5] The race groups, White, Black, Asian or Pacific Islander, and American Indian or Alaska Native, include persons of Hispanic and non-Hispanic origin. Persons of Hispanic origin may be of any race. Death rates for the American Indian or Alaska Native, Asian or Pacific Islander, and Hispanic populations are known to be underestimated.

[6] In 1950, rate is for the age group 75 years and over.

[7] Prior to 1997, excludes data from states lacking an Hispanic-origin item on the death certificate.

Table 2-32. Death Rates for Malignant Neoplasms of the Trachea, Bronchus, and Lung, by Sex, Race, Hispanic Origin, and Age, Selected Years, 1950–2015—*Continued*

(Deaths per 100,000 resident population.)

Sex, race, Hispanic origin, and age	2007[3]	2008[3]	2009[3]	2010[3]	2011[3]	2012[3]	2013[3]	2014[3]	2015[3]
75 to 84 years	339.5	361.5	249.4	325.8	333.2	259.8	299.3	292.1	276.2
85 years and over	422.6	333.6	*	276.4	328.3	310.7	369.4	193.3	229.9
Asian or Pacific Islander Male[5]									
All ages, age-adjusted[4]	35.9	36.1	34.8	33.8	32.9	32.7	30.6	29.6	29.5
All ages, crude	22.0	22.9	22.3	22.5	22.7	22.9	22.3	22.4	23.0
45 to 54 years	17.0	16.3	13.1	13.8	12.2	13.0	12.7	13.1	11.2
55 to 64 years	43.4	49.5	49.6	51.1	45.0	45.3	42.5	44.7	44.5
65 to 74 years	132.5	136.5	117.7	127.0	131.3	114.8	110.3	108.9	116.5
75 to 84 years	311.1	303.2	304.9	286.4	276.1	279.4	257.5	239.8	239.4
85 years and over	423.9	416.6	429.9	382.0	370.7	411.4	387.3	363.2	347.3
Hispanic or Latino Male[5,7]									
All ages, age-adjusted[4]	31.6	32.2	29.8	29.6	28.7	26.8	26.2	25.0	24.3
All ages, crude	12.0	12.4	11.8	11.9	12.0	11.7	11.8	11.6	11.7
45 to 54 years	10.4	9.8	10.3	9.0	8.3	8.5	8.0	7.2	6.0
55 to 64 years	42.3	43.5	38.5	40.1	39.4	35.6	35.6	31.4	32.8
65 to 74 years	142.4	137.2	128.6	126.2	120.2	116.4	110.8	107.0	103.4
75 to 84 years	260.0	278.1	263.3	256.3	240.6	237.3	225.4	216.1	211.0
85 years and over	335.3	337.7	290.7	307.9	330.3	258.0	282.7	276.0	267.7
White, Not Hispanic or Latino Male[7]									
All ages, age-adjusted[4]	67.2	65.9	63.9	62.7	60.3	58.5	56.3	54.4	52.2
All ages, crude	75.2	75.1	74.2	73.8	72.7	72.2	71.0	70.2	68.6
45 to 54 years	33.1	34.0	33.2	31.8	30.6	29.9	28.7	26.9	25.2
55 to 64 years	118.6	114.9	111.6	107.8	106.9	102.8	101.0	99.0	98.0
65 to 74 years	316.1	305.0	292.3	287.3	274.4	261.3	246.6	240.3	226.1
75 to 84 years	508.2	496.7	487.7	479.3	461.0	448.1	430.8	414.3	396.2
85 years and over	508.0	517.1	499.5	504.4	478.2	488.3	478.0	457.5	451.0
White Female[5]									
All ages, age-adjusted[4]	41.3	40.4	40.0	39.3	38.3	37.6	36.7	36.0	34.9
All ages, crude	51.0	50.5	50.4	50.0	49.3	49.4	48.9	48.7	48.1
45 to 54 years	24.8	24.7	25.2	24.3	23.9	23.0	22.6	21.7	19.7
55 to 64 years	77.6	73.1	70.1	68.9	67.2	68.0	66.0	66.3	64.8
65 to 74 years	202.5	195.6	193.6	187.4	179.6	174.3	169.0	161.4	156.2
75 to 84 years	293.1	294.1	289.8	290.5	284.9	280.7	274.1	275.3	263.0
85 years and over	250.5	253.1	257.3	258.3	256.3	254.5	250.9	247.7	260.2
Black or African American Female[5]									
All ages, age-adjusted[4]	37.9	36.8	35.8	36.5	35.4	34.7	34.1	32.7	30.7
All ages, crude	31.5	30.8	30.5	31.4	31.2	31.1	31.3	30.7	29.5
45 to 54 years	31.9	28.3	29.0	27.7	26.8	25.9	24.0	23.2	18.8
55 to 64 years	76.6	74.1	76.3	74.0	73.3	71.0	71.9	69.8	67.4
65 to 74 years	176.3	168.3	161.4	163.1	156.9	158.2	151.0	142.3	136.2
75 to 84 years[6]	250.1	249.0	243.2	249.2	240.5	239.8	235.8	227.5	209.6
85 years and over	212.0	226.3	197.6	249.3	236.8	211.2	224.9	220.8	218.6
American Indian or Alaska Native Female[5]									
All ages, age-adjusted[4]	27.4	27.4	25.1	26.3	23.9	25.6	22.9	22.7	22.5
All ages, crude	16.3	15.9	15.5	16.0	15.3	16.9	15.6	15.8	16.9
45 to 54 years	9.7	10.9	12.7	13.2	13.8	13.0	12.3	14.4	12.3
55 to 64 years	49.7	41.2	50.5	40.3	39.5	44.9	31.1	28.0	44.5
65 to 74 years	157.7	126.8	119.4	141.8	110.2	116.5	124.9	114.4	103.2
75 to 84 years	192.2	218.7	197.5	185.9	189.7	203.3	174.6	179.3	159.0
85 years and over	*	236.6	*	200.0	168.3	183.2	137.0	161.4	179.8
Asian or Pacific Islander Female[5]									
All ages, age-adjusted[4]	18.9	18.1	18.3	18.3	18.6	17.8	18.0	17.6	16.8
All ages, crude	14.8	14.2	14.5	14.9	15.8	15.5	16.0	16.0	15.8
45 to 54 years	10.3	9.5	8.7	8.8	8.5	10.9	9.3	9.0	9.7
55 to 64 years	31.8	25.8	25.1	28.0	29.0	25.1	24.3	25.2	24.2

NA = Not available.

* = Rates based on fewer than 20 deaths are considered unreliable and are not shown.

0.0 = Quantity more than zero but less than 0.05.

[3]Starting with 1999 data, cause of death is coded according to ICD-10.

[4]Age-adjusted rates are calculated using the year 2000 standard population. Prior to 2001, age-adjusted rates were calculated using standard million proportions based on rounded population numbers. Starting with 2001 data, unrounded population numbers are used to calculate age-adjusted rates.

[5]The race groups, White, Black, Asian or Pacific Islander, and American Indian or Alaska Native, include persons of Hispanic and non-Hispanic origin. Persons of Hispanic origin may be of any race. Death rates for the American Indian or Alaska Native, Asian or Pacific Islander, and Hispanic populations are known to be underestimated.

[6]In 1950, rate is for the age group 75 years and over.

[7]Prior to 1997, excludes data from states lacking an Hispanic-origin item on the death certificate.

Table 2-32. Death Rates for Malignant Neoplasms of the Trachea, Bronchus, and Lung, by Sex, Race, Hispanic Origin, and Age, Selected Years, 1950–2015—*Continued*

(Deaths per 100,000 resident population.)

Sex, race, Hispanic origin, and age	1950[1,2]	1960[1,2]	1970[2]	1980[2]	1985[2]	1990[2]	1995[2]	2000[3]	2005[3]	2006[3]
65 to 74 years	NA	NA	NA	62.4	60.7	71.6	84.2	77.0	73.9	74.2
75 to 84 years	NA	NA	NA	117.7	97.8	137.9	153.5	135.0	144.6	135.0
85 years and over	NA	NA	NA	*	*	172.9	235.5	175.3	184.4	190.7
Hispanic or Latina Female[5,7]										
All ages, age-adjusted[4]	NA	NA	NA	NA	10.9	14.1	14.3	14.7	14.8	14.0
All ages, crude	NA	NA	NA	NA	4.9	7.2	7.1	7.2	7.7	7.4
45 to 54 years	NA	NA	NA	NA	6.8	8.7	7.1	7.1	7.0	6.2
55 to 64 years	NA	NA	NA	NA	17.4	25.1	25.5	22.2	20.2	18.8
65 to 74 years	NA	NA	NA	NA	49.1	66.8	59.2	66.0	62.8	64.9
75 to 84 years	NA	NA	NA	NA	73.6	94.3	111.0	112.3	118.3	111.1
85 years and over	NA	NA	NA	NA	110.7	118.2	128.3	137.5	153.2	128.7
White, not Hispanic or Latina Female[7]										
All ages, age-adjusted[4]	NA	NA	NA	NA	31.7	39.0	42.5	44.1	43.8	43.5
All ages, crude	NA	NA	NA	NA	35.6	46.2	52.3	56.4	58.7	58.9
45 to 54 years	NA	NA	NA	NA	36.6	36.6	31.0	26.4	26.1	26.4
55 to 64 years	NA	NA	NA	NA	93.4	111.3	109.4	102.2	87.9	85.7
65 to 74 years	NA	NA	NA	NA	149.4	186.4	210.4	222.9	217.5	215.2
75 to 84 years	NA	NA	NA	NA	138.1	199.1	247.2	279.2	298.6	299.8
85 years and over	NA	NA	NA	NA	100.9	139.0	181.6	218.0	249.1	253.4

NA = Not available.

* = Rates based on fewer than 20 deaths are considered unreliable and are not shown.

0.0 = Quantity more than zero but less than 0.05.

[1] Includes deaths of persons who were not residents of the 50 states and the District of Columbia.

[2] Underlying cause of death was coded according to the 6th Revision of the International Classification of Diseases (ICD) in 1950, 7th Revision in 1960, 8th Revision in 1970, and 9th Revision in 1980-1998.

[3] Starting with 1999 data, cause of death is coded according to ICD-10.

[4] Age-adjusted rates are calculated using the year 2000 standard population. Prior to 2001, age-adjusted rates were calculated using standard million proportions based on rounded population numbers. Starting with 2001 data, unrounded population numbers are used to calculate age-adjusted rates.

[5] The race groups, White, Black, Asian or Pacific Islander, and American Indian or Alaska Native, include persons of Hispanic and non-Hispanic origin. Persons of Hispanic origin may be of any race. Death rates for the American Indian or Alaska Native, Asian or Pacific Islander, and Hispanic populations are known to be underestimated.

[7] Prior to 1997, excludes data from states lacking an Hispanic-origin item on the death certificate.

Table 2-32. Death Rates for Malignant Neoplasms of the Trachea, Bronchus, and Lung, by Sex, Race, Hispanic Origin, and Age, Selected Years, 1950–2015—*Continued*

(Deaths per 100,000 resident population.)

Sex, race, Hispanic origin, and age	2007[3]	2008[3]	2009[3]	2010[3]	2011[3]	2012[3]	2013[3]	2014[3]	2015[3]
65 to 74 years	73.0	73.8	68.0	67.0	70.6	68.6	63.9	59.3	64.4
75 to 84 years	145.2	148.6	153.9	160.3	149.1	142.8	150.2	149.3	134.7
85 years and over	193.6	168.3	203.9	171.1	200.8	181.7	207.4	199.6	183.2
Hispanic or Latina Female[6,7]									
All ages, age-adjusted[4]	14.9	14.2	13.6	13.8	13.3	13.6	13.2	13.3	12.9
All ages, crude	7.9	7.7	7.5	7.7	7.6	8.0	8.0	8.3	8.4
45 to 54 years	6.5	7.1	5.9	7.1	5.7	6.0	5.4	5.1	5.3
55 to 64 years	21.8	20.8	20.5	19.3	18.5	20.5	18.9	19.3	19.5
65 to 74 years	65.9	62.0	58.5	51.7	54.2	51.7	52.9	53.0	51.1
75 to 84 years	115.3	111.2	104.0	117.3	108.6	110.8	107.2	109.7	104.7
85 years and over	152.0	137.7	144.9	143.4	144.8	152.4	146.7	151.9	139.5
White, not Hispanic or Latina Female[7]									
All ages, age-adjusted[4]	43.5	42.7	42.3	41.7	40.7	39.9	39.0	38.4	37.3
All ages, crude	59.5	59.2	59.3	59.0	58.5	58.6	58.2	58.1	57.6
45 to 54 years	27.2	27.1	28.0	26.9	26.8	25.8	25.6	24.8	22.5
55 to 64 years	83.0	78.3	75.1	74.0	72.4	73.3	71.4	72.1	70.4
65 to 74 years	214.3	207.3	205.6	199.5	191.3	185.5	179.5	171.6	166.2
75 to 84 years	304.5	306.5	303.1	303.0	298.7	294.2	288.1	289.7	277.0
85 years and over	254.5	258.2	262.3	263.8	261.9	259.6	256.8	253.1	267.8

NA = Not available.

* = Rates based on fewer than 20 deaths are considered unreliable and are not shown.

0.0 = Quantity more than zero but less than 0.05.

[3]Starting with 1999 data, cause of death is coded according to ICD-10.

[4]Age-adjusted rates are calculated using the year 2000 standard population. Prior to 2001, age-adjusted rates were calculated using standard million proportions based on rounded population numbers. Starting with 2001 data, unrounded population numbers are used to calculate age-adjusted rates.

[6]The race groups, White, Black, Asian or Pacific Islander, and American Indian or Alaska Native, include persons of Hispanic and non-Hispanic origin. Persons of Hispanic origin may be of any race. Death rates for the American Indian or Alaska Native, Asian or Pacific Islander, and Hispanic populations are known to be underestimated.

[7]Prior to 1997, excludes data from states lacking an Hispanic-origin item on the death certificate.

Table 2-33. Death Rates for Motor Vehicle–Related Injuries, by Sex, Race, Hispanic Origin, and Age, Selected Years, 1950–2015

(Deaths per 100,000 resident population.)

Sex, race, Hispanic origin, and age	1950[1,2]	1960[1,2]	1970[2]	1980[2]	1985	1990[2]	1995	2000[3]	2005[3]	2006[3]
All Persons										
All ages, age-adjusted[4]	24.6	23.1	27.6	22.3	18.6	18.5	16.3	15.4	15.2	15.0
All ages, crude	23.1	21.3	26.9	23.5	19.3	18.8	16.3	15.4	15.3	15.2
Under 1 year	8.4	8.1	9.8	7.0	4.9	4.9	4.7	4.4	3.6	3.5
1 to 14 years	9.8	8.6	10.5	8.2	7.0	6.0	5.3	4.3	3.7	3.4
1 to 4 years	11.5	10.0	11.5	9.2	7.2	6.3	5.2	4.2	3.9	3.7
5 to 14 years	8.8	7.9	10.2	7.9	6.9	5.9	5.3	4.3	3.6	3.3
15 to 24 years	34.4	38.0	47.2	44.8	35.7	34.1	28.9	26.9	25.7	25.7
15 to 19 years	29.6	33.9	43.6	43.0	33.5	33.1	28.1	26.0	23.1	22.6
20 to 24 years	38.8	42.9	51.3	46.6	37.6	35.0	29.7	28.0	28.3	28.9
25 to 34 years	24.6	24.3	30.9	29.1	23.0	23.6	19.2	17.3	18.4	18.7
35 to 44 years	20.3	19.3	24.9	20.9	17.2	16.9	15.3	15.3	15.5	15.4
45 to 64 years	25.2	23.0	26.5	18.0	15.4	15.7	14.1	14.3	14.8	14.8
45 to 54 years	22.2	21.4	25.5	18.6	15.2	15.6	13.8	14.2	15.1	15.3
55 to 64 years	29.0	25.1	27.9	17.4	15.6	15.9	14.5	14.4	14.5	14.1
65 years and over	43.1	34.7	36.2	22.5	21.7	23.1	22.6	21.4	20.1	19.0
65 to 74 years	39.1	31.4	32.8	19.2	17.9	18.6	17.5	16.5	16.5	15.2
75 to 84 years	52.7	41.8	43.5	28.1	27.4	29.1	28.4	25.7	22.9	22.2
85 years and over	45.1	37.9	34.2	27.6	26.5	31.2	31.0	30.4	27.3	25.5
Male										
All ages, age-adjusted[4]	38.5	35.4	41.5	33.6	27.2	26.5	22.8	21.7	21.9	21.5
All ages, crude	35.4	31.8	39.7	35.3	28.0	26.7	22.4	21.3	21.8	21.6
Under 1 year	9.1	8.6	9.3	7.3	5.0	5.0	4.9	4.6	3.6	3.4
1 to 14 years	12.3	10.7	13.0	10.0	8.5	7.0	6.1	4.9	4.1	3.7
1 to 4 years	13.0	11.5	12.9	10.2	8.3	6.9	5.6	4.7	4.3	3.9
5 to 14 years	11.9	10.4	13.1	9.9	8.6	7.0	6.3	5.0	4.1	3.7
15 to 24 years	56.7	61.2	73.2	68.4	52.7	49.5	40.5	37.4	36.3	36.3
15 to 19 years	46.3	51.7	64.1	62.6	46.5	45.5	36.1	33.9	29.9	29.5
20 to 24 years	66.7	73.2	84.4	74.3	58.2	53.3	45.0	41.2	42.8	43.4
25 to 34 years	40.8	40.1	49.4	46.3	35.9	35.7	28.1	25.5	27.9	28.5
35 to 44 years	32.5	29.9	37.7	31.7	25.2	24.7	21.7	22.0	22.5	22.1
45 to 64 years	37.7	33.3	38.9	26.5	22.0	21.9	19.5	20.2	21.6	21.6
45 to 54 years	33.6	31.6	37.2	27.6	21.9	22.0	19.3	20.4	22.2	22.6
55 to 64 years	43.1	35.6	40.9	25.4	22.1	21.7	19.6	19.8	20.7	20.3
65 years and over	66.6	52.1	54.4	33.9	30.4	32.1	30.7	29.5	28.4	26.4
65 to 74 years	59.1	45.8	47.3	27.3	23.0	24.2	22.2	21.7	22.8	20.7
75 to 84 years	85.0	66.0	68.2	44.3	41.3	41.2	39.9	35.6	32.1	30.4
85 years and over	78.1	62.7	63.1	56.1	55.3	64.5	61.5	57.5	49.0	45.6
Female										
All ages, age-adjusted[4]	11.5	11.7	14.9	11.8	10.7	11.0	10.3	9.5	8.9	8.8
All ages, crude	10.9	11.0	14.7	12.3	11.0	11.3	10.4	9.7	9.1	9.0
Under 1 year	7.6	7.5	10.4	6.7	4.7	4.9	4.5	4.2	3.7	3.5
1 to 14 years	7.2	6.3	7.9	6.3	5.4	4.9	4.4	3.7	3.1	3.1
1 to 4 years	10.0	8.4	10.0	8.1	6.0	5.6	4.8	3.8	3.4	3.5
5 to 14 years	5.7	5.4	7.2	5.7	5.1	4.7	4.2	3.6	3.0	2.9
15 to 24 years	12.6	15.1	21.6	20.8	18.2	17.9	16.8	15.9	14.5	14.5
15 to 19 years	12.9	16.0	22.7	22.8	20.1	20.0	19.7	17.5	15.9	15.4
20 to 24 years	12.2	14.0	20.4	18.9	16.7	16.0	13.8	14.2	13.2	13.6
25 to 34 years	9.3	9.2	13.0	12.2	10.1	11.5	10.2	8.8	8.9	8.8
35 to 44 years	8.5	9.1	12.9	10.4	9.4	9.2	9.0	8.8	8.6	8.8
45 to 64 years	12.6	13.1	15.3	10.3	9.5	10.1	9.0	8.7	8.4	8.3
45 to 54 years	10.9	11.6	14.5	10.2	9.0	9.6	8.4	8.2	8.2	8.2
55 to 64 years	14.9	15.2	16.2	10.5	9.9	10.8	9.9	9.5	8.8	8.5
65 years and over	21.9	20.3	23.1	15.0	15.8	17.2	17.0	15.8	14.1	13.6
65 to 74 years	20.6	19.0	21.6	13.0	14.0	14.1	13.7	12.3	11.1	10.5
75 to 84 years	25.2	23.0	27.2	18.5	19.2	21.9	21.2	19.2	16.5	16.5
85 years and over	22.1	22.0	18.0	15.2	15.0	18.3	19.3	19.3	17.6	16.4
White Male[5]										
All ages, age-adjusted[4]	37.9	34.8	40.4	33.8	27.2	26.3	22.6	21.8	22.4	22.1
All ages, crude	35.1	31.5	39.1	35.9	28.3	26.7	22.4	21.6	22.5	22.2
Under 1 year	9.1	8.8	9.1	7.0	4.6	4.8	4.3	4.2	3.4	3.3
1 to 14 years	12.4	10.6	12.5	9.8	8.3	6.6	5.9	4.8	4.1	3.6
15 to 24 years	58.3	62.7	75.2	73.8	56.5	52.5	42.4	39.6	39.2	39.3
25 to 34 years	39.1	38.6	47.0	46.6	35.8	35.4	27.9	25.1	28.4	28.8
35 to 44 years	30.9	28.4	35.2	30.7	24.3	23.7	21.1	21.8	22.8	22.6

[1]Includes deaths of persons who were not residents of the 50 states and the District of Columbia.
[2]Underlying cause of death was coded according to the 6th Revision of the International Classification of Diseases (ICD) in 1950, 7th Revision in 1960, 8th Revision in 1970, and 9th Revision in 1980-1998.
[3]Starting with 1999 data, cause of death is coded according to ICD-10.
[4]Age-adjusted rates are calculated using the year 2000 standard population. Prior to 2001, age-adjusted rates were calculated using standard million proportions based on rounded population numbers. Starting with 2001 data, unrounded population numbers are used to calculate age-adjusted rates.
[5]The race groups, White, Black, Asian or Pacific Islander, and American Indian or Alaska Native, include persons of Hispanic and non-Hispanic origin. Persons of Hispanic origin may be of any race. Death rates for the American Indian or Alaska Native, Asian or Pacific Islander, and Hispanic populations are known to be underestimated.

Table 2-33. Death Rates for Motor Vehicle–Related Injuries, by Sex, Race, Hispanic Origin, and Age, Selected Years, 1950–2015—Continued

(Deaths per 100,000 resident population.)

Sex, race, Hispanic origin, and age	2007[3]	2008[3]	2009[3]	2010[3]	2011[3]	2012[3]	2013[3]	2014[3]	2015[3]
All Persons									
All ages, age-adjusted[4]	14.4	12.9	11.6	11.3	11.1	11.4	10.9	10.8	11.4
All ages, crude	14.6	13.1	11.8	11.4	11.3	11.6	11.2	11.1	11.7
Under 1 year	3.0	2.5	2.4	2.0	2.4	1.8	1.7	1.7	1.8
1 to 14 years	3.2	2.6	2.5	2.3	2.3	2.2	2.2	2.2	2.2
1 to 4 years	3.4	2.9	2.9	2.8	2.6	2.9	2.7	2.5	2.6
5 to 14 years	3.2	2.5	2.4	2.2	2.1	2.0	2.1	2.0	2.1
15 to 24 years	24.5	20.6	17.6	16.6	16.2	16.1	15.2	15.3	15.9
15 to 19 years	21.4	17.4	15.2	13.6	13.2	12.6	11.4	11.9	12.4
20 to 24 years	27.7	24.0	20.2	19.7	19.1	19.3	18.8	18.3	19.2
25 to 34 years	17.8	16.3	14.5	14.0	13.7	14.5	13.9	13.9	14.7
35 to 44 years	14.9	13.4	12.2	11.6	11.3	11.8	11.4	11.1	11.9
45 to 64 years	14.1	13.3	12.2	11.9	11.9	12.4	12.1	12.0	12.8
45 to 54 years	14.9	13.7	12.7	12.0	12.3	12.6	12.2	12.1	12.8
55 to 64 years	13.2	12.8	11.5	11.9	11.5	12.2	11.9	11.9	12.7
65 years and over	18.7	16.9	15.8	16.0	15.9	15.7	15.1	14.8	15.3
65 to 74 years	14.9	13.8	12.7	12.3	13.0	13.0	12.2	11.9	12.8
75 to 84 years	21.7	19.2	18.6	18.8	18.3	17.9	17.8	17.5	17.5
85 years and over	25.3	23.2	20.9	23.8	21.8	22.1	21.0	20.9	21.7
Male									
All ages, age-adjusted[4]	21.0	18.9	16.8	16.2	16.1	16.5	15.9	15.8	16.7
All ages, crude	21.0	18.9	16.9	16.3	16.3	16.6	16.1	16.0	17.0
Under 1 year	2.7	2.9	2.6	2.2	2.8	1.9	1.7	1.9	2.2
1 to 14 years	3.7	3.1	2.9	2.7	2.5	2.5	2.5	2.5	2.5
1 to 4 years	3.8	3.2	3.4	3.0	2.7	3.1	3.0	2.8	2.9
5 to 14 years	3.7	3.0	2.7	2.5	2.5	2.3	2.4	2.4	2.4
15 to 24 years	34.6	29.3	24.5	23.1	22.8	22.5	21.2	21.5	22.2
15 to 19 years	27.7	22.6	19.2	17.8	17.2	16.2	14.7	16.1	16.3
20 to 24 years	41.9	36.3	30.0	28.5	28.2	28.4	27.3	26.5	27.7
25 to 34 years	27.2	25.2	21.7	21.0	20.4	21.5	20.8	20.8	21.8
35 to 44 years	22.1	19.9	18.2	16.9	16.7	17.6	16.9	16.4	17.9
45 to 64 years	20.9	19.7	18.2	17.9	18.2	18.6	18.2	18.1	19.4
45 to 54 years	22.2	20.2	19.0	17.9	18.6	18.8	18.3	18.2	19.1
55 to 64 years	19.2	19.0	17.2	17.8	17.7	18.5	18.1	18.1	19.8
65 years and over	26.9	24.1	22.0	22.2	22.3	22.1	21.5	21.0	22.1
65 to 74 years	21.1	19.4	17.5	17.1	18.2	18.5	17.5	17.0	18.5
75 to 84 years	31.4	27.3	25.8	25.9	25.7	24.8	24.9	24.8	24.9
85 years and over	44.4	40.2	35.3	40.2	35.4	35.3	35.3	34.0	35.6
Female									
All ages, age-adjusted[4]	8.2	7.2	6.7	6.5	6.3	6.5	6.2	6.1	6.4
All ages, crude	8.4	7.4	6.9	6.8	6.5	6.7	6.4	6.3	6.7
Under 1 year	3.3	2.0	2.1	1.8	1.9	1.8	1.8	1.5	1.3
1 to 14 years	2.8	2.2	2.2	2.0	2.0	1.9	1.9	1.8	1.9
1 to 4 years	3.1	2.5	2.5	2.5	2.6	2.6	2.3	2.3	2.3
5 to 14 years	2.6	2.0	2.0	1.8	1.8	1.7	1.8	1.6	1.8
15 to 24 years	13.8	11.5	10.5	9.9	9.4	9.3	8.9	8.7	9.3
15 to 19 years	14.8	11.8	10.9	9.2	9.0	8.9	7.9	7.6	8.4
20 to 24 years	12.8	11.2	10.0	10.5	9.7	9.8	9.9	9.7	10.2
25 to 34 years	8.5	7.4	7.2	6.9	7.0	7.4	6.9	6.8	7.5
35 to 44 years	7.8	7.0	6.2	6.2	6.0	6.2	5.9	5.8	6.1
45 to 64 years	7.7	7.2	6.5	6.3	5.9	6.4	6.3	6.2	6.4
45 to 54 years	7.8	7.4	6.6	6.3	6.1	6.5	6.3	6.2	6.7
55 to 64 years	7.5	6.9	6.3	6.3	5.7	6.4	6.2	6.1	6.1
65 years and over	12.6	11.5	11.1	11.3	10.9	10.8	10.0	9.9	10.0
65 to 74 years	9.6	8.9	8.5	8.2	8.4	8.2	7.5	7.5	7.8
75 to 84 years	15.0	13.5	13.5	13.7	12.8	12.9	12.5	12.0	11.9
85 years and over	16.5	15.3	14.0	15.9	15.1	15.5	13.7	14.1	14.4
White Male[5]									
All ages, age-adjusted[4]	21.6	19.6	17.3	16.7	16.6	17.0	16.3	16.1	17.0
All ages, crude	21.7	19.7	17.5	17.0	16.9	17.3	16.7	16.5	17.4
Under 1 year	2.9	2.9	2.5	2.0	2.5	1.9	1.7	1.8	1.9
1 to 14 years	3.8	3.1	2.8	2.7	2.6	2.4	2.4	2.4	2.5
15 to 24 years	37.4	31.7	26.6	24.6	24.6	24.5	22.9	23.0	23.3
25 to 34 years	27.8	26.2	21.8	21.4	20.9	22.0	21.1	20.8	22.1
35 to 44 years	22.2	20.3	18.5	17.4	17.0	18.0	17.3	16.6	18.0

[3]Underlying cause of death was coded according to the 6th Revision of the International Classification of Diseases (ICD) in 1950, 7th Revision in 1960, 8th Revision in 1970, and 9th Revision in 1980-1998.

[3]Starting with 1999 data, cause of death is coded according to ICD-10.

[4]Age-adjusted rates are calculated using the year 2000 standard population. Prior to 2001, age-adjusted rates were calculated using standard million proportions based on rounded population numbers. Starting with 2001 data, unrounded population numbers are used to calculate age-adjusted rates.

[5]The race groups, White, Black, Asian or Pacific Islander, and American Indian or Alaska Native, include persons of Hispanic and non-Hispanic origin. Persons of Hispanic origin may be of any race. Death rates for the American Indian or Alaska Native, Asian or Pacific Islander, and Hispanic populations are known to be underestimated.

Table 2-33. Death Rates for Motor Vehicle–Related Injuries, by Sex, Race, Hispanic Origin, and Age, Selected Years, 1950–2015—Continued

(Deaths per 100,000 resident population.)

Sex, race, Hispanic origin, and age	1950[1,2]	1960[1,2]	1970[2]	1980[2]	1985	1990[2]	1995	2000[3]	2005[3]	2006[3]
45 to 64 years	36.2	31.7	36.5	25.2	20.8	20.6	18.7	19.7	21.7	21.6
65 years and over	67.1	52.1	54.2	32.7	29.9	31.4	30.1	29.4	28.7	26.6
Black or African American Male[5]										
All ages, age-adjusted[4]	34.8	39.6	51.0	34.2	29.0	29.9	26.1	24.4	22.5	22.6
All ages, crude	37.2	33.1	44.3	31.1	27.1	28.1	24.1	22.5	21.1	21.4
Under 1 year	NA	*	10.6	7.8	*	*	8.7	6.7	*	*
1 to 14 years[6]	10.4	11.2	16.3	11.4	9.7	8.9	7.5	5.5	4.4	4.8
15 to 24 years	42.5	46.4	58.1	34.9	32.0	36.1	33.9	30.2	27.8	26.9
25 to 34 years	54.4	51.0	70.4	44.9	37.7	39.5	32.2	32.6	32.1	34.4
35 to 44 years	46.7	43.6	59.5	41.2	34.7	33.5	28.7	27.2	25.8	25.1
45 to 64 years	54.6	47.8	61.7	39.5	32.9	33.3	26.2	27.1	24.1	25.2
65 years and over	52.6	48.2	53.4	42.4	35.2	36.3	36.9	32.1	29.1	26.1
American Indian or Alaska Native Male[5]										
All ages, age-adjusted[4]	NA	NA	NA	78.9	50.9	48.3	40.7	35.8	31.5	33.5
All ages, crude	NA	NA	NA	74.6	51.7	47.6	40.1	33.6	31.3	32.2
1 to 14 years	NA	NA	NA	15.1	16.2	11.6	7.6	7.8	9.6	4.6
15 to 24 years	NA	NA	NA	126.1	77.3	75.2	69.0	56.8	44.1	47.9
25 to 34 years	NA	NA	NA	107.0	84.0	78.2	67.8	49.8	49.0	45.2
35 to 44 years	NA	NA	NA	82.8	55.8	57.0	45.2	36.3	36.9	34.3
45 to 64 years	NA	NA	NA	77.4	52.2	45.9	38.8	32.0	31.9	41.4
65 years and over	NA	NA	NA	97.0	*	43.0	*	48.5	27.8	37.4
Asian or Pacific Islander Male[5]										
All ages, age-adjusted[4]	NA	NA	NA	19.0	17.3	17.9	14.5	10.6	9.5	9.3
All ages, crude	NA	NA	NA	17.1	16.0	15.8	12.6	9.8	8.7	8.6
1 to 14 years	NA	NA	NA	8.2	5.2	6.3	4.5	2.5	1.7	2.6
15 to 24 years	NA	NA	NA	27.2	28.1	25.7	18.5	17.0	14.5	14.9
25 to 34 years	NA	NA	NA	18.8	18.4	17.0	12.4	10.4	8.9	8.4
35 to 44 years	NA	NA	NA	13.1	12.0	12.2	9.9	6.9	6.6	6.0
45 to 64 years	NA	NA	NA	13.7	13.4	15.1	14.3	10.1	9.0	8.6
65 years and over	NA	NA	NA	37.3	37.3	33.6	32.1	21.1	20.8	19.7
Hispanic or Latino Male[5,6]										
All ages, age-adjusted[4]	NA	NA	NA	NA	25.4	29.5	24.4	21.3	21.4	21.4
All ages, crude	NA	NA	NA	NA	25.6	29.2	22.4	20.1	20.8	20.9
1 to 14 years	NA	NA	NA	NA	7.7	7.2	5.7	4.4	4.6	4.4
15 to 24 years	NA	NA	NA	NA	44.9	48.2	37.1	34.7	37.6	38.1
25 to 34 years	NA	NA	NA	NA	31.2	41.0	28.8	24.9	28.0	27.6
35 to 44 years	NA	NA	NA	NA	26.3	28.0	23.2	21.6	20.9	21.6
45 to 64 years	NA	NA	NA	NA	25.9	28.9	23.0	21.7	20.2	21.6
65 years and over	NA	NA	NA	NA	22.9	35.3	37.0	28.9	27.6	24.8
White, Not Hispanic or Latino Male[6]										
All ages, age-adjusted[4]	NA	NA	NA	NA	24.9	25.7	22.1	21.7	22.2	21.8
All ages, crude	NA	NA	NA	NA	25.9	26.0	21.9	21.5	22.5	22.1
1 to 14 years	NA	NA	NA	NA	7.8	6.4	5.8	4.9	3.9	3.2
15 to 24 years	NA	NA	NA	NA	53.3	52.3	42.7	40.3	38.8	38.8
25 to 34 years	NA	NA	NA	NA	33.2	34.0	27.1	24.7	27.8	28.5
35 to 44 years	NA	NA	NA	NA	21.6	23.1	20.3	21.6	22.9	22.4
45 to 64 years	NA	NA	NA	NA	18.0	19.8	18.1	19.3	21.7	21.4
65 years and over	NA	NA	NA	NA	27.6	31.1	29.4	29.3	28.6	26.6
White Female[5]										
All ages, age-adjusted[4]	11.4	11.7	14.9	12.2	10.9	11.2	10.4	9.8	9.3	9.2
All ages, crude	10.9	11.2	14.8	12.8	11.4	11.6	10.7	10.0	9.6	9.4
Under 1 year	7.8	7.5	10.2	7.1	3.9	4.7	4.5	3.5	3.0	3.1
1 to 14 years	7.2	6.2	7.5	6.2	5.4	4.8	4.3	3.7	3.2	3.1
15 to 24 years	12.6	15.6	22.7	23.0	20.0	19.5	18.1	17.1	15.7	15.9
25 to 34 years	9.0	9.0	12.7	12.2	10.1	11.6	10.2	8.9	9.4	9.1
35 to 44 years	8.1	8.9	12.3	10.6	9.4	9.2	8.9	8.9	9.0	9.2
45 to 64 years	12.7	13.1	15.1	10.4	9.5	9.9	8.9	8.7	8.6	8.3
65 years and over	22.2	20.8	23.7	15.3	16.2	17.4	17.5	16.2	14.5	14.0
Black or African American Female[5]										
All ages, age-adjusted[4]	9.3	10.4	14.1	8.5	8.5	9.6	9.0	8.4	7.6	7.7
All ages, crude	10.2	9.7	13.4	8.3	8.3	9.4	8.8	8.2	7.5	7.6
Under 1 year	NA	8.1	11.9	*	8.1	7.0	*	*	6.9	*
1 to 14 years[7]	7.2	6.9	10.2	6.3	5.1	5.3	4.9	3.9	3.4	3.4

NA = Not available.
* = Rates based on fewer than 20 deaths are considered unreliable and are not shown.
[1]Includes deaths of persons who were not residents of the 50 states and the District of Columbia.
[2]Underlying cause of death was coded according to the 6th Revision of the International Classification of Diseases (ICD) in 1950, 7th Revision in 1960, 8th Revision in 1970, and 9th Revision in 1980-1998.
[3]Starting with 1999 data, cause of death is coded according to ICD-10.
[4]Age-adjusted rates are calculated using the year 2000 standard population. Prior to 2001, age-adjusted rates were calculated using standard million proportions based on rounded population numbers. Starting with 2001 data, unrounded population numbers are used to calculate age-adjusted rates.
[5]The race groups, White, Black, Asian or Pacific Islander, and American Indian or Alaska Native, include persons of Hispanic and non-Hispanic origin. Persons of Hispanic origin may be of any race. Death rates for the American Indian or Alaska Native, Asian or Pacific Islander, and Hispanic populations are known to be underestimated.
[6]Prior to 1997, excludes data from states lacking an Hispanic-origin item on the death certificate.
[7]In 1950, rate is for the age group under 15 years.

Table 2-33. Death Rates for Motor Vehicle–Related Injuries, by Sex, Race, Hispanic Origin, and Age, Selected Years, 1950–2015—*Continued*

(Deaths per 100,000 resident population.)

Sex, race, Hispanic origin, and age	2007[3]	2008[3]	2009[3]	2010[3]	2011[3]	2012[3]	2013[3]	2014[3]	2015[3]
45 to 64 years	21.1	20.1	18.7	18.3	18.5	19.0	18.5	18.3	19.5
65 years and over	27.0	24.5	22.3	22.7	22.8	22.6	22.1	21.5	22.7
Black or African American Male[5]									
All ages, age-adjusted[4]	22.3	18.9	17.8	16.7	16.7	17.4	17.0	17.4	19.1
All ages, crude	21.0	18.0	16.7	15.9	15.8	16.6	16.4	16.8	18.7
Under 1 year	*	*	*	*	*	*	*	*	*
1 to 14 years[6]	4.0	3.1	3.5	3.0	2.7	3.2	3.3	2.9	3.2
15 to 24 years	26.9	22.4	18.5	19.4	17.7	17.5	17.6	18.7	21.8
25 to 34 years	32.0	27.0	26.9	24.9	22.4	25.6	25.1	25.7	26.7
35 to 44 years	27.2	23.0	21.9	19.4	20.8	20.8	20.5	21.2	23.7
45 to 64 years	24.0	21.5	19.3	19.1	20.2	20.8	21.1	21.1	24.5
65 years and over	27.4	22.9	22.8	20.0	21.3	21.8	18.5	19.8	19.6
American Indian or Alaska Native Male[5]									
All ages, age-adjusted[4]	28.6	24.1	22.7	21.1	22.5	22.2	20.0	23.4	22.8
All ages, crude	27.3	23.5	22.0	19.8	21.8	22.2	19.0	22.2	22.1
1 to 14 years	4.4	4.6	4.8	*	*	6.8	3.9	4.2	4.4
15 to 24 years	40.0	37.5	35.2	31.9	30.9	27.3	26.8	27.3	24.9
25 to 34 years	42.7	30.5	29.3	23.8	34.8	32.0	30.3	31.8	32.4
35 to 44 years	32.0	29.3	28.5	24.5	21.9	30.4	19.8	24.2	30.3
45 to 64 years	27.9	25.8	22.8	23.2	27.4	27.0	20.4	30.5	26.6
65 years and over	38.5	24.5	22.2	26.6	23.7	*	25.8	26.8	26.3
Asian or Pacific Islander Male[5]									
All ages, age-adjusted[4]	9.1	7.9	6.2	6.5	6.6	5.9	6.4	6.2	6.3
All ages, crude	8.3	7.5	5.8	6.2	6.2	5.6	5.9	6.0	6.1
1 to 14 years	1.8	1.6	1.5	*	*	*	1.5	1.2	*
15 to 24 years	15.7	11.6	8.8	9.6	9.3	8.9	8.1	8.6	9.7
25 to 34 years	7.0	8.5	7.3	7.8	6.6	5.8	5.9	8.0	6.7
35 to 44 years	6.1	6.4	4.5	4.1	4.8	3.5	5.3	4.1	3.8
45 to 64 years	7.7	7.4	5.6	6.0	6.5	6.3	5.9	5.7	6.4
65 years and over	20.9	16.1	11.9	14.6	14.9	12.5	14.3	13.1	13.5
Hispanic or Latino Male[5,7]									
All ages, age-adjusted[4]	19.4	16.7	14.7	14.0	13.7	13.9	14.2	14.3	15.2
All ages, crude	18.6	16.1	14.2	12.8	12.9	13.1	13.3	13.5	14.4
1 to 14 years	4.1	2.9	3.0	2.5	2.3	2.5	2.5	2.5	2.6
15 to 24 years	32.8	26.9	24.1	20.2	20.7	20.3	20.5	22.0	22.8
25 to 34 years	25.9	24.7	20.1	18.0	17.4	19.9	18.2	19.6	21.2
35 to 44 years	18.6	16.4	15.5	13.9	13.9	13.9	14.5	13.4	14.8
45 to 64 years	18.8	16.9	14.4	14.3	15.2	14.7	15.9	14.9	15.9
65 years and over	25.6	19.7	16.9	20.7	18.0	17.5	18.8	19.5	20.1
White, Not Hispanic or Latino Male[7]									
All ages, age-adjusted[4]	21.6	19.8	17.4	17.1	17.0	17.3	16.5	16.2	17.0
All ages, crude	22.0	20.2	17.9	17.6	17.6	18.0	17.2	16.9	17.9
1 to 14 years	3.5	3.1	2.6	2.7	2.7	2.2	2.3	2.3	2.4
15 to 24 years	37.9	32.5	26.6	25.4	25.3	25.3	23.0	22.6	22.8
25 to 34 years	27.6	26.1	21.8	21.9	21.5	22.0	21.4	20.7	21.7
35 to 44 years	22.7	20.9	18.9	18.0	17.5	18.9	17.8	17.2	18.6
45 to 64 years	21.1	20.2	19.0	18.6	18.7	19.3	18.6	18.6	19.8
65 years and over	27.0	24.7	22.6	22.7	23.0	22.9	22.3	21.5	22.8
White Female[5]									
All ages, age-adjusted[4]	8.6	7.5	6.9	6.8	6.6	6.8	6.4	6.3	6.6
All ages, crude	8.8	7.8	7.2	7.1	6.9	7.1	6.7	6.6	6.9
Under 1 year	2.9	1.8	1.5	1.9	1.4	1.6	1.7	1.5	*
1 to 14 years	2.7	2.1	2.1	2.1	2.0	1.9	1.8	1.8	1.8
15 to 24 years	15.1	12.6	11.3	10.8	10.1	10.0	9.5	9.2	9.8
25 to 34 years	9.0	7.6	7.4	7.1	7.3	7.6	7.1	7.1	7.7
35 to 44 years	8.1	7.4	6.5	6.5	6.4	6.6	6.1	6.1	6.4
45 to 64 years	7.8	7.3	6.6	6.4	6.1	6.5	6.4	6.3	6.6
65 years and over	13.0	11.8	11.4	11.5	11.3	11.3	10.4	10.3	10.3
Black or African American Female[5]									
All ages, age-adjusted[4]	7.0	6.4	6.2	5.9	5.7	5.9	5.7	5.6	6.1
All ages, crude	6.9	6.3	6.1	5.8	5.7	5.9	5.7	5.6	6.1
Under 1 year	*	*	*	*	*	*	*	*	*
1 to 14 years[6]	3.3	2.5	2.6	2.0	2.3	2.4	2.3	2.3	2.6

* = Rates based on fewer than 20 deaths are considered unreliable and are not shown.
[2]Underlying cause of death was coded according to the 6th Revision of the International Classification of Diseases (ICD) in 1950, 7th Revision in 1960, 8th Revision in 1970, and 9th Revision in 1980-1998.
[3]Starting with 1999 data, cause of death is coded according to ICD-10.
[4]Age-adjusted rates are calculated using the year 2000 standard population. Prior to 2001, age-adjusted rates were calculated using standard million proportions based on rounded population numbers. Starting with 2001 data, unrounded population numbers are used to calculate age-adjusted rates.
[5]The race groups, White, Black, Asian or Pacific Islander, and American Indian or Alaska Native, include persons of Hispanic and non-Hispanic origin. Persons of Hispanic origin may be of any race. Death rates for the American Indian or Alaska Native, Asian or Pacific Islander, and Hispanic populations are known to be underestimated.
[6]Prior to 1997, excludes data from states lacking an Hispanic-origin item on the death certificate.
[7]In 1950, rate is for the age group under 15 years.

Table 2-33. Death Rates for Motor Vehicle–Related Injuries, by Sex, Race, Hispanic Origin, and Age, Selected Years, 1950–2015—*Continued*

(Deaths per 100,000 resident population.)

Sex, race, Hispanic origin, and age	1950[1,2]	1960[1,2]	1970[2]	1980[2]	1985	1990[2]	1995	2000[3]	2005[3]	2006[3]
15 to 24 years	11.6	9.9	13.4	8.0	9.1	9.9	10.5	11.7	10.5	9.8
25 to 34 years	10.8	9.8	13.3	10.6	9.3	11.1	10.3	9.4	7.6	8.7
35 to 44 years	11.1	11.0	16.1	8.3	9.1	9.4	9.7	8.2	7.7	8.0
45 to 64 years	11.8	12.7	16.7	9.2	9.0	10.7	9.3	9.0	8.2	8.8
65 years and over	14.3	13.2	15.7	9.5	11.2	13.5	11.4	10.4	9.9	9.5
American Indian or Alaska Native Female[5]										
All ages, age-adjusted[4]	NA	NA	NA	32.0	19.8	17.5	18.2	19.5	14.0	15.1
All ages, crude	NA	NA	NA	32.0	20.6	17.3	18.8	18.6	13.8	14.9
1 to 14 years	NA	NA	NA	15.0	9.2	8.1	8.1	6.5	*	*
15 to 24 years	NA	NA	NA	42.3	29.5	31.4	30.4	30.3	22.0	24.5
25 to 34 years	NA	NA	NA	52.5	30.2	18.8	33.7	22.3	22.1	19.1
35 to 44 years	NA	NA	NA	38.1	27.0	18.2	17.2	22.0	15.7	17.7
45 to 64 years	NA	NA	NA	32.6	19.5	17.6	15.7	17.8	10.6	13.5
65 years and over	NA	NA	NA	*	*	*	*	24.0	*	17.1
Asian or Pacific Islander Female[5]										
All ages, age-adjusted[4]	NA	NA	NA	9.3	8.8	10.4	8.6	6.7	5.7	5.4
All ages, crude	NA	NA	NA	8.2	7.9	9.0	7.7	5.9	5.3	5.1
1 to 14 years	NA	NA	NA	7.4	5.0	3.6	3.2	2.3	1.5	1.7
15 to 24 years	NA	NA	NA	7.4	7.4	11.4	11.5	6.0	7.0	6.3
25 to 34 years	NA	NA	NA	7.3	8.4	7.3	4.8	4.5	3.4	3.2
35 to 44 years	NA	NA	NA	8.6	7.0	7.5	5.9	4.9	4.3	4.1
45 to 64 years	NA	NA	NA	8.5	8.6	11.8	10.4	6.4	6.4	6.0
65 years and over	NA	NA	NA	18.6	20.5	24.3	18.9	18.5	13.9	13.6
Hispanic or Latina Female[5,7]										
All ages, age-adjusted[4]	NA	NA	NA	NA	8.8	9.6	8.8	7.9	7.8	7.6
All ages, crude	NA	NA	NA	NA	7.9	8.9	8.0	7.2	7.3	7.0
1 to 14 years	NA	NA	NA	NA	4.8	4.8	4.3	3.9	3.3	3.1
15 to 24 years	NA	NA	NA	NA	10.1	11.6	11.8	10.6	12.7	10.9
25 to 34 years	NA	NA	NA	NA	7.5	9.4	7.2	6.5	7.1	6.8
35 to 44 years	NA	NA	NA	NA	8.8	8.0	7.9	7.3	7.3	7.1
45 to 64 years	NA	NA	NA	NA	9.4	11.4	9.3	8.3	7.4	8.0
65 years and over	NA	NA	NA	NA	14.8	14.9	14.6	13.4	11.4	12.0
White, not Hispanic or Latina Female[7]										
All ages, age-adjusted[4]	NA	NA	NA	NA	10.4	11.3	10.5	10.0	9.5	9.4
All ages, crude	NA	NA	NA	NA	10.9	11.7	10.9	10.3	9.9	9.8
1 to 14 years	NA	NA	NA	NA	4.9	4.7	4.2	3.5	3.0	3.0
15 to 24 years	NA	NA	NA	NA	20.2	20.4	19.0	18.4	16.3	16.9
25 to 34 years	NA	NA	NA	NA	9.8	11.7	10.5	9.3	9.9	9.6
35 to 44 years	NA	NA	NA	NA	8.6	9.3	8.9	9.0	9.2	9.4
45 to 64 years	NA	NA	NA	NA	8.6	9.7	8.6	8.7	8.6	8.3
65 years and over	NA	NA	NA	NA	15.3	17.5	17.5	16.3	14.7	14.1

NA = Not available.

* = Rates based on fewer than 20 deaths are considered unreliable and are not shown.

[1]Includes deaths of persons who were not residents of the 50 states and the District of Columbia.

[2]Underlying cause of death was coded according to the 6th Revision of the International Classification of Diseases (ICD) in 1950, 7th Revision in 1960, 8th Revision in 1970, and 9th Revision in 1980-1998.

[3]Starting with 1999 data, cause of death is coded according to ICD-10.

[4]Age-adjusted rates are calculated using the year 2000 standard population. Prior to 2001, age-adjusted rates were calculated using standard million proportions based on rounded population numbers. Starting with 2001 data, unrounded population numbers are used to calculate age-adjusted rates.

[5]The race groups, White, Black, Asian or Pacific Islander, and American Indian or Alaska Native, include persons of Hispanic and non-Hispanic origin. Persons of Hispanic origin may be of any race. Death rates for the American Indian or Alaska Native, Asian or Pacific Islander, and Hispanic populations are known to be underestimated.

[7]In 1950, rate is for the age group under 15 years.

Table 2-33. Death Rates for Motor Vehicle–Related Injuries, by Sex, Race, Hispanic Origin, and Age, Selected Years, 1950–2015—Continued

(Deaths per 100,000 resident population.)

Sex, race, Hispanic origin, and age	2007[3]	2008[3]	2009[3]	2010[3]	2011[3]	2012[3]	2013[3]	2014[3]	2015[3]
15 to 24 years	9.5	8.4	8.1	7.8	7.6	7.7	7.7	7.7	8.9
25 to 34 years	7.5	7.1	7.6	6.8	7.1	7.4	7.2	6.9	7.8
35 to 44 years	7.0	6.7	6.0	5.8	5.4	5.7	6.4	5.7	6.1
45 to 64 years	7.4	7.0	6.5	6.3	5.9	6.5	6.2	6.2	6.3
65 years and over	8.7	8.4	7.9	8.6	7.6	7.7	5.9	6.4	6.8
American Indian or Alaska Native Female[5]									
All ages, age-adjusted[4]	13.5	12.8	11.8	10.6	10.8	10.2	11.0	10.1	11.2
All ages, crude	13.5	12.4	11.7	10.0	10.5	10.1	10.7	10.0	11.2
1 to 14 years	*	*	*	*	*	*	4.9	*	*
15 to 24 years	21.4	17.4	19.8	13.4	14.7	16.2	13.6	16.5	13.8
25 to 34 years	19.4	19.2	13.8	17.7	18.0	15.1	17.0	13.4	21.2
35 to 44 years	18.8	15.3	16.9	13.1	11.3	11.6	14.2	12.0	12.6
45 to 64 years	10.8	10.3	11.7	8.4	8.7	10.5	8.7	9.7	11.9
65 years and over	*	17.8	*	14.8	14.4	*	*	*	*
Asian or Pacific Islander Female[5]									
All ages, age-adjusted[4]	5.0	4.2	3.8	3.9	3.3	3.3	3.4	3.2	3.6
All ages, crude	4.6	3.9	3.5	3.6	3.1	3.3	3.4	3.2	3.6
1 to 14 years	*	1.4	1.5	*	*	*	*	*	*
15 to 24 years	6.7	4.5	4.3	3.3	3.7	3.0	3.0	3.0	3.4
25 to 34 years	2.9	3.1	2.9	3.1	1.9	2.8	2.5	2.5	2.6
35 to 44 years	2.7	2.2	2.1	2.0	2.3	1.7	*	2.0	1.7
45 to 64 years	5.4	4.4	3.0	4.3	3.0	4.2	4.1	3.3	4.0
65 years and over	13.4	12.1	11.4	12.2	10.2	8.7	10.8	9.4	11.2
Hispanic or Latina Female[5,7]									
All ages, age-adjusted[4]	6.8	5.5	5.5	5.3	4.8	5.3	5.2	5.0	5.2
All ages, crude	6.3	5.0	5.1	4.9	4.5	4.9	4.8	4.7	5.0
1 to 14 years	2.7	2.1	2.3	2.0	1.7	1.9	1.7	1.9	1.8
15 to 24 years	10.1	7.8	7.8	7.7	6.3	7.2	7.4	7.5	7.7
25 to 34 years	6.6	5.4	5.5	5.0	5.1	5.4	5.1	5.3	6.1
35 to 44 years	6.7	4.8	4.6	4.5	4.6	4.5	4.7	4.1	4.6
45 to 64 years	6.7	5.1	5.5	5.6	4.8	5.6	5.3	5.3	5.2
65 years and over	10.5	10.7	9.5	9.4	8.6	9.2	9.0	8.1	8.3
White, not Hispanic or Latina Female[7]									
All ages, age-adjusted[4]	8.8	7.9	7.1	7.0	6.9	7.0	6.6	6.5	6.8
All ages, crude	9.2	8.3	7.5	7.5	7.3	7.5	7.1	7.0	7.3
1 to 14 years	2.6	2.1	1.9	2.0	2.1	1.8	1.8	1.7	1.8
15 to 24 years	16.2	13.7	12.0	11.4	11.0	10.7	10.0	9.6	10.3
25 to 34 years	9.5	8.1	7.7	7.6	7.7	8.2	7.5	7.5	8.0
35 to 44 years	8.3	7.9	6.8	6.9	6.7	7.0	6.4	6.6	6.8
45 to 64 years	7.9	7.6	6.7	6.4	6.2	6.6	6.5	6.4	6.7
65 years and over	13.1	11.8	11.5	11.6	11.5	11.4	10.5	10.4	10.5

* = Rates based on fewer than 20 deaths are considered unreliable and are not shown.

[2]Underlying cause of death was coded according to the 6th Revision of the International Classification of Diseases (ICD) in 1950, 7th Revision in 1960, 8th Revision in 1970, and 9th Revision in 1980-1998.

[3]Starting with 1999 data, cause of death is coded according to ICD-10.

[4]Age-adjusted rates are calculated using the year 2000 standard population. Prior to 2001, age-adjusted rates were calculated using standard million proportions based on rounded population numbers. Starting with 2001 data, unrounded population numbers are used to calculate age-adjusted rates.

[5]The race groups, White, Black, Asian or Pacific Islander, and American Indian or Alaska Native, include persons of Hispanic and non-Hispanic origin. Persons of Hispanic origin may be of any race. Death rates for the American Indian or Alaska Native, Asian or Pacific Islander, and Hispanic populations are known to be underestimated.

[7]In 1950, rate is for the age group under 15 years.

Table 2-34. Occupant and Alcohol-Impaired Driving Deaths, by State, 2005–2014

(Number.)

State	Alcohol-impaired driving deaths	Occupant deaths
United States..	113,001	255,297
Alabama..	2,997	7,754
Alaska..	205	439
Arizona...	1,636	4,526
Arkansas...	2,656	5,712
California..	9,791	20,733
Colorado...	1,599	3,521
Connecticut..	1,049	1,806
Delaware...	430	767
District of Columbia	96	130
Florida...	8,053	16,041
Georgia..	3,513	10,406
Hawaii...	453	587
Idaho..	661	1,725
Illinois...	3,554	7,348
Indiana..	2,171	5,966
Iowa...	967	2,970
Kansas..	1,142	3,248
Kentucky..	1,900	6,133
Louisiana..	2,875	6,073
Maine..	454	1,231
Maryland..	1,586	3,454
Massachusetts...	1,309	2,465
Michigan...	2,710	6,699
Minnesota...	1,274	3,248
Mississippi...	2,367	6,100
Missouri...	3,004	7,219
Montana...	897	1,778
Nebraska..	631	1,919
Nevada..	968	1,962
New Hampshire..	386	853
New Jersey	1,747	3,832
New Mexico	1,166	2,766
New York..	3,605	7,013
North Carolina...	3,996	10,093
North Dakota..	539	1,078
Ohio...	3,457	8,223
Oklahoma..	2,095	5,711
Oregon..	1,129	2,735
Pennsylvania..	4,355	9,656
Rhode Island..	265	429
South Carolina	3,723	6,648
South Dakota	469	1,107
Tennessee	3,154	8,357
Texas..	13,171	24,013
Utah	456	1,882
Vermont...	199	535
Virginia..	2,518	6,335
Washington..	1,799	3,542
West Virginia..	1,040	2,762
Wisconsin..	2,300	4,572
Wyoming	484	1,195

Note: Alcohol-Impaired Driving Fatalities 2003-2012; All persons killed in crashes involving a driver with BAC > = .08 g/dL. Occupant Fatalities 2003-2012; All occupants killed where body type = 1-79. Source: Fatality Analysis Reporting System (FARS) 2003-2011 and 2012 ARF.

Table 2-35. Death Rates for Drug Poisoning and Drug Poisoning Involving Opioid Analgesics and Heroin, by Sex, Race, Hispanic Origin, and Age, Selected Years, 1999–2015

(Deaths per 100,000 resident population.)

Sex, race, Hispanic origin, and age	1999	2000	2005	2006	2007	2008	2009	2010	2011	2012	2013	2014	2015
	Drug poisoning deaths per 100,000 resident population[1]												
All Persons													
All ages, age-adjusted[2]	6.1	6.2	10.1	11.5	11.9	11.9	11.9	12.3	13.2	13.1	13.8	14.7	16.3
All ages, crude	6.0	6.2	10.1	11.5	12.0	12.0	12.1	12.4	13.3	13.2	13.9	14.8	16.3
Under 15 years	0.1	0.1	0.2	0.2	0.2	0.2	0.2	0.2	0.2	0.2	0.2	0.2	0.2
15 to 24 years	3.2	3.7	6.9	8.1	8.2	8.0	7.7	8.2	8.6	8.0	8.3	8.6	9.7
25 to 34 years	8.1	7.9	13.6	16.1	16.8	16.8	17.2	18.4	20.2	20.1	20.9	23.1	26.9
35 to 44 years	14.0	14.3	19.6	21.7	21.4	21.1	20.5	20.8	22.5	22.1	23.0	25.0	28.3
45 to 54 years	11.1	11.6	21.1	24.1	25.1	25.2	25.4	25.1	26.7	26.9	27.5	28.2	30.0
55 to 64 years	4.2	4.2	9.0	10.5	12.2	12.9	13.7	15.0	15.9	16.6	19.2	20.3	21.8
65 to 74 years	2.4	2.0	3.2	3.5	4.0	4.6	4.7	4.7	5.4	5.8	6.4	6.9	7.2
75 to 84 years	2.8	2.4	3.1	3.3	3.2	3.3	3.8	3.4	3.4	3.4	3.6	3.6	3.6
85 years and over	3.8	4.4	4.1	4.4	4.5	4.1	4.4	4.7	4.2	4.3	4.3	4.1	4.4
Male													
All ages, age-adjusted[2]	8.2	8.3	12.8	14.8	14.9	14.9	14.8	15.0	16.1	16.1	17.0	18.3	20.8
All ages, crude	8.2	8.4	12.9	14.9	15.1	15.0	15.0	15.2	16.3	16.3	17.2	18.4	20.8
Under 15 years	0.1	0.2	0.2	0.2	0.3	0.2	0.2	0.3	0.2	0.2	0.2	0.2	0.2
15 to 24 years	4.5	5.3	10.0	12.0	12.0	11.9	11.3	11.6	12.4	11.4	11.7	12.1	13.3
25 to 34 years	11.5	11.3	18.7	22.7	23.4	23.6	24.0	25.0	27.5	27.0	28.6	31.9	37.9
35 to 44 years	19.2	19.5	24.4	27.5	26.7	25.6	25.2	24.9	26.8	27.1	28.1	30.8	36.3
45 to 54 years	15.2	15.7	25.8	29.7	29.2	29.6	29.1	28.5	30.4	30.4	31.5	32.9	35.3
55 to 64 years	4.9	4.4	10.6	12.3	14.0	14.8	16.0	17.3	18.5	19.4	22.7	23.5	26.2
65 to 74 years	2.7	2.1	3.3	3.5	4.4	4.8	4.8	4.5	5.4	6.2	6.9	7.3	8.5
75 to 84 years	2.5	2.5	3.4	3.2	3.2	3.2	3.5	3.6	3.4	3.2	3.7	3.8	3.9
85 years and over	4.4	5.9	5.2	4.7	4.9	4.4	5.2	5.1	4.3	5.3	5.9	4.3	5.0
Female													
All ages, age-adjusted[2]	3.9	4.1	7.3	8.2	8.8	8.9	9.1	9.6	10.2	10.2	10.6	11.1	11.8
All ages, crude	3.9	4.1	7.4	8.3	9.0	9.0	9.2	9.8	10.3	10.3	10.7	11.3	11.9
Under 15 years	0.1	0.1	0.2	0.2	0.2	0.2	0.2	0.2	0.2	0.2	0.2	0.2	0.3
15 to 24 years	1.8	1.9	3.5	3.9	4.2	4.0	4.1	4.6	4.6	4.4	4.8	5.0	5.9
25 to 34 years	4.6	4.6	8.5	9.5	10.1	9.9	10.4	11.9	12.8	13.1	13.0	14.1	15.7
35 to 44 years	8.7	9.2	14.8	15.9	16.1	16.5	16.0	16.8	18.2	17.1	18.0	19.2	20.5
45 to 54 years	7.2	7.7	16.5	18.6	21.0	21.0	21.8	21.8	23.1	23.4	23.6	23.7	24.9
55 to 64 years	3.5	3.9	7.5	8.8	10.5	11.1	11.6	12.9	13.5	14.0	15.9	17.2	17.6
65 to 74 years	2.1	2.0	3.1	3.6	3.7	4.4	4.6	4.8	5.3	5.5	5.9	6.5	6.1
75 to 84 years	3.0	2.3	2.9	3.3	3.2	3.3	3.9	3.3	3.4	3.5	3.4	3.5	3.3
85 years and over	3.5	3.9	3.7	4.2	4.3	4.0	3.9	4.5	4.2	3.8	3.5	4.0	4.1
All Ages, Age-Adjusted[2,3]													
White male	8.1	8.4	13.6	15.7	16.3	16.5	16.4	16.8	18.1	18.1	19.0	20.4	23.2
Black or African American male	11.5	10.8	12.8	15.2	13.0	11.3	10.8	10.1	11.0	11.3	12.9	13.8	16.8
American Indian or Alaska Native male	5.7	6.1	10.8	13.0	10.5	13.5	14.2	11.8	12.9	12.8	12.9	15.9	16.0
Asian or Pacific Islander male	1.5	1.4	2.2	2.3	2.2	2.1	2.8	2.5	3.2	3.1	3.2	3.3	4.1
Hispanic or Latino male	8.6	7.1	8.4	9.1	8.7	8.4	8.2	7.6	8.1	8.5	9.2	9.3	10.9
White, not Hispanic or Latino male	8.0	8.6	14.7	17.2	18.0	18.3	18.3	19.0	20.5	20.4	21.4	23.2	26.2
White female	4.0	4.3	8.0	9.0	9.8	10.1	10.3	10.9	11.7	11.6	12.1		
Black or African American female	3.9	4.1	6.0	6.3	6.3	5.4	5.6	5.7	5.9	6.0	6.3	12.7	13.6
American Indian or Alaska Native female	4.6	3.7	8.6	7.9	9.9	8.8	9.6	9.7	10.7	12.2	11.6	7.0	7.5
Asian or Pacific Islander female	1.0	0.8	1.3	1.4	1.6	1.3	1.3	1.5	1.6	1.4	1.5	11.2	11.3
Hispanic or Latina female	2.2	2.0	3.0	3.4	3.1	3.2	3.5	3.6	4.0	4.0	4.1	1.7	1.5
White, not Hispanic or Latina female	4.3	4.5	8.8	10.0	11.0	11.4	11.6	12.5	13.3	13.2	13.8	4.1	4.4

0.0 = Rate more than zero but less than 0.05.
[1] Drug poisoning was coded using underlying cause of death according to the 10th Revision of the International Classification of Diseases (ICD-10).
[2] Age-adjusted rates are calculated using the year 2000 standard population with unrounded population numbers.
[3] The race groups, White, Black, Asian or Pacific Islander, and American Indian or Alaska Native, include persons of Hispanic and non-Hispanic origin. Persons of Hispanic origin may be of any race. Death rates for the American Indian or Alaska Native, Asian or Pacific Islander, and Hispanic populations are known to be underestimated.

Table 2-35. Death Rates for Drug Poisoning and Drug Poisoning Involving Opioid Analgesics and Heroin, by Sex, Race, Hispanic Origin, and Age, Selected Years, 1999–2015—Continued

(Deaths per 100,000 resident population.)

Sex, race, Hispanic origin, and age	1999	2000	2005	2006	2007	2008	2009	2010	2011	2012	2013	2014	2015
	Drug poisoning deaths involving opioid analgesics per 100,000 resident population[4]												
All Persons													
All ages, age-adjusted[2]	1.4	1.5	3.7	4.6	4.8	4.8	5.0	5.4	5.4	5.1	5.1	5.9	7.0
All ages, crude	1.4	1.6	3.7	4.6	4.8	4.9	5.1	5.4	5.4	5.1	5.1	5.9	7.0
Under 15 years	*	0.0	0.1	0.1	0.1	0.1	0.1	0.1	0.1	0.1	0.1	0.1	0.1
15 to 24 years	0.7	0.8	2.7	3.8	3.9	3.7	3.6	3.9	3.6	2.8	2.6	3.1	3.9
25 to 34 years	1.9	1.9	5.3	6.9	7.3	7.2	7.6	8.5	8.5	7.7	7.5	9.0	11.8
35 to 44 years	3.5	3.7	6.9	8.3	8.3	8.4	8.6	9.1	9.3	8.8	8.6	10.3	12.6
45 to 54 years	2.9	3.2	7.9	9.6	9.8	10.4	10.6	10.9	11.2	10.6	10.6	11.7	12.9
55 to 64 years	1.0	1.1	3.1	3.9	4.7	4.9	5.8	6.2	6.3	6.6	7.5	8.5	9.5
65 to 74 years	0.4	0.4	1.0	1.1	1.2	1.4	1.7	1.5	1.8	2.0	2.3	2.7	2.9
75 to 84 years	0.3	0.2	0.6	0.6	0.6	0.6	0.8	0.7	0.7	0.9	0.8	0.9	1.0
85 years and over	*	*	0.9	0.7	0.9	0.6	0.7	1.1	0.8	0.8	0.9	0.9	0.9
Male													
All ages, age-adjusted[2]	2.0	2.0	4.6	5.8	5.9	6.0	6.2	6.5	6.5	6.0	5.9	6.9	8.7
All ages, crude	2.0	2.1	4.6	5.9	5.9	6.1	6.2	6.6	6.5	6.0	5.9	7.0	8.7
Under 15 years	*	*	0.1	0.1	0.1	0.1	0.1	0.2	0.1	0.1	0.1	0.1	0.1
15 to 24 years	1.0	1.2	4.2	5.8	5.8	5.6	5.3	5.6	5.3	4.2	3.9	4.4	5.4
25 to 34 years	2.7	2.7	7.2	9.7	10.2	10.2	10.6	11.7	11.4	10.0	10.0	12.2	16.7
35 to 44 years	5.0	4.9	8.3	10.4	10.0	10.0	10.4	10.9	10.9	10.3	9.6	11.9	15.7
45 to 54 years	3.9	4.3	9.4	11.3	10.8	11.8	11.6	12.0	12.1	11.1	11.1	12.5	14.2
55 to 64 years	1.1	1.0	3.5	4.2	5.1	5.3	6.3	7.0	6.9	7.3	8.0	9.2	10.7
65 to 74 years	0.5	0.3	0.7	1.0	1.1	1.5	1.6	1.2	1.7	2.0	2.2	2.5	3.4
75 to 84 years	*	*	0.6	0.6	0.5	0.5	0.6	0.7	0.7	0.7	0.9	0.8	1.0
85 years and over	*	*	*	*	1.3	*	1.2	1.3	*	1.0	1.3	*	*
Female													
All ages, age-adjusted[2]	0.9	1.1	2.8	3.3	3.6	3.7	3.9	4.2	4.3	4.2	4.3	4.9	5.4
All ages, crude	0.9	1.1	2.8	3.3	3.7	3.7	4.0	4.2	4.4	4.2	4.4	4.9	5.4
Under 15 years	*	*	*	0.1	0.1	0.1	0.1	0.1	0.1	0.1	0.1	0.1	0.1
15 to 24 years	0.3	0.4	1.2	1.6	1.8	1.6	1.7	2.1	1.9	1.5	1.4	1.7	2.3
25 to 34 years	1.1	1.2	3.4	4.0	4.4	4.2	4.7	5.3	5.5	5.3	5.0	5.7	6.9
35 to 44 years	2.1	2.5	5.6	6.2	6.6	6.8	6.9	7.3	7.8	7.3	7.6	8.7	9.6
45 to 54 years	1.9	2.2	6.5	8.0	8.9	9.0	9.7	9.8	10.2	10.1	10.1	10.9	11.6
55 to 64 years	0.8	1.1	2.8	3.6	4.2	4.6	5.2	5.5	5.7	6.0	6.9	7.8	8.4
65 to 74 years	0.3	0.4	1.2	1.1	1.2	1.4	1.7	1.7	1.8	2.0	2.4	2.9	2.4
75 to 84 years	0.4	*	0.6	0.6	0.7	0.7	0.9	0.7	0.7	0.9	0.7	1.0	1.0
85 years and over	*	*	0.8	0.8	0.7	0.8	*	1.1	0.8	0.7	0.8	1.0	0.9
All Ages, Age-Adjusted[2,3]													
White male	2.2	2.3	5.3	6.6	6.8	7.0	7.2	7.7	7.6	7.0	6.8	8.0	10.1
Black or African American male	1.2	1.2	2.1	3.5	2.3	2.2	2.4	2.2	2.4	2.3	2.7	3.9	5.3
American Indian or Alaska Native male	*	1.9	4.4	5.4	4.0	5.9	7.5	5.3	5.5	5.8	4.8	6.4	6.1
Asian or Pacific Islander male	*	*	0.5	0.6	0.4	0.5	0.7	0.8	1.0	0.7	0.9	0.9	1.0
Hispanic or Latino male	2.9	1.7	2.2	2.7	2.8	2.9	2.6	2.4	2.6	2.5	2.7	2.7	3.4
White, not Hispanic or Latino male	2.1	2.3	5.9	7.5	7.8	8.0	8.2	9.0	8.8	8.1	7.9	9.3	11.8
White female	1.0	1.2	3.2	3.8	4.2	4.3	4.5	4.8	5.1	4.9	5.0	5.6	6.3
Black or African American female	0.6	0.6	1.4	1.8	1.7	1.6	1.8	2.0	2.0	2.0	2.2	2.6	2.9
American Indian or Alaska Native female	*	*	3.8	3.2	4.5	4.6	4.7	4.9	4.6	5.4	5.4	4.6	4.7
Asian or Pacific Islander female	*	*	0.4	0.4	0.3	0.5	0.4	0.5	0.4	0.4	0.3	0.5	0.4
Hispanic or Latina female	0.5	0.5	1.0	1.3	1.2	1.2	1.3	1.3	1.4	1.5	1.5	1.6	1.6
White, not Hispanic or Latina female	1.1	1.3	3.5	4.2	4.8	4.8	5.2	5.6	5.8	5.6	5.8	6.5	7.4

0.0 = Rate more than zero but less than 0.05.
* = Rates based on fewer than 20 deaths are considered unreliable and are not shown.
[2]Age-adjusted rates are calculated using the year 2000 standard population with unrounded population numbers.
[3]The race groups, White, Black, Asian or Pacific Islander, and American Indian or Alaska Native, include persons of Hispanic and non-Hispanic origin. Persons of Hispanic origin may be of any race. Death rates for the American Indian or Alaska Native, Asian or Pacific Islander, and Hispanic populations are known to be underestimated.
[4]Opioid analgesics include opioids such as hydrocodone, codeine, and methadone, and synthetic narcotics such as fentanyl, tramadol, and propoxyphene (removed from the market in 2010). Drug poisoning deaths involving opioid analgesics include those with an underlying cause of drug poisoning and with an opioid analgesic mentioned in the ICD–10 multiple causes of death. Drug poisoning deaths involving heroin include those with an underlying cause of drug poisoning and with heroin mentioned in the ICD–10 multiple causes of death. Drug-poisoning deaths may involve multiple drugs. Deaths involving both opioid analgesics and heroin are included in the death rate for opioid analgesics and the death rate for heroin. Opioid analgesic death rates include deaths involving fentanyl, a synthetic opioid. A sharp increase in deaths involving synthetic opioids, other than methadone, in 2014 coincided with law enforcement reports of increased availability of illicitly manufactured, or non-pharmaceutical, fentanyl. Illicitly manufactured fentanyl cannot be distinguished from pharmaceutical fentanyl in death certificate data. Metabolic breakdown of heroin into morphine in the body can make it difficult to distinguish between deaths from heroin and deaths from morphine based on the information on the death certificate. Some deaths reported to involve morphine could be deaths from heroin. This may result in an undercount of heroin-related deaths. In 1999–2015, 17%–25% of drug poisoning deaths did not include specifc information on the death certifcate on the type of drug that was involved. Some of these deaths could have potentially involved heroin or opioid analgesics.

Table 2-35. Death Rates for Drug Poisoning and Drug Poisoning Involving Opioid Analgesics and Heroin, by Sex, Race, Hispanic Origin, and Age, Selected Years, 1999–2015—*Continued*

(Deaths per 100,000 resident population.)

Sex, race, Hispanic origin, and age	1999	2000	2005	2006	2007	2008	2009	2010	2011	2012	2013	2014	2015
	Drug poisoning deaths involving heroin per 100,000 resident population[4]												
All Persons													
All ages, age-adjusted[2]	0.7	0.7	0.6	0.7	0.7	0.6	0.7	1.0	1.4	1.9	2.7	3.4	4.1
All ages, crude	0.7	0.7	0.6	0.7	0.7	0.6	0.7	1.0	1.4	1.9	2.6	3.3	4.0
Under 15 years	*	*	*	*	*	*	*	*	*	*	*	*	*
15 to 24 years	0.5	0.6	0.5	0.6	0.6	0.6	0.7	1.2	1.8	2.2	2.9	3.3	3.8
25 to 34 years	1.0	1.0	1.0	1.1	1.1	1.1	1.2	2.2	3.4	4.6	6.3	8.0	9.7
35 to 44 years	1.8	1.5	1.5	1.7	1.5	1.2	1.2	1.6	2.2	3.1	4.4	5.9	7.4
45 to 54 years	1.3	1.2	1.2	1.4	1.5	1.2	1.4	1.4	2.0	2.8	3.7	4.7	5.6
55 to 64 years	0.3	0.3	0.3	0.3	0.3	0.4	0.4	0.7	1.0	1.3	2.1	2.7	3.4
65 to 74 years	*	*	*	*	*	*	*	*	*	0.2	0.1	0.3	0.5	0.6
75 to 84 years	*	*	*	*	*	*	*	*	*	*	*	*	*
85 years and over	*	*	*	*	*	*	*	*	*	*	*	*	*
Male													
All ages, age-adjusted[2]	1.2	1.1	1.0	1.2	1.2	1.1	1.1	1.6	2.3	3.1	4.2	5.2	6.3
All ages, crude	1.2	1.1	1.0	1.2	1.2	1.1	1.1	1.6	2.3	3.0	4.2	5.2	6.2
Under 15 years	*	*	*	*	*	*	*	*	*	*	*	*	*
15 to 24 years	0.8	0.9	0.8	0.9	1.0	1.0	1.0	1.9	2.8	3.2	4.2	4.8	5.2
25 to 34 years	1.6	1.7	1.6	1.7	1.9	1.9	2.0	3.5	5.4	7.1	9.9	12.3	14.8
35 to 44 years	3.0	2.6	2.3	2.8	2.4	2.0	1.9	2.8	3.6	5.1	6.9	9.2	11.4
45 to 54 years	2.3	2.2	2.0	2.5	2.6	2.0	2.3	2.4	3.2	4.5	6.0	7.2	8.7
55 to 64 years	0.5	0.4	0.5	0.6	0.6	0.6	0.7	1.1	1.7	2.3	3.6	4.4	5.6
65 to 74 years	*	*	*	*	*	*	*	*	0.3	0.3	0.5	0.9	1.1
75 to 84 years	*	*	*	*	*	*	*	*	*	*	*	*	*
85 years and over	*	*	*	*	*	*	*	*	*	*	*	*	*
Female													
All ages, age-adjusted[2]	0.2	0.2	0.2	0.2	0.2	0.2	0.3	0.4	0.6	0.8	1.2	1.6	2.0
All ages, crude	0.2	0.2	0.2	0.2	0.2	0.2	0.3	0.4	0.6	0.8	1.1	1.5	1.9
Under 15 years	*	*	*	*	*	*	*	*	*	*	*	*	*
15 to 24 years	0.2	0.2	0.2	0.3	0.3	0.3	0.3	0.6	0.9	1.1	1.5	1.7	2.2
25 to 34 years	0.3	0.4	0.3	0.4	0.3	0.4	0.5	0.9	1.4	2.0	2.6	3.7	4.6
35 to 44 years	0.6	0.5	0.6	0.6	0.5	0.5	0.5	0.6	0.8	1.1	1.9	2.6	3.5
45 to 54 years	0.3	0.3	0.3	0.4	0.5	0.4	0.5	0.5	0.8	1.1	1.6	2.2	2.7
55 to 64 years	*	*	*	*	*	0.1	*	0.3	0.3	0.4	0.7	1.0	1.5
65 to 74 years	*	*	*	*	*	*	*	*	*	*	*	*	0.2
75 to 84 years	*	*	*	*	*	*	*	*	*	*	*	*	*
85 years and over	*	*	*	*	*	*	*	*	*	*	*	*	*
All Ages, Age-Adjusted[2,3]													
White male	1.2	1.1	1.1	1.2	1.3	1.1	1.1	1.8	2.6	3.5	4.7	6.0	7.2
Black or African American male	1.4	1.6	1.3	1.6	1.3	1.1	1.3	1.2	1.6	2.1	3.4	4.1	5.0
American Indian or Alaska Native male	*	*	*	*	*	*	*	*	1.3	1.7	2.6	3.5	4.0
Asian or Pacific Islander male	*	*	*	*	*	*	*	*	0.3	0.3	0.5	0.6	0.8
Hispanic or Latino male	2.0	1.6	1.4	1.8	1.8	1.3	1.4	1.5	1.7	2.2	2.6	3.2	3.8
White, not Hispanic or Latino male	1.1	1.0	1.0	1.2	1.2	1.1	1.1	1.9	2.9	3.9	5.3	6.7	8.1
White female	0.2	0.2	0.2	0.2	0.3	0.2	0.3	0.4	0.6	0.9	1.3	1.8	2.3
Black or African American female	0.3	0.3	0.3	0.3	0.3	0.3	0.3	0.3	0.4	0.5	0.7	1.1	1.3
American Indian or Alaska Native female	*	*	*	*	*	*	*	*	1.0	*	1.0	1.2	1.8
Asian or Pacific Islander female	*	*	*	*	*	*	*	*	*	*	*	*	0.2
Hispanic or Latina female	0.2	0.1	0.2	0.3	0.2	0.2	0.2	0.2	0.3	0.4	0.5	0.7	0.8
White, not Hispanic or Latina female	0.2	0.2	0.2	0.3	0.3	0.3	0.3	0.5	0.7	1.1	1.5	2.1	2.7

0.0 = Rate more than zero but less than 0.05.

* = Rates based on fewer than 20 deaths are considered unreliable and are not shown.

[2]Age-adjusted rates are calculated using the year 2000 standard population with unrounded population numbers.

[3]The race groups, White, Black, Asian or Pacific Islander, and American Indian or Alaska Native, include persons of Hispanic and non-Hispanic origin. Persons of Hispanic origin may be of any race. Death rates for the American Indian or Alaska Native, Asian or Pacific Islander, and Hispanic populations are known to be underestimated.

[4]Opioid analgesics include opioids such as hydrocodone, codeine, and methadone, and synthetic narcotics such as fentanyl, tramadol, and propoxyphene (removed from the market in 2010). Drug poisoning deaths involving opioid analgesics include those with an underlying cause of drug poisoning and with an opioid analgesic mentioned in the ICD-10 multiple causes of death. Drug poisoning deaths involving heroin include those with an underlying cause of drug poisoning and with heroin mentioned in the ICD-10 multiple causes of death. Drug-poisoning deaths may involve multiple drugs. Deaths involving both opioid analgesics and heroin are included in the death rate for opioid analgesics and the death rate for heroin. Opioid analgesic death rates include deaths involving fentanyl, a synthetic opioid. A sharp increase in deaths involving synthetic opioids, other than methadone, in 2014 coincided with law enforcement reports of increased availability of illicitly manufactured, or non-pharmaceutical, fentanyl. Illicitly manufactured fentanyl cannot be distinguished from pharmaceutical fentanyl in death certificate data. Metabolic breakdown of heroin into morphine in the body can make it difficult to distinguish between deaths from heroin and deaths from morphine based on the information on the death certificate. Some deaths reported to involve morphine could be deaths from heroin. This may result in an undercount of heroin-related deaths. In 1999-2015, 17%–25% of drug poisoning deaths did not include specifc information on the death certifcate on the type of drug that was involved. Some of these deaths could have potentially involved heroin or opioid analgesics.

Table 2-36. Death Rates for Homicide, by Sex, Race, Hispanic Origin, and Age, Selected Years, 1950–2015

(Deaths per 100,000 resident population.)

Sex, race, Hispanic origin, and age	1950[1,2]	1960[1,2]	1970[2]	1980[2]	1985[2]	1990[2]	1995	2000[3]	2005[3]	2006[3]
All Persons										
All ages, age-adjusted[4]	5.1	5.0	8.8	10.4	7.9	9.4	8.3	5.9	6.1	6.2
All ages, crude	5.0	4.6	8.1	10.6	8.2	9.9	8.5	6.0	6.1	6.2
Under 1 year	4.4	4.8	4.3	5.9	5.4	8.4	8.2	9.2	7.6	8.3
1 to 14 years	0.6	0.6	1.1	1.5	1.6	1.8	1.9	1.3	1.3	1.3
1 to 4 years	0.6	0.7	1.9	2.5	2.5	2.5	2.9	2.3	2.4	2.3
5 to 14 years	0.5	0.5	0.9	1.2	1.2	1.5	1.5	0.9	0.8	1.0
15 to 24 years	5.8	5.6	11.3	15.4	11.7	19.7	19.6	12.6	12.9	13.3
15 to 19 years	3.9	3.9	7.7	10.5	8.4	16.9	17.8	9.5	9.7	10.5
20 to 24 years	8.5	7.7	15.6	20.2	14.6	22.2	21.5	16.0	16.2	16.3
25 to 44 years	8.9	8.5	14.9	17.5	13.1	14.7	11.9	8.7	9.5	9.4
25 to 34 years	9.3	9.2	16.2	19.3	14.6	17.4	14.4	10.4	12.1	12.0
35 to 44 years	8.4	7.8	13.5	14.9	11.1	11.6	9.4	7.1	7.1	7.0
45 to 64 years	5.0	5.3	8.7	9.0	6.9	6.3	5.4	4.0	4.0	4.3
45 to 54 years	5.9	6.1	10.0	11.0	8.1	7.5	6.0	4.7	4.8	5.1
55 to 64 years	3.9	4.1	7.1	7.0	5.7	5.0	4.4	3.0	2.8	3.2
65 years and over	3.0	2.7	4.6	5.5	4.3	4.0	3.1	2.4	2.3	2.1
65 to 74 years	3.2	2.8	4.9	5.7	4.3	3.8	3.2	2.4	2.3	2.1
75 to 84 years	2.5	2.3	4.0	5.2	4.3	4.3	3.0	2.4	2.2	2.1
85 years and over	2.3	2.4	4.2	5.3	4.1	4.6	3.2	2.4	2.3	2.1
Male										
All ages, age-adjusted[4]	7.9	7.5	14.3	16.6	12.2	14.8	12.8	9.0	9.7	9.8
All ages, crude	7.7	6.8	13.1	17.1	12.8	15.9	13.4	9.3	9.9	10.0
Under 1 year	4.5	4.7	4.5	6.3	5.6	8.8	9.0	10.4	8.4	9.6
1 to 14 years	0.6	0.6	1.2	1.6	1.8	2.0	2.2	1.5	1.4	1.6
1 to 4 years	0.5	0.7	1.9	2.7	2.5	2.7	3.1	2.5	2.6	2.6
5 to 14 years	0.6	0.5	1.0	1.2	1.4	1.7	1.9	1.1	1.0	1.2
15 to 24 years	8.6	8.4	18.2	24.0	18.2	32.5	32.8	20.9	21.9	22.7
15 to 19 years	5.5	5.7	12.1	15.9	12.8	27.8	29.1	15.5	16.4	17.8
20 to 24 years	13.5	11.8	25.6	32.2	23.0	36.9	36.5	26.7	27.5	27.8
25 to 44 years	13.8	12.8	24.4	28.9	20.6	23.5	18.2	13.3	15.3	15.1
25 to 34 years	14.4	13.9	26.8	31.9	22.8	27.7	22.5	16.7	20.3	20.1
35 to 44 years	13.2	11.7	21.7	24.5	17.6	18.6	14.0	10.3	10.7	10.5
45 to 64 years	8.1	8.1	14.8	15.2	11.0	10.2	8.3	6.0	6.2	6.5
45 to 54 years	9.5	9.4	16.8	18.4	12.7	11.9	9.2	6.9	7.6	7.7
55 to 64 years	6.3	6.4	12.1	11.8	9.1	8.0	7.0	4.6	4.3	4.8
65 years and over	4.8	4.3	7.7	8.8	6.2	5.8	4.2	3.3	3.0	2.8
65 to 74 years	5.2	4.6	8.5	9.2	6.5	5.8	4.5	3.4	3.2	2.9
75 to 84 years	3.9	3.7	5.9	8.1	5.7	5.7	3.7	3.2	2.6	2.6
85 years and over	2.5	3.6	7.4	7.5	5.0	6.7	4.1	3.3	3.0	2.5
Female										
All ages, age-adjusted[4]	2.4	2.6	3.7	4.4	3.8	4.0	3.7	2.8	2.5	2.6
All ages, crude	2.4	2.4	3.4	4.5	3.9	4.2	3.8	2.8	2.5	2.5
Under 1 year	4.2	4.9	4.1	5.6	5.2	8.0	7.4	7.9	6.8	6.9
1 to 14 years	0.6	0.5	1.0	1.4	1.4	1.6	1.5	1.1	1.1	1.1
1 to 4 years	0.7	0.7	1.9	2.2	2.4	2.3	2.6	2.1	2.1	2.0
5 to 14 years	0.5	0.4	0.7	1.1	1.0	1.2	1.0	0.7	0.7	0.7
15 to 24 years	3.0	2.8	4.6	6.6	5.1	6.2	5.9	3.9	3.4	3.5
15 to 19 years	2.4	1.9	3.2	4.9	3.9	5.4	5.8	3.1	2.5	2.8
20 to 24 years	3.7	3.8	6.2	8.2	6.1	7.0	6.0	4.7	4.3	4.2
25 to 44 years	4.2	4.3	5.8	6.4	5.7	6.0	5.6	4.0	3.7	3.6
25 to 34 years	4.5	4.6	6.0	6.9	6.4	7.1	6.3	4.1	3.8	3.8
35 to 44 years	3.8	4.0	5.7	5.7	4.9	4.8	4.9	4.0	3.6	3.5
45 to 64 years	1.9	2.5	3.1	3.4	3.2	2.8	2.6	2.1	1.9	2.2
45 to 54 years	2.3	2.9	3.7	4.1	3.7	3.2	2.9	2.5	2.2	2.6
55 to 64 years	1.4	2.0	2.5	2.8	2.7	2.3	2.1	1.6	1.4	1.7
65 years and over	1.4	1.3	2.3	3.3	3.0	2.8	2.4	1.8	1.7	1.6
65 to 74 years	1.3	1.3	2.2	3.0	2.6	2.2	2.1	1.6	1.5	1.3
75 to 84 years	1.4	1.3	2.7	3.5	3.4	3.4	2.6	2.0	1.9	1.8
85 years and over	2.1	1.6	2.5	4.3	3.8	3.8	2.9	2.0	2.0	1.9
White Male[5]										
All ages, age-adjusted[4]	3.8	3.9	7.2	10.4	7.7	8.3	7.3	5.2	5.4	5.5
All ages, crude	3.6	3.6	6.6	10.7	8.1	8.8	7.5	5.2	5.5	5.5
Under 1 year	4.3	3.8	2.9	4.3	3.8	6.4	7.1	8.2	6.9	7.6
1 to 14 years	0.4	0.5	0.7	1.2	1.3	1.3	1.5	1.2	1.0	1.1
15 to 24 years	3.2	5.0	7.6	15.1	10.7	15.2	15.9	9.9	10.6	10.7
25 to 44 years	5.4	5.5	11.6	17.2	12.7	13.0	10.4	7.4	8.2	8.0
25 to 34 years	4.9	5.7	12.5	18.5	13.7	14.7	12.1	8.4	10.2	9.8
35 to 44 years	6.1	5.2	10.8	15.2	11.3	11.1	8.7	6.5	6.5	6.5

[1]Includes deaths of persons who were not residents of the 50 states and the District of Columbia.
[2]Underlying cause of death was coded according to the 6th Revision of the International Classification of Diseases (ICD) in 1950, 7th Revision in 1960, 8th Revision in 1970, and 9th Revision in 1980-1998.
[3]Starting with 1999 data, cause of death is coded according to ICD-10.
[4]Age-adjusted rates are calculated using the year 2000 standard population. Prior to 2001, age-adjusted rates were calculated using standard million proportions based on rounded population numbers. Starting with 2001 data, unrounded population numbers are used to calculate age-adjusted rates.
[5]The race groups, White, Black, Asian or Pacific Islander, and American Indian or Alaska Native, include persons of Hispanic and non-Hispanic origin. Persons of Hispanic origin may be of any race. Death rates for the American Indian or Alaska Native, Asian or Pacific Islander, and Hispanic populations are known to be underestimated.

Table 2-36. Death Rates for Homicide, by Sex, Race, Hispanic Origin, and Age, Selected Years, 1950–2015—Continued

(Deaths per 100,000 resident population.)

Sex, race, Hispanic origin, and age	2007³	2008³	2009³	2010³	2011³	2012³	2013³	2014³	2015³
All Persons									
All ages, age-adjusted⁴	6.1	5.9	5.5	5.3	5.3	5.4	5.2	5.1	5.7
All ages, crude	6.1	5.9	5.5	5.3	5.2	5.3	5.1	5.0	5.5
Under 1 year	8.5	8.2	7.9	7.9	7.3	7.3	7.2	6.3	6.6
1 to 14 years	1.3	1.3	1.2	1.1	1.2	1.1	1.1	1.1	1.2
1 to 4 years	2.5	2.6	2.3	2.4	2.5	2.1	2.1	2.3	2.3
5 to 14 years	0.9	0.8	0.7	0.6	0.7	0.8	0.7	0.7	0.7
15 to 24 years	12.9	12.2	11.2	10.7	10.4	10.5	9.8	9.5	10.8
15 to 19 years	10.1	9.4	8.6	8.3	7.8	7.6	6.6	6.7	7.5
20 to 24 years	15.8	15.0	13.8	13.2	13.0	13.3	12.8	12.1	13.8
25 to 44 years	9.5	9.1	8.5	8.2	8.1	8.5	8.2	8.1	9.2
25 to 34 years	12.0	11.5	10.4	10.4	10.0	10.3	9.9	9.6	11.0
35 to 44 years	7.1	6.9	6.7	6.0	6.2	6.7	6.4	6.4	7.1
45 to 64 years	4.0	4.0	3.8	3.8	3.8	3.9	3.8	3.7	4.1
45 to 54 years	4.9	4.8	4.6	4.4	4.6	4.6	4.5	4.5	4.9
55 to 64 years	3.0	2.9	2.9	2.9	2.9	3.0	3.0	2.9	3.2
65 years and over	2.0	2.1	2.2	2.0	2.0	2.0	2.0	2.0	2.0
65 to 74 years	2.1	2.3	2.2	2.1	2.0	2.1	2.0	2.1	2.0
75 to 84 years	2.0	1.8	2.0	1.9	2.0	2.0	2.1	2.0	2.1
85 years and over	1.6	2.3	2.3	2.0	2.2	1.9	1.9	1.9	1.7
Male									
All ages, age-adjusted⁴	9.7	9.3	8.6	8.4	8.3	8.5	8.2	8.0	9.1
All ages, crude	9.8	9.5	8.7	8.4	8.3	8.5	8.2	8.0	9.0
Under 1 year	9.7	9.3	9.0	8.8	8.2	8.1	8.7	7.1	7.1
1 to 14 years	1.5	1.5	1.3	1.4	1.4	1.3	1.2	1.2	1.5
1 to 4 years	2.6	2.8	2.3	2.8	2.9	2.4	2.3	2.4	2.8
5 to 14 years	1.0	0.9	0.9	0.8	0.8	0.9	0.8	0.8	0.9
15 to 24 years	21.8	20.6	18.8	18.2	17.6	17.7	16.7	16.1	18.4
15 to 19 years	17.0	15.9	14.5	14.0	13.0	12.8	11.4	11.2	12.7
20 to 24 years	26.8	25.5	23.4	22.6	22.1	22.4	21.6	20.6	23.7
25 to 44 years	15.3	14.9	13.6	13.3	13.2	13.9	13.4	13.2	15.1
25 to 34 years	20.2	19.3	17.0	17.3	16.6	17.1	16.4	15.9	18.4
35 to 44 years	10.7	10.7	10.3	9.2	9.6	10.6	10.1	10.3	11.5
45 to 64 years	6.1	6.1	5.7	5.6	5.7	5.8	5.7	5.7	6.3
45 to 54 years	7.3	7.3	6.8	6.7	6.8	7.0	6.9	6.9	7.6
55 to 64 years	4.5	4.4	4.2	4.3	4.4	4.4	4.3	4.3	4.8
65 years and over	2.8	2.8	3.0	2.6	2.7	2.8	2.8	2.7	2.7
65 to 74 years	3.1	3.1	3.2	2.9	2.7	3.0	2.9	2.9	2.9
75 to 84 years	2.8	2.4	2.6	2.1	2.7	2.5	2.5	2.2	2.3
85 years and over	1.6	2.5	3.1	2.2	2.5	2.2	2.9	2.2	1.9
Female									
All ages, age-adjusted⁴	2.5	2.4	2.4	2.3	2.2	2.2	2.1	2.1	2.2
All ages, crude	2.5	2.4	2.4	2.2	2.2	2.2	2.1	2.1	2.2
Under 1 year	7.2	7.1	6.8	6.9	6.2	6.5	5.5	5.4	6.1
1 to 14 years	1.2	1.1	1.1	0.9	1.0	1.0	0.9	1.0	0.9
1 to 4 years	2.4	2.4	2.4	1.9	2.2	1.8	2.0	2.2	1.8
5 to 14 years	0.7	0.6	0.5	0.5	0.5	0.6	0.5	0.6	0.5
15 to 24 years	3.4	3.3	3.1	2.9	2.9	2.9	2.6	2.5	2.8
15 to 19 years	2.7	2.6	2.5	2.3	2.2	2.0	1.6	1.9	2.1
20 to 24 years	4.2	4.0	3.7	3.4	3.5	3.7	3.6	3.1	3.5
25 to 44 years	3.6	3.3	3.4	3.1	3.1	3.0	3.0	2.9	3.1
25 to 34 years	3.7	3.6	3.7	3.3	3.3	3.3	3.2	3.2	3.5
35 to 44 years	3.5	3.1	3.1	2.9	2.8	2.8	2.7	2.6	2.8
45 to 64 years	2.1	2.0	2.1	2.0	2.0	2.0	2.0	1.8	1.9
45 to 54 years	2.5	2.4	2.4	2.3	2.4	2.3	2.3	2.2	2.2
55 to 64 years	1.5	1.5	1.6	1.7	1.5	1.6	1.7	1.5	1.7
65 years and over	1.4	1.6	1.6	1.6	1.6	1.5	1.4	1.5	1.5
65 to 74 years	1.2	1.6	1.5	1.4	1.4	1.3	1.3	1.3	1.2
75 to 84 years	1.5	1.3	1.5	1.8	1.5	1.7	1.7	1.8	1.9
85 years and over	1.6	2.3	2.0	2.0	2.1	1.7	1.4	1.8	1.7
White Male⁵									
All ages, age-adjusted⁴	5.5	5.5	4.9	4.7	4.6	4.6	4.4	4.3	4.7
All ages, crude	5.5	5.5	4.9	4.7	4.6	4.6	4.4	4.3	4.6
Under 1 year	8.1	7.7	7.1	8.5	6.5	6.4	6.8	5.8	5.9
1 to 14 years	1.0	1.1	1.0	1.0	1.1	1.0	0.9	0.9	1.0
15 to 24 years	10.5	10.2	9.1	8.2	7.6	7.5	7.1	6.5	7.3
25 to 44 years	8.4	8.3	7.3	6.9	6.8	7.1	6.5	6.8	7.2
25 to 34 years	10.4	9.9	8.3	8.3	7.9	8.1	7.4	7.5	8.0
35 to 44 years	6.5	6.9	6.3	5.5	5.6	6.0	5.6	6.0	6.3

³Starting with 1999 data, cause of death is coded according to ICD-10.
⁴Age-adjusted rates are calculated using the year 2000 standard population. Prior to 2001, age-adjusted rates were calculated using standard million proportions based on rounded population numbers. Starting with 2001 data, unrounded population numbers are used to calculate age-adjusted rates.
⁵The race groups, White, Black, Asian or Pacific Islander, and American Indian or Alaska Native, include persons of Hispanic and non-Hispanic origin. Persons of Hispanic origin may be of any race. Death rates for the American Indian or Alaska Native, Asian or Pacific Islander, and Hispanic populations are known to be underestimated.

Table 2-36. Death Rates for Homicide, by Sex, Race, Hispanic Origin, and Age, Selected Years, 1950–2015—*Continued*

(Deaths per 100,000 resident population.)

Sex, race, Hispanic origin, and age	1950[1,2]	1960[1,2]	1970[2]	1980[2]	1985[2]	1990[2]	1995	2000[3]	2005[3]	2006[3]
45 to 64 years	4.8	4.6	8.3	9.8	7.4	6.9	5.5	4.1	4.3	4.4
65 years and over	3.8	3.1	5.4	6.7	4.4	4.1	2.9	2.5	2.2	2.1
Black or African American Male[5]										
All ages, age-adjusted[4]	47.0	42.3	78.2	69.4	48.4	63.1	51.1	35.4	37.6	38.0
All ages, crude	44.7	35.0	66.0	65.7	48.3	68.5	54.5	37.2	39.6	40.4
Under 1 year	NA	10.3	14.3	18.6	16.7	21.4	20.3	23.3	16.4	21.4
1 to 14 years[6]	1.8	1.5	4.4	4.1	4.2	5.8	5.8	3.1	3.9	4.0
15 to 24 years	53.8	43.2	98.3	82.6	64.8	137.1	129.4	85.3	83.5	87.3
25 to 44 years	92.8	80.5	140.2	130.0	86.1	105.4	75.8	55.8	64.6	64.2
25 to 34 years	104.3	86.4	154.5	142.9	94.0	123.7	95.1	73.9	89.8	89.9
35 to 44 years	80.0	74.4	124.0	109.3	74.0	81.2	54.9	38.5	40.5	39.5
45 to 64 years	46.0	44.6	82.3	70.6	46.0	41.4	33.4	21.9	21.6	22.5
65 years and over	16.5	17.3	33.3	30.9	26.1	25.7	20.3	12.8	11.8	9.9
American Indian or Alaska Native Male[5]										
All ages, age-adjusted[4]	NA	NA	NA	23.3	19.1	16.7	14.4	10.7	10.1	10.5
All ages, crude	NA	NA	NA	23.1	18.4	16.6	15.7	10.7	10.9	11.2
15 to 24 years	NA	NA	NA	35.4	27.1	25.1	28.0	17.0	19.3	19.2
25 to 44 years	NA	NA	NA	39.2	28.2	25.7	24.6	17.0	14.7	16.1
45 to 64 years	NA	NA	NA	22.1	21.2	14.8	12.0	*	10.0	8.4
Asian or Pacific Islander Male[5]										
All ages, age-adjusted[4]	NA	NA	NA	9.1	5.5	7.3	7.2	4.3	4.3	4.2
All ages, crude	NA	NA	NA	8.3	5.7	7.9	7.5	4.4	4.5	4.4
15 to 24 years	NA	NA	NA	9.3	8.0	14.9	17.2	7.8	9.7	10.2
25 to 44 years	NA	NA	NA	11.3	8.6	9.6	7.4	4.6	4.9	4.1
45 to 64 years	NA	NA	NA	10.4	5.2	7.0	7.7	6.1	4.1	4.7
Hispanic or Latino Male[5,7]										
All ages, age-adjusted[4]	NA	NA	NA	NA	24.9	27.4	20.4	11.8	12.1	11.7
All ages, crude	NA	NA	NA	NA	27.2	31.0	23.5	13.4	13.7	13.2
Under 1 year	NA	NA	NA	NA	*	8.7	5.9	6.6	6.0	9.7
1 to 14 years	NA	NA	NA	NA	1.5	3.1	3.2	1.7	1.5	1.6
15 to 24 years	NA	NA	NA	NA	42.1	55.4	54.7	28.5	29.0	28.7
25 to 44 years	NA	NA	NA	NA	46.7	46.4	28.8	17.2	19.0	17.6
25 to 34 years	NA	NA	NA	NA	50.6	50.9	33.0	19.9	23.7	21.3
35 to 44 years	NA	NA	NA	NA	39.8	39.3	22.8	13.5	13.2	13.1
45 to 64 years	NA	NA	NA	NA	19.6	20.5	14.7	9.1	8.3	8.4
65 years and over	NA	NA	NA	NA	8.9	9.4	5.8	4.4	4.6	3.3
White, not Hispanic or Latino Male[7]										
All ages, age-adjusted[4]	NA	NA	NA	NA	6.1	5.6	4.8	3.6	3.6	3.6
All ages, crude	NA	NA	NA	NA	6.2	5.8	4.9	3.6	3.6	3.7
Under 1 year	NA	NA	NA	NA	4.6	5.4	6.8	8.3	7.3	6.8
1 to 14 years	NA	NA	NA	NA	1.2	0.9	1.1	1.0	0.8	0.9
15 to 24 years	NA	NA	NA	NA	7.6	7.5	7.2	4.7	4.8	4.8
25 to 44 years	NA	NA	NA	NA	9.2	8.7	7.2	5.2	5.2	5.2
25 to 34 years	NA	NA	NA	NA	9.3	9.3	7.7	5.2	5.6	5.6
35 to 44 years	NA	NA	NA	NA	9.1	8.0	6.7	5.2	4.9	4.9
45 to 64 years	NA	NA	NA	NA	6.3	5.7	4.6	3.6	3.8	3.9
65 years and over	NA	NA	NA	NA	4.4	3.7	2.6	2.3	2.1	2.1
White Female[4]										
All ages, age-adjusted[4]	1.4	1.5	2.3	3.2	2.9	2.7	2.7	2.1	1.9	2.0
All ages, crude	1.4	1.4	2.1	3.2	2.9	2.8	2.7	2.1	1.9	1.9
Under 1 year	3.9	3.5	2.9	4.3	4.3	5.1	5.1	5.0	5.7	6.6
1 to 14 years	0.4	0.4	0.7	1.1	1.1	1.0	1.1	0.8	0.8	0.8
15 to 24 years	1.3	1.5	2.7	4.7	3.6	4.0	4.0	2.7	2.3	2.4
25 to 44 years	2.0	2.1	3.3	4.2	4.1	3.8	3.7	2.9	2.8	2.5
45 to 64 years	1.5	1.7	2.1	2.6	2.6	2.3	2.2	1.8	1.5	1.8
65 years and over	1.2	1.2	1.9	2.9	2.6	2.2	2.0	1.6	1.6	1.5
Black or African American Female[4]										
All ages, age-adjusted[4]	11.1	11.4	14.7	13.2	10.6	12.5	10.4	7.1	6.0	6.4
All ages, crude	11.5	10.4	13.2	13.5	11.0	13.4	10.9	7.2	6.1	6.5
Under 1 year	NA	13.8	10.7	12.8	10.7	22.8	20.1	22.2	12.9	11.3
1 to 14 years[6]	1.8	1.2	3.1	3.3	3.3	4.7	3.4	2.7	2.3	2.5
15 to 24 years	16.5	11.9	17.7	18.4	14.2	18.9	16.4	10.7	8.7	9.3
25 to 44 years	22.5	22.7	25.3	22.6	17.8	21.0	17.1	11.0	9.3	10.1
45 to 64 years	6.8	10.3	13.4	10.8	7.9	6.5	5.9	4.5	4.8	5.1
65 years and over	3.6	3.0	7.4	8.0	7.8	9.4	6.8	3.5	3.0	2.5

NA = Not available.
* = Rates based on fewer than 20 deaths are considered unreliable and are not shown.
[1]Includes deaths of persons who were not residents of the 50 states and the District of Columbia.
[2]Underlying cause of death was coded according to the 6th Revision of the International Classification of Diseases (ICD) in 1950, 7th Revision in 1960, 8th Revision in 1970, and 9th Revision in 1980-1998.
[3]Starting with 1999 data, cause of death is coded according to ICD-10.
[4]Age-adjusted rates are calculated using the year 2000 standard population. Prior to 2001, age-adjusted rates were calculated using standard million proportions based on rounded population numbers. Starting with 2001 data, unrounded population numbers are used to calculate age-adjusted rates.
[5]The race groups, White, Black, Asian or Pacific Islander, and American Indian or Alaska Native, include persons of Hispanic and non-Hispanic origin. Persons of Hispanic origin may be of any race. Death rates for the American Indian or Alaska Native, Asian or Pacific Islander, and Hispanic populations are known to be underestimated.
[6]In 1950, rate is for the age group under 15 years.
[7]Prior to 1997, excludes data from states lacking an Hispanic-origin item on the death certificate.

Table 2-36. Death Rates for Homicide, by Sex, Race, Hispanic Origin, and Age, Selected Years, 1950–2015—*Continued*

(Deaths per 100,000 resident population.)

Sex, race, Hispanic origin, and age	2007[3]	2008[3]	2009[3]	2010[3]	2011[3]	2012[3]	2013[3]	2014[3]	2015[3]
45 to 64 years	4.2	4.4	4.1	4.1	4.1	4.1	4.0	4.0	4.4
65 years and over	2.2	2.3	2.5	2.1	2.3	2.4	2.4	2.2	2.3
Black or African American Male[5]									
All ages, age-adjusted[4]	37.1	34.4	32.0	31.5	31.2	32.8	31.6	30.6	35.4
All ages, crude	39.3	36.5	33.8	33.4	33.0	34.5	33.1	32.1	37.3
Under 1 year	19.8	17.5	18.7	12.3	17.0	17.6	17.9	13.9	13.4
1 to 14 years[6]	3.9	3.7	3.2	3.4	3.1	3.2	2.6	3.1	3.7
15 to 24 years	83.9	76.7	70.7	71.0	69.4	70.8	66.6	65.0	74.9
25 to 44 years	63.3	60.1	56.4	55.9	55.4	59.2	57.9	54.8	65.5
25 to 34 years	86.2	82.2	74.1	76.1	72.5	73.9	73.2	67.7	81.4
35 to 44 years	40.7	38.0	38.0	34.5	36.5	42.6	40.4	39.7	46.4
45 to 64 years	21.5	19.9	18.0	17.6	18.4	18.8	18.4	18.2	20.4
65 years and over	10.6	8.4	8.8	8.0	6.8	7.5	7.3	8.4	7.2
American Indian or Alaska Native Male[5]									
All ages, age-adjusted[4]	7.9	9.2	8.9	8.8	8.9	9.0	8.2	9.1	9.8
All ages, crude	8.5	9.6	9.3	9.5	9.0	9.4	8.3	9.2	9.9
15 to 24 years	12.2	13.2	15.8	17.6	11.2	12.4	7.1	12.1	15.2
25 to 44 years	15.0	16.1	15.0	14.8	13.8	15.3	15.4	13.6	15.1
45 to 64 years	5.8	7.8	7.5	6.5	10.9	9.7	8.0	9.7	10.1
Asian or Pacific Islander Male[5]									
All ages, age-adjusted[4]	3.1	2.9	2.8	2.6	2.9	2.5	2.3	2.2	2.3
All ages, crude	3.3	3.1	3.0	2.7	2.9	2.7	2.3	2.3	2.4
15 to 24 years	6.3	5.9	4.4	4.0	4.2	3.8	3.5	3.4	2.9
25 to 44 years	3.9	3.5	3.2	3.3	4.1	3.7	2.7	3.0	3.1
45 to 64 years	3.3	2.8	3.7	3.1	2.0	2.9	2.5	2.5	2.8
Hispanic or Latino Male[5,7]									
All ages, age-adjusted[4]	11.1	10.3	9.7	8.7	7.9	7.9	7.3	7.2	7.9
All ages, crude	12.4	11.4	10.5	9.5	8.6	8.5	7.8	7.6	8.4
Under 1 year	8.1	7.4	5.7	7.0	5.8	5.0	6.8	4.5	*
1 to 14 years	1.2	1.2	1.2	1.1	1.3	0.9	0.9	0.7	1.2
15 to 24 years	27.1	24.5	22.9	19.7	17.6	17.1	15.3	14.2	16.5
25 to 44 years	16.9	15.8	14.2	13.2	12.0	12.3	11.0	11.6	12.2
25 to 34 years	21.3	18.8	16.5	16.8	14.6	14.7	13.3	13.1	14.3
35 to 44 years	11.7	12.3	11.5	8.9	9.0	9.5	8.4	9.9	9.9
45 to 64 years	7.7	7.5	6.9	6.9	5.9	5.9	6.1	5.6	6.3
65 years and over	3.9	3.1	4.9	3.2	3.5	3.3	2.9	3.3	2.9
White, not Hispanic or Latino Male[7]									
All ages, age-adjusted[4]	3.8	3.9	3.4	3.3	3.4	3.5	3.4	3.3	3.6
All ages, crude	3.7	3.9	3.4	3.3	3.4	3.5	3.3	3.3	3.5
Under 1 year	7.6	7.4	7.3	8.7	6.9	6.8	6.5	6.5	7.0
1 to 14 years	0.9	1.0	0.8	0.9	1.0	1.0	0.9	0.9	1.0
15 to 24 years	5.0	5.2	4.1	4.1	3.9	3.9	3.9	3.5	3.8
25 to 44 years	5.7	5.9	4.9	4.7	4.9	5.1	4.9	4.9	5.3
25 to 34 years	6.4	6.6	5.2	5.0	5.4	5.5	5.2	5.3	5.5
35 to 44 years	5.1	5.3	4.7	4.4	4.5	4.8	4.6	4.6	5.0
45 to 64 years	3.7	3.9	3.7	3.6	3.7	3.7	3.6	3.6	3.9
65 years and over	2.0	2.2	2.3	2.0	2.2	2.3	2.3	2.0	2.2
White Female[4]									
All ages, age-adjusted[4]	2.0	1.9	1.9	1.8	1.8	1.8	1.7	1.7	1.8
All ages, crude	1.9	1.9	1.9	1.8	1.8	1.8	1.7	1.7	1.7
Under 1 year	6.4	5.6	5.1	5.8	4.9	5.9	4.3	4.5	4.2
1 to 14 years	0.9	0.8	0.9	0.7	0.8	0.8	0.7	0.8	0.7
15 to 24 years	2.5	2.2	2.1	2.0	1.9	1.9	1.8	1.7	1.9
25 to 44 years	2.8	2.7	2.7	2.4	2.5	2.4	2.3	2.3	2.5
45 to 64 years	1.7	1.8	1.8	1.7	1.7	1.7	1.7	1.5	1.7
65 years and over	1.3	1.5	1.5	1.6	1.4	1.4	1.4	1.4	1.4
Black or African American Female[4]									
All ages, age-adjusted[4]	6.0	5.4	5.2	5.0	4.9	4.9	4.9	4.7	4.9
All ages, crude	6.1	5.5	5.3	5.1	5.0	4.9	4.9	4.7	4.9
Under 1 year	11.7	15.4	15.4	13.9	11.9	11.5	12.4	10.8	15.8
1 to 14 years[6]	2.7	2.5	2.2	2.0	2.2	2.0	2.1	2.2	1.9
15 to 24 years	8.6	9.3	8.0	7.5	8.1	8.0	6.9	7.0	7.5
25 to 44 years	9.1	7.6	7.8	7.4	7.0	7.1	7.2	6.7	7.4
45 to 64 years	4.8	3.7	4.0	4.2	3.9	3.9	4.3	3.7	3.7
65 years and over	2.6	2.3	2.2	1.8	2.3	2.2	2.0	2.4	2.0

NA = Not available.

* = Rates based on fewer than 20 deaths are considered unreliable and are not shown.

[3]Starting with 1999 data, cause of death is coded according to ICD-10.

[4]Age-adjusted rates are calculated using the year 2000 standard population. Prior to 2001, age-adjusted rates were calculated using standard million proportions based on rounded population numbers. Starting with 2001 data, unrounded population numbers are used to calculate age-adjusted rates.

[5]The race groups, White, Black, Asian or Pacific Islander, and American Indian or Alaska Native, include persons of Hispanic and non-Hispanic origin. Persons of Hispanic origin may be of any race. Death rates for the American Indian or Alaska Native, Asian or Pacific Islander, and Hispanic populations are known to be underestimated.

[6]In 1950, rate is for the age group under 15 years.

[7]Prior to 1997, excludes data from states lacking an Hispanic-origin item on the death certificate.

Table 2-36. Death Rates for Homicide, by Sex, Race, Hispanic Origin, and Age, Selected Years, 1950–2015—*Continued*

(Deaths per 100,000 resident population.)

Sex, race, Hispanic origin, and age	1950[1,2]	1960[1,2]	1970[2]	1980[2]	1985[2]	1990[2]	1995	2000[3]	2005[3]	2006[3]
American Indian or Alaska Native Female[4]										
All ages, age-adjusted[4]	NA	NA	NA	8.1	4.8	4.6	5.3	3.0	3.5	2.6
All ages, crude	NA	NA	NA	7.7	4.5	4.8	5.1	2.9	3.6	2.6
15 to 24 years	NA	NA	NA	*	*	*	*	*	*	*
25 to 44 years	NA	NA	NA	13.7	*	6.9	8.3	5.9	5.4	5.2
45 to 64 years	NA	NA	NA	*	*	*	*	*	*	*
Asian or Pacific Islander Female[5]										
All ages, age-adjusted[4]	NA	NA	NA	3.1	2.6	2.8	2.4	1.7	1.5	1.3
All ages, crude	NA	NA	NA	3.1	2.8	2.8	2.6	1.7	1.5	1.4
15 to 24 years	NA	NA	NA	*	*	*	*	*	2.5	*
25 to 44 years	NA	NA	NA	4.6	2.9	3.8	3.6	2.2	1.6	1.6
45 to 64 years	NA	NA	NA	*	*	*	2.2	2.0	1.2	1.9
Hispanic or Latina Female[5,7]										
All ages, age-adjusted[4]	NA	NA	NA	NA	4.1	4.3	4.0	2.8	2.3	2.3
All ages, crude	NA	NA	NA	NA	4.3	4.7	4.2	2.8	2.4	2.4
Under 1 year	NA	NA	NA	NA	*	*	*	7.4	6.2	6.2
1 to 14 years	NA	NA	NA	NA	1.5	1.9	1.8	1.0	1.0	1.0
15 to 24 years	NA	NA	NA	NA	5.7	8.1	6.4	3.7	3.4	3.6
25 to 44 years	NA	NA	NA	NA	6.8	6.1	5.6	3.7	3.3	3.1
45 to 64 years	NA	NA	NA	NA	3.2	3.3	3.4	2.9	1.9	1.8
65 years and over	NA	NA	NA	NA	*	*	2.4	2.4	*	*
White, not Hispanic or Latina Female[7]										
All ages, age-adjusted[4]	NA	NA	NA	NA	2.9	2.5	2.3	1.9	1.8	1.8
All ages, crude	NA	NA	NA	NA	2.9	2.5	2.3	1.9	1.8	1.8
Under 1 year	NA	NA	NA	NA	4.1	4.4	4.4	4.1	5.3	6.5
1 to 14 years	NA	NA	NA	NA	1.0	0.8	0.9	0.8	0.7	0.8
15 to 24 years	NA	NA	NA	NA	3.5	3.3	3.4	2.3	2.0	2.1
25 to 44 years	NA	NA	NA	NA	3.9	3.5	3.3	2.7	2.7	2.3
45 to 64 years	NA	NA	NA	NA	3.6	2.2	1.9	1.6	1.4	1.8
65 years and over	NA	NA	NA	NA	2.6	2.2	1.9	1.6	1.6	1.5

NA = Not available.

* = Rates based on fewer than 20 deaths are considered unreliable and are not shown.

[1]Includes deaths of persons who were not residents of the 50 states and the District of Columbia.

[2]Underlying cause of death was coded according to the 6th Revision of the International Classification of Diseases (ICD) in 1950, 7th Revision in 1960, 8th Revision in 1970, and 9th Revision in 1980-1998.

[3]Starting with 1999 data, cause of death is coded according to ICD-10.

[4]Age-adjusted rates are calculated using the year 2000 standard population. Prior to 2001, age-adjusted rates were calculated using standard million proportions based on rounded population numbers. Starting with 2001 data, unrounded population numbers are used to calculate age-adjusted rates.

[5]The race groups, White, Black, Asian or Pacific Islander, and American Indian or Alaska Native, include persons of Hispanic and non-Hispanic origin. Persons of Hispanic origin may be of any race. Death rates for the American Indian or Alaska Native, Asian or Pacific Islander, and Hispanic populations are known to be underestimated.

[7]Prior to 1997, excludes data from states lacking an Hispanic-origin item on the death certificate.

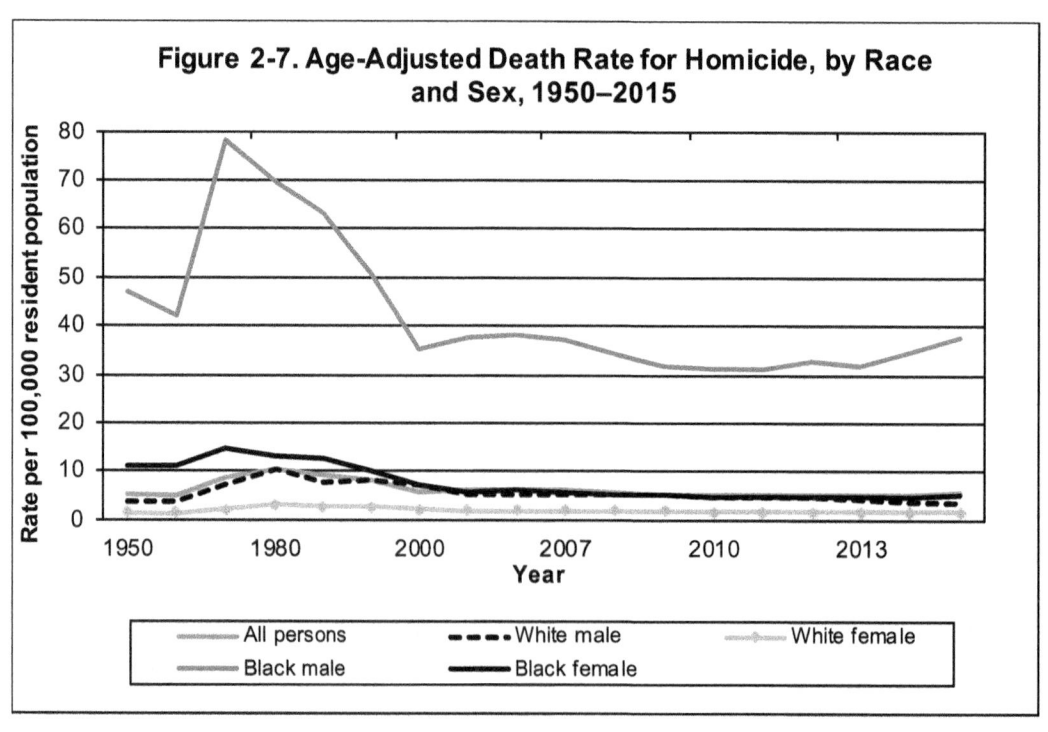

Figure 2-7. Age-Adjusted Death Rate for Homicide, by Race and Sex, 1950–2015

Table 2-36. Death Rates for Homicide, by Sex, Race, Hispanic Origin, and Age, Selected Years, 1950–2015—*Continued*

(Deaths per 100,000 resident population.)

Sex, race, Hispanic origin, and age	2007[3]	2008[3]	2009[3]	2010[3]	2011[3]	2012[3]	2013[3]	2014[3]	2015[3]
American Indian or Alaska Native Female[4]									
All ages, age-adjusted[4]	3.1	3.1	2.9	2.5	2.8	2.4	2.4	2.5	2.5
All ages, crude	3.0	3.2	3.0	2.5	2.7	2.6	2.4	2.4	2.5
15 to 24 years	*	*	*	*	*	*	*	*	*
25 to 44 years	4.4	3.9	*	4.7	*	3.6	3.7	4.2	4.1
45 to 64 years	*	*	*	*	*	*	*	*	*
Asian or Pacific Islander Female[5]									
All ages, age-adjusted[4]	1.3	1.2	1.3	1.2	1.3	1.2	0.9	1.0	1.0
All ages, crude	1.3	1.2	1.3	1.2	1.3	1.2	0.9	1.0	1.0
15 to 24 years	*	*	*	*	*	*	*	*	*
25 to 44 years	1.8	1.3	1.5	1.3	1.5	1.2	1.3	0.8	1.0
45 to 64 years	1.5	1.1	1.6	1.4	1.3	1.6	1.1	1.5	1.0
Hispanic or Latina Female[5,7]									
All ages, age-adjusted[4]	2.2	2.3	2.2	1.8	1.8	1.8	1.6	1.7	1.8
All ages, crude	2.4	2.4	2.2	1.8	1.9	1.8	1.6	1.8	1.8
Under 1 year	7.1	5.4	6.1	6.6	3.9	4.6	4.0	4.6	4.2
1 to 14 years	1.2	1.1	1.1	0.5	0.9	0.8	0.7	1.0	0.5
15 to 24 years	3.2	3.3	3.0	2.6	2.3	2.2	2.5	2.7	2.4
25 to 44 years	3.2	3.1	2.9	2.5	2.8	2.4	2.4	2.3	2.5
45 to 64 years	1.7	2.0	2.0	1.6	1.5	1.8	1.2	1.4	1.7
65 years and over	*	1.6	1.3	1.3	*	*	*	*	1.2
White, not Hispanic or Latina Female[7]									
All ages, age-adjusted[4]	1.9	1.8	1.8	1.8	1.7	1.7	1.7	1.6	1.7
All ages, crude	1.8	1.8	1.8	1.7	1.7	1.7	1.7	1.6	1.7
Under 1 year	5.9	5.7	4.2	5.3	5.0	6.1	4.4	4.4	4.4
1 to 14 years	0.8	0.7	0.8	0.7	0.7	0.8	0.7	0.7	0.7
15 to 24 years	2.2	1.8	1.7	1.8	1.7	1.7	1.6	1.3	1.7
25 to 44 years	2.6	2.5	2.5	2.4	2.3	2.4	2.2	2.3	2.4
45 to 64 years	1.7	1.7	1.7	1.7	1.7	1.7	1.8	1.5	1.7
65 years and over	1.3	1.5	1.5	1.6	1.5	1.4	1.5	1.5	1.4

NA = Not available.
* = Rates based on fewer than 20 deaths are considered unreliable and are not shown.
[3]Starting with 1999 data, cause of death is coded according to ICD-10.
[4]Age-adjusted rates are calculated using the year 2000 standard population. Prior to 2001, age-adjusted rates were calculated using standard million proportions based on rounded population numbers. Starting with 2001 data, unrounded population numbers are used to calculate age-adjusted rates.
[5]The race groups, White, Black, Asian or Pacific Islander, and American Indian or Alaska Native, include persons of Hispanic and non-Hispanic origin. Persons of Hispanic origin may be of any race. Death rates for the American Indian or Alaska Native, Asian or Pacific Islander, and Hispanic populations are known to be underestimated.
[7]Prior to 1997, excludes data from states lacking an Hispanic-origin item on the death certificate.

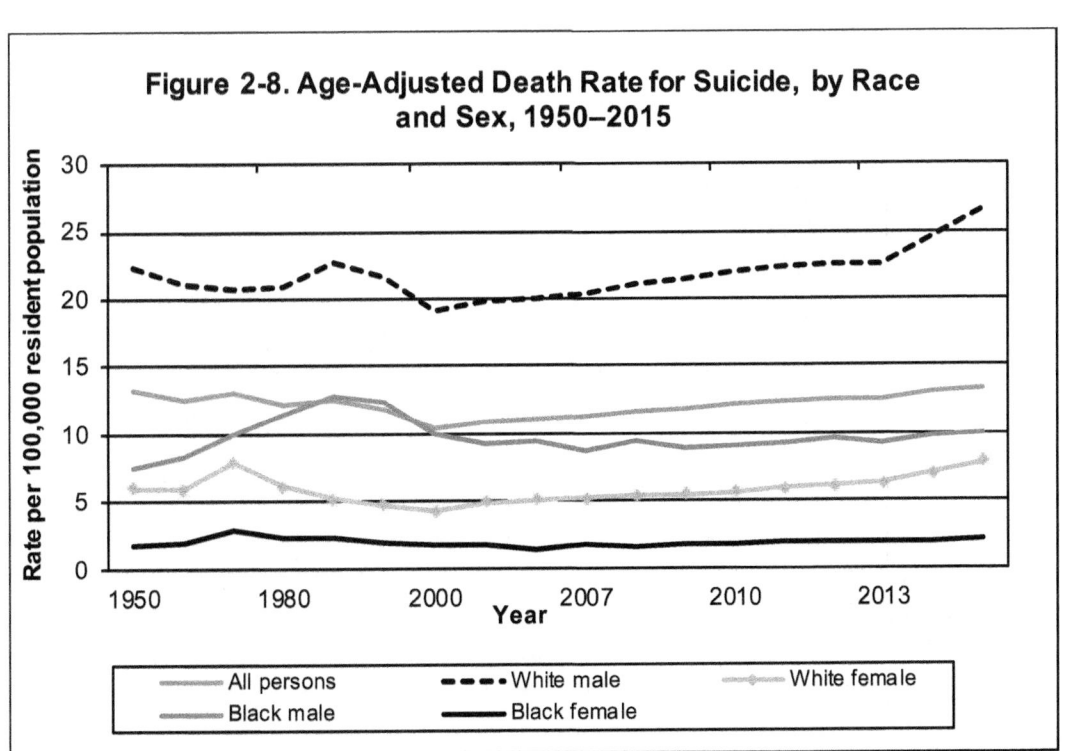

Figure 2-8. Age-Adjusted Death Rate for Suicide, by Race and Sex, 1950–2015

Table 2-37. Death Rates for Suicide, by Sex, Race, Hispanic Origin, and Age, Selected Years, 1950–2015

(Deaths per 100,000 resident population.)

Sex, race, Hispanic origin, and age	1950[1,2]	1960[1,2]	1970[2]	1980[2]	1985	1990[2]	1995	2000[3]	2005[3]	2006[3]
All Persons										
All ages, age-adjusted[4]	13.2	12.5	13.1	12.2	12.5	12.5	11.8	10.4	10.9	11.0
All ages, crude	11.4	10.6	11.6	11.9	12.4	12.4	11.7	10.4	11.0	11.2
Under 1 year	X	X	X	X	X	X	X	X	X	X
1 to 4 years	X	X	X	X	X	X	X	X	X	X
5 to 14 years	0.2	0.3	0.3	0.4	0.8	0.8	0.9	0.7	0.7	0.5
15 to 24 years	4.5	5.2	8.8	12.3	12.8	13.2	13.0	10.2	9.9	9.8
15 to 19 years	2.7	3.6	5.9	8.5	9.9	11.1	10.3	8.0	7.5	7.1
20 to 24 years	6.2	7.1	12.2	16.1	15.4	15.1	15.8	12.5	12.4	12.5
25 to 44 years	11.6	12.2	15.4	15.6	15.0	15.2	15.1	13.4	13.9	14.0
25 to 34 years	9.1	10.0	14.1	16.0	15.3	15.2	15.0	12.0	12.7	12.7
35 to 44 years	14.3	14.2	16.9	15.4	14.6	15.3	15.1	14.5	15.1	15.2
45 to 64 years	23.5	22.0	20.6	15.9	16.3	15.3	13.9	13.5	15.3	16.0
45 to 54 years	20.9	20.7	20.0	15.9	15.7	14.8	14.4	14.4	16.5	17.2
55 to 64 years	26.8	23.7	21.4	15.9	16.8	16.0	13.2	12.1	13.7	14.4
65 years and over	30.0	24.5	20.8	17.6	20.4	20.5	17.9	15.2	14.7	14.3
65 to 74 years	29.6	23.0	20.8	16.9	18.7	17.9	15.7	12.5	12.4	12.4
75 to 84 years	31.1	27.9	21.2	19.1	23.9	24.9	20.6	17.6	16.8	15.8
85 years and over	28.8	26.0	19.0	19.2	19.4	22.2	21.3	19.6	18.3	17.3
Male										
All ages, age-adjusted[4]	21.2	20.0	19.8	19.9	21.1	21.5	20.3	17.7	18.1	18.1
All ages, crude	17.8	16.5	16.8	18.6	20.0	20.4	19.5	17.1	17.8	17.9
Under 1 year	X	X	X	X	X	X	X	X	X	X
1 to 4 years	X	X	X	X	X	X	X	X	X	X
5 to 14 years	0.3	0.4	0.5	0.6	1.2	1.1	1.3	1.2	1.0	0.7
15 to 24 years	6.5	8.2	13.5	20.2	21.0	22.0	22.0	17.1	16.1	16.0
15 to 19 years	3.5	5.6	8.8	13.8	15.8	18.1	17.1	13.0	11.8	11.3
20 to 24 years	9.3	11.5	19.3	26.8	25.7	25.7	27.0	21.4	20.4	21.0
25 to 44 years	17.2	17.9	20.9	24.0	23.7	24.4	24.4	21.3	22.1	22.1
25 to 34 years	13.4	14.7	19.8	25.0	24.7	24.8	24.8	19.6	20.6	20.5
35 to 44 years	21.3	21.0	22.1	22.5	22.3	23.9	24.0	22.8	23.4	23.5
45 to 64 years	37.1	34.4	30.0	23.7	25.3	24.3	22.2	21.3	23.9	24.6
45 to 54 years	32.0	31.6	27.9	22.9	23.6	23.2	22.5	22.4	25.2	26.2
55 to 64 years	43.6	38.1	32.7	24.5	27.1	25.7	21.8	19.4	22.0	22.5
65 years and over	52.8	44.0	38.4	35.0	40.9	41.6	36.2	31.1	29.5	28.4
65 to 74 years	50.5	39.6	36.0	30.4	33.9	32.2	28.5	22.7	22.3	22.2
75 to 84 years	58.3	52.5	42.8	42.3	53.1	56.1	44.9	38.6	35.5	32.9
85 years and over	58.3	57.4	42.4	50.6	56.2	65.9	62.7	57.5	49.9	48.0
Female										
All ages, age-adjusted[4]	5.6	5.6	7.4	5.7	5.2	4.8	4.3	4.0	4.4	4.5
All ages, crude	5.1	4.9	6.6	5.5	5.2	4.8	4.3	4.0	4.5	4.6
Under 1 year	X	X	X	X	X	X	X	X	X	X
1 to 4 years	X	X	X	X	X	X	X	X	X	X
5 to 14 years	0.1	0.1	0.2	0.2	0.4	0.4	0.4	0.3	0.3	0.3
15 to 24 years	2.6	2.2	4.2	4.3	4.3	3.9	3.6	3.0	3.5	3.2
15 to 19 years	1.8	1.6	2.9	3.0	3.7	3.7	3.1	2.7	3.0	2.8
20 to 24 years	3.3	2.9	5.7	5.5	4.9	4.1	4.2	3.2	4.0	3.6
25 to 44 years	6.2	6.6	10.2	7.7	6.5	6.2	5.8	5.4	5.8	5.9
25 to 34 years	4.9	5.5	8.6	7.1	5.9	5.6	5.1	4.3	4.7	4.7
35 to 44 years	7.5	7.7	11.9	8.5	7.1	6.8	6.4	6.4	6.8	7.0
45 to 64 years	9.9	10.2	12.0	8.9	8.0	7.1	6.1	6.2	7.2	7.7
45 to 54 years	9.9	10.2	12.6	9.4	8.3	6.9	6.6	6.7	8.0	8.4
55 to 64 years	9.9	10.2	11.4	8.4	7.8	7.3	5.3	5.4	6.0	6.8
65 years and over	9.4	8.4	8.1	6.1	6.6	6.4	5.4	4.0	4.0	3.9
65 to 74 years	10.1	8.4	9.0	6.5	6.9	6.7	5.4	4.0	4.0	4.0
75 to 84 years	8.1	8.9	7.0	5.5	6.7	6.3	5.4	4.0	4.0	4.0
85 years and over	8.2	6.0	5.9	5.5	4.7	5.4	5.4	4.2	4.3	3.3
White Male[5]										
All ages, age-adjusted[4]	22.3	21.1	20.8	20.9	22.4	22.8	21.6	19.1	19.8	19.9
All ages, crude	19.0	17.6	18.0	19.9	21.6	22.0	21.1	18.8	19.9	20.0
15 to 24 years	6.6	8.6	13.9	21.4	22.3	23.2	23.1	17.9	17.3	17.2
25 to 44 years	17.9	18.5	21.5	24.6	24.8	25.4	25.8	22.9	24.2	24.2
45 to 64 years	39.3	36.5	31.9	25.0	27.0	26.0	23.9	23.2	26.6	27.5
65 years and over	55.8	46.7	41.1	37.2	43.7	44.2	38.5	33.3	32.0	30.8
65 to 74 years	53.2	42.0	38.7	32.5	35.8	34.2	30.1	24.3	24.5	24.3

X = Not applicable.

[1]Includes deaths of persons who were not residents of the 50 states and the District of Columbia.

[2]Underlying cause of death was coded according to the 6th Revision of the International Classification of Diseases (ICD) in 1950, 7th Revision in 1960, 8th Revision in 1970, and 9th Revision in 1980-1998.

[3]Starting with 1999 data, cause of death is coded according to ICD-10.

[4]Age-adjusted rates are calculated using the year 2000 standard population. Prior to 2001, age-adjusted rates were calculated using standard million proportions based on rounded population numbers. Starting with 2001 data, unrounded population numbers are used to calculate age-adjusted rates.

[5]The race groups, White, Black, Asian or Pacific Islander, and American Indian or Alaska Native, include persons of Hispanic and non-Hispanic origin. Persons of Hispanic origin may be of any race. Death rates for the American Indian or Alaska Native, Asian or Pacific Islander, and Hispanic populations are known to be underestimated.

Table 2-37. Death Rates for Suicide, by Sex, Race, Hispanic Origin, and Age, Selected Years, 1950–2015—*Continued*

(Deaths per 100,000 resident population.)

Sex, race, Hispanic origin, and age	2007[3]	2008[3]	2009[3]	2010[3]	2011[3]	2012[3]	2013[3]	2014[3]	2015[3]
All Persons									
All ages, age-adjusted[4]	11.3	11.6	11.8	12.1	12.3	12.6	12.6	13.0	13.3
All ages, crude	11.5	11.8	12.0	12.4	12.7	12.9	13.0	13.4	13.7
Under 1 year	X	X	X	X	X	X	X	X	X
1 to 4 years	X	X	X	X	X	X	X	X	X
5 to 14 years	0.5	0.5	0.6	0.7	0.7	0.8	1.0	1.0	1.0
15 to 24 years	9.6	9.9	10.0	10.5	11.0	11.1	11.1	11.6	12.5
15 to 19 years	6.7	7.2	7.5	7.5	8.3	8.3	8.3	8.7	9.8
20 to 24 years	12.6	12.7	12.6	13.6	13.6	13.7	13.7	14.2	15.1
25 to 44 years	14.5	14.6	14.6	15.0	15.4	15.7	15.5	15.8	16.4
25 to 34 years	13.3	13.2	13.1	14.0	14.6	14.7	14.8	15.1	15.7
35 to 44 years	15.7	15.9	16.1	16.0	16.2	16.7	16.2	16.6	17.1
45 to 64 years	16.7	17.5	17.9	18.6	18.6	19.1	19.0	19.5	19.6
45 to 54 years	17.7	18.6	19.2	19.6	19.8	20.0	19.7	20.2	20.3
55 to 64 years	15.3	16.0	16.4	17.5	17.1	18.0	18.1	18.8	18.9
65 years and over	14.3	14.8	14.8	14.9	15.3	15.4	16.1	16.7	16.6
65 to 74 years	12.4	13.6	13.7	13.7	14.1	14.0	15.0	15.6	15.2
75 to 84 years	16.2	16.1	15.8	15.7	16.5	16.8	17.1	17.5	17.9
85 years and over	17.0	16.4	16.4	17.6	16.9	17.8	18.6	19.3	19.4
Male									
All ages, age-adjusted[4]	18.5	19.0	19.2	19.8	20.0	20.4	20.3	20.7	21.1
All ages, crude	18.4	19.0	19.3	19.9	20.2	20.6	20.6	21.1	21.5
Under 1 year	X	X	X	X	X	X	X	X	X
1 to 4 years	X	X	X	X	X	X	X	X	X
5 to 14 years	0.6	0.7	0.8	0.9	1.0	1.1	1.2	1.3	1.2
15 to 24 years	15.7	16.0	16.1	16.9	17.6	17.4	17.3	18.2	19.4
15 to 19 years	10.8	11.3	11.6	11.7	12.9	12.5	12.4	13.0	14.2
20 to 24 years	20.9	21.0	20.8	22.2	22.3	22.0	21.9	22.9	24.2
25 to 44 years	22.9	22.8	23.0	23.6	24.0	24.5	24.1	24.4	25.2
25 to 34 years	21.5	21.2	21.0	22.5	23.1	23.4	23.4	23.8	24.7
35 to 44 years	24.2	24.4	24.9	24.6	24.9	25.7	24.8	25.0	25.9
45 to 64 years	25.7	27.4	27.9	29.2	28.9	29.5	29.0	29.7	29.5
45 to 54 years	27.0	28.6	29.3	30.4	30.1	30.2	29.6	30.0	30.1
55 to 64 years	23.9	25.8	26.1	27.7	27.3	28.7	28.3	29.4	28.9
65 years and over	28.4	29.2	29.1	29.0	29.4	29.5	30.9	31.4	31.0
65 to 74 years	22.0	24.3	24.3	23.9	24.4	24.1	26.0	26.6	26.2
75 to 84 years	33.8	33.5	32.9	32.3	33.8	34.2	34.7	34.9	35.2
85 years and over	46.6	43.0	44.0	47.3	44.1	46.9	48.5	49.9	48.2
Female									
All ages, age-adjusted[4]	4.6	4.8	4.9	5.0	5.2	5.4	5.5	5.8	6.0
All ages, crude	4.8	4.9	5.0	5.2	5.4	5.5	5.7	6.0	6.2
Under 1 year	X	X	X	X	X	X	X	X	X
1 to 4 years	X	X	X	X	X	X	X	X	X
5 to 14 years	0.3	0.3	0.5	0.4	0.4	0.4	0.7	0.7	0.8
15 to 24 years	3.1	3.5	3.6	3.9	4.0	4.5	4.5	4.6	5.3
15 to 19 years	2.4	3.0	3.2	3.1	3.5	3.9	3.9	4.2	5.1
20 to 24 years	3.9	4.0	4.1	4.7	4.5	4.9	5.2	5.0	5.5
25 to 44 years	6.2	6.3	6.2	6.4	6.8	6.8	6.8	7.2	7.5
25 to 34 years	5.0	5.1	5.1	5.3	6.0	5.9	6.1	6.3	6.6
35 to 44 years	7.3	7.4	7.4	7.5	7.6	7.7	7.6	8.2	8.4
45 to 64 years	8.1	8.1	8.5	8.6	8.8	9.1	9.4	9.8	10.2
45 to 54 years	8.7	9.0	9.3	9.0	9.8	10.2	10.0	10.7	10.7
55 to 64 years	7.2	6.9	7.4	8.0	7.6	8.0	8.7	8.9	9.7
65 years and over	3.9	4.1	4.0	4.2	4.5	4.5	4.6	5.0	5.1
65 to 74 years	4.2	4.4	4.6	4.8	5.2	5.2	5.4	5.9	5.7
75 to 84 years	3.8	3.8	3.6	3.7	3.8	3.9	3.9	4.3	4.6
85 years and over	3.4	3.8	3.2	3.3	3.5	3.2	3.3	3.4	4.2
White Male[6]									
All ages, age-adjusted[4]	20.4	21.1	21.4	22.0	22.3	22.6	22.6	23.3	23.6
All ages, crude	20.7	21.5	21.9	22.6	23.0	23.3	23.4	24.2	24.6
15 to 24 years	16.9	17.2	17.6	18.3	19.3	19.0	18.7	19.9	20.9
25 to 44 years	25.3	25.4	25.7	26.2	26.8	27.2	26.8	27.5	28.6
45 to 64 years	28.8	30.8	31.4	33.0	32.8	33.5	33.0	34.0	33.8
65 years and over	30.9	31.6	31.5	31.7	32.1	32.2	34.1	34.7	34.3
65 to 74 years	24.1	26.3	26.6	26.3	26.7	26.4	28.9	29.5	29.1

X = Not applicable.

[3]Starting with 1999 data, cause of death is coded according to ICD-10.

[4]Age-adjusted rates are calculated using the year 2000 standard population. Prior to 2001, age-adjusted rates were calculated using standard million proportions based on rounded population numbers. Starting with 2001 data, unrounded population numbers are used to calculate age-adjusted rates.

[5]The race groups, White, Black, Asian or Pacific Islander, and American Indian or Alaska Native, include persons of Hispanic and non-Hispanic origin. Persons of Hispanic origin may be of any race. Death rates for the American Indian or Alaska Native, Asian or Pacific Islander, and Hispanic populations are known to be underestimated.

[6]In 1950, rate is for the age group 75 years and over.

[7]Prior to 1997, excludes data from states lacking an Hispanic-origin item on the death certificate.

Table 2-37. Death Rates for Suicide, by Sex, Race, Hispanic Origin, and Age, Selected Years, 1950–2015—Continued

(Deaths per 100,000 resident population.)

Sex, race, Hispanic origin, and age	1950[1,2]	1960[1,2]	1970[2]	1980[2]	1985	1990[2]	1995	2000[3]	2005[3]	2006[3]
75 to 84 years	61.9	55.7	45.5	45.5	57.0	60.2	47.7	41.1	38.0	35.4
85 years and over	61.9	61.3	45.8	52.8	60.9	70.3	67.9	61.6	53.1	50.8
Black or African American Male[5]										
All ages, age-adjusted[4]	7.5	8.4	10.0	11.4	11.8	12.8	12.4	10.0	9.2	9.4
All ages, crude	6.3	6.4	8.0	10.3	11.0	12.0	11.7	9.4	8.7	8.8
15 to 24 years	4.9	4.1	10.5	12.3	13.3	15.1	17.8	14.2	11.4	10.5
25 to 44 years	9.8	12.6	16.1	19.2	17.8	19.6	18.3	14.3	14.0	14.5
45 to 64 years	12.7	13.0	12.4	11.8	12.9	13.1	11.5	9.9	9.1	9.5
65 years and over	9.0	9.9	8.7	11.4	15.8	14.9	14.6	11.5	10.2	10.3
65 to 74 years	10.0	11.3	8.7	11.1	16.7	14.7	13.8	11.1	8.1	8.4
75 to 84 years[6]	*	*	*	10.5	15.6	14.4	16.7	12.1	12.9	11.6
85 years and over	NA	*	*	*	*	*	*	*	*	*
American Indian or Alaska Native Male[5]										
All ages, age-adjusted[4]	NA	NA	NA	19.3	17.9	20.1	17.4	16.0	17.3	16.5
All ages, crude	NA	NA	NA	20.9	20.3	20.9	18.0	15.9	17.6	16.8
15 to 24 years	NA	NA	NA	45.3	42.0	49.1	30.8	26.2	28.6	30.6
25 to 44 years	NA	NA	NA	31.2	30.2	27.8	29.1	24.5	27.0	23.3
45 to 64 years	NA	NA	NA	*	*	*	13.6	15.4	15.6	16.5
65 years and over	NA	NA	NA	*	*	*	*	*	*	*
Asian or Pacific Islander Male[5]										
All ages, age-adjusted[4]	NA	NA	NA	10.7	9.3	9.6	9.6	8.6	7.3	7.8
All ages, crude	NA	NA	NA	8.8	8.4	8.7	9.0	7.9	7.1	7.8
15 to 24 years	NA	NA	NA	10.8	14.2	13.5	14.4	9.1	6.5	10.6
25 to 44 years	NA	NA	NA	11.0	9.3	10.6	10.8	9.9	9.6	9.3
45 to 64 years	NA	NA	NA	13.0	10.4	9.7	8.7	9.7	8.9	9.7
65 years and over	NA	NA	NA	18.6	16.7	16.8	18.9	15.4	11.2	10.8
Hispanic or Latino Male[5,7]										
All ages, age-adjusted[4]	NA	NA	NA	NA	11.0	13.7	12.7	10.3	9.6	9.0
All ages, crude	NA	NA	NA	NA	9.8	11.4	10.9	8.4	8.4	8.0
15 to 24 years	NA	NA	NA	NA	13.8	14.7	16.0	10.9	11.3	10.7
25 to 44 years	NA	NA	NA	NA	14.8	16.2	14.5	11.2	11.8	11.5
45 to 64 years	NA	NA	NA	NA	12.3	16.1	14.2	12.0	10.8	10.4
65 years and over	NA	NA	NA	NA	14.7	23.4	21.0	19.5	14.7	12.7
White, not Hispanic or Latino Male[7]										
All ages, age-adjusted[4]	NA	NA	NA	NA	22.9	23.5	22.3	20.2	21.4	21.6
All ages, crude	NA	NA	NA	NA	22.3	23.1	22.2	20.4	22.1	22.4
15 to 24 years	NA	NA	NA	NA	22.6	24.4	24.0	19.5	18.8	18.8
25 to 44 years	NA	NA	NA	NA	25.1	26.4	27.1	25.1	27.1	27.4
45 to 64 years	NA	NA	NA	NA	27.3	26.8	24.5	24.0	28.2	29.3
65 years and over	NA	NA	NA	NA	46.4	45.4	39.0	33.9	33.0	31.9
White Female[5]										
All ages, age-adjusted[4]	6.0	5.9	7.9	6.1	5.7	5.2	4.7	4.3	4.9	5.1
All ages, crude	5.5	5.3	7.1	5.9	5.6	5.3	4.8	4.4	5.0	5.3
15 to 24 years	2.7	2.3	4.2	4.6	4.7	4.2	3.8	3.1	3.7	3.4
25 to 44 years	6.6	7.0	11.0	8.1	7.0	6.6	6.3	6.0	6.6	6.9
45 to 64 years	10.6	10.9	13.0	9.6	8.7	7.7	6.7	6.9	8.1	8.8
65 years and over	9.9	8.8	8.5	6.4	6.9	6.8	5.7	4.3	4.2	4.1
Black or African American Female[5]										
All ages, age-adjusted[4]	1.8	2.0	2.9	2.4	2.3	2.4	2.0	1.8	1.8	1.4
All ages, crude	1.5	1.6	2.6	2.2	2.1	2.3	2.0	1.7	1.8	1.4
15 to 24 years	1.8	*	3.8	2.3	2.0	2.3	2.2	2.2	1.7	1.7
25 to 44 years	2.3	3.0	4.8	4.3	3.2	3.8	3.3	2.6	2.8	2.0
45 to 64 years	2.7	3.1	2.9	2.5	2.8	2.9	2.0	2.1	2.4	1.9
65 years and over	*	*	2.6	*	2.7	1.9	2.1	1.3	1.5	*
American Indian or Alaska Native Female[5]										
All ages, age-adjusted[4]	NA	NA	NA	4.7	4.1	3.6	3.9	3.8	4.2	4.5
All ages, crude	NA	NA	NA	4.7	4.4	3.7	3.8	4.0	4.4	4.7
15 to 24 years	NA	NA	NA	*	*	*	*	*	9.1	7.9
25 to 44 years	NA	NA	NA	10.7	*	*	6.4	7.2	6.6	6.9

NA = Not available.

* = Rates based on fewer than 20 deaths are considered unreliable and are not shown.

[1]Includes deaths of persons who were not residents of the 50 states and the District of Columbia.

[2]Underlying cause of death was coded according to the 6th Revision of the International Classification of Diseases (ICD) in 1950, 7th Revision in 1960, 8th Revision in 1970, and 9th Revision in 1980-1998.

[3]Starting with 1999 data, cause of death is coded according to ICD-10.

[4]Age-adjusted rates are calculated using the year 2000 standard population. Prior to 2001, age-adjusted rates were calculated using standard million proportions based on rounded population numbers. Starting with 2001 data, unrounded population numbers are used to calculate age-adjusted rates.

[5]The race groups, White, Black, Asian or Pacific Islander, and American Indian or Alaska Native, include persons of Hispanic and non-Hispanic origin. Persons of Hispanic origin may be of any race. Death rates for the American Indian or Alaska Native, Asian or Pacific Islander, and Hispanic populations are known to be underestimated.

[6]In 1950, rate is for the age group 75 years and over.

[7]Prior to 1997, excludes data from states lacking an Hispanic-origin item on the death certificate.

Table 2-37. Death Rates for Suicide, by Sex, Race, Hispanic Origin, and Age, Selected Years, 1950–2015—*Continued*

(Deaths per 100,000 resident population.)

	2007[3]	2008[3]	2009[3]	2010[3]	2011[3]	2012[3]	2013[3]	2014[3]	2015[3]
75 to 84 years	36.2	36.1	35.3	34.9	36.8	37.0	38.1	38.3	38.6
85 years and over	50.1	45.8	46.9	50.8	47.0	50.7	52.6	54.4	52.5
Black or African American Male[5]									
All ages, age-adjusted[4].....................	8.7	9.4	8.9	9.1	9.3	9.6	9.3	9.5	9.6
All ages, crude	8.3	9.0	8.5	8.7	9.0	9.2	9.0	9.2	9.4
15 to 24 years	10.1	12.0	10.4	11.1	11.5	11.4	11.5	12.0	12.9
25 to 44 years	13.9	13.9	13.2	14.5	14.4	15.3	14.4	14.4	14.8
45 to 64 years	9.0	9.8	9.6	9.5	9.5	9.6	10.0	9.9	9.7
65 years and over	8.5	10.8	9.6	9.6	8.3	9.4	9.6	8.9	8.6
65 to 74 years	7.9	10.4	8.0	7.6	9.1	8.4	7.8	7.7	7.3
75 to 84 years[6]	11.2	11.8	11.9	9.9	8.4	12.5	9.1	11.0	11.2
85 years and over	*	*	*	*	*	*	*	*	*
American Indian or Alaska Native Male[5]									
All ages, age-adjusted[4].....................	15.9	15.4	14.6	15.5	16.4	17.4	18.1	16.4	18.8
All ages, crude	16.2	15.4	15.1	16.1	16.1	17.5	17.9	16.0	18.5
15 to 24 years	26.8	29.0	28.9	30.6	27.6	29.3	29.1	23.5	29.5
25 to 44 years	24.9	22.7	20.4	20.9	24.2	24.3	26.6	26.2	27.3
45 to 64 years	14.4	11.1	15.4	17.8	14.9	19.1	18.3	15.1	20.8
65 years and over	*	*	*	*	*	*	*	13.4	13.2
Asian or Pacific Islander Male[5]									
All ages, age-adjusted[4].....................	8.8	7.9	8.7	9.5	8.7	9.4	9.1	8.9	9.1
All ages, crude	8.4	7.5	8.4	9.3	8.6	9.3	9.2	9.0	9.2
15 to 24 years	11.4	7.1	8.0	10.9	9.6	9.7	11.9	12.9	15.6
25 to 44 years	9.7	8.5	9.7	10.6	10.6	11.8	11.9	9.7	9.6
45 to 64 years	10.6	10.9	12.1	12.8	11.1	12.3	10.9	12.1	10.9
65 years and over	13.1	14.8	15.3	14.9	13.3	12.9	10.9	11.6	12.6
Hispanic or Latino Male[5,7]									
All ages, age-adjusted[4].....................	10.3	9.5	9.9	9.9	9.4	9.5	9.3	10.3	9.9
All ages, crude	8.8	8.0	8.5	8.5	8.4	8.5	8.3	9.2	9.0
15 to 24 years	10.4	9.5	10.7	10.7	10.7	11.5	10.1	11.6	12.8
25 to 44 years	12.5	11.2	11.4	11.2	11.7	11.4	11.5	12.6	12.2
45 to 64 years	13.1	11.6	12.6	12.9	11.6	12.0	11.4	12.4	11.4
65 years and over	16.6	16.7	16.0	15.7	13.7	13.5	14.2	15.9	14.5
White, not Hispanic or Latino Male[7]									
All ages, age-adjusted[4].....................	22.1	23.1	23.4	24.2	24.8	25.2	25.3	25.9	26.6
All ages, crude	23.1	24.3	24.7	25.7	26.2	26.7	26.9	27.7	28.3
15 to 24 years	18.6	19.2	19.4	20.4	21.9	21.2	21.4	22.4	23.4
25 to 44 years	28.6	29.1	29.5	30.3	31.0	31.7	31.2	31.8	33.5
45 to 64 years	30.5	33.0	33.6	35.4	35.5	36.3	36.1	37.2	37.2
65 years and over	31.8	32.5	32.5	32.7	33.4	33.6	35.6	36.1	35.9
White Female[5]									
All ages, age-adjusted[4].....................	5.2	5.4	5.5	5.6	5.9	6.1	6.3	6.6	6.9
All ages, crude	5.4	5.6	5.7	5.9	6.1	6.3	6.5	6.9	7.2
15 to 24 years	3.4	3.6	3.8	4.2	4.4	4.6	5.0	5.0	5.6
25 to 44 years	7.0	7.2	7.1	7.3	7.7	7.8	7.9	8.4	8.7
45 to 64 years	9.3	9.4	9.6	9.9	10.2	10.6	10.9	11.5	11.9
65 years and over	4.2	4.4	4.4	4.5	4.8	4.9	5.1	5.5	5.6
Black or African American Female[5]									
All ages, age-adjusted[4].....................	1.7	1.6	1.8	1.8	1.9	2.0	2.0	2.1	2.0
All ages, crude	1.7	1.6	1.8	1.8	1.9	2.0	2.0	2.1	2.1
15 to 24 years	1.6	2.4	2.1	2.0	2.3	2.8	2.6	2.6	3.6
25 to 44 years	2.7	2.5	2.7	2.8	3.1	3.1	2.9	2.9	2.7
45 to 64 years	2.2	1.6	2.5	2.1	2.0	2.4	2.7	2.7	2.6
65 years and over	*	1.2	1.0	*	1.2	*	*	1.3	0.9
American Indian or Alaska Native Female[5]									
All ages, age-adjusted[4].....................	4.3	4.9	5.4	6.1	5.0	4.3	5.3	5.5	6.5
All ages, crude	4.3	5.1	5.6	5.9	5.0	4.5	5.4	5.6	6.6
15 to 24 years	6.7	8.6	11.1	10.4	7.1	9.7	9.4	9.6	11.7
25 to 44 years	5.8	6.2	7.5	7.4	7.8	6.6	7.5	9.7	8.8

X = Not applicable.
* = Rates based on fewer than 20 deaths are considered unreliable and are not shown.
[3]Starting with 1999 data, cause of death is coded according to ICD-10.
[4]Age-adjusted rates are calculated using the year 2000 standard population. Prior to 2001, age-adjusted rates were calculated using standard million proportions based on rounded population numbers. Starting with 2001 data, unrounded population numbers are used to calculate age-adjusted rates.
[5]The race groups, White, Black, Asian or Pacific Islander, and American Indian or Alaska Native, include persons of Hispanic and non-Hispanic origin. Persons of Hispanic origin may be of any race. Death rates for the American Indian or Alaska Native, Asian or Pacific Islander, and Hispanic populations are known to be underestimated.
[6]In 1950, rate is for the age group 75 years and over.
[7]Prior to 1997, excludes data from states lacking an Hispanic-origin item on the death certificate.

Table 2-37. Death Rates for Suicide, by Sex, Race, Hispanic Origin, and Age, Selected Years, 1950–2015—*Continued*

(Deaths per 100,000 resident population.)

Sex, race, Hispanic origin, and age	1950[1,2]	1960[1,2]	1970[2]	1980[2]	1985	1990[2]	1995	2000[3]	2005[3]	2006[3]
45 to 64 years	NA	NA	NA	*	*	*	*	*	*	*
65 years and over	NA	NA	NA	*	*	*	*	*	*	*
Asian or Pacific Islander Female[5]										
All ages, age-adjusted[4]	NA	NA	NA	5.5	5.0	4.1	4.1	2.8	3.2	3.3
All ages, crude	NA	NA	NA	4.7	4.3	3.4	3.7	2.7	3.1	3.2
15 to 24 years	NA	NA	NA	*	5.8	3.9	4.8	2.7	3.2	3.5
25 to 44 years	NA	NA	NA	5.4	4.2	3.8	3.6	3.3	3.3	3.2
45 to 64 years	NA	NA	NA	7.9	5.4	5.0	4.7	3.2	3.7	4.1
65 years and over	NA	NA	NA	*	13.6	8.5	8.6	5.2	6.9	7.0
Hispanic or Latina Female[5,7]										
All ages, age-adjusted[4]	NA	NA	NA	NA	1.9	2.3	2.0	1.7	1.8	1.8
All ages, crude	NA	NA	NA	NA	1.6	2.2	1.8	1.5	1.6	1.7
15 to 24 years	NA	NA	NA	NA	2.1	3.1	2.4	2.0	2.5	2.5
25 to 44 years	NA	NA	NA	NA	2.1	3.1	2.5	2.1	2.2	2.3
45 to 64 years	NA	NA	NA	NA	3.2	2.5	2.8	2.5	2.1	2.4
65 years and over	NA	NA	NA	NA	*	*	*	*	2.0	1.7
White, not Hispanic or Latina Female[7]										
All ages, age-adjusted[4]	NA	NA	NA	NA	6.1	5.4	4.9	4.7	5.3	5.6
All ages, crude	NA	NA	NA	NA	6.2	5.6	5.1	4.9	5.6	5.9
15 to 24 years	NA	NA	NA	NA	4.7	4.3	4.0	3.3	4.0	3.5
25 to 44 years	NA	NA	NA	NA	7.7	7.0	6.6	6.7	7.5	7.9
45 to 64 years	NA	NA	NA	NA	9.2	8.0	6.9	7.3	8.7	9.5
65 years and over	NA	NA	NA	NA	7.5	7.0	5.8	4.4	4.4	4.3

NA = Not available.

* = Rates based on fewer than 20 deaths are considered unreliable and are not shown.

[1]Includes deaths of persons who were not residents of the 50 states and the District of Columbia.

[2]Underlying cause of death was coded according to the 6th Revision of the International Classification of Diseases (ICD) in 1950, 7th Revision in 1960, 8th Revision in 1970, and 9th Revision in 1980-1998.

[3]Starting with 1999 data, cause of death is coded according to ICD-10.

[4]Age-adjusted rates are calculated using the year 2000 standard population. Prior to 2001, age-adjusted rates were calculated using standard million proportions based on rounded population numbers. Starting with 2001 data, unrounded population numbers are used to calculate age-adjusted rates.

[5]The race groups, White, Black, Asian or Pacific Islander, and American Indian or Alaska Native, include persons of Hispanic and non-Hispanic origin. Persons of Hispanic origin may be of any race. Death rates for the American Indian or Alaska Native, Asian or Pacific Islander, and Hispanic populations are known to be underestimated.

[7]Prior to 1997, excludes data from states lacking an Hispanic-origin item on the death certificate.

Table 2-37. Death Rates for Suicide, by Sex, Race, Hispanic Origin, and Age, Selected Years, 1950–2015—*Continued*

(Deaths per 100,000 resident population.)

	2007[3]	2008[3]	2009[3]	2010[3]	2011[3]	2012[3]	2013[3]	2014[3]	2015[3]
45 to 64 years	*	6.5	5.9	6.2	5.8	*	6.6	*	6.9
65 years and over	*	*	*	*	*	*	*	*	*
Asian or Pacific Islander Female[5]									
All ages, age-adjusted[4]	3.4	3.5	3.5	3.4	3.4	3.6	3.0	3.4	4.0
All ages, crude	3.4	3.5	3.5	3.4	3.5	3.7	3.1	3.5	4.1
15 to 24 years	3.2	3.9	4.4	3.5	3.1	5.5	3.6	4.1	4.9
25 to 44 years	4.3	4.5	3.9	4.1	4.3	3.9	3.7	4.0	4.5
45 to 64 years	3.9	3.7	4.7	4.7	4.6	4.3	3.9	4.2	5.2
65 years and over	5.3	5.8	4.8	4.3	5.1	5.3	3.3	5.2	5.2
Hispanic or Latina Female[5,7]									
All ages, age-adjusted[4]	1.8	1.8	2.0	2.1	2.0	2.2	2.3	2.5	2.6
All ages, crude	1.7	1.7	1.8	2.0	1.9	2.1	2.2	2.4	2.6
15 to 24 years	2.0	2.2	2.3	3.1	2.9	2.9	3.3	3.4	3.9
25 to 44 years	2.6	2.2	2.5	2.4	2.6	2.7	2.8	3.0	3.2
45 to 64 years	2.7	2.7	2.5	2.8	2.7	3.2	3.2	3.5	3.8
65 years and over	*	1.6	2.3	2.2	1.6	2.1	1.2	2.1	1.9
White, not Hispanic or Latina Female[7]									
All ages, age-adjusted[4]	5.8	6.0	6.1	6.2	6.7	6.9	7.1	7.5	7.8
All ages, crude	6.1	6.3	6.5	6.7	7.0	7.2	7.5	7.9	8.3
15 to 24 years	3.7	3.9	4.1	4.4	4.8	5.1	5.4	5.4	6.1
25 to 44 years	8.1	8.4	8.3	8.6	9.1	9.2	9.3	9.8	10.3
45 to 64 years	10.0	10.1	10.5	10.7	11.1	11.6	12.0	12.6	13.1
65 years and over	4.4	4.6	4.5	4.7	5.1	5.1	5.4	5.8	6.0

* = Rates based on fewer than 20 deaths are considered unreliable and are not shown.
[3]Starting with 1999 data, cause of death is coded according to ICD-10.
[4]Age-adjusted rates are calculated using the year 2000 standard population. Prior to 2001, age-adjusted rates were calculated using standard million proportions based on rounded population numbers. Starting with 2001 data, unrounded population numbers are used to calculate age-adjusted rates.
[5]The race groups, White, Black, Asian or Pacific Islander, and American Indian or Alaska Native, include persons of Hispanic and non-Hispanic origin. Persons of Hispanic origin may be of any race. Death rates for the American Indian or Alaska Native, Asian or Pacific Islander, and Hispanic populations are known to be underestimated.
[7]Prior to 1997, excludes data from states lacking an Hispanic-origin item on the death certificate.

Table 2-38. Death Rates for Firearm-Related Injuries, by Sex, Race, Hispanic Origin, and Age, Selected Years, 1970–2015

(Deaths per 100,000 resident population.)

Sex, race, Hispanic origin, and age	1970[1]	1980[1]	1985	1990[1]	1995[1]	2000[2]	2005[2]	2006[2]
All Persons								
All ages, age-adjusted[3]	14.3	14.8	13.1	14.6	13.4	10.2	10.3	10.3
All ages, crude	13.1	14.9	13.3	14.9	13.5	10.2	10.4	10.4
Under 1 year	*	*	*	*	*	*	*	*
1 to 14 years	1.6	1.4	1.4	1.5	1.6	0.7	0.7	0.7
1 to 4 years	1.0	0.7	0.7	0.6	0.6	0.3	0.4	0.4
5 to 14 years	1.7	1.6	1.8	1.9	1.9	0.9	0.8	0.9
15 to 24 years	15.5	20.6	17.2	25.8	26.7	16.8	16.1	16.7
15 to 19 years	11.4	14.7	13.3	23.3	24.1	12.9	12.2	12.9
20 to 24 years	20.3	26.4	20.6	28.1	29.2	20.9	20.0	20.7
25 to 44 years	20.9	22.5	17.9	19.3	16.9	13.1	13.8	13.6
25 to 34 years	22.2	24.3	19.3	21.8	19.6	14.5	16.1	15.7
35 to 44 years	19.6	20.0	16.0	16.3	14.3	11.9	11.7	11.6
45 to 64 years	17.6	15.2	14.3	13.6	11.7	10.0	10.6	10.6
45 to 54 years	18.1	16.4	14.7	13.9	12.0	10.5	11.2	11.2
55 to 64 years	17.0	13.9	13.9	13.3	11.3	9.4	9.7	9.7
65 years and over	13.8	13.5	15.6	16.0	14.1	12.2	11.8	11.3
65 to 74 years	14.5	13.8	15.1	14.4	12.8	10.6	10.2	9.9
75 to 84 years	13.4	13.4	17.7	19.4	16.3	13.9	13.6	12.9
85 years and over	10.2	11.6	12.2	14.7	14.4	14.2	13.0	12.5
Male								
All ages, age-adjusted[3]	24.8	25.9	23.1	26.1	23.8	18.1	18.5	18.2
All ages, crude	22.2	25.7	22.8	26.2	23.6	17.8	18.4	18.2
Under 1 year	*	*	*	*	*	*	*	*
1 to 14 years	2.3	2.0	2.1	2.2	2.3	1.1	1.0	1.0
1 to 4 years	1.2	0.9	0.8	0.7	0.8	0.4	0.5	0.5
5 to 14 years	2.7	2.5	2.7	2.9	2.9	1.4	1.2	1.2
15 to 24 years	26.4	34.8	29.1	44.7	46.5	29.4	28.5	29.5
15 to 19 years	19.2	24.5	22.4	40.1	41.6	22.4	21.5	22.7
20 to 24 years	35.1	45.2	35.0	49.1	51.5	37.0	35.7	36.6
25 to 44 years	34.1	38.1	29.7	32.6	28.4	22.0	23.7	23.2
25 to 34 years	36.5	41.4	32.1	37.0	33.2	24.9	28.2	27.6
35 to 44 years	31.6	33.2	26.6	27.4	23.6	19.4	19.5	19.2
45 to 64 years	31.0	25.9	24.5	23.4	20.0	17.1	18.2	17.8
45 to 54 years	30.7	27.3	24.4	23.2	20.1	17.6	18.9	18.6
55 to 64 years	31.3	24.5	24.6	23.7	19.8	16.3	17.2	16.8
65 years and over	29.7	29.7	34.2	35.3	30.7	26.4	25.1	24.0
65 to 74 years	29.5	27.8	30.0	28.2	25.1	20.3	19.3	18.8
75 to 84 years	31.0	33.0	42.7	46.9	37.8	32.2	30.5	28.8
85 years and over	26.2	34.9	38.2	49.3	47.1	44.7	39.3	37.3
Female								
All ages, age-adjusted[3]	4.8	4.7	4.2	4.2	3.8	2.8	2.7	2.7
All ages, crude	4.4	4.7	4.2	4.3	3.8	2.8	2.7	2.8
Under 1 year	*	*	*	*	*	*	*	*
1 to 14 years	0.8	0.7	0.7	0.8	0.8	0.3	0.4	0.4
1 to 4 years	0.9	0.5	0.5	0.5	0.5	*	0.3	*
5 to 14 years	0.8	0.7	0.8	1.0	0.9	0.4	0.4	0.4
15 to 24 years	4.8	6.1	5.0	6.0	5.9	3.5	3.0	3.1
15 to 19 years	3.5	4.6	3.9	5.7	5.6	2.9	2.4	2.5
20 to 24 years	6.4	7.7	5.9	6.3	6.1	4.2	3.6	3.8
25 to 44 years	8.3	7.4	6.2	6.1	5.5	4.2	3.9	3.9
25 to 34 years	8.4	7.5	6.6	6.7	5.8	4.0	3.8	3.7
35 to 44 years	8.2	7.2	5.8	5.4	5.2	4.4	4.0	4.1
45 to 64 years	5.4	5.4	5.0	4.5	3.9	3.4	3.3	3.6
45 to 54 years	6.4	6.2	5.6	4.9	4.2	3.6	3.7	4.0
55 to 64 years	4.2	4.6	4.5	4.0	3.5	3.0	2.8	3.1
65 years and over	2.4	2.5	3.2	3.1	2.8	2.2	2.1	1.9
65 to 74 years	2.8	3.1	3.6	3.6	3.0	2.5	2.5	2.2
75 to 84 years	1.7	1.7	3.0	2.9	2.8	2.0	2.1	1.8
85 years and over	*	1.3	1.8	1.3	1.8	1.7	1.4	1.2
White Male[4]								
All ages, age-adjusted[3]	19.7	22.1	21.0	22.0	20.1	15.9	15.9	15.5
All ages, crude	17.6	21.8	20.7	21.8	19.9	15.6	16.0	15.6
1 to 14 years	1.8	1.9	2.1	1.9	1.9	1.0	0.8	0.8
15 to 24 years	16.9	28.4	24.1	29.5	30.8	19.6	18.3	18.4

* = Rates based on fewer than 20 deaths are considered unreliable and are not shown.
[1]Underlying cause of death was coded according to the 8th Revision of the International Classification of Diseases (ICD) in 1970 and 9th Revision in 1980–1998.
[2]Starting with 1999 data, cause of death is coded according to ICD–10.
[3]Age-adjusted rates are calculated using the year 2000 standard population. Prior to 2001, age-adjusted rates were calculated using standard million proportions based on rounded population numbers. Starting with 2001 data, unrounded population numbers are used to calculate age-adjusted rates.
[4]The race groups, White, Black, Asian or Pacific Islander, and American Indian or Alaska Native, include persons of Hispanic and non-Hispanic origin. Persons of Hispanic origin may be of any race. Death rates for the American Indian or Alaska Native, Asian or Pacific Islander, and Hispanic populations are known to be underestimated.

Table 2-38. Death Rates for Firearm-Related Injuries, by Sex, Race, Hispanic Origin, and Age, Selected Years, 1970–2015—*Continued*

(Deaths per 100,000 resident population.)

Sex, race, Hispanic origin, and age	2007²	2008²	2009²	2010²	2011²	2012²	2013²	2014²	2015²
All Persons									
All ages, age-adjusted³	10.3	10.3	10.1	10.1	10.2	10.5	10.4	10.3	11.1
All ages, crude	10.4	10.4	10.2	10.3	10.4	10.7	10.6	10.5	11.3
Under 1 year	*	*	*	*	*	*	*	*	*
1 to 14 years	0.7	0.6	0.6	0.6	0.7	0.7	0.7	0.8	0.8
1 to 4 years	0.4	0.5	0.4	0.4	0.5	0.4	0.4	0.4	0.5
5 to 14 years	0.8	0.7	0.7	0.7	0.8	0.8	0.8	0.9	0.9
15 to 24 years	16.0	15.4	14.4	14.2	14.4	14.7	14.1	14.0	15.7
15 to 19 years	12.1	11.7	11.1	10.6	10.7	10.7	9.7	9.9	11.3
20 to 24 years	20.1	19.3	18.0	17.9	18.0	18.5	18.1	17.7	19.8
25 to 44 years	13.8	13.5	13.2	13.3	13.4	13.8	13.9	13.4	15.0
25 to 34 years	15.9	15.4	14.5	15.0	15.0	15.3	15.3	14.7	16.8
35 to 44 years	12.0	11.8	11.9	11.7	11.7	12.4	12.3	12.1	13.1
45 to 64 years	10.6	11.2	11.4	11.6	11.7	12.0	11.9	11.8	12.0
45 to 54 years	11.1	11.5	11.8	12.0	12.2	12.4	12.3	12.2	12.4
55 to 64 years	10.1	10.8	10.8	11.1	11.0	11.6	11.5	11.4	11.7
65 years and over	11.3	11.8	11.9	11.7	12.1	12.2	12.5	12.7	12.7
65 to 74 years	9.8	10.7	10.9	10.7	10.9	10.8	11.3	11.5	11.3
75 to 84 years	13.1	13.2	13.3	12.7	13.7	14.1	14.1	13.9	14.5
85 years and over	12.7	12.5	12.5	13.2	13.1	13.6	13.9	15.0	14.5
Male									
All ages, age-adjusted³	18.3	18.3	17.8	17.9	18.0	18.5	18.3	18.0	19.4
All ages, crude	18.3	18.3	17.9	18.0	18.1	18.7	18.5	18.3	19.6
Under 1 year	*	*	*	*	*	*	*	*	*
1 to 14 years	1.0	0.9	0.9	1.0	1.0	1.0	1.0	1.1	1.1
1 to 4 years	0.5	0.6	0.5	0.6	0.6	0.5	0.6	0.5	0.6
5 to 14 years	1.1	1.0	1.0	1.1	1.1	1.1	1.2	1.3	1.2
15 to 24 years	28.2	27.0	25.3	25.0	25.0	25.6	24.4	24.3	27.4
15 to 19 years	21.2	20.4	19.3	18.4	18.4	18.5	17.0	17.2	19.5
20 to 24 years	35.5	34.0	31.6	31.8	31.5	32.4	31.2	30.8	34.7
25 to 44 years	23.8	23.3	22.4	22.9	22.7	23.6	23.7	22.8	25.6
25 to 34 years	28.0	27.1	25.0	26.4	25.9	26.4	26.3	25.2	28.8
35 to 44 years	19.8	19.6	19.9	19.3	19.4	20.7	20.8	20.1	22.1
45 to 64 years	18.2	19.2	19.3	19.9	19.8	20.5	20.1	19.8	20.2
45 to 54 years	18.6	19.4	19.6	20.3	20.1	20.4	20.4	19.9	20.5
55 to 64 years	17.7	19.0	19.1	19.3	19.5	20.5	19.8	19.8	19.9
65 years and over	24.0	24.7	24.8	24.1	24.8	25.0	25.3	25.7	25.5
65 to 74 years	18.7	20.3	20.6	20.0	20.3	20.2	20.9	21.5	21.1
75 to 84 years	29.0	29.0	28.8	27.5	29.5	30.1	29.8	29.2	30.2
85 years and over	37.4	35.5	35.7	37.4	36.1	37.5	38.3	40.7	38.9
Female									
All ages, age-adjusted³	2.7	2.7	2.8	2.7	2.9	3.0	3.0	3.0	3.2
All ages, crude	2.7	2.8	2.8	2.7	2.9	3.0	3.0	3.0	3.2
Under 1 year	*	*	*	*	*	*	*	*	*
1 to 14 years	0.4	0.4	0.3	0.3	0.4	0.4	0.4	0.5	0.5
1 to 4 years	0.4	0.4	0.4	0.3	0.3	0.3	0.3	0.4	0.4
5 to 14 years	0.4	0.4	0.3	0.3	0.4	0.5	0.4	0.5	0.5
15 to 24 years	3.2	3.2	3.1	2.9	3.2	3.2	3.2	3.1	3.4
15 to 19 years	2.5	2.4	2.4	2.3	2.5	2.4	2.0	2.3	2.7
20 to 24 years	3.9	4.0	3.7	3.5	3.8	3.9	4.3	3.9	4.1
25 to 44 years	3.9	3.8	3.9	3.8	4.0	4.0	4.0	4.0	4.4
25 to 34 years	3.6	3.6	3.9	3.5	3.9	4.0	4.1	3.9	4.5
35 to 44 years	4.2	4.0	3.9	4.1	4.0	4.1	4.0	4.1	4.3
45 to 64 years	3.4	3.6	3.8	3.7	3.9	4.0	4.1	4.1	4.3
45 to 54 years	3.7	3.9	4.3	3.8	4.5	4.6	4.5	4.7	4.5
55 to 64 years	3.0	3.1	3.2	3.4	3.1	3.3	3.8	3.6	4.0
65 years and over	2.0	2.1	2.2	2.2	2.3	2.3	2.4	2.5	2.5
65 to 74 years	2.2	2.4	2.6	2.6	2.7	2.6	2.8	2.7	2.7
75 to 84 years	2.0	2.0	2.2	2.1	2.1	2.3	2.3	2.4	2.6
85 years and over	1.2	1.6	1.3	1.5	1.7	1.6	1.5	1.6	1.7
White Male⁴									
All ages, age-adjusted³	15.8	16.1	15.9	16.1	16.2	16.5	16.5	16.3	17.0
All ages, crude	15.9	16.4	16.2	16.5	16.6	17.0	17.1	17.0	17.7
1 to 14 years	0.7	0.7	0.8	0.8	0.9	0.9	1.0	1.0	0.9
15 to 24 years	17.5	17.7	16.9	16.2	16.5	16.7	16.0	16.1	17.5

* = Rates based on fewer than 20 deaths are considered unreliable and are not shown.
²Starting with 1999 data, cause of death is coded according to ICD–10.
³Age-adjusted rates are calculated using the year 2000 standard population. Prior to 2001, age-adjusted rates were calculated using standard million proportions based on rounded population numbers. Starting with 2001 data, unrounded population numbers are used to calculate age-adjusted rates.
⁴The race groups, White, Black, Asian or Pacific Islander, and American Indian or Alaska Native, include persons of Hispanic and non-Hispanic origin. Persons of Hispanic origin may be of any race. Death rates for the American Indian or Alaska Native, Asian or Pacific Islander, and Hispanic populations are known to be underestimated.

Table 2-38. Death Rates for Firearm-Related Injuries, by Sex, Race, Hispanic Origin, and Age, Selected Years, 1970–2015—*Continued*

(Deaths per 100,000 resident population.)

Sex, race, Hispanic origin, and age	1970[1]	1980[1]	1985	1990[1]	1995[1]	2000[2]	2005[2]	2006[2]
25 to 44 years	24.2	29.5	25.0	25.7	23.2	18.0	18.4	17.9
25 to 34 years	24.3	31.1	26.3	27.8	25.2	18.1	19.4	18.5
35 to 44 years	24.1	27.1	23.3	23.3	21.2	17.9	17.5	17.3
45 to 64 years	27.4	23.3	23.6	22.8	19.5	17.4	19.0	18.4
65 years and over	29.9	30.1	35.4	36.8	32.2	28.2	27.0	25.8
Black or African American Male[4]								
All ages, age-adjusted[3]	70.8	60.1	40.9	56.3	49.2	34.2	36.7	37.6
All ages, crude	60.8	57.7	41.3	61.9	52.9	36.1	38.6	39.8
1 to 14 years	5.3	3.0	2.7	4.4	4.4	1.8	2.1	2.2
15 to 24 years	97.3	77.9	61.3	138.0	138.7	89.3	86.2	90.9
25 to 44 years	126.2	114.1	71.8	90.3	70.2	54.1	64.8	64.8
25 to 34 years	145.6	128.4	79.8	108.6	92.3	74.8	92.1	92.8
35 to 44 years	104.2	92.3	59.2	66.1	46.3	34.3	38.6	37.8
45 to 64 years	71.1	55.6	36.9	34.5	28.3	18.4	17.2	18.5
65 years and over	30.6	29.7	26.3	23.9	21.8	13.8	13.5	13.2
American Indian or Alaska Native Male[4]								
All ages, age-adjusted[3]	NA	24.0	23.6	19.4	19.4	13.1	14.4	13.3
All ages, crude	NA	27.5	24.4	20.5	20.9	13.2	14.9	13.7
15 to 24 years	NA	55.3	39.8	49.1	40.9	26.9	28.6	27.8
25 to 44 years	NA	43.9	40.3	25.4	31.2	16.6	21.3	19.0
45 to 64 years	NA	*	21.2	*	14.2	12.2	12.1	10.1
65 years and over	NA	*	*	*	*	*	*	*
Asian or Pacific Islander Male[4]								
All ages, age-adjusted[3]	NA	7.8	7.3	8.8	9.2	6.0	5.1	5.2
All ages, crude	NA	8.2	7.3	9.4	10.0	6.2	5.4	5.5
15 to 24 years	NA	10.8	12.6	21.0	24.3	9.3	10.9	12.9
25 to 44 years	NA	12.8	9.8	10.9	10.6	8.1	6.4	5.7
45 to 64 years	NA	10.4	6.7	8.1	8.2	7.4	5.7	5.6
65 years and over	NA	*	*	*	*	*	*	*
Hispanic or Latino Male[4,5]								
All ages, age-adjusted[3]	NA	NA	24.2	27.6	23.8	13.6	13.4	12.8
All ages, crude	NA	NA	26.0	29.9	26.2	14.2	14.3	13.8
1 to 14 years	NA	NA	1.4	2.6	2.8	1.0	0.7	1.1
15 to 24 years	NA	NA	42.0	55.5	61.7	30.8	30.8	31.1
25 to 44 years	NA	NA	43.2	42.7	31.4	17.3	19.7	18.5
25 to 34 years	NA	NA	47.3	47.3	36.4	20.3	24.4	22.5
35 to 44 years	NA	NA	35.9	35.4	24.2	13.2	13.9	13.5
45 to 64 years	NA	NA	19.2	21.4	17.2	12.0	9.2	8.6
65 years and over	NA	NA	12.4	19.1	16.5	12.2	10.2	8.0
White, not Hispanic or Latino Male[5]								
All ages, age-adjusted[3]	NA	NA	20.2	20.6	18.6	15.5	15.5	15.1
All ages, crude	NA	NA	19.9	20.4	18.5	15.7	16.1	15.8
1 to 14 years	NA	NA	2.0	1.6	1.6	1.0	0.9	0.7
15 to 24 years	NA	NA	22.0	24.1	23.5	16.2	14.1	14.1
25 to 44 years	NA	NA	23.0	23.3	21.4	17.9	17.7	17.4
25 to 34 years	NA	NA	23.7	24.7	22.5	17.2	17.4	16.7
35 to 44 years	NA	NA	22.0	21.6	20.4	18.4	17.9	18.0
45 to 64 years	NA	NA	23.0	22.7	19.5	17.8	20.0	19.5
65 years and over	NA	NA	37.3	37.4	32.5	29.0	28.1	27.0
White Female[4]								
All ages, age-adjusted[3]	4.0	4.2	3.9	3.8	3.5	2.7	2.6	2.6
All ages, crude	3.7	4.1	4.0	3.8	3.5	2.7	2.6	2.7
15 to 24 years	3.4	5.1	4.4	4.8	4.5	2.8	2.3	2.3
25 to 44 years	6.9	6.2	5.6	5.3	4.9	3.9	3.8	3.6
45 to 64 years	5.0	5.1	5.0	4.5	4.0	3.5	3.5	3.9
65 years and over	2.2	2.5	3.2	3.1	2.8	2.4	2.3	2.1
Black or African American Female[4]								
All ages, age-adjusted[3]	11.1	8.7	6.4	7.3	6.2	3.9	3.6	3.9
All ages, crude	10.0	8.8	6.5	7.8	6.5	4.0	3.7	4.1
15 to 24 years	15.2	12.3	8.3	13.3	13.2	7.6	6.6	7.5
25 to 44 years	19.4	16.1	11.4	12.4	9.8	6.5	6.0	6.9

NA = Not available.
* = Rates based on fewer than 20 deaths are considered unreliable and are not shown.
[1]Underlying cause of death was coded according to the 8th Revision of the International Classification of Diseases (ICD) in 1970 and 9th Revision in 1980–1998.
[2]Starting with 1999 data, cause of death is coded according to ICD-10.
[3]Age-adjusted rates are calculated using the year 2000 standard population. Prior to 2001, age-adjusted rates were calculated using standard million proportions based on rounded population numbers. Starting with 2001 data, unrounded population numbers are used to calculate age-adjusted rates.
[4]The race groups, White, Black, Asian or Pacific Islander, and American Indian or Alaska Native, include persons of Hispanic and non-Hispanic origin. Persons of Hispanic origin may be of any race. Death rates for the American Indian or Alaska Native, Asian or Pacific Islander, and Hispanic populations are known to be underestimated.
[5]Prior to 1997, data from states that did not report Hispanic origin on the death certificate were excluded.

Table 2-38. Death Rates for Firearm-Related Injuries, by Sex, Race, Hispanic Origin, and Age, Selected Years, 1970–2015—Continued

(Deaths per 100,000 resident population.)

Sex, race, Hispanic origin, and age	2007[2]	2008[2]	2009[2]	2010[2]	2011[2]	2012[2]	2013[2]	2014[2]	2015[2]
25 to 44 years	18.9	18.6	18.1	18.6	18.4	18.8	18.9	18.4	20.0
25 to 34 years	19.8	19.1	17.9	19.1	19.1	19.2	19.1	18.7	20.5
35 to 44 years	18.0	18.2	18.2	18.0	17.7	18.4	18.8	18.2	19.4
45 to 64 years	19.0	20.5	20.5	21.3	21.3	22.0	21.6	21.4	21.6
65 years and over	26.0	26.6	26.9	26.5	27.1	27.4	28.0	28.3	28.3
Black or African American Male[4]									
All ages, age-adjusted[3]	36.2	34.3	32.3	31.8	31.7	33.4	32.1	31.5	36.4
All ages, crude	38.5	36.2	33.7	33.4	33.2	34.8	33.5	32.9	38.1
1 to 14 years	2.2	2.0	1.6	1.9	1.4	1.5	1.4	1.9	2.1
15 to 24 years	87.7	79.7	72.8	73.2	72.4	74.2	69.9	68.9	79.7
25 to 44 years	63.3	60.8	57.2	57.3	57.4	61.1	60.2	57.4	68.1
25 to 34 years	88.5	85.3	76.0	78.2	75.5	77.1	76.6	71.3	84.9
35 to 44 years	38.4	36.2	37.7	35.2	37.5	43.1	41.5	41.0	47.9
45 to 64 years	18.1	16.9	17.1	16.5	16.3	17.0	16.7	16.9	18.7
65 years and over	10.9	13.2	12.1	9.4	10.7	11.1	8.8	10.9	10.0
American Indian or Alaska Native Male[4]									
All ages, age-adjusted[3]	11.0	11.7	11.4	11.7	11.9	13.5	12.9	12.9	14.4
All ages, crude	11.1	11.7	11.6	12.5	11.7	13.4	12.5	12.4	14.2
15 to 24 years	20.8	22.2	22.2	26.0	19.0	21.2	18.4	17.7	26.4
25 to 44 years	14.2	17.3	16.3	16.9	17.1	20.1	18.8	19.3	18.7
45 to 64 years	10.6	7.1	11.1	11.1	11.6	14.3	13.5	12.6	14.0
65 years and over	*	*	*	*	*	*	*	*	*
Asian or Pacific Islander Male[4]									
All ages, age-adjusted[3]	5.0	4.2	4.4	4.2	4.0	4.4	4.1	3.7	4.4
All ages, crude	5.1	4.4	4.5	4.4	4.1	4.6	4.3	3.8	4.7
15 to 24 years	9.7	7.5	5.4	6.8	5.7	6.3	5.9	6.3	8.0
25 to 44 years	5.9	5.2	6.2	6.0	5.7	6.4	6.4	4.8	6.0
45 to 64 years	5.6	4.7	5.2	4.4	4.4	5.0	4.6	4.1	5.0
65 years and over	4.5	4.4	4.7	3.9	4.0	4.0	*	3.4	3.7
Hispanic or Latino Male[4,5]									
All ages, age-adjusted[3]	12.9	11.7	11.4	10.5	9.8	10.1	9.4	9.4	10.1
All ages, crude	13.4	12.0	11.4	10.5	9.9	10.1	9.4	9.4	10.2
1 to 14 years	0.8	0.5	0.7	0.6	0.7	0.6	0.5	0.5	0.5
15 to 24 years	28.4	24.9	23.3	20.9	19.2	19.6	17.4	17.2	19.6
25 to 44 years	18.2	16.6	15.5	14.4	13.9	14.4	13.8	14.1	15.0
25 to 34 years	22.5	19.4	18.0	18.0	17.0	17.3	16.2	15.7	17.7
35 to 44 years	12.9	13.2	12.4	10.2	10.2	11.0	11.1	12.3	11.9
45 to 64 years	9.7	9.0	9.5	9.1	8.0	8.2	8.2	7.9	8.0
65 years and over	11.2	10.3	10.8	9.9	9.6	9.7	8.1	7.8	9.1
White, not Hispanic or Latino Male[5]									
All ages, age-adjusted[3]	15.5	16.2	16.1	16.6	16.9	17.2	17.5	17.3	18.0
All ages, crude	16.3	17.1	17.0	17.6	18.0	18.5	18.8	18.7	19.4
1 to 14 years	0.7	0.7	0.7	0.9	1.0	1.0	1.2	1.2	1.0
15 to 24 years	13.7	14.9	14.2	14.2	15.1	15.2	15.1	15.4	16.4
25 to 44 years	18.7	18.9	18.4	19.4	19.4	19.8	20.2	19.4	21.2
25 to 34 years	18.5	18.5	17.4	18.9	19.3	19.3	19.7	19.2	20.9
35 to 44 years	18.8	19.2	19.4	19.9	19.6	20.3	20.8	19.7	21.5
45 to 64 years	20.0	21.8	21.8	22.8	23.0	23.8	23.5	23.4	23.7
65 years and over	27.0	27.7	27.9	27.6	28.4	28.7	29.6	29.9	29.8
White Female[4]									
All ages, age-adjusted[3]	2.6	2.7	2.8	2.7	2.9	2.9	3.0	3.1	3.2
All ages, crude	2.7	2.8	2.9	2.8	3.0	3.0	3.1	3.2	3.3
15 to 24 years	2.6	2.3	2.4	2.3	2.6	2.4	2.7	2.6	2.8
25 to 44 years	3.8	3.8	3.8	3.7	3.9	4.0	3.9	4.0	4.4
45 to 64 years	3.7	4.0	4.2	4.1	4.3	4.4	4.7	4.7	4.9
65 years and over	2.1	2.3	2.5	2.5	2.6	2.5	2.7	2.7	2.8
Black or African American Female[4]									
All ages, age-adjusted[3]	3.8	3.4	3.4	3.3	3.3	3.6	3.4	3.2	3.6
All ages, crude	3.8	3.5	3.5	3.3	3.4	3.7	3.4	3.2	3.7
15 to 24 years	6.9	7.9	6.7	6.4	6.7	7.2	6.1	6.2	6.8
25 to 44 years	6.3	5.3	5.7	5.6	5.6	5.8	6.0	5.3	6.2

NA = Not available.

* = Rates based on fewer than 20 deaths are considered unreliable and are not shown.

[2]Starting with 1999 data, cause of death is coded according to ICD–10.

[3]Age-adjusted rates are calculated using the year 2000 standard population. Prior to 2001, age-adjusted rates were calculated using standard million proportions based on rounded population numbers. Starting with 2001 data, unrounded population numbers are used to calculate age-adjusted rates.

[4]The race groups, White, Black, Asian or Pacific Islander, and American Indian or Alaska Native, include persons of Hispanic and non-Hispanic origin. Persons of Hispanic origin may be of any race. Death rates for the American Indian or Alaska Native, Asian or Pacific Islander, and Hispanic populations are known to be underestimated.

[5]Prior to 1997, data from states that did not report Hispanic origin on the death certificate were excluded.

Table 2-38. Death Rates for Firearm-Related Injuries, by Sex, Race, Hispanic Origin, and Age, Selected Years, 1970–2015—*Continued*

(Deaths per 100,000 resident population.)

Sex, race, Hispanic origin, and age	1970[1]	1980[1]	1985	1990[1]	1995[1]	2000[2]	2005[2]	2006[2]
45 to 64 years	10.2	8.2	5.8	4.8	4.1	3.1	2.7	2.6
65 years and over	4.3	3.1	3.7	3.1	2.6	1.3	1.3	1.0
American Indian or Alaska Native Female[4]								
All ages, age-adjusted[3]	NA	5.8	3.9	3.3	3.8	2.9	2.2	2.1
All ages, crude	NA	5.8	4.1	3.4	4.1	2.9	2.3	2.1
15 to 24 years	NA	*	*	*	*	*	*	*
25 to 44 years	NA	10.2	*	*	7.0	5.5	*	*
45 to 64 years	NA	*	*	*	*	*	*	*
65 years and over	NA	*	*	*	*	*	*	*
Asian or Pacific Islander Female[4]								
All ages, age-adjusted[3]	NA	2.0	1.5	1.9	2.0	1.1	0.9	0.9
All ages, crude	NA	2.1	1.7	2.1	2.1	1.2	0.9	1.0
15 to 24 years	NA	*	*	*	3.9	*	2.0	*
25 to 44 years	NA	3.2	2.2	2.7	2.7	1.5	0.9	1.2
45 to 64 years	NA	*	*	*	*	*	*	1.2
65 years and over	NA	*	*	*	*	*	*	*
Hispanic or Latina Female[4,5]								
All ages, age-adjusted[3]	NA	NA	2.9	3.3	3.1	1.8	1.5	1.4
All ages, crude	NA	NA	3.2	3.6	3.3	1.8	1.5	1.5
15 to 24 years	NA	NA	5.1	6.9	6.1	2.9	2.4	2.5
25 to 44 years	NA	NA	5.5	5.1	4.7	2.5	2.6	2.2
45 to 64 years	NA	NA	2.2	2.4	2.4	2.2	1.2	1.3
65 years and over	NA	NA	*	*	*	*	*	*
White, not Hispanic or Latina Female[5]								
All ages, age-adjusted[3]	NA	NA	4.0	3.7	3.4	2.8	2.7	2.7
All ages, crude	NA	NA	4.1	3.7	3.5	2.9	2.8	2.9
15 to 24 years	NA	NA	4.5	4.3	4.1	2.7	2.2	2.2
25 to 44 years	NA	NA	5.6	5.1	4.8	4.2	4.0	3.8
45 to 64 years	NA	NA	5.1	4.6	4.1	3.6	3.8	4.2
65 years and over	NA	NA	3.4	3.2	2.8	2.4	2.4	2.2

NA = Not available.
* = Rates based on fewer than 20 deaths are considered unreliable and are not shown.
[1]Underlying cause of death was coded according to the 8th Revision of the International Classification of Diseases (ICD) in 1970 and 9th Revision in 1980–1998.
[2]Starting with 1999 data, cause of death is coded according to ICD-10.
[3]Age-adjusted rates are calculated using the year 2000 standard population. Prior to 2001, age-adjusted rates were calculated using standard million proportions based on rounded population numbers. Starting with 2001 data, unrounded population numbers are used to calculate age-adjusted rates.
[4]The race groups, White, Black, Asian or Pacific Islander, and American Indian or Alaska Native, include persons of Hispanic and non-Hispanic origin. Persons of Hispanic origin may be of any race. Death rates for the American Indian or Alaska Native, Asian or Pacific Islander, and Hispanic populations are known to be underestimated.
[5]Prior to 1997, data from states that did not report Hispanic origin on the death certificate were excluded.

Table 2-38. Death Rates for Firearm-Related Injuries, by Sex, Race, Hispanic Origin, and Age, Selected Years, 1970–2015—Continued

(Deaths per 100,000 resident population.)

Sex, race, Hispanic origin, and age	2007[2]	2008[2]	2009[2]	2010[2]	2011[2]	2012[2]	2013[2]	2014[2]	2015[2]
45 to 64 years	2.7	2.0	2.4	2.2	2.2	2.7	2.5	2.1	2.3
65 years and over	1.2	1.3	*	*	1.0	1.3	0.9	1.4	1.1
American Indian or Alaska Native Female[4]									
All ages, age-adjusted[3]	1.8	2.3	2.5	2.6	2.4	1.8	2.0	2.4	2.6
All ages, crude	1.7	2.3	2.4	2.4	2.3	1.8	2.0	2.4	2.5
15 to 24 years	*	*	*	*	*	*	*	*	*
25 to 44 years	*	3.5	3.6	3.7	3.3	*	*	5.6	4.3
45 to 64 years	*	*	*	*	*	*	*	*	*
65 years and over	*	*	*	*	*	*	*	*	*
Asian or Pacific Islander Female[4]									
All ages, age-adjusted[3]	0.7	0.7	0.9	0.6	0.8	0.9	0.9	0.7	0.8
All ages, crude	0.7	0.8	0.9	0.6	0.9	0.9	0.9	0.8	0.8
15 to 24 years	*	*	*	*	*	*	*	*	*
25 to 44 years	0.9	1.1	1.1	1.1	1.4	1.1	1.5	0.8	1.0
45 to 64 years	*	*	1.2	*	1.0	0.9	0.8	1.3	0.8
65 years and over	*	*	*	*	*	*	*	*	*
Hispanic or Latina Female[4,5]									
All ages, age-adjusted[3]	1.5	1.5	1.4	1.3	1.3	1.3	1.3	1.4	1.5
All ages, crude	1.5	1.5	1.4	1.3	1.3	1.3	1.3	1.4	1.5
15 to 24 years	2.6	2.6	2.6	2.1	2.1	1.9	2.3	2.6	2.5
25 to 44 years	2.2	1.9	1.9	1.8	2.0	2.0	2.0	1.9	2.2
45 to 64 years	1.4	1.6	1.4	1.5	1.3	1.4	1.2	1.2	1.6
65 years and over	*	*	*	*	*	*	*	*	*
White, not Hispanic or Latina Female[5]									
All ages, age-adjusted[3]	2.8	2.9	3.0	3.0	3.2	3.3	3.3	3.4	3.6
All ages, crude	2.9	3.0	3.1	3.1	3.3	3.4	3.5	3.6	3.7
15 to 24 years	2.5	2.2	2.2	2.3	2.6	2.5	2.8	2.6	2.9
25 to 44 years	4.1	4.2	4.3	4.2	4.4	4.5	4.4	4.6	5.0
45 to 64 years	3.9	4.2	4.5	4.4	4.7	4.9	5.2	5.2	5.4
65 years and over	2.2	2.4	2.6	2.6	2.7	2.7	2.9	2.9	3.0

NA = Not available.

* = Rates based on fewer than 20 deaths are considered unreliable and are not shown.

[2]Starting with 1999 data, cause of death is coded according to ICD–10.

[3]Age-adjusted rates are calculated using the year 2000 standard population. Prior to 2001, age-adjusted rates were calculated using standard million proportions based on rounded population numbers. Starting with 2001 data, unrounded population numbers are used to calculate age-adjusted rates.

[4]The race groups, White, Black, Asian or Pacific Islander, and American Indian or Alaska Native, include persons of Hispanic and non-Hispanic origin. Persons of Hispanic origin may be of any race. Death rates for the American Indian or Alaska Native, Asian or Pacific Islander, and Hispanic populations are known to be underestimated.

[5]Prior to 1997, data from states that did not report Hispanic origin on the death certificate were excluded.

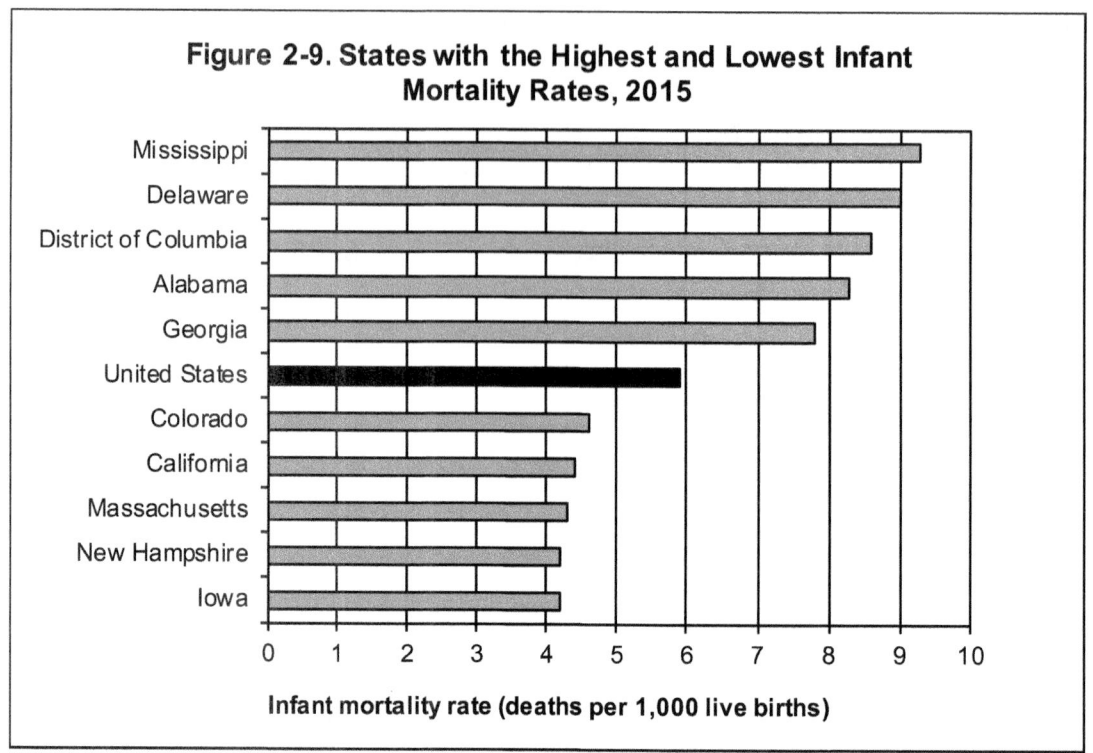

Figure 2-9. States with the Highest and Lowest Infant Mortality Rates, 2015

Table 2-39. Infant, Neonatal, and Postneonatal Mortality Rates, by Race and Sex, Selected Years, 1940–2015

(Rates are infant [under 1 year], neonatal [under 28 days], and postneonatal [28 days to 11 months]; deaths per 1,000 live births in specified group).

Year	All races			White[1]			All other[1] Total[1]			All other[1] Black[1]		
	Both sexes	Male	Female	Both sexes	Male	Female	Both sexes	Male	Female	Both sexes	Male	Female
INFANT MORTALITY RATE												
Race of Mother[2]												
1980	12.60	13.93	11.21	10.86	12.12	9.52	20.19	21.89	18.43	22.19	24.16	20.15
1981	11.93	13.14	10.66	10.34	11.50	9.12	18.82	20.36	17.24	20.81	22.54	19.03
1982	11.52	12.77	10.21	9.94	11.08	8.73	18.31	20.07	16.49	20.48	22.45	18.44
1983	11.16	12.31	9.96	9.61	10.66	8.49	17.80	19.44	16.11	19.98	21.95	17.96
1984	10.79	11.90	9.62	9.30	10.38	8.17	17.05	18.37	15.69	19.15	20.67	17.58
1985	10.64	11.91	9.32	9.17	10.39	7.88	16.84	18.33	15.28	19.01	20.76	17.22
1986	10.35	11.55	9.10	8.80	9.87	7.67	16.72	18.45	14.91	18.90	20.91	16.81
1987	10.08	11.17	8.94	8.48	9.45	7.45	16.46	18.06	14.80	18.75	20.63	16.83
1988	9.95	10.99	8.86	8.36	9.35	7.31	16.08	17.33	14.79	18.54	20.04	16.99
1989	9.81	10.81	8.77	8.08	9.01	7.10	16.33	17.60	15.02	18.61	20.02	17.15
1990	9.22	10.26	8.13	7.56	8.51	6.56	15.52	16.96	14.03	17.96	19.62	16.25
1991	8.94	10.00	7.84	7.30	8.26	6.30	15.07	16.53	13.57	17.57	19.38	15.71
1992	8.52	9.39	7.61	6.92	7.69	6.12	14.44	15.72	13.10	16.85	18.38	15.26
1993	8.37	9.25	7.43	6.82	7.56	6.05	14.07	15.58	12.52	16.52	18.33	14.67
1994	8.02	8.81	7.20	6.57	7.22	5.89	13.47	14.82	12.08	15.83	17.49	14.12
1995	7.59	8.33	6.81	6.29	6.99	5.55	12.61	13.53	11.65	15.12	16.34	13.86
1996	7.32	8.02	6.59	6.07	6.67	5.44	12.18	13.31	11.01	14.68	16.04	13.27
1997	7.23	7.95	6.47	6.03	6.67	5.36	11.76	12.83	10.65	14.16	15.47	12.82
1998	7.20	7.83	6.54	5.95	6.47	5.41	11.92	13.01	10.79	14.31	15.75	12.82
1999	7.06	7.72	6.36	5.77	6.35	5.15	11.94	12.94	10.90	14.56	15.92	13.16
2000	6.91	7.57	6.21	5.68	6.22	5.11	11.44	12.57	10.26	14.09	15.50	12.63
2001	6.85	7.52	6.14	5.65	6.21	5.06	11.33	12.44	10.18	14.02	15.48	12.52
2002	6.97	7.64	6.27	5.79	6.42	5.13	11.41	12.24	10.55	14.36	15.43	13.25
2003	6.85	7.60	6.07	5.72	6.36	5.05	11.09	12.24	9.90	14.01	15.53	12.43
2004	6.79	7.47	6.09	5.66	6.22	5.07	10.92	12.01	9.77	13.79	15.19	12.33
2005	6.87	7.56	6.15	5.73	6.32	5.11	10.92	11.98	9.82	13.73	15.15	12.27
2006	6.69	7.32	6.03	5.56	6.10	4.99	10.60	11.54	9.61	13.29	14.38	12.16
2007	6.75	7.38	6.09	5.64	6.17	5.08	10.55	11.51	9.54	13.24	14.49	11.94
2008	6.61	7.21	5.97	5.55	6.05	5.02	10.16	11.11	9.18	12.74	13.93	11.50
2009	6.39	7.01	5.75	5.30	5.79	4.78	10.02	11.06	8.94	12.64	14.08	11.15
2010	6.15	6.69	5.57	5.20	5.65	4.73	9.28	10.16	8.36	11.63	12.71	10.51
2011	6.07	6.58	5.52	5.12	5.54	4.67	9.13	9.96	8.27	11.51	12.61	10.37
2012	5.98	6.50	5.43	5.09	5.50	4.65	8.78	9.65	7.88	11.19	12.33	10.01
2013	5.96	6.52	5.38	5.07	5.59	4.52	8.79	9.46	8.08	11.22	12.03	10.39
2014	5.82	6.31	5.30	4.81	5.26	4.34	11.37	12.33	10.39	5.20	5.63	4.79
2015	5.90	6.39	5.38	4.82	5.27	4.36	11.73	12.75	10.67	5.20	5.56	4.83
Race of Child[3]												
1940	47.02	52.45	41.29	43.23	48.32	37.84	73.78	82.21	65.19	72.94	81.07	64.61
1950	29.21	32.75	25.48	26.77	30.21	23.13	44.46	48.87	39.93	43.91	48.27	39.44
1960	26.04	29.33	22.59	22.91	26.01	19.64	43.21	47.88	38.46	44.32	49.12	39.43
1970	20.01	22.37	17.52	17.75	19.95	15.42	30.92	34.20	27.53	32.65	36.18	29.01
1975	16.07	17.86	14.18	14.17	15.94	12.30	24.23	26.24	22.17	26.21	28.32	24.03
1976	15.24	16.82	13.57	13.31	14.81	11.71	23.50	25.51	21.42	25.54	27.83	23.19
1977	14.12	15.75	12.40	12.34	13.90	10.68	21.68	23.71	19.58	23.64	25.91	21.30
1978	13.78	15.26	12.23	12.01	13.37	10.58	21.06	23.15	18.90	23.11	25.39	20.77
1979	13.07	14.50	11.56	11.42	12.82	9.94	19.81	21.47	18.09	21.78	23.66	19.85
1980	12.60	13.93	11.21	11.00	12.27	9.65	19.12	20.73	17.47	21.37	23.27	19.43
NEONATAL MORTALITY RATE												
Race of Mother[2]												
1980	8.48	9.31	7.60	7.39	8.19	6.54	13.21	14.27	12.13	14.62	15.91	13.29
1981	8.02	8.81	7.20	6.99	7.73	6.20	12.51	13.52	11.48	13.98	15.16	12.77
1982	7.70	8.48	6.88	6.69	7.39	5.94	12.04	13.15	10.88	13.62	14.86	12.34
1983	7.28	8.01	6.52	6.31	6.98	5.61	11.41	12.46	10.33	12.93	14.20	11.63
1984	7.00	7.66	6.31	6.09	6.72	5.41	10.87	11.66	10.06	12.32	13.22	11.40
1985	6.96	7.75	6.13	6.00	6.75	5.21	11.00	12.00	9.95	12.62	13.81	11.39
1986	6.71	7.42	5.97	5.72	6.34	5.05	10.79	11.83	9.70	12.31	13.59	10.98
1987	6.46	7.11	5.79	5.40	5.96	4.82	10.68	11.72	9.61	12.30	13.52	11.05

[1]Multiple-race data were reported by 42 states and the District of Columbia in 2012 and 2013, by 38 states and the District of Columbia in 2011, by 37 states and the District of Columbia in 2010, by 34 states and the District of Columbia in 2008 and 2009, bby 27 states and the District of Columbia in 2007, by 25 states and the District of Columbia in 2006, by 21 states and the District of Columbia in 2005, by 15 states in 2004, and by 7 states in 2003. Multiple-race data were reported for births by 38 states and the District of Columbia in 2010, by 32 states and the District of Columbia in 2009, by 30 areas in 2008, by 27 areas in 2007, by 23 areas in 2006, by 19 areas in 2005, by 15 areas in 2004, and by 6 areas in 2003. The multiple-race data for these reporting areas were bridged to the single-race categories of the 1977 OMB standards for comparability with other reporting areas.
[2]Infant deaths are based on race of child as stated on the death certificate; live births are based on race of mother as stated on the birth certificate.
[3]Infant deaths are based on race of child as stated on the death certificate; live births are based on race of parents as stated on the birth certificate.

Table 2-39. Infant, Neonatal, and Postneonatal Mortality Rates, by Race and Sex, Selected Years, 1940–2015—*Continued*

(Rates are infant [under 1 year], neonatal [under 28 days], and postneonatal [28 days to 11 months]; deaths per 1,000 live births in specified group).

Year	All races			White[1]			All other[1] Total[1]			All other[1] Black[1]		
	Both sexes	Male	Female	Both sexes	Male	Female	Both sexes	Male	Female	Both sexes	Male	Female
1988	6.32	6.95	5.65	5.27	5.84	4.67	10.33	11.22	9.42	12.05	13.14	10.93
1989	6.23	6.79	5.63	5.15	5.66	4.60	10.30	11.08	9.49	11.92	12.84	10.97
1990	5.85	6.50	5.16	4.79	5.38	4.17	9.86	10.79	8.89	11.55	12.69	10.38
1991	5.59	6.17	4.98	4.53	5.01	4.04	9.52	10.54	8.47	11.25	12.56	9.89
1992	5.37	5.84	4.89	4.35	4.72	3.96	9.19	10.02	8.32	10.83	11.83	9.79
1993	5.29	5.75	4.81	4.29	4.64	3.92	9.02	9.90	8.11	10.69	11.76	9.59
1994	5.12	5.58	4.64	4.20	4.55	3.83	8.60	9.51	7.65	10.21	11.32	9.07
1995	4.91	5.36	4.44	4.08	4.50	3.64	8.13	8.71	7.53	9.85	10.63	9.05
1996	4.77	5.18	4.34	3.97	4.31	3.62	7.86	8.59	7.12	9.56	10.45	8.65
1997	4.77	5.20	4.32	3.99	4.37	3.59	7.74	8.36	7.09	9.40	10.12	8.65
1998	4.80	5.21	4.37	3.98	4.31	3.63	7.91	8.63	7.17	9.55	10.51	8.56
1999	4.73	5.11	4.33	3.88	4.19	3.56	7.94	8.60	7.25	9.77	10.72	8.79
2000	4.63	5.06	4.17	3.82	4.16	3.46	7.60	8.39	6.79	9.38	10.39	8.35
2001	4.54	4.97	4.08	3.78	4.15	3.39	7.37	8.06	6.65	9.21	10.15	8.25
2002	4.66	5.06	4.25	3.89	4.27	3.50	7.55	8.03	7.05	9.51	10.13	8.87
2003	4.62	5.08	4.14	3.87	4.26	3.46	7.40	8.14	6.64	9.40	10.40	8.37
2004	4.52	4.94	4.09	3.78	4.14	3.41	7.19	7.82	6.54	9.13	9.95	8.27
2005	4.54	4.93	4.12	3.79	4.10	3.46	7.18	7.88	6.47	9.07	9.96	8.14
2006	4.45	4.84	4.05	3.72	4.05	3.37	7.00	7.58	6.40	8.82	9.49	8.12
2007	4.42	4.79	4.02	3.70	4.01	3.37	6.86	7.49	6.22	8.65	9.48	7.78
2008	4.29	4.67	3.89	3.62	3.94	3.28	6.54	7.14	5.92	8.23	8.99	7.45
2009	4.18	4.53	3.81	3.48	3.76	3.19	6.48	7.10	5.83	8.17	9.04	7.28
2010	4.05	4.37	3.71	3.46	3.73	3.18	6.00	6.51	5.45	7.49	8.08	6.89
2011	4.06	4.36	3.73	3.46	3.71	3.20	5.99	6.49	5.46	7.53	8.17	6.88
2012	4.01	4.34	3.67	3.45	3.71	3.18	5.76	6.31	5.20	7.34	8.04	6.61
2013	4.04	4.37	3.68	3.47	3.79	3.13	5.83	6.22	5.43	7.43	7.93	6.92
2014	3.94	4.25	3.62	3.23	3.48	2.97	7.51	8.13	6.87	3.67	3.98	3.34
2015	3.93	4.22	3.64	3.16	3.37	2.92	7.60	8.16	7.02	3.73	4.02	3.42
Race of Child[3]												
1940	28.75	32.56	24.74	27.20	30.85	23.33	39.71	44.87	34.45	39.90	44.78	34.89
1950	20.50	23.34	17.50	19.37	22.18	16.40	27.54	30.76	24.23	27.80	31.09	24.44
1960	18.73	21.24	16.09	17.24	19.66	14.70	26.86	30.04	23.62	27.83	31.13	24.49
1970	15.08	16.96	13.10	13.77	15.55	11.88	21.43	23.87	18.91	22.76	25.37	20.07
1975	11.58	12.91	10.18	10.38	11.70	8.98	16.78	18.21	15.31	18.32	19.78	16.81
1976	10.92	12.03	9.75	9.66	10.73	8.52	16.31	17.68	14.90	17.92	19.47	16.32
1977	9.88	11.00	8.70	8.75	9.83	7.60	14.66	16.02	13.27	16.08	17.60	14.52
1978	9.49	10.54	8.38	8.39	9.34	7.38	14.01	15.54	12.43	15.47	17.17	13.72
1979	8.87	9.79	7.89	7.88	8.80	6.92	12.89	13.91	11.83	14.31	15.45	13.14
1980	8.48	9.31	7.60	7.48	8.29	6.62	12.52	13.51	11.49	14.08	15.32	12.81
POSTNEONATAL MORTALITY RATE												
Race of Mother[2]												
1980	4.13	4.62	3.61	3.47	3.93	2.98	6.97	7.62	6.30	7.57	8.25	6.87
1981	3.91	4.34	3.46	3.35	3.77	2.92	6.31	6.84	5.76	6.83	7.38	6.26
1982	3.82	4.29	3.33	3.25	3.68	2.79	6.28	6.92	5.61	6.86	7.59	6.10
1983	3.88	4.30	3.44	3.29	3.68	2.88	6.39	6.98	5.78	7.05	7.75	6.32
1984	3.79	4.23	3.31	3.22	3.65	2.76	6.18	6.71	5.63	6.83	7.46	6.18
1985	3.68	4.15	3.19	3.17	3.64	2.67	5.84	6.33	5.33	6.40	6.95	5.83
1986	3.64	4.13	3.13	3.08	3.53	2.62	5.93	6.62	5.21	6.59	7.33	5.83
1987	3.62	4.06	3.15	3.08	3.49	2.64	5.77	6.34	5.18	6.45	7.10	5.77
1988	3.64	4.04	3.21	3.09	3.51	2.65	5.75	6.11	5.37	6.49	6.90	6.07
1989	3.59	4.01	3.14	2.93	3.35	2.49	6.03	6.52	5.53	6.69	7.18	6.19
1990	3.38	3.76	2.97	2.78	3.14	2.39	5.66	6.16	5.13	6.41	6.93	5.87
1991	3.35	3.82	2.86	2.76	3.25	2.26	5.55	5.99	5.10	6.32	6.82	5.81
1992	3.14	3.55	2.72	2.58	2.97	2.16	5.25	5.69	4.78	6.02	6.54	5.47
1993	3.07	3.50	2.62	2.54	2.92	2.13	5.06	5.68	4.42	5.83	6.57	5.08
1994	2.90	3.22	2.56	2.37	2.67	2.06	4.88	5.32	4.42	5.61	6.17	5.04
1995	2.67	2.97	2.37	2.21	2.49	1.91	4.47	4.82	4.11	5.27	5.71	4.81
1996	2.55	2.84	2.24	2.09	2.36	1.81	4.32	4.72	3.90	5.11	5.60	4.62
1997	2.45	2.75	2.14	2.04	2.30	1.77	4.02	4.47	3.56	4.77	5.34	4.17

[1]Multiple-race data were reported by 42 states and the District of Columbia in 2012 and 2013, by 38 states and the District of Columbia in 2011, by 37 states and the District of Columbia in 2010, by 34 states and the District of Columbia in 2008 and 2009, bby 27 states and the District of Columbia in 2007, by 25 states and the District of Columbia in 2006, by 21 states and the District of Columbia in 2005, by 15 states in 2004, and by 7 states in 2003. Multiple-race data were reported for births by 38 states and the District of Columbia in 2010, by 32 states and the District of Columbia in 2009, by 30 areas in 2008, by 27 areas in 2007, by 23 areas in 2006, by 19 areas in 2005, by 15 areas in 2004, and by 6 areas in 2003. The multiple-race data for these reporting areas were bridged to the single-race categories of the 1977 OMB standards for comparability with other reporting areas.
[2]Infant deaths are based on race of child as stated on the death certificate; live births are based on race of mother as stated on the birth certificate.
[3]Infant deaths are based on race of child as stated on the death certificate; live births are based on race of parents as stated on the birth certificate.

Table 2-39. Infant, Neonatal, and Postneonatal Mortality Rates, by Race and Sex, Selected Years, 1940–2015—*Continued*

(Rates are infant [under 1 year], neonatal [under 28 days], and postneonatal [28 days to 11 months]; deaths per 1,000 live births in specified group).

Year	All races			White[1]			All other[1]					
							Total[1]			Black[1]		
	Both sexes	Male	Female	Both sexes	Male	Female	Both sexes	Male	Female	Both sexes	Male	Female
1998...	2.40	2.62	2.16	1.97	2.16	1.78	4.01	4.38	3.62	4.76	5.24	4.26
1999...	2.33	2.61	2.03	1.88	2.16	1.60	4.00	4.34	3.64	4.79	5.20	4.36
2000...	2.28	2.51	2.04	1.86	2.06	1.66	3.83	4.18	3.47	4.70	5.11	4.28
2001...	2.31	2.55	2.06	1.87	2.06	1.67	3.96	4.37	3.53	4.81	5.32	4.27
2002...	2.31	2.58	2.03	1.89	2.15	1.63	3.86	4.21	3.50	4.85	5.30	4.38
2003...	2.23	2.52	1.94	1.84	2.09	1.58	3.69	4.10	3.26	4.60	5.13	4.06
2004...	2.27	2.53	2.00	1.87	2.07	1.66	3.72	4.19	3.23	4.66	5.24	4.06
2005...	2.34	2.63	2.03	1.94	2.22	1.65	3.73	4.10	3.36	4.67	5.19	4.13
2006...	2.24	2.48	1.98	1.84	2.05	1.62	3.60	3.96	3.22	4.47	4.89	4.04
2007...	2.34	2.58	2.07	1.94	2.16	1.71	3.68	4.02	3.32	4.59	5.01	4.16
2008...	2.32	2.54	2.08	1.93	2.12	1.73	3.62	3.97	3.26	4.50	4.93	4.06
2009...	2.10	2.32	1.87	1.74	1.92	1.55	3.29	3.65	2.91	4.14	4.63	3.62
2010...	2.22	2.48	1.94	1.82	2.04	1.59	3.55	3.96	3.11	4.47	5.05	3.87
2011...	2.01	2.22	1.79	1.66	1.84	1.47	3.15	3.47	2.81	3.98	4.44	3.49
2012...	1.97	2.16	1.76	1.63	1.79	1.47	3.02	3.34	2.69	3.85	4.29	3.40
2013...	1.93	2.15	1.70	1.60	1.80	1.39	2.95	3.24	2.65	3.79	4.10	3.47
2014...	1.88	2.07	1.68	1.58	1.78	1.37	3.86	4.21	3.51	1.55	1.66	1.45
2015...	1.96	2.17	1.74	1.67	1.89	1.43	4.13	4.59	3.65	1.47	1.54	1.41
Race of Child[3]												
1940...	18.27	19.89	16.55	16.03	17.47	14.50	34.07	37.35	30.74	33.05	36.29	29.72
1950...	8.71	9.41	7.98	7.40	8.04	6.73	16.92	18.11	15.70	16.10	17.18	15.00
1960...	7.31	8.10	6.49	5.66	6.35	4.94	16.35	17.84	14.84	16.48	17.99	14.95
1970...	4.93	5.41	4.42	3.98	4.40	3.54	9.49	10.33	8.62	9.89	10.81	8.94
1975...	4.49	4.95	4.00	3.80	4.24	3.33	7.45	8.03	6.86	7.89	8.54	7.22
1976...	4.32	4.79	3.83	3.65	4.08	3.19	7.19	7.83	6.52	7.63	8.36	6.88
1977...	4.24	4.75	3.71	3.59	4.07	3.08	7.01	7.69	6.31	7.56	8.32	6.78
1978...	4.30	4.72	3.85	3.63	4.03	3.20	7.05	7.60	6.48	7.64	8.22	7.05
1979...	4.20	4.71	3.67	3.54	4.02	3.03	6.92	7.57	6.25	7.47	8.21	6.71
1980...	4.13	4.62	3.61	3.52	3.98	3.02	6.61	7.22	5.97	7.29	7.95	6.62

[1]Multiple-race data were reported by 42 states and the District of Columbia in 2012 and 2013, by 38 states and the District of Columbia in 2011, by 37 states and the District of Columbia in 2010, by 34 states and the District of Columbia in 2008 and 2009, by 27 states and the District of Columbia in 2007, by 25 states and the District of Columbia in 2006, by 21 states and the District of Columbia in 2005, by 15 states in 2004, and by 7 states in 2003. Multiple-race data were reported for births by 38 states and the District of Columbia in 2010, by 32 states and the District of Columbia in 2009, by 30 areas in 2008, by 27 areas in 2007, by 23 areas in 2006, by 19 areas in 2005, by 15 areas in 2004, and by 6 areas in 2003. The multiple-race data for these reporting areas were bridged to the single-race categories of the 1977 OMB standards for comparability with other reporting areas.
[3]Infant deaths are based on race of child as stated on the death certificate; live births are based on race of parents as stated on the birth certificate.

Table 2-40. Number of Infant Deaths and Mortality Rates, by Race, Hispanic Origin, Sex, State, and Territory, 2015

(Infant [under 1 year] and neonatal [under 28 days] deaths per 1,000 live births in specified group. Infant and neonatal deaths are based on race of decedent; live births are based on race of mother.)

Sex, state, and territory	Infant deaths							
	All races[1]		Non-Hispanic White[2]		Non-Hispanic Black[2]		Hispanic	
	Number	Rate	Number	Rate	Number	Rate	Number	Rate
United States[3]	23,455	5.9	10,277	4.8	6,907	11.7	4,805	5.2
Male	13,008	6.4	5,758	5.3	3,815	12.8	2,619	5.6
Female	10,447	5.4	4,519	4.4	3,092	10.7	2,186	4.8
Alabama	495	8.3	185	5.2	278	15.2	27	6.3
Alaska	78	6.9	36	5.5	2	*	2	*
Arizona	469	5.5	153	4.1	49	10.7	213	6.0
Arkansas	293	7.5	172	6.7	96	12.7	19	*
California	2,169	4.4	547	3.9	259	9.6	1,115	4.8
Colorado	309	4.6	157	3.8	36	10.4	102	5.6
Connecticut	200	5.6	73	3.6	56	12.6	64	7.7
Delaware	100	9.0	40	6.7	40	13.4	15	*
District of Columbia	82	8.6	6	*	65	13.5	8	*
Florida	1,400	6.2	464	4.5	537	10.8	307	4.8
Georgia	1,024	7.8	330	5.5	574	12.6	102	5.7
Hawaii	108	5.9	24	5.0	7	*	20	7.2
Idaho	106	4.6	89	4.9	–	*	15	*
Illinois	953	6.0	383	4.5	339	12.5	188	5.6
Indiana	611	7.3	396	6.2	135	13.1	65	8.5
Iowa	166	4.2	123	3.8	20	8.0	21	6.1
Kansas	232	5.9	135	4.8	37	12.7	49	7.8
Kentucky	375	6.7	299	6.5	51	9.7	20	6.7
Louisiana	498	7.7	176	5.2	285	11.8	29	6.0
Maine	83	6.6	76	6.6	4	*	1	*
Maryland	490	6.7	130	4.0	267	11.3	62	5.3
Massachusetts	309	4.3	167	3.8	57	8.1	61	4.7
Michigan	744	6.6	369	4.7	280	12.8	77	10.4
Minnesota	360	5.2	199	4.0	94	11.7	25	5.2
Mississippi	356	9.3	131	6.7	214	13.0	1	*
Missouri	490	6.5	314	5.5	144	12.7	19	*
Montana	75	6.0	48	4.7	3	*	7	*
Nebraska	153	5.7	99	5.2	16	*	28	6.6
Nevada	190	5.2	59	4.0	52	11.7	62	4.7
New Hampshire	52	4.2	47	4.3	1	*	3	*
New Jersey	487	4.7	171	3.6	162	10.9	130	4.7
New Mexico	131	5.1	37	5.2	3	*	67	4.6
New York	1,087	4.6	432	3.8	314	8.6	205	3.7
North Carolina	884	7.3	391	5.8	358	12.4	98	5.4
North Dakota	81	7.2	56	6.4	6	*	4	*
Ohio	1,005	7.2	590	5.7	359	15.1	42	6.0
Oklahoma	386	7.3	188	5.7	67	13.4	64	8.6
Oregon	232	5.1	152	4.7	20	15.0	45	5.3
Pennsylvania	862	6.1	467	4.8	255	12.7	94	6.3
Rhode Island	62	5.6	31	4.6	13	*	12	*
South Carolina	405	7.0	164	4.8	211	11.9	23	4.7
South Dakota	90	7.3	53	5.9	6	*	3	*
Tennessee	570	7.0	340	6.1	184	11.0	33	4.5
Texas	2,308	5.7	690	4.9	542	10.9	1,005	5.3
Utah	257	5.1	191	5.0	4	*	47	6.0
Vermont	27	4.6	24	4.5	1	*	1	*
Virginia	612	5.9	259	4.4	241	11.1	71	5.1
Washington	432	4.9	246	4.4	43	9.3	87	5.4
West Virginia	142	7.2	125	6.8	13	*	3	*
Wisconsin	386	5.8	209	4.3	107	15.1	41	6.2
Wyoming	39	5.0	34	5.5	–	*	3	*
Puerto Rico	218	7.00	-	*	1	*	217	*
Virgin Islands	4	*	-	*	-	*	2	*
Guam	47	14.00	-	*	-	*	-	*
American Samoa	10	*	-	*	-	*	-	*
Northern Marianas	5	*	-	*	-	*	-	*

NA = Not available.
- = Quantity zero.
* = Figure does not meet standards of reliability or precision.
[1]Includes races and origins not shown separately.
[2]Multiple-race data reported according to 1997 OMB standards were bridged to the single-race categories of 1977 OMB standards.
[3]Excludes data for Puerto Rico, Virgin Islands, Guam, American Samoa, and Northern Marianas.

NOTES AND DEFINITIONS

Sources of Data

Several different publications were used to obtain the mortality data. A significant amount of notes and information are derived from Murphy SL, Xu JQ, Kochanek KD, Curtin SC, Arias E. *Deaths: Final Data for 2015.* National Vital Statistics Reports; vol 66 no 6. Hyattsville, MD: National Center for Health Statistics. 2017.

In these tables, the asterisks (*) preceding the cause-of-death codes indicate that they are not part of the *International Classification of Diseases, Tenth Revision (ICD–10), Second Edition.* Updated tables were accessed via https://www.cdc.gov/nchs/data/nvsr/nvsr66/nvsr66_06.pdf.

Tables 2-22 through 2-24 come from the Census of Fatal Occupational Injuries, which can be found on the Web site of the U.S. Department of Commerce's Bureau of Labor Statistics.

Table 2-34 can be found at https://data.cdc.gov/Motor-Vehicle/Occupant-and-Alcohol-Impaired-Driving-Deaths-in-St/haed-k2ka.

Notes on the Data

Final data in Part B are based on information from all resident death certificates filed in the 50 states and the District of Columbia. It is believed that more than 99 percent of all deaths that occur in the United States are registered.

Data shown for geographic areas are by place of residence. Beginning with 1970, mortality statistics for the United States exclude deaths of nonresidents of the United States. All data exclude fetal deaths. Mortality statistics for Puerto Rico, Virgin Islands, American Samoa, and Northern Marianas exclude deaths of nonresidents for each area. For Guam, however, mortality statistics exclude deaths that occurred to a resident of any place other than Guam or the United States.

Race and Hispanic origin are reported separately on the death certificate. Therefore, data shown by race include persons of Hispanic and non-Hispanic origin, and data for Hispanic origin include persons of any race. Unless otherwise specified, deaths of Hispanic origin are included in the totals for each race group—White, Black, American Indian or Alaska Native (AIAN), and Asian or Pacific Islander (API)—according to the decedent's race as reported on the death certificate. Data shown for Hispanic persons include all persons of Hispanic origin of any race.

Age-adjusted rates are used to compare relative mortality risks among groups and over time. However, they should be viewed as relative indexes rather than as actual measures of mortality risk. They were computed by the direct method—that is, by applying age-specific death rates to the U.S. standard population age distribution. Beginning with the 1999 data year, NCHS adopted a new population standard for use in age-adjusting death rates. Based on the projected year 2000 population of the United States, the new standard replaced the 1940 standard population that had been used for more than 50 years. The new population standard affects levels of mortality and, to some extent, trends and group comparisons. Of particular note are the effects on race mortality comparisons. Beginning with 2003 data, the traditional standard million population along with corresponding standard weights to six decimal places were replaced by the projected year 2000 population age distribution. The effect of the change is negligible and does not significantly affect comparability with age-adjusted rates calculated using the previous method. All age-adjusted rates shown in this report are based on the 2000 U.S. standard population.

Infant mortality rates are the most commonly used index for measuring the risk of dying during the first year of life. The rates presented in this report are calculated by dividing the number of infant deaths in a calendar year by the number of live births registered for the same period and are presented as rates per 1,000 or per 100,000 live births. In contrast to infant mortality rates based on live births, infant death rates are based on the estimated population under age 1 year. Infant death rates that appear in tabulations of age-specific death rates in this report are calculated by dividing the number of infant deaths by the April 1, 2010, population estimate of persons under age 1, based on 2010 census populations. These rates are presented per 100,000 population in this age group. Because of differences in the denominators, infant death rates may differ from infant mortality rates.

Race and Hispanic origin are reported separately on the death certificate. Therefore, data shown by race include persons of Hispanic and non-Hispanic origin, and data for Hispanic origin include persons of any race. In this report, unless otherwise specified, deaths of persons of Hispanic origin are included in the totals for each race group (White, Black, American Indian and Alaska Native, and Asian or Pacific Islander) according to the decedent's race as reported on the death certificate. Mortality data for the Hispanic-origin population are based on deaths of residents of all 50 states and the District of Columbia. Death rates for Hispanic, American Indian and Alaska Native, and Asian or Pacific Islander persons should be interpreted with caution because of inconsistencies in reporting Hispanic origin or race on the death certificate compared with censuses, surveys, and birth certificates. Studies have shown underreporting on death certificates of American Indian and Alaska Native, Asian or Pacific Islander, and Hispanic decedents, as well as under-counts of these groups in censuses.

Cause of death statistics are in accordance with the *International Classification of Diseases, Tenth Revision (ICD-10).*

Concepts and Definitions

Age-adjusted death rate—the death rate used to make comparisons of relative mortality risks across groups and over time. This rate should be viewed as a construct or an index rather than as a direct or actual measure of mortality risk. Statistically, it is a weighted average of the age-specific death rates, where the weights represent the fixed population proportions by age.

Age-specific death rate—deaths per 100,000 population in a specified age group, such as 1–4 years or 5–9 years for a specified period.

Cause of death—for the purpose of national mortality statistics, every death is attributed to one underlying condition, based on information reported on the death certificate and using the international rules for selecting the underlying cause of death from the conditions stated on the death certificate. The underlying cause is defined by the World Health Organization as the disease or injury that initiated the train of events leading directly to death, or the circumstances of the accident or violence that produced the fatal injury. Generally more medical information is reported on death certificates than is directly reflected in the underlying cause of death. The conditions that are not selected as underlying cause of death constitute the nonunderlying causes of death, also known as multiple cause of death.

Cause-of-death ranking—selected causes of death of public health and medical importance comprise tabulation lists and are ranked according to the number of deaths assigned to these causes. The top-ranking causes determine the leading causes of death. Certain causes on the tabulation lists are not ranked if, for example, the category title represents a group title (such as major cardiovascular diseases and symptoms, signs, and abnormal clinical and laboratory findings, not elsewhere classified); or the category title begins with the words "other" and "all other". In addition, when one of the titles that represents a subtotal (such as malignant neoplasms) is ranked, its component parts are not ranked.

Crude death rate—total deaths per 100,000 population for a specified period. The crude death rate represents the average chance of dying during a specified period for persons in the entire population.

Fetal death rate—the number of fetal deaths with stated or presumed gestation of 20 weeks or more, divided by the sum of live births plus fetal deaths, per 1,000 live births plus fetal deaths.

Infant deaths—deaths of infants under 1 year of age.

International Classification of Diseases (ICD)—used to code and classify cause-of-death data. It is developed collaboratively by the World Health Organization and 10 international centers, one of which is housed at NCHS. The purpose of it is to promote international comparability in the collection, classification, processing, and presentation of health statistics. Since 1900, it has been modified about once every 10 years, except for the 20-year interval between the ninth and tenth editions. The purpose of the revisions is to stay abreast with advances in medical science. New revisions usually introduce major disruptions in time series of mortality statistics.

Hispanic origin—includes persons of Mexican, Puerto Rican, Cuban, Central and South American, and other or unknown Latin American or Spanish origins. Persons of Hispanic origin may be of any race.

Late fetal death rate—the number of fetal deaths with stated or presumed gestation of 28 weeks or more, divided by the sum of live births plus late fetal deaths per 1,000 live births plus late fetal deaths.

Life expectancy—the average number of years of life remaining to a person at a particular age and is based on a given set of age-specific death rates, generally the mortality conditions existing in the period mentioned.

Maternal mortality rate—the number of maternal deaths per 100,000 live births. The maternal mortality rate is the measure of the likelihood that a pregnant woman will die from maternal causes.

Neonatal deaths—deaths of infants aged 0–27 days.

Perinatal mortality rate—the sum of late fetal deaths plus infant deaths within 7 days of birth divided by the sum of live births plus late fetal deaths, per 1,000 live births plus late fetal deaths.

Perinatal mortality ratio—the sum of late fetal deaths plus infant deaths within 7 days of birth divided by the number of live births, per 1,000 live births.

Postneonatal deaths—deaths of infants aged 28 days–1 year old.

Years of potential life lost (YPLL)—a measure of premature mortality. YPLL is presented for persons under 75 years of age because the average life expectancy in the United States is over 75 years. YPLL-75 is calculated using the following eight age groups: under 1 year, 1–14 years, 15–24 years, 25–34 years, 35–44 years, 45–54 years, 55–64 years, and 65–74 years. The number of deaths for each age group is multiplied by years of life lost, calculated as the difference between age 75 years and the midpoint of the age group. For the eight age groups, the midpoints are 0.5, 7.5, 19.5, 29.5, 39.5, 49.5, 59.5, and 69.5. For example, the death of a person 15–24 years of age counts as 55.5 years of life lost. Years of potential life lost is derived by summing years of life lost over all age groups.

PART III: HEALTH

PART III: HEALTH

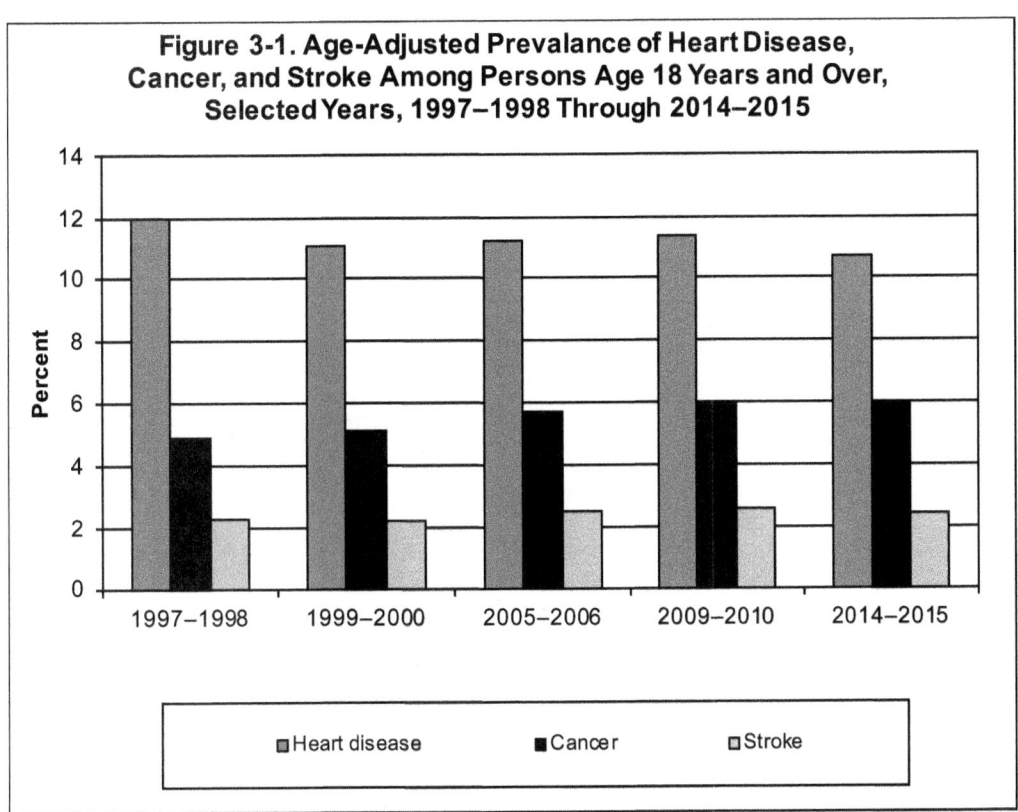

Figure 3-1. Age-Adjusted Prevalance of Heart Disease, Cancer, and Stroke Among Persons Age 18 Years and Over, Selected Years, 1997–1998 Through 2014–2015

HIGHLIGHTS

- In 2014–2015, according to age-adjusted data, 10.7 percent of people suffered from heart disease, a decline from 12.0 percent in 1997–1998. Although the percent of people with heart disease declined, the percent of people suffering from cancer increased from 4.9 percent to 5.9 percent (a rate that has been static since 2011–2012), while the percentage of people suffering from a stroke increased from 2.3 percent to 2.4 percent. (Table 3-5)

- Approximately 9.5 percent of adults age 18 years and over, when surveyed in 2013, had five or more drinks in one day on at least 12 days in the past year. This percentage was down from 21.1 percent in 1997. (Table 3-25)

- Approximately 20.1 percent of American Indian or Alaska Natives had no usual source of health care in 2014 to 2015, compared to 17.0 percent of Whites. (Table 3-31)

- The mean annual wage for healthcare practitioners and technical occupations in May 2016 was $79,160. Anesthesiologists earned the most at $269,900, while home health aides earned the least at $23,600. (Table 3-57)

- In 2015, 10.9 percent of people in the United States did not have health insurance. Massachusetts had the highest percentage of insured residents, with only 3.2 percent lacking insurance, while Texas had the highest percentage of uninsured residents at 19.0 percent. (Table 3-75)

DETERMINANTS AND MEASURES OF HEALTH

Table 3-1. Selected Notifiable Disease Rates and Number of New Cases, Selected Years, 1950–2015

(Cases per 100,000 population; number.)

Disease	1950	1960	1970	1980	1985	1988	1989	1990	1991	1992	1993
Rate											
Acute hepatitis A viral infection	NA	NA	27.87	12.84	10.03	11.60	14.43	12.64	9.67	9.06	9.40
Acute hepatitis B viral infection	NA	NA	4.08	8.39	11.50	9.43	9.43	8.48	7.14	6.32	5.18
Acute hepatitis C viral infection[1]	NA	NA	NA	NA	NA	NA	NA	1.03	1.42	2.36	1.86
Diphtheria	3.83	0.51	0.21	0.00	0.00	0.00	0.00	0.00	0.00	0.00	-
Haemophilus influenzae, invasive	NA	NA	NA	NA	NA	NA	NA	NA	1.10	0.55	0.55
Lyme disease[2]	NA	NA	NA	NA	NA	NA	NA	NA	NA	NA	NA
Measles (Rubeola)	211.01	245.42	23.23	5.96	1.18	1.38	7.33	11.17	3.82	0.88	0.12
Meningococcal disease	NA	NA	1.23	1.25	1.04	1.21	1.10	0.99	0.84	0.84	1.02
Mumps	NA	NA	55.55	3.86	1.30	2.05	2.34	2.17	1.72	1.03	0.66
Pertussis (whooping cough)	79.82	8.23	2.08	0.76	1.50	1.40	1.67	1.84	1.08	1.60	2.55
Poliomyelitis, paralytic[3]	NA	1.40	0.02	0.00	0.00	0.00	0.00	0.00	0.00	0.00	0.00
Rubella (German measles)	NA	NA	27.75	1.72	0.26	0.09	0.16	0.45	0.56	0.06	0.07
Salmonellosis, excluding typhoid fever	NA	3.85	10.84	14.88	27.37	19.91	19.26	19.54	19.10	16.04	16.15
Shigellosis	15.45	6.94	6.79	8.41	7.14	12.46	10.07	10.89	9.34	9.38	12.48
Spotted fever rickettsiosis[4]	NA	NA	0.19	0.52	0.30	0.25	0.25	0.26	0.25	0.20	0.18
Tuberculosis[5]	NA	30.83	18.28	12.25	9.30	9.13	9.46	10.33	10.42	10.46	9.82
Sexually transmitted diseases[6]											
Syphilis[7]	146.02	68.78	44.80	30.30	28.39	42.75	46.63	54.32	50.88	44.73	39.48
Primary and secondary	16.73	9.06	10.80	12.00	11.40	16.55	18.57	20.26	16.98	13.26	10.21
Early latent	39.71	10.11	8.00	8.90	9.11	14.71	18.39	22.19	21.29	19.46	16.13
Late and late latent[8]	70.22	45.91	24.70	9.20	7.74	11.19	8.93	10.32	10.87	10.42	11.83
Congenital[9]	368.30	103.70	52.30	7.70	8.75	18.95	45.46	92.95	107.62	100.05	85.49
Chlamydia[10]	NA	NA	NA	NA	17.42	87.13	102.45	160.19	179.66	182.35	178.05
Gonorrhea[11]	192.50	145.40	294.20	442.10	382.98	301.86	297.09	276.43	245.84	196.04	171.07
Chancroid	3.34	0.94	0.70	0.30	0.87	2.00	1.90	1.69	1.37	0.74	0.50
Number											
Acute hepatitis A viral infection	NA	NA	56,797	29,087	23,210	28,507	35,821	31,441	24,378	23,112	24,238
Acute hepatitis B viral infection	NA	NA	8,310	19,015	26,611	23,117	23,419	21,102	18,003	16,126	13,361
Acute hepatitis C viral infection[1]	NA	NA	NA	NA	NA	NA	NA	2,553	3,582	6,010	4,786
Diphtheria	5,796	918	435	3	3	2	3	4	5	4	-
Haemophilus influenzae, invasive	NA	NA	NA	NA	NA	NA	NA	NA	2,764	1,412	1,419
Lyme disease[2]	NA	NA	NA	NA	NA	NA	NA	NA	NA	NA	NA
Measles (Rubeola)	319,124	441,703	47,351	13,506	2,822	3,396	18,193	27,786	9,643	2,237	312
Meningococcal disease	NA	NA	2,505	2,840	2,479	2,964	2,727	2,451	2,130	2,134	2,637
Mumps	NA	NA	104,953	8,576	2,982	4,866	5,712	5,292	4,264	2,572	1,692
Pertussis (whooping cough)	120,718	14,809	4,249	1,730	3,589	3,450	4,157	4,570	2,719	4,083	6,586
Poliomyelitis, paralytic[3]	NA	2,525	31	4	8	9	11	6	10	6	4
Rubella (German measles)	NA	NA	56,552	3,904	630	225	396	1,125	1,401	160	192
Salmonellosis, excluding typhoid fever	NA	6,929	22,096	33,715	65,347	48,948	47,812	48,603	48,154	40,912	41,641
Shigellosis	23,367	12,487	13,845	19,041	17,057	30,617	25,010	27,077	23,548	23,931	32,198
Spotted fever rickettsiosis[4]	464	NA	380	1,163	714	609	623	651	628	502	456
Tuberculosis[5]	NA	55,494	37,137	27,749	22,201	22,436	23,495	25,701	26,283	26,673	25,313
Sexually transmitted diseases[6]											
Syphilis[7]	217,558	122,538	91,382	68,832	67,563	104,546	115,089	135,590	128,719	114,730	102,612
Primary and secondary	23,939	16,145	21,982	27,204	27,131	40,474	45,826	50,578	42,950	34,009	26,527
Early latent	59,256	18,017	16,311	20,297	21,689	35,968	45,394	55,397	53,855	49,929	41,919
Late and late latent[8]	113,569	81,798	50,348	20,979	18,414	27,363	22,032	25,750	27,490	26,725	30,746
Congenital[9]	13,377	4,416	1,953	277	329	741	1,837	3,865	4,424	4,067	3,420
Chlamydia[10]	NA	NA	NA	NA	25,848	157,854	200,904	323,663	381,228	409,694	405,332
Gonorrhea[11]	286,746	258,933	600,072	1,004,029	911,419	738,160	733,294	690,042	621,918	502,858	444,649
Chancroid	4,977	1,680	1,416	788	2,067	4,891	4,697	4,212	3,476	1,906	1,292

- = Quantity zero.
NA = Not available.
0.00 = Rate more than zero but less than 0.005.
[1]Anti-HCV antibody test became available May 1990.
[2]Not nationally notifiable. National surveillance case definition revised in 2008; probable cases not previously reported.
[3]Cases of vaccine-associated paralytic poliomyelitis caused by polio vaccine virus.
[4]Prior to 2010 data, cases of spotted fever rickettsiosis were reported as Rocky Mountain spotted fever (RMSF). Because serologic tests commonly used to diagnose RMSF exhibit cross-reactivity between spotted fever rickettsial pathogens, some cases reported as RMSF might actually be disease caused by other spotted fever rickettsial infections, and therefore are more correctly referred to as spotted fever rickettsiosis starting with 2010 data.
[5]Case reporting for tuberculosis began in 1953. Data prior to 1975 are not comparable with subsequent years because of changes in reporting criteria effective in 1975.
[6]For 1950, data for Alaska and Hawaii were not included. Starting with 1991, data include both civilian and military cases. Cases and rates shown do not include U.S. outlying areas of Guam, Puerto Rico, and the Virgin Islands.
[7]Includes stage of syphilis not stated.
[8]Includes cases of unknown duration.
[9]Rates include all cases of congenitally acquired syphilis per 100,000 live births. Cases of congenitally acquired syphilis were reported through 1994. Starting with 1995 data, only congenital syphilis for cases under 1 year of age were reported.
[10]Prior to 1994, chlamydia was not notifiable. In 1994–1999, cases for New York were exclusively reported by New York City. Starting with 2000 data, cases for New York include the entire state.
[11]Data for 1994 do not include cases from Georgia.

Table 3-1. Selected Notifiable Disease Rates and Number of New Cases, Selected Years, 1950–2015—*Continued*

(Cases per 100,000 population; number.)

Disease	1994	1995	1996	1997	1998	1999	2000	2001	2002	2003	2004
Rate											
Acute hepatitis A viral infection	10.29	12.13	11.70	11.22	8.59	6.25	4.91	3.77	3.13	2.66	1.95
Acute hepatitis B viral infection	4.81	4.19	4.01	3.90	3.80	2.82	2.95	2.79	2.84	2.61	2.14
Acute hepatitis C viral infection[1]	1.78	1.78	1.41	1.43	1.30	1.14	1.17	1.41	0.65	0.38	0.31
Diphtheria	0.00	-	0.01	0.01	0.00	0.00	0.00	0.00	0.00	0.00	-
Haemophilus influenzae, invasive	0.45	0.45	0.45	0.44	0.44	0.48	0.51	0.57	0.62	0.70	0.72
Lyme disease[2]	NA	NA	NA	NA	NA	NA	NA	NA	NA	NA	NA
Measles (Rubeola)	0.37	0.12	0.20	0.06	0.04	0.04	0.03	0.04	0.02	0.02	0.01
Meningococcal disease	1.11	1.25	1.30	1.24	1.01	0.92	0.83	0.83	0.64	0.61	0.47
Mumps	0.60	0.35	0.29	0.27	0.25	0.14	0.13	0.10	0.10	0.08	0.09
Pertussis (whooping cough)	1.77	1.97	2.94	2.46	2.74	2.67	2.88	2.69	3.47	4.04	8.88
Poliomyelitis, paralytic[3]	0.00	0.00	0.03	0.02	0.01	0.00	-	-	-	-	-
Rubella (German measles)	0.09	0.05	0.10	0.07	0.13	0.10	0.06	0.01	0.01	0.00	0.00
Salmonellosis, excluding typhoid fever	16.64	17.66	17.15	15.66	16.17	14.89	14.51	14.39	15.73	15.16	14.47
Shigellosis	11.44	12.32	9.80	8.64	8.74	6.43	8.41	7.19	8.37	8.19	4.99
Spotted fever rickettsiosis[4]	0.18	0.23	0.32	0.16	0.14	0.21	0.18	0.25	0.39	0.38	0.60
Tuberculosis[5]	9.36	8.70	8.04	7.42	6.79	6.43	6.01	5.68	5.36	5.17	5.09
Sexually transmitted diseases[6]											
Syphilis[7]	31.43	26.05	19.76	17.13	13.88	12.68	11.20	11.32	11.42	11.79	11.38
Primary and secondary	7.84	6.21	4.23	3.14	2.54	2.37	2.12	2.14	2.38	2.47	2.72
Early latent	12.17	10.01	7.49	6.10	4.60	4.13	3.35	3.05	2.92	2.88	2.65
Late and late latent[8]	10.49	9.12	7.56	7.50	6.43	5.97	5.53	5.95	5.95	6.30	5.89
Congenital[9]	62.03	47.77	32.94	27.88	21.39	14.62	14.29	12.52	11.44	10.56	9.12
Chlamydia[10]	192.49	187.84	190.57	205.49	231.83	247.16	251.38	274.52	289.41	301.74	316.51
Gonorrhea[11]	163.93	147.46	121.82	120.18	129.23	129.31	128.67	126.77	122.01	115.23	112.42
Chancroid	0.30	0.23	0.14	0.09	0.07	0.04	0.03	0.01	0.02	0.02	0.01
Number											
Acute hepatitis A viral infection	26,796	31,582	31,032	30,021	23,229	17,047	13,397	10,609	8,795	7,653	5,683
Acute hepatitis B viral infection	12,517	10,805	10,637	10,416	10,258	7,694	8,036	7,843	7,996	7,526	6,212
Acute hepatitis C viral infection[1]	4,470	4,576	3,716	3,816	3,518	3,111	3,197	3,976	1,835	1,102	720
Diphtheria	2	-	2	4	1	1	1	2	1	1	-
Haemophilus influenzae, invasive	1,174	1,180	1,170	1,162	1,194	1,309	1,398	1,597	1,743	2,013	2,085
Lyme disease[2]	NA	NA	NA	NA	NA	NA	NA	NA	NA	NA	NA
Measles (Rubeola)	963	309	508	138	100	100	86	116	44	56	37
Meningococcal disease	2,886	3,243	3,437	3,308	2,725	2,501	2,256	2,333	1,814	1,756	1,361
Mumps	1,537	906	751	683	666	387	338	266	270	231	258
Pertussis (whooping cough)	4,617	5,137	7,796	6,564	7,405	7,288	7,867	7,580	9,771	11,647	25,827
Poliomyelitis, paralytic[3]	8	7	7	6	3	2	-	-	-	-	-
Rubella (German measles)	227	128	238	181	364	267	176	23	18	7	10
Salmonellosis, excluding typhoid fever	43,323	45,970	45,471	41,901	43,694	40,596	39,574	40,495	44,264	43,657	42,197
Shigellosis	29,769	32,080	25,978	23,117	23,626	17,521	22,922	20,221	23,541	23,581	14,627
Spotted fever rickettsiosis[4]	465	590	831	409	365	579	495	695	1,104	1,091	1,713
Tuberculosis[5]	24,361	22,860	21,337	19,851	18,361	17,531	16,377	15,989	15,075	14,874	14,517
Sexually transmitted diseases[6]											
Syphilis[7]	82,713	69,359	53,240	46,716	38,289	35,385	31,618	32,286	32,919	34,289	33,423
Primary and secondary	20,641	16,543	11,405	8,556	7,007	6,617	5,979	6,103	6,862	7,177	7,980
Early latent	32,017	26,657	20,187	16,631	12,696	11,534	9,465	8,701	8,429	8,361	7,768
Late and late latent[8]	27,603	24,296	20,366	20,447	17,743	16,655	15,594	16,976	17,168	18,319	17,300
Congenital[9]	2,452	1,863	1,282	1,082	843	580	580	506	460	432	375
Chlamydia[10]	451,785	478,577	492,631	537,904	614,250	662,647	709,452	783,242	834,555	877,478	929,462
Gonorrhea[11]	419,602	392,651	328,169	327,665	356,492	360,813	363,136	361,705	351,852	335,104	330,132
Chancroid	782	607	386	246	189	110	78	38	48	54	30

- = Quantity zero.
NA = Not available.
0.00 = Rate more than zero but less than 0.005.
[1]Anti-HCV antibody test became available May 1990.
[2]Not nationally notifiable. National surveillance case definition revised in 2008; probable cases not previously reported.
[3]Cases of vaccine-associated paralytic poliomyelitis caused by polio vaccine virus.
[4]Prior to 2010 data, cases of spotted fever rickettsiosis were reported as Rocky Mountain spotted fever (RMSF). Because serologic tests commonly used to diagnose RMSF exhibit cross-reactivity between spotted fever rickettsial pathogens, some cases reported as RMSF might actually be disease caused by other spotted fever rickettsial infections, and therefore are more correctly referred to as spotted fever rickettsiosis starting with 2010 data.
[5]Case reporting for tuberculosis began in 1953. Data prior to 1975 are not comparable with subsequent years because of changes in reporting criteria effective in 1975.
[6]For 1950, data for Alaska and Hawaii were not included. Starting with 1991, data include both civilian and military cases. Cases and rates shown do not include U.S. outlying areas of Guam, Puerto Rico, and the Virgin Islands.
[7]Includes stage of syphilis not stated.
[8]Includes cases of unknown duration.
[9]Rates include all cases of congenitally acquired syphilis per 100,000 live births. Cases of congenitally acquired syphilis were reported through 1994. Starting with 1995 data, only congenital syphilis for cases under 1 year of age were reported.
[10]Prior to 1994, chlamydia was not notifiable. In 1994–1999, cases for New York were exclusively reported by New York City. Starting with 2000 data, cases for New York include the entire state.
[11]Data for 1994 do not include cases from Georgia.

Table 3-1. Selected Notifiable Disease Rates and Number of New Cases, Selected Years, 1950–2015—*Continued*

(Cases per 100,000 population; number.)

Disease	2005	2006	2007	2008	2009	2010	2011	2012	2013	2014	2015
Rate											
Acute hepatitis A viral infection	1.53	1.21	1.00	0.86	0.65	0.54	0.45	0.50	0.57	0.39	-
Acute hepatitis B viral infection	1.78	1.62	1.51	1.34	1.12	1.10	0.94	0.93	0.97	0.88	-
Acute hepatitis C viral infection[1]	0.23	0.26	0.28	0.29	0.27	0.29	0.42	0.59	0.71	0.73	-
Diphtheria	-	-	-	-	-	-	-	0.00	-	0.00	-
Haemophilus influenzae, invasive	0.78	0.82	0.85	0.96	0.99	1.03	1.15	1.10	1.21	1.11	-
Lyme disease[2]	NA	NA	NA	11.67	12.71	9.86	10.78	9.96	11.62	10.54	-
Measles (Rubeola)	0.02	0.02	0.01	0.05	0.02	0.02	0.06	0.02	0.06	0.21	-
Meningococcal disease	0.42	0.40	0.36	0.39	0.32	0.27	0.25	0.18	0.18	0.14	-
Mumps	0.11	2.22	0.27	0.15	0.65	0.85	0.13	0.07	0.19	0.38	-
Pertussis (whooping cough)	8.72	5.27	3.49	4.40	5.54	8.97	6.06	15.49	9.12	10.34	-
Poliomyelitis, paralytic[3]	-	-	-	-	0.00	-	-	-	-	0.00	-
Rubella (German measles)	0.00	0.00	0.00	0.01	0.00	0.00	0.00	0.00	0.00	0.00	-
Salmonellosis, excluding typhoid fever	15.43	15.45	16.03	16.92	16.18	17.73	16.79	17.27	16.13	16.14	-
Shigellosis	5.51	5.23	6.60	7.50	5.24	4.82	4.32	4.90	4.06	6.51	-
Spotted fever rickettsiosis[4]	0.66	0.80	0.77	0.85	0.60	0.65	0.91	1.44	1.08	1.18	-
Tuberculosis[5]	4.80	4.65	4.44	4.28	3.80	3.64	3.41	3.19	3.05	2.95	-
Sexually transmitted diseases[6]											
Syphilis[7]	11.23	12.34	13.57	15.22	14.74	14.93	14.91	16.02	17.87	19.90	23.43
Primary and secondary	2.94	3.26	3.80	4.44	4.60	4.49	4.52	5.03	5.50	6.27	7.49
Early latent	2.76	3.07	3.57	4.08	4.30	4.43	4.25	4.65	5.36	6.10	7.58
Late and late latent[8]	5.41	5.89	6.05	6.56	5.70	5.89	6.02	6.23	6.90	7.38	8.21
Congenital[9]	8.19	8.72	10.20	10.43	10.01	8.73	8.48	7.80	9.11	11.72	12.38
Chlamydia[10]	329.42	344.33	367.47	398.12	409.19	426.01	457.59	456.68	443.46	452.17	478.79
Gonorrhea[11]	114.57	119.70	118.03	110.75	99.05	100.76	104.24	107.46	105.34	109.79	123.95
Chancroid	0.01	0.01	0.01	0.01	0.01	0.01	0.00	0.00	0.00	0.00	0.00
Number											
Acute hepatitis A viral infection	4,488	3,579	2,979	2,585	1,987	1,670	1,398	1,562	1,781	1,239	-
Acute hepatitis B viral infection	5,119	4,713	4,519	4,033	3,405	3,374	2,903	2,895	3,050	2,791	-
Acute hepatitis C viral infection[1]	662	766	845	877	782	849	1,229	1,782	2,138	2,204	-
Diphtheria	-	-	-	-	-	-	-	1	-	1	-
Haemophilus influenzae, invasive	2,304	2,496	2,541	2,886	3,022	3,151	3,539	3,418	3,792	3,541	-
Lyme disease[2]	NA	NA	NA	35,198	38,468	30,158	33,097	30,831	36,307	33,461	-
Measles (Rubeola)	66	55	43	140	71	63	55	220	187	667	-
Meningococcal disease	1,245	1,194	1,077	1,172	980	833	759	551	556	433	-
Mumps	314	6,584	800	454	1,991	2,612	404	229	584	1,223	-
Pertussis (whooping cough)	25,616	15,632	10,454	13,278	16,858	27,550	18,719	48,277	28,639	32,971	-
Poliomyelitis, paralytic[3]	-	-	-	-	1	-	-	-	1	-	-
Rubella (German measles)	11	11	12	16	3	5	4	9	9	6	-
Salmonellosis, excluding typhoid fever	45,322	45,808	47,995	51,040	49,192	54,424	51,887	53,800	50,634	51,455	-
Shigellosis	16,168	15,503	19,758	22,625	15,931	14,786	13,352	15,283	12,729	20,745	-
Spotted fever rickettsiosis[4]	1,936	2,288	2,221	2,563	1,815	1,985	4,470	2,802	3,359	3,757	-
Tuberculosis[5]	14,097	13,779	13,299	12,904	11,545	11,182	10,528	9,945	9,582	9,421	-
Sexually transmitted diseases[6]											
Syphilis[7]	33,288	36,958	40,925	46,292	44,830	45,844	46,040	49,903	56,482	63,450	74,702
Primary and secondary	8,724	9,756	11,466	13,500	13,997	13,774	13,970	15,667	17,375	19,999	23,872
Early latent	8,176	9,186	10,768	12,401	13,066	13,604	13,136	14,503	16,929	19,452	24,173
Late and late latent[8]	16,049	17,644	18,256	19,945	17,338	18,079	18,576	19,411	21,819	23,541	26,170
Congenital[9]	339	372	435	446	429	387	358	322	359	458	487
Chlamydia[10]	976,445	1,030,911	1,108,374	1,210,523	1,244,180	1,307,893	1,412,791	1,422,976	1,401,906	1,441,789	1,526,658
Gonorrhea[11]	339,593	358,366	355,991	336,742	301,174	309,341	321,849	334,826	333,004	350,062	395,216
Chancroid	17	19	23	25	28	24	8	15	10	6	11

- = Quantity zero.
NA = Not available.
0.00 = Rate more than zero but less than 0.005.
[1]Anti-HCV antibody test became available May 1990.
[2]Not nationally notifiable. National surveillance case definition revised in 2008; probable cases not previously reported.
[3]Cases of vaccine-associated paralytic poliomyelitis caused by polio vaccine virus.
[4]Prior to 2010 data, cases of spotted fever rickettsiosis were reported as Rocky Mountain spotted fever (RMSF). Because serologic tests commonly used to diagnose RMSF exhibit cross-reactivity between spotted fever rickettsial pathogens, some cases reported as RMSF might actually be disease caused by other spotted fever rickettsial infections, and therefore are more correctly referred to as spotted fever rickettsiosis starting with 2010 data.
[5]Case reporting for tuberculosis began in 1953. Data prior to 1975 are not comparable with subsequent years because of changes in reporting criteria effective in 1975.
[6]For 1950, data for Alaska and Hawaii were not included. Starting with 1991, data include both civilian and military cases. Cases and rates shown do not include U.S. outlying areas of Guam, Puerto Rico, and the Virgin Islands.
[7]Includes stage of syphilis not stated.
[8]Includes cases of unknown duration.
[9]Rates include all cases of congenitally acquired syphilis per 100,000 live births. Cases of congenitally acquired syphilis were reported through 1994. Starting with 1995 data, only congenital syphilis for cases under 1 year of age were reported.
[10]Prior to 1994, chlamydia was not notifiable. In 1994–1999, cases for New York were exclusively reported by New York City. Starting with 2000 data, cases for New York include the entire state.
[11]Data for 1994 do not include cases from Georgia.

Table 3-2. Human Immunodeficiency Virus (HIV) Diagnoses, by Year of Diagnosis and Selected Characteristics, 2010–2015

(Number, percent distribution.)

Characteristic	Year of diagnosis[1]					
	2010	2011	2012	2013	2014	2015
Estimated number of HIV diagnoses[2]						
All persons[3]..	43,978	42,120	41,265	39,632	40,234	39,513
Sex and Age						
Male, 13 years and over................................	34,100	33,051	32,720	31,720	32,390	31,991
Female, 13 years and over.............................	9,642	8,868	8,303	7,723	7,668	7,402
Age at Diagnosis						
Under 13 years..	236	201	242	189	176	120
13-14 years...	42	43	48	42	35	25
15-19 years...	2,087	2,005	1,881	1,693	1,726	1,698
20-24 years...	7,082	7,078	7,181	7,040	7,312	7,084
25-29 years...	6,353	6,381	6,476	6,676	7,156	7,510
30-34 years...	5,527	5,282	5,481	5,185	5,458	5,437
35-39 years...	5,080	4,476	4,161	3,989	4,283	4,194
40-44 years...	5,239	4,814	4,456	3,946	3,787	3,418
45-49 years...	4,887	4,583	4,319	3,938	3,633	3,302
50-54 years...	3,507	3,371	3,215	2,987	2,916	3,010
55-59 years...	2,082	1,990	1,929	2,017	1,952	1,860
60-64 years...	1,062	1,074	1,059	1,072	977	996
65 years and over	794	822	817	858	823	859
Hispanic Origin and Race[4]						
Not Hispanic or Latino						
White	11,802	11,311	11,198	10,758	10,769	10,509
Black or African American.........................	20,447	19,323	18,583	17,698	17,842	17,670
American Indian or Alaska Native.............	168	151	182	168	200	209
Asian..	697	764	803	816	949	955
Native Hawaiian or Other Pacific Islander	55	56	56	52	43	79
Multiple race	1,643	1,518	1,437	1,318	1,080	801
Hispanic or Latino[5]......................................	9,166	8,997	9,006	8,822	9,351	9,290
Region of Residence						
Northeast...	8,362	7,798	7,608	7,052	7,039	6,516
Midwest...	5,551	5,411	5,477	5,302	5,090	5,157
South..	22,008	21,333	20,477	20,015	20,343	20,408
West..	8,057	7,578	7,703	7,263	7,762	7,432
Estimated Number of HIV Diagnoses per 100,000 Resident Population[2]						
All persons..	14.2	13.5	13.1	12.5	12.6	12.3
Sex and Age						
Male, 13 years and over................................	27.3	26.2	25.7	24.6	24.9	24.4
Female, 13 years and over.............................	7.3	6.7	6.2	5.7	5.6	5.4
Age at Diagnosis						
Under 13 years..	0.4	0.4	0.5	0.4	0.3	0.2
13-14 years...	0.5	0.5	0.6	0.5	0.4	0.3
15-19 years...	9.5	9.3	8.8	8.0	8.2	8.0
20-24 years...	32.6	31.9	31.8	30.8	31.9	31.2
25-29 years...	30.0	30.0	30.3	30.9	32.5	33.4
30-34 years...	27.5	25.7	26.2	24.3	25.3	25.1
35-39 years...	25.3	22.8	21.3	20.3	21.5	20.6
40-44 years...	25.1	22.9	21.2	18.9	18.4	16.9
45-49 years...	21.6	20.7	19.9	18.5	17.4	15.8
50-54 years...	15.7	14.9	14.2	13.2	12.9	13.5
55-59 years...	10.5	9.8	9.3	9.5	9.1	8.5
60-64 years...	6.3	6.0	5.9	5.9	5.3	5.2
65 years and over	2.0	2.0	1.9	1.9	1.8	1.8
Hispanic Origin and Race[4]						
Not Hispanic or Latino						
White	6.0	5.7	5.7	5.4	5.4	5.3
Black or African American.........................	53.8	50.3	47.9	45.2	45.1	44.3
American Indian or Alaska Native.............	7.4	6.6	7.9	7.2	8.5	8.8
Asian..	4.7	5.0	5.1	5.0	5.6	5.5
Native Hawaiian or Other Pacific Islander	11.0	11.0	10.7	9.7	7.9	14.1
Multiple race	29.1	26.0	23.9	21.3	16.9	12.2
Hispanic or Latino[5]......................................	18.1	17.3	17.0	16.3	16.9	16.4
Region of Residence						
Northeast...	15.1	14.0	13.6	12.6	12.5	11.6
Midwest...	8.3	8.1	8.1	7.8	7.5	7.6
South..	19.2	18.4	17.5	16.9	17.0	16.8
West..	11.2	10.4	10.5	9.8	10.3	9.8

Note: Data for 2015 are preliminary; CDC cautions against using the 2015 data in this report for assessments of trends.
- =Quantity zero.
[1]Based on diagnoses during 2010–2015 that were reported to CDC through June 30, 2016. Includes persons with a diagnosis of HIV infection regardless of the stage of disease (stage 0, 1, 2, 3 [AIDS], or unknown). In 2014, the criteria used to define HIV diagnoses changed. Cases diagnosed before 2014 were classified according to the 2008 HIV case definition. Starting with 2014 data, cases were classified according to the new definition. Because of the change in case definition, HIV diagnoses prior to 2014 are not strictly comparable to HIV diagnoses for 2014. The vertical line in the table represents the discontinuity in the HIV diagnosis trend.
[2]Numbers and rates are point estimates that result from statistical adjustments for reporting delays and missing risk factor information. The estimates do not include adjustments for incomplete reporting.
[3]All persons totals were calculated independent of values for subpopulations. Consequently, sums of subpopulations may not equal totals for all persons.
[4]Hispanic origin and race categories are mutually exclusive.
[5]Persons of Hispanic origin may be of any race.

Table 3-3. Age-Adjusted Cancer Incidence Rates for Selected Cancer Sites, by Sex, Race, and Hispanic Origin, Selected Geographic Areas, Selected Years, 1990–2013

(Number of new cases per 100,000 population.[1])

Site, sex, race, and Hispanic origin	1990	1991	1992	1993	1994	1995	1996	1997	1998	1999	2000	2001	2002
All Sites													
All persons	475.8	495.2	503.3	487.0	475.3	471.4	473.1	478.6	480.3	481.4	475.2	478.7	474.3
White	483.3	504.2	510.9	491.2	480.5	477.4	479.8	485.8	488.8	490.3	485.8	490.2	484.7
Black or African American	515.2	538.4	554.9	560.0	544.5	539.4	538.4	541.5	536.2	538.9	525.9	518.1	524.8
American Indian or Alaska Native[3]	348.1	357.8	363.1	384.7	362.3	371.7	376.9	396.3	376.6	414.0	365.9	396.1	359.0
Asian or Pacific Islander	335.4	341.1	359.3	354.0	348.5	340.6	336.9	349.0	343.0	345.8	341.5	347.4	346.8
Hispanic or Latino[4]	356.1	365.6	377.5	369.0	360.0	359.9	363.9	359.5	374.3	372.7	362.0	366.1	372.2
White, not Hispanic or Latino[4]	495.2	517.5	524.1	503.8	493.6	491.2	494.1	502.1	504.2	506.8	503.6	508.7	502.1
Male	584.1	626.9	649.0	611.4	579.8	564.7	563.7	565.8	563.4	568.5	565.6	566.8	558.6
White	591.1	635.1	654.6	609.3	578.9	563.5	565.4	566.1	565.4	570.5	569.8	572.9	564.1
Black or African American	688.5	753.9	792.3	795.5	751.1	742.9	723.1	729.8	721.3	720.2	707.2	692.0	689.6
American Indian or Alaska Native[3]	395.1	413.5	409.0	492.3	417.3	424.0	406.9	455.6	400.8	474.8	374.7	459.3	384.7
Asian or Pacific Islander	386.0	401.3	431.9	426.1	414.2	398.9	387.9	399.8	387.7	398.6	400.4	394.8	390.0
Hispanic or Latino[4]	417.5	440.3	471.5	459.1	442.4	440.7	438.2	431.4	443.3	444.2	436.6	437.6	443.7
White, not Hispanic or Latino[4]	606.7	653.0	672.1	623.9	593.4	577.3	580.5	582.7	581.1	587.3	588.9	591.8	581.7
Female	411.5	413.5	409.4	405.6	407.3	410.6	414.2	421.8	426.6	423.8	414.0	418.6	417.1
White	421.3	424.5	419.9	415.6	417.8	423.2	425.5	434.9	440.7	438.4	430.0	434.6	431.4
Black or African American	406.5	404.7	401.9	406.2	409.8	403.2	417.1	417.5	416.2	419.2	404.0	400.1	415.0
American Indian or Alaska Native[3]	316.5	318.4	331.4	304.4	322.0	338.6	358.1	354.8	361.5	374.3	366.2	355.5	339.1
Asian or Pacific Islander	295.7	293.2	303.0	298.3	299.2	297.8	300.5	313.4	313.0	310.2	300.9	316.0	319.9
Hispanic or Latina[4]	322.7	322.9	320.9	312.9	310.2	310.5	319.1	315.8	332.2	329.7	317.9	321.7	328.3
White, not Hispanic or Latina[4]	430.7	434.3	429.8	426.6	429.5	436.7	438.9	450.7	455.8	454.2	446.0	452.2	448.1
Lung and Bronchus													
Male	95.0	94.2	93.1	89.7	87.2	86.9	84.4	82.6	83.3	80.4	77.8	77.3	75.7
White	94.1	92.8	90.9	88.2	86.6	85.0	82.9	80.9	82.1	78.8	76.3	76.2	75.0
Black or African American	134.2	141.9	142.6	130.9	123.2	137.0	130.1	125.3	124.1	121.3	111.7	113.5	109.2
American Indian or Alaska Native[3]	77.3	45.0	54.2	94.2	77.2	82.8	67.8	75.1	69.2	54.6	62.6	82.7	46.2
Asian or Pacific Islander	64.4	63.0	69.4	64.6	60.7	60.1	60.9	62.4	61.9	62.6	63.9	57.9	57.8
Hispanic or Latino[4]	59.4	54.2	54.3	51.1	49.0	52.4	48.6	48.0	50.7	44.6	45.2	43.1	49.1
White, not Hispanic or Latino[4]	97.4	96.5	94.5	91.8	90.3	88.4	86.6	84.5	85.6	82.9	80.2	80.6	78.4
Female	47.2	48.3	48.7	48.8	48.9	49.3	50.1	50.3	51.0	50.4	48.6	48.9	49.4
White	48.5	49.8	50.4	50.7	50.5	51.7	52.2	52.9	53.0	52.4	50.7	50.8	51.5
Black or African American	52.9	54.7	52.0	53.1	55.3	50.0	54.8	50.8	57.6	58.5	55.1	55.3	55.4
American Indian or Alaska Native[3]	30.4	21.7	35.9	33.1	35.7	46.1	35.2	35.9	26.9	34.0	38.5	35.5	39.9
Asian or Pacific Islander	28.4	26.3	29.4	26.5	29.1	27.6	28.1	30.0	29.3	29.2	27.3	30.2	29.7
Hispanic or Latina[4]	26.2	28.0	26.1	28.1	22.7	25.2	26.2	25.2	26.5	26.2	24.3	25.4	25.1
White, not Hispanic or Latina[4]	50.8	52.2	53.2	53.2	53.6	54.8	55.4	56.4	56.6	55.9	54.4	54.3	55.4
Colon and Rectum													
Male	72.3	71.4	69.0	66.5	65.3	63.2	64.6	66.4	66.0	64.2	62.6	61.8	60.1
White	73.0	71.6	69.3	66.1	65.2	62.5	64.9	66.0	65.6	64.1	62.0	61.2	58.9
Black or African American	73.1	79.0	75.8	76.7	73.4	75.2	68.7	75.1	78.6	73.4	73.6	72.2	72.5
American Indian or Alaska Native[3]	61.9	60.4	52.0	58.9	61.0	66.2	61.1	72.2	48.6	81.9	48.7	61.9	49.4
Asian or Pacific Islander	60.9	60.1	58.2	58.8	58.1	58.8	56.6	59.8	58.0	55.2	58.0	56.9	59.0
Hispanic or Latino[4]	47.7	51.6	49.2	45.9	45.9	46.0	49.8	51.0	52.4	49.3	50.5	49.9	46.0
White, not Hispanic or Latino[4]	75.0	73.2	71.0	67.8	66.9	63.9	66.2	67.3	66.9	65.7	63.4	62.5	60.3
Female	50.2	49.2	48.1	47.6	46.5	45.9	46.0	47.2	48.6	47.0	46.1	45.4	45.2
White	49.7	48.8	47.4	47.1	45.7	45.4	45.5	46.9	48.2	46.2	45.6	44.4	44.1
Black or African American	61.3	56.8	57.1	55.7	58.1	54.9	54.7	58.3	56.7	58.6	58.1	57.0	56.3
American Indian or Alaska Native[3]	45.8	40.5	54.1	34.4	47.2	47.9	43.4	54.0	61.5	56.4	39.1	50.4	51.5
Asian or Pacific Islander	37.8	42.0	41.2	41.1	39.3	38.9	39.4	36.3	40.8	40.2	37.5	41.2	41.8
Hispanic or Latina[4]	34.5	34.0	33.2	32.8	33.2	31.9	33.8	32.6	34.5	35.5	34.1	32.8	32.1
White, not Hispanic or Latina[4]	50.9	50.0	48.6	48.4	46.7	46.7	46.7	48.3	49.7	47.3	46.7	45.8	45.5
Prostate													
Male	166.9	210.3	234.2	207.2	177.5	166.6	166.8	172.0	169.9	180.4	179.0	180.2	178.0
White	168.5	212.5	234.8	201.1	171.0	161.3	162.3	167.7	164.7	175.6	174.9	177.5	174.7
Black or African American	219.5	281.4	324.4	339.0	304.3	279.7	276.8	280.6	288.1	290.0	291.6	273.5	281.1
American Indian or Alaska Native[3]	98.3	114.9	123.5	147.4	86.8	93.5	111.7	106.4	84.3	102.6	71.5	102.5	96.9
Asian or Pacific Islander	88.6	108.4	125.9	124.4	114.0	104.7	95.8	97.4	94.3	107.5	108.1	110.3	104.2
Hispanic or Latino[4]	119.2	138.8	162.4	163.5	150.7	141.2	141.4	143.6	149.9	152.4	150.6	148.6	153.0
White, not Hispanic or Latino[4]	172.2	218.6	241.2	204.6	173.2	163.6	165.3	171.0	167.1	179.1	178.7	181.5	177.7
Breast													
Female	129.4	130.7	130.0	127.2	128.8	130.9	132.1	136.1	139.1	138.5	134.2	135.8	132.8
White	134.2	136.2	134.3	131.9	134.1	136.3	137.1	141.3	144.9	144.9	140.6	142.5	138.7
Black or African American	117.4	116.4	122.2	118.0	122.4	123.0	124.1	126.5	126.3	125.6	122.8	118.3	124.3
American Indian or Alaska Native[3]	69.6	73.1	98.7	98.2	87.4	96.7	118.4	85.1	92.6	85.9	100.2	97.1	82.1
Asian or Pacific Islander	88.1	83.2	90.7	86.8	83.5	88.4	91.8	101.5	101.3	100.5	94.9	101.8	100.8
Hispanic or Latina[4]	91.0	93.9	91.0	83.3	86.1	89.4	93.0	91.0	95.1	95.1	97.0	91.5	93.4
White, not Hispanic or Latina[4]	138.6	140.6	138.8	137.3	139.6	141.9	142.7	148.1	151.7	152.1	147.0	150.4	145.8
Cervix Uteri													
Female	11.9	10.8	11.0	10.7	10.5	9.9	10.7	9.8	9.8	9.4	8.9	8.8	8.4
White	11.2	10.2	10.5	10.1	9.8	9.2	9.9	9.2	9.3	9.1	8.9	8.4	8.3

Note: Estimates are based on 13 SEER areas, November 2015 submission and differ from published estimates based on 9 SEER areas or other submission dates. The site variable distinguishes Kaposi Sarcoma and Mesothelioma as individual cancer sites. As a result, Kaposi Sarcoma and Mesothelioma cases do not contribute to other cancer sites.
[1] Age adjusted by 5-year age groups to the year 2000 U.S. standard population. Age-adjusted rates are based on at least 16 cases.
[3] Estimates for the American Indian or Alaska Native populations are based on the Contract Health Service Delivery Area (CHSDA) counties within SEER areas.
[4] Hispanic data exclude cases from Alaska. The race groups White, Black, Asian or Pacific Islander, and American Indian or Alaska Native, include persons of Hispanic and non-Hispanic origin. Persons of Hispanic origin may be of any race. The North American Association of Central Cancer Registries (NAACCR) Hispanic Identification Algorithm was used on a combination of variables to classify cases as Hispanic for analytic purposes.

Table 3-3. Age-Adjusted Cancer Incidence Rates for Selected Cancer Sites, by Sex, Race, and Hispanic Origin, Selected Geographic Areas, Selected Years, 1990–2013—*Continued*

(Number of new cases per 100,000 population.[1])

Site, sex, race, and Hispanic origin	2003	2004	2005	2006	2007	2008	2009	2010	2011	2012	2013	1990–2013 APC[2]
All Sites												
All persons	463.4	465.0	460.8	461.4	468.6	462.3	460.6	450.7	443.0	429.3	419.5	-0.5†
White	474.1	475.3	473.1	474.3	480.5	474.4	472.3	462.0	454.8	439.5	429.9	-0.4†
Black or African American	514.3	519.8	505.3	500.8	508.9	503.5	503.4	483.9	476.8	464.4	444.2	-0.7†
American Indian or Alaska Native[3]	380.6	404.5	404.1	391.8	372.4	391.0	392.4	406.8	377.7	357.0	367.6	0.1
Asian or Pacific Islander	334.4	338.5	331.9	327.0	339.4	332.3	327.8	324.1	321.8	310.5	305.3	-0.5†
Hispanic or Latino[4]	358.3	367.4	365.0	356.8	363.4	360.4	358.1	348.9	351.3	336.7	327.4	-0.3†
White, not Hispanic or Latino[4]	492.4	492.8	491.3	494.3	501.0	494.5	493.0	482.7	474.6	459.5	451.1	-0.3†
Male	545.9	546.1	534.9	537.9	549.9	531.7	525.0	512.8	498.3	468.5	454.4	-1.0†
White	550.9	552.2	543.6	546.4	557.5	539.3	532.4	519.9	506.6	475.1	460.4	-1.0†
Black or African American	669.6	671.4	637.6	630.2	649.8	642.3	627.8	596.0	571.6	548.4	523.1	-1.5†
American Indian or Alaska Native[3]	448.0	410.1	426.4	400.8	410.2	429.0	432.7	456.7	403.9	350.0	377.3	-0.3
Asian or Pacific Islander	387.5	385.0	371.8	372.1	380.8	362.4	353.1	347.2	343.9	317.3	309.9	-1.1†
Hispanic or Latino[4]	423.9	438.0	426.9	416.6	427.4	414.9	413.3	398.8	392.1	365.6	343.9	-0.9†
White, not Hispanic or Latino[4]	569.3	569.7	561.8	566.9	579.0	559.8	552.8	540.8	526.9	495.4	483.2	-0.9†
Female	407.1	409.1	409.8	407.6	410.7	413.5	415.5	406.6	404.6	403.7	397.6	-0.1†
White	422.3	422.5	424.8	423.7	425.6	429.1	430.2	421.2	419.1	417.2	412.0	0.0
Black or African American	410.1	418.8	416.2	411.9	412.7	408.6	419.1	406.0	411.6	406.8	389.9	0.0
American Indian or Alaska Native[3]	336.1	406.7	389.0	390.0	351.5	370.9	369.6	378.3	364.1	370.2	365.7	0.6†
Asian or Pacific Islander	299.7	308.9	306.9	298.3	313.0	314.8	314.3	312.0	310.0	310.3	307.3	0.2†
Hispanic or Latina[4]	318.0	323.9	326.3	319.5	323.4	326.8	323.6	318.4	327.6	321.9	322.7	0.1
White, not Hispanic or Latina[4]	439.9	439.3	442.4	442.6	444.4	448.0	450.5	440.8	437.8	436.3	431.5	0.1
Lung and Bronchus												
Male	75.5	71.7	71.5	70.0	69.2	67.3	66.4	63.1	60.8	58.8	55.9	-2.1†
White	74.3	70.4	70.8	68.8	68.5	66.1	65.4	62.8	60.3	58.0	55.1	-2.1†
Black or African American	112.1	103.0	98.0	98.5	95.5	96.3	96.2	82.2	82.7	81.6	74.1	-2.6†
American Indian or Alaska Native[3]	74.2	60.9	67.4	63.6	61.5	69.5	62.0	67.1	55.6	45.2	53.2	-1.2†
Asian or Pacific Islander	58.7	59.6	58.2	57.4	55.4	55.9	52.7	51.0	50.0	48.8	48.5	-1.3†
Hispanic or Latino[4]	46.5	41.1	43.9	39.8	44.6	40.0	38.8	34.5	35.6	33.9	33.8	-2.1†
White, not Hispanic or Latino[4]	77.9	74.5	74.6	73.0	72.2	70.0	69.4	67.2	64.2	62.0	58.8	-1.9†
Female	49.8	49.0	50.0	49.2	49.3	47.8	48.4	46.1	44.9	44.4	43.2	-0.4†
White	52.4	50.6	51.9	51.2	52.0	50.4	50.3	48.1	46.6	46.1	45.1	-0.3†
Black or African American	55.5	57.9	58.4	57.3	54.3	53.4	55.7	52.9	50.0	52.0	48.1	-0.1
American Indian or Alaska Native[3]	41.4	57.0	45.5	45.8	34.9	45.0	35.3	37.2	42.1	34.6	27.5	0.5
Asian or Pacific Islander	29.1	31.0	30.8	30.0	29.0	27.6	31.1	29.2	31.3	29.0	29.2	0.3†
Hispanic or Latina[4]	24.4	25.8	22.9	24.2	25.4	24.8	25.9	24.8	23.8	22.8	24.5	-0.4†
White, not Hispanic or Latina[4]	56.6	54.5	56.4	55.6	56.4	54.7	54.6	52.0	50.8	50.3	49.1	-0.1
Colon and Rectum												
Male	58.4	56.8	54.7	53.4	53.1	51.7	49.1	46.9	45.4	43.6	42.3	-2.1†
White	57.1	55.7	54.1	52.2	51.8	50.5	47.6	45.4	43.6	42.1	40.3	-2.3†
Black or African American	76.3	74.7	67.0	65.7	66.3	67.2	61.8	57.7	57.0	55.7	55.8	-1.4†
American Indian or Alaska Native[3]	70.4	54.5	65.6	50.1	51.5	48.6	64.7	64.7	65.0	57.7	53.6	-0.2
Asian or Pacific Islander	53.3	50.3	47.7	51.1	49.1	46.7	46.5	45.5	45.6	42.3	42.5	-1.6†
Hispanic or Latino[4]	47.4	48.3	47.4	47.1	46.1	47.7	45.9	42.0	43.5	40.2	38.2	-0.9†
White, not Hispanic or Latino[4]	58.1	56.5	54.8	52.9	52.4	50.7	47.7	46.0	43.6	42.4	40.8	-2.4†
Female	43.6	42.1	41.4	41.2	40.2	39.8	38.1	36.0	34.7	33.6	32.1	-1.6†
White	42.9	41.0	40.3	40.3	39.2	39.0	36.7	34.5	33.8	32.8	31.5	-1.7†
Black or African American	55.4	54.1	54.2	54.1	52.7	49.1	50.8	46.5	42.5	41.5	38.6	-1.4†
American Indian or Alaska Native[3]	45.1	66.4	48.3	47.6	45.0	47.0	45.9	42.9	46.0	45.4	48.9	-0.2
Asian or Pacific Islander	36.4	37.3	36.9	35.5	35.3	35.6	34.4	34.6	31.6	28.8	27.5	-1.4†
Hispanic or Latina[4]	33.6	33.2	33.7	32.9	34.5	32.1	31.6	30.7	29.3	28.1	26.8	-0.7†
White, not Hispanic or Latina[4]	44.0	42.0	41.3	41.4	39.8	40.1	37.4	35.0	34.6	33.7	32.5	-1.7†
Prostate												
Male	165.5	165.5	154.1	164.7	168.0	153.6	150.3	143.8	137.2	111.5	104.6	-2.0†
White	161.7	162.4	150.1	161.5	163.3	150.0	145.8	139.3	132.9	105.6	99.6	-2.1†
Black or African American	253.7	253.0	243.8	244.4	255.3	240.1	236.6	219.9	208.2	181.4	170.0	-2.0†
American Indian or Alaska Native[3]	113.1	90.1	94.4	92.0	100.2	83.7	92.1	83.8	66.6	62.0	58.9	-2.2†
Asian or Pacific Islander	105.2	103.6	95.8	97.8	101.5	87.9	84.7	79.2	79.6	63.9	56.7	-2.1†
Hispanic or Latino[4]	139.3	150.7	132.8	134.0	133.2	127.1	124.0	118.9	110.2	94.5	83.1	-1.8†
White, not Hispanic or Latino[4]	165.3	164.4	152.7	165.9	168.8	154.2	150.0	143.2	137.3	108.3	103.4	-2.0†
Breast												
Female	124.2	124.9	124.5	122.9	126.1	126.2	127.7	123.5	126.7	126.3	126.2	-0.3†
White	129.1	129.0	129.6	127.4	130.3	129.9	132.1	127.3	130.5	129.3	129.1	-0.3†
Black or African American	123.3	124.0	119.3	124.7	126.6	126.0	128.7	123.5	129.2	130.8	126.4	0.3†
American Indian or Alaska Native[3]	94.1	102.0	105.6	89.2	89.8	90.2	99.3	91.7	105.3	97.2	89.7	0.3
Asian or Pacific Islander	92.2	97.3	95.7	92.8	100.0	102.5	99.9	100.7	102.7	104.3	107.4	0.7†
Hispanic or Latina[4]	88.0	91.3	93.0	91.2	90.9	93.0	91.3	87.3	96.0	91.7	93.4	0.1
White, not Hispanic or Latina[4]	135.8	135.6	136.2	133.7	137.5	136.7	140.1	135.5	137.4	137.1	137.0	-0.2
Cervix Uteri												
Female	8.2	7.9	7.9	7.6	7.5	7.6	7.4	7.2	7.0	6.9	6.6	-2.4†
White	7.9	7.8	7.8	7.7	7.4	7.5	7.5	7.2	7.2	6.8	6.5	-2.1†

Note: Estimates are based on 13 SEER areas, November 2015 submission and differ from published estimates based on 9 SEER areas or other submission dates. The site variable distinguishes Kaposi Sarcoma and Mesothelioma as individual cancer sites. As a result, Kaposi Sarcoma and Mesothelioma cases do not contribute to other cancer sites.
[1]Age adjusted by 5-year age groups to the year 2000 U.S. standard population. Age-adjusted rates are based on at least 16 cases.
[2]APC has been calculated by fitting a linear regression model to the natural logarithm of the yearly rates from 1990–2011.
[3]Estimates for the American Indian or Alaska Native populations are based on the Contract Health Service Delivery Area (CHSDA) counties within SEER areas.
[4]Hispanic data exclude cases from Alaska. The race groups White, Black, Asian or Pacific Islander, and American Indian or Alaska Native, include persons of Hispanic and non-Hispanic origin. Persons of Hispanic origin may be of any race. The North American Association of Central Cancer Registries (NAACCR) Hispanic Identification Algorithm was used on a combination of variables to classify cases as Hispanic for analytic purposes.

Table 3-3. Age-Adjusted Cancer Incidence Rates for Selected Cancer Sites, by Sex, Race, and Hispanic Origin, Selected Geographic Areas, Selected Years, 1990–2013—Continued

(Number of new cases per 100,000 population.[1])

Site, sex, race, and Hispanic origin	1990	1991	1992	1993	1994	1995	1996	1997	1998	1999	2000	2001	2002
Black or African American	16.7	16.1	14.3	14.8	13.7	14.9	14.3	13.3	12.8	13.0	10.7	10.8	10.1
American Indian or Alaska Native[3]	14.7	16.9	*	*	*	*	14.7	15.4	*	*	*	10.1	*
Asian or Pacific Islander	12.2	10.9	12.3	11.8	14.2	11.2	13.2	11.2	10.8	8.4	8.0	9.8	8.2
Hispanic or Latina[4]	21.3	19.7	21.2	20.1	20.1	17.4	18.5	16.6	15.5	17.0	17.1	15.1	14.5
White, not Hispanic or Latina[4]	9.7	8.6	8.8	8.5	8.1	7.8	8.5	7.9	8.1	7.6	7.1	6.9	7.0
Corpus and Uterus, Not Otherwise Specified													
Female	24.7	24.3	24.4	23.9	24.3	24.9	24.5	25.3	24.9	24.6	23.9	24.8	24.0
White	26.4	25.9	26.2	25.4	25.7	26.4	25.9	26.9	26.4	26.2	25.6	26.1	24.8
Black or African American	17.0	17.1	16.1	17.8	18.3	17.9	19.3	18.2	18.8	18.5	17.4	20.6	22.5
American Indian or Alaska Native[3]	19.3	*	*	*	17.3	*	16.7	14.8	19.7	18.7	18.5	21.1	19.2
Asian or Pacific Islander	13.5	15.8	15.3	15.3	16.0	17.8	16.8	17.7	18.1	17.9	16.6	17.9	18.9
Hispanic or Latina[4]	17.7	18.2	16.6	16.4	16.2	16.5	16.5	17.3	18.0	16.9	15.8	17.3	17.3
White, not Hispanic or Latina[4]	27.1	26.7	27.1	26.4	26.8	27.5	27.0	28.0	27.5	27.4	26.9	27.3	25.8
Ovary													
Female	15.6	15.3	14.9	15.2	14.4	14.6	14.0	14.2	14.1	14.3	14.2	14.2	13.9
White	16.4	16.2	15.8	16.0	15.1	15.4	15.1	15.0	15.0	15.2	15.0	15.4	14.7
Black or African American	11.3	10.4	10.5	11.8	11.6	10.8	9.3	10.5	10.8	10.5	10.9	9.5	10.0
American Indian or Alaska Native[3]	21.9	28.9	*	*	*	*	*	19.5	*	13.7	18.9	19.6	*
Asian or Pacific Islander	11.1	10.6	10.1	11.3	10.1	10.4	9.4	11.5	10.5	11.1	10.4	9.8	12.2
Hispanic or Latina[4]	12.2	12.0	12.8	11.7	12.2	11.7	12.3	11.3	12.2	11.1	10.6	13.6	13.8
White, not Hispanic or Latina[4]	16.8	16.6	16.0	16.4	15.4	15.9	15.4	15.5	15.4	15.7	15.6	15.7	14.7
Oral Cavity and Pharynx													
Male	18.5	17.7	18.0	17.7	17.2	16.5	17.2	16.8	16.4	15.4	15.8	15.1	15.7
White	18.0	17.6	17.7	17.4	16.7	16.4	16.8	16.7	16.2	15.2	15.6	15.4	15.9
Black or African American	25.4	21.4	23.5	23.0	23.7	22.3	22.8	19.5	21.5	20.0	19.4	18.4	18.1
American Indian or Alaska Native[3]	*	*	*	*	25.4	*	*	19.4	21.7	19.3	*	*	*
Asian or Pacific Islander	14.9	13.0	13.7	12.6	13.9	11.8	14.2	14.7	13.0	11.5	13.7	10.1	12.9
Hispanic or Latino[4]	10.7	11.1	11.3	10.5	11.4	12.3	11.6	11.0	10.0	10.1	9.1	9.1	9.7
White, not Hispanic or Latino[4]	18.8	18.3	18.4	18.2	17.3	16.9	17.5	17.4	16.9	16.0	16.6	16.3	16.9
Female	7.3	7.3	6.8	7.2	6.8	7.0	6.9	6.9	6.7	6.3	6.2	6.7	6.5
White	7.4	7.3	6.8	7.3	6.8	7.1	6.8	6.9	6.8	6.2	6.2	6.7	6.5
Black or African American	6.4	7.0	6.5	7.3	7.1	6.7	7.5	7.1	6.7	6.1	5.4	6.6	6.3
American Indian or Alaska Native[3]	*	*	*	*	*	*	*	*	*	*	*	*	*
Asian or Pacific Islander	6.1	6.7	6.3	6.0	5.7	5.2	6.0	6.6	4.6	6.6	6.3	5.8	6.0
Hispanic or Latina[4]	4.0	3.9	4.3	5.3	4.6	3.7	4.0	4.1	3.7	4.8	3.7	4.2	3.7
White, not Hispanic or Latina[4]	7.8	7.7	7.1	7.5	7.1	7.5	7.2	7.3	7.2	6.5	6.6	7.0	7.0
Stomach													
Male	14.6	14.7	14.3	14.3	14.2	13.5	13.7	13.4	12.8	12.8	12.6	11.9	12.0
White	12.8	12.7	12.4	12.3	12.2	11.9	11.8	11.3	11.0	11.2	10.6	10.3	10.4
Black or African American	21.5	24.4	20.8	20.6	23.0	18.6	22.5	22.2	20.5	17.0	18.6	17.6	15.9
American Indian or Alaska Native[3]	*	*	*	25.2	*	24.1	*	23.3	24.2	25.9	20.2	23.6	25.3
Asian or Pacific Islander	26.8	25.8	28.0	28.3	24.6	24.5	23.4	25.0	21.3	22.6	23.0	19.2	20.5
Hispanic or Latino[4]	20.2	19.8	19.4	20.2	21.6	19.3	17.3	19.1	19.2	20.1	16.1	15.9	16.4
White, not Hispanic or Latino[4]	12.1	12.0	11.6	11.4	11.2	11.1	11.2	10.4	10.1	10.1	10.0	9.4	9.6
Female	6.7	7.0	6.6	6.4	6.2	6.2	6.1	6.1	6.4	6.6	6.1	5.8	6.2
White	5.7	5.9	5.6	5.4	5.0	5.1	5.1	4.9	5.2	5.5	5.0	4.7	5.1
Black or African American	10.0	11.2	9.2	9.1	9.9	9.8	9.1	10.9	10.9	10.6	8.7	9.0	9.9
American Indian or Alaska Native[3]	*	*	*	*	*	*	*	*	*	18.2	*	*	17.2
Asian or Pacific Islander	15.4	15.4	14.7	15.4	15.1	13.0	13.8	12.1	13.0	12.1	12.9	12.3	11.5
Hispanic or Latina[4]	10.8	11.1	11.1	10.9	9.2	11.2	10.3	10.0	11.0	9.6	10.6	10.2	10.7
White, not Hispanic or Latina[4]	5.1	5.4	5.0	4.7	4.5	4.5	4.4	4.3	4.5	4.9	4.2	3.8	4.2
Pancreas													
Male	13.0	12.7	12.8	12.6	13.1	12.8	12.5	12.9	12.9	12.5	12.8	12.8	12.8
White	12.7	12.6	12.6	12.2	12.4	12.4	12.2	12.6	12.8	12.4	12.6	12.9	13.0
Black or African American	19.3	17.9	18.8	18.4	19.0	19.1	18.9	18.1	17.5	18.4	18.2	15.6	13.9
American Indian or Alaska Native[3]	*	*	*	*	*	*	*	*	*	*	*	*	*
Asian or Pacific Islander	11.0	10.3	10.7	11.9	14.3	10.3	10.6	12.1	10.6	9.2	10.7	10.0	9.9
Hispanic or Latino[4]	10.7	9.9	11.3	10.4	9.7	12.0	11.4	11.7	9.9	9.3	12.2	9.6	10.9
White, not Hispanic or Latino[4]	12.8	12.8	12.7	12.3	12.7	12.4	12.3	12.7	13.1	12.7	12.7	13.3	13.2
Female	10.0	10.3	10.0	9.9	9.9	9.9	10.1	10.1	10.1	9.6	9.9	9.8	10.5
White	9.7	10.0	9.7	9.5	9.7	9.6	9.7	9.7	9.9	9.3	9.6	9.5	10.1
Black or African American	12.9	15.7	16.0	15.9	15.0	15.5	15.3	16.8	13.7	13.4	12.8	13.7	15.9
American Indian or Alaska Native[3]	*	*	*	*	*	*	*	20.2	*	*	20.4	*	*
Asian or Pacific Islander	9.9	8.5	7.2	8.1	6.7	8.1	7.9	8.4	8.6	8.6	9.2	9.3	9.1
Hispanic or Latina[4]	9.9	10.7	9.3	10.0	9.8	9.0	9.0	9.9	10.1	9.8	9.1	10.0	11.1
White, not Hispanic or Latina[4]	9.7	9.8	9.7	9.5	9.7	9.7	9.8	9.6	9.8	9.3	9.6	9.4	10.0

Note: Estimates are based on 13 SEER areas, November 2015 submission and differ from published estimates based on 9 SEER areas or other submission dates. The site variable distinguishes Kaposi Sarcoma and Mesothelioma as individual cancer sites. As a result, Kaposi Sarcoma and Mesothelioma cases do not contribute to other cancer sites.

*Estimates are considered unreliable. Data not shown if the rate is based on fewer than 16 cases for the time interval.

[1]Age adjusted by 5-year age groups to the year 2000 U.S. standard population. Age-adjusted rates are based on at least 16 cases.

[3]Estimates for the American Indian or Alaska Native populations are based on the Contract Health Service Delivery Area (CHSDA) counties within SEER areas.

[4]Hispanic data exclude cases from Alaska. The race groups White, Black, Asian or Pacific Islander, and American Indian or Alaska Native, include persons of Hispanic and non-Hispanic origin. Persons of Hispanic origin may be of any race. The North American Association of Central Cancer Registries (NAACCR) Hispanic Identification Algorithm was used on a combination of variables to classify cases as Hispanic for analytic purposes.

Table 3-3. Age-Adjusted Cancer Incidence Rates for Selected Cancer Sites, by Sex, Race, and Hispanic Origin, Selected Geographic Areas, Selected Years, 1990–2013—Continued

(Number of new cases per 100,000 population.[1])

Site, sex, race, and Hispanic origin	2003	2004	2005	2006	2007	2008	2009	2010	2011	2012	2013	1990–2013 APC[2]
Black or African American	10.8	9.8	9.3	8.1	8.3	9.2	8.0	8.5	7.8	7.7	8.1	-3.5†
American Indian or Alaska Native[3]	*	*	10.7	9.8	*	9.6	11.6	8.3	9.5	*	9.4	-1.9†
Asian or Pacific Islander	8.1	7.2	7.8	7.0	7.0	6.3	6.6	6.5	5.4	6.7	5.7	-3.8†
Hispanic or Latina[4]	14.0	13.4	13.7	11.9	10.7	11.8	10.1	10.5	9.3	9.4	8.2	-3.9†
White, not Hispanic or Latina[4]	6.5	6.6	6.4	6.7	6.5	6.4	6.6	6.2	6.5	6.0	5.9	-1.9†
Corpus and Uterus, Not Otherwise Specified												
Female	23.6	24.0	24.1	24.1	24.5	25.3	26.5	26.7	26.6	27.0	26.4	0.4†
White	25.0	25.2	25.4	25.5	25.5	26.3	27.4	27.6	27.2	28.0	26.9	0.2†
Black or African American	20.3	20.8	21.5	19.2	23.2	24.0	25.7	24.6	27.7	25.1	27.0	2.2†
American Indian or Alaska Native[3]	19.5	17.1	14.4	23.0	21.6	20.4	28.7	27.6	20.5	19.3	27.1	*
Asian or Pacific Islander	16.6	19.0	18.9	17.9	19.2	20.3	21.3	22.5	21.7	22.3	22.4	1.8†
Hispanic or Latina[4]	17.8	19.8	19.3	18.2	19.2	19.1	20.9	20.4	22.1	23.9	23.3	1.6†
White, not Hispanic or Latina[4]	26.0	25.8	26.2	26.6	26.4	27.4	28.3	28.6	27.7	28.4	27.2	0.1
Ovary												
Female	13.6	13.2	13.2	12.9	13.1	13.0	12.7	12.5	12.2	12.3	11.4	-1.1†
White	14.3	13.9	13.9	13.7	13.7	13.8	13.6	13.4	12.9	13.0	11.9	-1.1†
Black or African American	11.6	11.2	10.8	9.1	11.6	10.0	10.2	9.6	10.0	10.6	8.8	-0.5†
American Indian or Alaska Native[3]	13.4	12.1	12.2	15.5	13.1	11.1	16.6	11.9	11.6	15.7	10.9	*
Asian or Pacific Islander	10.2	10.0	11.0	10.5	10.6	10.2	9.6	9.8	9.6	9.6	9.7	-0.5†
Hispanic or Latina[4]	11.6	11.9	11.8	10.9	11.0	12.3	10.5	11.8	11.2	12.2	10.0	-0.4
White, not Hispanic or Latina[4]	14.7	14.1	14.1	14.2	14.2	13.9	13.9	13.4	13.1	13.0	12.1	-1.1†
Oral Cavity and Pharynx												
Male	15.2	15.3	15.1	14.9	15.4	15.8	15.9	15.5	15.9	15.6	16.3	-0.6†
White	15.3	15.7	15.5	15.1	15.9	16.2	16.5	16.1	16.9	16.4	16.9	-0.3
Black or African American	17.6	16.0	15.9	16.2	15.9	14.6	15.2	13.8	13.9	14.0	14.2	-2.7†
American Indian or Alaska Native[3]	16.3	*	10.4	*	13.0	*	10.0	21.3	16.0	15.4	12.8	*
Asian or Pacific Islander	11.9	11.3	11.5	11.1	11.1	13.0	11.8	11.7	10.9	10.7	12.5	-0.9†
Hispanic or Latino[4]	8.8	10.3	9.8	7.7	9.5	10.4	11.4	8.9	10.8	10.0	8.9	-0.6†
White, not Hispanic or Latino[4]	16.3	16.7	16.4	16.4	17.2	17.4	17.6	17.5	18.1	17.6	18.5	0.0
Female	6.0	6.1	6.1	6.2	6.1	6.3	6.1	6.1	6.1	6.3	6.1	-0.8†
White	5.9	6.1	6.0	6.3	6.1	6.4	6.2	6.3	6.3	6.5	6.3	-0.7†
Black or African American	6.7	6.0	6.9	5.5	5.7	5.0	6.1	5.4	5.2	4.5	5.2	-1.5†
American Indian or Alaska Native[3]	*	*	*	*	*	*	*	*	*	7.4	8.8	*
Asian or Pacific Islander	5.1	5.9	5.9	5.4	5.4	5.7	4.7	5.2	4.8	5.9	5.2	-0.8†
Hispanic or Latina[4]	3.9	3.4	3.5	4.0	4.2	4.4	4.2	4.2	3.7	3.9	4.1	-0.3
White, not Hispanic or Latina[4]	6.2	6.6	6.4	6.7	6.5	6.8	6.6	6.7	6.9	7.0	6.8	-0.6†
Stomach												
Male	11.8	11.9	11.4	11.3	11.4	10.6	11.3	10.5	10.6	10.1	10.0	-1.7†
White	10.1	10.3	9.6	9.8	9.8	9.3	9.9	9.3	9.5	8.8	8.7	-1.6†
Black or African American	18.7	16.5	17.4	16.6	17.3	16.8	15.7	13.3	14.1	14.8	14.2	-2.1†
American Indian or Alaska Native[3]	*	25.3	20.8	20.8	21.0	12.7	16.6	20.7	21.2	16.1	22.8	-0.3
Asian or Pacific Islander	19.2	20.2	20.2	18.1	18.0	15.7	17.1	15.3	14.2	14.9	14.3	-2.9†
Hispanic or Latino[4]	16.2	17.0	15.5	15.6	17.3	16.0	16.1	14.9	14.2	13.0	12.1	-1.9†
White, not Hispanic or Latino[4]	9.2	9.3	8.7	8.7	8.6	8.2	8.7	8.3	8.5	7.9	7.8	-1.9†
Female	6.0	6.0	5.7	5.9	5.6	5.6	5.8	5.7	5.6	5.9	5.4	-0.8†
White	5.0	5.0	4.7	5.0	4.6	4.6	4.5	4.7	4.8	5.0	4.5	-0.8†
Black or African American	9.5	7.6	8.1	9.6	7.7	8.1	8.9	8.5	9.4	8.1	6.9	-1.2†
American Indian or Alaska Native[3]	*	*	*	*	11.5	*	9.9	13.0	*	12.1	12.3	*
Asian or Pacific Islander	11.1	11.5	10.3	9.1	10.5	9.9	10.8	8.9	7.8	8.8	8.8	-2.7†
Hispanic or Latina[4]	10.3	10.2	10.2	9.8	9.2	8.5	8.3	9.4	8.8	9.6	8.8	-1.0†
White, not Hispanic or Latina[4]	4.1	4.1	3.8	4.1	3.7	3.7	3.8	3.6	3.9	3.9	3.5	-1.5†
Pancreas												
Male	12.5	13.5	13.7	13.7	13.9	14.0	14.1	13.7	14.2	14.0	14.1	0.6†
White	12.3	13.2	13.4	13.9	13.9	13.7	14.1	13.5	14.2	14.5	14.0	0.7†
Black or African American	17.4	18.2	18.3	17.2	16.4	18.5	18.9	18.6	17.0	16.1	17.8	-0.3
American Indian or Alaska Native[3]	*	*	21.2	*	16.8	16.0	13.7	17.4	17.7	*	13.0	*
Asian or Pacific Islander	10.2	12.1	11.8	10.4	11.8	11.9	10.7	11.4	12.2	10.3	12.1	0.2
Hispanic or Latino[4]	10.1	11.4	12.3	12.9	11.9	11.6	13.5	11.5	13.4	10.7	11.8	0.7†
White, not Hispanic or Latino[4]	12.7	13.4	13.6	14.0	14.2	14.1	14.2	13.8	14.3	15.0	14.3	0.7†
Female	10.4	10.4	10.8	10.9	10.7	10.9	11.3	11.2	10.6	11.3	11.0	0.6†
White	10.2	10.2	10.6	10.6	10.5	10.6	11.1	10.9	10.4	11.0	11.0	0.7†
Black or African American	14.4	14.6	16.4	15.5	14.6	15.3	14.7	15.1	15.1	15.1	13.3	-0.1
American Indian or Alaska Native[3]	*	*	12.4	20.1	13.2	12.6	11.4	12.9	*	12.1	*	*
Asian or Pacific Islander	8.1	9.1	8.0	9.5	8.8	9.3	9.7	10.5	9.1	10.3	9.4	1.0†
Hispanic or Latina[4]	8.6	9.3	11.1	9.7	10.6	9.6	9.6	9.9	10.2	10.4	11.2	0.3
White, not Hispanic or Latina[4]	10.5	10.3	10.6	10.7	10.4	10.8	11.4	11.1	10.4	11.1	10.9	0.7†

Note: Estimates are based on 13 SEER areas, November 2015 submission and differ from published estimates based on 9 SEER areas or other submission dates. The site variable distinguishes Kaposi Sarcoma and Mesothelioma as individual cancer sites. As a result, Kaposi Sarcoma and Mesothelioma cases do not contribute to other cancer sites.

*Estimates are considered unreliable. Data not shown if the rate is based on fewer than 16 cases for the time interval.

[1] Age adjusted by 5-year age groups to the year 2000 U.S. standard population. Age-adjusted rates are based on at least 16 cases.

[2] APC has been calculated by fitting a linear regression model to the natural logarithm of the yearly rates from 1990–2011.

[3] Estimates for the American Indian or Alaska Native populations are based on the Contract Health Service Delivery Area (CHSDA) counties within SEER areas.

[4] Hispanic data exclude cases from Alaska. The race groups White, Black, Asian or Pacific Islander, and American Indian or Alaska Native, include persons of Hispanic and non-Hispanic origin. Persons of Hispanic origin may be of any race. The North American Association of Central Cancer Registries (NAACCR) Hispanic Identification Algorithm was used on a combination of variables to classify cases as Hispanic for analytic purposes.

Table 3-3. Age-Adjusted Cancer Incidence Rates for Selected Cancer Sites, by Sex, Race, and Hispanic Origin, Selected Geographic Areas, Selected Years, 1990–2013—*Continued*

(Number of new cases per 100,000 population.[1])

Site, sex, race, and Hispanic origin	1990	1991	1992	1993	1994	1995	1996	1997	1998	1999	2000	2001	2002
Urinary Bladder													
Male	37.2	37.4	36.9	36.8	36.1	35.4	35.9	36.0	36.8	36.6	36.8	37.0	35.8
White	40.7	41.2	40.5	39.9	39.6	38.8	39.5	39.7	40.7	40.2	40.8	41.2	39.3
Black or African American	19.7	21.3	18.4	23.9	19.9	19.7	20.0	21.6	21.0	22.2	20.2	19.7	21.0
American Indian or Alaska Native[3]	*	*	*	*	*	*	*	*	*	25.8	*	*	*
Asian or Pacific Islander	15.4	12.9	17.0	16.8	15.9	17.2	16.1	15.7	16.2	17.6	16.9	17.1	19.7
Hispanic or Latino[4]	22.4	19.9	20.2	20.9	21.5	17.8	18.5	18.8	18.3	19.8	20.4	22.0	21.2
White, not Hispanic or Latino[4]	42.4	43.1	42.4	41.7	41.4	40.9	41.6	42.0	43.2	42.4	43.2	43.5	41.6
Female	9.5	9.2	9.4	9.4	9.1	9.3	9.0	9.3	9.0	9.3	9.1	9.1	9.1
White	10.0	9.8	10.1	10.1	9.8	10.1	9.8	10.0	9.8	10.0	10.0	10.0	10.0
Black or African American	8.7	8.5	7.2	7.7	6.9	7.3	7.0	8.6	6.7	8.8	7.8	7.2	8.5
American Indian or Alaska Native[3]	*	*	*	*	*	*	*	*	*	*	*	*	*
Asian or Pacific Islander	5.2	4.0	4.9	3.9	4.0	4.5	3.7	5.1	4.7	4.1	4.3	4.6	3.4
Hispanic or Latina[4]	5.8	5.4	5.9	5.5	5.5	5.3	5.9	5.4	5.1	4.8	5.8	5.2	6.4
White, not Hispanic or Latina[4]	10.3	10.3	10.5	10.6	10.3	10.6	10.3	10.6	10.3	10.6	10.5	10.6	10.5
Non-Hodgkin's Lymphoma													
Male	22.6	23.2	23.3	23.4	24.8	25.1	24.6	23.9	23.0	24.4	23.6	24.0	23.8
White	23.6	24.5	24.4	24.5	25.8	26.2	25.8	24.8	24.2	25.4	25.0	25.2	25.1
Black or African American	17.7	17.2	19.1	17.7	20.5	21.7	19.3	23.0	17.6	18.7	17.6	18.2	18.0
American Indian or Alaska Native[3]	*	*	*	*	*	*	*	*	*	15.9	15.3	20.9	16.6
Asian or Pacific Islander	16.7	16.0	16.4	15.9	18.2	16.5	16.9	16.7	15.7	19.2	16.4	18.1	16.5
Hispanic or Latino[4]	17.3	17.9	21.9	17.9	19.0	21.0	21.5	18.5	20.2	18.2	20.5	18.6	20.6
White, not Hispanic or Latino[4]	24.3	25.2	24.6	25.0	26.5	26.7	26.2	25.5	24.7	26.3	25.5	26.0	25.7
Female	14.5	14.4	14.6	14.5	15.3	15.2	15.2	16.0	16.4	16.2	16.0	16.2	16.5
White	15.4	15.1	15.6	15.3	16.2	15.9	16.0	16.8	17.2	17.3	16.9	17.0	17.5
Black or African American	10.4	10.4	9.3	10.1	8.8	10.3	11.8	12.0	13.2	11.3	11.9	12.6	11.9
American Indian or Alaska Native[3]	*	*	*	*	*	*	*	*	*	15.1	13.5	*	*
Asian or Pacific Islander	9.5	10.1	9.1	11.0	12.3	12.2	9.8	11.0	11.2	11.6	11.5	13.0	12.4
Hispanic or Latina[4]	13.6	11.7	12.4	13.6	13.9	13.1	13.7	14.9	14.5	14.6	13.8	14.4	13.6
White, not Hispanic or Latina[4]	15.6	15.5	15.9	15.4	16.3	16.2	16.4	17.1	17.6	17.6	17.3	17.5	18.1
Leukemia													
Male	17.2	16.8	17.6	16.8	16.8	17.7	16.9	17.2	17.3	16.8	17.2	18.0	17.2
White	18.0	17.8	18.7	17.8	17.9	19.0	17.7	18.4	18.5	17.8	18.2	19.3	18.6
Black or African American	16.2	12.5	14.4	14.1	11.8	13.4	14.9	14.3	13.6	14.1	14.3	13.7	12.8
American Indian or Alaska Native[3]	*	*	*	*	*	*	*	*	*	*	*	10.9	7.9
Asian or Pacific Islander	8.4	11.1	9.1	9.8	10.2	10.2	11.2	9.3	10.6	10.8	10.6	10.5	9.6
Hispanic or Latino[4]	12.2	11.8	11.8	10.7	10.8	14.6	12.5	12.6	12.5	12.0	13.3	11.3	12.3
White, not Hispanic or Latino[4]	18.3	18.2	19.2	18.2	18.3	19.3	18.0	18.8	18.9	18.3	18.7	20.0	19.2
Female	9.9	10.3	9.7	10.1	9.9	10.3	10.2	10.0	10.1	9.5	10.4	10.6	10.1
White	10.3	10.8	10.1	10.4	10.5	10.9	10.7	10.7	10.8	10.0	11.0	11.4	10.9
Black or African American	8.5	9.4	8.1	10.0	7.7	8.4	8.6	8.3	7.7	8.1	9.8	9.1	7.5
American Indian or Alaska Native[3]	*	*	*	*	*	*	*	*	*	*	*	*	*
Asian or Pacific Islander	5.7	5.8	7.0	7.4	6.9	6.4	6.5	5.8	6.7	6.6	6.4	5.3	6.4
Hispanic or Latina[4]	8.5	8.3	8.2	7.5	8.4	8.2	7.4	8.9	9.1	8.2	7.8	7.8	8.7
White, not Hispanic or Latina[4]	10.3	10.8	10.1	10.4	10.6	11.1	10.9	10.9	10.7	10.2	11.1	11.8	10.9

Note: Estimates are based on 13 SEER areas, November 2015 submission and differ from published estimates based on 9 SEER areas or other submission dates. The site variable distinguishes Kaposi Sarcoma and Mesothelioma as individual cancer sites. As a result, Kaposi Sarcoma and Mesothelioma cases do not contribute to other cancer sites.
^ = Annual percent change (APC) is significantly different from 0 (p<0.05).
*Estimates are considered unreliable. Data not shown if the rate is based on fewer than 16 cases for the time interval.
[1]Age adjusted by 5-year age groups to the year 2000 U.S. standard population. Age-adjusted rates are based on at least 16 cases.
[3]Estimates for the American Indian or Alaska Native populations are based on the Contract Health Service Delivery Area (CHSDA) counties within SEER areas.
[4]Hispanic data exclude cases from Alaska. The race groups White, Black, Asian or Pacific Islander, and American Indian or Alaska Native, include persons of Hispanic and non-Hispanic origin. Persons of Hispanic origin may be of any race. The North American Association of Central Cancer Registries (NAACCR) Hispanic Identification Algorithm was used on a combination of variables to classify cases as Hispanic for analytic purposes.

Table 3-3. Age-Adjusted Cancer Incidence Rates for Selected Cancer Sites, by Sex, Race, and Hispanic Origin, Selected Geographic Areas, Selected Years, 1990–2013—*Continued*

(Number of new cases per 100,000 population.[1])

Site, sex, race, and Hispanic origin	2003	2004	2005	2006	2007	2008	2009	2010	2011	2012	2013	1990–2013 APC[2]
Urinary Bladder												
Male	37.0	37.1	37.0	36.1	37.5	35.7	35.2	35.9	33.9	34.2	32.7	-0.3†
White	40.8	41.0	40.9	39.8	41.6	39.2	38.6	40.0	38.1	38.0	36.2	-0.2†
Black or African American	23.2	23.2	23.2	20.5	21.9	22.9	22.4	22.2	20.7	23.3	22.6	0.5†
American Indian or Alaska Native[3]	*	14.5	16.8	14.0	*	23.0	20.2	17.4	17.7	*	13.7	*
Asian or Pacific Islander	18.1	17.4	17.5	18.9	18.4	18.4	17.9	17.3	14.9	16.4	15.5	0.2
Hispanic or Latino[4]	20.2	20.0	20.2	20.7	20.8	17.5	19.3	18.5	19.9	18.8	18.1	-0.4
White, not Hispanic or Latino[4]	43.4	43.8	43.6	42.4	44.5	42.3	41.5	43.2	41.0	41.0	39.3	-0.1
Female	9.2	9.2	9.0	8.8	8.6	8.8	8.4	8.6	8.3	8.3	7.8	-0.6†
White	10.0	10.1	9.7	9.6	9.4	9.7	9.2	9.4	9.1	9.3	8.5	-0.5†
Black or African American	7.8	8.3	7.9	8.6	7.6	6.5	7.0	7.0	7.1	6.0	7.7	-0.5
American Indian or Alaska Native[3]	*	*	*	*	*	*	*	*	*	*	*	*
Asian or Pacific Islander	5.0	3.9	5.2	3.9	3.8	5.1	4.0	4.7	4.4	4.1	3.8	-0.3
Hispanic or Latina[4]	4.7	5.6	5.9	5.6	5.3	5.6	5.1	4.7	5.6	4.8	4.4	-0.6†
White, not Hispanic or Latina[4]	10.8	10.7	10.3	10.2	10.1	10.4	9.9	10.2	9.8	10.1	9.3	-0.3†
Non-Hodgkin's Lymphoma												
Male	24.3	25.1	24.7	24.0	25.1	24.8	24.9	25.4	23.7	23.6	23.6	0.1
White	25.7	26.3	25.9	25.6	26.8	26.2	26.3	26.6	25.0	24.9	24.7	0.2†
Black or African American	19.4	22.3	19.6	19.6	18.3	18.9	19.3	21.4	17.4	17.4	17.6	-0.1
American Indian or Alaska Native[3]	*	*	23.2	13.9	15.0	13.7	20.3	19.6	10.8	13.8	10.4	*
Asian or Pacific Islander	16.4	16.8	17.9	15.5	16.8	18.3	17.2	17.5	18.1	17.6	17.9	0.3
Hispanic or Latino[4]	19.5	21.5	19.9	19.2	20.9	21.0	20.4	22.8	19.9	19.4	19.6	0.3
White, not Hispanic or Latino[4]	26.5	26.9	27.0	26.5	27.8	27.0	27.4	27.2	25.7	25.9	25.7	0.3†
Female	17.2	17.4	16.5	16.9	16.8	16.6	17.1	17.0	15.8	16.1	15.6	0.5†
White	18.0	18.4	17.7	18.1	17.9	17.4	18.1	18.1	16.6	17.1	16.5	0.6†
Black or African American	13.5	13.6	13.3	12.5	13.2	13.5	12.4	12.7	12.9	13.6	12.8	1.2†
American Indian or Alaska Native[3]	*	14.7	12.2	17.7	*	12.1	16.1	13.0	16.5	11.1	12.8	*
Asian or Pacific Islander	12.7	12.3	9.7	11.3	11.6	12.3	12.3	11.9	12.0	11.4	10.8	0.4
Hispanic or Latina[4]	15.3	15.5	15.0	15.7	14.8	14.9	17.4	15.5	14.6	15.2	14.5	0.7†
White, not Hispanic or Latina[4]	18.4	18.9	18.1	18.6	18.5	17.7	18.2	18.4	17.0	17.2	16.9	0.6†
Leukemia												
Male	17.4	17.4	17.5	16.8	17.5	17.6	17.5	18.1	17.7	17.3	16.8	0.1
White	18.5	18.5	19.1	18.2	19.0	18.9	18.6	19.6	19.0	18.2	18.1	0.2†
Black or African American	15.1	17.0	12.9	14.0	13.4	14.1	15.1	13.7	14.3	14.9	14.0	0.1
American Indian or Alaska Native[3]	*	11.9	12.3	12.1	*	14.1	*	*	9.8	14.6	11.4	*
Asian or Pacific Islander	10.5	10.2	9.4	9.1	9.7	10.1	10.1	10.1	10.4	10.5	8.7	-0.1
Hispanic or Latino[4]	12.3	13.1	13.2	13.8	12.3	12.5	12.8	13.2	13.8	11.5	12.7	0.3
White, not Hispanic or Latino[4]	19.1	19.0	19.5	18.4	19.6	19.4	19.3	20.1	19.6	19.0	18.6	0.2†
Female	10.1	10.5	10.1	10.9	10.1	10.9	10.3	10.7	10.5	10.6	10.3	0.3†
White	10.7	11.0	10.7	11.9	11.0	11.5	11.0	11.5	11.4	11.3	11.2	0.4†
Black or African American	9.1	9.9	9.6	8.5	7.7	8.3	8.1	9.1	9.4	9.2	8.4	0.1
American Indian or Alaska Native[3]	*	*	*	*	*	11.0	*	8.7	*	7.0	8.1	*
Asian or Pacific Islander	6.5	6.7	6.4	6.3	6.2	7.2	6.9	6.1	6.4	6.6	6.2	0.0
Hispanic or Latina[4]	7.2	8.8	8.3	9.0	8.3	9.7	8.5	8.7	8.7	8.8	9.6	0.6†
White, not Hispanic or Latina[4]	11.2	11.3	10.7	12.2	11.3	11.5	11.1	11.8	11.6	11.4	11.2	0.5†

Note: Estimates are based on 13 SEER areas, November 2015 submission and differ from published estimates based on 9 SEER areas or other submission dates. The site variable distinguishes Kaposi Sarcoma and Mesothelioma as individual cancer sites. As a result, Kaposi Sarcoma and Mesothelioma cases do not contribute to other cancer sites.
*Estimates are considered unreliable. Data not shown if the rate is based on fewer than 16 cases for the time interval.
† = Difference not statistically significant.
[1]Age adjusted by 5-year age groups to the year 2000 U.S. standard population. Age-adjusted rates are based on at least 16 cases.
[2]APC has been calculated by fitting a linear regression model to the natural logarithm of the yearly rates from 1990–2011.
[3]Estimates for the American Indian or Alaska Native populations are based on the Contract Health Service Delivery Area (CHSDA) counties within SEER areas.
[4]Hispanic data exclude cases from Alaska. The race groups White, Black, Asian or Pacific Islander, and American Indian or Alaska Native, include persons of Hispanic and non-Hispanic origin. Persons of Hispanic origin may be of any race. The North American Association of Central Cancer Registries (NAACCR) Hispanic Identification Algorithm was used on a combination of variables to classify cases as Hispanic for analytic purposes.

Table 3-4. Five-Year Relative Cancer Survival Rates for Selected Cancer Sites, by Sex and Selected Race, Selected Geographic Areas, Selected Years 1975–1977 Through 2006–2012

(Percent of patients.)

Sex and site	White										
	1975–1977	1978–1980	1981–1983	1984–1986	1987–1989	1990–1992	1993–1995	1996–1998	1999–2001	2002–2005	2006–2012
Both Sexes											
All sites	49.8	50.0	51.3	53.6	56.7	61.4	62.4	64.3	67.2	68.5	70.0
Oral cavity and pharynx	54.1	55.3	54.0	56.3	55.9	57.9	60.0	59.9	62.2	65.7	68.7
Esophagus	5.5	5.3	7.3	10.2	10.5	12.9	13.4	14.1	18.8	19.4	21.7
Stomach	14.1	15.4	16.2	16.8	18.3	18.8	19.9	20.3	22.3	25.9	30.2
Colon	50.9	52.4	55.4	59.0	60.6	62.7	60.4	62.8	66.6	66.0	66.7
Rectum	48.3	49.7	52.0	57.0	58.7	59.9	60.6	63.5	66.5	69.0	68.0
Pancreas	2.5	2.5	2.5	2.6	3.2	4.4	3.9	4.1	5.0	5.9	8.5
Lung and bronchus	12.2	12.9	13.3	13.0	13.3	13.9	14.6	14.8	15.5	16.9	19.0
Urinary bladder	73.3	74.7	77.4	77.2	79.8	80.2	81.1	79.8	81.0	80.8	78.9
Non-Hodgkin's lymphoma	46.8	47.8	50.8	52.0	51.3	51.5	53.2	59.4	64.9	71.5	73.6
Leukemia	34.6	36.7	38.0	41.6	43.9	46.4	48.5	49.5	51.8	59.4	63.5
Male											
All sites	42.7	44.3	46.6	48.6	52.8	60.8	62.0	64.0	67.5	69.0	70.3
Oral cavity and pharynx	53.8	54.4	52.8	54.8	54.1	56.4	59.4	59.1	62.0	65.7	68.3
Esophagus	4.8	5.3	6.5	9.0	11.0	12.3	13.6	13.9	18.6	19.2	21.8
Stomach	13.1	13.6	15.4	14.4	15.5	16.0	18.9	18.6	21.0	24.3	28.8
Colon	50.5	51.3	56.1	59.6	61.4	63.1	60.7	62.9	67.8	66.1	67.0
Rectum	47.3	49.3	51.0	56.4	58.9	59.0	59.5	62.8	66.5	69.4	67.6
Pancreas	2.7	2.6	2.1	2.1	3.1	4.2	3.6	4.7	5.5	5.5	8.9
Lung and bronchus	11.1	11.5	11.7	11.2	12.0	12.4	12.6	13.0	13.3	14.6	16.4
Prostate gland	68.5	71.2	73.1	76.4	84.4	94.1	95.9	97.8	99.7	99.8	99.7
Urinary bladder	74.3	75.4	78.5	78.5	82.0	82.6	82.5	81.1	81.5	82.4	80.2
Non-Hodgkin's lymphoma	46.3	46.2	50.5	50.6	48.1	47.5	49.7	57.6	62.8	70.5	72.9
Leukemia	33.6	35.8	37.8	41.3	45.5	46.2	49.4	49.4	52.7	60.1	64.7
Female											
All sites	56.5	55.6	56.0	58.5	60.6	62.0	62.8	64.7	66.8	67.9	69.7
Colon	51.3	53.4	54.8	58.5	59.9	62.4	60.2	62.8	65.5	65.9	66.3
Rectum	49.4	50.1	53.2	57.7	58.4	61.0	61.9	64.4	66.4	68.5	68.7
Pancreas	2.3	2.5	3.0	3.1	3.3	4.5	4.2	3.6	4.4	6.3	8.0
Lung and bronchus	15.4	16.2	16.6	16.3	15.3	16.2	17.1	17.0	18.0	19.3	21.8
Melanoma of skin	86.2	87.8	87.2	90.9	91.3	91.7	92.6	92.7	94.6	95.6	95.1
Breast	75.6	75.1	77.1	80.0	85.1	86.5	87.7	89.3	90.8	91.6	92.0
Cervix uteri	69.7	68.1	67.8	68.8	72.5	70.9	74.2	73.7	73.4	70.1	70.6
Corpus uteri, not otherwise specified	88.0	83.7	82.2	84.0	83.9	85.8	84.9	85.2	85.9	85.2	85.6
Ovary	35.3	36.8	38.4	37.5	38.1	40.4	40.6	43.3	43.5	43.5	46.0
Non-Hodgkin's lymphoma	47.3	49.5	51.1	53.6	55.2	56.4	57.6	61.4	67.5	72.6	74.5

Note: Rates are based on follow-up of patients through 2013. The rate is the ratio of the observed survival rate for the patient group to the expected survival rate for persons in the general population similar to the patient group with respect to age, sex, race, and calendar year of observation. It estimates the chance of surviving the effects of cancer. The site variable distinguishes Kaposi Sarcoma and Mesothelioma as individual cancer sites. As a result, Kaposi Sarcoma and Mesothelioma cases are excluded from each of the sites shown except all sites combined. The race groups White and Black include persons of Hispanic and non-Hispanic origin. Due to death certificate race-ethnicity classification and other methodological issues related to developing life tables, survival rates for race-ethnicity groups other than White and Black are not calculated.

Table 3-4. Five-Year Relative Cancer Survival Rates for Selected Cancer Sites, by Sex and Selected Race, Selected Geographic Areas, Selected Years 1975–1977 Through 2006–2012—*Continued*

(Percent of patients.)

Sex and site	Black or African American										
	1975–1977	1978–1980	1981–1983	1984–1986	1987–1989	1990–1992	1993–1995	1996–1998	1999–2001	2002–2005	2006–2012
Both Sexes											
All sites	39.0	39.0	38.8	40.2	43.0	47.8	52.8	55.2	57.9	59.5	62.7
Oral cavity and pharynx	36.0	34.9	30.8	35.0	34.0	32.9	37.9	36.1	44.6	45.8	47.2
Esophagus	3.5	4.3	4.3	8.7	6.6	9.1	7.6	10.2	12.5	12.9	12.5
Stomach	16.1	16.4	16.4	19.1	18.8	22.7	19.3	22.6	23.0	28.6	30.3
Colon	44.7	48.9	48.5	49.1	52.3	53.4	51.1	53.6	52.5	54.9	56.9
Rectum	44.4	34.6	40.3	45.9	52.3	51.2	53.8	55.1	59.2	60.2	64.7
Pancreas	2.3	5.7	3.6	4.7	5.5	3.6	3.6	3.4	5.6	4.3	8.0
Lung and bronchus	11.2	11.7	11.3	11.1	10.9	10.5	12.8	12.3	12.6	13.5	15.9
Urinary bladder	50.3	54.5	59.5	59.4	62.6	63.1	60.5	62.7	67.4	63.2	66.1
Non-Hodgkin's lymphoma	48.6	51.3	49.5	46.8	46.0	42.2	42.1	54.6	55.7	63.3	65.2
Leukemia	33.4	28.2	33.9	32.7	35.0	35.9	41.3	38.6	43.2	52.7	57.5
Male											
All sites	32.7	33.3	34.2	35.5	38.9	47.6	54.4	57.9	61.0	63.2	65.6
Oral cavity and pharynx	29.7	29.8	25.3	29.5	30.0	28.2	33.0	31.2	39.4	42.0	44.5
Esophagus	2.0	3.4	3.7	8.2	5.3	9.4	7.8	8.5	10.6	11.2	10.5
Stomach	16.1	15.6	16.2	16.9	16.6	22.0	17.5	20.4	25.0	24.5	24.1
Colon	44.0	47.5	44.6	48.9	50.7	54.6	51.2	55.8	53.6	52.9	56.8
Rectum	41.4	33.5	38.1	43.4	47.7	53.7	51.4	53.6	60.0	56.5	59.4
Pancreas	2.5	4.5	3.7	3.9	5.1	3.2	3.3	3.1	3.7	2.9	8.6
Lung and bronchus	10.5	9.7	10.1	10.3	10.8	9.3	11.2	10.7	10.8	12.8	13.3
Prostate gland	60.7	62.1	62.8	65.6	71.1	84.4	91.7	94.9	97.3	97.7	97.3
Urinary bladder	56.5	62.6	64.9	62.3	67.5	65.7	67.7	65.6	71.6	67.4	70.9
Non-Hodgkin's lymphoma	42.6	47.3	49.2	44.5	41.7	38.2	35.7	53.0	48.9	59.3	61.3
Leukemia	30.4	27.3	33.4	31.5	32.7	30.9	41.6	39.0	44.2	54.5	60.1
Female											
All sites	46.2	45.6	44.4	45.5	47.7	48.2	50.6	52.1	54.3	55.5	59.5
Colon	45.3	49.8	51.5	49.3	53.7	52.3	51.0	51.9	51.6	56.5	57.0
Rectum	46.8	35.5	42.5	48.2	56.9	48.5	56.4	56.4	58.2	63.8	70.1
Pancreas	1.9	7.0	3.2	5.3	5.8	4.0	3.7	3.5	7.4	5.5	7.4
Lung and bronchus	13.8	17.8	14.9	12.8	11.1	12.7	15.7	14.9	15.2	14.5	19.0
Melanoma of skin	*	*	*	*	89.5	*	*	78.6	76.1	77.7	76.2
Breast	62.2	63.4	63.4	65.1	71.1	71.5	72.7	76.2	78.8	77.8	81.5
Cervix uteri	64.6	61.0	59.2	57.9	57.0	57.9	62.8	64.8	66.0	62.7	58.4
Corpus uteri, not otherwise specified	60.0	54.9	50.7	56.2	56.7	54.0	58.5	61.4	61.4	60.2	65.7
Ovary	41.9	38.8	37.5	39.4	33.7	35.5	41.5	39.2	35.6	36.8	38.1
Non-Hodgkin's lymphoma	55.3	56.7	49.8	49.9	51.0	47.7	54.0	56.9	63.8	67.9	69.2

Note: Rates are based on follow-up of patients through 2013. The rate is the ratio of the observed survival rate for the patient group to the expected survival rate for persons in the general population similar to the patient group with respect to age, sex, race, and calendar year of observation. It estimates the chance of surviving the effects of cancer. The site variable distinguishes Kaposi Sarcoma and Mesothelioma as individual cancer sites. As a result, Kaposi Sarcoma and Mesothelioma cases are excluded from each of the sites shown except all sites combined. The race groups White and Black include persons of Hispanic and non-Hispanic origin. Due to death certificate race-ethnicity classification and other methodological issues related to developing life tables, survival rates for race-ethnicity groups other than White and Black are not calculated.
*Data for population groups with fewer than 25 cases are not shown because estimates are considered unreliable.

Table 3-5. Respondent-Reported Prevalence of Heart Disease, Cancer, and Stroke Among Adults 18 Years of Age and Over, by Selected Characteristics, Selected Years, 1997–1998 Through 2014–2015

(Percent.)

Characteristic	Heart disease[1]													
	1997–1998	1999–2000	2000–2001	2001–2002	2003–2004	2005–2006	2007–2008	2008–2009	2009–2010	2010–2011	2011–2012	2012–2013	2013–2014	2014–2015
18 years and over, age adjusted[4,5]	12.0	11.1	11.5	11.5	11.3	11.2	11.3	11.5	11.4	11.1	10.8	10.6	10.7	10.7
18 years and over, crude[5]	11.6	10.9	11.3	11.3	11.3	11.4	11.6	11.8	11.8	11.6	11.4	11.4	11.5	11.6
Age														
18 to 44 years	4.6	4.3	4.4	4.3	4.1	4.0	4.4	4.5	4.4	4.0	3.7	3.8	4.0	4.3
18 to 24 years	3.2	3.3	3.4	3.3	3.0	3.2	3.1	3.3	3.4	3.0	2.6	2.6	2.8	3.3
25 to 44 years	5.0	4.6	4.7	4.6	4.5	4.2	4.8	4.9	4.8	4.4	4.0	4.2	4.5	4.7
45 to 64 years	13.5	12.6	12.9	12.9	12.5	12.9	12.2	12.7	13.1	13.0	12.5	12.1	12.0	11.9
45 to 54 years	10.9	10.0	10.2	10.0	9.4	9.4	8.8	9.5	10.1	9.6	9.2	8.9	8.6	8.5
55 to 64 years	17.4	16.6	17.1	17.4	17.0	17.8	16.8	16.8	17.0	17.1	16.2	15.8	15.8	15.5
65 years and over	31.8	29.6	30.9	31.3	31.8	31.2	31.8	31.7	30.4	30.5	30.3	29.8	29.4	29.2
65 to 74 years	27.8	25.8	26.6	26.6	27.3	26.5	26.9	26.2	25.1	25.6	25.5	25.0	25.1	25.3
75 years and over	37.0	34.3	36.0	36.8	36.8	36.6	37.5	38.0	37.0	36.5	36.4	36.3	35.4	34.8
Sex[4]														
Male	12.3	11.9	12.3	12.4	12.3	12.2	12.5	12.8	12.8	12.4	12.1	11.9	11.9	11.9
Female	11.8	10.5	10.9	10.8	10.7	10.5	10.5	10.5	10.3	10.2	9.7	9.6	9.6	9.8
Sex and Age														
Male														
18 to 44 years	3.7	3.6	3.6	3.6	3.6	3.3	3.8	4.4	4.3	3.7	3.6	3.8	3.9	4.2
45 to 54 years	11.0	10.0	10.2	10.1	8.7	9.8	9.2	10.0	10.4	9.5	9.6	9.8	9.0	8.4
55 to 64 years	18.7	19.7	19.4	19.9	20.4	20.5	18.3	18.8	19.0	19.1	18.5	17.9	17.9	17.4
65 to 74 years	32.0	30.4	31.4	31.9	33.1	31.6	32.0	30.5	30.8	31.3	30.7	30.1	30.9	31.2
75 years and over	40.8	39.2	42.7	43.6	42.6	43.1	46.5	46.6	45.3	44.7	43.5	41.7	41.4	41.5
Female														
18 to 44 years	5.5	4.9	5.1	4.9	4.7	4.7	4.9	4.7	4.5	4.3	3.8	3.7	4.1	4.4
45 to 54 years	10.8	9.9	10.1	9.9	10.1	9.1	8.4	9.0	9.8	9.6	8.9	8.1	8.2	8.6
55 to 64 years	16.2	13.8	14.9	15.2	13.9	15.4	15.4	14.9	15.1	15.3	14.1	13.8	14.0	13.9
65 to 74 years	24.5	22.0	22.7	22.2	22.5	22.2	22.5	22.6	20.2	20.6	21.0	20.5	20.0	20.2
75 years and over	34.6	31.2	31.9	32.6	33.1	32.4	31.7	32.3	31.3	30.9	31.5	32.6	31.1	30.1
Race[4,6]														
White only	12.2	11.3	11.7	11.7	11.6	11.5	11.7	11.9	11.6	11.2	10.8	10.8	10.9	11.0
Black or African American only	11.4	10.6	10.9	10.6	9.8	10.1	10.2	10.7	11.0	10.7	10.7	10.5	10.1	9.7
American Indian or Alaska Native only	18.6	14.7	14.2	11.4	12.8	15.9	11.1	10.2	10.3	12.5	12.1	10.1	10.8	13.4
Asian only	6.9	6.3	7.3	8.8	6.3	6.8	6.0	5.7	6.7	7.2	7.0	6.4	6.0	6.5
Native Hawaiian or Other Pacific Islander only	NA	*	*	*	*	*	*	*	*	*	*	*	*	*
Two or more races	NA	17.0	16.8	16.5	12.5	14.7	16.9	15.2	15.5	16.7	16.8	15.5	15.9	16.5
Hispanic Origin and Race[4,6]														
Hispanic or Latino	8.7	8.0	8.0	8.0	8.5	8.0	8.5	8.4	8.3	8.4	8.2	8.0	8.0	8.0
Mexican	7.5	7.4	7.5	7.8	8.9	7.5	8.3	8.4	8.4	8.4	8.1	8.0	7.9	7.7
Not Hispanic or Latino	12.2	11.4	11.8	11.8	11.6	11.6	11.7	11.9	11.8	11.4	11.1	11.0	11.0	11.1
White only	12.5	11.6	12.0	12.1	12.0	12.0	12.1	12.4	12.1	11.7	11.3	11.3	11.4	11.5
Black or African American only	11.4	10.5	10.9	10.5	9.8	10.2	10.2	10.8	11.1	10.8	10.8	10.5	10.2	9.8
Education[7,8]														
No high school diploma or GED	15.1	13.8	14.3	14.3	14.3	14.2	14.9	14.5	14.5	14.6	13.9	13.7	13.7	13.8
High school diploma or GED	12.8	11.9	12.3	12.4	12.3	12.6	11.9	12.7	12.7	12.4	11.9	12.1	12.3	12.0
Some college or more	12.7	12.0	12.5	12.4	12.2	11.9	12.4	12.4	12.2	12.2	11.9	11.6	11.3	11.5
Percent of Poverty Level[4,9]														
Below 100 percent	15.3	13.6	14.7	14.4	14.3	14.6	14.0	14.1	14.5	13.9	13.3	13.8	13.7	13.7
100 percent to 199 percent	13.2	12.0	12.5	12.4	12.8	12.5	13.0	13.2	12.8	12.3	11.9	12.0	11.9	12.0
200 percent to 399 percent	11.5	11.0	11.3	11.3	11.4	11.0	11.7	11.6	11.3	11.3	10.7	10.5	10.6	10.7
400 percent or more	11.0	10.2	10.6	10.9	10.0	10.1	10.0	10.1	10.0	9.8	9.5	9.3	9.3	9.5
Hispanic Origin and Race and Percent of Poverty Level[4,6,9]														
Hispanic or Latino														
Below 100 percent	9.7	9.7	8.8	8.7	11.3	11.0	11.0	10.3	10.3	9.4	9.4	10.0	10.2	10.2
100 percent to 199 percent	8.7	8.4	8.9	9.0	8.0	8.1	9.6	8.8	7.9	8.3	8.5	8.4	7.9	8.0
200 percent to 399 percent	8.4	8.2	7.3	6.5	8.2	6.9	7.1	7.7	8.4	8.5	7.9	7.0	7.0	6.8
400 percent or more	8.4	5.6	6.6	6.9	5.4	5.1	8.0	7.1	7.2	7.5	7.3	7.2	7.6	7.8
Not Hispanic or Latino														
White only														
Below 100 percent	17.8	15.2	16.9	16.5	15.9	16.9	16.0	15.9	16.3	15.8	15.1	16.1	16.0	16.2
100 percent to 199 percent	14.1	12.8	13.6	13.5	14.8	14.3	14.7	15.6	15.1	13.8	13.3	13.7	13.6	13.7
200 percent to 399 percent	12.2	11.6	12.0	12.1	12.3	11.9	12.9	12.8	12.1	11.8	11.3	11.1	11.6	11.8
400 percent or more	11.3	10.6	11.0	11.3	10.3	10.6	10.5	10.6	10.6	10.5	10.2	9.9	9.8	9.9

NA = Not available.

* = Figure does not meet standards of reliability or precision. Data preceded by an asterisk have a relative standard error (RSE) of 20 percent to 30 percent. Data not shown have an RSE of greater than 30 percent.

[1]Heart disease is based on self-reported responses to questions about whether respondents had ever been told by a doctor or other health professional that they had coronary heart disease, angina (angina pectoris), a heart attack (myocardial infarction), or any other kind or heart disease or heart condition.

[4]Estimates are age-adjusted to the year 2000 standard population using five age groups: 18 to 44 years, 45 to 54 years, 55 to 64 years, 65 to 74 years, and 75 years and over. Age-adjusted estimates in this table may differ from other age-adjusted estimates based on the same data and presented elsewhere if different age groups are used in the adjustment procedure.

[5]Includes all other races not shown separately and unknown education level.

[6]The race groups White, Black, American Indian or Alaska Native, Asian, Native Hawaiian or Other Pacific Islander, and two or more races, include persons of Hispanic and non-Hispanic origin. Persons of Hispanic origin may be of any race.

[7]Estimates are for persons 25 years of age and over and are age-adjusted to the year 2000 standard population using five age groups: 25 to 44 years, 45 to 54 years, 55 to 64 years, 65 to 74 years, and 75 years and over.

[8]GED is General Educational Development high school equivalency diploma.

[9]Percent of poverty level is based on family income and family size and composition using U.S. Census Bureau poverty thresholds.

Table 3-5. Respondent-Reported Prevalence of Heart Disease, Cancer, and Stroke Among Adults 18 Years of Age and Over, by Selected Characteristics, Selected Years, 1997–1998 Through 2014–2015—Continued

(Percent.)

Characteristic	Cancer[2]													
	1997–1998	1999–2000	2000–2001	2001–2002	2003–2004	2005–2006	2007–2008	2008–2009	2009–2010	2010–2011	2011–2012	2012–2013	2013–2014	2014–2015
18 years and over, age adjusted[4,5]	4.9	5.1	5.1	5.3	5.2	5.7	5.6	5.9	6.0	6.0	5.9	5.9	5.9	5.9
18 years and over, crude[5]	4.8	4.9	5.0	5.2	5.2	5.7	5.8	6.1	6.3	6.3	6.2	6.4	6.4	6.5
Age														
18 to 44 years	1.7	1.7	1.7	1.7	1.5	1.8	1.7	1.6	1.6	1.7	1.6	1.6	1.6	1.6
18 to 24 years	0.8	1.0	0.8	0.8	0.7	0.9	0.8	0.8	0.7	0.7	*0.7	*0.5	*0.6	*0.5
25 to 44 years	2.0	1.9	2.0	2.1	1.7	2.2	2.0	1.9	2.0	2.0	1.9	1.9	2.0	2.0
45 to 64 years	5.4	5.2	5.3	5.7	5.8	6.0	6.3	6.7	7.1	6.9	6.5	6.7	6.7	6.6
45 to 54 years	4.0	4.0	4.1	4.2	4.2	4.4	4.6	4.9	5.3	4.9	4.4	4.4	4.3	4.2
55 to 64 years	7.4	7.2	7.3	7.9	8.1	8.2	8.6	9.2	9.3	9.3	8.9	9.3	9.3	9.1
65 years and over	14.1	15.2	15.2	15.6	15.9	17.1	17.0	17.7	18.1	18.5	18.5	18.4	18.2	18.4
65 to 74 years	12.4	13.1	13.1	13.9	13.8	14.3	14.6	15.8	16.1	15.9	16.2	16.2	15.6	15.0
75 years and over	16.2	17.7	17.8	17.6	18.3	20.2	19.8	20.0	20.5	21.7	21.5	21.4	21.8	23.2
Sex[4]														
Male	4.1	4.4	4.4	4.7	4.7	5.1	4.8	5.0	5.5	5.5	5.3	5.4	5.3	5.3
Female	5.8	5.8	5.8	6.0	5.9	6.4	6.5	6.8	6.6	6.6	6.5	6.5	6.5	6.5
Sex and Age														
Male														
18 to 44 years	0.8	0.8	0.8	0.7	0.7	0.8	0.8	0.7	0.8	0.9	0.8	0.7	0.7	0.9
45 to 54 years	2.0	2.0	2.0	2.2	2.7	2.6	2.6	2.9	3.3	3.1	2.9	2.9	2.9	2.7
55 to 64 years	5.8	5.9	5.7	6.5	6.7	6.8	7.2	7.0	7.8	7.5	7.0	8.2	8.2	7.4
65 to 74 years	12.8	13.9	14.0	16.1	14.3	15.5	14.3	16.2	17.6	16.9	17.3	17.3	15.9	14.6
75 years and over	18.3	20.3	21.6	20.8	22.1	24.3	21.9	22.2	24.8	26.1	24.7	24.6	25.2	26.1
Female														
18 to 44 years	2.6	2.5	2.6	2.7	2.3	2.9	2.5	2.5	2.4	2.5	2.3	2.4	2.4	2.2
45 to 54 years	6.0	5.9	6.0	6.1	5.7	6.2	6.4	6.8	7.3	6.6	5.8	5.9	5.7	5.6
55 to 64 years	8.8	8.4	8.7	9.1	9.5	9.5	10.0	11.2	10.7	10.9	10.7	10.4	10.4	10.6
65 to 74 years	12.1	12.5	12.3	12.1	13.4	13.3	14.8	15.6	14.9	15.0	15.2	15.2	15.3	15.3
75 years and over	14.9	16.1	15.4	15.5	15.9	17.6	18.5	18.5	17.6	18.7	19.3	19.2	19.4	21.2
Race[4,6]														
White only	5.2	5.4	5.4	5.6	5.5	6.0	6.0	6.2	6.3	6.3	6.1	6.2	6.2	6.3
Black or African American only	3.5	3.5	3.4	3.3	4.0	3.9	4.4	4.3	4.7	5.1	4.9	4.8	4.6	4.5
American Indian or Alaska Native only	*6.5	*5.7	*	*	7.0	*7.4	*4.3	*5.4	7.0	6.5	*	*4.3	*4.8	5.3
Asian only	2.4	*2.3	*2.0	*1.6	3.0	2.9	3.1	3.0	2.9	3.0	3.7	3.4	2.8	2.9
Native Hawaiian or Other Pacific Islander only	NA	*	*	*	*	*	*	*	*	*	*	*	*	*
Two or more races	NA	*4.7	*4.5	7.1	*3.4	7.8	5.8	9.1	9.8	7.9	7.5	8.9	7.8	6.0
Hispanic Origin and Race[4,6]														
Hispanic or Latino	2.9	3.0	2.9	2.9	3.0	3.5	3.7	3.6	3.4	3.4	3.3	3.6	4.0	3.9
Mexican	3.0	2.8	2.6	2.9	2.6	3.1	3.6	3.3	3.2	3.2	2.9	3.3	3.6	3.7
Not Hispanic or Latino	5.1	5.2	5.3	5.5	5.5	5.9	5.9	6.1	6.3	6.3	6.2	6.2	6.1	6.1
White only	5.4	5.5	5.7	5.9	5.8	6.3	6.3	6.5	6.7	6.7	6.5	6.6	6.5	6.6
Black or African American only	3.6	3.6	3.4	3.3	3.9	3.9	4.3	4.2	4.7	5.1	4.8	4.8	4.6	4.4
Education[7,8]														
No high school diploma or GED	5.3	5.5	5.2	5.4	5.6	5.7	5.8	6.1	5.9	5.8	5.4	5.3	5.6	5.8
High school diploma or GED	5.5	5.8	6.1	6.3	5.7	6.4	6.1	6.4	6.7	6.8	6.8	7.0	7.1	6.8
Some college or more	6.0	5.9	6.0	6.2	6.4	6.9	6.9	7.1	7.4	7.4	7.0	7.0	6.8	7.1
Percent of Poverty Level[4,9]														
Below 100 percent	4.9	4.9	5.4	5.4	5.6	5.3	6.2	6.2	5.4	5.3	5.8	5.8	5.2	5.8
100 percent to 199 percent	4.8	5.3	5.0	5.0	5.6	5.7	5.8	6.0	6.1	5.9	5.3	5.5	5.7	5.5
200 percent to 399 percent	4.9	5.1	5.3	5.6	5.2	5.5	5.4	5.5	5.9	6.2	5.9	5.9	6.1	5.9
400 percent or more	5.2	5.1	5.1	5.2	5.0	6.1	5.8	6.0	6.3	6.2	6.2	6.2	6.0	6.2
Hispanic Origin and Race and Percent of Poverty Level[4,6,9]														
Hispanic or Latino														
Below 100 percent	2.2	2.3	2.7	2.9	2.9	3.5	5.0	3.8	2.8	2.9	3.4	3.8	3.7	4.3
100 percent to 199 percent	2.8	3.2	2.2	2.3	3.7	3.3	3.2	3.2	2.5	2.6	2.7	2.8	3.4	3.4
200 percent to 399 percent	2.7	2.7	*3.5	3.5	2.8	3.6	3.2	3.3	4.3	4.7	3.9	4.2	4.7	4.6
400 percent or more	*5.5	*4.5	*	*3.1	*1.9	*3.4	3.6	4.2	4.2	3.3	3.5	4.0	4.7	3.8
Not Hispanic or Latino														
White only														
Below 100 percent	6.3	6.2	7.1	7.2	6.9	6.9	8.0	8.1	6.9	6.8	7.5	7.4	6.8	7.4
100 percent to 199 percent	5.6	6.2	6.0	5.9	6.6	6.7	7.4	7.4	7.3	7.3	6.5	6.9	6.9	6.7
200 percent to 399 percent	5.2	5.5	5.8	6.1	5.7	6.0	6.0	6.1	6.5	6.8	6.3	6.3	6.5	6.5
400 percent or more	5.4	5.3	5.3	5.5	5.3	6.5	6.0	6.2	6.6	6.6	6.6	6.6	6.5	6.7

NA = Not available.
* = Figure does not meet standards of reliability or precision. Data preceded by an asterisk have a relative standard error (RSE) of 20 percent to 30 percent. Data not shown have an RSE of greater than 30 percent.
[2]Cancer is based on self-reported responses to a question about whether respondents had ever been told by a doctor or other health professional that they had cancer or a malignancy of any kind. Excludes squamous cell and basal cell carcinomas.
[4]Estimates are age-adjusted to the year 2000 standard population using five age groups: 18 to 44 years, 45 to 54 years, 55 to 64 years, 65 to 74 years, and 75 years and over. Age-adjusted estimates in this table may differ from other age-adjusted estimates based on the same data and presented elsewhere if different age groups are used in the adjustment procedure.
[5]Includes all other races not shown separately and unknown education level.
[6]The race groups White, Black, American Indian or Alaska Native, Asian, Native Hawaiian or Other Pacific Islander, and two or more races, include persons of Hispanic and non-Hispanic origin. Persons of Hispanic origin may be of any race.
[7]Estimates are for persons 25 years of age and over and are age-adjusted to the year 2000 standard population using five age groups: 25 to 44 years, 45 to 54 years, 55 to 64 years, 65 to 74 years, and 75 years and over.
[8]GED is General Educational Development high school equivalency diploma.
[9]Percent of poverty level is based on family income and family size and composition using U.S. Census Bureau poverty thresholds.

Table 3-5. Respondent-Reported Prevalence of Heart Disease, Cancer, and Stroke Among Adults 18 Years of Age and Over, by Selected Characteristics, Selected Years, 1997–1998 Through 2014–2015—*Continued*

(Percent.)

Characteristic	Heart disease[1]													
	1997–1998	1999–2000	2000–2001	2001–2002	2003–2004	2005–2006	2007–2008	2008–2009	2009–2010	2010–2011	2011–2012	2012–2013	2013–2014	2014–2015
Black or African American only														
Below 100 percent	14.6	13.0	14.5	14.1	14.1	13.2	13.2	15.2	15.7	14.7	14.3	14.0	13.2	12.8
100 percent to 199 percent..........................	12.9	11.2	11.9	12.3	10.5	10.7	11.3	10.9	10.5	11.2	11.8	11.0	11.2	11.4
200 percent to 399 percent..........................	9.2	10.2	9.8	9.0	8.0	9.1	9.3	9.3	10.2	10.5	9.4	9.6	9.7	8.5
400 percent or more	9.5	8.9	8.1	8.0	7.7	8.5	7.7	8.9	8.7	7.3	8.7	8.4	7.0	7.4
Geographic Region[4]														
Northeast	11.6	10.6	10.8	10.9	10.8	11.0	10.9	11.1	10.8	10.1	9.8	9.7	9.7	10.1
Midwest..........................	12.1	11.4	12.2	12.1	11.8	12.3	12.4	12.4	12.1	11.5	11.2	11.8	11.8	12.3
South..........................	12.5	11.5	11.9	11.7	11.7	11.5	11.7	12.3	12.3	12.1	11.7	11.2	11.2	10.9
West..........................	11.1	10.4	10.5	10.9	10.5	9.8	9.9	9.7	9.8	9.9	9.5	9.3	9.4	9.3
Location of Residence[4]														
Within MSA[10]..........................	11.7	10.7	11.1	11.2	10.9	10.9	10.8	11.2	11.2	10.8	10.4	10.3	10.3	10.3
Outside MSA[10]..........................	12.8	12.5	12.9	12.7	13.0	13.0	14.1	13.1	12.5	13.0	12.7	12.5	12.4	13.1

[1]Heart disease is based on self-reported responses to questions about whether respondents had ever been told by a doctor or other health professional that they had coronary heart disease, angina (angina pectoris), a heart attack (myocardial infarction), or any other kind or heart disease or heart condition.

[4]Estimates are age-adjusted to the year 2000 standard population using five age groups: 18 to 44 years, 45 to 54 years, 55 to 64 years, 65 to 74 years, and 75 years and over. Age-adjusted estimates in this table may differ from other age-adjusted estimates based on the same data and presented elsewhere if different age groups are used in the adjustment procedure.

[10]MSA = metropolitan statistical area.

Table 3-5. Respondent-Reported Prevalence of Heart Disease, Cancer, and Stroke Among Adults 18 Years of Age and Over, by Selected Characteristics, Selected Years, 1997–1998 Through 2014–2015—*Continued*

(Percent.)

Characteristic	Cancer[2]													
	1997–1998	1999–2000	2000–2001	2001–2002	2003–2004	2005–2006	2007–2008	2008–2009	2009–2010	2010–2011	2011–2012	2012–2013	2013–2014	2014–2015
Black or African American only														
Below 100 percent	4.4	4.0	3.8	3.2	4.6	3.6	4.6	4.9	4.9	4.5	4.3	4.1	3.8	4.5
100 percent to 199 percent	3.3	3.2	3.6	3.2	4.1	4.3	3.5	3.6	4.9	5.2	4.5	4.3	5.0	4.4
200 percent to 399 percent	3.2	3.7	3.0	3.6	3.5	4.2	4.4	4.0	4.3	5.3	5.5	5.7	5.2	4.4
400 percent or more	4.0	4.3	*3.7	*3.3	4.5	3.6	5.4	5.0	5.2	5.6	5.0	4.7	3.8	4.3
Geographic Region[4]														
Northeast	4.5	5.0	4.9	5.0	5.3	5.6	6.1	6.2	5.9	5.6	5.7	6.1	5.9	5.6
Midwest	5.1	5.2	5.2	5.7	5.3	5.7	5.5	5.8	6.4	6.7	6.4	6.4	6.1	5.9
South	5.0	5.0	5.2	5.3	5.2	5.6	5.8	5.9	6.1	6.2	5.8	5.8	6.0	6.1
West	5.1	5.0	5.0	5.1	5.2	5.7	5.3	5.6	5.6	5.5	5.6	5.5	5.5	5.8
Location of Residence[4]														
Within MSA[10]	4.9	5.0	5.0	5.1	5.1	5.6	5.6	5.7	5.9	5.9	5.7	5.8	5.8	5.8
Outside MSA[10]	5.1	5.5	5.5	6.0	5.7	6.0	6.2	7.0	6.8	6.7	6.8	6.7	6.4	6.3

* = Figure does not meet standards of reliability or precision. Data preceded by an asterisk have a relative standard error (RSE) of 20 percent to 30 percent. Data not shown have an RSE of greater than 30 percent.
[2]Cancer is based on self-reported responses to a question about whether respondents had ever been told by a doctor or other health professional that they had cancer or a malignancy of any kind. Excludes squamous cell and basal cell carcinomas.
[4]Estimates are age-adjusted to the year 2000 standard population using five age groups: 18 to 44 years, 45 to 54 years, 55 to 64 years, 65 to 74 years, and 75 years and over. Age-adjusted estimates in this table may differ from other age-adjusted estimates based on the same data and presented elsewhere if different age groups are used in the adjustment procedure.
[10]MSA = metropolitan statistical area.

Table 3-5. Respondent-Reported Prevalence of Heart Disease, Cancer, and Stroke Among Adults 18 Years of Age and Over, by Selected Characteristics, Selected Years, 1997–1998 Through 2014–2015—Continued

(Percent.)

Characteristic	Stroke[3]													
	1997–1998	1999–2000	2000–2001	2001–2002	2003–2004	2005–2006	2007–2008	2008–2009	2009–2010	2010–2011	2011–2012	2012–2013	2013–2014	2014–2015
18 years and over, age adjusted[4,5]	2.3	2.2	2.3	2.4	2.5	2.5	2.6	2.7	2.6	2.6	2.5	2.5	2.5	2.4
18 years and over, crude[5]	2.2	2.1	2.3	2.4	2.5	2.5	2.7	2.8	2.7	2.7	2.7	2.7	2.7	2.7
Age														
18 to 44 years	0.4	0.4	0.4	0.4	0.4	0.4	0.5	0.6	0.6	0.6	0.5	0.5	0.5	0.5
18 to 24 years	*	*	*	*	*	*	*	*	*	*	*	*	*	*
25 to 44 years	0.4	0.5	0.5	0.5	0.5	0.5	0.6	0.7	0.7	0.7	0.7	0.6	0.6	0.7
45 to 64 years	2.3	2.0	2.2	2.4	2.4	2.3	2.9	2.7	2.8	2.9	2.8	2.8	2.9	2.8
45 to 54 years	1.4	1.3	1.5	1.8	1.5	1.5	2.0	1.8	1.9	2.1	2.1	2.0	1.8	1.8
55 to 64 years	3.8	3.1	3.3	3.3	3.7	3.5	4.0	3.8	3.8	3.9	3.7	3.8	4.2	3.9
65 years and over	8.1	8.1	8.6	8.8	9.2	9.2	8.8	9.2	8.6	8.2	8.3	8.3	7.9	7.5
65 to 74 years	6.7	6.2	6.7	6.6	7.1	6.9	6.9	6.3	6.3	6.3	6.4	6.4	6.0	5.5
75 years and over	9.8	10.3	10.9	11.2	11.6	11.8	11.8	12.5	11.4	10.6	10.6	11.1	10.5	10.5
Sex[4]														
Male	2.6	2.4	2.5	2.6	2.7	2.6	2.5	2.7	2.7	2.6	2.5	2.6	2.6	2.5
Female	2.1	2.1	2.2	2.3	2.4	2.4	2.6	2.7	2.6	2.6	2.6	2.5	2.4	2.3
Sex and Age														
Male														
18 to 44 years	0.3	0.3	0.3	0.4	0.4	0.4	*0.3	0.5	0.5	0.5	0.6	0.5	0.4	0.5
45 to 54 years	1.2	1.3	1.6	1.9	1.5	1.5	2.0	1.6	1.6	1.9	1.9	2.0	1.9	1.7
55 to 64 years	4.6	3.7	3.6	3.5	4.2	3.9	4.2	4.4	4.1	4.0	3.5	3.8	4.3	4.1
65 to 74 years	8.1	6.7	7.2	7.2	8.3	7.7	7.0	6.7	6.9	6.6	6.4	7.0	6.7	6.6
75 years and over	11.2	11.3	12.0	12.6	12.5	12.5	11.1	12.8	12.1	10.6	10.3	11.6	11.2	10.6
Female														
18 to 44 years	0.4	0.4	0.5	0.5	0.5	0.5	0.6	0.8	0.6	0.6	0.5	0.6	0.6	0.6
45 to 54 years	1.5	1.4	1.4	1.6	1.5	1.4	2.1	2.1	2.3	2.2	2.3	1.9	1.7	1.9
55 to 64 years	3.2	2.6	2.9	3.2	3.3	3.1	3.8	3.3	3.5	3.9	3.8	3.7	4.0	3.8
65 to 74 years	5.5	5.8	6.2	6.1	6.1	6.3	5.7	6.0	5.7	6.1	6.4	6.0	5.3	4.6
75 years and over	9.0	9.6	10.3	10.4	11.0	11.5	12.2	12.3	10.9	10.6	10.8	10.7	10.1	10.3
Race[4,6]														
White only	2.2	2.1	2.2	2.3	2.4	2.3	2.5	2.6	2.5	2.3	2.3	2.4	2.3	2.3
Black or African American only	3.3	3.5	3.4	3.3	3.4	4.0	3.6	3.7	3.9	4.1	4.1	3.7	3.8	3.8
American Indian or Alaska Native only	*5.0	*5.4	*2.6	*	*	*	*	*	*	*4.7	*4.3	*3.3	*2.8	*2.6
Asian only	*1.2	*1.2	*2.7	*3.1	*2.2	1.9	2.1	1.5	1.6	2.4	2.3	1.8	1.6	1.4
Native Hawaiian or Other Pacific Islander only	NA	*	*	*	*	*	*	*	*	*	*	*	*	*
Two or more races	NA	*4.0	*4.4	*4.9	4.0	*4.6	*4.1	*3.5	*3.3	*3.9	5.1	4.7	3.3	3.7
Hispanic Origin and Race[4,6]														
Hispanic or Latino	2.1	1.9	2.5	2.5	2.6	2.1	2.6	2.3	2.3	2.7	2.7	2.6	2.5	2.4
Mexican	2.5	2.0	2.8	2.7	2.9	2.5	2.5	2.5	2.4	2.6	2.7	2.7	2.6	2.7
Not Hispanic or Latino	2.3	2.2	2.3	2.4	2.5	2.5	2.6	2.7	2.6	2.6	2.5	2.5	2.5	2.4
White only	2.2	2.1	2.2	2.3	2.4	2.3	2.4	2.7	2.5	2.3	2.2	2.4	2.3	2.3
Black or African American only	3.3	3.5	3.5	3.3	3.4	4.1	3.6	3.7	3.9	4.2	4.2	3.7	3.8	3.9
Education[7,8]														
No high school diploma or GED	3.9	3.8	3.7	3.8	4.4	4.1	4.4	4.5	4.2	4.4	4.5	4.5	4.1	4.1
High school diploma or GED	2.5	2.5	2.7	2.9	2.8	2.9	3.2	3.3	3.2	3.4	3.2	3.1	3.1	3.1
Some college or more	2.1	1.9	2.2	2.3	2.3	2.3	2.3	2.5	2.5	2.3	2.3	2.4	2.3	2.2
Percent of Poverty Level[4,9]														
Below 100 percent	4.3	3.7	3.6	3.7	4.4	4.1	4.4	4.4	4.4	4.6	4.6	4.7	4.3	4.3
100 percent to 199 percent	3.1	3.2	3.4	3.3	3.5	3.2	3.9	3.6	3.5	3.7	3.6	3.4	3.6	3.6
200 percent to 399 percent	2.1	2.1	2.2	2.4	2.3	2.4	2.5	2.7	2.6	2.5	2.4	2.5	2.4	2.4
400 percent or more	1.6	1.5	1.7	1.9	1.8	1.8	1.6	1.8	1.7	1.5	1.5	1.5	1.4	1.4
Hispanic Origin and Race and Percent of Poverty Level[4,6,9]														
Hispanic or Latino														
Below 100 percent	3.0	2.0	2.3	2.7	3.9	3.1	3.8	2.6	2.9	3.4	3.6	3.8	3.5	3.5
100 percent to 199 percent	2.2	2.2	3.0	3.2	2.8	1.8	2.6	2.6	2.3	3.2	3.4	2.6	2.3	2.7
200 percent to 399 percent	*1.8	*2.3	*2.6	2.0	*2.0	*2.0	*2.2	2.4	2.0	2.2	2.4	2.5	2.2	*2.0
400 percent or more	*	*	*	*	*	*	*2.7	*	*2.6	*2.1	*	*	*1.9	*1.1
Not Hispanic or Latino														
White only														
Below 100 percent	4.4	3.8	3.5	3.6	4.3	4.1	4.3	4.4	4.4	4.4	4.3	5.0	4.4	4.2
100 percent to 199 percent	3.2	3.0	3.3	3.2	3.5	3.2	4.1	4.0	3.9	3.6	3.4	3.6	3.6	3.6
200 percent to 399 percent	2.1	2.1	2.2	2.3	2.3	2.3	2.6	2.8	2.5	2.3	2.3	2.4	2.4	2.4
400 percent or more	1.6	1.5	1.7	1.8	1.8	1.8	1.5	1.8	1.7	1.4	1.5	1.5	1.4	1.4

NA = Not available.

* = Figure does not meet standards of reliability or precision. Data preceded by an asterisk have a relative standard error (RSE) of 20 percent to 30 percent. Data not shown have an RSE of greater than 30 percent.

[3]Stroke is based on self-reported responses to a question about whether respondents had ever been told by a doctor or other health professional that they had a stroke.

[4]Estimates are age-adjusted to the year 2000 standard population using five age groups: 18 to 44 years, 45 to 54 years, 55 to 64 years, 65 to 74 years, and 75 years and over. Age-adjusted estimates in this table may differ from other age-adjusted estimates based on the same data and presented elsewhere if different age groups are used in the adjustment procedure.

[5]Includes all other races not shown separately and unknown education level.

[6]The race groups White, Black, American Indian or Alaska Native, Asian, Native Hawaiian or Other Pacific Islander, and two or more races, include persons of Hispanic and non-Hispanic origin. Persons of Hispanic origin may be of any race.

[7]Estimates are for persons 25 years of age and over and are age-adjusted to the year 2000 standard population using five age groups: 25 to 44 years, 45 to 54 years, 55 to 64 years, 65 to 74 years, and 75 years and over.

[8]GED is General Educational Development high school equivalency diploma.

[9]Percent of poverty level is based on family income and family size and composition using U.S. Census Bureau poverty thresholds.

Table 3-5. Respondent-Reported Prevalence of Heart Disease, Cancer, and Stroke Among Adults 18 Years of Age and Over, by Selected Characteristics, Selected Years, 1997–1998 Through 2014–2015—*Continued*

(Percent.)

Characteristic	Stroke[3]													
	1997–1998	1999–2000	2000–2001	2001–2002	2003–2004	2005–2006	2007–2008	2008–2009	2009–2010	2010–2011	2011–2012	2012–2013	2013–2014	2014–2015
Black or African American only														
Below 100 percent	5.0	4.5	4.5	4.8	5.6	5.3	5.5	6.4	6.2	6.2	6.5	5.4	5.0	5.8
100 percent to 199 percent	4.2	5.1	4.6	3.9	3.8	4.6	4.7	4.0	3.9	4.6	4.6	3.9	5.1	5.0
200 percent to 399 percent	2.5	2.7	3.1	2.8	2.4	4.1	2.7	2.8	3.7	3.9	3.3	3.0	3.0	2.9
400 percent or more	*	*	*	*	*2.0	*2.6	*2.6	*2.5	*2.6	*2.1	2.8	3.0	2.3	2.4
Geographic Region[4]														
Northeast	1.8	1.8	1.7	2.1	2.2	1.9	2.4	2.3	2.1	2.0	1.9	2.1	2.2	1.9
Midwest	2.3	2.2	2.4	2.4	2.5	2.5	2.5	2.6	2.6	2.6	2.4	2.5	2.5	2.7
South	2.6	2.5	2.7	2.5	2.8	2.9	3.0	3.2	3.0	2.9	3.0	2.9	2.7	2.6
West	2.1	2.0	2.4	2.7	2.4	2.1	2.2	2.2	2.3	2.4	2.4	2.4	2.2	2.2
Location of Residence[4]														
Within MSA[10]	2.2	2.1	2.3	2.4	2.4	2.4	2.5	2.6	2.4	2.4	2.4	2.4	2.3	2.3
Outside MSA[10]	2.7	2.5	2.5	2.5	2.8	2.9	2.9	3.0	3.3	3.4	3.2	3.3	3.1	2.9

* = Figure does not meet standards of reliability or precision. Data preceded by an asterisk have a relative standard error (RSE) of 20 percent to 30 percent. Data not shown have an RSE of greater than 30 percent.
[3]Stroke is based on self-reported responses to a question about whether respondents had ever been told by a doctor or other health professional that they had a stroke.
[4]Estimates are age-adjusted to the year 2000 standard population using five age groups: 18 to 44 years, 45 to 54 years, 55 to 64 years, 65 to 74 years, and 75 years and over. Age-adjusted estimates in this table may differ from other age-adjusted estimates based on the same data and presented elsewhere if different age groups are used in the adjustment procedure.
[10]MSA = metropolitan statistical area.

Table 3-6. Diabetes Prevalence and Glycemic Control Among Adults 20 Years of Age and Over, by Sex, Age, Race and Hispanic Origin, Selected Years 1988–1994 Through 2011–2014

(Percent.)

Age, race, sex, and Hispanic origin	Physician-diagnosed and undiagnosed diabetes[1,2]								Physician-diagnosed diabetes[1]							
	1988–1994	1999–2002	2001–2004	2003–2006	2005–2008	2007–2010	2009–2012	2011–2014	1988–1994	1999–2002	2001–2004	2003–2006	2005–2008	2007–2010	2009–2012	2011–2014
20 Years and Over, Age-Adjusted[3]																
All persons[4]	8.8	9.9	10.8	10.6	10.9	11.4	11.7	11.9	5.2	6.6	7.4	7.7	7.9	8.1	8.4	9.0
Sex																
Male	9.6	11.2	12.4	11.1	11.4	13.2	13.2	12.8	5.5	7.3	7.9	7.0	7.4	8.8	9.0	9.4
Female	8.2	8.6	9.3	10.2	10.5	9.8	10.3	11.2	5.1	5.9	6.9	8.2	8.2	7.4	7.8	8.7
Hispanic Origin																
Not Hispanic or Latino																
White only	7.7	8.5	9.0	8.9	9.2	9.6	9.1	9.6	4.8	5.5	6.1	6.2	6.6	6.7	6.6	7.6
Black or African American only	16.3	14.0	15.9	16.7	18.9	18.4	17.9	18.0	9.1	9.2	11.7	13.0	13.2	13.2	13.3	13.4
Mexican[5]	15.6	13.9	16.1	17.1	17.7	18.9	20.5	18.0	10.7	10.8	12.7	12.9	12.6	13.4	13.9	13.0
Percent of Poverty Level[6]																
Below 100 percent	14.2	14.6	14.5	14.8	15.7	13.8	17.1	17.4	8.8	9.0	9.7	12.4	12.0	10.1	12.1	13.4
100 percent or more	8.1	9.3	10.1	10.1	10.4	10.9	10.8	11.2	4.8	6.4	7.0	7.1	7.3	7.6	7.8	8.5
100 percent to 199 percent	9.7	13.1	13.5	13.9	14.8	14.8	14.8	15.0	5.2	9.4	9.8	9.5	10.2	11.0	11.4	10.5
200 percent or more	7.8	8.2	9.1	8.9	9.3	10.0	9.4	9.7	4.7	5.5	6.1	6.3	6.6	6.8	6.5	7.7
200 percent to 399 percent	7.8	10.5	10.7	10.5	10.7	12.3	11.5	11.4	4.3	7.3	7.0	7.5	7.8	8.9	8.4	8.6
400 percent or more	7.8	6.7	8.0	7.0	7.3	7.9	7.7	8.6	5.3	4.3	5.8	5.2	5.1	4.9	*5.2	7.2
20 Years and Over, Crude																
All persons[4]	8.3	9.8	10.6	10.9	11.4	12.0	12.3	12.6	4.9	6.6	7.3	7.9	8.2	8.5	8.9	9.6
Sex																
Male	8.6	10.8	11.8	11.0	11.4	13.4	13.5	13.2	4.9	7.1	7.5	6.9	7.5	8.9	9.1	9.7
Female	8.0	8.9	9.5	10.8	11.3	10.7	11.2	12.1	5.0	6.1	7.1	8.7	9.0	8.2	8.7	9.5
Hispanic Origin																
Not Hispanic or Latino																
White only	7.6	8.9	9.4	9.6	10.3	10.9	10.5	11.0	4.7	5.6	6.3	6.7	7.3	7.6	7.6	8.7
Black or African American only	13.3	12.5	14.6	15.8	17.9	17.0	17.1	17.5	7.2	8.3	10.9	12.3	12.8	12.3	12.5	13.0
Mexican	10.4	9.3	10.8	12.6	12.8	13.7	15.8	14.3	6.3	7.2	7.9	8.8	8.9	9.4	10.1	10.1
Percent of Poverty Level[6]																
Below 100 percent	11.6	13.4	12.2	12.7	13.8	11.4	14.3	15.0	7.2	8.4	8.4	10.6	10.3	8.3	9.8	11.2
100 percent or more	7.6	9.2	10.1	10.5	10.8	11.8	11.8	12.3	4.5	6.3	7.0	7.3	7.7	8.3	8.6	9.4
100 percent to 199 percent	9.1	12.9	13.3	14.9	16.3	15.8	15.8	16.8	5.2	9.3	9.6	10.2	11.2	11.7	12.3	12.1
200 percent or more	7.1	8.0	9.0	9.1	9.3	10.6	10.4	10.8	4.3	5.4	6.1	6.5	6.7	7.2	7.3	8.4
200 percent to 399 percent	6.8	10.2	10.6	11.0	11.2	13.0	12.3	12.3	3.7	7.0	7.0	7.7	8.1	9.4	9.0	9.3
400 percent or more	7.6	6.4	7.7	7.4	7.7	8.7	8.9	9.5	5.2	4.1	5.5	5.3	5.4	5.4	*5.8	7.7
Age																
20 to 44 years	*2.1	4.4	4.2	3.9	3.7	3.3	3.7	4.0	*	3.2	3.1	2.8	2.6	2.1	2.1	2.6
45 to 64 years	14.0	12.8	13.5	13.7	13.8	15.3	16.2	16.6	7.9	8.3	9.3	10.1	10.6	11.4	11.4	12.3
65 years and over	19.4	20.4	24.8	24.9	26.9	28.1	26.8	26.3	12.7	13.7	16.4	17.5	18.3	19.3	21.2	21.9

Note: Pregnant women are excluded. Fasting weights were used to obtain estimates of total, physician-diagnosed, and undiagnosed diabetes prevalence. Examination weights were used to obtain the poor glycemic control estimates. Estimates in this table may differ from other estimates based on the same data and presented elsewhere if different weights, age adjustment groups, definitions, or trend adjustments are used.

*Estimates are considered unreliable. Data preceded by an asterisk have a relative standard error (RSE) of 20 percent–30 percent. Data not shown have an RSE greater than 30 percent.

[1]Physician-diagnosed diabetes was obtained by self-report and excludes women who are pregnant.

[2]Undiagnosed diabetes is defined as a fasting plasma glucose (FPG) of at least 126 mg/dL or a hemoglobin A1c of at least 6.5 percent and no reported physician diagnosis. Respondents had fasted for at least 8 hours and less than 24 hours. Pregnant females are excluded. Estimates in some prior editions of Health, United States included data from respondents who had fasted for at least 9 hours and less than 24 hours. Starting in 2005–2006, testing was performed at a different laboratory and using different instruments than testing in earlier years. The National Health and Nutrition Examination Survey (NHANES) conducted crossover studies to evaluate the impact of these changes on FPG and A1c measurements and recommended adjustments to the FPG data. The adjustments recommended by NHANES were incorporated into the data presented here. For more information, see http://www.cdc.gov/nchs/nhanes/nhanes2005-2006/GLU_D.htm.

[3]Estimates are age-adjusted to the year 2000 standard population using three age groups: 20–44 years, 45–64 years, and 65 years and over. Age-adjusted estimates in this table may differ from other age-adjusted estimates based on the same data and presented elsewhere if different age groups are used in the adjustment procedure.

[4]Includes all other races and Hispanic origins not shown separately.

[5]Persons of Mexican origin may be of any race. Starting with 1999 data, race-specific estimates are tabulated according to the 1997 Revisions to the Standards for the Classification of Federal Data on Race and Ethnicity and are not strictly comparable with estimates for earlier years. The two non-Hispanic race categories shown in the table conform to the 1997 Standards. Starting with 1999 data, race-specific estimates are for persons who reported only one racial group. Prior to data year 1999, estimates were tabulated according to the 1977 Standards. Estimates for single-race categories prior to 1999 included persons who reported one race or, if they reported more than one race, identified one race as best representing their race.

[6]Percent of poverty level was calculated by dividing family income by the U.S. Department of Health and Human Services' poverty guideline specific to family size, as well as the appropriate year, and state. Persons with unknown percent of poverty level are excluded (7 percent in 2009–2012).

Table 3-6. Diabetes Prevalence and Glycemic Control Among Adults 20 Years of Age and Over, by Sex, Age, Race and Hispanic Origin, Selected Years 1988–1994 Through 2011–2014—Continued

(Percent.)

Age, race, sex, and Hispanic origin¹	Undiagnosed diabetes²								Poor glycemic control (A1c greater than 9%) among persons with physician-diagnosed diabetes							
	1988–1994	1999–2002	2001–2004	2003–2006	2005–2008	2007–2010	2009–2012	2011–2014	1988–1994	1999–2002	2001–2004	2003–2006	2005–2008	2007–2010	2009–2012	2011–2014
20 Years and Over, Age-Adjusted³																
All persons⁴	3.6	3.2	3.4	3.0	3.1	3.3	3.3	2.9	26.3	24.7	17.4	18.8	20.3	18.3	21.3	20.6
Sex																
Male	4.1	3.9	4.5	4.1	4.0	4.4	4.2	3.3	22.4	27.7	22.5	20.7	21.6	20.8	26.2	24.1
Female	3.2	2.7	2.4	2.0	2.2	2.4	2.5	2.4	29.4	*20.3	11.6	17.1	19.2	15.8	16.5	18.0
Hispanic Origin																
Not Hispanic or Latino																
White only	2.9	3.0	2.9	2.7	2.6	2.8	2.5	2.0	23.7	*22.9	*18.1	*14.9	*15.2	*11.2	*	*16.6
Black or African American only	7.2	4.8	4.2	3.8	5.7	5.1	4.7	4.6	38.9	25.4	*15.5	25.7	31.8	30.4	28.8	23.9
Mexican⁵	5.0	3.1	3.5	4.2	5.1	5.5	6.6	5.1	29.8	28.0	23.7	*26.3	*25.5	*24.3	32.5	27.6
Percent of Poverty Level⁶																
Below 100 percent	*5.4	5.6	4.8	*	*3.7	3.7	5.0	3.9	37.2	30.6	*17.8	*19.9	23.2	22.9	23.6	27.3
100 percent or more	3.3	2.9	3.1	3.0	3.1	3.3	3.0	2.7	22.8	*22.6	*18.1	19.8	20.0	17.2	21.2	18.3
100 percent to 199 percent	4.4	*3.6	3.7	4.4	4.6	3.8	3.4	4.5	*	*	*19.2	*22.0	*	*20.0		21.7
200 percent or more	3.1	2.7	2.9	2.6	2.7	3.2	2.9	2.1	21.2	*25.6	*22.6	20.8	19.4	18.0	*22.0	*16.6
200 percent to 399 percent	3.6	3.2	3.6	*3.1	*2.9	3.3	3.1	2.8	*24.2	*27.0	*22.9	*19.1	*16.3	*20.2	*21.4	*13.5
400 percent or more	2.5	2.3	*2.3	*	*2.2	3.0	2.5	*1.4	*	*	*	*	*22.4	*	*	*
20 Years and Over, Crude																
All persons⁴	3.4	3.2	3.3	3.0	3.2	3.5	3.5	3.0	23.3	18.4	14.5	13.0	13.9	12.5	13.8	15.6
Sex																
Male	3.7	3.7	4.3	4.0	3.9	4.5	4.4	3.5	20.2	20.2	17.5	14.8	14.9	14.0	14.8	15.4
Female	3.1	2.8	2.4	2.1	2.4	2.5	2.6	2.5	25.8	16.7	11.6	11.5	12.9	11.0	12.8	15.7
Hispanic Origin																
Not Hispanic or Latino																
White only	2.9	3.2	3.1	3.0	3.0	3.2	2.8	2.3	20.6	13.6	11.5	8.7	10.5	9.5	9.5	12.0
Black or African American only	6.1	4.2	3.7	3.5	5.1	4.6	4.6	4.6	34.2	25.4	20.0	21.0	21.0	19.0	19.6	19.0
Mexican	4.1	2.0	*2.9	*3.8	3.9	4.3	5.7	4.2	29.2	26.8	23.0	24.0	21.7	19.6	23.5	22.9
Percent of Poverty Level⁶																
Below 100 percent	4.4	5.1	3.9	*	*3.5	3.1	4.5	3.7	30.2	25.6	16.3	17.6	20.3	18.5	19.8	23.2
100 percent or more	3.1	2.9	3.1	3.1	3.2	3.6	3.3	2.9	21.4	15.9	13.9	12.2	12.8	11.1	11.9	13.6
100 percent to 199 percent	3.9	*3.6	3.7	4.7	5.1	4.1	3.5	4.7	24.2	*14.9	*10.6	*11.5	*11.8	9.8	12.4	13.9
200 percent or more	2.8	2.6	2.9	2.7	2.7	3.4	3.2	2.3	20.0	16.4	15.5	12.5	13.3	11.8	11.7	13.4
200 percent to 399 percent	3.1	*3.1	3.6	*3.2	*3.1	3.5	3.3	3.0	*21.2	*17.5	15.6	*10.7	*11.2	12.4	12.3	13.1
400 percent or more	*2.5	2.3	*2.3	*2.2	2.3	3.2	*3.1	*1.8	*18.3	*	15.5	14.8	*15.6	*11.2	*11.1	*13.8
Age																
20 to 44 years	1.1	*	*1.1	*1.1	*1.1	1.1	1.6	1.4	29.5	*32.7	*20.0	25.2	28.1	24.9	30.1	26.2
45 to 64 years	6.0	4.5	4.2	3.5	3.2	3.9	4.8	4.3	26.0	19.9	19.5	16.6	15.4	14.1	14.4	17.8
65 years and over	6.7	6.7	8.5	7.4	8.6	8.8	5.5	4.3	18.0	*10.2	*6.3	*4.1	6.2	6.8	8.0	9.2

Note: Pregnant women are excluded. Fasting weights were used to obtain estimates of total, physician-diagnosed, and undiagnosed diabetes prevalence. Examination weights were used to obtain the poor glycemic control estimates. Estimates in this table may differ from other estimates based on the same data and presented elsewhere if different weights, age adjustment groups, definitions, or trend adjustments are used.

*Estimates are considered unreliable. Data preceded by an asterisk have a relative standard error (RSE) of 20 percent–30 percent. Data not shown have an RSE greater than 30 percent.

¹Physician-diagnosed diabetes was obtained by self-report and excludes women who are pregnant.

²Undiagnosed diabetes is defined as a fasting plasma glucose (FPG) of at least 126 mg/dL or a hemoglobin A1c of at least 6.5 percent and no reported physician diagnosis. Respondents had fasted for at least 8 hours and less than 24 hours. Pregnant females are excluded. Estimates in some prior editions of Health, United States included data from respondents who had fasted for at least 9 hours and less than 24 hours. Starting in 2005–2006, testing was performed at a different laboratory and using different instruments than testing in earlier years. The National Health and Nutrition Examination Survey (NHANES) conducted crossover studies to evaluate the impact of these changes on FPG and A1c measurements and recommended adjustments to the FPG data. The adjustments recommended by NHANES were incorporated into the data presented here. For more information, see http://www.cdc.gov/nchs/nhanes/nhanes2005-2006/GLU_D.htm.

³Estimates are age-adjusted to the year 2000 standard population using three age groups: 20–44 years, 45–64 years, and 65 years and over. Age-adjusted estimates in this table may differ from other age-adjusted estimates based on the same data and presented elsewhere if different age groups are used in the adjustment procedure.

⁴Includes all other races and Hispanic origins not shown separately.

⁵Persons of Mexican origin may be of any race. Starting with 1999 data, race-specific estimates are tabulated according to the 1997 Revisions to the Standards for the Classification of Federal Data on Race and Ethnicity and are not strictly comparable with estimates for earlier years. The two non-Hispanic race categories shown in the table conform to the 1997 Standards. Starting with 1999 data, race-specific estimates are for persons who reported only one racial group. Prior to data year 1999, estimates were tabulated according to the 1977 Standards. Estimates for single-race categories prior to 1999 included persons who reported one race or, if they reported more than one race, identified one race as best representing their race.

⁶Percent of poverty level was calculated by dividing family income by the U.S. Department of Health and Human Services' poverty guideline specific to family size, as well as the appropriate year, and state. Persons with unknown percent of poverty level are excluded (7 percent in 2009–2012).

Table 3-7. End-Stage Renal Disease Patients, by Selected Characteristics, Selected Years, 2000–2012

(Number, rate per million population.)

Characteristic	Incidence — Number of new patients				Prevalence — Number of patients alive on December 31			
	2000	2010	2011	2012	2000	2010	2011	2012
Total	91,241	113,380	111,209	112,596	378,074	577,675	597,620	620,136
Age								
Under 20 years..	1,148	1,167	1,172	1,113	6,039	7,015	7,066	7,020
20 to 44 years...	12,687	13,050	12,734	12,836	86,043	96,067	96,936	98,142
45 to 64 years...	31,736	43,456	43,294	44,120	154,117	259,855	268,220	275,940
65 to 74 years...	23,148	27,100	26,318	27,409	75,480	119,941	127,391	136,859
75 years and over	22,522	28,607	27,691	27,118	56,395	94,797	98,007	102,175
Sex								
Male..	48,769	64,553	63,600	64,524	206,248	327,379	339,676	353,372
Female	42,472	48,827	47,609	48,072	171,826	250,296	257,944	266,764
Race[1]								
White..	59,472	75,214	73,229	74,667	231,829	353,938	364,579	377,797
Black or African American...............................	26,204	31,828	31,530	31,148	123,654	185,683	192,745	199,632
American Indian or Alaska Native....................	*	1,233	1,234	1,260	*	7,571	7,840	8,080
Asian or Pacific Islander	3,460	5,105	5,216	5,521	16,064	30,483	32,456	34,627
Hispanic Origin[1]								
Hispanic...	10,053	15,251	15,582	15,399	40,627	85,228	90,856	95,819
Not Hispanic[2]	81,188	98,129	95,627	97,197	337,447	492,447	506,764	524,317
Primary Diagnosis...................................								
Diabetes..	40,489	50,020	49,151	49,258	133,128	217,165	225,110	234,160
Hypertension..	24,490	32,317	31,506	32,293	92,817	143,951	149,710	156,595
Glomerulonephritis...	9,958	9,311	9,218	8,988	75,477	98,822	101,103	103,312
Cystic kidney...	2,140	2,582	2,476	2,495	17,685	27,492	28,407	29,389
Other urologic	1,610	526	429	533	7,996	7,499	7,287	7,253
Other cause...	8,486	13,662	13,633	12,157	33,250	54,967	57,266	58,717
Unknown cause..	3,712	4,262	4,026	3,469	15,539	24,232	24,733	24,923
Missing disease	356	700	770	3,403	2,182	3,547	4,004	5,787

Characteristic	New patients per million population				Patients alive on December 31 per million population			
	2000	2010	2011	2012	2000	2010	2011	2012
Total	323.3	366.5	356.9	358.6	1,333.2	1,860.7	1,910.8	1,968.2
Age								
Under 20 years..	14.2	14.0	14.1	13.4	74.7	84.5	85.4	85.2
20 to 44 years...	121.8	125.6	121.7	121.7	825.8	921.5	923.2	927.4
45 to 64 years...	508.3	531.4	522.8	532.4	2,428.5	3,157.8	3,238.2	3,329.3
65 to 74 years...	1,259.1	1,239.8	1,170.4	1,142.7	4,105.7	5,409.7	5,482.5	5,532.9
75 years and over	1,349.7	1,536.3	1,466.1	1,415.3	3,357.6	5,054.8	5,151.9	5,294.9
Sex								
Male..	352.2	424.4	414.9	417.6	1,482.0	2,144.2	2,207.4	2,278.2
Female	295.5	310.5	300.7	301.5	1,189.9	1,586.3	1,623.5	1,667.5
Race[1]								
White..	257.9	306.0	296.5	300.8	1,001.9	1,436.7	1,472.4	1,518.1
Black or African American...............................	713.4	754.2	738.4	720.9	3,342.9	4,374.5	4,487.7	4,593.7
American Indian or Alaska Native....................	*	288.3	284.5	286.4	*	1,758.1	1,795.0	1,824.2
Asian or Pacific Islander	290.9	298.3	296.4	305.2	1,320.9	1,756.7	1,819.1	1,888.6
Hispanic Origin[1]								
Hispanic...	281.8	300.5	300.3	290.3	1,116.0	1,660.8	1,732.0	1,787.6
Not Hispanic[2]	329.3	379.4	368.2	372.5	1,365.2	1,900.2	1,946.8	2,005.2
Primary Diagnosis...................................								
Diabetes..	143.4	161.7	157.7	156.9	469.4	699.5	719.7	743.1
Hypertension..	86.7	104.4	101.1	102.8	327.3	463.6	478.6	497.0
Glomerulonephritis...	35.2	30.1	29.5	28.6	266.1	318.3	323.2	327.8
Cystic kidney...	7.5	8.3	7.9	7.9	62.3	88.5	90.8	93.2
Other urologic	5.7	1.7	1.3	1.6	28.1	24.1	23.2	23.0
Other cause...	30.0	44.1	43.7	38.7	117.2	177.0	183.1	186.3
Unknown cause..	13.1	13.7	12.9	11.0	54.7	78.0	79.0	79.1
Missing disease	1.2	2.2	2.4	10.8	7.6	11.4	12.8	18.3

*Data are considered unreliable and are not shown.
[1]The race groups White, Black, American Indian or Alaska Native, and Asian or Pacific Islander, include persons of Hispanic and non-Hispanic origin. Persons of Hispanic origin may be of any race.
[2]Not Hispanic includes unknown ethnicity.

Table 3-8. Severe Headache or Migraine, Low Back Pain, and Neck Pain Among Adults 18 Years of Age and Over, by Selected Characteristics, 1997, 2000, 2010, and 2015

(Percent of adults with pain in the last 3 months.)

Characteristic	Severe headache or migraine[1]				Low back pain[1]				Neck pain[1]			
	1997	2000	2010	2015	1997	2000	2010	2015	1997	2000	2010	2015
18 years and over, age-adjusted[2,3]	15.8	14.7	16.6	15.4	28.2	27.3	28.4	29.1	14.7	14.4	15.4	15.7
18 years and over, crude[3]	16.0	14.8	16.4	15.0	28.1	27.2	28.8	29.8	14.6	14.4	15.8	16.1
Age												
18 to 44 years	18.7	17.2	20.4	17.9	26.1	24.6	25.2	23.9	13.3	12.6	13.1	12.9
18 to 24 years	18.7	16.1	19.6	15.4	21.9	20.9	19.4	16.2	9.8	8.7	8.3	7.8
25 to 44 years	18.7	17.6	20.7	18.8	27.3	25.8	27.2	26.7	14.3	13.9	14.8	14.8
45 to 64 years	15.8	14.8	15.6	15.9	31.3	30.4	32.4	35.4	17.0	17.7	20.0	20.1
45 to 54 years	17.8	16.3	16.7	17.6	31.3	29.4	31.3	34.6	17.3	17.8	19.1	19.8
55 to 64 years	12.7	12.3	14.1	14.2	31.2	32.0	33.8	36.1	16.6	17.6	21.0	20.5
65 years and over	7.0	7.0	6.4	6.4	29.5	30.0	31.8	34.4	15.0	14.0	14.8	16.6
65 to 74 years	8.2	7.9	7.4	7.3	30.2	29.6	32.5	34.0	15.0	13.9	15.5	16.9
75 years and over	5.4	6.0	5.1	5.1	28.6	30.6	30.9	34.9	15.0	14.2	14.0	16.2
Sex[2]												
Male	9.9	8.9	11.0	9.7	26.5	25.5	26.3	27.6	12.6	12.1	13.1	13.9
Female	21.4	20.3	22.1	20.9	29.6	28.8	30.3	30.4	16.6	16.5	17.6	17.4
Sex and Age												
Male												
18 to 44 years	11.9	10.4	13.5	11.0	24.8	23.4	23.2	22.3	11.6	10.6	11.0	11.2
45 to 54 years	10.3	9.1	10.4	10.7	29.4	27.4	29.6	34.1	13.9	14.8	16.3	17.4
55 to 64 years	8.8	7.6	9.6	10.5	30.7	29.6	32.8	35.5	14.6	15.1	17.6	19.1
65 to 74 years	5.0	5.1	5.5	5.0	29.0	27.5	28.4	31.7	13.6	12.0	12.8	14.4
75 years and over	*2.4	4.5	4.0	3.4	22.5	26.3	27.4	32.1	12.6	12.4	13.0	14.9
Female												
18 to 44 years	25.4	23.9	27.3	24.7	27.3	25.7	27.1	25.5	14.9	14.6	15.2	14.6
45 to 54 years	24.9	23.2	22.9	24.2	33.1	31.3	33.0	35.2	20.6	20.7	21.8	22.0
55 to 64 years	16.3	16.7	18.2	17.6	31.7	34.2	34.7	36.7	18.4	19.8	24.1	21.8
65 to 74 years	10.7	10.1	9.1	9.3	31.1	31.2	36.1	35.9	16.1	15.5	17.8	19.0
75 years and over	7.4	6.9	5.8	6.3	32.4	33.2	33.2	36.9	16.5	15.2	14.6	17.0
Race[2,4]												
White only	15.9	15.0	16.7	15.5	28.7	28.0	29.1	29.9	15.1	15.0	16.0	16.3
Black or African American only	16.7	13.9	18.2	16.3	26.9	24.3	27.2	28.1	13.3	10.7	13.3	13.8
American Indian or Alaska Native only	18.9	21.1	18.8	18.7	33.3	31.4	33.6	34.1	16.2	19.6	16.9	20.4
Asian only	11.7	12.0	10.1	11.3	21.0	19.0	19.1	19.3	9.2	11.0	9.6	11.5
Native Hawaiian or Other Pacific Islander only	NA	*	*	*	NA	*	*	*	NA	*	*	*
2 or more races	NA	19.9	21.5	20.7	NA	41.8	35.6	33.7	NA	22.1	22.0	19.0
Hispanic Origin and Race[2,4]												
Hispanic or Latino	15.5	13.5	16.2	14.9	26.4	25.0	27.4	27.4	13.9	13.4	15.1	14.2
Mexican	14.6	12.3	15.7	14.1	25.2	21.5	26.5	26.4	12.9	11.6	14.7	12.9
Not Hispanic or Latino	15.9	15.0	16.8	15.6	28.4	27.7	28.7	29.4	14.9	14.7	15.5	16.1
White only	16.1	15.4	17.0	16.0	29.1	28.4	29.7	30.5	15.4	15.4	16.3	17.1
Black or African American only	16.8	13.8	18.4	16.1	26.9	24.2	27.1	27.9	13.3	10.6	13.3	13.6
Education[5,6]												
25 years and over												
No high school diploma or GED	19.2	17.9	18.2	19.4	33.6	32.4	34.5	34.6	16.5	15.9	18.9	18.1
High school diploma or GED	16.0	14.8	17.4	14.9	30.2	29.4	31.9	34.8	15.5	15.4	16.8	17.3
Some college or more	13.8	13.4	15.1	14.9	26.9	26.3	28.0	29.3	14.6	15.0	15.8	16.5
Percent of Poverty Level[2,7]												
Below 100 percent	23.3	19.9	22.7	21.8	35.4	32.4	34.9	36.8	18.6	16.5	20.2	19.9
100 percent to 199 percent	18.9	17.7	19.5	19.0	30.8	30.6	32.5	33.8	16.1	15.3	17.7	18.3
200 percent to 399 percent	15.5	15.4	16.6	15.5	27.9	27.4	28.5	28.7	14.8	14.7	15.2	14.9
400 percent or more	12.4	11.8	13.3	11.9	24.8	24.5	24.7	25.1	12.8	13.4	13.1	14.3
Hispanic Origin and Race and Percent of Poverty Level[2,4,7]												
Hispanic or Latino												
Below 100 percent	18.9	18.1	19.6	19.9	29.5	28.4	29.0	33.4	16.4	15.6	17.4	17.8
100 percent to 199 percent	15.7	12.9	15.1	14.2	26.8	24.8	27.2	25.9	12.9	13.3	15.7	15.9
200 percent to 399 percent	14.0	13.6	16.5	13.6	25.0	23.5	27.5	25.0	13.8	13.6	12.9	11.4
400 percent or more	13.0	9.6	14.0	12.9	21.6	24.1	25.6	27.5	12.1	11.6	15.3	12.0
Not Hispanic or Latino												
White only												
Below 100 percent	26.1	21.3	24.8	25.5	38.9	36.6	40.5	42.0	20.5	18.7	23.7	23.6
100 percent to 199 percent	20.4	20.3	22.0	22.8	33.3	34.6	35.9	38.6	18.0	17.6	19.9	21.5

NA = Not available.
* = Figure does not meet standards of reliability or precision. Data preceded by an asterisk have a relative standard error (RSE) of 20 percent to 30 percent. Data not shown have an RSE of greater than 30 percent.
[1] In three separate questions, respondents were asked, "During the past 3 months, did you have a severe headache or migraine? ...low back pain? ...neck pain?" Respondents were instructed to report pain that had lasted a whole day or more, and not to report fleeting or minor aches or pains. Persons may be represented in more than one column.
[2] Estimates are age adjusted to the year 2000 standard population using five age groups: 18 to 44 years, 45 to 54 years, 55 to 64 years, 65 to 74 years, and 75 years and over. Age-adjusted estimates in this table may differ from other age-adjusted estimates based on the same data and presented elsewhere if different age groups are used in the adjustment procedure.
[3] Includes all other races not shown separately, unknown education level, and unknown disability status.
[4] The race groups White, Black, American Indian or Alaska Native, Asian, Native Hawaiian or Other Pacific Islander, and two or more races, include persons of Hispanic and non-Hispanic origin. Persons of Hispanic origin may be of any race.
[5] Estimates are for persons 25 years of age and over and are age-adjusted to the year 2000 standard population using five age groups: 25 to 44 years, 45 to 54 years, 55 to 64 years, 65 to 74 years, and 75 years and over.
[6] GED is General Educational Development high school equivalency diploma.
[7] Percent of poverty level is based on family income and family size and composition using U.S. Census Bureau poverty thresholds.

Table 3-8. Severe Headache or Migraine, Low Back Pain, and Neck Pain Among Adults 18 Years of Age and Over, by Selected Characteristics, 1997, 2000, 2010, and 2015—*Continued*

(Percent of adults with pain in the last 3 months.)

Characteristic	Severe headache or migraine[1]				Low back pain[1]				Neck pain[1]			
	1997	2000	2010	2015	1997	2000	2010	2015	1997	2000	2010	2015
200 percent to 399 percent	16.3	16.5	16.9	16.4	29.1	28.5	30.5	30.9	15.9	16.0	16.8	16.8
400 percent or more	12.5	12.3	13.8	11.8	25.4	25.2	25.2	25.9	13.1	14.0	13.6	15.1
Black or African American only												
Below 100 percent	22.7	21.1	24.0	19.8	34.5	27.5	32.5	33.1	17.9	13.7	18.6	17.3
100 percent to 199 percent	17.6	16.3	19.6	16.4	27.7	26.2	31.2	33.7	14.0	11.1	14.4	15.1
200 percent to 399 percent	14.0	11.4	17.6	15.7	24.3	23.8	23.7	24.9	10.2	9.8	11.7	12.0
400 percent or more	12.9	8.2	12.2	13.6	21.5	20.3	21.0	22.2	11.9	8.1	8.5	11.8
Disability Measure[2,8]												
Any basic actions difficulty or complex activity limitation	29.3	28.3	30.1	29.5	48.0	49.0	49.5	51.7	27.2	29.0	28.1	30.1
Any basic actions difficulty	30.0	29.3	30.9	30.4	49.3	50.0	51.1	53.0	27.9	29.9	29.0	30.7
Any complex activity limitation	34.6	32.7	36.0	34.6	55.1	54.3	54.5	57.5	33.1	33.9	34.3	37.1
No disability	11.0	10.4	11.7	10.6	19.4	18.7	19.0	19.4	9.1	9.1	9.7	9.7
Geographic Region[2]												
Northeast	14.5	12.7	15.4	14.6	27.1	26.0	28.0	28.8	14.0	13.5	14.9	15.8
Midwest	15.6	15.1	16.8	15.9	28.7	28.2	28.1	29.0	15.3	14.5	16.0	14.9
South	17.1	14.9	18.2	15.8	27.5	26.5	28.3	28.6	13.9	13.7	14.6	14.9
West	15.3	15.9	15.1	15.2	30.0	28.6	29.3	29.9	16.1	16.5	16.5	17.5
Location of Residence[2]												
Within MSA[9]	15.2	14.4	16.3	15.1	27.0	26.6	27.5	28.2	14.2	14.3	14.9	15.3
Outside MSA[9]	18.1	16.1	18.6	17.9	32.5	29.6	33.8	34.5	16.4	14.9	18.1	18.2

[1]In three separate questions, respondents were asked, "During the past 3 months, did you have a severe headache or migraine? ...low back pain? ...neck pain?" Respondents were instructed to report pain that had lasted a whole day or more, and not to report fleeting or minor aches or pains. Persons may be represented in more than one column.

[2]Estimates are age adjusted to the year 2000 standard population using five age groups: 18 to 44 years, 45 to 54 years, 55 to 64 years, 65 to 74 years, and 75 years and over. Age-adjusted estimates in this table may differ from other age-adjusted estimates based on the same data and presented elsewhere if different age groups are used in the adjustment procedure.

[8]Any basic actions difficulty or complex activity limitation is defined as having one or more of the following limitations or difficulties: movement difficulty, emotional difficulty, sensory (seeing or hearing) difficulty, cognitive difficulty, self-care (activities of daily living or instrumental activities of daily living) limitation, social limitation, or work limitation.

[9]MSA = metropolitan statistical area.

Table 3-9. Joint Pain Among Adults 18 Years of Age and Over, by Selected Characteristics, Selected Years, 2002–2010

(Percent.)

Characteristic	Any joint pain[1]			Knee pain[1]			Shoulder pain[1]			Finger pain[1]			Hip pain[1]		
	2002	2005	2010	2002	2005	2010	2002	2005	2010	2002	2005	2010	2002	2005	2010
18 years and over, age-adjusted[2,3]	29.5	30.7	32.1	16.5	18.2	19.6	8.6	9.2	9.0	7.5	7.4	7.1	6.6	7.1	7.0
18 years and over, crude[3]	29.5	31.1	33.3	16.5	18.5	20.3	8.7	9.3	9.4	7.5	7.6	7.5	6.6	7.2	7.3
Age															
18 to 44 years	19.3	19.1	20.6	10.5	11.6	12.6	4.9	4.9	5.2	3.4	2.8	3.1	3.2	3.2	3.2
18 to 24 years	14.2	14.0	15.2	8.3	8.8	9.8	3.4	2.4	3.5	2.0	*1.0	1.7	1.6	2.1	*1.5
25 to 44 years	21.0	20.9	22.6	11.2	12.6	13.6	5.4	5.8	5.8	3.9	3.5	3.6	3.8	3.6	3.8
45 to 64 years	37.5	39.9	42.9	20.4	23.2	26.1	12.3	12.9	13.2	11.0	11.2	10.5	9.1	9.7	10.0
45 to 54 years	34.3	35.8	39.3	18.4	20.6	23.5	10.5	11.5	12.0	9.1	9.2	8.4	7.8	7.6	9.0
55 to 64 years	42.3	45.7	47.3	23.4	26.9	29.3	15.1	14.9	14.8	13.9	14.0	13.2	11.0	12.6	11.3
65 years and over	47.2	50.9	49.6	28.6	30.2	30.5	14.1	16.0	13.6	13.9	15.2	14.2	12.9	14.6	13.5
65 to 74 years	46.0	49.3	49.5	27.6	29.7	30.2	14.0	15.7	13.5	14.4	14.9	15.3	12.6	13.7	13.3
75 years and over	48.7	52.6	49.8	29.7	30.8	30.9	14.1	16.2	13.7	13.3	15.4	12.8	13.3	15.7	13.7
Sex[2]															
Male	28.0	28.9	30.8	15.2	16.8	18.7	8.4	9.3	9.3	5.8	6.0	5.8	5.1	5.4	5.3
Female	30.7	32.2	33.2	17.6	19.4	20.3	8.8	9.0	8.6	8.9	8.7	8.2	8.0	8.6	8.6
Sex and Age															
Male															
18 to 44 years	20.1	19.3	21.6	10.7	12.0	12.9	5.5	5.4	6.1	3.0	2.6	3.0	2.5	2.4	2.0
45 to 54 years	31.1	33.4	37.3	16.2	18.9	22.3	9.5	11.4	12.2	6.6	7.5	7.3	5.6	5.7	6.8
55 to 64 years	37.3	40.7	42.5	20.1	23.1	27.4	13.7	14.7	15.3	10.5	10.4	9.9	8.0	9.5	8.7
65 to 74 years	41.7	45.1	42.9	24.1	25.1	25.3	13.3	15.7	11.8	11.2	11.4	10.9	10.5	10.8	10.3
75 years and over	43.9	47.0	46.6	25.7	25.7	28.7	11.4	15.1	13.1	10.0	12.1	9.5	10.1	12.7	12.9
Female															
18 to 44 years	18.4	18.9	19.7	10.2	11.2	12.2	4.2	4.5	4.3	3.8	3.0	3.1	3.9	4.0	4.5
45 to 54 years	37.3	38.2	41.3	20.5	22.3	24.8	11.4	11.5	11.8	11.5	10.9	9.4	9.9	9.5	11.1
55 to 64 years	46.8	50.4	51.8	26.4	30.5	31.0	16.3	15.1	14.3	17.0	17.4	16.2	13.7	15.4	13.7
65 to 74 years	49.6	52.9	55.2	30.5	33.6	34.4	14.7	15.7	15.0	17.1	17.9	19.0	14.2	16.2	15.8
75 years and over	51.6	56.2	51.9	32.1	34.0	32.4	15.7	16.9	14.1	15.3	17.5	15.1	15.2	17.5	14.3
Race[2,4]															
White only	29.8	31.3	32.6	16.3	18.5	19.7	8.8	9.5	9.1	7.6	7.8	7.4	6.9	7.4	7.2
Black or African American only	30.8	28.5	32.0	20.2	18.2	21.0	8.3	7.6	8.9	6.5	4.6	5.6	5.6	6.1	6.0
American Indian or Alaska Native only	36.7	34.8	38.1	24.5	15.0	26.9	*11.3	*8.1	10.1	*12.9	*13.0	*7.2	*10.4	*	*9.9
Asian only	18.1	18.5	20.4	8.5	10.2	12.8	3.9	5.3	6.9	*3.2	4.1	3.3	*2.3	*2.1	*2.4
Native Hawaiian or Other Pacific Islander only	*	*	*	*	*	*	*	*	*	*	*	*	*	*	*
2 or more races........................	42.7	46.2	43.5	28.1	28.6	27.1	15.4	18.9	13.9	12.8	10.5	12.2	10.0	13.7	11.7
Hispanic Origin and Race[2,4]															
Hispanic or Latino............................	23.4	24.2	25.4	13.6	14.9	15.5	7.6	8.2	7.4	6.8	6.0	6.0	3.8	4.1	4.3
Mexican...............................	24.6	23.8	25.0	14.1	14.9	15.4	8.3	8.5	7.3	7.8	7.0	6.3	4.0	4.1	3.9
Not Hispanic or Latino	30.4	31.7	33.3	17.0	18.9	20.3	8.9	9.4	9.3	7.6	7.6	7.3	6.9	7.4	7.3
White only.................................	30.8	32.8	34.3	16.9	19.4	20.7	9.1	9.8	9.5	7.8	8.2	7.7	7.3	7.8	7.7
Black or African American only	30.8	28.5	32.1	20.1	18.1	21.0	8.3	7.6	8.9	6.5	4.7	5.6	5.7	6.2	6.1
Education[5,6]															
25 years and over															
No high school diploma or GED.....	33.0	33.3	33.8	19.5	20.7	22.0	10.8	11.7	10.9	9.5	8.8	8.5	7.3	8.5	7.9
High school diploma or GED.........	32.9	33.1	36.8	18.6	19.7	22.7	10.2	10.5	10.9	8.3	8.8	9.1	7.3	7.5	9.0
Some college or more....................	31.1	33.2	34.0	16.9	19.2	20.1	8.8	9.7	9.1	8.2	8.1	7.4	7.5	7.8	7.3
Percent of Poverty Level[2,7]															
Below 100 percent	31.7	33.7	35.6	19.9	21.4	22.9	11.2	11.2	11.1	9.8	8.0	9.1	8.5	8.9	9.7
100 percent to 199 percent..............	31.7	31.9	34.0	19.0	19.8	21.9	10.4	10.5	10.9	8.9	8.2	8.3	7.5	8.1	8.5
200 percent to 399 percent...............	30.1	31.0	32.2	16.4	18.4	19.3	8.8	9.2	9.0	7.9	7.9	7.2	6.8	6.9	6.8
400 percent or more..........................	27.6	29.3	30.5	14.9	16.6	18.1	7.3	8.1	7.7	6.2	6.6	6.0	5.8	6.3	5.7
Hispanic Origin and Race and Percent of Poverty Level[2,4,7] ...															
Hispanic or Latino............................															
Below 100 percent	26.8	24.5	25.3	16.1	15.7	15.9	11.5	10.5	7.6	8.6	6.4	6.4	5.9	4.4	5.6
100 percent to 199 percent...........	24.5	24.1	25.4	14.4	15.2	16.1	8.2	8.3	8.0	8.2	5.7	5.2	3.9	3.9	4.5

* = Figure does not meet standards of reliability or precision. Data preceded by an asterisk have a relative standard error (RSE) of 20 percent to 30 percent. Data not shown have an RSE of greater than 30 percent.
[1]Starting with 2002 data, respondents were asked, "During the past 30 days, have you had any symptoms of pain, aching, or stiffness in or around a joint?" Respondents were instructed not to include the back or neck. To facilitate their responses, respondents were shown a card illustrating the body joints. Respondents reporting more than one type of joint pain were included in each response category. This table shows the most commonly reported joints.
[2]Estimates are age adjusted to the year 2000 standard population using five age groups: 18 to 44 years, 45 to 54 years, 55 to 64 years, 65 to 74 years, and 75 years and over. Age-adjusted estimates in this table may differ from other age-adjusted estimates based on the same data and presented elsewhere if different age groups are used in the adjustment procedure.
[3]Includes all other races not shown separately, unknown education level, and unknown disability status.
[4]The race groups White, Black, American Indian or Alaska Native, Asian, Native Hawaiian or Other Pacific Islander, and two or more races, include persons of Hispanic and non-Hispanic origin. Persons of Hispanic origin may be of any race.
[5]Estimates are for persons 25 years of age and over and are age-adjusted to the year 2000 standard population using five age groups: 25 to 44 years, 45 to 54 years, 55 to 64 years, 65 to 74 years, and 75 years and over.
[6]GED is General Educational Development high school equivalency diploma.
[7]Percent of poverty level is based on family income and family size and composition using U.S. Census Bureau poverty thresholds.
[8]MSA = metropolitan statistical area.

Table 3-9. Joint Pain Among Adults 18 Years of Age and Over, by Selected Characteristics, Selected Years, 2002–2010—*Continued*

(Percent.)

Characteristic	Any joint pain[1]			Knee pain[1]			Shoulder pain[1]			Finger pain[1]			Hip pain[1]		
	2002	2005	2010	2002	2005	2010	2002	2005	2010	2002	2005	2010	2002	2005	2010
200 percent to 399 percent...........	21.6	23.6	24.8	11.7	13.1	14.5	5.7	8.2	6.8	6.2	6.5	6.8	3.2	4.2	3.1
400 percent or more	21.9	24.7	27.4	12.3	15.6	16.3	4.9	*6.4	7.4	*5.3	*5.1	5.8	*1.8	*4.3	*5.2
Not Hispanic or Latino															
White only...................................															
Below 100 percent	34.2	39.3	40.1	21.3	24.7	25.2	12.4	13.4	12.6	10.9	9.9	11.1	9.9	11.6	12.0
100 percent to 199 percent.......	34.9	36.2	38.7	20.3	22.8	24.8	11.6	12.0	12.2	9.9	9.6	9.8	9.1	9.8	10.6
200 percent to 399 percent........	32.0	33.6	34.8	17.0	20.1	20.9	9.6	10.1	10.0	8.5	8.9	7.8	7.5	7.8	7.8
400 percent or more	28.2	30.1	31.8	15.1	17.0	18.8	7.6	8.4	8.0	6.5	7.0	6.3	6.2	6.8	6.0
Black or African American only															
Below 100 percent	31.6	33.0	37.6	20.8	22.5	25.1	9.1	9.0	11.9	7.9	5.7	7.8	8.1	7.7	9.0
100 percent to 199 percent.......	34.0	28.6	33.0	23.2	18.3	22.6	10.9	8.3	10.0	7.4	6.0	6.2	6.4	6.3	5.9
200 percent to 399 percent........	29.1	27.2	30.8	19.1	16.6	19.8	7.4	7.2	7.8	6.0	3.9	4.3	4.7	6.0	5.2
400 percent or more	29.8	25.8	26.8	18.2	15.8	15.7	*8.0	*5.7	6.5	*4.8	*2.8	*4.2	*4.5	*5.5	4.7
Disability Measure[2,8]															
Any basic actions difficulty or															
complex activity limitation	52.5	54.8	54.6	32.1	35.7	35.9	17.8	18.8	16.8	14.5	14.2	12.8	13.8	14.6	14.2
Any basic actions difficulty	54.0	56.7	56.2	33.4	37.3	37.3	18.3	19.5	17.2	14.9	14.8	13.3	14.4	15.2	14.6
Any complex activity limitation	56.4	57.8	56.5	35.2	38.2	37.5	22.0	23.5	20.6	17.8	16.9	15.0	17.8	19.7	18.7
No disability	19.6	20.3	21.5	9.4	10.4	11.6	4.6	4.8	4.9	4.0	4.1	4.2	3.1	3.3	3.1
Geographic Region[2]															
Northeast	27.5	28.6	28.9	15.8	16.7	17.9	7.9	8.1	8.3	6.6	6.2	5.5	5.7	6.4	5.5
Midwest	32.1	34.8	35.7	18.4	21.6	22.3	8.6	10.1	10.0	7.5	8.5	7.9	6.9	7.9	8.5
South	29.3	29.8	32.4	16.7	17.9	19.8	9.1	8.9	9.0	7.6	7.3	7.4	7.0	7.1	7.2
West..	28.4	29.2	30.6	14.6	16.3	17.9	8.6	9.6	8.5	8.0	7.5	7.1	6.4	6.6	6.3
Location of Residence[2]															
Within MSA[9]	28.3	29.2	31.1	16.0	17.2	19.0	8.1	8.4	8.3	7.2	7.0	7.0	6.2	6.5	6.5
Outside MSA[9]................................	33.9	36.3	37.4	18.7	22.3	23.0	10.8	12.2	12.3	8.4	9.1	7.9	8.0	9.3	9.4

* = Figure does not meet standards of reliability or precision. Data preceded by an asterisk have a relative standard error (RSE) of 20 percent to 30 percent. Data not shown have an RSE of greater than 30 percent.
[1]Starting with 2002 data, respondents were asked, "During the past 30 days, have you had any symptoms of pain, aching, or stiffness in or around a joint?" Respondents were instructed not to include the back or neck. To facilitate their responses, respondents were shown a card illustrating the body joints. Respondents reporting more than one type of joint pain were included in each response category. This table shows the most commonly reported joints.
[2]Estimates are age adjusted to the year 2000 standard population using five age groups: 18 to 44 years, 45 to 54 years, 55 to 64 years, 65 to 74 years, and 75 years and over. Age-adjusted estimates in this table may differ from other age-adjusted estimates based on the same data and presented elsewhere if different age groups are used in the adjustment procedure.
[8]Any basic actions difficulty or complex activity limitation is defined as having one or more of the following limitations or difficulties: movement difficulty, emotional difficulty, sensory (seeing or hearing) difficulty, cognitive difficulty, self-care (activities of daily living or instrumental activities of daily living) limitation, social limitation, or work limitation.
[9]MSA = metropolitan statistical area.

Table 3-10. Basic Actions Difficulty and Complex Activity Limitation Among Adults 18 Years of Age and Over, by Selected Characteristics, Selected Years, 1997–2013

(Number, percent.)

Characteristic	18 years and over					18 to 64 years					65 years and over				
	1997	2000	2005	2010[1]	2013[1]	1997	2000	2005	2010[1]	2013[1]	1997	2000	2005	2010[1]	2013[1]
Number in Millions															
At least one basic actions difficulty or complex activity limitation[2,3]	60.9	59.0	66.5	73.7	75.4	41.3	39.3	45.4	50.7	49.8	19.6	19.7	21.1	23.0	25.6
At least one basic actions difficulty[2]	56.7	55.2	62.4	69.2	70.9	38.1	36.4	42.1	47.2	46.3	18.6	18.7	20.3	22.0	24.6
At least one complex activity limitation[3]	29.0	27.2	31.3	35.0	37.5	18.1	16.7	19.9	22.9	23.9	11.0	10.5	11.5	12.1	13.6
Percent with At Least One Basic Actions Difficulty or Complex Activity Limitation[2,3]															
Total, age-adjusted[4,5]	32.5	29.9	31.0	31.9	31.4	X	X	X	X	X	X	X	X	X	X
Total, crude[4]	31.8	29.5	31.2	32.8	32.9	25.8	23.5	25.3	27.1	26.6	62.2	60.8	62.4	61.7	61.1
Percent with At Least One Basic Actions Difficulty[2]															
Total, age-adjusted[4,5]	30.1	27.9	29.1	29.9	29.5	X	X	X	X	X	X	X	X	X	X
Total, crude[4]	29.4	27.5	29.3	30.8	30.9	23.6	21.7	23.5	25.1	24.7	58.8	58.1	60.1	59.3	58.9
Sex															
Male	25.6	23.8	25.2	26.3	26.3	20.7	18.9	20.3	21.4	21.0	54.5	53.4	55.2	53.8	52.8
Female	32.9	31.0	33.1	35.1	35.2	26.4	24.3	26.6	28.8	28.3	61.9	61.5	63.7	63.6	63.7
Race[6]															
White only	29.6	28.1	29.7	31.2	31.4	23.5	21.8	23.5	25.1	24.7	58.5	58.0	60.0	59.2	58.4
Black or African American only	31.4	27.2	30.4	32.3	33.6	26.9	22.7	26.1	28.4	29.0	64.4	60.6	63.2	62.9	63.8
American Indian or Alaska Native only	43.8	36.8	25.6	41.6	35.7	41.9	34.1	25.2	38.5	30.4	66.0	70.2	*	74.0	74.3
Asian only	15.5	15.5	15.7	17.5	17.6	13.0	12.6	11.8	12.8	12.3	46.4	44.7	46.2	50.1	53.4
Native Hawaiian or Other Pacific Islander only	NA	*	*	*	*	NA	*	*	*	*	NA	*	*	*	*
Two or more races	NA	38.0	40.0	36.3	34.7	NA	34.4	34.9	33.9	30.8	NA	70.7	90.4	65.4	71.6
Hispanic Origin and Race[6]															
Hispanic or Latino	23.8	19.6	21.6	24.7	23.3	21.0	16.6	18.7	21.2	19.9	54.6	57.5	56.2	61.5	56.9
Not Hispanic or Latino	30.0	28.5	30.4	31.8	32.3	23.9	22.4	24.3	25.9	25.7	59.0	58.2	60.3	59.1	59.1
White only	30.3	29.1	31.1	32.4	33.0	23.8	22.5	24.5	26.0	25.9	58.7	58.2	60.3	59.0	58.7
Black or African American only	31.5	27.3	30.7	32.6	34.1	27.0	22.9	26.3	28.6	29.5	64.4	60.4	63.5	63.2	63.7
Percent of Poverty Level[7]															
Below 100 percent	41.9	38.4	40.2	40.6	43.7	36.2	31.9	34.9	36.3	38.9	74.1	71.6	73.1	72.7	75.0
100 percent to 199 percent	38.2	37.1	38.4	38.7	39.4	29.2	26.5	29.6	30.5	30.6	66.6	69.4	68.5	69.5	70.2
200 percent to 399 percent	28.4	28.2	29.7	31.1	30.2	22.0	22.1	22.8	24.1	22.7	56.1	53.9	59.0	58.9	59.5
400 percent or more	21.0	19.4	21.4	23.0	22.4	18.2	16.8	18.1	19.3	18.0	45.5	44.7	48.2	47.0	45.4
Location of Residence															
Within MSA[8]	27.7	25.9	27.5	29.2	29.3	22.3	20.3	22.1	23.6	23.3	56.6	56.7	58.3	59.2	58.3
Outside MSA[8]	35.6	33.6	36.3	39.3	40.0	28.6	26.8	29.5	33.8	33.2	65.8	62.6	65.5	59.9	61.3
Percent with At Least One Complex Activity Limitation[3]															
Total, age-adjusted[4,5]	15.6	13.7	14.5	14.9	15.2	X	X	X	X	X	X	X	X	X	X
Total, crude[4]	15.1	13.4	14.6	15.5	16.0	11.2	9.8	11.0	12.1	12.4	35.1	32.0	33.6	32.3	32.0
Sex															
Male	13.7	12.0	12.9	14.0	14.8	10.6	9.4	10.1	11.3	12.0	31.9	28.1	29.4	30.1	29.1
Female	16.5	14.7	16.1	16.8	17.0	11.9	10.3	11.8	12.9	12.9	37.4	34.9	36.7	34.0	34.3
Race[6]															
White only	15.0	13.6	14.4	15.2	16.0	10.9	9.8	10.7	11.7	12.2	34.3	31.5	33.1	31.7	31.4
Black or African American only	19.0	15.0	17.1	19.7	19.0	15.2	11.7	14.0	17.0	15.9	47.1	40.4	40.9	39.9	39.7
American Indian or Alaska Native only	23.7	20.6	14.2	15.4	22.2	22.1	17.8	13.0	14.5	19.4	*42.6	*54.9	*	*	42.7
Asian only	5.7	4.7	6.6	7.7	7.4	4.9	3.6	4.7	5.0	4.7	*14.8	*15.5	*20.8	26.7	26.0
Native Hawaiian or Other Pacific Islander only	NA	*	*	*	*	NA	*	*	*	*	NA	*	*	*	*
Two or more races	NA	22.5	26.2	19.6	19.7	NA	20.3	21.8	17.0	17.8	NA	*42.2	69.7	53.6	37.9
Hispanic Origin and Race[6]															
Hispanic or Latino	11.9	9.1	9.8	10.4	10.5	9.8	7.3	7.6	7.9	8.3	33.9	32.4	35.0	37.6	32.9
Not Hispanic or Latino	15.5	14.0	15.3	16.3	16.9	11.4	10.2	11.5	12.9	13.3	35.1	32.0	33.5	31.9	31.9
White only	15.4	14.1	15.2	16.1	17.1	11.1	10.1	11.3	12.5	13.2	34.4	31.5	32.9	31.1	31.4
Black or African American only	18.8	15.1	17.3	20.0	19.4	15.0	11.7	14.1	17.3	16.3	46.8	40.3	40.9	40.0	39.7
Percent of Poverty Level[7]															
Below 100 percent	30.0	26.0	27.3	27.5	29.6	25.2	22.0	23.4	24.0	26.1	56.9	46.7	51.5	54.5	52.7
100 percent to 199 percent	23.3	22.0	22.7	23.7	23.9	16.7	15.1	17.2	18.4	17.9	43.9	42.8	41.3	43.7	45.1
200 percent to 399 percent	13.3	12.8	14.0	14.5	14.9	9.3	9.2	9.9	10.8	10.7	30.6	27.5	31.8	29.3	31.6
400 percent or more	7.3	6.4	7.3	7.7	7.8	5.8	5.0	5.5	5.8	6.0	20.2	19.6	21.5	19.8	17.2
Location of Residence															
Within MSA[8]	14.1	12.1	13.2	14.2	14.8	10.6	8.9	9.9	10.9	11.5	32.7	29.8	31.7	31.6	31.2
Outside MSA[8]	19.0	18.2	20.0	22.2	22.3	13.6	13.4	15.4	18.8	18.2	42.8	38.8	39.7	35.2	35.3

NA = Not available.
X = Not applicable.
* = Figure does not meet standards of reliability or precision. Data preceded by an asterisk have a relative standard error (RSE) of 20 percent to 30 percent. Data not shown have an RSE of greater than 30 percent.
[1]Starting with 2007 data, the hearing question, a component of the basic actions difficulty measure, was revised. Consequently, data for basic actions difficulty prior to 2007 are not comparable with 2007 data and beyond.
[2]A basic actions difficulty is defined as having one or more of the following difficulties: movement, emotional, sensory (seeing or hearing), or cognitive.
[3]A complex activity limitation is defined as having one or more of the following limitations: self-care (activities of daily living or instrumental activities of daily living), social, or work.
[4]Includes all other races not shown separately.
[5]Estimates are for persons 25 years of age and over and are age-adjusted to the year 2000 standard population using five age groups: 25 to 44 years, 45 to 54 years, 55 to 64 years, 65 to 74 years, and 75 years and over.
[6]The race groups, White, Black, American Indian or Alaska Native, Asian, Native Hawaiian or Other Pacific Islander, and 2 or more races, include persons of Hispanic and non-Hispanic origin. Persons of Hispanic origin may be of any race.
[7]Percent of poverty level is based on family income and family size and composition using U.S. Census Bureau poverty thresholds.
[8]MSA = metropolitan statistical area.

Table 3-11. Selected Vision and Hearing Limitations Among Adults 18 Years of Age and Over, by Selected Characteristics, Selected Years, 1997–2015

(Percent.)

Characteristic	Any trouble seeing, even with glasses or contacts[1]					A lot of trouble hearing or deaf[2]				
	1997	2000	2005	2010	2015	2007	2010	2011	2012	2015
Percent of Adults										
18 years and over, age-adjusted[3,4]	10.0	9.0	9.2	9.1	9.0	2.3	2.1	2.2	2.0	2.0
18 years and over, crude[4]	9.8	8.9	9.3	9.4	9.4	2.3	2.2	2.2	2.0	2.1
Age										
18 to 44 years	6.2	5.3	5.5	6.2	5.6	0.4	0.5	0.6	0.4	0.4
18 to 24 years	5.4	4.2	5.0	5.8	4.9	*	*	*	*	*
25 to 44 years	6.5	5.7	5.7	6.3	5.8	0.5	0.5	0.7	0.5	0.4
45 to 64 years	12.0	10.7	11.2	11.6	11.6	2.0	1.9	1.9	1.7	1.5
45 to 54 years	12.2	10.9	11.0	10.7	11.2	1.2	1.2	1.5	1.3	1.1
55 to 64 years	11.6	10.5	11.5	12.7	12.1	3.0	2.7	2.4	2.0	1.9
65 years and over	18.1	17.4	17.4	13.9	14.9	8.7	7.6	7.7	7.0	7.4
65 to 74 years	14.2	13.6	13.2	12.2	11.9	4.7	4.6	4.6	4.0	4.2
75 years and over	23.1	21.9	22.0	16.1	19.1	13.3	11.1	11.6	11.1	11.9
Sex[3]										
Male	8.8	7.9	7.9	7.9	7.4	3.1	2.8	2.7	2.6	2.6
Female	11.1	10.1	10.5	10.3	10.6	1.6	1.6	1.7	1.5	1.5
Sex and Age										
Male										
18 to 44 years	5.3	4.4	4.5	5.2	4.0	*0.5	*0.7	*0.6	*0.5	*0.3
45 to 54 years	10.1	8.8	8.8	9.1	8.9	1.5	*1.1	*1.8	1.6	*1.6
55 to 64 years	10.5	9.5	10.5	10.7	10.2	4.7	3.9	3.2	2.8	2.9
65 to 74 years	13.2	12.8	11.4	10.5	10.0	7.0	6.7	6.0	5.9	5.8
75 years and over	21.4	20.7	20.4	15.7	18.8	16.9	14.5	14.7	14.2	15.8
Female										
18 to 44 years	7.1	6.2	6.5	7.1	7.1	*0.3	*0.3	0.5	0.4	*0.5
45 to 54 years	14.2	12.8	13.2	12.3	13.4	*1.0	*1.3	1.1	*1.1	*0.7
55 to 64 years	12.6	11.5	12.4	14.6	13.8	*1.3	1.6	1.6	1.3	*1.0
65 to 74 years	15.0	14.4	14.8	13.6	13.5	2.8	2.9	3.3	*2.2	2.9
75 years and over	24.2	22.7	23.0	16.4	19.4	11.1	8.9	9.5	9.0	9.1
Race[3,5]										
White only	9.7	8.8	9.1	8.8	9.0	2.4	2.3	2.3	2.1	2.1
Black or African American only	12.8	10.6	10.9	12.1	10.3	1.2	1.1	1.2	1.1	0.9
American Indian or Alaska Native only	19.2	16.6	*14.9	15.0	*10.9	*3.8	*	*	*	*6.3
Asian only	6.2	6.3	5.5	5.3	6.3	*	*1.0	*1.8	*1.2	*1.4
Native Hawaiian or Other Pacific Islander only	NA	*	*	*	*	*	*	*	*	*
Two or more races	NA	16.2	16.4	13.1	12.4	*4.9	*	*	*	*
Hispanic Origin and Race[3,5]										
Hispanic or Latino	10.0	9.7	9.6	9.2	9.3	2.5	1.4	1.4	2.0	1.3
Mexican	10.2	8.3	9.9	9.0	9.3	2.5	*1.5	1.6	*2.0	1.5
Not Hispanic or Latino	10.0	9.1	9.2	9.2	9.0	2.3	2.2	2.3	2.0	2.0
White only	9.8	8.9	9.1	8.9	9.1	2.5	2.4	2.4	2.1	2.2
Black or African American only	12.8	10.6	10.9	12.2	10.2	1.2	1.1	1.2	1.1	*0.9
Education[6,7]										
25 years of age and over										
No high school diploma or GED	15.0	12.2	13.5	14.1	13.4	4.1	3.2	3.1	2.5	2.9
High school diploma or GED	10.6	9.5	10.3	10.5	9.5	2.8	2.5	2.8	2.6	2.8
Some college or more	8.9	8.9	8.6	8.0	8.9	1.9	2.0	2.0	1.9	1.8
Percent of Poverty Level[3,8]										
Below 100 percent	17.0	12.9	15.3	14.8	14.2	3.4	2.7	2.7	2.7	2.3
100 percent to 199 percent	12.9	11.6	11.5	12.2	11.8	2.8	2.5	2.5	2.3	2.6
200 percent to 399 percent	9.1	8.8	8.9	9.0	9.4	2.4	2.1	2.4	1.9	2.2
400 percent or more	7.3	7.1	6.9	6.4	6.3	1.6	1.8	1.7	1.7	1.4
Hispanic Origin and Race and Percent of Poverty Level[3,5,8]										
Hispanic or Latino										
Below 100 percent	12.8	11.0	13.6	10.8	15.1	*	*	*1.3	*1.8	*1.7
100 percent to 199 percent	11.2	9.4	8.8	10.8	10.1	*2.1	*2.3	*1.8	*	*1.8
200 percent to 399 percent	8.1	9.2	8.2	8.9	7.2	*	*	*1.3	*2.0	*
400 percent or more	*8.1	10.5	8.0	5.3	5.2	*	*	*	*	*
Not Hispanic or Latino										
White only										
Below 100 percent	17.9	13.1	16.2	16.8	14.8	4.3	3.7	3.6	3.6	3.2

NA = Not available.
* = Figure does not meet standards of reliability or precision. Data preceded by an asterisk have a relative standard error (RSE) of 20 percent to 30 percent.
[1]Respondents were asked, "Do you have any trouble seeing, even when wearing glasses or contact lenses?" Respondents were also asked, "Are you blind or unable to see at all?" In this analysis, any trouble seeing and blind are combined into one category. In 2011, 0.4 percent of adults 18 years of age and over identified themselves as blind.
[2]Starting in 2007, respondents were asked, "WITHOUT the use of hearing aids or other listening devices,is your hearing excellent, good, a little trouble hearing, moderate trouble, a lot of trouble, or are you deaf?"
[3]Estimates are age adjusted to the year 2000 standard population using five age groups: 18 to 44 years, 45 to 54 years, 55 to 64 years, 65 to 74 years, and 75 years and over. Age-adjusted estimates in this table may differ from other age-adjusted estimates based on the same data and presented elsewhere if different age groups are used in the adjustment procedure.
[4]Includes all other races not shown separately and unknown education level.
[5]The race groups White, Black, American Indian or Alaska Native, Asian, Native Hawaiian or Other Pacific Islander, and two or more races, include persons of Hispanic and non-Hispanic origin. Persons of Hispanic origin may be of any race.
[6]Estimates are for persons 25 years of age and over and are age-adjusted to the year 2000 standard population using five age groups: 25 to 44 years, 45 to 54 years, 55 to 64 years, 65 to 74 years, and 75 years and over.
[7]GED is General Educational Development high school equivalency diploma.
[8]Percent of poverty level is based on family income and family size and composition using U.S. Census Bureau poverty thresholds.

Table 3-11. Selected Vision and Hearing Limitations Among Adults 18 Years of Age and Over, by Selected Characteristics, Selected Years, 1997–2015—*Continued*

(Percent.)

Characteristic	Any trouble seeing, even with glasses or contacts[1]					A lot of trouble hearing or deaf[2]				
	1997	2000	2005	2010	2015	2007	2010	2011	2012	2015
100 percent to 199 percent	13.1	12.0	12.7	12.6	12.9	3.3	3.0	2.8	2.7	3.2
200 percent to 399 percent	9.2	9.2	9.0	8.8	10.3	2.6	2.3	2.8	2.0	2.6
400 percent or more	7.3	7.0	6.9	6.7	6.4	1.7	2.0	1.8	1.8	1.4
Black or African American only										
Below 100 percent	17.9	13.6	16.0	15.8	13.6	*	*1.5	*1.6	*2.1	*
100 percent to 199 percent	16.0	12.9	11.3	14.9	12.4	*	*0.7	*1.5	*1.2	*
200 percent to 399 percent	9.3	7.7	9.7	12.0	9.5	*	*	*1.0	*	*
400 percent or more	7.7	8.3	6.4	6.6	6.1	*	*	*	*	*
Geographic Region[3]										
Northeast	8.6	7.4	8.1	7.8	7.9	1.7	1.4	2.3	1.6	1.4
Midwest	9.5	9.6	9.7	9.1	9.3	2.3	2.3	1.9	2.0	2.2
South	11.4	9.2	9.8	10.6	9.4	2.5	2.6	2.4	2.2	2.1
West	9.7	9.9	8.6	8.0	8.9	2.4	1.9	2.1	1.9	1.9
Location of Residence[3]										
Within MSA[9]	9.5	8.5	8.6	8.6	8.7	2.1	1.9	2.0	1.9	1.9
Outside MSA[9]	12.0	11.1	11.7	11.6	11.0	3.3	3.0	3.0	2.4	2.6

* = Figure does not meet standards of reliability or precision. Data preceded by an asterisk have a relative standard error (RSE) of 20 percent to 30 percent.
[1]Respondents were asked, "Do you have any trouble seeing, even when wearing glasses or contact lenses?" Respondents were also asked, "Are you blind or unable to see at all?" In this analysis, any trouble seeing and blind are combined into one category. In 2011, 0.4 percent of adults 18 years of age and over identified themselves as blind.
[2]Starting in 2007, respondents were asked, "WITHOUT the use of hearing aids or other listening devices, is your hearing excellent, good, a little trouble hearing, moderate trouble, a lot of trouble, or are you deaf?"
[3]Estimates are age adjusted to the year 2000 standard population using five age groups: 18 to 44 years, 45 to 54 years, 55 to 64 years, 65 to 74 years, and 75 years and over. Age-adjusted estimates in this table may differ from other age-adjusted estimates based on the same data and presented elsewhere if different age groups are used in the adjustment procedure.
[9]MSA = metropolitan statistical area.

Table 3-12. Respondent-Assessed Fair-Poor Health Status, by Selected Characteristics, Selected Years, 1991–2015

(Percent.)

Characteristic	1991[1]	1995[1]	2000	2005	2006	2007	2008	2009	2010	2011	2012	2013	2014	2015
Percent of Persons with Fair or Poor Health[2]														
All ages, age-adjusted[3,4]	10.4	10.6	9.0	9.2	9.2	9.5	9.5	9.4	9.6	9.8	9.5	9.4	8.9	9.2
All ages, crude[4]	10.0	10.1	8.9	9.3	9.5	9.8	9.9	9.9	10.1	10.4	10.3	10.2	9.8	10.1
Age														
Under 18 years	2.6	2.6	1.7	1.8	1.9	1.7	1.8	1.8	2.0	2.0	2.1	1.7	1.6	1.8
Under 6 years	2.7	2.7	1.5	1.6	1.9	1.5	1.2	1.3	1.8	1.5	1.5	1.6	1.3	1.2
6 to 17 years	2.6	2.5	1.8	1.9	1.9	1.7	2.1	2.0	2.2	2.2	2.4	1.8	1.8	2.1
18 to 44 years	6.1	6.6	5.1	5.5	5.7	5.9	6.3	6.3	6.3	6.5	6.4	6.2	6.1	6.3
18 to 24 years	4.8	4.5	3.3	3.3	3.7	3.3	4.0	3.6	3.9	4.2	3.8	3.6	3.7	3.8
25 to 44 years	6.4	7.2	5.7	6.3	6.3	6.8	7.2	7.2	7.2	7.3	7.4	7.2	7.0	7.2
45 to 54 years	13.4	13.4	11.9	11.6	12.9	13.3	12.9	13.1	13.3	14.1	14.2	14.1	12.8	13.5
55 to 64 years	20.7	21.4	17.9	18.3	18.8	17.9	18.8	19.1	19.4	19.1	19.3	19.2	18.4	18.7
65 years and over	29.0	28.3	26.9	26.6	24.8	26.8	24.9	24.0	24.4	24.7	22.7	23.1	21.7	21.8
65 to 74 years	26.0	25.6	22.5	23.4	21.9	23.4	21.8	19.9	21.2	21.5	19.6	19.7	19.5	19.0
75 years and over	33.6	32.2	32.1	30.2	28.1	30.7	28.4	28.9	28.3	28.6	26.6	27.6	24.9	25.8
Sex[3]														
Male	10.0	10.1	8.8	8.8	9.0	9.1	9.1	9.1	9.2	9.4	9.2	9.0	8.7	8.9
Female	10.8	11.1	9.3	9.5	9.5	9.9	9.8	9.7	10.0	10.1	9.9	9.8	9.2	9.5
Race[3,5]														
White only	9.6	9.7	8.2	8.6	8.6	8.8	8.9	8.7	8.8	9.0	8.8	8.7	8.3	8.5
Black or African American only	16.8	17.2	14.6	14.3	14.4	14.2	14.6	14.2	14.9	15.0	14.9	14.3	13.6	13.6
American Indian or Alaska Native only	18.3	18.7	17.2	13.2	12.1	17.1	14.5	16.3	17.8	14.4	16.5	15.3	14.1	16.6
Asian only	7.8	9.3	7.4	6.8	6.9	7.1	6.7	8.4	8.1	8.7	7.9	7.7	7.3	7.8
Native Hawaiian or Other Pacific Islander only	NA	NA	*	*	*	*	*	*	*	*	*	*	*	*
Two or more races	NA	NA	16.2	14.5	13.1	16.8	12.9	15.3	15.6	14.2	13.0	13.9	12.8	14.4
Black or African American; White	NA	NA	*14.5	8.3	*15.0	*16.6	20.2	18.0	*16.7	16.7	16.3	*19.0	11.9	*13.7
American Indian and Alaska Native; White	NA	NA	18.7	17.2	13.9	19.2	14.6	15.2	19.0	16.5	14.4	16.2	17.6	18.2
Hispanic Origin and Race[3,5]														
Hispanic or Latino	15.6	15.1	12.8	13.3	13.0	13.0	12.8	13.3	13.1	13.2	13.3	12.7	12.2	12.7
Mexican	17.0	16.7	12.8	14.3	14.1	13.2	13.4	13.7	13.7	14.0	13.6	13.3	13.0	12.7
Not Hispanic or Latino	10.0	10.1	8.7	8.7	8.8	9.1	9.1	8.9	9.2	9.4	9.1	9.0	8.5	8.7
White only	9.1	9.1	7.9	8.0	8.0	8.3	8.4	8.0	8.2	8.4	8.1	8.2	7.7	7.9
Black or African American only	16.8	17.3	14.6	14.4	14.4	14.1	14.6	14.2	14.9	15.0	15.0	14.2	13.6	13.4
Percent of Poverty Level[3,6]														
Below 100 percent	22.8	23.7	19.6	20.4	20.3	21.0	21.8	21.8	20.9	21.5	21.6	21.8	19.8	21.2
100 percent to 199 percent	14.7	15.5	14.1	14.4	14.4	15.3	15.4	14.9	15.2	15.0	14.9	14.4	14.2	14.9
200 percent to 399 percent	7.9	7.9	8.4	8.3	8.1	9.0	8.7	8.6	8.3	8.7	8.4	8.2	7.9	8.4
400 percent or more	4.9	4.7	4.5	4.7	4.5	4.7	4.4	4.3	4.3	4.3	3.9	4.0	3.9	4.0
Hispanic Origin and Race and Percent of Poverty Level[3,5,6]														
Hispanic or Latino														
Below 100 percent	23.6	22.7	18.7	20.2	20.6	21.0	21.0	22.1	19.2	21.0	20.9	20.3	18.7	21.3
100 percent to 199 percent	18.0	16.9	15.3	15.3	14.4	15.1	14.6	16.2	15.6	14.4	14.5	14.3	14.1	14.4
200 percent to 399 percent	10.3	10.1	10.3	10.3	10.5	10.5	10.7	9.7	10.3	10.8	10.0	10.3	9.4	9.7
400 percent or more	6.6	4.0	5.5	7.6	5.7	7.2	5.6	5.6	6.4	5.0	6.7	5.3	5.5	5.7
Not Hispanic or Latino														
White only														
Below 100 percent	21.9	22.8	18.8	20.1	19.5	20.9	22.1	20.5	20.9	21.2	21.1	22.2	20.3	20.7
100 percent to 199 percent	14.0	14.8	13.4	13.8	14.2	15.2	15.7	14.6	14.8	15.0	15.3	14.4	14.1	15.0
200 percent to 399 percent	7.5	7.3	7.9	7.9	7.5	8.4	8.3	8.1	7.7	8.1	7.7	7.7	7.4	8.0
400 percent or more	4.7	4.6	4.2	4.3	4.2	4.3	4.1	4.0	4.0	4.1	3.5	3.8	3.5	3.7
Black or African American only														
Below 100 percent	25.8	27.7	23.8	23.3	23.0	22.6	25.1	25.2	23.9	24.7	25.0	24.8	21.8	23.3
100 percent to 199 percent	17.0	19.3	18.2	17.6	16.9	17.7	18.1	16.6	18.3	18.5	16.9	17.5	16.8	17.0
200 percent to 399 percent	12.0	11.4	11.7	11.2	11.0	11.3	11.2	11.0	11.2	10.7	11.9	9.8	9.8	9.8
400 percent or more	5.9	6.5	7.3	7.1	7.0	7.2	6.9	5.9	6.8	6.9	6.6	5.0	5.7	6.3
Disability Measure Among Adults 18 Years and Over[3,7]														
Any basic actions difficulty or complex activity limitation	NA	NA	27.6	28.5	27.2	31.2	28.5	30.3	28.7	30.1	30.2	30.5	28.8	29.1

NA = Not available.
* = Figure does not meet standards of reliability or precision. Data preceded by an asterisk have a relative standard error (RSE) of 20 percent to 30 percent. Data not shown have an RSE of greater than 30 percent.
[1]Data prior to 1997 are not strictly comparable with data for later years due to the 1997 questionnaire redesign.
[2]See Appendix II, Health status, respondent-assessed, in Health, United States, 2014.
[3]Estimates are age-adjusted to the year 2000 standard population using six age groups: under 18 years, 18 to 44 years, 45 to 54 years, 55 to 64 years, 65 to 74 years, and 75 years and over. The disability measure is age-adjusted using the five adult age groups.
[4]Includes all other races not shown separately and unknown disability status.
[5]The race groups White, Black, American Indian or Alaska Native, Asian, Native Hawaiian or Other Pacific Islander, and two or more races, include persons of Hispanic and non-Hispanic origin. Persons of Hispanic origin may be of any race.
[6]Percent of poverty level is based on family income and family size and composition using U.S. Census Bureau poverty thresholds.
[7]Any basic actions difficulty or complex activity limitation is defined as having one or more of the following limitations or difficulties: movement difficulty, emotional difficulty, sensory (seeing or hearing) difficulty, cognitive difficulty, self-care (activities of daily living or instrumental activities of daily living) limitation, social limitation, or work limitation.

Table 3-12. Respondent-Assessed Fair-Poor Health Status, by Selected Characteristics, Selected Years, 1991–2015—*Continued*

(Percent.)

Characteristic	1991[1]	1995[1]	2000	2005	2006	2007	2008	2009	2010	2011	2012	2013	2014	2015
Any basic actions difficulty	NA	NA	27.7	29.1	27.6	31.6	28.7	30.9	28.9	30.6	30.6	30.7	29.1	29.9
Any complex activity limitation	NA	NA	45.6	46.3	45.4	50.8	47.9	48.8	46.0	48.3	46.6	47.8	47.6	46.3
No disability	NA	NA	3.8	3.6	4.0	4.0	4.2	3.6	3.5	3.6	3.6	3.8	3.8	3.5
Geographic Region[3]														
Northeast	8.3	9.1	7.6	7.5	8.2	8.4	8.0	8.4	7.9	8.4	8.0	8.2	7.2	8.2
Midwest	9.1	9.7	8.0	8.3	8.8	8.6	8.8	8.6	9.0	8.8	9.1	8.8	8.5	8.8
South	13.1	12.3	10.7	11.0	10.4	11.0	11.0	10.9	11.1	11.2	10.8	10.6	10.2	10.0
West	9.7	10.1	8.8	8.6	8.5	9.0	9.0	8.8	9.2	9.5	9.1	9.1	8.6	9.1
Location of Residence[3]														
Within MSA	9.9	10.1	8.5	8.7	8.7	9.0	9.1	9.1	9.2	9.4	9.0	9.1	8.5	8.8
Outside MSA	11.9	12.6	11.1	11.2	11.7	12.0	11.7	11.2	11.9	11.7	12.3	11.4	11.4	11.8

NA = Not available.
* = Figure does not meet standards of reliability or precision. Data preceded by an asterisk have a relative standard error (RSE) of 20 percent to 30 percent. Data not shown have an RSE of greater than 30 percent.
[1]Data prior to 1997 are not strictly comparable with data for later years due to the 1997 questionnaire redesign.
[2]See Appendix II, Health status, respondent-assessed, in Health, United States, 2014.
[3]Estimates are age-adjusted to the year 2000 standard population using six age groups: under 18 years, 18 to 44 years, 45 to 54 years, 55 to 64 years, 65 to 74 years, and 75 years and over. The disability measure is age-adjusted using the five adult age groups. The disability measure is age-adjusted using the five adult age groups.
[4]Includes all other races not shown separately and unknown disability status.
[5]The race groups White, Black, American Indian or Alaska Native, Asian, Native Hawaiian or Other Pacific Islander, and two or more races, include persons of Hispanic and non-Hispanic origin. Persons of Hispanic origin may be of any race.
[6]Percent of poverty level is based on family income and family size and composition using U.S. Census Bureau poverty thresholds.
[7]Any basic actions difficulty or complex activity limitation is defined as having one or more of the following limitations or difficulties: movement difficulty, emotional difficulty, sensory (seeing or hearing) difficulty, cognitive difficulty, self-care (activities of daily living or instrumental activities of daily living) limitation, social limitation, or work limitation.

Table 3-13. Serious Psychological Distress in the Past 30 Days Among Adults 18 Years of Age and Over, by Selected Characteristics, Annual Average, Selected Years, 1997–1998 Through 2014–2015

(Percent of persons with serious psychological distress[1].)

Characteristic	1997–1998	1999–2000	2000–2001	2001–2002	2002–2003	2003–2004	2004–2005	2006–2007	2007–2008	2008–2009	2009–2010	2010–2011	2011–2012	2013–2014[2]	2014–2015[2]
18 years and over, age-adjusted[3,4]	3.2	2.6	3.0	3.1	3.1	3.1	3.0	2.8	2.9	3.2	3.2	3.3	3.1	3.4	3.3
18 years and over, crude[4]	3.2	2.6	3.0	3.1	3.1	3.1	3.0	2.9	2.9	3.2	3.3	3.4	3.2	3.5	3.4
Age	2.9	2.3	2.7	2.9	2.9	2.9	2.8	2.5	2.7	3.1	3.1	2.9	2.8		
18 to 44 years	2.7	2.2	2.6	2.8	2.8	2.8	2.5	2.0	2.3	2.5	2.4	2.4	2.3	3.1	3.3
18 to 24 years	3.0	2.4	2.8	3.0	2.9	2.9	2.9	2.7	2.8	3.3	3.4	3.1	3.0	2.5	3.2
25 to 44 years	3.7	3.2	3.6	3.9	4.0	3.9	3.7	3.7	3.6	3.7	4.1	4.5	4.2	3.4	3.3
45 to 64 years	3.9	3.5	3.7	4.2	4.2	3.9	3.9	3.7	3.6	3.9	4.1	4.2	4.0	4.5	4.1
45 to 54 years	3.4	2.6	3.4	3.4	3.6	3.9	3.4	3.8	3.6	3.6	4.0	4.7	4.4	4.6	3.9
55 to 64 years	3.1	2.4	2.7	2.4	2.3	2.4	2.5	2.1	2.4	2.4	2.1	2.4	2.3	4.5	4.3
65 years and over	2.5	2.3	2.8	2.4	2.3	2.3	2.2	2.1	2.4	2.2	2.0	2.6	2.5	2.5	2.2
65 to 74 years	3.8	2.5	2.5	2.4	2.3	2.5	2.9	2.0	2.4	2.6	2.3	2.1	1.9	2.7	2.4
75 years and over														2.2	1.9
Sex[3]	2.5	2.0	2.4	2.4	2.3	2.3	2.3	2.1	2.2	2.7	2.8	2.8	2.5		
Male	3.8	3.1	3.5	3.8	3.9	3.9	3.7	3.4	3.5	3.6	3.7	3.7	3.7	2.9	2.7
Female														3.9	3.9
Race[3,5]	3.1	2.5	2.9	3.0	3.0	3.1	2.9	2.7	2.9	3.2	3.2	3.2	3.1		
White only	4.0	2.9	3.1	3.5	3.4	3.4	3.6	3.2	3.2	3.7	3.8	3.7	3.3	3.4	3.3
Black or African American only	7.8	*7.2	*7.4	8.1	*7.1	*5.5	*3.5	*3.9	*	*3.8	*5.2	5.6	6.5	3.5	3.4
American Indian or Alaska Native only	2.0	*1.4	*2.0	*1.8	*1.9	*1.8	1.7	2.0	*1.0	*1.1	1.6	1.7	1.9	*5.4	*11.8
Asian only														1.9	1.9
Native Hawaiian or Other Pacific Islander only	NA	*	*	*	*	*	*	*	*	*	*	*	*	*	*
Two or more races	NA	4.8	5.5	5.0	7.3	9.1	7.9	6.5	5.9	*4.9	5.2	5.6	6.7	8.6	8.4
Hispanic Origin and Race[3,5]															
Hispanic or Latino	5.0	3.5	4.0	4.0	3.9	3.9	3.7	3.4	3.6	3.4	3.6	4.0	3.8	4.5	4.4
Mexican	5.2	2.9	3.4	3.8	3.7	3.6	3.6	3.2	3.3	2.9	2.8	3.6	3.4	4.6	4.3
Not Hispanic or Latino	3.0	2.5	2.9	3.1	3.1	3.1	3.0	2.8	2.8	3.1	3.2	3.2	3.1	3.3	3.2
White only	2.9	2.4	2.9	3.0	3.0	3.0	2.9	2.7	2.9	3.2	3.1	3.2	3.1	3.2	3.1
Black or African American only	3.9	2.9	3.1	3.5	3.4	3.3	3.6	3.2	3.1	3.7	3.8	3.7	3.3	3.4	3.4
Percent of Poverty Level[3,6]															
Below 100 percent	9.1	6.8	7.7	8.4	8.6	8.8	8.6	7.2	8.3	9.0	8.4	8.2	8.2	9.1	8.3
100 percent to 199 percent	5.0	4.4	5.0	5.2	5.2	5.2	5.0	5.0	4.7	4.9	4.8	5.0	4.9	5.5	5.3
200 percent to 399 percent	2.5	2.3	2.7	2.8	2.6	2.5	2.5	2.1	2.4	2.7	2.8	2.9	2.6	2.6	2.8
400 percent or more	1.3	1.2	1.2	1.3	1.3	1.2	1.1	1.2	1.1	1.1	1.2	1.2	1.1	1.2	1.3
Hispanic Origin and Race and Percent of Poverty Level[3,5,6]															
Hispanic or Latino															
Below 100 percent	8.6	6.1	6.9	7.5	7.6	7.4	6.6	6.0	7.0	6.7	6.4	7.5	7.4	8.2	7.4
100 percent to 199 percent	5.4	3.8	4.4	4.1	3.8	3.7	3.9	2.9	4.5	4.5	4.1	4.3	3.9	5.0	5.1
200 percent to 399 percent	3.4	2.1	3.0	3.5	3.0	2.5	2.6	2.8	2.2	1.8	2.6	3.1	2.3	3.2	3.0
400 percent or more	*	2.3	*1.6	*	*	*1.8	*1.9	*2.2	*1.6	*1.0	*1.5	*1.4	*1.4	*1.8	2.7
Not Hispanic or Latino															
White only															
Below 100 percent	9.6	7.8	8.9	9.2	9.6	10.4	10.2	8.8	10.7	11.2	10.1	9.6	9.4	10.7	9.8
100 percent to 199 percent	5.2	4.9	5.5	5.9	6.1	6.1	5.6	6.0	5.4	5.7	5.5	5.6	5.8	6.5	6.0
200 percent to 399 percent	2.5	2.3	2.9	2.9	2.7	2.6	2.6	2.1	2.6	3.1	3.2	3.2	2.8	2.7	2.9
400 percent or more	1.3	1.1	1.2	1.3	1.3	1.2	1.1	1.1	1.0	1.0	1.1	1.1	1.0	1.2	1.2
Black or African American only															
Below 100 percent	8.7	6.0	6.3	7.2	7.1	7.4	7.6	6.2	6.2	8.0	8.3	7.7	7.3	7.4	6.9
100 percent to 199 percent	4.3	3.6	4.3	4.9	4.5	4.1	4.8	4.3	3.6	3.1	3.5	4.4	3.5	3.5	3.2
200 percent to 399 percent	2.2	*1.7	1.9	2.3	2.0	1.9	2.1	2.0	2.4	2.9	2.5	1.9	2.0	2.3	2.6
400 percent or more	*	*1.0	*	*	*1.2	*	*	*	*	*	*1.6	*1.5	*1.0	*0.7	*1.0
Geographic Region															
Northeast	2.7	1.9	2.5	2.8	3.0	2.9	2.5	2.6	2.6	2.9	3.1	3.0	2.7	2.8	2.7
Midwest	2.6	2.5	2.8	2.9	2.7	2.7	2.7	2.9	2.7	3.2	3.3	3.1	3.0	3.5	3.3
South	3.8	2.9	3.2	3.5	3.5	3.5	3.7	3.1	3.3	3.5	3.5	3.6	3.5	3.7	3.4
West	3.3	2.8	3.2	3.0	3.0	3.0	2.8	2.5	2.7	2.8	2.9	3.3	3.1	3.4	3.7
Location of Residence[3,7]															
Within MSA	3.0	2.3	2.8	3.0	2.9	2.9	2.8	2.6	2.7	3.0	3.1	3.1	3.0	3.3	3.2
Outside MSA	3.9	3.5	3.6	3.8	3.9	3.8	4.0	3.7	3.7	4.0	4.1	4.0	4.1	4.3	4.3

NA = Not available.

* = Figure does not meet standards of reliability or precision. Data preceded by an asterisk have a relative standard error (RSE) of 20 percent to 30 percent. Data not shown have an RSE of greater than 30 percent.

[1]Serious psychological distress is measured by a six-question scale that asks respondents how often they experienced each of six symptoms of psychological distress in the past 30 days.

[2]Starting in 2013, the six psychological distress questions were moved to the adult selected items section of the sample adult questionnaire. Observed differences between the 2012 and earlier estimates and the 2013 and later estimates may be partially or fully attributable to this change in question placement within the sample adult questionnaire.

[3]Estimates are age adjusted to the year 2000 standard population using five age groups: 18 to 44 years, 45 to 54 years, 55 to 64 years, 65 to 74 years, and 75 years and over.

[4]Includes all other races not shown separately.

[5]The race groups White, Black, American Indian or Alaska Native, Asian, Native Hawaiian or Other Pacific Islander, and two or more races, include persons of Hispanic and non-Hispanic origin. Persons of Hispanic origin may be of any race.

[6]Percent of poverty level is based on family income and family size and composition using U.S. Census Bureau poverty thresholds.

[7]MSA = metropolitan statistical area.

Table 3-14. Children Under 18 Years of Age Who Suffer from Asthma, by Selected Characteristics, Annual Average, Selected Years, 1997–1999 Through 2011–2013

(Percent of children.)

Characteristic	Current asthma[1]									Asthma attack in the past 12 months[2]								
	1997–1999	2000–2002	2003–2005	2006–2008	2007–2009	2008–2010	2009–2011	2010–2012	2011–2013	1997–1999	2000–2002	2003–2005	2006–2008	2007–2009	2008–2010	2009–2011	2010–2012	2011–2013
Children Under 18 Years[3]	NA	NA	8.7	9.3	9.4	9.5	9.5	9.4	9.0	5.4	5.7	5.4	5.5	5.4	5.6	5.6	5.5	5.3
Age																		
0 to 4 years..............................	NA	NA	6.1	6.2	6.4	6.2	6.4	6.1	5.5	4.3	4.7	4.2	4.3	4.3	4.4	4.5	4.2	3.6
5 to 17 years............................	NA	NA	9.6	10.5	10.6	10.8	10.7	10.7	10.4	5.7	6.1	5.8	5.9	5.9	6.1	6.0	6.1	5.9
5 to 9 years............................	NA	NA	9.1	10.6	10.2	10.7	10.2	10.3	9.8	5.6	6.3	6.1	6.8	6.2	6.5	6.2	6.6	6.2
10 to 17 years........................	NA	NA	9.9	10.4	10.8	10.9	11.1	10.9	10.8	5.8	5.9	5.7	5.4	5.7	5.8	5.8	5.7	5.7
Sex																		
Male.......................................	NA	NA	9.9	10.7	10.8	11.1	10.7	10.2	9.8	6.2	6.6	6.3	6.2	6.2	6.5	6.3	6.3	5.9
Female	NA	NA	7.3	7.8	7.9	7.8	8.3	8.5	8.2	4.5	4.7	4.4	4.7	4.6	4.6	4.8	4.8	4.7
Hispanic Origin and Race[4]																		
Race[4]																		
White only................................	NA	NA	7.7	8.2	8.0	8.2	8.1	8.1	7.8	5.0	5.2	4.9	4.9	4.7	4.9	4.8	4.9	4.7
Black or African American only	NA	NA	13.0	14.6	16.0	16.0	16.4	16.0	15.3	7.0	8.0	7.6	8.1	8.6	8.7	8.8	8.9	8.5
American Indian or Alaska Native only .	NA	NA	12.2	*10.4	*10.8	*10.3	*6.6	9.4	9.5	6.4	*8.7	*6.1	*	*	*	*3.5	*5.5	*5.8
Asian only	NA	NA	4.8	5.8	6.3	6.7	7.7	6.8	5.6	4.3	4.7	3.3	3.9	4.1	4.8	5.2	4.4	3.2
Native Hawaiian or Other Pacific Islander only	NA	NA	*	*	*	*	*	*	*	NA	*	*	*	*	*	*	*	*
Two or more races	NA	NA	13.5	13.6	13.9	12.8	13.3	12.7	13.1	NA	7.3	8.8	8.2	9.3	9.0	8.0	7.1	7.1
Hispanic Origin																		
Hispanic or Latino	NA	NA	7.6	8.3	7.9	7.5	8.5	8.8	8.6	4.8	4.2	4.6	5.0	4.6	4.4	4.7	4.9	4.6
Not Hispanic or Latino	NA	NA	8.9	9.6	9.8	10.0	9.8	9.6	9.2	5.5	6.0	5.6	5.6	5.7	5.9	5.8	5.7	5.5
White only............................	NA	NA	7.9	8.2	8.2	8.5	8.2	8.0	7.7	5.1	5.5	5.0	4.9	4.8	5.1	5.0	5.0	4.8
Black or African American only	NA	NA	13.0	14.6	16.0	16.2	16.4	16.1	15.2	7.0	7.9	7.5	8.0	8.5	8.8	8.8	9.0	8.5
Percent of Poverty Level[5]																		
Below 100 percent	NA	NA	10.4	11.7	12.2	12.4	12.7	12.5	12.4	6.1	7.1	6.5	6.8	6.9	7.4	7.5	7.5	7.2
100 percent to 199 percent	NA	NA	8.6	9.9	9.8	9.9	9.9	9.9	9.2	5.3	5.4	5.2	5.8	5.7	6.0	5.9	6.0	5.2
200 percent to 399 percent	NA	NA	8.3	8.8	8.2	8.2	8.3	8.7	8.3	5.0	5.3	5.2	4.9	4.7	4.6	4.6	4.7	4.7
400 percent or more	NA	NA	7.9	7.6	8.4	8.2	7.8	7.0	6.7	5.2	5.5	4.9	4.8	5.0	5.0	4.7	4.4	4.3
Health Insurance Status at the Time of Interview[6]																		
Insured.....................................	NA	NA	9.0	9.7	9.7	9.8	9.7	9.6	9.2	5.6	5.9	5.6	5.7	5.6	5.8	5.7	5.7	5.4
Private...................................	NA	NA	8.0	8.6	8.3	8.4	8.2	8.1	7.7	5.0	5.3	5.0	5.0	5.1	5.1	4.9	4.8	4.6
Medicaid	NA	NA	11.4	12.4	12.1	12.0	12.0	11.9	11.4	7.7	7.7	7.1	7.0	6.7	7.0	6.9	7.0	6.4
Uninsured	NA	NA	5.6	6.0	6.3	6.6	6.8	6.7	6.9	3.9	4.3	3.3	3.7	3.5	3.6	3.6	4.0	4.3

NA = Not available.

* = Figure does not meet standards of reliability or precision. Data preceded by an asterisk have a relative standard error (RSE) of 20 percent to 30 percent. Data not shown have an RSE of greater than 30 percent.

[1]Based on parent or knowledgeable adult responding to both questions, "Has a doctor or other health professional ever told you that your child had asthma?" and "Does your child still have asthma?"

[2]Based on parent or knowledgeable adult responding to both questions, "Has a doctor or other health professional ever told you that your child had asthma?" and "During the past 12 months, did your child have an episode of asthma or an asthma attack?"

[3]Includes all other races not shown separately, unknown poverty level, and unknown health insurance status.

[4]The race groups White, Black, American Indian or Alaska Native, Asian, Native Hawaiian or Other Pacific Islander, and two or more races, include persons of Hispanic and non-Hispanic origin. Persons of Hispanic origin may be of any race.

[5]Percent of poverty level is based on family income and family size and composition using U.S. Census Bureau poverty thresholds. Missing family income data were imputed for 1997 and beyond.

[6]Health insurance categories are mutually exclusive. Persons who reported both Medicaid and private coverage are classified as having private coverage. Starting with 1997 data, state-sponsored health plan coverage is included as Medicaid coverage. Starting with 1999 data, coverage by the Children's Health Insurance Program (CHIP) is included as Medicaid coverage. In addition to private and Medicaid, the insured category also includes military, other government, and Medicare coverage. Persons not covered by private insurance, Medicaid, CHIP, state-sponsored or other government-sponsored health plans, Medicare, or military plans are considered to have no health insurance coverage. Persons with only Indian Health Service coverage are considered to have no health insurance coverage.

Table 3-15. Hypertension Among Persons 20 Years of Age and Over, by Selected Characteristics, Selected Years, 1988–1994 Through 2011–2014

(Percent.)

Sex, age, race and Hispanic origin,[1] and percent of poverty level	Hypertension[2,3]			Uncontrolled high blood pressure among persons with hypertension[4]		
	1988–1994	2001–2004	2011–2014	1988–1994	2001–2004	2011–2014
20 Years and Over, Age-Adjusted[5]						
Both Sexes[6]	25.5	30.9	30.4	77.2	66.0	52.8
Male	26.4	30.3	31.0	83.2	68.3	58.1
Female	24.4	31.0	29.7	68.5	57.6	45.5
Not Hispanic or Latino						
White only, male	25.6	29.3	30.2	82.6	67.8	53.5
White only, female	23.0	29.0	28.0	67.0	52.7	40.2
Black or African American only, male	37.5	41.5	42.4	84.0	70.8	66.2
Black or African American only, female	38.3	44.3	44.0	71.1	65.4	52.8
Mexican origin, male	26.9	26.1	27.5	87.9	76.4	71.4
Mexican origin, female	25.0	29.7	29.4	77.6	63.8	40.7
Percent of Poverty Level[7]						
Below 100 percent	31.7	35.5	34.1	75.0	66.1	54.8
100 percent to 199 percent	26.6	34.0	33.4	76.0	70.1	56.4
200 percent to 399 percent	24.7	31.4	30.0	76.2	67.8	51.5
400 percent or more	22.6	27.9	27.7	81.5	60.8	53.5
20 Years and Over, Crude						
Both Sexes[6]	24.1	30.8	33.0	73.9	63.0	47.0
Male	23.8	29.0	32.6	79.3	62.1	49.9
Female	24.4	32.5	33.4	68.8	63.7	44.3
Not Hispanic or Latino						
White only, male	24.3	29.9	34.6	78.0	59.4	46.0
White only, female	24.6	32.9	34.5	67.8	63.8	42.5
Black or African American only, male	31.1	36.7	40.9	83.3	68.7	58.3
Black or African American only, female	32.5	41.6	44.8	70.0	61.9	48.1
Mexican male	16.4	15.8	20.2	86.5	73.6	62.6
Mexican female	15.9	19.0	22.5	80.6	69.8	47.8
Percent of Poverty Level[7]						
Below 100 percent	25.7	28.3	29.1	74.0	67.3	52.4
100 percent to 199 percent	26.7	34.6	36.5	75.1	64.5	48.3
200 percent to 399 percent	22.4	31.5	33.2	73.4	63.4	46.7
400 percent or more	22.0	28.4	32.2	74.3	59.2	44.2
Male						
20 to 44 years	10.9	12.3	11.5	90.5	71.0	67.8
20 to 34 years	7.1	7.0	6.9	92.6	87.1	74.1
35 to 44 years	17.1	19.2	18.8	89.0	63.2	64.2
45 to 64 years	34.2	39.9	43.8	73.1	61.1	49.7
45 to 54 years	29.2	35.9	33.0	76.2	64.9	46.3
55 to 64 years	40.6	47.5	54.9	70.3	55.5	51.7
65 to 74 years	54.4	61.7	63.4	74.3	49.5	38.2
75 years and over	60.4	67.1	72.3	82.5	68.3	46.5
Female						
20 to 44 years	6.5	7.7	10.2	63.4	51.0	41.9
20 to 34 years	2.9	*2.7	4.3	82.2	*50.2	55.5
35 to 44 years	11.2	14.0	18.6	56.8	51.2	37.7
45 to 64 years	32.8	42.6	39.5	62.1	60.9	36.8
45 to 54 years	23.9	35.2	28.1	58.5	66.1	40.3
55 to 64 years	42.6	54.4	52.1	64.3	55.6	34.8
65 to 74 years	56.2	72.9	64.3	68.7	67.2	44.5
75 years and over	73.6	82.0	79.9	81.9	72.4	61.5

* = Figure does not meet standards of reliability or precision. Data preceded by an asterisk have a relative standard error (RSE) of 20 percent to 30 percent.
[1]Persons of Mexican origin may be of any race.
[2]Hypertension is defined as having measured high blood pressure and/or taking antihypertensive medication. High blood pressure is defined as having measured systolic pressure of at least 140 mmHg or diastolic pressure of at least 90 mmHg. Those with high blood pressure also may be taking prescribed medicine for high blood pressure. Those taking antihypertensive medication may not have measured high blood pressure but are still classified as having hypertension.
[3]Respondents were asked, "Are you now taking prescribed medicine for your high blood pressure?"
[4]Uncontrolled high blood pressure among persons with hypertension is defined as measured systolic pressure of at least 140 mmHg or diastolic pressure of at least 90 mmHg, among those with measured high blood pressure or reporting taking antihypertensive medication.
[5]Age-adjusted to the 2000 standard population using five age groups: 20 to 34 years, 35 to 44 years, 45 to 54 years, 55 to 64 years, and 65 years and over.
[6]Includes persons of all races and Hispanic origins, not just those shown separately.
[7]Percent of poverty level is based on family income and family size. Persons with unknown percent of poverty level are excluded (8 percent in 2007-2010).

Table 3-16. Cholesterol Among Persons 20 Years of Age and Over, by Selected Characteristics, Selected Years, 1988–1994 Through 2011–2014

(Percent, number.)

Sex, age, race and Hispanic origin,[1] and percent of poverty level	1988–1994	1999–2002	2003–2006	2007–2010	2009–2012	2011–2014
PERCENT OF POPULATION WITH HYPERCHOLESTER-OLEMIA (SERUM TOTAL CHOLESTEROL GREATER THAN OR EQUAL TO 240 MG/DL OR TAKING CHOLESTEROL-LOWERING MEDICATIONS)[2]						
20 Years and Over, Age-Adjusted[3]						
Both Sexes[4]	22.8	25.0	27.7	27.4	27.8	27.8
Male	21.1	25.3	27.7	28.0	27.9	28.4
Female	24.0	24.3	27.4	26.7	27.5	27.3
Not Hispanic or Latino						
White only, male	21.1	26.0	28.7	28.1	28.1	29.4
White only, female	24.2	25.1	28.2	27.4	28.2	28.0
Black or African American only, male	18.6	20.1	22.8	25.4	25.6	24.5
Black or African American only, female	23.1	22.0	23.3	25.6	26.3	25.7
Mexican origin, male	19.9	21.6	24.2	28.6	27.2	26.6
Mexican origin, female	19.8	19.3	24.1	25.5	26.2	22.7
Percent of Poverty Level[5]						
Below 100 percent	23.0	25.0	27.9	26.5	28.7	29.2
100 percent to 199 percent	22.1	25.9	27.6	27.6	27.1	25.4
200 percent to 399 percent	23.1	26.5	27.5	28.9	28.1	29.0
400 percent or more	21.7	23.1	27.9	26.6	27.4	28.1
20 Years and Over, Crude						
Both Sexes[4]	21.5	25.0	28.0	28.7	29.5	29.8
Male	19.6	25.1	27.5	28.7	28.8	29.5
Female	23.2	24.8	28.5	28.7	30.1	30.1
Not Hispanic or Latino						
White only, male	20.0	26.8	29.7	30.4	30.9	32.6
White only, female	24.5	27.0	30.8	31.4	33.4	33.5
Black or African American only, male	16.0	18.5	21.3	24.1	24.4	24.0
Black or African American only, female	19.7	19.9	21.9	24.7	25.5	25.4
Mexican origin, male	16.2	17.0	19.3	23.7	21.9	21.2
Mexican origin, female	14.9	13.8	18.7	21.0	19.4	16.8
Percent of Poverty Level[5]						
Below 100 percent	19.4	21.6	24.1	22.3	24.1	25.3
100 percent to 199 percent	21.3	25.4	28.3	28.7	28.2	27.4
200 percent to 399 percent	21.3	26.2	28.1	30.6	30.5	31.6
400 percent or more	21.9	24.2	28.7	29.6	31.6	32.2
Male						
20 to 44 years	13.1	16.1	16.5	14.3	12.6	12.3
20 to 34 years	8.2	10.4	10.2	8.5	6.6	6.7
35 to 44 years	21.0	23.1	25.2	22.5	21.2	21.1
45 to 64 years	30.1	36.0	35.7	39.0	39.8	39.3
45 to 54 years	29.6	34.1	32.4	34.0	35.7	32.9
55 to 64 years	30.8	39.1	41.6	46.2	44.5	46.0
65 to 74 years	27.4	36.3	49.4	48.9	50.7	55.8
75 years and over	24.4	29.0	37.1	45.2	51.2	54.4
Female						
20 to 44 years	9.9	11.4	12.9	10.6	9.4	9.0
20 to 34 years	7.3	9.1	10.8	6.8	6.3	6.1
35 to 44 years	13.5	14.4	15.8	15.7	14.0	13.2
45 to 64 years	36.4	31.7	37.3	39.1	42.4	40.6
45 to 54 years	28.2	27.2	29.6	29.1	31.2	31.2
55 to 64 years	45.8	39.2	49.2	51.4	55.3	51.2
65 to 74 years	46.9	51.9	55.3	53.3	57.7	58.1
75 years and over	41.2	44.0	47.3	52.5	53.3	59.1
PERCENT OF POPULATION WITH HIGH CHOLESTEROL (SERUM TOTAL CHOLESTEROL GREATER THAN OR EQUAL TO 240 MG/DL)[6]						
20 Years and Over, Age-Adjusted[3]						
Both Sexes[4]	20.8	17.3	16.3	13.7	12.9	11.9
Male	19.0	16.4	15.1	12.6	11.7	10.8
Female	22.0	17.8	17.1	14.4	14.0	12.7
Not Hispanic or Latino						

[1]Persons of Mexican origin may be of any race.
[2]Hypercholesterolemia is defined as measured serum total cholesterol greater than or equal to 240 mg/dL or reporting taking cholesterol-lowering medications. Respondents were asked, "Are you now following this advice [from a doctor or health professional] to take prescribed medicine [to lower your cholesterol]?"
[3]Age adjusted to the 2000 standard population using five age groups: 20 to 34 years, 35 to 44 years, 45 to 54 years, 55 to 64 years, and 65 years and over.
[4]Includes persons of all races and Hispanic origins, not just those shown separately.
[5]Percent of poverty level is based on family income and family size. Persons with unknown percent of poverty level are excluded (8 percent in 2007–2010).
[6]High cholesterol is defined as serum total cholesterol greater than or equal to 240 mg/dL (6.20 mmol/L), regardless of whether the respondent reported taking cholesterol-lowering medications.

Table 3-16. Cholesterol Among Persons 20 Years of Age and Over, by Selected Characteristics, Selected Years, 1988–1994 Through 2011–2014—Continued

(Percent, number.)

Sex, age, race and Hispanic origin,[1] and percent of poverty level	1988–1994	1999–2002	2003–2006	2007–2010	2009–2012	2011–2014
White only, male	18.8	16.5	15.5	12.2	11.6	11.2
White only, female	22.2	18.1	18.0	15.3	14.7	13.3
Black or African American only, male	16.9	12.4	10.9	10.8	9.0	7.7
Black or African American only, female	21.4	17.7	13.3	11.5	10.8	9.4
Mexican origin, male	18.5	17.4	17.6	15.1	13.5	12.8
Mexican origin, female	18.7	13.8	14.4	13.6	12.8	9.3
Percent of Poverty Level[5]						
Below 100 percent	20.6	18.3	18.1	14.4	13.4	12.3
100 percent to 199 percent	20.6	19.1	16.7	15.0	13.2	11.3
200 percent to 399 percent	20.8	18.9	15.8	14.4	13.2	13.0
400 percent or more	19.5	14.4	15.9	12.3	12.3	11.5
20 Years and Over, Crude						
Both Sexes[4]	19.6	17.3	16.4	14.1	13.4	12.1
Male	17.7	16.5	15.2	12.9	11.8	10.7
Female	21.3	18.0	17.5	15.2	14.9	13.5
Not Hispanic or Latino						
White only, male	18.0	16.9	15.7	12.6	11.8	10.8
White only, female	22.5	19.1	18.9	16.7	16.5	14.9
Black or African American only, male	14.7	12.2	10.8	10.9	8.8	7.4
Black or African American only, female	18.2	16.1	12.5	11.3	10.6	9.5
Mexican origin, male	15.4	15.0	15.7	14.7	13.0	12.3
Mexican origin, female	14.3	10.7	12.6	12.3	10.9	8.8
Percent of Poverty Level[5]						
Below 100 percent	17.6	16.4	16.8	12.8	12.0	11.3
100 percent to 199 percent	19.8	18.2	16.0	14.6	12.9	11.1
200 percent to 399 percent	19.3	18.7	15.8	14.6	13.9	13.4
400 percent or more	19.9	15.5	17.1	13.7	13.6	12.5
Male						
20 to 44 years	12.5	14.2	14.1	11.1	10.0	10.0
20 to 34 years	8.2	9.8	9.5	7.6	6.0	6.0
35 to 44 years	19.4	19.7	20.5	16.2	15.8	16.2
45 to 64 years	27.2	22.2	19.1	17.7	16.2	13.6
45 to 54 years	26.6	23.6	20.8	18.7	18.0	15.7
55 to 64 years	28.0	19.9	16.0	16.3	14.1	11.5
65 to 74 years	21.9	13.7	10.9	7.5	8.1	7.6
75 years and over	20.4	10.2	9.6	6.8	*5.5	*3.6
Female						
20 to 44 years	9.4	10.4	11.3	8.4	7.6	7.2
20 to 34 years	7.3	8.9	10.3	5.8	5.7	5.4
35 to 44 years	12.3	12.4	12.7	11.9	10.4	9.8
45 to 64 years	33.4	23.0	23.9	21.3	22.4	19.9
45 to 54 years	26.7	21.4	19.7	17.7	18.7	18.0
55 to 64 years	40.9	25.6	30.5	25.6	26.6	22.1
65 to 74 years	41.3	32.3	24.2	20.6	19.6	15.8
75 years and over	38.2	26.5	18.6	20.2	16.2	16.1
MEAN SERUM TOTAL CHOLESTEROL LEVEL, MG/DL						
20 Years and Over, Age-Adjusted[3]						
Both Sexes[4]	206	203	200	196	195	192
Male	204	202	198	194	192	189
Female	207	204	202	198	198	195
Not Hispanic or Latino						
White only, male	205	202	198	193	192	189
White only, female	208	205	203	199	199	196
Black or African American only, male	202	195	193	191	188	183
Black or African American only, female	207	202	195	192	192	189
Mexican origin, male	206	204	203	200	197	194
Mexican origin, female	206	199	200	196	194	191
Percent of Poverty Level[5]						
Below 100 percent	205	201	203	196	196	191

[1]Persons of Mexican origin may be of any race.
[3]Age adjusted to the 2000 standard population using five age groups: 20 to 34 years, 35 to 44 years, 45 to 54 years, 55 to 64 years, and 65 years and over.
[4]Includes persons of all races and Hispanic origins, not just those shown separately.
[5]Percent of poverty level is based on family income and family size. Persons with unknown percent of poverty level are excluded (8 percent in 2007–2010).

Table 3-16. Cholesterol Among Persons 20 Years of Age and Over, by Selected Characteristics, Selected Years, 1988–1994 Through 2011–2014—*Continued*

(Percent, number.)

Sex, age, race and Hispanic origin,[1] and percent of poverty level	1988–1994	1999–2002	2003–2006	2007–2010	2009–2012	2011–2014
100 percent to 199 percent	205	204	201	198	194	191
200 percent to 399 percent	207	205	199	196	195	193
400 percent or more	205	202	201	195	196	194
20 Years and Over, Crude						
Both Sexes[4]	204	203	200	197	196	192
Male	202	202	198	194	193	188
Female	206	204	202	199	199	196
Not Hispanic or Latino						
White only, male	203	203	198	193	193	188
White only, female	208	206	205	201	202	199
Black or African American only, male	198	194	192	191	187	183
Black or African American only, female	201	199	194	191	191	189
Mexican origin, male	199	200	200	200	198	194
Mexican origin, female	198	194	196	195	193	189
Percent of Poverty Level[5]						
Below 100 percent	200	198	200	194	192	189
100 percent to 199 percent	202	202	199	197	193	190
200 percent to 399 percent	205	204	199	197	196	193
400 percent or more	206	204	203	198	199	196
Male						
20 to 44 years	194	196	196	194	191	188
20 to 34 years	186	188	186	186	182	179
35 to 44 years	206	207	209	205	204	202
45 to 64 years	216	213	206	202	200	196
45 to 54 years	216	215	208	204	203	200
55 to 64 years	216	212	202	199	198	192
65 to 74 years	212	202	191	182	184	180
75 years and over	205	195	187	176	173	168
Female						
20 to 44 years	189	191	192	187	187	184
20 to 34 years	184	185	188	181	180	179
35 to 44 years	195	198	197	195	196	193
45 to 64 years	225	215	213	211	212	209
45 to 54 years	217	211	208	208	209	207
55 to 64 years	235	221	219	214	216	210
65 to 74 years	233	224	214	207	206	200
75 years and over	229	217	206	203	201	199

[1]Persons of Mexican origin may be of any race.
[4]Includes persons of all races and Hispanic origins, not just those shown separately.
[5]Percent of poverty level is based on family income and family size. Persons with unknown percent of poverty level are excluded (8 percent in 2007–2010).

Table 3-17. Mean Macronutrient Intake Among Persons 20 Years of Age and Over, by Sex and Age, Selected Years, 1988–1994 Through 2011–2014

(Number, percent.)

Characteristic	1988–1994	1999–2002	2003–2006	2007–2010	2009–2012	2011–2014
Percent kcal from carbohydrates						
Both sexes, age-adjusted[1]	49.8	50.7	48.9	49.5	49.5	48.6
Both sexes, crude	49.8	50.7	48.9	49.4	49.4	48.5
20-44 years	49.2	51.3	49.3	50.1	49.9	48.8
45-64 years	49.7	49.3	47.5	48.2	48.5	47.9
65-74 years	51.1	50.5	49.2	49.0	49.0	48.2
75 years and over	53.0	52.6	51.5	51.1	51.0	50.5
Male, age-adjusted[1]	48.5	49.5	47.8	48.0	48.1	47.5
Male, crude	48.4	49.4	47.7	47.9	48.0	47.4
20-44 years	48.1	50.2	48.4	48.7	48.5	47.5
45-64 years	48.3	48.0	46.3	46.4	47.2	47.2
65-74 years	49.4	49.4	47.6	47.5	47.0	46.6
75 years and over	50.9	51.0	50.3	50.4	50.3	49.0
Female, age-adjusted[1]	51.0	51.9	49.9	50.8	50.8	49.7
Female, crude	51.0	51.9	49.9	50.7	50.7	49.6
20-44 years	50.3	52.5	50.2	51.4	51.3	50.0
45-64 years	51.0	50.6	48.7	49.8	49.8	48.6
65-74 years	52.5	51.4	50.6	50.4	50.9	49.6
75 years and over	54.2	53.7	52.4	51.6	51.6	51.6
Percent kcal from protein						
Both sexes, age-adjusted[1]	15.5	15.3	15.6	15.8	15.7	15.8
Both sexes, crude	15.4	15.3	15.6	15.8	15.7	15.8
20-44 years	15.0	14.9	15.3	15.6	15.6	15.7
45-64 years	15.9	15.6	16.0	16.0	15.8	15.8
65-74 years	16.2	16.3	15.9	16.2	16.4	16.3
75 years and over	16.0	15.4	15.6	15.8	15.8	15.7
Male, age-adjusted[1]	15.5	15.4	15.6	16.0	16.0	16.1
Male, crude	15.4	15.4	15.6	16.0	16.0	16.1
20-44 years	15.0	15.0	15.4	15.8	15.8	16.1
45-64 years	15.9	15.7	15.8	16.3	16.0	16.0
65-74 years	15.9	16.3	16.0	16.3	16.6	16.6
75 years and over	16.3	15.7	15.8	15.9	16.0	16.1
Female, age-adjusted[1]	15.5	15.2	15.6	15.6	15.5	15.5
Female, crude	15.4	15.2	15.6	15.6	15.5	15.6
20-44 years	14.9	14.8	15.2	15.4	15.3	15.3
45-64 years	15.9	15.5	16.1	15.8	15.5	15.7
65-74 years	16.5	16.3	15.9	16.1	16.2	16.1
75 years and over	15.9	15.3	15.5	15.7	15.6	15.3
Percent kcal from total fat						
Both sexes, age-adjusted[1]	33.5	33.0	33.7	33.1	32.9	33.6
Both sexes, crude	33.5	33.0	33.7	33.2	33.0	33.7
20-44 years	34.0	32.4	33.1	32.3	32.3	33.2
45-64 years	33.4	33.9	34.6	34.1	33.5	34.0
65-74 years	32.3	33.4	34.3	34.1	33.7	34.4
75 years and over	32.0	32.8	33.1	33.3	33.3	33.7
Male, age-adjusted[1]	33.8	33.0	33.5	33.1	33.0	33.6
Male, crude	33.9	33.0	33.6	33.2	33.0	33.6
20-44 years	34.1	32.2	32.6	32.2	32.2	33.0
45-64 years	33.9	34.0	34.8	34.3	33.8	34.1
65-74 years	33.0	33.4	34.5	34.4	34.1	34.5
75 years and over	33.0	33.2	33.3	33.2	33.1	34.1
Female, age-adjusted[1]	33.2	33.1	33.8	33.1	32.8	33.7
Female, crude	33.2	33.1	33.9	33.2	32.9	33.7
20-44 years	33.9	32.6	33.6	32.4	32.4	33.5
45-64 years	32.9	33.9	34.4	33.9	33.2	33.9
65-74 years	31.6	33.3	34.1	33.9	33.3	34.2
75 years and over	31.5	32.6	32.9	33.4	33.5	33.4
Percent kcal from saturated fat						
Both sexes, age-adjusted[1]	11.2	10.7	11.2	10.8	10.6	10.8
Both sexes, crude	11.2	10.7	11.2	10.9	10.6	10.8
20-44 years	11.5	10.8	11.1	10.6	10.5	10.7
45-64 years	11.1	10.8	11.4	11.1	10.8	10.8
65-74 years	10.7	10.5	11.2	11.1	10.7	10.8
75 years and over	10.7	10.3	11.0	10.9	10.8	11.1
Male, age-adjusted[1]	11.3	10.7	11.1	10.8	10.6	10.8
Male, crude	11.4	10.7	11.1	10.9	10.6	10.8
20-44 years	11.5	10.8	11.0	10.6	10.4	10.6
45-64 years	11.2	10.7	11.3	11.2	10.9	10.9
65-74 years	10.9	10.6	11.2	11.0	10.8	11.0
75 years and over	11.2	10.7	11.2	10.9	10.7	11.1
Female, age-adjusted[1]	11.1	10.7	11.2	10.9	10.6	10.8
Female, crude	11.1	10.7	11.3	10.9	10.6	10.8
20-44 years	11.4	10.8	11.2	10.7	10.5	10.8
45-64 years	10.9	10.9	11.5	11.0	10.6	10.7
65-74 years	10.4	10.4	11.3	11.2	10.7	10.6
75 years and over	10.5	10.1	10.8	11.0	10.9	11.0

[1]Age adjusted to the 2000 standard population using four age groups: 20 to 44 years, 45 to 64 years, 65 to 74 years, and 75 years and over. Age-adjusted estimates in this table may differ from other age-adjusted estimates based on the same data and presented elsewhere if different age groups are used in the adjustment procedure.

Table 3-18. Participation in Leisure-Time Aerobic and Muscle-Strengthening Activities That Meet the 2008 Federal Physical Activity Guidelines for Adults 18 Years of Age and Over, by Selected Characteristics, 2000 and 2015

(Percent.)

Characteristic	2008 Physical Activity Guidelines for Americans[1]							
	Met both aerobic activity and muscle-strengthening guidelines		Met neither aerobic activity nor muscle-strengthening guideline		Met aerobic activity guideline		Met muscle-strengthening guideline	
	2000	2015	2000	2015	2000	2015	2000	2015
18 years and over, age-adjusted[2,3]	15.0	21.6	54.7	46.8	42.2	49.8	18.0	25.0
18 years and over, crude[3]	15.1	20.9	54.6	47.5	42.4	49.0	18.1	24.4
Age								
18 to 44 years	18.9	26.4	49.1	40.7	47.7	56.4	22.1	29.3
18 to 24 years	23.8	29.8	44.5	37.8	52.2	59.0	27.2	32.9
25 to 44 years	17.3	25.2	50.6	41.7	46.3	55.5	20.5	27.9
45 to 64 years	12.8	18.1	57.6	50.5	39.7	45.9	15.5	21.8
45 to 54 years	14.5	19.3	55.4	49.0	42.1	47.9	17.0	22.5
55 to 64 years	10.1	16.9	61.0	52.2	36.1	43.8	13.1	21.0
65 years and over	6.8	12.7	67.0	58.8	30.1	36.6	9.8	17.3
65 to 74 years	8.4	15.5	60.3	52.4	36.8	43.3	11.3	19.8
75 years and over	4.9	8.7	75.0	67.8	22.1	27.2	8.0	13.8
Sex[2]								
Male	17.9	25.3	49.6	43.5	47.4	53.0	20.8	28.8
Female	12.3	18.0	59.4	49.9	37.6	46.9	15.4	21.2
Sex and Age								
Male								
18 to 44 years	23.0	32.1	43.0	36.8	53.6	60.0	26.3	35.2
45 to 54 years	16.0	21.6	52.7	47.5	45.2	49.3	18.0	25.0
55 to 64 years	11.3	18.9	58.7	50.3	38.9	46.5	13.8	22.1
65 to 74 years	9.4	15.7	55.3	48.4	41.8	47.2	12.2	20.1
75 years and over	7.1	9.4	66.7	63.2	30.7	31.1	10.1	15.0
Female								
18 to 44 years	15.0	20.9	55.0	44.5	42.0	52.9	17.9	23.5
45 to 54 years	13.1	17.1	57.9	50.4	39.1	46.6	16.1	20.1
55 to 64 years	9.0	15.0	63.1	53.9	33.5	41.2	12.4	19.9
65 to 74 years	7.7	15.3	64.3	55.9	32.6	39.9	10.5	19.5
75 years and over	3.6	8.2	80.0	71.1	16.8	24.4	6.7	12.9
Race[2,4]								
White only	15.7	22.0	53.1	45.7	44.1	51.0	18.5	25.3
Black or African American only	12.2	19.8	64.6	54.5	31.7	42.0	16.0	23.5
American Indian or Alaska Native only	*10.6	18.8	67.1	47.0	29.7	46.9	13.9	24.4
Asian only	14.1	19.1	55.0	45.1	41.7	51.4	17.2	22.6
Native Hawaiian or Other Pacific Islander only	*	*	*	*	*	*	*	*
Two or more races	19.0	22.7	52.8	47.8	43.9	49.0	22.2	26.3
Hispanic Origin and Race[2,4]								
Hispanic or Latino	9.2	16.8	66.5	53.5	30.8	43.3	11.9	20.0
Mexican	8.1	16.4	67.0	55.0	30.0	42.3	11.3	19.2
Not Hispanic or Latino	15.8	22.6	53.2	45.4	43.7	51.2	18.8	26.0
White only	16.5	23.5	51.4	43.6	45.7	53.1	19.3	26.7
Black or African American only	12.2	19.9	64.6	54.3	31.7	42.1	16.0	23.7
Education[5,6]								
No high school diploma or GED	4.3	8.1	74.0	67.0	23.9	30.1	6.6	11.0
High school diploma or GED	9.5	13.2	61.7	58.1	35.7	39.0	12.1	16.2
Some college or more	18.9	25.2	47.1	40.7	49.4	55.5	22.4	29.0
Percent of Poverty Level[2,7]								
Below 100 percent	9.3	13.1	68.0	60.1	29.3	37.1	12.3	16.0
100 percent to 199 percent	9.0	12.7	65.5	58.3	32.0	38.5	11.5	15.9
200 percent to 399 percent	13.2	20.1	56.8	49.2	39.9	47.4	16.5	23.6
400 percent or more	20.5	29.7	45.0	35.8	52.0	60.7	23.4	33.2
Hispanic Origin and Race and Percent of Poverty Level[2,4,7]								
Hispanic or Latino								
Below 100 percent	4.4	10.3	75.2	64.2	22.1	33.1	7.2	13.4
100 percent to 199 percent	5.0	11.8	72.2	58.9	25.8	38.9	7.1	14.2
200 percent to 399 percent	10.2	18.9	63.1	50.6	33.0	45.3	14.0	22.8
400 percent or more	19.6	28.4	52.8	38.7	45.1	57.4	21.7	32.2
Not Hispanic or Latino								
White only								
Below 100 percent	11.7	15.0	63.5	55.1	34.0	41.8	14.7	18.1

* = Figure does not meet standards of reliability or precision. Data preceded by an asterisk have a relative standard error (RSE) of 20 percent to 30 percent. Data not shown have an RSE of greater than 30 percent.
[1]Starting with Health, United States, 2010, measures of physical activity shown in this table changed to reflect the 2008 federal Physical Activity Guidelines for Americans (available from http://www.health.gov/PAGuidelines/).
[2]Estimates are age adjusted to the year 2000 standard population using five age groups: 18 to 44 years, 45 to 54 years, 55 to 64 years, 65 to 74 years, and 75 years and over.
[3]Includes all other races not shown separately, unknown education level, and unknown disability status.
[4]The race groups White, Black, American Indian or Alaska Native, Asian, Native Hawaiian or Other Pacific Islander, and two or more races, include persons of Hispanic and non-Hispanic origin. Persons of Hispanic origin may be of any race.
[5]Estimates are for persons 25 years of age and over and are age-adjusted to the year 2000 standard population using five age groups: 25–44 years, 45–54 years, 55–64 years, 65–74 years, and 75 years and over.
[6]GED is General Educational Development high school equivalency diploma.
[7]Percent of poverty level is based on family income and family size and composition using U.S. Census Bureau poverty thresholds.
[8]Any basic actions difficulty or complex activity limitation is defined as having one or more of the following limitations or difficulties: movement difficulty, emotional difficulty, sensory (seeing or hearing) difficulty, cognitive difficulty, self-care (activities of daily living or instrumental activities of daily living) limitation, social limitation, or work limitation.
[9]MSA = metropolitan statistical area.

Table 3-18. Participation in Leisure-Time Aerobic and Muscle-Strengthening Activities That Meet the 2008 Federal Physical Activity Guidelines for Adults 18 Years of Age and Over, by Selected Characteristics, 2000 and 2015—Continued

(Percent.)

Characteristic	2008 Physical Activity Guidelines for Americans[1]							
	Met both aerobic activity and muscle-strengthening guidelines		Met neither aerobic activity nor muscle-strengthening guideline		Met aerobic activity guideline		Met muscle-strengthening guideline	
	2000	2015	2000	2015	2000	2015	2000	2015
100 percent to 199 percent	10.3	12.5	62.6	58.4	34.8	38.0	12.9	15.9
200 percent to 399 percent	13.9	20.2	54.7	48.6	42.3	48.3	16.9	23.3
400 percent or more	21.0	30.6	43.7	34.1	53.4	62.5	23.8	33.9
Black or African American only								
Below 100 percent	9.5	13.0	72.1	64.8	25.4	32.9	12.1	15.3
100 percent to 199 percent	9.5	14.6	69.2	59.6	28.0	37.3	12.3	18.0
200 percent to 399 percent	11.8	20.7	64.3	50.8	31.4	45.2	16.2	25.3
400 percent or more	17.6	30.1	54.9	44.9	40.3	50.7	22.4	34.5
Disability Measure[2,8]								
Any basic actions difficulty or complex activity limitation	10.3	14.0	62.2	59.0	34.2	37.4	14.0	17.4
Any basic actions difficulty	10.3	13.7	62.1	59.6	34.0	36.9	14.2	17.1
Any complex activity limitation	7.2	9.6	71.2	68.5	24.9	27.6	11.3	13.4
No disability	17.0	25.3	50.6	39.9	46.6	56.9	19.8	28.5
Geographic Region[2]								
Northeast	17.0	22.1	51.8	46.8	45.3	49.8	20.0	25.5
Midwest	16.4	21.0	53.4	48.2	43.5	48.3	19.3	24.5
South	12.1	20.7	59.7	48.4	37.3	48.1	15.1	24.1
West	16.7	23.2	50.1	42.8	46.9	54.2	19.7	26.3
Location of residence[2,9]								
Within MSA	15.7	22.4	54.1	45.5	42.9	51.2	18.6	25.8
Outside MSA	12.3	16.1	56.9	55.1	39.9	41.1	15.5	19.7

* = Figure does not meet standards of reliability or precision. Data preceded by an asterisk have a relative standard error (RSE) of 20 percent to 30 percent. Data not shown have an RSE of greater than 30 percent.
[1]Starting with Health, United States, 2010, measures of physical activity shown in this table changed to reflect the 2008 federal Physical Activity Guidelines for Americans (available from http://www.health.gov/PAGuidelines/).
[2]Estimates are age adjusted to the year 2000 standard population using five age groups: 18 to 44 years, 45 to 54 years, 55 to 64 years, 65 to 74 years, and 75 years and over.
[8]Any basic actions difficulty or complex activity limitation is defined as having one or more of the following limitations or difficulties: movement difficulty, emotional difficulty, sensory (seeing or hearing) difficulty, cognitive difficulty, self-care (activities of daily living or instrumental activities of daily living) limitation, social limitation, or work limitation.
[9]MSA = metropolitan statistical area.

Table 3-19. Healthy Weight, Overweight, and Obesity Among Persons 20 Years of Age and Over, by Selected Characteristics, Selected Years, 1988–1994 Through 2011–2014

(Percent.)

Sex, age, race and Hispanic origin,[1] and percent of poverty level	Healthy weight (BMI from 18.5 to 24.9)[2]							
	1988–1994	1999–2002	2001–2004	2003–2006	2005–2008	2007–2010	2009–2012	2011–2014
20 Years and Over, Age-Adjusted[3]								
Both Sexes[4]	41.6	33.0	32.3	31.6	30.8	29.8	29.6	28.9
Male	37.9	30.2	28.3	26.6	26.1	25.7	26.2	26.0
Female	45.0	35.7	36.1	36.5	35.2	33.7	32.8	31.7
Not Hispanic or Latino								25.6
White only, male	37.3	29.6	28.0	26.8	26.0	25.5	26.2	34.3
White only, female	48.7	39.5	39.8	39.6	37.8	36.9	36.0	29.0
Black or African American only, male	40.1	34.7	30.8	27.0	26.7	28.5	28.0	16.0
Black or African American only, female	29.2	21.6	18.9	19.2	20.4	17.9	16.4	16.5
Mexican origin, male	30.2	26.5	25.3	23.8	21.8	18.5	17.5	19.1
Mexican origin, female	29.7	27.5	26.5	25.1	24.1	21.3	20.9	
Percent of Poverty Level[5]								28.1
Below 100 percent	37.5	32.7	34.3	32.1	29.1	27.3	27.3	24.6
100 percent to 199 percent	39.3	30.5	31.9	31.3	28.3	27.6	26.5	27.5
200 percent to 399 percent	41.8	29.6	29.4	29.7	30.0	29.7	30.0	33.4
400 percent or more	45.5	36.5	35.1	33.7	33.5	32.1	32.0	
20 Years and Over, Crude								
Both Sexes[4]	42.6	32.9	32.2	31.4	30.5	29.6	29.2	28.6
Male	39.4	30.4	28.4	26.6	26.1	25.8	26.2	26.2
Female	45.7	35.4	35.8	35.9	34.8	33.2	31.9	31.0
Not Hispanic or Latino								
White only, male	38.2	29.2	27.4	26.2	25.4	24.8	25.6	25.1
White only, female	48.8	38.7	38.8	38.2	36.9	35.7	34.2	32.8
Black or African American only, male	41.5	35.9	31.5	27.1	27.4	29.4	28.5	29.3
Black or African American only, female	31.2	21.8	19.3	19.2	20.3	17.6	16.1	15.8
Mexican origin, male	35.2	29.4	28.1	25.2	22.8	19.5	17.9	17.0
Mexican origin, female	32.4	29.5	28.0	25.8	24.7	22.3	22.2	19.9
Percent of Poverty Level[5]								
Below 100 percent	39.8	34.5	36.2	33.2	30.9	29.2	29.2	29.8
100 percent to 199 percent	41.5	31.5	32.6	31.7	28.8	28.0	26.8	25.2
200 percent to 399 percent	42.9	29.7	29.3	29.6	30.0	29.5	29.6	27.4
400 percent or more	44.6	35.3	33.5	32.1	31.8	30.5	30.3	31.3
Male								
20 to 34 years	51.1	40.3	38.3	35.9	38.0	37.5	37.5	37.6
35 to 44 years	33.4	29.0	26.5	24.1	20.9	19.8	21.0	20.5
45 to 54 years	33.6	24.0	21.2	20.8	21.7	21.8	20.0	18.7
55 to 64 years	28.6	23.8	22.2	22.2	19.3	19.4	21.9	22.7
65 to 74 years	30.1	22.8	23.1	21.2	20.2	21.6	22.4	22.2
75 years and over	40.9	32.0	32.1	33.1	28.1	25.4	28.2	28.1
Female								
20 to 34 years	57.9	42.5	44.2	45.1	40.5	41.1	40.8	38.1
35 to 44 years	47.1	37.1	38.3	37.6	36.2	34.4	35.2	32.5
45 to 54 years	37.2	33.1	31.0	31.1	32.1	30.7	27.3	27.8
55 to 64 years	31.5	27.6	29.2	29.5	29.9	26.7	23.8	24.2
65 to 74 years	37.0	26.4	27.0	28.5	28.8	23.9	23.5	26.9
75 years and over	43.0	36.9	34.6	35.4	36.3	35.4	35.3	32.9

NA = Not available.
* = Figure does not meet standards of reliability or precision. Data preceded by an asterisk have a relative standard error (RSE) of 20 percent to 30 percent. Data not shown have an RSE of greater than 30 percent.
[1]Persons of Mexican origin may be of any race.
[2]Body mass index (BMI) equals weight in kilograms divided by height in meters squared.
[3]Age adjusted to the year 2000 standard population using five age groups: 20 to 34 years, 35 to 44 years, 45 to 54 years, 55 to 64 years, and 65 years and over (65 to 74 years for estimates for 20 to 74 years).
[4]Includes all other races and origins not shown separately.
[5]Percent of poverty level is based on family income and family size. Persons with unknown percent of poverty level are excluded (6 percent in 2011–2014).

Table 3-19. Healthy Weight, Overweight, and Obesity Among Persons 20 Years of Age and Over, by Selected Characteristics, Selected Years, 1988–1994 Through 2011–2014—*Continued*

(Percent.)

Sex, age, race and Hispanic origin,[1] and percent of poverty level	Overweight (includes obesity; BMI greater than or equal to 25.0)[2]							
	1988–1994	1999–2002	2001–2004	2003–2006	2005–2008	2007–2010	2009–2012	2011–2014
20 Years and Over, Age-Adjusted[3]								
Both Sexes[4]	56.0	65.1	66.0	66.7	67.5	68.5	68.7	69.5
Male	60.9	68.8	70.5	72.1	72.9	73.3	72.9	73.0
Female	51.4	61.6	61.6	61.3	62.5	63.9	64.6	66.2
Not Hispanic or Latino								
White only, male	61.6	69.4	71.0	71.8	72.9	73.6	73.2	73.7
White only, female	47.5	57.2	57.6	57.9	59.6	60.3	60.9	63.5
Black or African American only, male	57.8	62.6	67.0	71.6	71.7	70.0	70.2	69.6
Black or African American only, female	68.2	77.2	79.6	79.8	78.0	80.0	81.8	82.0
Mexican origin, male	68.9	73.2	74.6	75.8	77.7	81.3	81.9	82.7
Mexican origin, female	68.9	71.2	73.0	73.9	74.8	78.0	78.3	80.3
Percent of Poverty Level[5]								
Below 100 percent	59.6	64.7	63.4	65.7	67.7	69.7	70.0	69.1
100 percent to 199 percent	58.0	67.3	66.2	66.5	69.6	70.5	71.7	73.9
200 percent to 399 percent	56.0	68.6	68.8	69.0	68.7	68.6	68.3	71.6
400 percent or more	52.4	62.2	63.7	64.7	65.3	66.9	66.8	65.6
20 Years and Over, Crude								
Both Sexes[4]	54.9	65.2	66.1	66.9	67.8	68.7	69.1	69.8
Male	59.4	68.6	70.4	72.1	72.8	73.2	72.9	72.8
Female	50.7	62.0	61.9	61.9	63.0	64.5	65.5	67.0
Not Hispanic or Latino								
White only, male	60.6	69.9	71.6	72.5	73.4	74.2	73.8	74.2
White only, female	47.4	58.2	58.7	59.4	60.7	61.7	62.9	65.2
Black or African American only, male	56.7	61.7	66.3	71.6	71.1	69.1	69.6	69.1
Black or African American only, female	66.0	76.9	79.1	79.7	78.1	80.2	82.1	82.3
Mexican origin, male	63.9	70.1	71.8	74.6	76.8	80.2	81.4	82.3
Mexican origin, female	65.9	69.3	71.4	73.0	73.9	77.1	76.9	79.5
Percent of Poverty Level[5]								
Below 100 percent	56.8	62.5	61.4	64.4	65.9	67.8	68.0	67.1
100 percent to 199 percent	55.7	66.2	65.3	66.0	69.1	70.1	71.4	73.1
200 percent to 399 percent	54.9	68.5	69.0	69.0	68.7	68.8	68.8	71.8
400 percent or more	53.3	63.7	65.5	66.5	67.2	68.5	68.6	67.7
Male								
20 to 34 years	47.5	57.4	59.0	61.6	60.5	61.1	60.9	60.4
35 to 44 years	65.5	70.5	72.9	75.2	78.8	80.2	78.9	79.3
45 to 54 years	66.1	75.7	78.5	78.5	76.8	76.8	79.3	80.8
55 to 64 years	70.5	75.4	77.3	79.7	80.5	79.8	77.4	76.7
65 to 74 years	68.5	76.2	76.1	78.0	79.1	77.5	76.9	76.1
75 years and over	56.5	67.4	66.8	65.8	70.8	73.2	70.4	71.0
Female								
20 to 34 years	37.0	52.9	51.6	50.9	55.6	55.4	55.2	58.5
35 to 44 years	49.6	60.6	60.1	60.7	62.1	63.9	62.4	65.6
45 to 54 years	60.3	65.1	67.4	67.3	65.8	66.2	70.5	71.4
55 to 64 years	66.3	72.2	69.9	69.6	69.4	72.2	75.1	74.3
65 to 74 years	60.3	70.9	71.5	70.5	69.6	74.2	73.8	71.2
75 years and over	52.3	59.9	63.7	62.6	61.3	63.2	62.4	64.6

NA = Not available.

* = Figure does not meet standards of reliability or precision. Data preceded by an asterisk have a relative standard error (RSE) of 20 percent to 30 percent. Data not shown have an RSE of greater than 30 percent.

[1]Persons of Mexican origin may be of any race.

[2]Body mass index (BMI) equals weight in kilograms divided by height in meters squared.

[3]Age adjusted to the year 2000 standard population using five age groups: 20 to 34 years, 35 to 44 years, 45 to 54 years, 55 to 64 years, and 65 years and over (65 to 74 years for estimates for 20 to 74 years).

[4]Includes all other races and origins not shown separately.

[5]Percent of poverty level is based on family income and family size. Persons with unknown percent of poverty level are excluded (6 percent in 2011–2014).

Table 3-19. Healthy Weight, Overweight, and Obesity Among Persons 20 Years of Age and Over, by Selected Characteristics, Selected Years, 1988–1994 Through 2011–2014—Continued

(Percent.)

Sex, age, race and Hispanic origin,[1] and percent of poverty level	Obesity (BMI greater than or equal to 30.0)[2]							
	1988–1994	1999–2002	2001–2004	2003–2006	2005–2008	2007–2010	2009–2012	2011–2014
20 Years and Over, Age-Adjusted[3]								
Both Sexes[4]	22.9	30.4	31.4	33.4	34.0	34.7	35.3	36.4
Male	20.2	27.5	29.5	32.4	32.7	33.9	34.6	34.5
Female	25.5	33.2	33.2	34.3	35.4	35.5	35.9	38.1
Not Hispanic or Latino								
White only, male	20.3	28.0	30.2	32.4	32.6	34.1	34.4	34.0
White only, female	22.9	30.7	30.7	31.6	33.1	32.5	32.3	35.3
Black or African American only, male	20.9	27.8	30.8	35.7	37.5	38.3	38.1	37.9
Black or African American only, female	38.3	48.6	51.1	53.4	51.0	54.0	57.5	56.5
Mexican origin, male	23.8	27.8	29.1	29.5	32.0	36.3	40.2	43.3
Mexican origin, female	35.2	38.0	39.4	41.8	43.3	44.6	46.3	49.6
Percent of Poverty Level[5]								
Below 100 percent	28.1	34.7	33.7	35.0	35.9	37.2	38.3	39.2
100 percent to 199 percent	26.1	34.1	33.6	35.9	38.0	37.3	40.1	42.6
200 percent to 399 percent	22.7	32.1	33.3	35.7	35.7	36.8	37.0	38.8
400 percent or more	18.7	25.5	27.3	28.9	29.4	31.3	30.2	29.7
20 Years and Over, Crude								
Both Sexes[4]	22.3	30.5	31.5	33.5	34.3	34.9	35.5	36.5
Male	19.5	27.5	29.5	32.4	32.8	33.9	34.6	34.5
Female	25.0	33.4	33.3	34.6	35.6	35.9	36.4	38.5
Not Hispanic or Latino								
White only, male	19.9	28.4	30.5	32.6	33.1	34.4	34.7	34.3
White only, female	22.7	31.3	31.2	32.2	33.3	33.2	33.5	36.2
Black or African American only, male	20.7	27.5	30.7	35.8	37.2	38.1	37.9	37.6
Black or African American only, female	36.7	48.7	51.1	53.2	51.0	54.2	57.6	56.9
Mexican origin, male	20.6	26.0	27.8	29.0	30.9	35.6	40.2	43.5
Mexican origin, female	33.3	37.0	38.5	41.2	42.9	44.2	45.2	48.6
Percent of Poverty Level[5]								
Below 100 percent	25.9	33.0	33.0	34.6	35.4	36.5	37.0	38.1
100 percent to 199 percent	24.3	32.8	32.6	35.0	37.0	36.8	40.0	41.9
200 percent to 399 percent	22.1	31.8	33.2	35.5	35.6	36.8	37.1	38.8
400 percent or more	19.3	27.2	28.6	30.7	31.7	32.4	31.7	31.1
Male								
20 to 34 years	14.1	21.7	23.2	26.2	25.4	27.1	28.9	28.5
35 to 44 years	21.5	28.5	33.8	37.0	35.9	37.2	38.1	39.8
45 to 54 years	23.2	30.6	31.8	34.6	35.9	36.6	38.1	36.6
55 to 64 years	27.2	35.5	36.0	39.3	40.4	37.3	38.1	38.1
65 to 74 years	24.1	31.9	32.1	33.0	36.2	41.5	36.4	36.2
75 years and over	13.2	18.0	19.9	24.0	25.6	26.6	27.4	26.8
Female								
20 to 34 years	18.5	28.3	28.6	28.4	31.4	30.4	30.0	33.4
35 to 44 years	25.5	32.1	33.3	36.1	36.7	37.1	36.0	39.1
45 to 54 years	32.4	36.9	38.0	40.0	39.1	36.9	38.3	41.7
55 to 64 years	33.7	42.1	39.0	41.0	42.3	43.4	42.9	44.4
65 to 74 years	26.9	39.3	37.9	36.4	35.6	40.3	44.2	40.7
75 years and over	19.2	23.6	23.2	24.2	25.9	28.7	29.8	30.5

NA = Not available.
* = Figure does not meet standards of reliability or precision. Data preceded by an asterisk have a relative standard error (RSE) of 20 percent to 30 percent. Data not shown have an RSE of greater than 30 percent.
[1]Persons of Mexican origin may be of any race.
[2]Body mass index (BMI) equals weight in kilograms divided by height in meters squared.
[3]Age adjusted to the year 2000 standard population using five age groups: 20 to 34 years, 35 to 44 years, 45 to 54 years, 55 to 64 years, and 65 years and over (65 to 74 years for estimates for 20 to 74 years).
[4]Includes all other races and origins not shown separately.
[5]Percent of poverty level is based on family income and family size. Persons with unknown percent of poverty level are excluded (6 percent in 2011–2014).

Table 3-20. Obesity Among Children and Adolescents 2 to 19 Years of Age, by Selected Characteristics, Selected Years, 1988–1994 Through 2011–2014

(Percent.)

Sex, age, race and Hispanic origin,[1] and percent of poverty level	1988–1994	1999–2002	2001–2004	2003–2006	2005–2008	2007–2010	2009–2012	2011–2014
2 to 5 Years								
Both sexes[2]	7.2	10.3	12.4	12.5	10.5	11.1	10.2	8.9
Not Hispanic or Latino								
White only	5.2	8.7	10.2	10.8	9.3	9.0	6.4	*5.2
Black or African American only	7.7	8.8	11.0	14.9	14.0	15.0	14.7	10.4
Mexican origin	12.3	13.1	17.7	16.7	14.1	14.6	15.7	15.3
Boys	6.1	10.0	13.1	12.8	9.8	11.9	12.0	9.2
Not Hispanic or Latino								
White only	*4.5	*8.2	*11.5	11.1	*7.4	8.8	*9.3	*
Black or African American only	7.7	*8.0	9.7	13.3	13.7	15.7	*14.3	*9.0
Mexican origin	12.4	14.1	19.8	18.8	17.1	19.1	17.6	*14.5
Girls	8.2	10.6	11.7	12.2	11.2	10.2	8.4	8.6
Not Hispanic or Latino								
White only	5.9	*9.0	*9.1	10.4	11.3	*9.2	*	*4.4
Black or African American only	7.6	9.6	12.2	16.6	14.3	*14.2	15.3	11.9
Mexican origin	12.3	*12.2	*15.7	14.5	10.8	*9.9	*13.8	*16.1
Percent of Poverty Level[3]								
Below 100 percent	9.7	10.9	14.4	14.3	12.3	13.2	12.3	11.6
100 percent to 199 percent	7.2	*13.8	13.3	12.7	10.0	11.8	11.6	10.2
200 percent to 399 percent	5.6	*7.6	13.6	11.9	11.6	13.9	11.0	*7.7
400 percent or more	*	*	*	*10.0	*	*5.8	*5.0	*
6 to 11 Years								
Both sexes[2]	11.3	15.9	17.5	17.0	17.4	18.8	17.9	17.5
Not Hispanic or Latino								
White only								13.6
Black or African American only								21.4
Mexican origin								25.3
Boys	11.6	16.9	18.7	18.0	18.7	20.7	18.3	17.6
Not Hispanic or Latino								
White only	10.7	14.0	16.9	15.5	16.5	18.6	12.9	13.0
Black or African American only	12.3	17.0	17.2	18.6	18.7	23.3	27.6	21.2
Mexican origin	17.5	26.5	25.6	27.5	28.4	24.3	25.0	25.3
Girls	11.0	14.7	16.3	15.8	16.0	16.9	17.4	17.5
Not Hispanic or Latino								
White only	*9.8	13.1	15.6	14.4	14.5	14.0	14.2	14.4
Black or African American only	17.0	22.8	24.8	24.0	21.3	24.5	24.8	21.6
Mexican origin	15.3	17.1	16.6	19.7	21.2	22.4	23.1	25.3
Percent of Poverty Level[3]								
Below 100 percent	11.4	19.1	20.0	22.0	21.5	22.2	24.6	21.5
100 percent to 199 percent	11.1	16.4	18.4	19.2	22.2	20.7	18.5	20.4
200 percent to 399 percent	11.7	15.3	18.2	16.7	16.8	18.9	15.8	15.7
400 percent or more	*	12.9	11.4	9.2	*9.5	*12.5	*12.2	*12.2
12 to 19 Years								
Both sexes[2]	10.5	16.0	17.0	17.6	17.9	18.2	19.4	20.5
Not Hispanic or Latino								
White only								19.6
Black or African American only								22.6
Mexican origin								23.5
Boys	11.3	16.7	17.9	18.2	18.7	19.4	20.0	20.1
Not Hispanic or Latino								
White only	11.6	14.6	17.9	17.3	16.1	17.1	17.9	18.7
Black or African American only	10.7	18.8	17.6	18.4	19.1	21.2	22.0	20.9
Mexican origin	14.1	24.7	20.0	22.1	26.2	27.9	27.0	22.8
Girls	9.7	15.3	16.0	16.8	17.0	16.9	18.9	21.0
Not Hispanic or Latino								
White only	8.9	12.6	14.6	14.5	14.0	14.6	17.8	20.4
Black or African American only	16.3	23.5	23.8	27.7	29.5	27.1	23.7	24.4
Mexican origin	*13.4	19.6	17.1	19.9	21.3	18.0	20.2	24.2
Percent of Poverty Level[3]								
Below 100 percent	15.8	19.8	18.2	19.3	23.1	24.3	23.2	22.4
100 percent to 199 percent	11.2	15.1	17.0	18.4	19.8	20.1	22.5	25.7
200 percent to 399 percent	9.4	15.7	19.0	19.3	17.2	16.3	17.9	19.7
400 percent or more	*	13.9	13.2	12.6	14.0	14.0	13.8	*13.7

* = Figure does not meet standards of reliability or precision. Data preceded by an asterisk have a relative standard error (RSE) of 20 percent to 30 percent.
Data not shown have an RSE of greater than 30 percent.
[1]Persons of Mexican origin may be of any race.
[2]Includes persons of all races and Hispanic origins, not just those shown separately.
[3]Percent of poverty level is based on family income and family size. Persons with unknown percent of poverty level are excluded (6 percent in 2011–2014).

Table 3-21. Untreated Dental Caries, by Selected Characteristics, Selected Years, 1988–1994 Through 2011–2014

(Percent.)

Sex, race and Hispanic origin,[1] and percent of poverty level	Age 5–19 years		Age 20–44 years		Age 45-64 years		Age 65 years and over	
	1988–1994	2011–2014	1988–1994	2011–2014	1988–1994	2011–2014	1988–1994	2011–2014
Total[2]	24.3	18.6	29.5	31.6	25.4	27.2	27.1	21.8
Sex								
Male	23.6	19.7	32.8	32.8	28.5	31.8	31.2	24.7
Female	25.0	17.4	26.4	30.3	22.6	22.9	24.1	19.4
Race and Hispanic Origin								
Not Hispanic or Latino								
White only	19.4	16.7	24.8	27.1	21.7	23.4	24.6	18.6
Black or African American only	33.9	23.4	49.2	46.1	46.2	45.4	51.2	40.7
Mexican origin	37.9	23.8	40.0	40.0	41.4	40.8	46.3	46.3
Percent of Poverty Level[3]								
Below 100 percent	39.0	24.7	47.8	47.0	49.5	54.2	46.8	44.0
100 percent to 199 percent	29.6	22.3	43.7	40.8	42.5	45.0	37.6	36.8
200 percent to 399 percent	16.6	16.0	24.5	28.1	25.0	29.2	24.1	18.3
400 percent or more	*10.4	9.1	12.5	14.8	13.0	12.6	15.6	*9.5
Race and Hispanic Origin, and Percent of Poverty Level[3]								
Not Hispanic or Latino								
White only								
Below 100% of poverty level	33.8	24.5	42.9	47.4	47.6	52.2	38.5	46.7
100% or more of poverty level	17.3	14.8	22.7	23.0	19.7	20.9	23.9	17.2
Black or African American only				56.0		71.7		52.9
Below 100% of poverty level	37.4	27.5	60.0	41.3	62.9	37.9	56.3	38.6
100% or more of poverty level	31.2	19.3	44.8		41.2		47.8	
				44.4		49.9		58.7
				35.8		38.5		42.3
Mexican origin								
Below 100% of poverty level	47.5	23.1	52.7	38.0	52.7	*45.7	62.8	*56.7
100% or more of poverty level	28.0	23.7	31.2	35.1	34.5	43.4	35.4	*45.0

Note: Root caries are not included. Persons without at least one primary or one permanent tooth or one root tip were classified as edentulous and were excluded from this analysis. The majority of edentulous persons are 65 years of age and over. Estimates of edentulism among persons 65 years of age and over are 46 percent in 1971–1974, 33 percent in 1988–1994, and 23 percent in 2005–2008. For estimates prior to 2005–2008, only dental caries in primary teeth was evaluated for children 2–5 years of age. Caries in both permanent and primary teeth was evaluated for children 6–11 years of age. For children 12–19 years of age and adults, only dental caries in permanent teeth was evaluated. Starting with 2005–2006 data, dental caries data were collected using a simplified examination process that used health technologists to screen for caries instead of using dentists to conduct a comprehensive caries exam. In addition, dental caries data were not collected on children younger than 5 years of age. Because of this change in the examination process and because 2005–2008 dental caries data are based on both primary and permanent teeth, regardless of age, data for 2005–2008 need to be interpreted with caution, especially when comparing with earlier data.
* = Figure does not meet standards of reliability or precision. Data preceded by an asterisk have a relative standard error (RSE) of 20 percent to 30 percent. Data not shown have an RSE of greater than 30 percent.
[1]Persons of Mexican origin may be of any race.
[2]Includes persons of all races and Hispanic origins, not just those shown separately, and those with unknown percent of poverty level.
[3]Percent of poverty level is based on family income and family size. Persons with unknown percent of poverty level are excluded (6 percent in 2011–2014).

Table 3-22. Selected Health Conditions and Risk Factors, Selected Years, 1988–1994 Through 2013–2014

(Percent.)

Health condition	1988–1994	1999–2000	2001–2002	2003–2004	2005–2006	2007–2008	2009–2010	2011–2012	2013–2014
Diabetes[1]									
Total, age-adjusted[2]	9.1	9.0	10.5	10.8	10.4	NA	NA	11.9	11.9
Total, crude	8.4	8.5	10.1	10.8	10.7	NA	NA	12.5	12.7
Hypercholesterolemia[3]									
Total, age-adjusted[4]	22.8	25.0	24.4	27.5	27.0	27.2	26.7	28.2	27.4
Total, crude	21.5	24.0	23.9	27.5	27.6	28.3	27.9	30.4	29.3
High Cholesterol[5]									
Total, age-adjusted[4]	20.8	18.3	16.5	16.9	15.6	14.2	13.2	12.7	11.1
Total, crude	19.6	17.7	16.4	17.0	15.9	14.6	13.6	13.1	11.1
Hypertension[6]									
Total, age-adjusted[4]	25.5	30.0	29.7	32.1	30.5	31.2	30.0	30.0	30.8
Total, crude	24.1	28.9	28.9	32.5	31.7	32.6	31.9	32.5	33.5
Uncontrolled High Blood Pressure Among Persons with Hypertension[7]									
Total, age-adjusted[4]	77.2	71.9	68.3	63.8	63.0	56.2	55.7	54.6	51.3
Total, crude	73.9	69.1	65.4	60.8	56.6	51.8	46.7	48.0	46.1
Overweight (Includes Obesity)[8]									
Total, age-adjusted[4]	56.0	64.5	65.6	66.4	66.9	68.1	68.8	68.6	70.4
Total, crude	54.9	64.1	65.6	66.5	67.3	68.3	69.2	69.0	70.7
Obesity[9]									
Total, age-adjusted[4]	22.9	30.5	30.5	32.3	34.4	33.7	35.7	34.9	37.8
Total, crude	22.3	30.3	30.6	32.3	34.7	33.9	35.9	35.1	37.9
Untreated Dental Caries[10]									
Total, age-adjusted[4]	27.7	24.3	21.3	30.0	24.4	21.7	NA	25.5	31.5
Total, crude	28.2	25.0	21.6	30.3	24.5	21.8	NA	25.5	31.3
Percent of Persons Under 20 Years of Age									
Obesity[11]									
2 to 5 years	7.2	10.3	10.6	14.0	11.0	10.1	12.1	8.4	9.4
6 to 11 years	11.3	15.1	16.3	18.8	15.1	19.6	18.0	17.7	17.4
12 to 19 years	10.5	14.8	16.7	17.4	17.8	18.1	18.4	20.5	20.6
Untreated Dental Caries[10]									
5 to 19 years	23.6	22.7	20.6	25.2	NA	16.2	NA	17.5	19.6

NA = Not available.

[1]Includes physician-diagnosed and undiagnosed diabetes. Estimates were obtained using fasting weights, and obtained by self-report and excludes women who reported having diabetes only during pregnancy. Undiagnosed diabetes is defined as a fasting plasma glucose (FPG) of at least 126 mg/dL or a hemoglobin A1c of at least 6.5% and no reported physician diagnosis.
[2]Age adjusted to the 2000 standard population using three age groups: 20 to 44 years, 45 to 64 years, and 65 years and over.
[3]Hypercholesterolemia is defined as measured serum total cholesterol greater than or equal to 240 mg/dL or reporting taking cholesterol-lowering medication. Respondents were asked, "Are you now following this advice [from a doctor or health professional] to take prescribed medicine [to lower your cholesterol]?"
[4]Age adjusted to the 2000 standard population using five age groups: 20 to 34 years, 35 to 44 years, 45 to 54 years, 55 to 64 years, and 65 years and over.
[5]Highcholesterol is defined as greater than or equal to 240 mg/dL (6.20 mmol/L).
[6]Hypertension is defined as having measured high blood pressure and/or taking antihypertensive medication. High blood pressure is defined as having measured systolic pressure of at least 140 mmHg or diastolic pressure of at least 90 mmHg. Those with high blood pressure also may be taking prescribed medicine for high blood pressure. For antihypertensive medication use, respondents were asked, "Are you now taking prescribed medicine for your high blood pressure?"
[7]Uncontrolled high blood pressure among persons with hypertension is defined as measured systolic pressure of at least 140 mmHg or diastolic pressure of at least 90 mmHg, among those with measured high blood pressure or reporting taking antihypertensive medication.
[8]Excludes pregnant women. Overweight is defined as body mass index (BMI) greater than or equal to 25.0.
[9]Excludes pregnant women. Obesity is defined as body mass index (BMI) greater than or equal to 30.0.
[10]Untreated dental caries refers to decay on the crown or enamel surface of a tooth (i.e., coronal caries) that has not been treated or filled. The presence of caries was evaluated in primary and permanent teeth for persons aged 5 and older. The third molars were not included. Persons without at least one natural tooth (primary or permanent) were excluded.
[11]Obesity is defined as body mass index (BMI) at or above the sex- and age-specific 95th percentile BMI cutoff points from the 2000 CDC growth charts for the United States.

Table 3-23. Health Risk Behaviors Among Students in Grades 9 to 12, by Sex, Grade Level, Race, and Hispanic Origin, Selected Years, 1991–2015

(Percent.)

Sex, grade level, race, and Hispanic origin	Seriously considered suicide[1]			In a physical fight[1]			Carried a weapon[2,3]		
	1991	1999	2015	1991	1999	2015	1991	1999	2015
Total	29.0	19.3	17.7	42.5	35.7	22.6	26.1	17.3	16.2
Male									
Total	20.8	13.7	12.2	50.2	44.0	28.4	40.6	28.6	24.3
9th grade	17.6	11.9	10.7	57.8	49.5	32.5	44.4	28.7	24.6
10th grade	19.5	13.7	10.8	50.2	46.0	29.4	41.5	30.7	25.5
11th grade	25.3	13.7	13.3	51.0	38.9	27.1	44.0	26.9	23.0
12th grade	20.7	15.6	14.0	42.3	39.0	22.9	33.1	27.3	23.4
Not Hispanic or Latino									
White	21.7	12.5	11.5	49.1	43.2	26.6	41.2	28.6	28.0
Black or African American	13.3	11.7	11.0	58.4	44.4	38.6	43.4	23.1	17.6
Hispanic or Latino	18.0	13.6	12.4	48.5	50.5	27.3	40.0	29.5	20.2
Female									
Total	37.2	24.9	23.4	34.4	27.3	16.5	10.9	6.0	7.5
9th grade	40.3	24.4	26.5	42.9	32.5	22.6	10.4	6.5	6.6
10th grade	39.7	30.1	25.7	35.4	29.4	17.6	11.1	7.1	7.2
11th grade	38.4	23.0	22.1	34.5	23.4	12.8	12.9	5.2	8.0
12th grade	30.7	21.2	18.6	25.4	21.9	12.0	9.5	4.8	8.0
Not Hispanic or Latina									
White	38.6	23.2	22.8	32.2	22.3	13.5	7.5	3.6	8.1
Black or African American	29.4	18.8	18.7	43.8	38.6	25.4	23.6	11.7	6.2
Hispanic or Latina	34.6	26.1	25.6	34.8	29.7	18.6	12.9	8.4	7.1

Sex, grade level, race, and Hispanic origin	Ever had sexual intercourse			Did not use a condom at last sex[4]			Physically forced to have sex		
	1991	1999	2015	1991	1999	2015	1991	1999	2015
Total	54.1	49.9	41.2	53.8	42.0	43.1	NA	8.8	6.7
Male									
Total	57.4	52.2	43.2	45.5	34.5	38.5	NA	5.2	3.1
9th grade	45.6	44.5	27.3	44.1	30.5	36.7	NA	5.6	2.1
10th grade	50.9	51.1	37.9	43.1	30.0	34.4	NA	4.6	3.9
11th grade	64.5	51.4	51.2	43.2	30.7	37.5	NA	5.0	2.8
12th grade	68.3	63.9	59.0	49.3	44.1	42.6	NA	5.6	3.5
Not Hispanic or Latino									
White	52.7	45.4	39.5	44.8	37.0	41.9	NA	3.5	2.0
Black or African American	88.1	75.7	58.8	43.0	24.7	26.4	NA	9.7	4.4
Hispanic or Latino	64.1	62.9	45.1	53.0	33.9	37.5	NA	5.9	4.0
Female									
Total	50.8	47.7	39.2	62.0	49.3	48.0	NA	12.5	10.3
9th grade	32.2	32.5	20.7	49.7	36.9	43.3	NA	10.4	9.4
10th grade	45.3	42.6	33.5	63.6	44.7	46.0	NA	12.4	7.9
11th grade	60.2	53.8	48.2	59.3	50.0	47.1	NA	14.5	12.0
12th grade	65.1	65.8	57.2	67.4	58.9	51.2	NA	12.8	11.9
Not Hispanic or Latina									
White	47.1	44.8	40.3	62.0	52.4	44.1	NA	10.1	9.9
Black or African American	75.9	66.9	37.4	60.6	35.5	53.3	NA	13.5	10.3
Hispanic or Latina	43.3	45.5	39.8	73.1	57.0	51.7	NA	15.1	10.1

Note: Only youths attending school participated in the survey. Persons of Hispanic origin may be of any race.
NA = Data not available.
[1] During the last 12 months.
[2] During the last 30 days.
[3] Such as a gun, knife, or club.
[4] Among students who were currently sexually active.

Table 3-23. Health Risk Behaviors Among Students in Grades 9 to 12, by Sex, Grade Level, Race, and Hispanic Origin, Selected Years, 1991–2015—Continued

(Percent.)

Sex, grade level, race, and Hispanic origin	Did not eat breakfast on all 7 days[8]			Got fewer than 8 hours of sleep[9]		
	1991	1999	2015	1991	1999	2015
Total	NA	NA	63.7	NA	NA	72.7
Male						
Total	NA	NA	59.5	NA	NA	69.9
9th grade	NA	NA	53.4	NA	NA	60.7
10th grade	NA	NA	57.7	NA	NA	66.2
11th grade	NA	NA	62.9	NA	NA	77.1
12th grade	NA	NA	65.3	NA	NA	77.4
Not Hispanic or Latino						
White	NA	NA	56.7	NA	NA	68.9
Black or African American	NA	NA	69.2	NA	NA	74.4
Hispanic or Latino	NA	NA	60.5	NA	NA	67.1
Female						
Total	NA	NA	67.9	NA	NA	75.6
9th grade	NA	NA	68.1	NA	NA	70.9
10th grade	NA	NA	68.9	NA	NA	76.9
11th grade	NA	NA	67.6	NA	NA	77.0
12th grade	NA	NA	67.1	NA	NA	77.8
Not Hispanic or Latina						
White	NA	NA	65.2	NA	NA	75.1
Black or African American	NA	NA	75.3	NA	NA	79.4
Hispanic or Latina	NA	NA	69.9	NA	NA	73.2

Note: Only youths attending school participated in the survey. Persons of Hispanic origin may be of any race.
NA = Data not available.
[8]During the past 7 days. Data prior to 2011 are not available.
[9]On an average school night. Data prior to 2007 are not available.

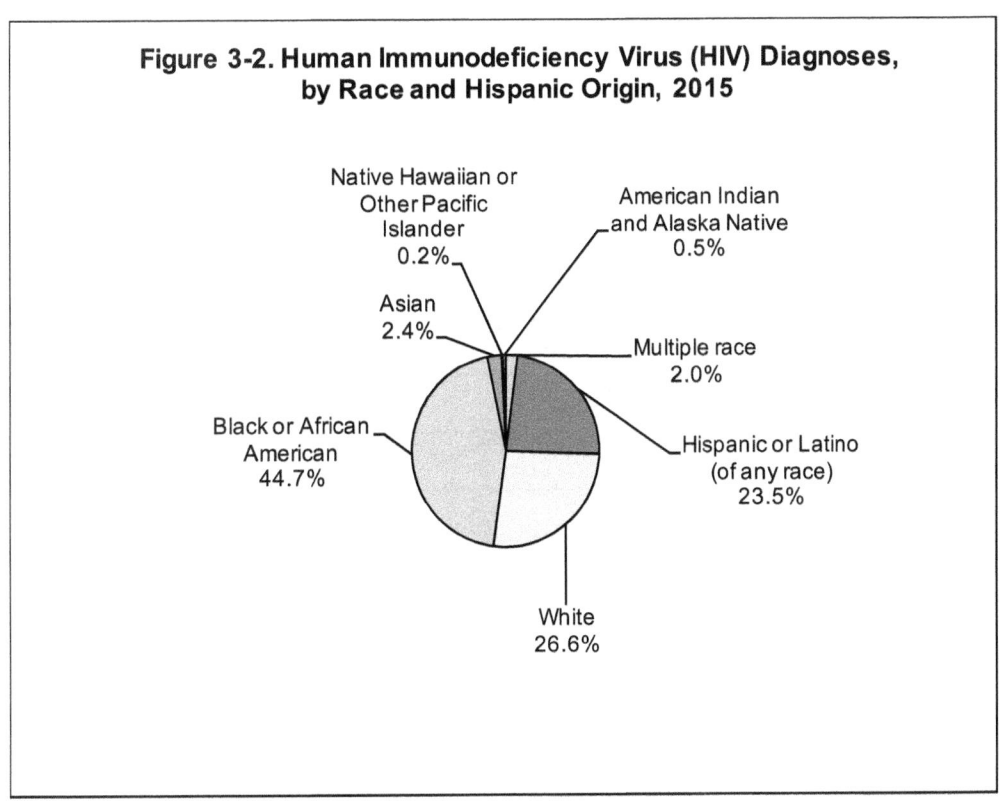

Figure 3-2. Human Immunodeficiency Virus (HIV) Diagnoses, by Race and Hispanic Origin, 2015

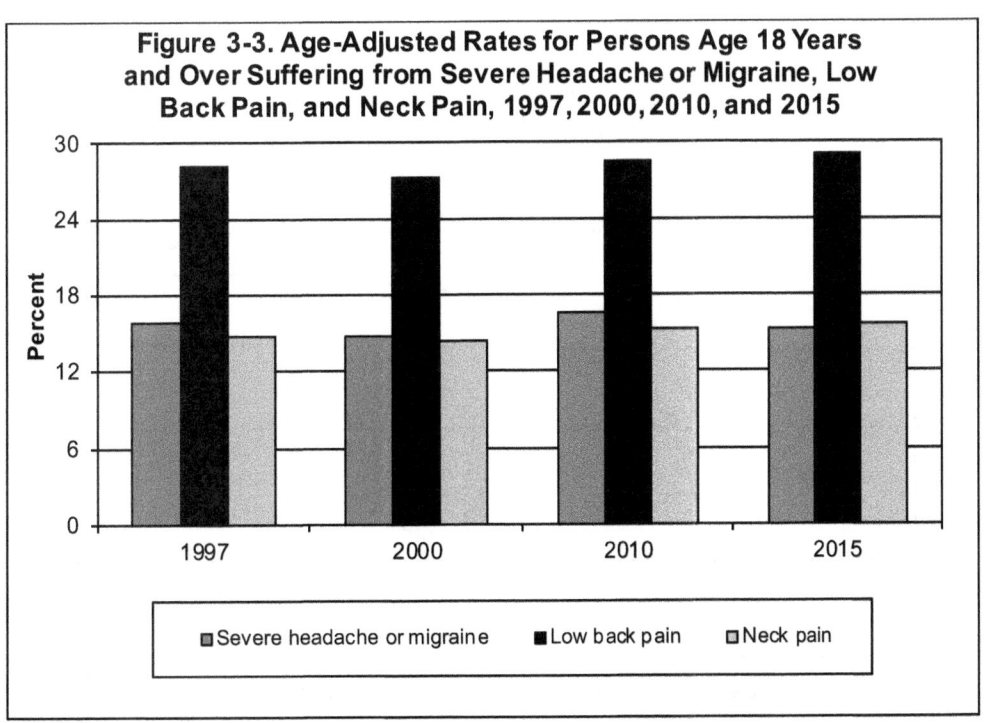

Figure 3-3. Age-Adjusted Rates for Persons Age 18 Years and Over Suffering from Severe Headache or Migraine, Low Back Pain, and Neck Pain, 1997, 2000, 2010, and 2015

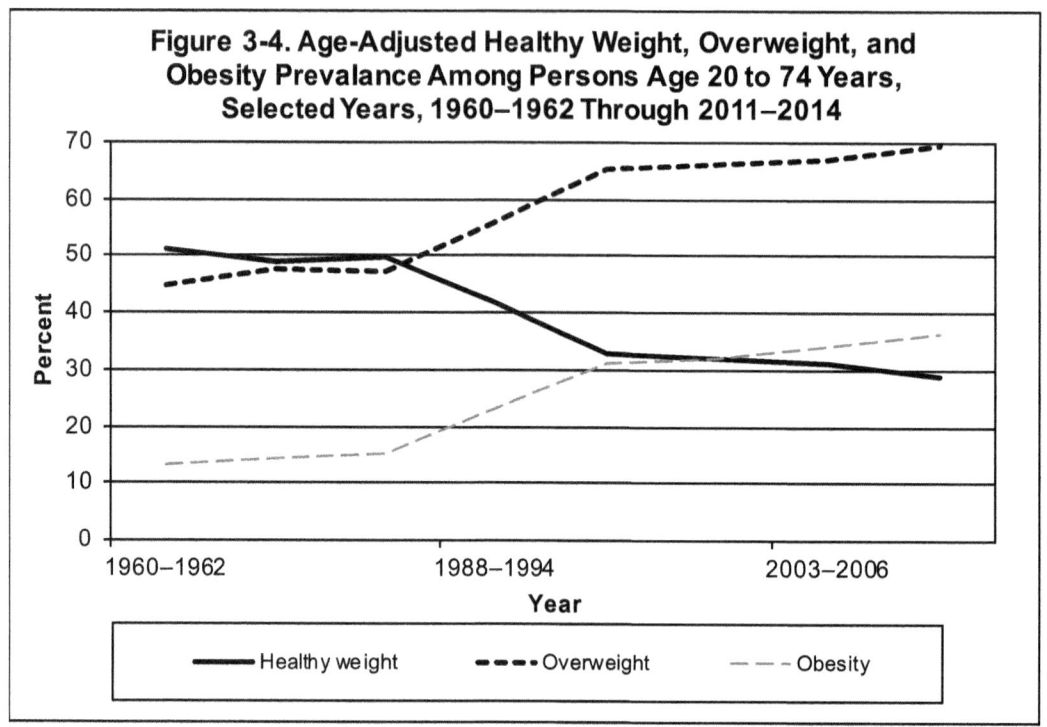

Figure 3-4. Age-Adjusted Healthy Weight, Overweight, and Obesity Prevalance Among Persons Age 20 to 74 Years, Selected Years, 1960–1962 Through 2011–2014

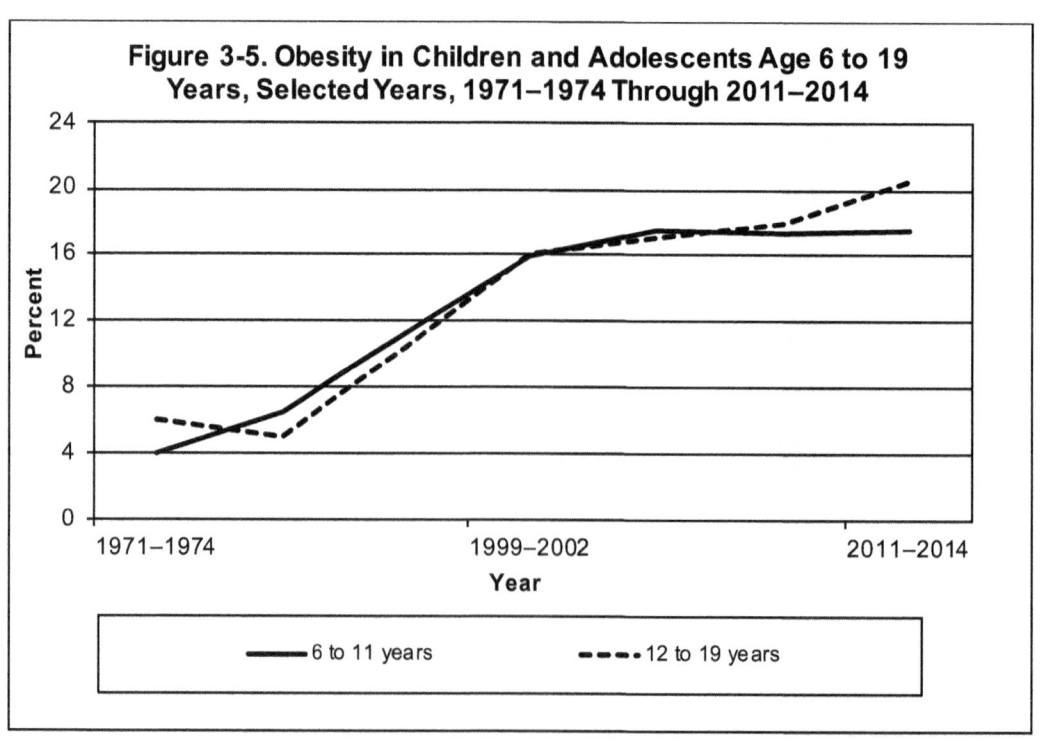

Figure 3-5. Obesity in Children and Adolescents Age 6 to 19 Years, Selected Years, 1971–1974 Through 2011–2014

USE OF ADDICTIVE SUBSTANCES

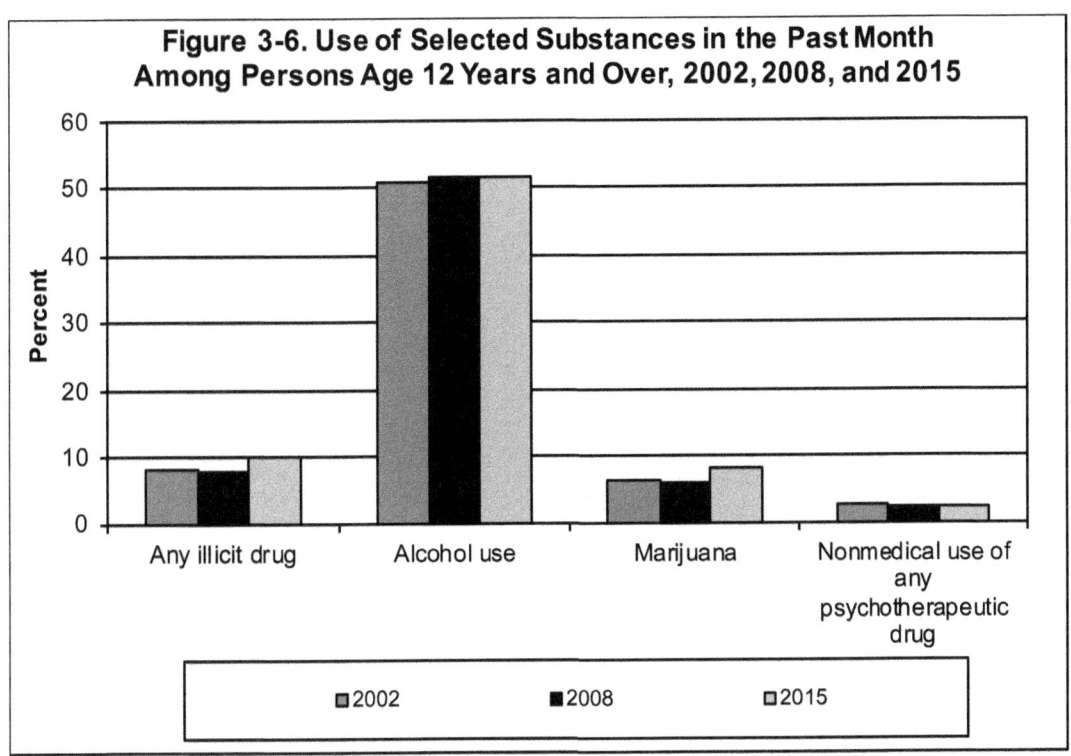

Figure 3-6. Use of Selected Substances in the Past Month Among Persons Age 12 Years and Over, 2002, 2008, and 2015

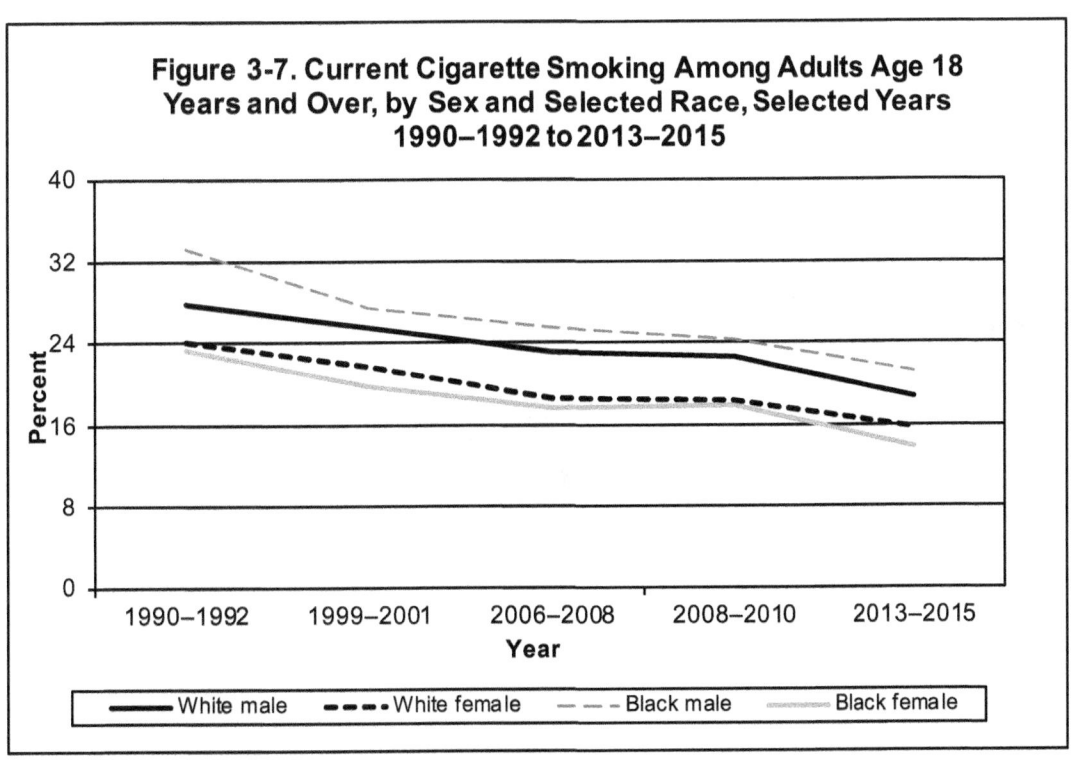

Figure 3-7. Current Cigarette Smoking Among Adults Age 18 Years and Over, by Sex and Selected Race, Selected Years 1990–1992 to 2013–2015

Table 3-24. Use of Selected Substances in the Past Month Among Persons 12 Years of Age and Over, by Age, Sex, Race, and Hispanic Origin, Selected Years, 2002–2015

(Percent.)

Age, sex, race, and Hispanic origin	Any illicit drug[1]			Marijuana			Nonmedical use of any psychotherapeutic drug[2]		
	2002	2008	2015	2002	2008	2015	2002	2008	2015
Total, 12 Years and Over	8.3	8.0	10.1	6.2	6.1	8.3	2.7	2.5	2.4
Age									
12 to 13 years	4.2	3.3	2.6	1.4	1.0	0.8	1.7	1.5	0.9
14 to 15 years	11.2	8.6	7.2	7.6	5.7	5.7	4.0	3.0	1.7
16 to 17 years	19.8	15.2	16.3	15.7	12.7	14.2	6.3	4.0	3.3
18 to 25 years	20.2	19.6	22.3	17.3	16.5	19.8	5.5	5.9	5.1
26 to 34 years	10.5	11.2	15.4	7.7	8.8	12.9	3.7	3.2	3.7
35 years and over	4.6	4.7	6.6	3.1	3.2	5.1	1.6	1.6	1.6
Sex									
Male	10.3	9.9	12.5	8.1	7.9	10.6	2.8	2.6	2.6
Female	6.4	6.3	7.9	4.4	4.4	6.2	2.6	2.4	2.2
Age and Sex									
12 to 17 years	11.6	9.3	8.8	8.2	6.7	7.0	4.0	2.9	2.0
Male	12.3	9.5	8.8	9.1	7.3	7.5	3.6	2.5	1.7
Female	10.9	9.1	8.8	7.2	6.0	6.5	4.4	3.3	2.3
Hispanic Origin and Race[3]									
Not Hispanic or Latino									
White only	8.5	8.2	10.2	6.5	6.2	8.4	2.8	2.8	2.6
Black or African American only	9.7	10.1	12.5	7.4	8.3	10.7	2.0	1.8	1.8
American Indian or Alaska Native only	10.1	9.5	14.2	6.7	8.2	11.2	3.2	3.0	2.6
Native Hawaiian or Other Pacific Islander only	7.9	7.3	9.8	4.4	5.5	9.2	3.8	1.7	1.7
Asian only	3.5	3.6	4.0	1.8	2.0	3.0	0.7	1.0	0.7
Two or more races	11.4	14.7	17.2	9.0	13.1	13.4	3.5	2.7	4.8
Hispanic or Latino	7.2	6.2	9.2	4.3	4.2	7.2	2.9	1.8	2.3

Age, sex, race, and Hispanic origin	Alcohol use			Binge alcohol use[4]			Heavy alcohol use[5]		
	2002	2008	2015	2002	2008	2015	2002	2008	2015
Total, 12 Years and Over	51.0	51.6	51.7	22.9	23.3	24.9	6.7	6.9	6.5
Age									
12 to 13 years	4.3	3.4	1.3	1.8	1.5	0.7	0.3	0.2	0.0
14 to 15 years	16.6	13.1	7.4	9.2	6.9	3.8	1.9	1.1	0.3
16 to 17 years	32.6	26.2	19.7	21.4	17.2	12.6	5.6	4.4	2.3
18 to 25 years	60.5	61.2	58.3	40.9	41.0	39.0	14.9	14.5	10.9
26 to 34 years	61.4	63.5	65.0	33.1	36.4	38.3	9.0	10.6	9.7
35 years and over	52.1	52.8	53.5	18.6	18.8	21.8	5.2	5.3	5.6
Sex									
Male	57.4	57.7	56.2	31.2	31.6	29.6	10.8	10.6	8.9
Female	44.9	45.9	47.4	15.1	15.4	20.5	3.0	3.4	4.2
Age and Sex									
12 to 17 years	17.6	14.6	9.6	10.7	8.8	5.8	2.5	2.0	0.9
Male	17.4	14.2	9.3	11.4	8.9	5.8	3.1	2.3	1.1
Female	17.9	15.0	9.9	9.9	8.7	5.8	1.9	1.6	0.7
Hispanic Origin and Race[3]									
Not Hispanic or Latino									
White only	55.0	56.2	57.0	23.4	24.0	26.0	7.5	7.7	7.6
Black or African American only	39.9	41.9	43.8	21.0	20.4	23.4	4.4	5.6	4.8
American Indian or Alaska Native only	44.7	43.3	37.9	27.9	24.4	24.1	8.7	5.7	4.7
Native Hawaiian or Other Pacific Islander only	*	*	33.8	25.2	*	17.8	8.3	3.5	3.0
Asian only	37.1	37.0	39.7	12.4	11.9	14.0	2.6	2.4	2.2
Two or more races	49.9	47.5	42.8	19.8	22.0	22.9	7.5	7.4	6.8
Hispanic or Latino	42.8	43.2	42.4	24.8	25.6	25.7	5.9	5.7	4.8

* = Figure does not meet standards of reliability or precision. Data not shown if the relative standard error is greater than 17.5 percent of the log transformation of the proportion, the minimum effective sample size is less than 68, the minimum nominal sample size is less than 100, or the prevalence is close to 0 percent or 100 percent.
[1]Any illicit drug includes marijuana/hashish, cocaine (including crack), heroin, hallucinogens (including LSD and PCP), inhalants, or any prescription-type psychotherapeutic drug used nonmedically.
[2]Nonmedical use of prescription-type psychotherapeutic drugs includes the nonmedical use of pain relievers, tranquilizers, stimulants, or sedatives and does not include over-the-counter drugs.
[3]Persons of Hispanic origin may be of any race.
[4]Binge alcohol use is defined as drinking five or more drinks on the same occasion on at least 1 day in the past 30 days. Occasion is defined as at the same time or within a couple of hours of each other.
[5]Heavy alcohol use is defined as drinking five or more drinks on the same occasion on each of 5 or more days in the past 30 days. By definition, all heavy alcohol users are also binge alcohol users.

Table 3-24. Use of Selected Substances in the Past Month Among Persons 12 Years of Age and Over, by Age, Sex, Race, and Hispanic Origin, Selected Years, 2002–2015—*Continued*

(Percent.)

Age, sex, race, and Hispanic origin	Any tobacco[6]			Cigarettes			Cigars		
	2002	2008	2015	2002	2008	2015	2002	2008	2015
Total, 12 Years and Over...........................	30.4	28.4	23.9	26.0	23.9	19.4	5.4	5.3	4.7
Age									
12 to 13 years......................................	3.8	2.5	0.6	3.2	2.1	0.5	0.7	0.6	0.2
14 to 15 years......................................	13.4	9.7	4.6	11.2	7.6	3.1	3.8	3.1	1.2
16 to 17 years......................................	29.0	21.1	12.4	24.9	16.8	8.7	9.3	7.3	4.8
18 to 25 years......................................	45.3	41.4	33.0	40.8	35.7	26.7	11.0	11.3	8.9
26 to 34 years......................................	38.2	38.3	35.1	32.7	33.6	29.3	6.6	7.2	7.8
35 years and over.................................	27.9	26.1	22.1	23.4	21.6	17.9	4.1	3.8	3.5
Sex									
Male..	37.0	34.5	29.6	28.7	26.3	21.8	9.4	9.0	7.6
Female..	24.3	22.5	18.5	23.4	21.7	17.1	1.7	1.7	2.0
Age and Sex									
12 to 17 years......................................	15.2	11.4	6.0	13.0	9.1	4.2	4.5	3.8	2.1
Male..	16.0	12.6	7.0	12.3	9.0	4.6	6.2	5.3	2.6
Female..	14.4	10.2	4.9	13.6	9.2	3.8	2.7	2.2	1.5
Hispanic Origin and Race[3]									
Not Hispanic or Latino..........................									
White only.....................................	32.0	30.4	25.9	26.9	25.2	20.7	5.5	5.3	4.5
Black or African American only............	28.8	28.6	26.0	25.3	24.8	21.3	6.8	7.0	8.0
American Indian or Alaska Native only....	44.3	48.7	37.0	37.1	44.1	29.5	5.2	5.6	6.4
Native Hawaiian or Other Pacific Islander only..	28.8	*	19.2	*	*	16.3	4.1	2.2	4.2
Asian only......................................	18.6	13.9	11.4	17.7	11.9	10.0	1.1	1.2	2.2
Two or more races..........................	38.1	37.3	31.9	35.0	32.2	26.8	5.5	7.2	5.9
Hispanic or Latino.................................	25.2	21.3	17.7	23.0	19.4	15.3	5.0	4.5	3.7

* = Figure does not meet standards of reliability or precision. Data not shown if the relative standard error is greater than 17.5 percent of the log transformation of the proportion, the minimum effective sample size is less than 68, the minimum nominal sample size is less than 100, or the prevalence is close to 0 percent or 100 percent.
[3]Persons of Hispanic origin may be of any race.
[6]Any tobacco product includes cigarettes, smokeless tobacco (i.e., chewing tobacco or snuff), cigars, or pipe tobacco.

Table 3-25. Heavier Drinking and Drinking Five or More Drinks in a Day Among Adults 18 Years of Age and Over, by Selected Characteristics, Selected Years, 1997–2013

(Percent.)

Characteristic	Heavier drinker[1]				Five or more drinks in a day on at least 1 day in the past year[1]				Five or more drinks in a day on at least 12 days in the past year[1]			
	1997	2000	2010	2013	1997	2000	2010	2013	1997	2000	2010	2013
BOTH SEXES												
18 years and over, age-adjusted[2]	4.9	4.3	5.2	5.3	21.1	19.2	23.8	23.6	9.7	8.7	10.1	9.5
18 years and over, crude	5.0	4.3	5.2	5.3	21.5	19.3	23.2	22.6	9.8	8.7	9.9	9.2
Age												
All persons												
18 to 44 years	5.2	4.7	5.7	5.2	29.2	26.9	32.5	31.9	13.2	12.2	13.7	12.5
18 to 24 years	5.3	5.8	6.2	5.2	31.8	30.3	34.0	31.3	15.2	15.5	16.2	12.8
25 to 44 years	5.2	4.3	5.5	5.1	28.5	25.8	31.9	32.2	12.6	11.1	12.7	12.4
45 to 64 years	5.5	4.6	5.4	6.0	15.9	14.4	19.0	18.6	7.6	6.4	8.1	8.0
45 to 54 years	5.5	4.4	5.9	5.9	19.0	16.4	22.9	21.7	8.7	7.0	9.3	9.3
55 to 64 years	5.4	5.0	4.7	6.1	11.1	11.3	14.1	15.1	5.8	5.4	6.7	6.6
65 years and over	3.1	2.6	3.7	4.3	4.9	3.8	5.5	6.4	2.2	1.8	2.6	3.0
65 to 74 years	3.9	3.1	4.4	5.4	6.7	5.2	7.9	9.1	3.0	2.5	3.5	4.2
75 years and over	2.1	2.0	2.8	2.9	2.4	2.1	2.7	2.6	1.1	*0.9	*1.4	*1.4
Race[2,3]												
White only	5.2	4.5	5.6	5.7	22.9	20.8	26.3	26.0	10.3	9.2	11.1	10.5
Black or African American only	4.0	3.5	4.1	3.5	11.7	11.6	14.0	14.4	6.5	6.5	6.1	5.7
American Indian or Alaska Native only	*	*	*	*7.8	29.2	23.7	15.3	23.3	17.4	*12.1	*9.5	*12.4
Asian only	*1.9	*2.3	*1.3	*2.5	11.4	8.8	12.1	11.7	*4.8	3.6	4.3	4.2
Native Hawaiian or Other Pacific Islander only	NA	*	*	*	NA	*	*	*	NA	*	*	*
Two or more races	NA	*7.5	*5.9	*6.5	NA	28.0	25.7	26.3	NA	15.9	12.5	10.9
Hispanic Origin and Race[2,3]												
Hispanic or Latino	3.9	3.2	2.8	3.3	20.4	17.3	19.7	20.9	11.2	9.0	9.2	9.0
Mexican	4.4	3.8	3.1	3.8	21.2	19.9	21.4	21.8	12.6	10.8	10.1	10.0
Not Hispanic or Latino	5.1	4.5	5.6	5.6	21.3	19.7	24.7	24.2	9.5	8.8	10.3	9.6
White only	5.4	4.7	6.2	6.2	23.5	21.5	27.9	27.5	10.3	9.3	11.5	11.0
Black or African American only	3.9	3.4	4.2	3.5	11.6	11.5	13.9	14.3	6.5	6.5	6.1	5.5
Percent of Poverty Level[2,4]												
Below 100 percent	4.8	4.3	4.7	4.9	17.3	15.0	17.6	19.1	9.7	8.6	8.5	9.1
100 percent to 199 percent	4.9	4.2	4.9	4.5	18.4	15.7	20.9	20.3	9.8	8.0	9.8	8.4
200 percent to 399 percent	4.9	4.2	4.8	5.2	21.0	18.7	23.3	23.4	9.8	8.9	10.1	10.0
400 percent or more	5.1	4.4	6.0	5.9	24.3	22.1	28.1	26.7	9.7	8.9	10.9	9.9
Disability Measure[2,5]												
Any basic actions difficulty or complex activity limitation	5.7	5.2	5.5	4.9	20.2	18.8	21.9	20.7	10.2	9.3	9.5	8.6
Any basic actions difficulty	5.8	5.3	5.5	4.9	20.6	19.1	22.3	21.1	10.5	9.4	9.7	8.6
Any complex activity limitation	4.5	4.3	5.5	3.7	16.4	14.3	16.2	16.1	8.8	7.3	7.8	7.0
No disability	4.9	4.1	5.3	5.6	21.8	19.7	25.0	24.9	9.6	8.7	10.4	9.9
MALE												
18 years and over, age-adjusted[2]	6.1	5.1	5.7	5.7	30.7	28.3	32.4	32.1	15.8	14.4	15.6	15.1
18 years and over, crude	6.1	5.2	5.7	5.7	31.7	29.0	32.2	31.3	16.3	14.7	15.6	14.7
Age												
All persons												
18 to 44 years	6.5	5.6	6.1	5.5	40.6	37.8	42.5	41.4	21.1	19.6	20.6	19.1
18 to 24 years	6.0	6.3	6.0	5.4	40.6	38.0	39.9	37.7	22.9	22.9	21.5	17.9
25 to 44 years	6.6	5.3	6.2	5.6	40.6	37.7	43.5	42.8	20.6	18.5	20.2	19.6
45 to 64 years	6.6	5.5	5.8	6.3	25.3	23.5	27.3	27.0	12.7	11.3	13.2	13.0
45 to 54 years	6.6	5.7	5.9	6.4	29.4	26.3	32.0	30.3	14.5	12.3	14.5	14.3
55 to 64 years	6.6	5.4	5.7	6.3	18.9	19.0	21.4	23.5	10.0	9.8	11.6	11.5
65 years and over	3.7	3.1	4.0	5.2	9.3	7.4	9.8	11.4	4.7	3.7	4.7	6.0
65 to 74 years	4.8	3.9	4.4	6.3	12.2	9.5	13.5	15.2	6.1	4.9	6.3	7.6
75 years and over	*2.1	*2.0	*3.5	*3.4	5.1	4.4	4.6	5.4	*2.5	*2.0	*2.5	*3.4
Race[2,3]												
White only	6.3	5.1	6.1	6.0	32.8	29.9	35.3	34.9	16.7	14.9	17.1	16.5
Black or African American only	5.3	5.4	4.6	4.2	18.4	19.8	20.2	21.0	11.0	12.4	9.8	9.6
American Indian or Alaska Native only	*	*	*	*	45.7	29.2	*20.5	34.7	30.4	*14.0	*15.7	*19.4
Asian only	*2.3	*3.5	*1.4	*	17.8	14.1	17.2	17.0	*7.5	*5.9	6.8	6.5
Native Hawaiian or Other Pacific Islander only	NA	*	*	*	NA	*	*	*	NA	*	*	*
Two or more races	NA	*12.1	*8.4	*6.3	NA	39.2	37.6	34.8	NA	23.7	20.3	15.7
Hispanic Origin and Race[2,3]												
Hispanic or Latino	5.7	5.2	3.9	4.9	30.9	27.9	28.8	31.1	18.8	15.9	14.6	15.3
Mexican	6.9	6.6	4.4	5.4	34.2	32.2	32.2	33.4	21.9	19.1	16.3	17.3

NA = Not available.

* = Figure does not meet standards of reliability or precision. Data preceded by an asterisk have a relative standard error (RSE) of 20 percent to 30 percent. Data not shown have an RSE of greater than 30 percent.

[1]Heavier drinking is based on self-reported responses to questions about average alcohol consumption and is defined as more than 14 drinks per week for men and more than seven drinks per week for women on average. Respondents were also asked, "In the past year, on how many days did you have five or more drinks of any alcoholic beverage?"

[2]Estimates are age adjusted to the year 2000 standard population using four age groups: 18 to 24 years, 25 to 44 years, 45 to 64 years, and 65 years and over. Age-adjusted estimates in this table may differ from other age-adjusted estimates based on the same data and presented elsewhere if different age groups are used in the adjustment procedure.

[3]The race groups White, Black, American Indian or Alaska Native, Asian, Native Hawaiian or Other Pacific Islander, and two or more races, include persons of Hispanic and non–Hispanic origin. Persons of Hispanic origin may be of any race.

[4]Percent of poverty level is based on family income and family size and composition using U.S. Census Bureau poverty thresholds. Missing family income data were imputed for 1997 and beyond.

[5]Any basic actions difficulty or complex activity limitation is defined as having one or more of the following limitations or difficulties: movement difficulty, emotional difficulty, sensory (seeing or hearing) difficulty, cognitive difficulty, self–care (activities of daily living or instrumental activities of daily living) limitation, social limitation, or work limitation.

Table 3-25. Heavier Drinking and Drinking Five or More Drinks in a Day Among Adults 18 Years of Age and Over, by Selected Characteristics, Selected Years, 1997–2013—*Continued*

(Percent.)

Characteristic	Heavier drinker[1]				Five or more drinks in a day on at least 1 day in the past year[1]				Five or more drinks in a day on at least 12 days in the past year[1]			
	1997	2000	2010	2013	1997	2000	2010	2013	1997	2000	2010	2013
Not Hispanic or Latino	6.1	5.2	6.0	5.8	30.7	28.6	33.3	32.3	15.5	14.3	15.9	15.0
White only	6.4	5.2	6.5	6.3	33.3	30.6	36.9	36.1	16.6	15.0	17.6	16.8
Black or African American only	5.3	5.4	4.7	4.1	18.4	19.7	20.3	20.6	11.1	12.3	9.9	9.2
Percent of Poverty Level[2,4]												
Below 100 percent	6.8	6.4	6.5	6.8	26.9	24.8	26.0	27.3	16.5	15.7	14.1	15.5
100 percent to 199 percent	7.1	5.8	5.8	5.6	27.3	23.6	29.1	28.9	16.4	13.3	14.8	13.5
200 percent to 399 percent	6.6	5.3	5.8	6.1	30.4	27.4	31.8	31.0	16.0	14.7	16.4	15.6
400 percent or more	5.0	4.4	5.4	5.3	33.6	31.3	36.4	35.1	15.4	14.4	15.8	15.0
Disability Measure[2,5]												
Any basic actions difficulty or complex activity limitation	7.2	6.8	6.6	5.8	29.4	28.9	30.6	29.0	17.0	16.5	14.8	14.0
Any basic actions difficulty	7.5	6.8	6.7	5.8	30.4	29.8	31.8	30.2	17.7	16.8	15.5	14.6
Any complex activity limitation	5.4	5.8	6.6	4.3	23.1	20.5	21.1	21.3	14.2	11.9	11.3	10.7
No disability	5.8	4.8	5.4	5.7	31.5	28.5	33.5	33.3	15.6	14.1	15.9	15.4
FEMALE												
18 years and over, age-adjusted[2]	3.9	3.5	4.8	4.9	12.2	10.8	15.6	15.7	3.9	3.4	4.8	4.3
18 years and over, crude	3.9	3.5	4.8	4.9	12.1	10.6	14.9	14.6	3.9	3.3	4.6	4.1
Age												
All persons												
18 to 44 years	4.0	3.8	5.2	4.8	18.3	16.5	22.6	22.8	5.5	5.2	6.9	6.1
18 to 24 years	4.5	5.2	6.4	5.0	23.0	22.8	28.1	25.0	7.6	8.3	10.9	7.7
25 to 44 years	3.9	3.4	4.8	4.7	16.9	14.5	20.6	22.1	4.9	4.2	5.4	5.5
45 to 64 years	4.4	3.8	4.9	5.7	7.2	6.0	11.1	10.6	2.9	1.9	3.4	3.4
45 to 54 years	4.5	3.2	5.9	5.4	9.2	7.1	14.3	13.6	3.3	2.1	4.3	4.6
55 to 64 years	4.4	4.6	3.8	6.0	4.1	4.4	7.3	7.4	2.1	1.5	2.3	2.0
65 years and over	2.6	2.2	3.4	3.7	1.6	1.2	2.3	2.4	*0.4	*0.4	*	*0.7
65 to 74 years	3.1	2.5	4.5	4.6	2.3	1.7	*3.1	3.8	*	*	*	*1.2
75 years and over	2.0	1.9	2.3	2.5	*0.7	*	*1.4	*0.7	*	*	*	*
Race[2,3]												
White only	4.2	4.0	5.2	5.3	13.5	12.1	17.4	17.5	4.2	3.7	5.2	4.8
Black or African American only	2.9	2.0	3.8	3.0	6.5	5.2	9.0	9.2	2.9	1.9	3.1	2.6
American Indian or Alaska Native only	*	*	*	*4.0	18.1	*19.0	*11.7	*13.3	*	*	*	*
Asian only	*	*	*	*2.3	*5.2	*3.7	7.3	7.0	*	*	*	*2.2
Native Hawaiian or Other Pacific Islander only	NA	*	*	*	NA	*	*	*	NA	*	*	*
Two or more races	NA	*	*	*	NA	17.0	16.4	18.8	NA	*8.2	*6.3	*6.4
Hispanic Origin and Race[2,3]												
Hispanic or Latina	2.2	1.2	1.7	1.9	9.7	6.8	10.3	10.8	3.5	2.1	3.6	2.8
Mexican	*1.9	*1.1	*1.7	2.1	8.2	7.1	10.4	10.4	3.2	*2.2	3.7	2.7
Not Hispanic or Latina	4.1	3.8	5.3	5.4	12.6	11.5	16.6	16.7	4.0	3.6	5.0	4.6
White only	4.4	4.3	5.9	6.1	14.2	13.0	19.1	19.4	4.3	4.0	5.6	5.3
Black or African American only	2.9	2.0	3.8	3.1	6.2	5.2	8.9	9.2	2.9	1.9	3.0	2.6
Percent of Poverty Level[2,4]												
Below 100 percent	3.6	2.8	3.4	3.5	10.8	8.2	11.3	13.2	5.1	3.6	4.2	4.4
100 percent to 199 percent	3.1	2.9	4.1	3.6	10.5	9.0	13.5	13.3	4.0	3.5	5.1	4.1
200 percent to 399 percent	3.3	3.2	3.9	4.4	12.1	10.7	15.3	15.9	4.0	3.5	4.2	4.4
400 percent or more	5.2	4.5	6.7	6.6	14.2	12.6	19.2	17.8	3.4	3.3	5.6	4.6
Disability Measure[2,5]												
Any basic actions difficulty or complex activity limitation	4.5	4.1	4.7	4.3	13.1	11.3	15.2	14.5	5.0	4.1	5.4	4.5
Any basic actions difficulty	4.5	4.2	4.7	4.3	13.2	11.6	15.4	14.9	5.1	4.1	5.4	4.5
Any complex activity limitation	3.7	*3.2	4.6	3.2	10.8	9.1	12.3	11.5	4.2	*3.1	5.0	3.7
No disability	3.9	3.5	5.1	5.4	12.0	10.9	16.1	16.3	3.6	3.3	4.7	4.3

NA = Not available.

* = Figure does not meet standards of reliability or precision. Data preceded by an asterisk have a relative standard error (RSE) of 20 percent to 30 percent. Data not shown have an RSE of greater than 30 percent.

[1]Heavier drinking is based on self–reported responses to questions about average alcohol consumption and is defined as more than 14 drinks per week for men and more than seven drinks per week for women on average. Respondents were also asked, "In the past year, on how many days did you have five or more drinks of any alcoholic beverage?"

[2]Estimates are age adjusted to the year 2000 standard population using four age groups: 18 to 24 years, 25 to 44 years, 45 to 64 years, and 65 years and over. Age-adjusted estimates in this table may differ from other age–adjusted estimates based on the same data and presented elsewhere if different age groups are used in the adjustment procedure.

[3]The race groups White, Black, American Indian or Alaska Native, Asian, Native Hawaiian or Other Pacific Islander, and two or more races, include persons of Hispanic and non–Hispanic origin. Persons of Hispanic origin may be of any race.

[4]Percent of poverty level is based on family income and family size and composition using U.S. Census Bureau poverty thresholds. Missing family income data were imputed for 1997 and beyond.

[5]Any basic actions difficulty or complex activity limitation is defined as having one or more of the following limitations or difficulties: movement difficulty, emotional difficulty, sensory (seeing or hearing) difficulty, cognitive difficulty, self–care (activities of daily living or instrumental activities of daily living) limitation, social limitation, or work limitation.

Table 3-26. Age-Adjusted Prevalence of Current Cigarette Smoking[1] Among Adults 25 Years of Age and Over, by Sex, Race, and Education Level, Selected Years, 1974–2015

(Percent.)

Sex, race, and education level	1974[2]	1979[2]	1985[2]	1990[2]	1995[2]	2000	2005	2006	2007
25 YEARS AND OVER, AGE-ADJUSTED[3]..									
All Persons[4].....................................	36.9	33.1	30.0	25.4	24.5	22.6	20.3	20.3	19.3
No high school diploma or GED....................	43.7	40.7	40.8	36.7	35.6	31.6	28.2	28.8	26.9
High school diploma or GED......................	36.2	33.6	32.0	29.1	29.1	29.2	27.0	26.5	26.6
Some college, no bachelor's degree..............	35.9	33.2	29.5	23.4	22.6	21.7	21.8	22.1	20.1
Bachelor's degree or higher	27.2	22.6	18.5	13.9	13.6	10.9	9.1	8.2	9.0
All Males[4].....................................	42.9	37.3	32.8	28.2	26.4	24.7	22.7	22.9	21.4
No high school diploma or GED....................	52.3	47.6	45.7	42.0	39.7	36.0	31.7	31.6	30.8
High school diploma or GED......................	42.4	38.9	35.5	33.1	32.7	32.1	29.9	29.7	29.4
Some college, no bachelor's degree..............	41.8	36.5	32.9	25.9	23.7	23.3	24.9	25.2	21.6
Bachelor's degree or higher	28.3	22.7	19.6	14.5	13.8	11.6	9.7	9.2	10.4
White Males[4,5]................................	41.9	36.7	31.7	27.6	25.9	24.7	22.4	22.7	21.6
No high school diploma or GED....................	51.5	47.6	45.0	41.8	38.7	38.2	31.6	31.4	30.8
High school diploma or GED......................	42.0	38.5	34.8	32.9	32.9	32.4	30.0	29.2	29.9
Some college, no bachelor's degree..............	41.6	36.4	32.2	25.4	23.3	23.5	24.5	25.8	21.8
Bachelor's degree or higher	27.8	22.5	19.1	14.4	13.4	11.3	9.3	8.9	10.5
Black or African American Males[4,5]..........	53.4	44.4	42.1	34.5	31.6	26.4	26.5	25.4	23.7
No high school diploma or GED....................	58.1	49.7	50.5	41.6	41.9	38.2	35.9	35.2	30.4
High school diploma or GED......................	*50.7	48.6	41.8	37.4	36.6	29.0	30.1	31.3	29.6
Some college, no bachelor's degree..............	*45.3	39.2	41.8	28.1	26.4	19.9	27.4	21.0	23.6
Bachelor's degree or higher	*41.4	*36.8	*32.0	*20.8	*17.3	14.6	10.0	12.9	*13.5
All Females[4]..................................	32.0	29.5	27.5	22.9	22.9	20.5	18.0	17.9	17.2
No high school diploma or GED....................	36.6	34.8	36.5	31.8	31.7	27.1	24.6	26.0	22.7
High school diploma or GED......................	32.2	29.8	29.5	26.1	26.4	26.6	24.1	23.4	23.8
Some college, no bachelor's degree..............	30.1	30.0	26.3	21.0	21.6	20.4	19.1	19.6	18.9
Bachelor's degree or higher	25.9	22.5	17.1	13.3	13.3	10.1	8.5	7.2	7.7
White Females[4,5]..............................	31.7	29.7	27.3	23.3	23.1	21.0	18.6	18.5	18.0
No high school diploma or GED....................	36.8	35.8	36.7	33.4	32.4	28.4	24.6	25.9	23.8
High school diploma or GED......................	31.9	29.9	29.4	26.5	26.8	27.8	25.9	24.6	25.2
Some college, no bachelor's degree..............	30.4	30.7	26.7	21.2	22.2	21.1	19.5	20.5	19.6
Bachelor's degree or higher	25.5	21.9	16.5	13.4	13.5	10.2	9.1	7.7	8.2
Black or African American Females[4,5]	35.6	30.3	32.0	22.4	25.7	21.6	17.5	19.1	16.6
No high school diploma or GED....................	36.1	31.6	39.4	26.3	32.3	31.1	27.8	31.2	23.1
High school diploma or GED......................	40.9	32.6	32.1	24.1	27.8	25.4	18.2	18.6	19.8
Some college, no bachelor's degree..............	32.3	*28.9	23.9	22.7	20.8	20.4	17.5	18.9	17.2
Bachelor's degree or higher	*36.3	*43.3	26.6	17.0	17.3	10.8	*6.6	*8.5	*6.0

* = Figure does not meet standards of reliability or precision. Data preceded by an asterisk have a relative standard error of 20 percent to 30 percent.
[1]Starting with 1993 data, current cigarette smokers were defined as ever smoking 100 cigarettes in their lifetime and smoking now every day or some days.
[2]Data prior to 1997 are not strictly comparable with data for later years due to the 1997 questionnaire redesign.
[3]Estimates are age adjusted to the year 2000 standard population using four age groups: 25 to 34 years, 35 to 44 years, 45 to 64 years, and 65 years and over.
[4]Includes unknown education level. Education categories shown are for 1997 and subsequent years. GED is General Educational Development high school equivalency diploma.
[5]The race groups White and Black include persons of Hispanic and non-Hispanic origin.

Table 3-26. Age-Adjusted Prevalence of Current Cigarette Smoking[1] Among Adults 25 Years of Age and Over, by Sex, Race, and Education Level, Selected Years, 1974–2015—Continued

(Percent.)

Sex, race, and education level	2008	2009	2010	2011	2012	2013	2014	2015
25 YEARS AND OVER, AGE-ADJUSTED[3]..								
All Persons[4]...............	20.5	20.4	19.2	19.0	18.3	17.8	17.1	15.6
No high school diploma or GED................	29.8	28.9	26.9	27.2	26.3	25.8	24.4	25.6
High school diploma or GED................	28.1	28.7	27.0	27.4	26.3	25.6	25.9	22.9
Some college, no bachelor's degree................	22.1	21.4	21.3	20.7	19.6	19.5	18.6	17.9
Bachelor's degree or higher	8.5	9.0	8.3	7.5	7.8	7.7	7.0	5.9
All Males[4]...............	22.6	22.4	21.0	21.2	20.6	20.3	19.1	17.1
No high school diploma or GED................	32.5	32.3	29.7	31.6	30.3	31.6	27.7	28.6
High school diploma or GED................	31.4	31.4	29.3	29.8	29.6	28.8	28.2	24.3
Some college, no bachelor's degree................	24.3	23.0	23.2	22.6	21.0	20.4	20.2	18.7
Bachelor's degree or higher	9.1	9.6	8.7	7.9	8.5	8.7	7.9	6.6
White Males[4,5]...............	22.6	22.7	21.0	21.3	20.5	20.1	18.6	16.9
No high school diploma or GED................	33.1	32.2	29.4	32.0	29.6	30.2	26.0	27.1
High school diploma or GED................	31.9	32.4	29.6	29.9	29.8	28.4	27.9	25.3
Some college, no bachelor's degree................	23.7	22.4	23.4	22.4	20.3	20.3	20.3	18.0
Bachelor's degree or higher	9.1	9.6	8.8	7.9	8.9	8.8	7.4	6.6
Black or African American Males[4,5]..........	25.9	23.7	23.9	23.9	23.3	23.1	22.9	20.9
No high school diploma or GED................	35.0	39.1	34.4	32.3	34.1	41.5	38.7	38.1
High school diploma or GED................	28.3	26.0	28.8	29.4	28.0	31.9	28.7	22.1
Some college, no bachelor's degree................	29.5	26.5	24.2	24.7	24.9	18.0	18.8	23.0
Bachelor's degree or higher	*10.0	9.9	8.1	7.9	*7.3	7.7	9.8	*6.9
All Females[4]...............	18.4	18.5	17.5	16.8	16.1	15.5	15.2	14.3
No high school diploma or GED................	27.0	24.8	23.7	22.7	22.2	19.8	21.2	22.6
High school diploma or GED................	25.0	26.1	24.9	24.7	22.6	22.0	23.5	21.2
Some college, no bachelor's degree................	20.1	20.0	19.6	19.0	18.4	18.8	17.3	17.2
Bachelor's degree or higher	8.1	8.4	7.9	7.1	7.2	6.8	6.2	5.3
White Females[4,5]...............	19.4	19.0	18.3	17.6	16.9	16.2	16.0	15.3
No high school diploma or GED................	28.4	24.4	24.0	22.7	22.4	19.0	21.0	23.8
High school diploma or GED................	27.1	26.5	25.8	26.8	24.0	23.5	25.4	22.7
Some college, no bachelor's degree................	21.6	21.2	21.0	20.0	19.0	19.8	18.3	18.6
Bachelor's degree or higher	8.5	9.1	8.7	7.5	7.7	7.3	6.6	5.9
Black or African American Females[4,5]......	17.5	19.3	17.0	16.1	15.2	15.3	14.0	13.9
No high school diploma or GED................	28.9	31.0	25.8	29.6	25.8	26.5	22.5	24.0
High school diploma or GED................	20.0	27.3	22.9	16.9	17.0	17.0	15.9	18.0
Some college, no bachelor's degree................	15.9	16.2	15.0	15.0	16.9	15.3	14.4	14.5
Bachelor's degree or higher	*9.3	*7.3	*6.6	7.2	7.1	7.3	6.9	*4.5

* = Figure does not meet standards of reliability or precision. Data preceded by an asterisk have a relative standard error of 20 percent to 30 percent.
[1]Starting with 1993 data, current cigarette smokers were defined as ever smoking 100 cigarettes in their lifetime and smoking now every day or some days.
[3]Estimates are age adjusted to the year 2000 standard population using four age groups: 25 to 34 years, 35 to 44 years, 45 to 64 years, and 65 years and over.
[4]Includes unknown education level. Education categories shown are for 1997 and subsequent years. GED is General Educational Development high school equivalency diploma.
[5]The race groups White and Black include persons of Hispanic and non-Hispanic origin.

Table 3-27. Current Cigarette Smoking[1] Among Adults, by Sex, Race, Hispanic Origin, Age, and Education Level, Average Annual, Selected Years 1990–1992 Through 2013–2015

(Percent.)

Characteristic	Male					Female				
	1990–1992[2]	1999–2001	2006–2008	2008–2010	2013–2015	1990–1992[2]	1999–2001	2006–2008	2008–2010	2013–2015
18 Years and Over, Age-Adjusted[3]										
All persons[4]	27.9	25.0	22.8	22.4	18.8	23.7	21.1	18.0	18.0	14.8
Race[5]										
White only	27.4	25.1	22.9	22.6		24.3	22.2	18.9	18.8	15.7
Black or African American only	33.9	27.2	24.8	23.7	18.7	23.1	19.7	17.2	17.5	13.8
American Indian or Alaska Native only	34.2	30.3	31.5	25.1	21.2	36.7	34.7	22.2	21.0	19.8
Asian only	24.8	20.3	15.6*	15.3	20.6	6.3	6.7	4.4*	5.5	4.4
Native Hawaiian or Other Pacific Islander only	NA	*	*	*	13.4*	NA	*	*	*	*
2 or more races	NA	34.4	25.1	27.7		NA	30.7	24.6	20.9	21.2
American Indian or Alaska Native; White	NA	38.7	34.6	34.6	27.2 / 30.5	NA	38.9	28.6	26.5	27.6
Hispanic Origin and Race[5]										
Hispanic or Latino	25.7	22.2	18.6	17.3		15.8	12.1	9.5	9.6	7.2
Mexican	26.2	21.9	18.7	17.5	14.4	14.8	10.6	8.8	8.4	6.7
Not Hispanic or Latino	28.1	25.5	23.7	23.4	14.6	24.4	22.3	19.4	19.5	16.4
White only	27.7	25.5	24.0	23.9	19.8	25.2	23.5	20.9	20.9	17.9
Black or African American only	33.9	27.2	25.1	24.0	19.9 / 21.4	23.2	19.7	17.2	17.7	14.0
18 Years and Over, Crude										
All persons[4]	28.4	25.5	23.1	22.7	18.7	23.6	21.0	17.9	17.8	14.6
Race[5]										
White only	27.8	25.4	23.0	22.7		24.1	21.7	18.5	18.4	15.3
Black or African American only	33.2	27.5	25.6	24.4	18.4	23.3	19.8	17.5	17.9	13.9
American Indian or Alaska Native only	35.5	31.8	30.7	25.6	21.4	37.3	36.9	23.0	21.6	20.3
Asian only	24.9	21.4	16.5*	15.7	20.5	6.3	6.9	4.6*	5.6	4.4
Native Hawaiian or Other Pacific Islander only	NA	*	*	*	13.8*	NA	*	*	*	*
2 or more races	NA	35.9	27.0	29.2		NA	31.5	25.3	21.9	20.6
American Indian or Alaska Native; White	NA	41.1	33.5	33.9	27.1 / 28.0	NA	40.1	30.0	27.5	27.6
Hispanic Origin and Race[5]										
Hispanic or Latino	26.5	23.2	19.6	18.4		16.6	12.6	9.7	9.8	7.2
Mexican	27.1	22.8	19.4	18.6	15.0	15.0	11.0	8.8	8.5	6.6
Not Hispanic or Latino	28.5	25.8	23.7	23.4	15.0	24.2	21.9	19.1	19.0	15.9
White only	28.0	25.5	23.7	23.6	19.4	24.8	22.7	20.1	20.0	17.0
Black or African American only	33.3	27.5	26.0	24.7	19.2 / 21.6	23.3	19.8	17.6	18.0	14.1
Age and Hispanic Origin and Race[5]										
18 to 24 Years										
Hispanic or Latino	19.3	22.6	18.4	19.3	13.6	12.8	12.9	8.0	8.0	5.0
Not Hispanic or Latino										
White only	28.9	32.7	29.1	28.2	21.9	28.7	30.8	24.1	21.2	18.4
Black or African American only	17.7	21.9	23.6	18.4	14.2	10.8	13.0	13.5	14.9	10.1
25 to 34 Years										
Hispanic or Latino	29.9	23.2	20.4	20.1	18.7	19.2	12.5	9.5	9.6	7.0
Not Hispanic or Latino										
White only	32.7	30.8	31.6	30.8	24.4	30.9	27.4	26.7	26.5	21.4
Black or African American only	34.6	23.3	28.5	25.7	27.2	29.2	16.9	16.2	19.1	15.7
35 to 44 Years										
Hispanic or Latino	32.1	25.3	20.5	18.2	13.9	19.9	14.1	10.2	10.4	7.7
Not Hispanic or Latino										
White only	32.3	29.6	25.9	26.5	22.9	27.3	28.3	24.1	24.7	20.9
Black or African American only	44.1	32.0	20.9	23.2	22.2	31.3	27.5	19.4	19.0	16.4
45 to 64 Years										
Hispanic or Latino	26.6	24.7	21.4	19.2	15.0	17.1	13.5	12.5	12.2	9.5
Not Hispanic or Latino										
White only	28.4	25.1	23.5	24.1	20.1	26.1	22.1	20.7	21.0	19.1
Black or African American only	38.0	34.0	31.8	31.7	24.0	26.1	23.6	23.2	21.6	16.3
65 Years and Over										
Hispanic or Latino	16.1	12.6	9.4	8.2	9.9	6.6	5.9	4.7	5.5	4.1
Not Hispanic or Latino										
White only	14.2	10.0	10.5	9.8	9.6	12.3	9.8	8.6	9.5	8.0
Black or African American only	25.2	17.6	16.3	13.7	15.0	10.7	11.0	7.8	9.8	8.1
Percent of Poverty Level[2,6]										
Below 100 percent	40.5	36.5	32.1	32.5	31.8	30.7	29.1	28.1	28.6	24.6
100 percent to 199 percent	35.0	32.8	29.4	29.3	26.0	26.9	25.6	22.4	22.8	19.8

NA = Not available.
* = Figure does not meet standards of reliability or precision. Data preceded by an asterisk have a relative standard error (RSE) of 20 percent to 30 percent. Data not shown have an RSE of greater than 30 percent.
[1]Starting with 1993 data, current cigarette smokers were defined as ever smoking 100 cigarettes in their lifetime and smoking now every day or some days.
[2]Data prior to 1997 are not strictly comparable with data for later years due to the 1997 questionnaire redesign.
[3]Estimates are age adjusted to the year 2000 standard population using five age groups: 18 to 24 years, 25 to 34 years, 35 to 44 years, 45 to 64 years, and 65 years and over. For age groups where smoking is 0 percent or 100 percent, the age-adjustment procedure was modified to substitute the percentage smoking from the previous 3-year period.
[4]Includes all other races not shown separately, unknown education level, and unknown disability measure.
[5]The race groups White, Black, American Indian or Alaska Native, Asian, Native Hawaiian or Other Pacific Islander, and two or more races include persons of Hispanic and non–Hispanic origin. Persons of Hispanic origin may be of any race.
[6]Percent of poverty level is based on family income and family size and composition using U.S. Census Bureau poverty thresholds. Missing family income data were imputed for 1990 and beyond.

Table 3-27. Current Cigarette Smoking[1] Among Adults, by Sex, Race, Hispanic Origin, Age, and Education Level, Average Annual, Selected Years 1990–1992 Through 2013–2015—Continued

(Percent.)

Characteristic	Male					Female				
	1990–1992[2]	1999–2001	2006–2008	2008–2010	2013–2015	1990–1992[2]	1999–2001	2006–2008	2008–2010	2013–2015
200 percent to 399 percent	26.5	27.3	24.8	24.3	19.6	22.6	22.3	18.5	18.5	14.7
400 percent or more	22.5	18.8	17.0	16.0	11.9	19.0	15.9	12.5	11.8	8.5
Hispanic Origin and Race and Percent of Poverty Level[2,4,6]										
Hispanic or Latino										
Below 100 percent	29.2	25.3	20.8	20.2	18.0	16.3	14.4	11.9	11.4	10.3
100 percent to 199 percent	29.5	22.0	18.4	17.8	14.7	16.0	11.8	8.3	8.7	7.3
200 percent to 399 percent	23.7	23.6	19.7	16.6	14.2	15.9	12.0	8.6	10.2	5.8
400 percent or more	19.7	18.1	15.7	15.1	11.0	13.6	9.4	9.9	7.9	5.5
Not Hispanic or Latino										
White only										
Below 100 percent	44.2	40.7	38.6	40.6	41.2	37.8	38.3	38.0	39.4	36.8
100 percent to 199 percent	36.3	37.5	35.0	35.3	33.3	31.1	32.0	30.7	30.7	28.6
200 percent to 399 percent	26.4	28.5	27.0	27.4	21.0	23.7	24.8	22.1	21.9	18.5
400 percent or more	22.5	19.1	17.4	16.3	12.5	19.5	17.1	13.6	13.1	9.7
Black or African American only										
Below 100 percent	43.5	40.6	38.2	36.5	35.8	28.9	27.7	27.0	29.1	23.8
100 percent to 199 percent	36.0	33.9	30.9	30.4	25.5	20.3	21.3	18.6	19.6	15.0
200 percent to 399 percent	31.4	24.9	21.8	20.7	20.3	21.4	17.3	13.5	13.2	9.6
400 percent or more	24.3	17.9	18.4	15.6	10.3	19.2	12.6	10.3	8.2	6.3
Disability Measure[7]										
Any basic actions difficulty or complex activity limitation	NA	33.1	32.1	30.3	27.9	NA	28.1	26.8	26.8	22.9
Any basic actions difficulty	NA	33.2	32.5	30.5	28.0	NA	28.2	27.0	27.0	23.1
Any complex activity limitation	NA	37.6	34.2	33.2	32.0	NA	30.6	31.8	31.5	27.4
No disability	NA	22.8	20.1	19.8	15.9	NA	18.8	14.9	14.6	11.6
Education, Hispanic Origin, and Race[5,8] 25 years and over, age-adjusted[9]										
No high school diploma or GED										
Hispanic or Latino	30.2	24.3	19.5	18.5	17.2	15.8	12.1	8.6	8.6	7.2
Not Hispanic or Latino										
White only	46.1	43.5	42.0	45.1	42.2	40.4	39.3	42.9	44.0	41.5
Black or African American only	45.4	40.0	35.9	37.2	40.5	31.3	29.4	28.7	29.9	26.0
High school diploma or GED										
Hispanic or Latino	29.6	24.1	21.7	20.3	15.2	18.4	12.5	10.7	11.4	8.0
Not Hispanic or Latino										
White only	32.9	31.8	32.7	34.4	30.5	28.4	29.2	28.8	30.3	29.2
Black or African American only	38.2	31.4	29.5	27.8	28.3	25.4	23.0	19.8	23.7	16.9
Some college or more										
Hispanic or Latino	20.4	17.1	15.8	12.9	10.8	14.3	11.1	10.3	9.9	7.5
Not Hispanic or Latino										
White only	19.3	17.6	16.2	15.9	13.4	18.1	16.7	14.7	15.5	13.0
Black or African American only	25.6	19.2	19.3	19.8	15.3	22.8	16.9	13.7	12.7	11.5

NA = Not available.

* = Figure does not meet standards of reliability or precision. Data preceded by an asterisk have a relative standard error (RSE) of 20 percent to 30 percent. Data not shown have an RSE of greater than 30 percent.

[1]Starting with 1993 data, current cigarette smokers were defined as ever smoking 100 cigarettes in their lifetime and smoking now every day or some days.

[2]Data prior to 1997 are not strictly comparable with data for later years due to the 1997 questionnaire redesign.

[4]Includes all other races not shown separately, unknown education level, and unknown disability measure.

[5]The race groups White, Black, American Indian or Alaska Native, Asian, Native Hawaiian or Other Pacific Islander, and two or more races include persons of Hispanic and non–Hispanic origin. Persons of Hispanic origin may be of any race.

[6]Percent of poverty level is based on family income and family size and composition using U.S. Census Bureau poverty thresholds. Missing family income data were imputed for 1990 and beyond.

[7]Any basic actions difficulty or complex activity limitation is defined as having one or more of the following limitations or difficulties: movement difficulty, emotional difficulty, sensory (seeing or hearing) difficulty, cognitive difficulty, self–care (activities of daily living or instrumental activities of daily living) limitation, social limitation, or work limitation.

[8]Education categories shown are for 1997 and subsequent years. GED is General Educational Development high school equivalency diploma.

[9]Estimates are age adjusted to the year 2000 standard using four age groups: 25 to 34 years, 35 to 44 years, 45 to 64 years, and 65 years and over.

Table 3-28. Current Cigarette Smoking[1] Among Adults 18 Years of Age and Over, by Sex, Race, and Age, Selected Years, 1965–2015

(Percent.)

Sex, race, and age	1965[2]	1974[2]	1983[2]	1985[2]	1990[2]	1995[2]	2000	2005	2006	2007	2008	2009	2010	2011	2012	2013	2014	2015
18 Years and Over, Age-Adjusted[3]																		
All persons	41.9	37.0	31.9	29.9	25.3	24.6	23.1	20.8	20.8	19.7	20.6	20.6	19.3	19.0	18.2	17.9	17.0	15.3
Male	51.2	42.8	34.8	32.2	28.0	26.5	25.2	23.4	23.6	22.0	22.8	23.2	21.2	21.2	20.6	20.5	19.0	16.8
Female	33.7	32.2	29.4	27.9	22.9	22.7	21.1	18.3	18.1	17.5	18.5	18.1	17.5	16.8	15.9	15.5	15.1	13.8
White male[4]	50.4	41.7	34.2	31.3	27.6	26.2	25.4	23.3	23.5	22.2	23.0	23.6	21.4	21.4	20.7	20.5	18.8	16.8
Black or African American male[4]	58.8	53.6	41.7	40.2	32.8	29.4	25.7	25.9	26.1	23.4	24.7	23.1	23.3	23.2	22.0	21.8	21.7	20.3
White female[4]	33.9	32.0	29.6	27.9	23.5	23.4	22.0	19.1	18.8	18.5	19.5	18.7	18.3	17.7	16.9	16.3	16.0	14.8
Black or African American female[4]	31.8	35.6	31.3	30.9	20.8	23.5	20.7	17.1	18.5	15.6	17.4	18.5	16.6	15.2	14.2	14.9	13.4	13.2
18 Years and Over, Crude																		
All persons	42.4	37.1	32.1	30.1	25.5	24.7	23.2	20.9	20.8	19.8	20.6	20.6	19.3	19.0	18.1	17.8	16.8	15.1
Male	51.9	43.1	35.1	32.6	28.4	27.0	25.6	23.9	23.9	22.3	23.1	23.5	21.5	21.6	20.5	20.5	18.8	16.7
Female	33.9	32.1	29.5	27.9	22.8	22.6	20.9	18.1	18.0	17.4	18.3	17.9	17.3	16.5	15.8	15.3	14.8	13.6
White male[4]	51.1	41.9	34.5	31.7	28.0	26.6	25.7	23.6	23.6	22.3	23.1	23.6	21.4	21.6	20.3	20.3	18.5	16.5
Black or African American male[4]	60.4	54.3	40.6	39.9	32.5	28.5	26.2	26.5	27.0	24.6	25.3	23.7	24.3	23.8	22.0	21.9	21.8	20.6
White female[4]	34.0	31.7	29.4	27.7	23.4	23.1	21.4	18.7	18.4	18.1	19.1	18.3	17.9	17.2	16.6	15.9	15.5	14.3
Black or African American female[4]	33.7	36.4	32.2	31.0	21.2	23.5	20.8	17.3	18.8	15.9	17.8	18.8	17.0	15.3	14.7	15.1	13.5	13.1
All Males																		
18 to 44 years	57.9	47.9	37.7	35.2	31.4	29.9	29.2	27.1	26.7	25.8	25.6	26.9	23.9	23.6	24.0	22.9	21.7	18.5
18 to 24 years	54.1	42.1	32.9	28.0	26.6	27.8	28.1	28.0	28.5	25.4	23.6	28.0	22.8	21.3	20.1	21.9	18.5	15.0
25 to 34 years	60.7	50.5	38.8	38.2	31.6	29.5	28.9	27.7	27.4	28.8	28.5	27.6	26.1	27.5	28.0	24.4	23.7	21.3
35 to 44 years	58.2	51.0	41.0	37.6	34.5	31.5	30.2	26.0	24.8	23.2	24.3	25.4	22.5	21.2	22.8	22.1	22.0	18.3
45 to 64 years	51.9	42.6	35.9	33.4	29.3	27.1	26.4	25.2	24.5	22.6	24.8	24.5	23.2	24.4	20.2	21.9	19.4	17.9
45 to 54 years	55.9	46.8	39.0	34.9	32.1	27.2	28.8	28.1	26.6	24.8	26.4	27.3	25.2	27.0	21.4	21.4	19.9	18.3
55 to 64 years	46.6	37.7	32.6	31.9	25.9	26.9	22.6	21.1	21.5	19.6	22.6	20.8	20.7	21.4	18.8	22.6	18.8	17.5
65 years and over	28.5	24.8	22.0	19.6	14.6	14.9	10.2	8.9	12.6	9.3	10.5	9.5	9.7	8.9	10.6	10.6	9.8	9.7
White Male[4]																		
18 to 44 years	57.1	46.8	37.5	34.6	31.3	30.1	30.2	27.7	27.1	26.6	26.7	28.1	24.6	24.3	24.8	23.4	21.7	18.9
18 to 24 years	53.0	40.8	32.5	28.4	27.4	28.4	30.4	29.7	28.9	26.5	25.2	30.0	23.8	22.1	21.9	23.5	20.0	15.6
25 to 34 years	60.1	49.5	38.6	37.3	31.6	29.9	29.7	27.7	27.9	29.0	29.5	28.4	26.6	28.6	28.4	24.6	23.4	20.9
35 to 44 years	57.3	50.1	40.8	36.6	33.5	31.2	30.6	26.3	25.3	24.4	24.9	26.3	23.1	21.4	23.3	21.9	21.2	19.1
45 to 64 years	51.3	41.2	35.0	32.1	28.7	26.3	25.8	24.5	23.4	22.1	24.0	24.0	22.5	24.0	19.4	21.7	19.0	17.3
45 to 54 years	55.3	45.0	38.0	33.7	31.3	25.9	28.0	27.4	25.7	24.4	26.1	27.1	24.5	26.6	20.7	21.2	19.7	17.8
55 to 64 years	46.1	36.6	31.9	30.5	25.6	27.0	22.5	20.4	20.4	19.1	21.2	20.1	20.1	20.8	17.9	22.2	18.2	16.9
65 years and over	27.7	24.3	20.6	18.9	13.7	14.1	9.8	7.9	12.6	8.9	9.9	9.3	9.6	8.6	10.3	10.0	9.4	9.3
Black or African American Male[4]																		
18 to 44 years	66.3	58.1	39.4	39.6	32.9	26.4	25.5	25.1	26.2	24.2	22.0	22.5	22.6	22.7	21.3	20.9	22.2	20.2
18 to 24 years	62.8	54.9	34.2	27.2	21.3	*	20.9	21.6	31.2	21.4	*17.0	18.9	18.8	18.4	13.2	*13.2	*13.9	*15.9
25 to 34 years	68.4	58.5	39.9	45.6	33.8	25.1	23.2	29.8	26.3	32.3	25.9	24.1	25.7	25.0	24.9	24.8	28.0	26.0
35 to 44 years	67.3	61.5	45.5	45.0	42.0	36.3	30.7	23.3	22.2	17.4	21.8	24.0	22.6	24.3	24.7	24.0	24.0	17.9
45 to 64 years	57.9	57.8	44.8	46.1	36.7	33.9	32.2	32.4	32.6	28.3	33.6	28.9	31.8	28.9	24.6	25.7	24.0	22.8
45 to 54 years	62.4	63.6	47.8	47.7	42.0	36.9	35.6	33.9	32.0	29.3	31.7	28.1	33.2	29.2	23.3	25.7	22.5	20.5
55 to 64 years	51.8	50.1	41.1	44.4	30.2	29.1	26.3	29.8	33.5	26.8	36.6	30.1	29.6	28.4	26.4	25.6	25.9	25.5
65 years and over	36.4	29.7	38.9	27.7	21.5	28.5	14.2	16.8	16.0	14.3	17.5	14.0	10.0	13.7	17.4	15.5	13.9	16.0
All Females																		
18 to 44 years	42.1	37.5	33.8	31.4	25.6	25.6	24.5	21.2	20.6	19.5	20.6	20.0	19.1	18.8	16.9	16.6	16.6	14.5
18 to 24 years	38.1	34.1	35.5	30.4	22.5	21.8	24.9	20.7	19.3	19.1	19.0	15.6	17.4	16.4	14.5	15.4	14.8	11.0
25 to 34 years	43.7	38.8	32.6	32.0	28.2	26.4	22.3	21.5	21.5	19.6	21.4	21.8	20.6	19.5	19.4	17.9	17.5	15.0
35 to 44 years	43.7	39.8	33.8	31.5	24.8	27.1	26.2	21.3	20.6	19.6	20.9	21.2	19.0	19.9	16.1	16.3	17.0	16.5
45 to 64 years	32.0	33.4	31.0	29.9	24.8	24.0	21.7	18.8	19.3	19.5	20.5	19.5	19.1	18.5	18.9	18.1	16.8	16.1
45 to 54 years	37.5	36.0	34.1	32.4	28.5	24.3	22.2	20.9	22.5	22.1	23.7	22.3	21.3	21.6	21.3	20.6	18.7	18.4
55 to 64 years	25.0	30.4	28.0	27.4	20.5	23.7	20.9	16.1	14.9	16.2	16.3	16.1	16.5	15.0	16.2	15.2	14.8	13.7
65 years and over	9.6	12.0	13.1	13.5	11.5	11.5	9.3	8.3	8.3	7.6	8.3	9.5	9.3	7.1	7.5	7.5	7.5	7.3
White Female[4]																		
18 to 44 years	42.2	37.3	34.2	31.6	26.5	26.6	26.5	22.6	22.2	21.2	22.1	21.2	20.5	20.3	18.6	17.8	17.8	15.7
18 to 24 years	38.4	34.0	36.5	31.8	25.4	24.9	28.5	22.6	20.7	21.6	20.1	16.7	18.4	18.4	16.9	17.0	16.5	11.2
25 to 34 years	43.4	38.6	32.2	32.0	28.5	27.3	24.9	23.1	23.7	21.4	23.1	22.7	22.0	20.6	20.7	19.2	18.6	16.3
35 to 44 years	43.9	39.3	34.8	31.0	25.0	27.0	26.6	22.2	21.7	20.7	22.6	22.9	20.5	21.5	17.6	17.0	18.0	18.3
45 to 64 years	32.7	33.0	30.6	29.7	25.4	24.3	21.4	18.9	18.8	19.6	20.9	19.4	19.5	19.0	19.4	18.4	17.6	17.1
45 to 54 years	38.2	34.9	33.3	32.4	29.1	24.6	21.9	21.0	22.1	22.2	24.2	22.4	22.4	22.5	22.7	21.2	19.9	20.2
55 to 64 years	25.7	30.6	28.1	27.2	21.2	23.8	20.6	16.2	14.4	16.2	16.8	15.8	15.9	15.1	15.8	15.5	15.3	14.0
65 years and over	9.8	12.3	13.2	13.3	11.5	11.7	9.1	8.4	8.4	8.0	8.6	9.6	9.4	7.0	7.5	7.9	7.6	7.5
Black or African American Female[4]																		
18 to 44 years	42.9	41.1	34.6	33.5	22.8	24.0	20.8	16.9	17.3	14.2	18.0	18.3	17.1	15.0	12.3	15.1	13.9	13.3
18 to 24 years	37.1	35.6	32.0	23.7	10.0	*8.8	14.2	14.2	14.8	*8.7	16.6	13.3	14.2	9.1	*7.4	11.8	*9.3	*8.6
25 to 34 years	47.8	42.2	38.0	36.2	29.1	26.7	15.5	16.9	15.4	14.9	17.6	20.1	19.3	17.5	17.3	16.4	15.1	14.9
35 to 44 years	42.8	46.4	32.7	40.2	25.5	31.9	30.2	19.0	21.0	17.7	19.6	20.0	17.2	17.4	11.2	16.4	16.4	15.4
45 to 64 years	25.7	38.9	36.3	33.4	22.6	27.5	25.6	21.0	25.5	22.6	21.3	22.7	19.8	18.3	20.4	18.8	15.0	14.5
45 to 54 years	32.3	46.2	43.6	36.4	26.5	28.3	26.5	22.2	29.3	26.3	24.9	23.5	20.4	20.1	20.1	22.2	15.7	14.7
55 to 64 years	16.5	29.3	28.0	29.8	17.6	26.3	24.2	19.1	19.5	17.0	15.9	21.4	18.9	16.0	20.8	14.8	14.2	14.3
65 years and over	7.1	*8.9	*13.1	14.5	11.1	13.3	10.2	10.0	9.3	6.4	8.1	11.5	9.4	9.1	9.1	6.5	8.1	9.7

* = Figure does not meet standards of reliability or precision. Data preceded by an asterisk have a relative standard error (RSE) of 20 percent to 30 percent. Data not shown have an RSE of greater than 30 percent.
[1]Starting with 1993 data, current cigarette smokers were defined as ever smoking 100 cigarettes in their lifetime and smoking now every day or some days.
[2]Data prior to 1997 are not strictly comparable with data for later years due to the 1997 questionnaire redesign.
[3]Estimates are age adjusted to the year 2000 standard population using five age groups: 18 to 24 years, 25 to 34 years, 35 to 44 years, 45 to 64 years, and 65 years and over. For age groups where smoking is 0 percent or 100 percent, the age-adjustment procedure was modified to substitute the percentage smoking from the previous 3-year period.
[4]The race groups White, Black, American Indian or Alaska Native, Asian, Native Hawaiian or Other Pacific Islander, and two or more races include persons of Hispanic and non–Hispanic origin. Persons of Hispanic origin may be of any race.

Table 3-29. Use of Selected Substances Among 12th Graders, 10th Graders, and 8th Graders, by Sex and Race, Selected Years, 1980–2015

(Percent.)

Substance, grade in school, sex, and race	1980	1985	1990	1995	2000	2005	2006	2007	2008	2009	2010	2011	2012	2013	2014	2015
Cigarettes																
All 12th graders	30.5	30.1	29.4	33.5	31.4	23.2	21.6	21.6	20.4	20.1	19.2	18.7	17.1	16.3	13.6	11.4
Male	26.8	28.2	29.1	34.5	32.8	24.8	22.4	23.1	21.5	22.1	21.9	21.5	19.3	18.4	15.2	13.0
Female	33.4	31.4	29.2	32.0	29.7	20.7	20.1	19.6	19.1	17.6	15.7	15.1	14.5	13.2	11.6	9.1
White	31.0	31.7	32.5	37.3	36.6	27.0	24.7	25.2	24.1	23.7	22.2	22.2	20.1	18.5	16.5	13.4
Black or African American	25.2	18.7	12.0	15.0	13.6	10.0	11.0	10.6	10.1	9.3	10.7	8.7	8.4	10.8	7.5	6.4
All 10th graders	NA	NA	NA	27.9	23.9	14.9	14.5	14.0	12.3	13.1	13.6	11.8	10.8	9.1	7.2	6.3
Male	NA	NA	NA	27.7	23.8	14.5	13.4	14.6	12.7	13.7	15.0	13.4	12.0	10.5	7.7	6.1
Female	NA	NA	NA	27.9	23.6	15.1	15.5	13.3	11.9	12.5	12.1	10.0	9.6	7.5	6.6	6.3
White	NA	NA	NA	31.2	27.3	17.0	16.3	16.1	14.1	14.6	14.8	13.7	12.2	10.4	8.5	7.3
Black or African American	NA	NA	NA	12.2	11.3	7.7	8.5	5.8	7.1	6.4	7.0	7.2	6.2	4.2	4.2	3.5
All 8th graders	NA	NA	NA	19.1	14.6	9.3	8.7	7.1	6.8	6.5	7.1	6.1	4.9	4.5	4.0	3.6
Male	NA	NA	NA	18.8	14.3	8.7	8.1	7.5	6.7	6.7	7.4	6.2	4.6	4.0	3.5	3.3
Female	NA	NA	NA	19.0	14.7	9.7	8.9	6.4	6.7	6.0	6.8	5.7	4.9	4.7	4.2	3.7
White	NA	NA	NA	21.7	16.4	9.5	9.1	7.1	7.3	7.3	7.9	6.5	5.0	4.3	4.6	3.8
Black or African American	NA	NA	NA	8.2	8.4	6.7	5.4	4.8	4.4	4.5	4.0	4.2	3.8	3.3	2.0	2.4
E-Cigarettes																
All 12th graders	NA	NA	NA	NA	NA	NA	NA	NA	NA	NA	NA	NA	NA	NA	17.1	16.2
Male	NA	NA	NA	NA	NA	NA	NA	NA	NA	NA	NA	NA	NA	NA	20.1	21.5
Female	NA	NA	NA	NA	NA	NA	NA	NA	NA	NA	NA	NA	NA	NA	13.7	10.9
White	NA	NA	NA	NA	NA	NA	NA	NA	NA	NA	NA	NA	NA	NA	19.5	19.0
Black or African American	NA	NA	NA	NA	NA	NA	NA	NA	NA	NA	NA	NA	NA	NA	7.1	7.4
All 10th graders	NA	NA	NA	NA	NA	NA	NA	NA	NA	NA	NA	NA	NA	NA	16.2	14.0
Male	NA	NA	NA	NA	NA	NA	NA	NA	NA	NA	NA	NA	NA	NA	19.2	15.9
Female	NA	NA	NA	NA	NA	NA	NA	NA	NA	NA	NA	NA	NA	NA	13.1	12.0
White	NA	NA	NA	NA	NA	NA	NA	NA	NA	NA	NA	NA	NA	NA	16.8	15.7
Black or African American	NA	NA	NA	NA	NA	NA	NA	NA	NA	NA	NA	NA	NA	NA	9.8	8.3
All 8th graders	NA	NA	NA	NA	NA	NA	NA	NA	NA	NA	NA	NA	NA	NA	8.7	9.5
Male	NA	NA	NA	NA	NA	NA	NA	NA	NA	NA	NA	NA	NA	NA	9.8	10.2
Female	NA	NA	NA	NA	NA	NA	NA	NA	NA	NA	NA	NA	NA	NA	7.1	8.6
White	NA	NA	NA	NA	NA	NA	NA	NA	NA	NA	NA	NA	NA	NA	7.3	8.8
Black or African American	NA	NA	NA	NA	NA	NA	NA	NA	NA	NA	NA	NA	NA	NA	5.1	6.9
Marijuana																
All 12th graders	33.7	25.7	14.0	21.2	21.6	19.8	18.3	18.8	19.4	20.6	21.4	22.6	22.9	22.7	21.2	21.3
Male	37.8	28.7	16.1	24.6	24.7	23.6	19.7	22.3	22.2	24.3	25.2	26.4	26.5	26.4	24.3	23.1
Female	29.1	22.4	11.5	17.2	18.3	15.8	16.4	15.0	16.2	16.8	16.9	18.4	18.8	18.7	17.9	19.2
White	34.2	26.4	15.6	21.5	22.0	21.7	19.2	19.9	20.4	21.2	21.6	22.9	22.3	21.3	21.4	20.6
Black or African American	26.5	21.7	5.2	17.8	17.5	15.1	16.7	15.4	17.1	20.6	19.7	22.2	22.4	25.7	20.7	20.9
All 10th graders	NA	NA	NA	17.2	19.7	15.2	14.2	14.2	13.8	15.9	16.7	17.6	17.0	18.0	16.6	14.8
Male	NA	NA	NA	19.2	23.3	16.7	15.7	15.8	15.2	18.7	20.1	20.8	19.8	20.6	17.4	15.6
Female	NA	NA	NA	15.0	16.2	13.4	12.6	12.5	12.3	13.2	13.3	14.5	14.4	15.3	15.7	13.7
White	NA	NA	NA	17.7	20.1	15.7	14.7	14.8	13.5	15.6	15.9	16.9	16.6	16.5	15.8	13.7
Black or African American	NA	NA	NA	15.1	17.0	13.5	14.2	11.0	12.3	15.1	15.9	20.0	17.6	20.7	17.4	17.5
All 8th graders	NA	NA	NA	9.1	9.1	6.6	6.5	5.7	5.8	6.5	8.0	7.2	6.5	7.0	6.5	6.5
Male	NA	NA	NA	9.8	10.2	7.6	6.7	6.2	6.6	7.5	9.2	8.5	7.0	6.7	6.9	6.6
Female	NA	NA	NA	8.2	7.8	5.7	6.0	4.9	4.8	5.3	6.8	5.7	6.0	7.2	5.9	6.2
White	NA	NA	NA	9.0	8.3	6.0	5.7	5.1	4.9	5.9	7.1	5.9	4.7	4.8	4.7	4.5
Black or African American	NA	NA	NA	7.0	8.5	8.2	6.7	6.0	6.2	7.2	8.2	8.0	7.1	9.3	6.5	7.9
Cocaine																
All 12th graders	5.2	6.7	1.9	1.8	2.1	2.3	2.5	2.0	1.9	1.3	1.3	1.1	1.1	1.1	1.0	1.1
Male	6.0	7.7	2.3	2.2	2.7	2.6	3.0	2.4	2.3	1.5	1.9	1.5	1.5	1.4	1.5	1.4
Female	4.3	5.6	1.3	1.3	1.6	1.8	2.1	1.5	1.3	0.9	0.7	0.7	0.6	0.5	0.5	0.8
White	5.4	7.0	1.8	1.7	2.2	2.3	2.6	2.3	2.0	1.2	1.2	1.2	1.0	0.7	0.8	1.0
Black or African American	2.0	2.7	0.5	0.4	1.0	0.5	1.0	0.5	0.5	0.2	0.9	0.8	0.5	0.6	1.4	0.4
All 10th graders	NA	NA	NA	1.7	1.8	1.5	1.5	1.3	1.2	0.9	0.9	0.7	0.8	0.8	0.6	0.8
Male	NA	NA	NA	1.8	2.1	1.9	1.6	1.4	1.4	1.0	1.1	0.8	0.8	1.2	0.8	0.9
Female	NA	NA	NA	1.5	1.4	1.2	1.3	1.1	1.0	0.8	0.5	0.5	0.7	0.5	0.4	0.6
White	NA	NA	NA	1.7	1.7	1.5	1.5	1.2	1.0	0.7	0.7	0.5	0.5	0.6	0.5	0.7
Black or African American	NA	NA	NA	0.4	0.4	0.8	0.7	0.4	0.7	0.5	0.6	0.6	1.2	0.9	0.5	0.7
All 8th graders	NA	NA	NA	1.2	1.2	1.0	1.0	0.9	0.8	0.8	0.6	0.8	0.5	0.5	0.5	0.5
Male	NA	NA	NA	1.1	1.3	0.9	1.0	0.7	0.9	0.8	0.6	0.7	0.5	0.4	0.5	0.5
Female	NA	NA	NA	1.2	1.1	1.0	0.9	1.0	0.7	0.7	0.6	0.7	0.4	0.5	0.4	0.4
White	NA	NA	NA	1.0	1.1	0.9	0.8	0.6	0.6	0.6	0.5	0.5	0.3	0.4	0.2	0.3
Black or African American	NA	NA	NA	0.4	0.5	0.3	0.4	0.6	0.4	0.7	0.3	0.5	0.5	0.5	0.4	0.5
Inhalants																
All 12th graders	1.4	2.2	2.7	3.2	2.2	2.0	1.5	1.2	1.4	1.2	1.4	1.0	0.9	1.0	0.7	0.7
Male	1.8	2.8	3.5	3.9	2.9	2.4	1.5	1.5	1.6	1.2	2.1	1.1	0.9	1.2	1.0	0.8
Female	1.0	1.7	2.0	2.5	1.7	1.6	1.4	0.9	1.2	1.0	0.7	0.9	0.8	0.7	0.5	0.6
White	1.4	2.4	3.0	3.7	2.1	2.1	1.5	1.2	1.5	1.1	1.1	0.9	0.6	0.6	0.6	0.5
Black or African American	1.0	0.8	1.5	1.1	2.1	1.4	1.2	0.9	1.0	1.1	1.5	1.3	0.9	1.3	1.4	0.8

NA = Not available.

Table 3-29. Use of Selected Substances Among 12th Graders, 10th Graders, and 8th Graders, by Sex and Race, Selected Years, 1980–2015—Continued

(Percent.)

Substance, grade in school, sex, and race	1980	1985	1990	1995	2000	2005	2006	2007	2008	2009	2010	2011	2012	2013	2014	2015
All 10th graders	NA	NA	NA	3.5	2.6	2.2	2.3	2.5	2.1	2.2	2.0	1.7	1.4	1.3	1.1	1.2
Male	NA	NA	NA	3.8	3.0	1.9	2.2	2.7	1.9	1.8	1.6	1.5	1.2	1.4	0.9	1.1
Female	NA	NA	NA	3.2	2.2	2.5	2.4	2.4	2.3	2.6	2.4	2.0	1.6	1.3	1.2	1.2
White	NA	NA	NA	3.9	2.8	2.2	2.4	2.6	1.6	1.9	1.7	1.4	1.1	1.0	0.9	0.8
Black or African American	NA	NA	NA	1.2	1.5	1.4	1.8	1.5	1.9	1.3	1.8	1.6	1.2	1.9	1.4	1.4
All 8th graders	NA	NA	NA	6.1	4.5	4.2	4.1	3.9	4.1	3.8	3.6	3.2	2.7	2.3	2.2	2.0
Male	NA	NA	NA	5.6	4.1	3.1	3.6	3.4	2.9	3.3	2.8	2.5	1.9	1.6	1.6	1.8
Female	NA	NA	NA	6.6	4.8	5.3	4.7	4.3	5.3	4.3	4.4	3.9	3.4	2.9	2.6	2.1
White	NA	NA	NA	7.0	4.8	4.0	4.2	3.6	3.8	3.7	3.2	2.7	2.1	1.7	1.7	1.6
Black or African American	NA	NA	NA	2.3	2.3	2.9	2.7	2.8	2.8	3.4	2.2	2.8	3.0	2.4	2.4	2.1
MDMA (Ecstasy)[1]																
All 12th graders	NA	NA	NA	NA	3.6	1.0	1.3	1.6	1.8	1.8	1.4	2.3	0.9	1.5	1.5	1.1
Male	NA	NA	NA	NA	4.1	1.0	1.5	1.5	2.3	2.4	1.5	2.8	1.2	2.1	2.2	1.2
Female	NA	NA	NA	NA	3.1	1.0	1.1	1.6	1.2	1.2	1.2	1.8	0.6	0.9	0.9	1.0
White	NA	NA	NA	NA	3.9	1.0	1.4	1.7	1.7	1.7	0.9	2.1	0.9	1.5	0.7	1.0
Black or African American	NA	NA	NA	NA	1.9	0.9	0.6	0.8	1.1	1.8	1.1	1.1	0.4	0.7	2.6	1.2
All 10th graders	NA	NA	NA	NA	2.6	1.0	1.2	1.2	1.1	1.3	1.9	1.6	1.0	1.2	1.1	0.9
Male	NA	NA	NA	NA	2.5	1.0	1.5	1.3	1.6	1.6	2.3	1.7	1.1	1.5	1.4	1.0
Female	NA	NA	NA	NA	2.5	0.9	0.8	1.1	0.7	1.0	1.5	1.3	1.0	1.0	0.9	0.6
White	NA	NA	NA	NA	2.5	1.0	1.3	1.4	1.0	1.0	1.5	1.1	1.0	0.9	1.3	0.8
Black or African American	NA	NA	NA	NA	1.8	0.3	1.0	0.4	0.1	0.6	1.1	1.1	1.1	0.4	1.3	0.7
All 8th graders	NA	NA	NA	NA	1.4	0.6	0.7	0.6	0.8	0.6	1.1	0.6	0.5	0.5	0.7	0.5
Male	NA	NA	NA	NA	1.6	0.8	0.5	0.7	0.7	0.5	1.2	0.7	0.4	0.4	1.0	0.4
Female	NA	NA	NA	NA	1.2	0.4	0.8	0.6	0.9	0.6	1.1	0.5	0.6	0.5	0.5	0.5
White	NA	NA	NA	NA	1.4	0.6	0.5	0.5	0.7	0.6	1.0	0.4	0.4	0.3	0.6	0.4
Black or African American	NA	NA	NA	NA	0.8	0.9	0.7	0.8	0.3	0.1	0.5	0.2	0.5	0.6	0.7	0.3
Alcohol[2]																
All 12th graders	72.0	65.9	57.1	51.3	50.0	47.0	45.3	44.4	43.1	43.5	41.2	40.0	41.5	39.2	37.4	35.3
Male	77.4	69.8	61.3	55.7	54.0	50.7	47.3	47.1	45.8	47.8	44.2	42.1	43.8	41.8	37.4	36.0
Female	66.8	62.1	52.3	47.0	46.1	43.3	43.0	41.4	40.9	38.9	37.9	37.5	38.8	36.3	37.1	35.0
White	75.8	70.2	62.2	54.8	55.3	52.2	49.1	49.4	47.8	46.6	44.1	43.4	44.3	42.8	42.1	39.7
Black or African American	47.7	43.6	32.9	37.4	29.3	28.8	29.5	27.9	29.3	32.2	30.8	29.4	29.8	27.0	24.9	23.2
All 10th graders	NA	NA	NA	38.8	41.0	33.2	33.8	33.4	28.8	30.4	28.9	27.2	27.6	25.7	23.5	21.5
Male	NA	NA	NA	39.7	43.3	32.8	33.8	33.4	28.6	31.0	30.1	28.2	28.0	26.0	23.0	20.6
Female	NA	NA	NA	37.8	38.6	33.6	33.8	33.3	29.0	29.8	27.7	26.0	27.1	25.3	23.9	22.5
White	NA	NA	NA	41.3	44.3	36.7	36.0	35.7	30.5	32.4	29.2	28.9	29.2	26.9	25.9	23.6
Black or African American	NA	NA	NA	24.9	24.7	20.8	22.4	21.0	20.4	20.1	21.3	20.3	20.1	17.7	15.5	14.8
All 8th graders	NA	NA	NA	24.6	22.4	17.1	17.2	15.9	15.9	14.9	13.8	12.7	11.0	10.2	9.0	9.7
Male	NA	NA	NA	25.0	22.5	16.2	16.3	15.6	15.4	14.7	13.2	12.1	10.3	9.3	8.2	9.1
Female	NA	NA	NA	24.0	22.0	17.9	17.6	16.0	16.4	14.9	14.3	12.8	11.5	11.2	9.5	9.9
White	NA	NA	NA	25.4	23.9	17.3	16.5	14.7	15.8	15.1	12.8	11.8	9.6	9.4	8.7	9.2
Black or African American	NA	NA	NA	17.3	15.1	13.9	12.4	12.3	13.5	11.1	12.7	10.5	9.4	9.9	7.9	8.5
Binge Drinking[3]																
All 12th graders	41.2	36.7	32.2	29.8	30.0	27.1	25.4	25.9	24.6	NA	NA	NA	NA	NA	19.4	17.2
Male	52.1	45.3	39.1	36.9	36.7	32.6	28.9	30.7	28.4	30.5	28.0	25.5	27.2	26.1	22.3	19.3
Female	30.5	28.2	24.4	23.0	23.5	21.6	21.5	21.5	21.3	20.2	18.4	17.6	19.7	18.1	16.6	14.9
White	44.6	40.1	36.2	32.9	34.4	31.8	28.9	30.5	29.3	28.7	26.5	25.3	26.2	25.0	22.5	19.8
Black or African American	17.0	16.7	11.6	15.5	11.0	10.9	11.9	11.0	10.8	13.7	12.6	10.0	13.0	12.0	10.6	9.1
All 10th graders	NA	NA	NA	22.0	24.1	19.0	19.9	19.6	16.0	17.5	16.3	14.7	15.6	13.7	12.6	10.9
Male	NA	NA	NA	24.1	27.6	19.9	21.0	20.9	16.6	18.8	17.9	16.5	16.4	14.7	13.1	11.3
Female	NA	NA	NA	19.7	20.6	17.9	18.9	18.3	15.4	16.1	14.6	12.7	14.8	12.5	12.2	10.6
White	NA	NA	NA	24.1	26.6	21.5	21.8	21.7	17.4	18.4	16.0	16.1	16.5	14.7	14.1	12.1
Black or African American	NA	NA	NA	9.6	10.6	8.4	9.9	10.0	9.6	10.0	11.5	7.3	9.3	7.9	7.2	6.6
All 8th graders	NA	NA	NA	12.3	11.7	8.4	8.7	8.3	8.1	7.8	7.2	6.4	5.1	5.1	4.1	4.6
Male	NA	NA	NA	12.5	11.7	8.2	8.6	8.2	8.1	7.8	6.5	6.1	4.6	4.5	3.5	4.6
Female	NA	NA	NA	12.1	11.3	8.6	8.5	8.2	8.0	7.7	7.8	6.5	5.5	5.7	4.6	4.6
White	NA	NA	NA	12.6	12.5	8.4	8.4	7.7	8.0	7.4	6.7	5.8	3.9	4.6	3.7	4.2
Black or African American	NA	NA	NA	7.8	6.2	5.8	5.5	5.7	5.7	4.8	5.9	4.4	4.2	4.8	4.1	4.1

NA = Not available.
[1]Starting in 2014, a revised question on the use of MDMA (ecstasy) including "Molly," a nickname for MDMA, was added to the questionnaire for each grade. The 2014 and 2015 data reported here are only for the revised question, which includes "Molly."
[2]In 1993, the alcohol question was changed to indicate that a drink meant more than a few sips.
[3]Five or more alcoholic drinks in a row at least once in the prior 2-week period.

AMBULATORY CARE

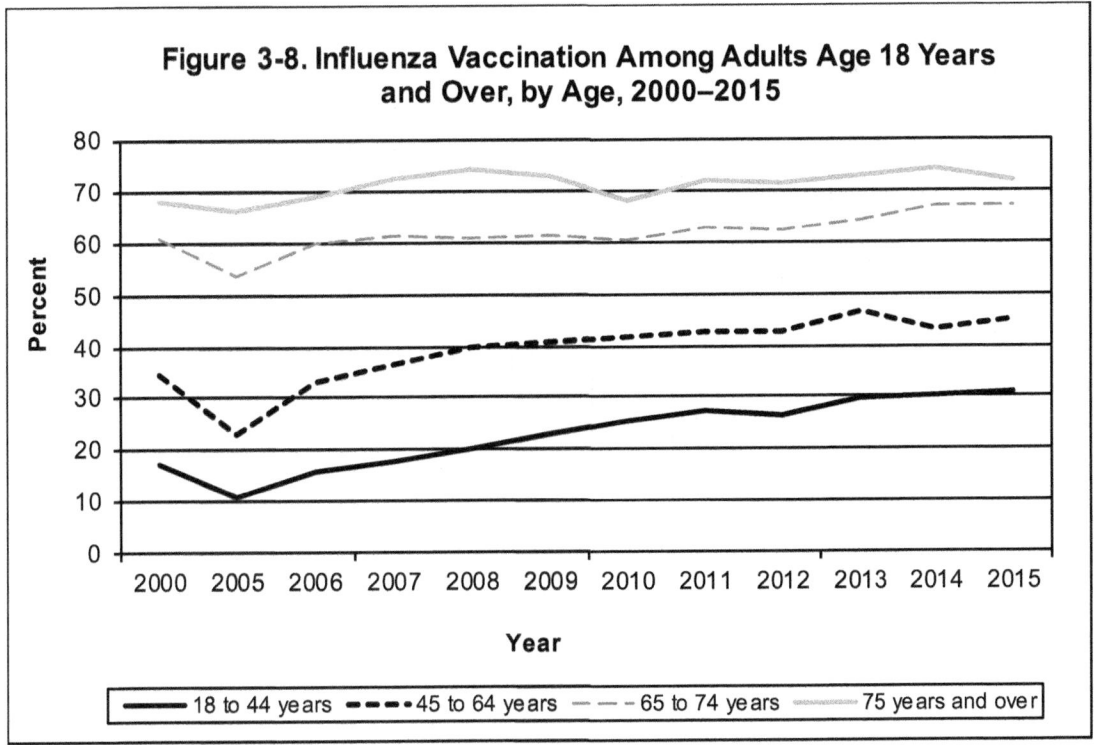

Figure 3-8. Influenza Vaccination Among Adults Age 18 Years and Over, by Age, 2000–2015

Table 3-30. No Usual Source of Health Care Among Children Under 18 Years of Age, by Selected Characteristics, Annual Average, Selected Years, 1993–1994 Through 2014–2015

(Percent.)

Characteristic	Under 18 years				Under 6 years				6 to 17 years			
	1993–1994[1]	1999–2000	2009–2010	2014–2015	1993–1994[1]	1999–2000	2009–2010	2014–2015	1993–1994[1]	1999–2000	2009–2010	2014–2015
Percent of Children without a Usual Source of Health Care[2]												
All Children[3]	7.7	6.9	5.4	4.0	5.2	4.6	4.1	2.7	9.0	8.0	6.2	4.6
Sex												
Male	8.1	6.7	5.5	3.9	5.3	4.5	4.2	2.4	9.6	7.8	6.1	4.6
Female	7.3	7.1	5.4	4.1	5.0	4.7	4.0	3.0	8.5	8.2	6.2	4.6
Race[4]												
White only	7.0	6.3	5.3	3.7	4.7	4.4	3.8	2.4	8.3	7.2	6.1	4.3
Black or African American only	10.3	7.7	5.6	4.8	7.6	4.4	4.3	4.0	11.9	9.1	6.3	5.1
American Indian or Alaska Native only	*9.3	*9.4	*	*	*	*	*	*	*8.7	*9.4	*9.2	*
Asian only	9.7	10.0	6.1	5.0	*3.4	*5.8	*3.9	*4.2	13.5	12.2	7.3	5.4
Native Hawaiian or Other Pacific Islander only	NA	*	*	*	NA	*	*	*	NA	*	*	*
Two or more races	NA	*4.9	4.6	4.8	NA	*	*4.2	*3.3	NA	*7.2	*4.9	5.8
Hispanic Origin and Race[4]												
Hispanic or Latino	14.3	14.2	9.5	6.2	9.3	9.0	5.8	3.9	17.7	17.2	11.8	7.5
Not Hispanic or Latino	6.7	5.5	4.3	3.3	4.4	3.6	3.5	2.3	7.8	6.3	4.7	3.7
White only	5.7	4.7	3.8	2.6	3.7	3.3	2.9	1.7	6.7	5.4	4.1	3.0
Black or African American only	10.2	7.6	5.4	4.5	7.7	4.5	4.3	3.8	11.6	9.0	6.0	4.8
Percent of Poverty Level[5]												
Below 100 percent	13.9	13.1	8.3	6.5	9.4	7.6	6.6	4.4	16.8	16.2	9.3	7.6
100 percent to 199 percent	9.8	10.6	7.5	5.4	6.7	7.5	4.8	3.7	11.6	12.2	9.0	6.2
200 percent to 399 percent	3.7	4.8	4.7	3.4	1.9	3.2	*3.1	2.3	4.5	5.6	5.5	3.9
400 percent or more	3.7	2.6	2.1	1.4	*1.6	1.5	*1.9	*0.8	5.0	3.0	2.2	1.7
Hispanic Origin and Race and Percent of Poverty Level[4,5]												
Hispanic or Latino												
Below 100 percent	19.6	19.4	10.7	7.6	12.7	11.6	7.1	*4.8	24.8	24.5	13.4	9.3
100 percent to 199 percent	15.3	17.1	10.6	6.9	9.9	11.3	6.3	*4.0	18.9	20.4	13.2	8.3
200 percent to 399 percent	5.2	8.3	8.5	5.0	*	*5.0	*4.1	*3.5	6.7	10.1	10.9	5.8
400 percent or more	*	*3.8	*3.6	*2.4	*	*	*	*	*	*5.0	*4.1	*3.0
Not Hispanic or Latino												
White only												
Below 100 percent	10.2	10.7	6.1	4.9	6.5	*6.3	*5.0	*	12.7	13.1	*6.8	*5.4
100 percent to 199 percent	8.7	7.8	5.7	4.0	6.3	5.7	*4.0	*3.2	10.1	8.8	6.6	4.5
200 percent to 399 percent	3.3	4.0	3.7	2.6	1.6	2.7	*	*1.3	4.0	4.6	4.2	3.3
400 percent or more	4.0	2.3	2.1	1.1	*1.7	*1.5	*1.9	*	5.4	2.6	2.1	1.4
Black or African American only												
Below 100 percent	13.7	9.4	6.3	5.0	10.9	*4.7	*6.2	*4.8	15.5	11.8	6.4	5.1
100 percent to 199 percent	9.1	9.7	6.2	5.3	*6.0	*6.4	*	*	10.8	11.2	8.1	6.1
200 percent to 399 percent	5.0	5.0	5.1	*4.1	*	*	*	*	6.2	5.7	5.4	*4.2
400 percent or more	*	*3.5	*	*	*	*	*	*	*	*4.0	*	*
Health Insurance Status at the Time of Interview[6]												
Insured	5.0	3.9	3.4	2.8	3.3	2.6	2.8	2.1	5.9	4.5	3.7	3.1
Private	3.8	3.4	2.6	2.1	1.9	2.2	1.7	1.5	4.6	3.9	3.0	2.3
Medicaid	8.9	5.3	4.4	3.7	6.4	3.5	3.7	2.8	11.3	6.7	4.9	4.3
Uninsured	23.5	29.3	28.8	27.9	18.0	20.8	21.4	20.3	26.0	32.9	31.5	30.3
Health Insurance Status Prior to Interview[6]												
Insured continuously all 12 months	4.6	3.6	3.2	2.5	3.1	2.3	2.7	1.9	5.5	4.2	3.4	2.8
Uninsured for any period up to 12 months	15.3	15.0	11.7	13.5	10.9	12.5	10.4	10.8	18.1	16.4	12.4	14.8
Uninsured more than 12 months	27.6	35.8	36.2	34.9	21.4	26.8	27.5	*23.5	30.0	39.1	38.5	37.5
Geographic Region												
Northeast				1.7				*1.4				1.8
Midwest	8.6	5.7	4.5	3.5	5.8	*2.7	4.1	2.7	10.7	7.5	4.7	3.8
South	21.7	19.8	*14.7	4.5	18.0	*16.0	*14.0	3.0	23.7	21.9	*15.2	5.3
West	31.2	42.7	43.0	5.1	25.5	31.0	41.9	3.1	33.4	47.1	43.3	6.1
Location of Residence												
Within MSA[7]	7.7	6.8	5.5	4.0	5.0	4.7	4.2	2.7	9.2	7.8	6.2	4.7
Outside MSA[7]	7.8	7.4	5.0	3.8	6.0	4.2	3.3	3.1	8.7	8.7	5.8	4.1

NA = Not available.

* = Figure does not meet standards of reliability or precision. Data preceded by an asterisk have a relative standard error (RSE) of 20 percent to 30 percent. Data not shown have an RSE of greater than 30 percent.

[1]Data prior to 1997 are not strictly comparable with data for later years due to the 1997 questionnaire redesign.

[2]Persons who report the emergency department as their usual source of care are defined as having no usual source of care.

[3]Includes all other races not shown separately and unknown health insurance status.

[4]The race groups White, Black, American Indian or Alaska Native, Asian, Native Hawaiian or Other Pacific Islander, and two or more races include persons of Hispanic and non-Hispanic origin. Persons of Hispanic origin may be of any race.

[5]Percent of poverty level is based on family income and family size and composition using U.S. Census Bureau poverty thresholds. Missing family income data were imputed starting in 1993.

[6]Health insurance categories are mutually exclusive. Persons who reported both Medicaid and private coverage are classified as having private coverage. Medicaid includes other public assistance through 1996. Starting with 1997 data, state-sponsored health plan coverage is included as Medicaid coverage. Starting with 1999 data, coverage by the Children's Health Insurance Program (CHIP) is included with Medicaid coverage. Persons not covered by private insurance, Medicaid, CHIP, public assistance (through 1996), state-sponsored or other government-sponsored health plans (starting in 1997), Medicare, or military plans are considered to have no health insurance coverage. Persons with only Indian Health Service coverage are considered to have no health insurance coverage. Health insurance status was unknown for 8 to 9 percent of children in 1993-1996 and about 1 percent in 1997-2015.

[7]MSA = metropolitan statistical area.

Table 3-31. No Usual Source of Health Care Among Adults 18 to 64 Years of Age, by Selected Characteristics, Annual Average, Selected Years, 1993–1994 Through 2014–2015

(Percent.)

Characteristic	1993 to 1994[1]	1995 to 1996[1]	1997 to 1998	1999 to 2000	2001 to 2002	2003 to 2004	2004 to 2005	2005 to 2006	2006 to 2007	2007 to 2008	2008 to 2009	2009 to 2010	2010 to 2011	2011 to 2012	2012 to 2013	2014 to 2015
PERCENT OF ADULTS WITHOUT A USUAL SOURCE OF HEALTH CARE[2]																
Total, 18 to 64 years[3]...............................	18.9	16.9	17.7	17.8	16.4	17.3	18.0	18.4	18.5	18.5	19.5	20.3	19.6	19.5	19.7	17.3
Age																
18 to 44 years......................................	21.7	19.6	21.1	21.6	20.6	21.7	22.8	23.5	23.5	23.6	25.0	26.0	25.2	25.0	25.4	22.5
18 to 24 years..................................	26.6	22.6	27.0	27.2	27.2	28.0	29.9	29.8	28.7	28.6	29.6	29.8	28.1	27.8	28.7	24.2
19 to 25 years..................................	28.0	24.2	28.6	29.0	28.5	29.7	31.3	31.8	30.9	30.0	32.0	33.1	30.9	30.3	30.8	26.9
25 to 44 years..................................	20.3	18.8	19.3	19.9	18.5	19.5	20.3	21.3	21.8	21.8	23.4	24.7	24.1	23.9	24.2	21.9
45 to 64 years......................................	12.8	11.3	11.2	10.9	9.2	10.4	10.6	10.7	11.2	11.0	11.6	12.3	11.8	12.0	12.0	10.2
45 to 54 years..................................	14.1	12.2	12.6	12.0	10.3	11.7	11.9	12.3	13.3	13.1	13.6	14.7	14.0	14.2	14.0	12.1
55 to 64 years..................................	11.1	9.8	9.0	9.2	7.6	8.7	8.8	8.4	8.3	8.3	9.0	9.3	9.0	9.6	9.6	8.1
Sex																
Male..	23.9	21.4	23.6	24.1	21.6	22.5	23.3	23.9	23.9	23.9	25.3	25.9	24.6	24.4	24.5	22.3
Female	14.1	12.6	12.0	11.8	11.4	12.4	12.9	13.0	13.3	13.1	13.8	14.8	14.7	14.8	15.1	12.4
Race[3]																
White only..	18.4	16.5	17.0	16.7	15.4	17.0	17.7	18.1	18.3	18.0	18.9	19.7	18.9	18.9	19.2	17.0
Black or African American only....................	20.0	18.3	19.4	19.2	16.9	18.4	19.3	19.8	19.8	20.5	21.5	22.4	22.5	21.9	21.4	18.0
American Indian or Alaska Native only............	19.7	16.5	21.3	19.2	16.3	21.5	22.8	21.9	24.4	24.4	24.8	26.7	22.4	23.6	26.6	20.1
Asian only...	24.8	21.5	21.7	22.1	20.1	19.3	18.8	17.9	17.3	17.8	19.4	20.8	20.8	20.8	19.9	17.5
Native Hawaiian or Other Pacific Islander only..................	NA	NA	NA	*	*	*	*	*	*	*	*	*	*	*	*	*
Two or more races...................................	NA	NA	NA	21.0	20.1	18.4	18.1	20.9	20.4	21.4	26.1	27.5	24.4	22.3	23.5	23.1
American Indian or Alaska Native; White	NA	NA	NA	25.8	18.1	17.8	19.1	21.4	19.3	20.9	25.9	27.1	23.9	19.0	19.7	23.9
Hispanic Origin and Race[4]																
Hispanic or Latino...................................	30.3	27.4	30.4	32.6	32.5	32.9	34.0	35.1	34.3	32.5	32.8	33.3	33.3	33.6	32.6	26.2
Mexican..	32.4	29.8	35.9	36.5	36.5	36.4	37.8	39.3	39.0	36.6	36.1	35.7	35.2	35.6	34.5	27.5
Not Hispanic or Latino...............................	17.7	15.7	16.2	15.8	14.0	14.9	15.4	15.6	15.9	16.0	17.1	17.9	17.0	16.8	17.1	15.4
White only..	17.1	15.0	15.4	14.9	13.1	14.0	14.6	14.8	15.2	15.1	16.0	16.8	15.8	15.5	16.0	14.6
Black or African American only.....................	19.7	18.1	19.3	19.2	16.8	18.1	19.0	19.2	18.9	20.2	21.4	22.2	22.1	21.6	21.3	18.0
Percent of Poverty Level[5]																
Below 100 percent...................................	29.5	26.1	29.1	29.6	29.3	28.9	31.8	32.1	30.6	30.4	32.7	33.8	32.8	32.1	32.9	27.3
100 percent to 199 percent........................	25.4	22.9	25.6	27.1	25.6	26.6	27.1	27.8	28.6	29.1	30.3	30.5	30.4	30.2	29.4	24.2
200 percent to 399 percent........................	15.6	13.4	16.6	17.2	16.0	17.3	17.9	17.8	18.5	18.9	19.7	20.5	19.3	19.3	19.3	18.1
400 percent or more................................	13.4	13.8	11.6	11.6	9.6	10.1	10.3	10.4	10.4	10.2	10.6	10.8	9.7	9.6	10.1	9.9
Hispanic Origin and Race and Percent of Poverty Level[4,5]																
Hispanic or Latino...................................																
Below 100 percent	40.0	34.3	42.8	44.4	46.3	42.8	44.5	46.7	46.7	43.7	44.1	45.5	44.3	42.9	43.5	35.4
100 percent to 199 percent.....................	36.9	32.9	35.4	40.6	40.0	39.7	40.7	41.8	42.1	40.6	40.7	39.7	40.4	40.0	37.7	30.1
200 percent to 399 percent.....................	20.7	19.5	23.6	26.9	27.9	28.2	30.1	31.2	29.5	28.0	27.9	29.1	28.9	29.4	28.8	23.3
400 percent or more.............................	13.8	16.3	14.4	16.1	13.7	16.4	16.2	16.4	15.9	16.9	16.6	14.0	13.4	15.4	15.1	13.1
Not Hispanic or Latino...............................																
White only..																
Below 100 percent	28.2	23.6	25.0	24.2	23.4	23.0	26.8	26.2	25.0	25.2	27.8	28.8	27.5	27.0	28.9	24.2
100 percent to 199 percent..................	23.3	20.7	22.4	23.0	20.7	22.0	22.8	23.5	24.5	24.9	26.0	26.6	26.0	25.7	25.5	22.2
200 percent to 399 percent..................	14.8	12.5	15.4	15.3	13.6	15.4	15.6	15.3	16.2	16.7	17.7	18.6	17.2	16.9	16.8	16.4
400 percent or more..........................	13.4	13.7	11.3	11.2	9.1	9.4	9.6	9.8	10.0	9.5	9.9	10.3	9.1	8.8	9.5	9.4
Black or African American only....................																
Below 100 percent	24.7	21.9	23.9	23.7	22.8	24.3	28.3	29.5	26.5	27.1	29.4	30.1	30.3	29.9	28.3	24.8
100 percent to 199 percent..................	22.3	22.1	25.3	24.4	20.4	22.8	22.1	22.6	23.4	25.7	27.6	28.5	29.6	28.2	27.3	20.3
200 percent to 399 percent..................	16.5	14.5	17.6	18.2	16.2	16.3	16.6	16.2	18.0	19.7	19.9	20.1	18.1	18.5	19.7	17.8
400 percent or more..........................	11.7	12.6	11.2	12.0	9.6	11.3	11.3	10.3	9.1	10.2	11.2	10.5	10.6	10.1	9.7	9.0
Health Insurance Status at the Time of Interview[6]																
Insured...	13.3	11.4	11.4	10.9	9.1	9.4	9.7	9.7	9.9	9.9	10.1	10.4	10.6	10.2	10.5	10.9	11.2
Private..	13.1	11.3	11.5	11.1	9.0	9.5	9.5	9.6	9.8	10.0	10.3	10.6	10.1	10.1	10.6	11.1
Medicaid..	16.3	13.0	10.3	9.9	11.1	9.9	12.1	11.6	11.5	11.7	12.1	12.5	12.3	13.1	13.2	13.1
Uninsured	43.1	41.8	46.7	49.2	49.1	50.2	52.5	53.0	52.8	52.1	54.1	55.6	54.2	54.1	54.2	52.6
Health Insurance Status Prior to Interview[6]																
Insured continuously all 12 months...............	12.7	10.8	10.6	10.3	8.3	8.7	8.9	8.9	9.0	9.1	9.5	9.8	9.3	9.6	10.0	10.0

NA = Not available.
* = Figure does not meet standards of reliability or precision. Data not shown have an RSE of greater than 30 percent.
[1]Data prior to 1997 are not strictly comparable with data for later years due to the 1997 questionnaire redesign.
[2]Persons who report the emergency department as their usual source of care are defined as having no usual source of care.
[3]Includes all other races not shown separately, unknown health insurance status, and unknown disability status.
[4]The race groups White, Black, American Indian or Alaska Native, Asian, Native Hawaiian or Other Pacific Islander, and two or more races include persons of Hispanic and non-Hispanic origin. Persons of Hispanic origin may be of any race.
[5]Percent of poverty level is based on family income and family size and composition using U.S. Census Bureau poverty thresholds. Missing family income data were imputed starting in 1993.
[6]Health insurance categories are mutually exclusive. Persons who reported both Medicaid and private coverage are classified as having private coverage. Medicaid includes other public assistance through 1996. Starting with 1997 data, state-sponsored health plan coverage is included as Medicaid coverage. Starting with 1999 data, coverage by the Children's Health Insurance Program (CHIP) is included with Medicaid coverage. Persons not covered by private insurance, Medicaid, CHIP, public assistance (through 1996), state-sponsored or other government-sponsored health plans (starting in 1997), Medicare, or military plans are considered to have no health insurance coverage. Persons with only Indian Health Service coverage are considered to have no health insurance coverage. Health insurance status was unknown for 8 to 9 percent of children in 1993-1996 and about 1 percent in 1997-2011.

Table 3-31. No Usual Source of Health Care Among Adults 18 to 64 Years of Age, by Selected Characteristics, Annual Average, Selected Years, 1993–1994 Through 2014–2015—*Continued*

(Percent.)

Characteristic	1993 to 1994[1]	1995 to 1996[1]	1997 to 1998	1999 to 2000	2001 to 2002	2003 to 2004	2004 to 2005	2005 to 2006	2006 to 2007	2007 to 2008	2008 to 2009	2009 to 2010	2010 to 2011	2011 to 2012	2012 to 2013	2014 to 2015
Uninsured for any period up to 12 months	30.9	29.6	30.7	31.2	33.3	32.1	34.0	33.4	33.6	35.1	36.7	36.5	33.6	33.2	34.1	32.4
Uninsured more than 12 months	46.9	44.8	51.4	54.8	54.6	55.0	57.4	58.0	57.9	56.1	57.2	59.5	58.3	57.8	57.9	56.9
Percent of Poverty Level and Health Insurance Status Prior to Interview[5,6]																
Below 100 percent	16.7	13.3	13.1	11.6	11.5	11.2	12.7	12.0	11.6	12.7	13.5	13.0	13.4	14.0	14.3	14.3
Insured continuously all 12 months	33.6	28.5	33.0	31.9	36.5	36.2	39.4	36.5	34.5	37.4	38.9	37.8	36.6	35.6	38.7	34.6
Uninsured for any period up to 12 months	50.1	46.1	54.3	57.1	58.8	57.2	61.6	63.2	62.6	61.1	63.4	65.3	62.6	61.3	62.3	56.1
Uninsured more than 12 months																
100 percent to 199 percent	14.7	12.2	13.0	12.3	11.0	10.5	10.7	10.4	10.5	11.9	13.0	12.5	11.9	12.8	13.0	12.0
Insured continuously all 12 months	30.9	31.1	31.1	34.6	35.1	34.2	37.1	37.8	36.6	35.9	37.1	38.1	37.0	35.9	35.0	31.9
Uninsured for any period up to 12 months	47.6	43.8	51.1	54.9	54.5	55.1	56.0	57.0	58.4	56.8	58.3	58.5	58.2	57.9	56.8	58.6
Uninsured more than 12 months																
200 percent to 399 percent	11.7	9.4	10.6	10.6	8.3	9.4	9.5	9.4	9.5	9.4	9.9	10.6	10.0	10.0	10.4	10.8
Insured continuously all 12 months	29.2	28.3	30.1	29.0	32.0	30.9	31.9	31.3	33.4	36.3	37.0	37.6	33.7	33.2	34.2	32.9
Uninsured for any period up to 12 months	44.5	44.7	50.9	53.6	53.4	54.2	55.6	55.5	55.3	54.2	54.1	56.6	55.4	55.3	56.1	57.2
Uninsured more than 12 months																
400 percent or more	11.8	11.8	9.5	9.3	7.2	7.5	7.4	7.7	7.8	7.5	7.6	7.9	7.3	7.4	8.0	7.9
Insured continuously all 12 months	31.5	32.3	28.6	30.2	30.7	27.5	28.8	28.6	29.1	30.3	33.8	31.2	24.6	25.6	25.9	29.8
Uninsured for any period up to 12 months	36.5	45.5	44.6	51.8	47.0	51.6	56.5	54.2	51.5	47.9	48.1	53.8	52.5	52.9	52.7	51.7
Uninsured more than 12 months																
Disability Measure[7]																
Any basic actions difficulty or complex activity limitation	NA	NA	15.5	14.1	13.2	14.3	15.0	15.2	15.7	16.6	17.1	16.8	16.2	16.5	16.1	14.1
Any basic actions difficulty	NA	NA	15.7	14.1	13.1	14.5	15.2	15.4	15.8	16.5	17.1	16.7	16.2	16.5	15.9	14.1
Any complex activity limitation	NA	NA	13.1	11.6	10.4	10.7	11.5	11.1	12.6	13.6	13.8	13.5	13.1	13.5	13.0	10.9
No disability	NA	NA	18.2	18.8	17.5	18.2	18.8	19.4	19.5	19.1	20.3	21.5	20.7	20.5	20.9	18.4
Geographic Region																
Northeast	14.7	13.4	13.3	12.8	11.9	12.1	11.7	12.2	13.1	12.5	12.9	14.0	13.9	13.1	12.8	11.5
Midwest	16.2	14.7	15.1	17.0	14.1	14.7	15.4	15.8	16.2	16.6	17.3	17.5	16.7	17.1	18.0	16.3
South	21.8	18.7	20.7	19.7	18.3	19.7	21.0	21.4	21.4	21.4	22.5	23.5	22.3	22.2	22.3	19.6
West	21.1	19.9	20.2	20.1	19.9	21.0	21.2	21.1	20.5	20.0	21.8	22.9	22.4	22.8	22.6	18.7
Location of Residence																
Within MSA[8]	19.3	17.3	17.9	18.1	16.6	17.6	18.3	18.7	18.9	18.7	19.5	20.3	19.8	19.8	19.9	17.5
Outside MSA[8]	17.5	15.4	17.0	16.8	15.4	16.2	16.6	16.7	16.5	16.9	19.4	20.4	18.4	17.8	18.4	16.0

NA = Not available.
* = Figure does not meet standards of reliability or precision. Data not shown have an RSE of greater than 30 percent.
[1]Data prior to 1997 are not strictly comparable with data for later years due to the 1997 questionnaire redesign.
[5]Percent of poverty level is based on family income and family size and composition using U.S. Census Bureau poverty thresholds. Missing family income data were imputed starting in 1993.
[6]Health insurance categories are mutually exclusive. Persons who reported both Medicaid and private coverage are classified as having private coverage. Medicaid includes other public assistance through 1996. Starting with 1997 data, state-sponsored health plan coverage is included as Medicaid coverage. Starting with 1999 data, coverage by the Children's Health Insurance Program (CHIP) is included with Medicaid coverage. Persons not covered by private insurance, Medicaid, CHIP, public assistance (through 1996), state-sponsored or other government-sponsored health plans (starting in 1997), Medicare, or military plans are considered to have no health insurance coverage. Persons with only Indian Health Service coverage are considered to have no health insurance coverage. Health insurance status was unknown for 8 to 9 percent of children in 1993-1996 and about 1 percent in 1997-2011.
[7]Any basic actions difficulty or complex activity limitation is defined as having one or more of the following limitations or difficulties: movement difficulty, emotional difficulty, sensory (seeing or hearing) difficulty, cognitive difficulty, self-care (activities of daily living or instrumental activities of daily living) limitation, social limitation, or work limitation.
[8]MSA = metropolitan statistical area.

Table 3-32. Delay or Nonreceipt of Needed Medical Care, Nonreceipt of Needed Prescription Drugs, or Nonreceipt of Needed Dental Care During the Past 12 Months Due to Cost, by Selected Characteristics, Selected Years 1997–2015

(Percent.)

Characteristic	Delay or nonreceipt of needed medical care due to cost[1]				Delay or nonreceipt of needed prescription drugs due to cost[2]				Delay or nonreceipt of needed dental care due to cost[3]			
	1997	2005	2010	2015	1997	2005	2010	2015	1997	2005	2010	2015
TOTAL[4]	8.3	8.5	10.9	7.3	4.8	7.2	8.3	5.2	8.6	10.7	13.5	9.4
Age												
Under 19 years	4.5	4.3	4.5	2.8	2.1	3.0	2.8	1.6	6.0	7.3	6.6	4.1
Under 18 years	4.4	4.2	4.4	2.7	2.2	2.9	2.7	1.6	6.0	7.3	6.6	4.1
Under 6 years	3.3	3.3	3.7	2.2	1.6	2.5	2.5	1.4	3.9	3.7	3.9	1.9
6 to 17 years	4.9	4.7	4.8	2.9	2.4	3.1	2.8	1.7	6.8	8.4	7.5	4.9
18 to 64 years	10.7	11.0	14.7	9.8	6.3	9.4	11.2	6.9	10.6	13.0	17.3	11.8
18 to 44 years	11.0	11.3	14.5	9.5	6.9	9.8	11.2	6.2	11.7	14.1	17.9	11.6
18 to 24 years	10.2	11.3	13.5	7.5	6.7	9.6	9.7	4.5	11.6	13.7	17.4	9.4
25 to 34 years	11.4	11.8	15.3	10.3	6.9	10.2	12.0	6.6	12.3	15.1	18.3	12.4
35 to 44 years	11.0	10.8	14.4	10.1	7.1	9.6	11.3	6.9	11.2	13.3	17.8	12.4
19 to 25 years	11.1	12.5	14.8	8.4	7.7	10.3	10.9	5.5	13.1	14.8	18.9	10.9
45 to 64 years	10.1	10.6	14.9	10.3	5.1	8.7	11.3	8.0	8.4	11.5	16.5	12.1
45 to 54 years	10.6	10.8	15.0	10.3	5.6	9.2	11.5	8.0	9.4	12.1	17.8	12.1
55 to 64 years	9.3	10.4	14.6	10.2	4.2	8.0	11.0	8.0	7.0	10.7	14.9	12.2
65 years and over	4.6	4.6	5.0	4.1	2.8	5.1	4.7	3.9	3.5	5.2	6.9	7.0
65 to 74 years	5.0	5.4	6.3	4.9	3.4	6.4	6.3	4.8	4.2	6.2	9.0	7.8
75 years and over	4.1	3.7	3.4	3.0	2.0	3.6	2.8	2.8	2.6	4.0	4.3	5.8
18 TO 64 YEARS												
Sex												
Male	9.3	10.0	13.5	8.9	5.1	7.2	8.8	5.4	8.8	10.8	15.2	10.0
Female	12.0	12.1	15.7	10.7	7.4	11.4	13.5	8.4	12.4	15.2	19.4	13.6
Race[5]												
White only	10.8	11.1	14.5	9.9	5.9	9.1	10.8	6.5	10.6	12.8	17.1	11.7
Black or African American only	10.8	12.0	17.4	11.0	9.5	11.6	15.6	10.1	10.8	15.2	20.7	13.6
American Indian or Alaska Native only	14.5	13.2	*15.7	9.8	*10.1	*14.1	18.6	*13.4	18.8	19.2	23.1	17.7
Asian only	6.3	5.0	8.0	4.8	*2.8	*3.5	4.2	3.4	7.8	6.8	8.7	7.4
Native Hawaiian or Other Pacific Islander only	NA	*	*	*	NA	*	*	*	NA	*	*	*
Two or more races	NA	19.9	24.0	15.2	NA	22.9	16.6	10.9	NA	23.0	25.6	14.3
Hispanic Origin and Race[5]												
Hispanic or Latino	10.5	11.5	15.4	10.8	6.7	11.2	13.0	8.3	11.5	15.5	21.6	14.5
Mexican origin	9.7	11.4	15.6	11.0	6.5	12.0	13.5	8.6	11.3	16.3	22.0	16.0
Not Hispanic or Latino	10.7	11.0	14.5	9.6	6.3	9.0	10.9	6.6	10.5	12.6	16.6	11.3
White only	10.9	11.1	14.3	9.7	5.9	8.7	10.3	6.1	10.5	12.3	16.2	11.1
Black or African American only	10.8	12.0	17.5	11.1	9.5	11.4	15.6	10.2	10.8	15.3	20.8	13.7
Education[6]												
No high school diploma or GED	16.2	16.2	20.6	14.0	11.5	16.4	18.1	13.9	14.5	20.3	26.3	20.3
High school diploma or GED	11.1	11.7	16.1	11.4	7.0	10.5	13.8	9.2	11.4	14.6	20.1	14.2
Some college or more	9.2	9.8	13.4	9.2	4.3	7.1	9.2	5.6	8.8	10.4	14.4	10.2
Percent of Poverty Level[7]												
Below 100 percent	19.6	20.0	23.4	16.6	14.8	19.5	21.5	12.9	19.4	24.4	30.4	21.2
100 percent to 199 percent	17.9	18.9	24.0	15.9	11.6	16.3	18.4	12.7	18.3	21.0	29.2	20.9
200 percent to 399 percent	10.5	11.8	15.2	10.8	5.5	9.5	11.4	7.0	10.2	13.7	17.3	12.9
400 percent or more	4.6	5.0	6.8	4.2	1.7	3.3	3.9	2.3	4.5	5.9	7.0	4.0
Hispanic Origin and Race and Percent of Poverty Level[5,7]												
Hispanic or Latino												
Below 100 percent	14.6	14.8	19.0	16.0	10.6	17.3	18.9	13.1	16.1	23.5	30.5	20.9
100 percent to 199 percent	12.2	14.5	18.6	12.5	8.1	13.0	14.7	10.8	13.5	18.2	25.2	18.8
200 percent to 399 percent	8.0	9.6	13.9	8.9	4.4	9.1	11.5	6.3	9.2	12.5	18.1	12.1
400 percent or more	5.1	6.2	7.7	5.6	*	*4.2	4.6	*2.1	4.5	5.8	9.1	4.8
Not Hispanic or Latino												
White only												
Below 100 percent	24.3	23.6	26.1	19.0	17.3	20.5	24.6	12.9	23.4	25.1	31.8	22.9
100 percent to 199 percent	20.9	21.8	27.6	18.7	12.4	18.2	19.9	13.5	20.6	22.9	31.7	23.3
200 percent to 399 percent	11.4	13.1	16.0	11.7	5.4	10.0	11.3	6.7	10.6	14.4	18.0	13.5
400 percent or more	4.6	5.0	6.9	4.3	1.7	3.2	3.8	2.4	4.5	5.9	6.9	4.1
Black or African American only												
Below 100 percent	16.1	20.1	24.4	15.2	14.9	21.7	21.1	13.8	14.8	25.5	29.7	19.6
100 percent to 199 percent	14.3	16.2	22.9	14.0	13.9	14.3	21.3	14.3	16.4	19.0	28.2	18.7

NA = Not available.
* = Figure does not meet standards of reliability or precision. Data preceded by an asterisk have a relative standard error (RSE) of 20 percent to 30 percent. Data not shown have an RSE of greater than 30 percent.
[1]Based on persons responding to the question, "During the past 12 months was there any time when person needed medical care but did not get it because person couldn't afford it?" and "During the past 12 months has medical care been delayed because of worry about the cost?"
[2]Based on persons responding to the question, "During the past 12 months was there any time when person needed prescription medicine but didn't get it because person couldn't afford it?"
[3]Based on persons responding to the question, "During the past 12 months was there any time when person needed dental care (including checkups) but didn't get it because person couldn't afford it?"
[4]Includes all other races not shown separately, unknown health insurance status, unknown education level, and unknown disability status.
[5]The race groups White, Black, American Indian or Alaska Native, Asian, Native Hawaiian or Other Pacific Islander, and two or more races include persons of Hispanic and non-Hispanic origin. Persons of Hispanic origin may be of any race.
[6]Estimates are for persons 25 to 64 years of age. GED is General Educational Development high school equivalency diploma.
[7]Percent of poverty level is based on family income and family size and composition using U.S. Census Bureau poverty thresholds. Missing family income data were imputed for 1997 and beyond.

Table 3-32. Delay or Nonreceipt of Needed Medical Care, Nonreceipt of Needed Prescription Drugs, or Nonreceipt of Needed Dental Care During the Past 12 Months Due to Cost, by Selected Characteristics, Selected Years 1997–2015—Continued

(Percent.)

Characteristic	Delay or nonreceipt of needed medical care due to cost[1]				Delay or nonreceipt of needed prescription drugs due to cost[2]				Delay or nonreceipt of needed dental care due to cost[3]			
	1997	2005	2010	2015	1997	2005	2010	2015	1997	2005	2010	2015
200 percent to 399 percent	8.8	9.2	14.6	11.2	7.0	7.9	13.7	9.9	8.6	12.0	16.1	13.8
400 percent or more	4.6	5.5	8.1	4.7	*2.9	*4.1	5.6	*	4.3	*7.0	9.1	*3.7
Health Insurance Status at the Time of Interview[8]												
Insured	6.8	6.8	9.1	7.4	3.7	6.0	7.3	5.4	7.2	8.7	11.8	9.4
Private	6.0	5.9	8.2	6.4	2.9	4.7	6.0	4.0	6.2	6.7	9.2	6.9
Medicaid	11.9	12.0	12.5	10.8	11.1	14.0	13.5	10.7	14.8	21.8	24.2	18.9
Uninsured	27.6	29.5	34.5	32.4	18.0	23.1	25.7	17.3	26.1	30.7	37.7	28.2
Health Insurance Status Prior to Interview[8]												
Insured continuously all 12 months	5.5	5.5	7.6	6.2	2.8	5.0	6.2	4.4	6.0	7.5	10.5	8.2
Uninsured for any period up to 12 months	28.7	31.7	35.1	31.8	17.7	23.5	25.1	19.6	25.2	30.3	33.6	27.6
Uninsured more than 12 months	30.6	31.1	35.9	33.8	18.9	24.5	26.2	17.4	28.0	32.1	39.4	29.6
Disability Measure[9]												
Any basic actions difficulty or complex activity limitation	23.3	24.8	28.9	26.3	14.8	20.0	22.6	16.0	19.8	23.8	28.8	22.8
Any basic actions difficulty	24.2	26.1	28.9	27.4	15.3	20.5	23.3	16.4	20.1	24.4	29.2	23.2
Any complex activity limitation	25.7	26.9	30.8	27.7	19.4	25.3	27.3	19.8	23.2	27.3	33.7	27.6
No disability	9.0	9.8	13.2	10.5	3.4	5.7	7.0	3.7	7.5	9.4	13.1	7.9
Geographic Region												
Northeast	8.8	8.7	10.2	9.0	4.9	7.2	7.7	5.2	8.9	10.6	12.9	9.1
Midwest	10.5	10.6	14.8	12.1	5.9	9.0	11.6	6.5	9.7	11.9	16.0	10.9
South	11.8	12.6	16.5	13.6	7.3	11.3	13.5	8.4	10.9	14.7	19.6	13.0
West	10.8	11.1	15.1	13.6	6.3	8.2	10.0	6.2	13.1	13.6	18.4	12.9
Location of Residence												
Within MSA[10]	10.2	10.6	14.2	12.1	5.9	8.8	10.8	6.7	10.0	12.7	17.0	11.4
Outside MSA[10]	12.5	12.8	17.4	14.6	7.9	11.8	13.6	8.3	12.9	14.6	19.1	14.5

NA = Not available.

* = Figure does not meet standards of reliability or precision. Data preceded by an asterisk have a relative standard error (RSE) of 20 percent to 30 percent. Data not shown have an RSE of greater than 30 percent.

[1]Based on persons responding to the question, "During the past 12 months was there any time when person needed medical care but did not get it because person couldn't afford it?" and "During the past 12 months has medical care been delayed because of worry about the cost?"

[2]Based on persons responding to the question, "During the past 12 months was there any time when person needed prescription medicine but didn't get it because person couldn't afford it?"

[3]Based on persons responding to the question, "During the past 12 months was there any time when person needed dental care (including checkups) but didn't get it because person couldn't afford it?"

[8]For information on the health insurance categories, see Appendix II, Health insurance coverage, in Health: United States, 2014.

[9]Any basic actions difficulty or complex activity limitation is defined as having one or more of the following limitations or difficulties: movement difficulty, emotional difficulty, sensory (seeing or hearing) difficulty, cognitive difficulty, self-care (activities of daily living or instrumental activities of daily living) limitation, social limitation, or work limitation.

[10]MSA = metropolitan statistical area.

Table 3-33. Reduced Access to Medical Care During the Past 12 Months Due to Cost, 25 Largest States, Selected Annual Averages, 1997–1998 Through 2010–2011

(Percent for the 25 states with the largest populations in 2010–2011.)

State	Did not get or delayed medical care due to cost[1]			Did not get prescription drugs due to cost[2]			Did not get dental care[3]		
	1997–1998	2000–2001	2010–2011	1997–1998	2000–2001	2010–2011	1997–1998	2000–2001	2010–2011
United States	7.9	7.5	10.6	4.5	5.3	8.0	8.1	8.4	13.2
Alabama	7.6	7.7	11.9	6.8	8.3	12.3	8.7	10.3	15.0
Arizona	8.0	7.4	14.4	4.1	4.6	11.1	9.4	8.4	20.6
California	6.8	6.6	10.4	3.9	4.7	7.2	8.3	8.1	15.0
Colorado	6.4	8.1	12.2	3.1	5.5	6.9	8.9	11.5	13.5
Florida	9.8	9.6	13.2	4.8	5.8	10.1	7.2	8.4	17.4
Georgia	8.0	7.7	12.1	4.2	4.0	9.7	5.8	5.3	13.8
Illinois	6.1	6.5	8.7	3.0	4.2	6.0	5.7	6.8	9.9
Indiana	9.0	8.6	12.0	5.1	6.8	11.9	7.2	6.9	12.2
Louisiana	9.8	11.1	11.4	8.7	9.8	12.0	11.3	16.4	18.0
Maryland	8.0	7.4	8.5	5.8	5.2	5.7	9.8	7.8	9.1
Massachusetts	5.1	4.3	5.1	*1.7	4.2	4.7	5.0	5.2	7.9
Michigan	7.2	7.0	11.4	3.8	5.1	9.8	7.5	7.9	15.9
Minnesota	8.1	7.0	10.3	3.6	3.9	6.0	8.7	8.3	10.7
Missouri	7.1	6.4	12.4	4.3	5.2	8.4	7.3	7.1	14.7
New Jersey	7.2	6.1	7.1	3.8	3.5	4.7	7.3	5.9	9.9
New York	6.4	5.8	6.9	2.8	3.8	5.4	5.6	7.5	7.8
North Carolina	7.8	7.9	11.3	4.0	5.8	7.9	8.2	7.9	12.4
Ohio	9.2	7.6	10.5	5.0	5.1	8.1	8.8	8.1	10.5
Pennsylvania	5.9	5.9	9.1	4.3	3.5	7.0	7.4	6.0	11.4
South Carolina	7.6	6.3	11.2	5.2	4.4	8.4	5.7	5.2	11.3
Tennessee	10.0	8.6	13.1	8.0	8.5	10.7	10.5	10.4	15.3
Texas	7.9	8.1	12.0	4.7	6.6	9.9	8.8	10.4	16.4
Virginia	6.2	7.2	9.3	4.1	5.2	6.9	8.3	7.4	9.6
Washington	8.6	9.2	13.0	4.8	6.8	8.3	11.6	11.9	17.6
Wisconsin	6.5	5.9	8.2	3.0	4.0	5.0	5.5	6.6	10.6

* = Figure does not meet standards of reliability or precision. Data preceded by an asterisk have a relative standard error (RSE) of 20 percent to 30 percent.

[1]Based on persons responding to the question, "During the past 12 months was there any time when person needed medical care but did not get it because person couldn't afford it?" and "During the past 12 months has medical care been delayed because of worry about the cost?"

[2]Based on persons responding to the question, "During the past 12 months was there any time when you needed prescription medicine but didn't get it because you couldn't afford it?"

[3]Based on persons responding to the question, "During the past 12 months was there any time when you needed dental care (including check ups) but didn't get it because you couldn't afford it?"

Table 3-34. No Health Care Visits[1] to an Office or Clinic Within the Past 12 Months Among Children Under 18 Years of Age, by Selected Characteristics, Selected Annual Averages, 1997–1998 Through 2014–2015

(Percent.)

Characteristic	Under 18 years				Under 6 years				6 to 17 years			
	1997–1998	2005–2006	2009–2010	2014–2015	1997–1998	2005–2006	2009–2010	2014–2015	1997–1998	2005–2006	2009–2010	2014–2015
ALL CHILDREN[2]	12.8	11.7	9.6	8.5	5.7	6.1	4.9	5.1	16.3	14.4	12.1	10.2
Sex												
Male	12.9	12.0	9.8	8.5	4.9	6.2	5.0	5.0	16.8	14.7	12.4	10.2
Female	12.7	11.4	9.4	8.5	6.5	6.1	4.8	5.2	15.8	14.0	11.8	10.2
Race[3]												
White only	12.2	11.3	9.4	8.2	5.5	6.3	4.5	5.0	15.5	13.8	11.8	9.7
Black or African American only	14.3	11.7	10.1	9.8	6.5	4.6	6.4	6.1	18.1	15.1	12.1	11.6
American Indian or Alaska Native only	13.8	*15.7	*12.4	15.6	*	*	*	*	*	*17.6	*17.7	*14.7	20.0
Asian only	16.3	17.5	12.7	9.6	*5.6	10.5	*4.8	*6.0	22.1	20.8	17.0	11.5
Native Hawaiian or Other Pacific Islander only	NA	*	*	*	NA	*	*	*	NA	*	*	*
Two or more races	NA	10.4	8.3	6.5	NA	*	*5.7	*	NA	14.8	10.1	9.2
Hispanic Origin and Race[3]												
Hispanic or Latino	19.3	17.4	13.5	11.3	9.7	9.6	7.7	5.9	25.3	21.9	17.2	14.2
Not Hispanic or Latino	11.6	10.3	8.5	7.6	4.8	5.1	4.0	4.8	14.9	12.6	10.7	8.9
White only	10.7	9.4	7.7	6.8	4.3	5.0	3.1	4.6	13.7	11.4	9.8	7.9
Black or African American only	14.5	11.7	10.3	9.7	6.5	*4.4	6.4	6.2	18.3	15.1	12.4	11.3
Percent of Poverty Level[4]												
Below 100 percent	17.6	14.2	12.4	10.3	8.1	7.7	6.9	6.7	23.6	18.2	16.0	12.3
100 percent to 199 percent	16.2	14.9	12.7	10.4	7.2	8.4	6.4	5.9	20.8	18.2	16.2	12.6
200 percent to 399 percent	11.7	11.1	9.0	8.8	4.9	6.1	4.2	5.3	14.8	13.4	11.4	10.5
400 percent or more	7.4	7.8	5.3	5.2	3.0	2.8	*2.3	2.6	9.5	10.0	6.7	6.3
Hispanic Origin and Race and Percent of Poverty Level[3,4]												
Hispanic or Latino												
Below 100 percent	23.2	20.0	14.6	11.1	11.7	11.5	9.0	6.8	31.1	25.6	18.5	13.7
100 percent to 199 percent	20.9	19.1	15.7	13.3	9.7	10.1	9.5	6.5	28.1	24.4	19.4	16.5
200 percent to 399 percent	15.7	14.6	10.9	11.3	8.0	8.1	*4.2	5.9	19.7	17.9	14.6	14.1
400 percent or more	7.8	10.9	8.5	6.2	*	*	*	*	9.3	14.1	11.3	8.9
Not Hispanic or Latino												
White only												
Below 100 percent	14.0	9.4	9.4	8.3	*5.6	*5.6	*	*6.6	19.7	11.8	13.1	9.2
100 percent to 199 percent	14.1	13.2	11.7	8.7	6.0	8.5	*3.6	6.5	18.0	15.4	16.1	9.8
200 percent to 399 percent	10.9	9.7	8.2	7.5	4.3	5.8	4.2	4.8	13.9	11.4	10.1	8.9
400 percent or more	7.2	7.1	4.6	4.8	*2.8	*2.2	*	*2.5	9.1	9.2	5.7	5.8
Black or African American only												
Below 100 percent	15.8	12.1	11.2	10.5	7.6	*	*6.4	*7.1	20.5	16.4	14.2	12.4
100 percent to 199 percent	16.4	13.1	11.3	9.1	*7.7	*	*	*	20.4	16.2	13.1	11.4
200 percent to 399 percent	13.3	11.7	9.4	10.6	*4.9	*	*	*	16.7	14.8	10.8	11.6
400 percent or more	8.3	*7.4	6.9	*6.5	*	*	*	*	10.7	*9.9	*8.4	*6.7
Health Insurance Status at the Time of Interview[5]												
Insured	10.4	9.5	7.7	7.5	4.5	4.9	4.3	4.8	13.4	11.9	9.6	8.9
Private	10.4	9.4	7.0	7.2	4.3	4.4	3.5	4.0	13.1	11.6	8.6	8.6
Medicaid	10.1	9.5	8.8	7.9	5.0	5.8	5.3	5.4	14.4	12.2	11.1	9.3
Uninsured	28.8	31.7	31.0	27.1	14.6	20.6	14.4	13.1	34.9	35.6	37.3	31.6
Health Insurance Status Prior to Interview[5]												
Insured continuously all 12 months	10.3	9.5	7.4	7.3	4.4	4.9	4.1	4.7	13.2	11.9	9.2	8.7
Uninsured for any period up to 12 months	15.9	15.8	16.3	14.6	7.7	9.3	7.7	*8.1	20.9	18.8	20.9	17.8
Uninsured more than 12 months	34.9	39.0	38.6	35.1	19.9	28.0	22.8	*18.2	40.2	42.2	42.9	39.0
Geographic Region												
Northeast	7.0	6.8	5.6	5.1	3.1	4.0	3.3	*3.2	8.9	8.1	6.7	6.0
Midwest	12.2	9.8	8.6	7.5	5.9	5.2	3.5	4.9	15.3	12.0	11.2	8.8
South	14.3	12.4	9.9	9.2	5.6	6.2	5.2	6.0	18.5	15.5	12.4	10.7
West	16.3	16.5	12.9	10.5	7.9	8.8	6.9	5.0	20.7	20.3	16.1	13.3
Location of Residence												
Within MSA[6]	12.3	11.4	9.4	8.2	5.4	5.9	4.7	5.1	15.9	14.1	11.9	9.8
Outside MSA[6]	14.6	12.9	10.8	10.2	6.9	7.4	6.0	5.3	17.9	15.4	13.1	12.6

NA = Not available.

* = Figure does not meet standards of reliability or precision. Data preceded by an asterisk have a relative standard error (RSE) of 20 percent to 30 percent. Data not shown have an RSE of greater than 30 percent.

[1] Respondents were asked how many times a doctor or other health care professional was seen in the past 12 months at a doctor's office, clinic, or some other place. Excluded are visits to emergency rooms, hospitalizations, home visits, and telephone calls. Starting with 2000 data, dental visits were also excluded.

[2] Includes all other races not shown separately and unknown health insurance status.

[3] The race groups White, Black, American Indian or Alaska Native, Asian, Native Hawaiian or Other Pacific Islander, and two or more races include persons of Hispanic and non-Hispanic origin. Persons of Hispanic origin may be of any race.

[4] Percent of poverty level is based on family income and family size and composition using U.S. Census Bureau poverty thresholds. Missing family income data were imputed starting in 1993.

[5] Health insurance categories are mutually exclusive. Persons who reported both Medicaid and private coverage are classified as having private coverage. Medicaid includes other public assistance through 1996. Starting with 1997 data, state-sponsored health plan coverage is included as Medicaid coverage. Starting with 1999 data, coverage by the Children's Health Insurance Program (CHIP) is included with Medicaid coverage. Persons not covered by private insurance, Medicaid, CHIP, public assistance (through 1996), state-sponsored or other government-sponsored health plans (starting in 1997), Medicare, or military plans are considered to have no health insurance coverage. Persons with only Indian Health Service coverage are considered to have no health insurance coverage.

[6] MSA = metropolitan statistical area.

Table 3-35. Health Care Visits to Doctors' Offices, Emergency Departments, and Home Visits within the Past 12 Months, by Selected Characteristics, Selected Years, 1997–2015

(Percent distribution of health care visits to doctors' offices, emergency departments, and home visits during a 12-month period.)

Characteristic	None				1 to 3 visits				4 to 9 visits				10 or more visits			
	1997	2005	2010	2015	1997	2005	2010	2015	1997	2005	2010	2015	1997	2005	2010	2015
Total, age-adjusted[1,2]	16.5	15.5	15.6	15.0	46.2	45.9	45.4	48.4	23.6	25.1	25.8	23.7	13.7	13.6	13.2	12.8
Total, crude[1]	16.5	15.4	15.4	14.6	46.5	45.9	45.2	47.8	23.5	25.1	26.0	24.1	13.5	13.6	13.5	13.5
Age																
Under 18 years	11.8	10.2	8.1	7.9	54.1	56.0	55.6	59.7	25.2	26.5	28.2	25.7	8.9	7.4	8.2	6.7
Under 6 years	5.0	5.1	3.7	4.7	44.9	47.4	48.9	52.2	37.0	38.0	36.8	35.7	13.0	9.5	10.6	7.5
6 to 17 years	15.3	12.6	10.4	9.5	58.7	60.1	59.1	63.3	19.3	20.9	23.6	20.9	6.8	6.3	6.9	6.4
18 to 44 years	21.7	22.9	24.2	23.3	46.7	45.8	43.9	46.9	19.0	19.2	20.6	18.7	12.6	12.0	11.3	11.1
18 to 24 years	22.0	24.2	25.9	24.5	46.8	44.4	43.4	47.2	20.0	19.6	21.1	19.6	11.2	11.8	9.6	8.8
25 to 44 years	21.6	22.5	23.6	22.9	46.7	46.3	44.1	46.8	18.7	19.1	20.5	18.3	13.0	12.1	11.9	11.9
45 to 64 years	16.9	14.0	14.8	13.7	42.9	42.9	42.8	45.5	24.7	26.8	26.1	24.5	15.5	16.3	16.4	16.3
45 to 54 years	17.9	15.8	17.6	16.1	43.9	44.8	43.5	47.0	23.4	24.3	23.9	23.3	14.8	15.0	15.0	13.6
55 to 64 years	15.3	11.4	11.1	11.2	41.3	40.2	41.9	43.8	26.7	30.3	28.8	25.9	16.7	18.2	18.2	19.1
65 years and over	8.9	5.6	5.3	5.5	34.7	30.7	33.8	35.5	32.5	37.5	36.7	33.9	23.8	26.2	24.2	25.1
65 to 74 years	9.8	5.9	6.3	6.4	36.9	34.4	36.1	37.9	31.6	35.8	35.7	33.7	21.6	23.9	21.9	22.0
75 years and over	7.7	5.2	4.1	4.2	31.8	26.4	31.0	32.0	33.8	39.5	38.0	34.2	26.6	28.8	27.0	29.6
Sex[2]																
Male	21.3	20.4	20.4	19.5	47.1	46.7	46.4	49.8	20.6	22.2	22.7	20.3	11.0	10.7	10.5	10.5
Female	11.8	10.7	10.9	10.8	45.4	45.1	44.4	47.1	26.5	27.9	28.8	26.9	16.3	16.3	15.9	15.2
Race[2,3]																
White only	16.0	15.1	15.3	14.8	46.1	45.6	44.9	47.8	23.9	25.4	26.1	24.0	14.0	13.9	13.7	13.4
Black or African American only	16.8	15.9	15.7	14.5	46.1	47.4	47.2	50.2	23.2	23.8	24.7	24.1	13.9	12.9	12.4	11.2
American Indian or Alaska Native only	17.1	20.4	19.4	20.6	38.0	36.4	40.3	39.0	24.2	29.8	28.1	23.3	20.7	13.4	12.2	17.1
Asian only	22.8	21.5	20.4	18.2	49.1	49.3	49.9	54.7	19.7	20.8	22.1	18.7	8.3	8.4	7.6	8.5
Native Hawaiian and Other Pacific Islander only	NA	*	*	*	NA	*	*	*	NA	*	*	*	NA	*	*	*
Two or more races	NA	15.4	13.9	17.3	NA	37.3	42.3	41.5	NA	27.6	25.2	25.0	NA	19.7	18.6	16.2
Hispanic Origin and Race[2,3]																
Hispanic or Latino	24.9	23.9	23.5	22.3	42.3	42.1	43.2	45.9	20.3	22.2	22.6	21.9	12.5	11.8	10.7	9.9
Mexican	28.9	26.6	25.2	24.8	40.8	41.5	43.3	44.8	18.5	20.8	21.4	20.7	11.8	11.1	10.1	9.7
Not Hispanic or Latino	15.4	13.9	14.0	13.4	46.7	46.5	45.8	49.0	24.0	25.7	26.5	24.1	13.9	13.9	13.7	13.5
White only	14.7	13.0	13.2	12.7	46.6	46.4	45.3	48.1	24.4	26.2	27.1	24.7	14.3	14.5	14.4	14.5
Black or African American only	16.9	15.9	15.6	14.7	46.1	47.4	47.3	50.5	23.1	23.8	24.9	23.8	13.8	12.9	12.2	11.0
Percent of Poverty Level[2,4]																
Below 100 percent	20.6	20.7	20.4	19.0	37.8	37.3	37.5	39.9	22.7	24.7	25.1	23.9	18.9	17.3	17.0	17.1
100 percent to 199 percent	20.1	20.2	20.8	18.4	43.3	42.0	42.1	45.1	21.7	23.4	23.1	22.9	14.9	14.4	13.9	13.6
200 percent to 399 percent	16.4	15.9	16.2	15.9	47.2	47.3	46.3	49.5	23.6	24.0	25.4	22.8	12.8	12.8	12.1	11.8
400 percent or more	12.8	11.0	10.2	11.2	49.8	49.2	49.4	51.8	24.9	27.0	27.6	24.7	12.5	12.8	12.7	12.3
Hispanic Origin and Race and Percent of Poverty Level[2,3,4]																
Hispanic or Latino																
Below 100 percent	32.3	27.9	28.7	26.3	33.3	37.2	36.5	38.3	19.2	20.2	22.5	22.7	15.1	14.6	12.3	12.7
100 percent to 199 percent	30.5	27.6	27.7	25.1	40.6	38.8	42.7	45.1	17.6	22.6	19.9	21.0	11.3	11.1	9.8	8.8
200 percent to 399 percent	24.2	22.7	21.6	22.2	45.5	44.9	45.0	49.5	19.9	23.1	23.1	20.2	10.3	9.2	10.3	8.2
400 percent or more	17.0	13.4	11.3	13.3	47.2	50.4	51.1	50.2	26.3	23.0	26.1	25.1	9.5	13.2	11.5	11.4
Not Hispanic or Latino																
White only																
Below 100 percent	18.0	16.4	15.0	15.2	36.9	36.1	37.0	38.3	25.3	28.0	27.4	25.6	19.8	19.5	20.6	20.9
100 percent to 199 percent	18.5	17.5	18.4	15.7	41.5	41.8	40.4	43.6	24.1	24.0	24.7	23.7	15.9	16.8	16.5	17.0
200 percent to 399 percent	15.3	13.8	14.7	13.7	44.6	47.3	46.0	48.6	26.1	24.7	26.3	24.0	13.9	14.2	13.0	13.7
400 percent or more	11.8	10.3	9.9	10.6	47.8	48.9	48.2	51.1	27.6	27.6	28.4	25.2	12.8	13.1	13.5	13.2
Black or African American only																
Below 100 percent	18.3	17.8	18.4	16.2	40.0	40.1	39.8	42.9	24.9	24.8	25.0	25.1	16.7	17.3	16.8	15.7
100 percent to 199 percent	20.8	16.1	17.6	14.6	44.2	47.0	45.7	47.6	20.7	24.3	24.3	25.2	14.3	12.6	12.5	12.6
200 percent to 399 percent	17.1	17.2	15.1	15.6	48.5	49.0	49.0	54.0	24.4	22.9	25.7	22.3	10.1	10.9	10.2	8.0
400 percent or more	11.3	12.1	10.0	11.7	52.2	52.0	58.2	55.9	24.8	24.7	22.5	23.2	11.7	11.2	9.3	9.2
Health Insurance Status at the Time of Interview[5,6]																
Under 65 years																
Insured	14.0	12.4	12.3	13.3	48.2	49.6	48.5	51.7	25.1	25.0	26.1	23.3	12.7	13.0	13.1	11.7

Note: This table presents a summary measure of the number of visits to hospital emergency departments, home visits by a nurse or other health care professional, and visits to doctor offices/clinics during a 12-month period.
NA = Not applicable.
* = Figure does not meet standards of reliability or precision. Data preceded by an asterisk have a relative standard error (RSE) of 20 percent to 30 percent. Data not shown have an RSE of greater than 30 percent.
[1]Includes all other races not shown separately, unknown health insurance status, and unknown disability status.
[2]Estimates are age adjusted to the year 2000 standard population using six age groups: under 18 years, 18 to 44 years, 45 to 54 years, 55 to 64 years, 65 to 74 years, and 75 years and over.
[3]The race groups White, Black, American Indian or Alaska Native, Asian, Native Hawaiian or Other Pacific Islander, and 2 or more races, include persons of Hispanic and non-Hispanic origin. Persons of Hispanic origin may be of any race.
[4]Percent of poverty level is based on family income and family size and composition. Missing family income data were imputed for 1997 and beyond.
[5]Estimates for persons under 65 years of age are age adjusted to the year 2000 standard population using four age groups: under 18 years, 18 to 44 years, 45 to 54 years, and 55 to64 years.
[6]Health insurance categories are mutually exclusive. Persons who reported both Medicaid and private coverage are classified as having private coverage. Medicaid includes other public assistance through 1996. Starting with 1997 data, state-sponsored health plan coverage is included as Medicaid coverage. Starting with 1999 data, coverage by the Children's Health Insurance Program (CHIP) is included with Medicaid coverage. Persons not covered by private insurance, Medicaid, CHIP, public assistance (through 1996), state-sponsored or other government-sponsored health plans (starting in 1997), Medicare, or military plans are considered to have no health insurance coverage. Persons with only Indian Health Service coverage are considered to have no health insurance coverage. Health insurance status was unknown for 8 to 9 percent of children in 1993-1996 and about 1 percent in 1997-2011.

Table 3-35. Health Care Visits to Doctors' Offices, Emergency Departments, and Home Visits within the Past 12 Months, by Selected Characteristics, Selected Years, 1997–2015—Continued

(Percent distribution of health care visits to doctors' offices, emergency departments, and home visits during a 12-month period.)

Characteristic	None				1 to 3 visits				4 to 9 visits				10 or more visits			
	1997	2005	2010	2015	1997	2005	2010	2015	1997	2005	2010	2015	1997	2005	2010	2015
Private	14.3	12.8	12.4	13.7	49.9	51.5	51.0	53.8	24.8	24.5	25.5	22.7	11.0	11.2	11.1	9.9
Medicaid	10.4	9.9	10.9	12.4	32.4	37.8	38.2	43.4	27.6	26.8	28.0	25.4	29.6	25.5	23.0	18.8
Uninsured	36.8	37.5	37.2	39.8	41.9	42.0	42.2	41.4	14.1	14.7	15.2	13.7	7.2	5.8	5.4	5.1
Health Insurance Status Prior to Interview[5,6]																
Under 65 years																
Insured continuously all 12 months	13.9	12.3	12.1	12.9	48.5	49.8	48.6	52.0	25.1	25.0	26.2	23.4	12.6	12.9	13.0	11.7
Uninsured for any period up to 12 months	20.4	18.9	18.5	21.5	44.1	44.9	47.8	46.9	21.5	22.5	22.0	20.0	13.9	13.7	11.6	11.6
Uninsured more than 12 months	43.1	43.5	43.8	48.7	39.5	40.0	39.7	37.8	12.3	12.3	12.6	10.4	5.1	4.2	3.9	3.1
Percent of Poverty Level and Health Insurance Status Prior to Interview (Under 65 Years)[4,5,6]																
Below 100 percent																
Insured continuously all 12 months	13.8	12.6	12.7	14.3	39.7	40.4	39.5	42.3	25.2	26.2	27.5	25.9	21.4	20.8	20.3	17.5
Uninsured for any period up to 12 months	19.7	18.9	16.9	21.8	37.6	37.4	43.0	45.6	21.9	23.7	25.0	19.0	20.9	20.0	15.1	13.7
Uninsured more than 12 months	41.2	46.0	45.0	48.8	39.9	35.2	38.1	36.9	12.2	14.4	13.6	10.6	6.6	4.3	3.3	*3.8
100 percent to 199 percent																
Insured continuously all 12 months	16.0	14.8	14.8	13.3	46.4	45.7	44.4	49.1	21.9	24.3	24.8	23.8	15.8	15.2	16.0	13.8
Uninsured for any period up to 12 months	18.8	19.2	21.0	25.6	45.1	44.7	46.0	41.9	21.0	22.1	20.6	19.4	15.0	14.0	12.4	13.0
Uninsured more than 12 months	38.7	43.5	43.2	48.8	41.0	39.2	39.4	37.6	14.0	12.9	12.4	11.1	6.3	4.4	5.0	*
200 percent to 399 percent																
Insured continuously all 12 months	15.1	13.3	13.6	14.0	49.4	50.7	49.4	53.5	23.4	23.7	25.3	22.0	12.1	12.3	11.7	10.5
Uninsured for any period up to 12 months	17.9	19.9	18.8	19.8	49.3	45.7	49.7	49.0	20.0	22.3	19.7	21.1	12.8	12.2	11.8	10.0
Uninsured more than 12 months	37.0	42.0	43.8	50.7	43.8	44.0	40.7	38.5	12.6	10.3	13.3	8.7	6.6	3.7	*2.2	*2.2
400 percent or more																
Insured continuously all 12 months	12.4	10.6	9.7	11.4	52.2	52.1	51.8	54.3	23.9	25.9	26.8	23.5	11.5	11.4	11.6	10.8
Uninsured for any period up to 12 months	17.2	16.1	16.6	16.6	50.0	51.9	53.5	54.1	24.2	22.8	23.9	20.2	*8.5	9.2	*6.0	9.0
Uninsured more than 12 months	35.1	39.3	39.2	39.3	44.1	46.6	46.0	41.1	15.1	9.6	*8.8	*	*5.7	*	*	*
Respondent-Assessed Health Status[2]																
Fair or poor	7.8	9.0	8.4	8.0	23.3	21.5	24.0	25.3	29.0	28.1	30.2	28.7	39.9	41.3	37.3	38.0
Good to excellent	17.2	16.1	16.3	15.7	48.4	48.2	47.5	50.6	23.3	24.8	25.5	23.3	11.1	10.8	10.7	10.3
Disability Measure Among Adults 18 Years of Age and Over[2,7]																
Any basic actions difficulty or complex activity limitation	11.1	9.6	11.5	10.6	32.0	29.7	30.9	31.2	27.9	29.6	29.3	29.0	29.1	31.1	28.3	29.2
Any basic actions difficulty	11.1	9.7	11.5	10.5	31.9	29.4	30.3	31.1	27.5	29.6	29.2	28.9	29.4	31.3	29.0	29.5
Any complex activity limitation	7.1	5.9	6.9	6.8	23.7	21.1	23.0	22.4	27.5	27.8	29.1	28.8	41.7	45.2	41.0	41.9
No disability	20.9	19.8	20.5	20.1	49.6	48.8	47.5	50.9	20.8	22.7	23.4	20.8	8.7	8.6	8.5	8.2
Geographic Region[2]																
Northeast	13.2	11.3	12.6	10.9	45.9	46.8	46.3	50.9	26.0	27.0	26.4	24.2	14.9	14.9	14.7	14.0
Midwest	15.9	13.8	13.4	14.5	47.7	47.2	46.8	48.9	22.8	25.2	26.4	23.3	13.6	13.9	13.3	13.3
South	17.2	16.0	16.1	15.9	46.1	45.7	44.2	47.2	23.3	25.1	26.6	24.4	13.5	13.3	13.2	12.5
West	19.1	20.0	19.1	17.1	44.8	44.2	45.2	48.3	22.8	23.3	23.5	22.5	13.3	12.5	12.2	12.1
Location of Residence[2]																
Within MSA[8]	16.2	15.5	15.6	14.9	46.4	46.2	45.8	49.0	23.7	24.9	25.6	23.4	13.7	13.3	13.0	12.6
Outside MSA[8]	17.3	15.3	15.9	15.7	45.4	44.5	42.7	44.5	23.3	25.6	27.0	25.1	13.9	14.6	14.4	14.7

Note: This table presents a summary measure of the number of visits to hospital emergency departments, home visits by a nurse or other health care professional, and visits to doctor offices/clinics during a 12-month period.

* = Figure does not meet standards of reliability or precision. Data preceded by an asterisk have a relative standard error (RSE) of 20 percent to 30 percent. Data not shown have an RSE of greater than 30 percent.

[2]Estimates are age adjusted to the year 2000 standard population using six age groups: under 18 years, 18 to 44 years, 45 to 54 years, 55 to 64 years, 65 to 74 years, and 75 years and over.

[4]Percent of poverty level is based on family income and family size and composition. Missing family income data were imputed for 1997 and beyond.

[5]Estimates for persons under 65 years of age are age adjusted to the year 2000 standard population using four age groups: under 18 years, 18 to 44 years, 45 to 54 years, and 55 to64 years.

[6]Health insurance categories are mutually exclusive. Persons who reported both Medicaid and private coverage are classified as having private coverage. Medicaid includes other public assistance through 1996. Starting with 1997 data, state-sponsored health plan coverage is included as Medicaid coverage. Starting with 1999 data, coverage by the Children's Health Insurance Program (CHIP) is included with Medicaid coverage. Persons not covered by private insurance, Medicaid, CHIP, public assistance (through 1996), state-sponsored or other government-sponsored health plans (starting in 1997), Medicare, or military plans are considered to have no health insurance coverage. Persons with only Indian Health Service coverage are considered to have no health insurance coverage. Health insurance status was unknown for 8 to 9 percent of children in 1993-1996 and about 1 percent in 1997-2011.

[7]Any basic actions difficulty or complex activity limitation is defined as having one or more of the following limitations or difficulties: movement difficulty, emotional difficulty, sensory (seeing or hearing) difficulty, cognitive difficulty, self-care (activities of daily living or instrumental activities of daily living) limitation, social limitation, or work limitation.

[8]MSA = metropolitan statistical area.

Table 3-36. Vaccination Coverage Among Children 19 to 35 Months of Age for Selected Diseases, by Race, Hispanic Origin, Poverty Level, and Location of Residence in Metropolitan Statistical Area, Selected Years, 1998–2015

(Percent.)

| Vaccination and year | All | Race and Hispanic origin[1] | | | | | | | Poverty level[2] | | Location of residence | | |
| | | Not Hispanic or Latino | | | | | | Hispanic or Latino | Below poverty level | At or above poverty level | Inside MSA[3] | | Outside MSA[3] |
		White	Black or African American	American Indian or Alaska Native	Asian[4]	Native Hawaiian or Other Pacific Islander	Two or more races				Central city	Remaining area	
Combined Series (4:3:1:3*:3:1:4)[5]													
2009	44.3	45.2	39.6	*	38.6	*	40.7	45.9	41.3	45.7	44.8	44.6	42.4
2010	56.6	56.9	54.5	64.1	59.3	*	61.3	55.5	52.8	58.7	56.5	57.2	55.2
2011	68.5	68.8	63.7	65.9	70.8	*	70.9	69.5	63.6	71.6	69.5	67.9	67.4
2012	68.4	69.3	64.8	*	71.6	*	71.5	67.8	63.4	71.6	67.6	69.4	68.0
2013	70.4	72.1	65.0	70.1	72.7	*	71.8	69.3	64.4	73.8	68.8	72.5	69.1
2014	71.6	72.6	65.4	*	69.5	*	68.5	74.3	65.7	75.4	70.8	72.7	71.2
2015	72.2	72.7	69.1	68.2	77.9	*	73.7	71.7	68.7	74.7	72.5	72.5	70.2
DTP/DT/DTaP (4 Doses or More)[6]													
1998	83.9	86.6	77.3	82.9	89.1	NA	NA	80.5	79.5	86.1	81.6	85.4	85.1
1999	83.3	85.5	79.0	80.2	86.8	NA	NA	80.2	78.5	85.4	82.1	84.3	83.3
2000	81.7	84.4	76.1	77.8	84.5	*	81.5	78.6	76.2	83.5	79.9	82.8	82.9
2001	82.1	83.5	76.5	76.9	83.6	*	81.2	82.5	76.5	83.6	80.5	83.4	82.2
2002	81.6	84.4	75.8	*	88.0	*	77.6	79.2	75.4	83.5	79.3	84.0	80.2
2003	84.8	87.5	79.9	80.1	88.5	*	83.5	81.9	79.7	86.8	84.1	86.2	82.9
2004	85.5	87.7	79.5	76.7	89.6	*	86.0	84.1	81.2	87.4	83.9	87.2	84.5
2005	85.7	87.1	84.0	*	88.8	*	86.3	83.6	81.8	87.4	84.8	87.0	84.7
2006	85.2	86.6	81.2	82.7	86.0	86.2	83.8	84.5	81.0	86.8	84.4	86.3	84.5
2007	84.5	85.3	82.3	86.4	87.5	*	84.2	83.8	81.1	85.9	84.5	85.1	82.9
2008	84.6	85.0	80.1	82.0	92.3	*	87.6	84.9	79.9	86.8	85.0	85.3	81.8
2009	83.9	85.8	78.6	82.1	86.6	93.1	81.8	82.9	80.1	85.7	83.8	84.2	84.2
2010	84.4	84.5	83.7	81.8	88.3	*	82.8	84.4	80.8	86.1	84.0	85.0	83.7
2011	84.6	85.0	81.3	72.7	92.0	93.0	87.1	84.1	81.0	86.8	86.1	83.8	82.2
2012	82.5	83.6	79.6	88.2	88.1	*	85.6	80.8	78.5	85.0	82.4	83.4	80.5
2013	83.1	85.3	74.7	78.1	89.0	*	83.1	82.3	77.8	86.0	81.8	84.7	82.4
2014	84.2	85.5	79.1	*	87.4	*	79.6	85.4	79.1	87.4	83.6	85.3	83.1
2015	84.6	85.2	82.0	79.6	90.0	*	82.5	84.5	80.2	87.1	85.4	84.3	82.7
Polio (3 Doses or More)													
1998	90.8	92.2	87.8	85.1	93.4	NA	NA	88.9	89.9	91.7	89.3	91.3	92.9
1999	89.6	90.3	87.0	88.2	90.1	NA	NA	89.4	87.4	90.5	88.7	90.1	89.7
2000	89.5	90.6	86.6	90.8	92.7	91.2	91.2	87.9	86.9	89.9	88.1	90.1	91.1
2001	89.4	90.1	85.2	87.5	89.6	*	86.5	90.7	87.4	90.1	87.9	90.2	90.6
2002	90.2	91.2	87.4	*	91.6	95.3	86.9	90.4	88.3	90.6	88.7	91.4	90.4
2003	91.6	93.0	89.2	91.3	91.3	90.2	91.0	90.1	89.1	92.5	90.7	92.1	91.9
2004	91.6	92.1	90.4	86.5	92.8	*	91.9	91.2	89.8	92.2	91.3	91.5	92.1
2005	91.7	91.4	91.0	*	92.9	*	93.8	92.3	89.7	92.4	90.6	92.6	92.2
2006	92.8	93.3	90.4	91.0	92.4	96.0	91.7	93.3	92.1	93.1	92.6	93.1	93.2
2007	92.6	92.6	91.1	94.8	95.0	87.4	92.3	93.0	91.9	92.8	92.0	92.7	93.8
2008	93.6	93.6	91.5	90.6	96.5	*	94.3	94.3	91.8	94.4	93.7	94.0	92.5
2009	92.8	93.3	90.9	92.2	94.0	97.3	92.8	92.5	92.0	93.3	93.5	92.1	92.1
2010	93.3	93.2	94.0	94.6	92.8	95.1	90.2	93.8	92.4	93.6	92.7	94.1	93.1
2011	93.9	93.9	93.9	88.1	96.5	96.6	93.5	93.8	93.6	94.2	94.3	93.4	94.2
2012	92.8	93.0	92.9	95.2	92.3	*	93.3	92.5	91.8	93.4	92.6	92.9	92.8
2013	92.7	93.7	91.2	92.2	95.5	*	90.8	91.6	89.2	94.4	91.9	93.2	93.4
2014	93.3	93.3	92.0	93.8	93.2	93.8	94.0	93.8	92.0	94.5	92.7	94.2	92.7
2015	93.7	93.1	93.3	91.8	96.9	92.8	92.4	94.5	91.8	94.6	93.9	94.0	91.7
Measles, Mumps, Rubella													
1998	92.0	93.1	88.8	91.4	92.2	NA	NA	91.0	90.1	93.1	91.3	92.4	92.4
1999	91.5	92.4	89.8	91.7	92.7	NA	NA	90.2	90.0	92.4	91.3	92.1	90.4
2000	90.5	91.6	87.7	89.4	89.3	94.5	88.1	90.0	88.9	90.9	89.7	91.0	90.8
2001	91.4	91.8	89.4	93.2	90.1	*	89.2	92.1	89.1	91.9	90.9	92.0	90.8
2002	91.6	92.6	90.3	84.3	94.6	94.3	89.1	90.5	90.2	91.9	90.2	93.3	90.2

Note: Final estimates from the National Immunization Survey include an adjustment for children with missing immunization provider data.

NA = Not available.

* = Estimates are considered unreliable. For data prior to 2007, percents not shown if the unweighted sample size for the numerator was less than 30, or the confidence interval half-width divided by the estimate was greater than 50 percent, or the confidence interval half-width was greater than 10. Starting with 2007 data, percents not shown if the unweighted sample size for the denominator was less than 30, or the confidence interval half-width divided by the estimate was greater than 60 percent, or the confidence interval half-width was greater than 10.

[1] Persons of Hispanic origin may be of any race.

[2] Poverty level is based on family income and family size using U.S. Census Bureau poverty thresholds. In 2015, 3.5% of the 15,167 children with provider-reported vaccination history data, 5.8% of Hispanic, 2.3% of non-Hispanic White, and 5.9% of non-Hispanic Black children, were missing information about poverty level and were omitted from the estimates of vaccination coverage by poverty level (unweighted percentages).

[3] MSA = metropolitan statistical area.

[4] Prior to data year 2000, the category Asian included Native Hawaiian and Other Pacific Islander.

[5] The 4:3:1:3:3:1:4 combined series consists of 4 or more doses of diphtheria and tetanus toxoids and pertussis vaccine (DTP), diphtheria and tetanus toxoids (DT), or diphtheria and tetanus toxoids and acellular pertussis vaccine (DTaP); 3 or more doses of any poliovirus vaccine; 1 or more doses of a measles-containing vaccine (MCV); 3 or more doses of Haemophilus influenzae type b vaccine (Hib); 3 or more doses of hepatitis B vaccine; 1 or more doses of varicella vaccine; and 4 or more doses of pneumococcal conjugate vaccine (PCV).

[6] Diphtheria and tetanus toxoids and pertussis vaccine (DTP), diphtheria and tetanus toxoids (DT), and diphtheria and tetanus toxoids and acellular pertussis vaccine (DTaP).

Table 3-36. Vaccination Coverage Among Children 19 to 35 Months of Age for Selected Diseases, by Race, Hispanic Origin, Poverty Level, and Location of Residence in Metropolitan Statistical Area, Selected Years, 1998–2015—Continued

(Percent.)

| | | Race and Hispanic origin[1] | | | | | | | Poverty level[2] | | Location of residence | | |
| | | Not Hispanic or Latino | | | | | | | | | Inside MSA[3] | | |
Vaccination and year	All	White	Black or African American	American Indian or Alaska Native	Asian[4]	Native Hawaiian or Other Pacific Islander	Two or more races	Hispanic or Latino	Below poverty level	At or above poverty level	Central city	Remaining area	Outside MSA[3]
2003	93.0	93.2	92.1	91.8	96.0	*	93.7	92.7	92.0	93.4	93.2	93.1	92.3
2004	93.0	93.5	90.7	88.8	94.1	*	93.5	93.2	91.3	93.5	92.8	93.5	92.4
2005	91.5	91.4	91.9	89.7	91.9	90.3	93.7	91.1	89.3	92.1	91.6	91.8	90.4
2006	92.3	92.8	90.9	89.3	94.7	94.3	91.0	92.0	91.1	93.1	92.5	92.5	91.5
2007	92.3	92.1	91.5	96.2	93.9	87.6	94.6	92.6	91.3	92.6	91.8	92.8	92.3
2008	92.1	91.3	92.0	95.8	94.7	97.0	94.0	92.8	92.3	92.0	92.6	92.3	90.4
2009	90.0	90.8	88.2	94.9	90.7	96.9	88.5	89.3	88.8	90.6	91.1	88.6	88.6
2010	91.5	90.6	92.1	93.4	91.7	96.9	89.7	92.9	91.3	91.4	92.4	90.5	91.4
2011	91.6	91.1	90.8	94.8	93.9	98.7	91.1	92.4	91.3	91.7	92.0	91.2	91.5
2012	90.8	90.9	90.9	92.0	89.8	*	92.3	90.7	89.9	91.4	90.1	91.0	92.4
2013	91.9	91.5	90.9	96.3	96.7	90.4	91.5	92.1	90.5	92.5	91.5	92.4	91.3
2014	91.5	91.2	90.3	96.5	95.7	95.7	90.5	91.9	89.5	92.8	91.9	91.2	91.2
2015	91.9	91.8	90.7	88.5	92.5	92.0	93.0	92.3	90.3	92.9	92.4	91.7	90.7
Hib (full series)[7]													
2009	54.8	55.3	51.2	*	54.6	*	53.7	55.4	51.4	56.5	55.5	54.9	53.0
2010	66.8	67.5	65.4	77.1	69.5	*	70.1	64.8	61.3	69.7	66.5	68.4	63.4
2011	80.4	81.0	74.6	73.7	83.5	*	82.0	81.6	75.5	83.4	81.4	80.3	77.8
2012	80.9	82.2	77.5	84.7	86.1	*	82.5	79.5	76.4	84.0	80.5	81.8	79.9
2013	82.0	84.2	74.9	82.9	82.0	*	84.9	80.9	75.8	85.3	80.6	84.3	79.7
2014	82.0	83.8	75.2	83.8	83.1	*	78.7	82.8	76.3	85.5	81.4	82.7	81.6
2015	82.7	83.0	78.9	81.4	87.0	*	82.4	83.0	78.1	85.5	82.3	83.6	80.9
Hepatitis A (2 Doses or More)													
2008	40.4	NA	NA	NA	NA	NA	NA	NA	NA	NA	NA	NA	NA
2009	46.6	46.2	41.3	33.2	50.9	*	47.8	49.3	47.3	46.2	48.2	46.9	42.0
2010	49.7	45.8	48.6	*	50.8	*	49.8	57.0	51.0	49.1	52.4	48.8	45.1
2011	52.2	50.0	50.9	*	56.9	*	50.2	56.3	50.7	53.4	55.0	50.9	47.6
2012	53.0	52.6	52.0	*	57.5	*	49.4	54.4	49.4	55.4	54.7	53.0	48.2
2013	54.7	53.4	49.1	*	67.3	*	57.8	56.6	53.5	56.1	55.5	55.2	50.1
2014	57.5	55.4	56.7	*	67.7	*	53.7	61.6	54.0	59.2	58.9	58.1	51.2
2015	59.6	58.7	59.3	61.3	67.8	*	54.1	60.9	56.0	61.7	60.5	59.6	55.7
Hepatitis B (3 Doses or More)													
1998	87.0	88.3	83.7	81.6	89.0	NA	NA	85.7	85.3	87.7	85.3	88.3	87.4
1999	88.1	88.9	86.5	*	88.2	NA	NA	87.3	86.5	89.0	87.0	89.1	88.0
2000	90.3	91.4	88.8	91.9	89.5	93.1	92.6	88.2	87.3	91.4	89.4	90.3	92.3
2001	88.9	89.6	85.0	86.6	88.8	93.9	88.0	89.8	86.5	89.5	87.5	90.0	88.9
2002	89.9	90.9	88.0	*	93.8	94.1	83.7	89.5	87.7	90.3	88.5	91.1	89.5
2003	92.4	93.2	91.6	90.3	93.6	*	93.3	91.2	91.1	93.2	91.6	92.8	92.9
2004	92.4	93.0	90.8	91.2	93.0	*	94.4	91.9	91.4	92.8	91.6	92.7	93.1
2005	92.9	93.1	92.7	90.1	92.7	*	94.4	92.7	91.4	93.5	91.8	93.9	93.4
2006	93.3	93.8	91.5	95.1	91.5	97.0	91.7	93.6	92.9	93.5	92.9	94.0	92.9
2007	92.7	92.5	91.2	96.7	93.8	*	92.1	93.6	92.1	92.9	92.2	92.8	93.5
2008	93.5	93.4	92.1	91.5	97.5	*	94.9	93.7	91.4	94.4	93.4	94.1	92.6
2009	92.4	92.3	91.6	92.5	93.1	96.2	93.3	92.6	92.3	92.7	92.8	91.8	91.8
2010	91.8	91.4	92.1	97.2	91.7	96.7	89.9	92.5	91.5	92.0	91.2	92.0	92.7
2011	91.1	90.3	92.1	92.6	95.5	91.1	90.7	91.5	91.8	91.2	91.0	90.7	92.5
2012	89.7	89.3	89.7	94.0	93.2	*	92.2	89.4	89.4	89.8	89.5	89.6	90.7
2013	90.8	91.0	91.1	96.1	92.0	94.9	90.7	89.7	88.3	92.0	89.6	91.8	91.4
2014	91.6	90.7	92.3	98.5	92.9	95.2	92.9	91.9	91.3	92.0	90.5	92.5	91.9
2015	92.6	92.0	93.3	92.4	95.5	94.1	91.4	93.2	92.5	92.7	92.9	92.5	92.1
Varicella[8]													
1998	43.2	41.9	42.4	28.0	52.6	NA	NA	46.9	40.5	44.1	45.1	45.2	34.3
1999	57.5	56.0	57.6	*	64.0	NA	NA	60.5	55.4	58.2	58.9	60.5	47.2
2000	67.8	66.3	67.6	65.8	76.3	*	69.7	70.2	63.5	69.2	69.0	69.8	60.2
2001	76.3	74.7	75.7	69.1	82.3	*	75.3	80.3	74.0	77.1	78.0	78.2	68.4

Note: Final estimates from the National Immunization Survey include an adjustment for children with missing immunization provider data.

NA = Not available.

* = Estimates are considered unreliable. For data prior to 2007, percents not shown if the unweighted sample size for the numerator was less than 30, or the confidence interval half-width divided by the estimate was greater than 50 percent, or the confidence interval half-width was greater than 10. Starting with 2007 data, percents not shown if the unweighted sample size for the denominator was less than 30, or the confidence interval half-width divided by the estimate was greater than 60 percent, or the confidence interval half-width was greater than 10.

[1]Persons of Hispanic origin may be of any race.

[2]Poverty level is based on family income and family size using U.S. Census Bureau poverty thresholds. In 2015, 3.5% of the 15,167 children with provider-reported vaccination history data, 5.8% of Hispanic, 2.3% of non-Hispanic White, and 5.9% of non-Hispanic Black children, were missing information about poverty level and were omitted from the estimates of vaccination coverage by poverty level (unweighted percentages).

[3]MSA = metropolitan statistical area.

[4]Prior to data year 2000, the category Asian included Native Hawaiian and Other Pacific Islander.

[7]Haemophilus influenzae type b vaccine (Hib) full series includes primary series plus the booster dose. Before January 2009, NIS did not distinguish between Hib vaccine product types; therefore, children who received 3 doses of a vaccine product that requires 4 doses were misclassified as fully vaccinated. In addition, there was a Hib vaccine shortage during December 2007-September 2009.

[8]Recommended in 1996. Data collection for varicella began in July 1996.

Table 3-36. Vaccination Coverage Among Children 19 to 35 Months of Age for Selected Diseases, by Race, Hispanic Origin, Poverty Level, and Location of Residence in Metropolitan Statistical Area, Selected Years, 1998–2015—Continued

(Percent.)

Vaccination and year	All	Race and Hispanic origin[1] — Not Hispanic or Latino — White	Black or African American	American Indian or Alaska Native	Asian[4]	Native Hawaiian or Other Pacific Islander	Two or more races	Hispanic or Latino	Poverty level[2] — Below poverty level	At or above poverty level	Location of residence — Inside MSA[3] — Central city	Remaining area	Outside MSA[3]
2002	80.6	79.4	82.7	70.8	87.2	*	79.2	81.8	78.9	80.9	81.0	82.5	74.8
2003	84.8	83.8	85.4	81.4	91.1	*	86.1	85.7	84.4	85.0	85.9	85.8	80.2
2004	87.5	86.5	86.3	84.0	91.1	*	89.4	89.1	86.4	87.5	87.5	88.5	84.8
2005	87.9	86.1	90.6	82.2	91.9	*	90.1	89.2	87.3	87.7	88.4	88.2	85.7
2006	89.2	88.7	89.1	85.4	92.7	90.4	91.2	89.6	88.6	90.0	90.0	90.0	86.1
2007	90.0	89.2	89.8	94.9	93.7	88.6	91.6	90.6	89.2	90.1	90.1	90.4	88.7
2008	90.7	89.8	90.4	93.8	94.2	92.3	90.9	91.8	90.1	91.1	91.9	90.4	88.4
2009	89.6	89.2	88.2	89.2	89.5	97.5	90.6	90.7	89.0	90.2	90.6	88.5	88.5
2010	90.4	88.9	91.5	95.7	92.5	92.7	88.9	92.3	89.6	90.6	90.8	90.1	90.0
2011	90.8	89.6	91.2	90.1	93.5	99.0	91.9	92.0	90.2	90.9	90.9	91.0	89.8
2012	90.2	89.8	90.4	92.5	91.9	*	90.9	90.9	89.7	90.6	90.1	90.0	91.3
2013	91.2	90.0	92.1	95.4	96.0	88.7	91.0	92.0	90.3	91.6	91.1	91.6	90.3
2014	91.0	90.3	90.1	95.7	95.3	94.9	90.0	92.1	89.9	91.9	91.4	91.1	89.8
2015	91.8	91.2	91.8	87.8	93.4	91.8	92.1	92.7	90.6	92.5	92.5	91.5	89.9
PCV (4 doses or more)[9]													
2005	53.7	57.3	46.2	*	56.2	*	54.2	50.5	44.6	57.1	51.7	57.7	48.4
2006	68.4	70.9	60.5	62.7	64.8	*	71.3	67.4	61.8	71.1	68.9	70.5	61.8
2007	75.3	76.6	70.3	80.4	75.0	*	74.1	75.4	72.8	76.3	74.8	77.3	71.0
2008	80.1	81.4	76.4	70.6	82.3	*	85.4	78.6	74.2	82.8	80.7	81.4	75.1
2009	80.4	83.4	73.2	76.2	72.5	*	73.1	80.6	74.8	83.2	79.7	81.8	81.8
2010	83.3	84.2	79.7	85.3	78.9	*	83.0	83.9	78.7	85.6	82.6	84.3	82.6
2011	84.4	85.3	81.3	75.3	84.9	93.1	84.0	84.6	80.6	86.9	85.0	84.6	82.3
2012	81.9	83.5	77.1	*	80.7	*	84.1	82.1	76.7	85.3	80.4	84.0	80.8
2013	82.0	84.1	76.1	79.0	85.6	*	83.0	80.4	74.5	86.1	80.7	84.1	79.9
2014	82.9	84.5	78.0	*	80.9	93.1	82.1	83.2	76.9	86.9	81.4	84.5	82.9
2015	84.1	85.0	81.4	77.1	85.0	*	83.7	84.0	78.9	87.2	83.9	85.5	80.4
Rotavirus vaccine[10]													
2009	43.9	46.4	38.0	*	41.7	*	38.4	43.7	37.7	47.1	44.6	46.6	35.6
2010	59.2	60.2	52.7	*	62.6	*	57.7	60.5	51.5	62.9	59.2	62.2	51.6
2011	67.3	68.3	62.5	57.7	66.9	*	67.8	68.3	61.1	71.1	68.9	67.4	62.7
2012	68.6	70.5	60.4	*	69.9	*	69.3	70.0	63.0	72.5	68.8	70.5	62.5
2013	72.6	74.8	62.1	*	74.9	*	72.8	73.7	64.3	76.9	72.4	74.7	66.7
2014	71.7	74.8	61.6	*	72.4	*	73.9	71.3	62.8	76.9	71.2	73.2	68.4
2015	73.2	74.6	69.7	*	75.6	*	70.6	72.9	66.8	76.8	72.7	75.1	68.6

Vaccination and year (percent of children age 19 to 35 months)	Not Hispanic or Latino — White — Below poverty level	At or above poverty level	Not Hispanic or Latino — Black or African American — Below poverty level	At or above poverty level	Hispanic or Latino — Below poverty level	At or above poverty level
Combined Series (4:3:1:3*:3:1:4)[5]						
2009	43.2	45.6	37.8	43.5	43.5	48.5
2010	48.7	59.0	53.4	56.3	55.0	55.2
2011	59.8	71.8	61.0	68.0	67.9	71.1
2012	58.2	72.1	62.7	68.5	68.1	68.3
2013	61.3	74.9	60.4	69.1	68.6	70.2
2014	61.2	75.4	61.5	71.0	71.8	79.4
2015	64.1	75.4	65.8	73.2	72.9	70.1

Note: Final estimates from the National Immunization Survey include an adjustment for children with missing immunization provider data.

NA = Not available.

* = Estimates are considered unreliable. For data prior to 2007, percents not shown if the unweighted sample size for the numerator was less than 30, or the confidence interval half-width divided by the estimate was greater than 50 percent, or the confidence interval half-width was greater than 10. Starting with 2007 data, percents not shown if the unweighted sample size for the denominator was less than 30, or the confidence interval half-width divided by the estimate was greater than 60 percent, or the confidence interval half-width was greater than 10.

[1]Persons of Hispanic origin may be of any race.

[2]Poverty level is based on family income and family size using U.S. Census Bureau poverty thresholds. In 2015, 3.5% of the 15,167 children with provider-reported vaccination history data, 5.8% of Hispanic, 2.3% of non-Hispanic White, and 5.9% of non-Hispanic Black children, were missing information about poverty level and were omitted from the estimates of vaccination coverage by poverty level (unweighted percentages).

[3]MSA = metropolitan statistical area.

[4]Prior to data year 2000, the category Asian included Native Hawaiian and Other Pacific Islander.

[5]The 4:3:1:3:3:1:4 combined series consists of 4 or more doses of diphtheria and tetanus toxoids and pertussis vaccine (DTP), diphtheria and tetanus toxoids (DT), or diphtheria and tetanus toxoids and acellular pertussis vaccine (DTaP);3 or more doses of any poliovirus vaccine; 1 or more doses of a measles-containing vaccine (MCV); 3 or more doses of Haemophilus influenzae type b vaccine (Hib); 3 or more doses of hepatitis B vaccine; 1 or more doses of varicella vaccine; and 4 or more doses of pneumococcal conjugate vaccine (PCV).

[9]PCV is pneumococcal conjugate vaccine. Recommended in 2000.

[10]Rotavirus vaccine includes 2 or more or 3 or more doses, depending on the product type received.

Table 3-37. Vaccination Coverage Among Adolescents 13 to 17 Years of Age for Selected Diseases, by Selected Characteristics, 2008–2013

(Percent.)

Vaccination coverage	2008	2009	2010	2011	2012	2013
Percent of Adolescents, 13 to 17 Years						
Measles, mumps, rubella (2 doses or more)	89.3	89.1	90.5	91.1	91.4	91.8
Hepatitis B (3 doses or more)	87.9	89.9	91.6	92.3	92.8	93.2
History of varicella or received varicella vaccine (2 doses or more)[1]	73.5	75.7	76.8	79.9	82.6	84.0
Tdap (1 dose or more)[2]	40.8	55.6	68.7	78.2	84.6	86.0
Meningococcal conjugate vaccine (MenACWY) (1 dose or more)[3]	41.8	53.6	62.7	70.5	74.0	77.8
Human papillomavirus (HPV) (3 doses or more among females)[4]	17.9	26.7	32.0	34.8	33.4	37.6
Human papillomavirus (HPV) (3 doses or more among males)[4]	X	X	X	1.3	6.8	13.9

| | Race and Hispanic origin[5] | | | | | Poverty level[6] | | Location of residence | | |
| | Not Hispanic or Latino | | | | | | | Inside MSA[7] | | |
Vaccination coverage, 2013	White	Black or African American	American Indian or Alaska Native	Asian	Hispanic or Latino	Below poverty level	At or above poverty level	Central city	Remaining area	Outside MSA[7]
Percent of Adolescents, 13 to 17 Years										
Measles, mumps, rubella (2 doses or more)	92.8	91.1	93.5	90.8	90.2	91.7	91.8	91.2	92.1	92.6
Hepatitis B (3 doses or more)	93.8	93.2	93.4	87.8	92.8	93.2	93.1	92.9	93.3	93.8
History of varicella or received varicella vaccine (2 doses or more)[1]	77.7	77.9	78.7	85.2	80.3	77.3	79.0	79.1	80.4	69.5
Tdap (1 dose or more)[2]	85.9	84.1	85.3	89.7	87.1	85.2	86.4	86.2	87.1	81.7
Meningococcal conjugate vaccine (MenACWY) (1 dose or more)[3]	75.6	77.0	71.7	83.8	83.4	78.4	77.5	80.5	79.7	63.1
Human papillomavirus (HPV) (3 doses or more among females)[4]	34.9	34.2	43.2	40.4	44.8	41.5	36.4	39.5	37.7	31.6
Human papillomavirus (HPV) (3 doses or more among males)[4]	11.1	15.7	*	9.1	20.3	16.7	13.0	16.9	13.0	8.0

X = Not applicable.
* = Estimates are not reliable and not shown if the unweighted sample size for the denominator is less than 30 or the confidence interval half-width divided by the estimate is greater than 0.588.
[1]Varicella is chickenpox.
[2]Tdap refers to tetanus toxoid-diphtheria vaccine (Td) or tetanus toxoid, reduced diphtheria toxoid, and acellular pertussis vaccine (Tdap) or tetanus-unknown type vaccine received since the age of 10 years.
[3]Includes persons receiving MenACWY or meningococcal-unknown type vaccine.
[4]For 2008, refers to HPV vaccine quadrivalent; for 2009 and beyond, refers to HPV vaccine quadrivalent or bivalent.
[5]Persons of Hispanic origin may be of any race.
[6]Poverty level is based on family income and family size using U.S. Census Bureau poverty thresholds. In 2011, less than 4 percent (unweighted) of adolescents with provider-reported vaccination data were missing information about poverty level and were not included in the estimates of vaccination coverage by poverty level.
[7]MSA = metropolitan statistical area.

Table 3-38. Influenza Vaccination[1] Among Adults 18 Years of Age and Over, by Selected Characteristics, Selected Years, 1989–2015

(Percent.)

Characteristic	1989	1995	2000	2005	2006	2007	2008	2009	2010	2011	2012	2013	2014	2015
18 years and over, age-adjusted[2,3]	9.6	23.7	28.7	21.6	27.5	29.9	32.2	34.2	35.3	37.2	36.8	39.9	41.0	41.7
18 years and over, crude[3]	9.1	23.0	28.4	21.4	27.6	30.1	32.6	34.7	35.8	37.9	37.7	41.0	42.2	43.2
Age														
18 to 44 years	3.3	12.0	15.6	10.1	14.6	16.5	18.8	22.2	24.6	26.0	25.6	28.5	30.2	30.9
45 to 64 years	8.8	24.5	31.6	20.2	29.2	32.5	35.9	36.8	37.8	40.0	39.4	43.7	43.3	45.1
65 years and over	30.4	58.2	64.4	59.7	64.3	66.7	67.2	66.8	63.9	66.9	66.5	67.9	70.1	69.1
65 to 74 years	28.0	54.9	61.1	53.7	60.1	61.6	60.9	61.5	60.5	63.0	62.6	64.4	67.1	67.0
75 years and over	34.2	63.0	68.4	66.3	69.2	72.6	74.3	73.2	68.2	71.9	71.7	72.8	74.3	72.1
18 YEARS AND OVER														
Sex														
Male	8.5	21.5	26.7	18.4	24.8	27.1	28.9	31.2	31.3	34.1	33.4	37.0	37.9	39.2
Female	9.7	24.4	30.0	24.2	30.1	32.9	36.2	37.9	40.0	41.5	41.7	44.7	46.1	46.8
Race[4]														
White only	9.6	23.7	30.1	22.5	28.6	31.4	33.8	35.9	36.9	39.0	38.7	42.2	43.4	44.2
Black or African American only	6.4	19.0	19.8	15.5	21.1	22.5	25.8	27.6	28.1	30.8	30.6	33.0	34.1	35.7
American Indian or Alaska Native only	10.9	*16.5	31.1	16.2	26.7	30.8	26.9	26.9	36.3	38.1	37.2	37.9	42.6	39.3
Asian only	4.3	20.0	27.0	16.9	26.4	27.9	31.7	36.2	38.6	39.1	40.9	43.9	45.0	47.0
Native Hawaiian or Other Pacific Islander only	---	---	*	*	*	*	*	*	*	*	*	*	*	*
Two or more races	---	---	25.3	15.9	23.7	25.4	29.3	25.2	28.9	30.8	30.1	34.7	34.3	40.8
Hispanic Origin and Race[4]														
Hispanic or Latino	5.9	16.1	17.7	12.0	16.0	19.2	20.8	23.7	26.5	28.9	28.1	28.9	31.0	31.2
Mexican	5.2	16.0	16.6	10.9	15.2	18.2	19.2	22.7	25.1	27.6	26.8	29.2	31.2	30.4
Not Hispanic or Latino	9.4	23.7	29.8	22.8	29.3	31.8	34.5	36.4	37.3	39.4	39.4	43.1	44.2	45.4
White only	9.9	24.6	31.4	24.3	30.8	33.6	36.2	38.1	38.8	41.0	40.9	44.9	46.0	46.9
Black or African American only	6.4	19.2	19.9	15.6	21.6	22.3	25.7	27.8	28.0	30.9	30.9	33.2	34.4	36.0
Percent of Poverty Level[5]														
Below 100 percent	8.9	20.6	23.1	16.9	21.3	22.7	24.8	25.9	25.0	28.1	29.2	30.1	32.0	33.6
100 percent to 199 percent	11.5	23.4	28.1	22.0	26.7	28.3	30.2	31.0	31.3	32.7	32.3	35.5	36.7	37.0
200 percent to 399 percent	8.0	22.8	29.6	22.9	27.8	29.5	32.2	34.1	34.8	38.0	36.8	40.1	40.8	41.2
400 percent or more	9.0	24.3	29.2	21.3	30.0	33.6	36.4	39.8	42.7	44.1	44.5	48.6	49.7	50.4
Hispanic Origin and Race and Percent of Poverty Level[4,5]														
Hispanic or Latino														
Below 100 percent	5.1	13.3	14.5	9.5	13.7	20.5	17.9	19.5	21.9	25.3	25.4	25.8	26.8	29.9
100 percent to 199 percent	7.5	17.8	15.8	11.9	13.7	17.9	19.6	20.3	23.3	27.2	25.7	25.4	29.6	27.7
200 percent to 399 percent	6.3	15.7	19.3	11.8	17.2	17.4	19.7	25.2	27.5	29.3	28.6	29.4	30.8	30.0
400 percent or more	6.0	19.8	22.2	15.5	20.3	22.5	26.4	32.1	36.4	36.0	35.5	37.6	39.8	40.0
Not Hispanic or Latino														
White only														
Below 100 percent	10.6	23.9	27.8	20.6	25.0	24.4	28.4	30.3	26.5	29.3	31.3	32.4	35.1	34.9
100 percent to 199 percent	13.2	25.6	33.1	27.4	32.1	33.8	35.7	36.2	35.0	34.9	35.8	40.7	41.2	41.7
200 percent to 399 percent	8.3	23.8	32.5	26.3	30.9	32.9	35.8	36.5	37.5	40.7	38.9	42.9	44.0	44.4
400 percent or more	9.4	25.5	30.5	22.4	31.5	35.7	38.1	41.4	43.8	45.9	46.2	50.4	51.3	52.2
Black or African American only														
Below 100 percent	7.5	19.8	20.0	17.0	20.0	18.9	23.4	24.5	24.0	27.5	27.7	28.3	29.4	30.2
100 percent to 199 percent	6.4	18.8	21.3	15.4	21.4	20.5	24.3	26.6	28.6	30.7	29.9	30.9	33.0	33.9
200 percent to 399 percent	6.9	20.4	19.5	15.1	21.1	24.5	25.9	28.9	27.4	31.6	31.8	35.2	34.6	36.1
400 percent or more	5.6	15.6	19.2	15.3	23.8	24.2	28.8	31.1	32.9	33.9	34.2	38.2	41.6	43.3
Disability Measure[6]														
Any basic actions difficulty or complex activity limitation	NA	NA	40.8	34.1	39.8	42.5	44.0	44.9	44.6	47.6	47.3	50.6	51.4	52.2
Any basic actions difficulty	NA	NA	41.0	34.4	40.2	43.1	44.6	45.3	45.1	48.1	47.8	51.3	51.8	52.5
Any complex activity limitation	NA	NA	44.7	40.3	45.1	45.6	48.5	49.4	47.7	50.8	50.9	52.3	54.7	53.9
No disability	NA	NA	23.2	15.6	21.9	24.3	27.2	29.8	31.6	33.2	33.2	36.7	37.9	38.8
Geographic Region														
Northeast	8.6	21.2	28.0	23.2	27.4	31.2	34.0	37.0	39.1	40.8	40.1	44.5	45.0	46.6
Midwest	8.8	22.7	28.5	22.6	30.5	32.6	35.4	35.9	37.6	37.9	38.4	41.4	43.6	43.1
South	9.5	24.7	28.7	20.3	26.5	29.1	31.8	34.5	35.1	38.2	37.2	40.1	41.5	42.4
West	9.4	22.3	28.1	20.2	26.3	28.2	30.1	31.8	32.6	35.4	36.0	39.4	39.7	41.8
Location of Residence														
Within MSA[7]	8.5	22.3	27.5	20.4	26.5	28.8	31.7	34.1	35.7	37.7	37.7	40.8	41.9	43.4
Outside MSA[7]	11.4	25.7	31.8	25.1	32.3	36.4	37.2	37.4	36.1	39.2	37.9	42.2	44.1	41.9

NA = Not available.
* = Figure does not meet standards of reliability or precision.
NA = Data not available.
[1] Questions concerning use of influenza vaccination differed slightly on the National Health Interview Survey across the years for which data are shown.
[2] Estimates are age adjusted to the year 2000 standard population using four age groups: 18 to 49 years, 50 to 64 years, 65 to 74 years, and 75 years and over.
[3] Includes all other races not shown separately, unknown disability status, and unknown poverty level in 1989.
[4] The race groups White, Black, American Indian or Alaska Native, Asian, Native Hawaiian or Other Pacific Islander, and two or more races, include persons of Hispanic and non-Hispanic origin. Persons of Hispanic origin may be of any race.
[5] Percent of poverty level is based on family income and family size and composition using U.S. Census Bureau poverty thresholds. Poverty level was unknown for 11 percent of persons 18 years of age and over in 1989. Missing family income data were imputed for 1991 and beyond.
[6] Any basic actions difficulty or complex activity limitation is defined as having one or more of the following limitations or difficulties: movement difficulty, emotional difficulty, sensory (seeing or hearing) difficulty, cognitive difficulty, self-care (activities of daily living or instrumental activities of daily living) limitation, social limitation, or work limitation.
[7] MSA = metropolitan statistical area.

Table 3-39. Pneumococcal Vaccination[1] Among Adults 18 Years of Age and Over, by Selected Characteristics, Selected Years, 1989–2015

(Percent.)

Characteristic	1989	1995	2000	2005	2006	2007	2008	2009	2010	2011	2012	2013	2014	2015
18 years and over, age-adjusted[2,3]	4.6	12.0	15.4	16.7	17.1	16.8	18.3	19.0	19.2	20.6	19.9	19.9	20.5	21.2
18 years and over, crude[3]	4.4	11.7	15.1	16.5	17.0	16.7	18.5	19.3	19.6	21.1	20.7	21.0	21.8	22.9
Age														
18 to 44 years	2.1	6.6	5.1	5.3	5.4	4.9	6.3	6.8	6.9	8.3	7.9	7.5	8.3	8.8
45 to 64 years	3.7	8.8	12.2	14.3	14.9	14.4	15.9	16.8	17.7	18.4	18.0	18.8	18.4	18.8
65 years and over	14.1	34.0	53.1	56.2	57.1	57.7	60.0	60.6	59.7	62.3	59.9	59.7	61.3	63.6
65 to 74 years	13.1	31.4	48.2	49.4	52.0	51.8	52.5	54.6	54.6	56.0	55.0	55.0	55.8	60.2
75 years and over	15.7	37.8	59.1	63.9	63.0	64.4	68.7	68.0	66.0	70.0	66.4	67.1	69.3	68.5
High-Risk Group[4]														
Total, 18 to 64 years	NA	NA	18.3	22.6	23.1	24.4	24.9	17.4	18.3	20.0	19.9	21.0	20.2	23.0
18 to 49 years	NA	NA	11.3	13.8	11.7	14.3	13.8	9.5	9.8	12.4	11.3	11.7	11.3	12.8
50 to 64 years	NA	NA	23.3	27.9	29.5	29.6	31.3	25.4	26.7	27.3	28.0	29.4	28.3	31.6
65 YEARS AND OVER														
Sex														
Male	13.9	34.6	52.1	53.4	54.3	55.1	56.4	59.2	57.6	59.5	55.8	57.1	58.4	62.9
Female	14.3	33.6	53.9	58.4	59.2	59.6	62.8	61.7	61.3	64.5	63.1	61.8	63.7	64.2
Race[5]														
White only	14.8	35.3	55.6	58.4	60.0	60.1	62.5	63.1	61.6	64.7	62.3	61.7	63.1	65.8
Black or African American only	6.4	21.9	30.6	40.2	35.5	43.7	44.1	44.2	45.5	47.5	46.0	48.4	49.2	49.9
American Indian or Alaska Native only	31.2	*	70.1	*	*57.5	*	66.9	*	*48.5	53.0	*36.3	52.9	57.1	60.3
Asian only	*	*23.4	40.9	35.0	35.6	33.4	45.7	44.8	47.9	40.3	41.1	45.0	47.7	49.3
Native Hawaiian or Other Pacific Islander only	NA	NA	*	*	*	*	*	*	*	*	*	*	*	*
Two or more races	NA	NA	55.6	64.8	63.6	55.8	*35.9	67.9	65.5	77.1	45.4	50.8	71.2	60.4
Hispanic Origin and Race[5]														
Hispanic or Latino	9.8	23.2	30.4	27.5	33.3	31.8	36.4	40.1	39.0	43.1	43.4	39.2	45.2	41.7
Mexican	12.9	*18.8	32.0	31.3	29.3	34.3	39.5	42.8	41.4	47.1	45.5	47.4	47.8	49.1
Not Hispanic or Latino	14.3	34.5	54.4	58.1	58.7	59.6	61.8	62.2	61.3	63.8	61.2	61.4	62.7	65.5
White only	15.0	35.9	56.8	60.6	62.0	62.2	64.5	64.8	63.5	66.5	64.0	63.6	64.7	68.1
Black or African American only	6.2	21.8	30.6	40.4	35.6	44.0	44.5	44.7	46.2	47.6	46.1	48.7	49.8	50.2
Percent of Poverty Level[6]														
Below 100 percent	11.2	28.7	40.6	46.7	45.4	48.7	46.5	48.5	42.6	49.6	39.5	50.5	47.3	48.7
100 percent to 199 percent	15.1	30.7	51.4	54.5	55.8	55.6	59.5	60.6	57.2	60.3	59.8	58.0	59.5	61.7
200 percent to 399 percent	15.1	36.1	55.8	60.8	59.9	59.8	61.4	62.9	62.2	63.4	63.6	61.7	64.5	64.8
400 percent or more	15.5	39.5	56.9	55.3	59.3	59.8	62.8	61.5	64.0	66.4	61.4	61.6	63.2	67.1
Hispanic Origin and Race and Percent of Poverty Level[5,6]														
Hispanic or Latino														
Below 100 percent	*	*14.1	23.8	20.9	24.5	*22.4	*25.7	32.6	30.2	34.8	30.9	35.3	34.1	31.0
100 percent to 199 percent	*11.0	*15.6	32.3	26.9	30.9	37.9	32.9	41.8	36.9	49.3	42.0	39.1	44.4	45.2
200 percent to 399 percent	*11.1	*34.4	37.6	35.2	42.3	29.6	44.8	40.0	45.8	39.2	54.5	36.1	52.1	43.9
400 percent or more	*	*55.1	*26.4	*25.2	*38.2	*33.7	42.4	49.1	43.0	49.1	46.4	49.1	54.0	44.3
Not Hispanic or Latino														
White only														
Below 100 percent	13.3	32.5	47.9	55.6	56.0	59.7	60.4	61.0	51.1	60.3	46.5	59.1	55.4	54.1
100 percent to 199 percent	16.0	33.5	56.1	60.5	61.6	60.8	66.3	66.3	61.3	64.6	66.1	63.3	64.1	67.4
200 percent to 399 percent	15.7	37.1	57.6	64.1	62.6	63.4	64.5	66.3	64.9	66.9	65.9	65.2	66.9	68.4
400 percent or more	15.9	39.3	59.5	57.4	63.0	62.4	64.1	62.9	66.0	68.6	63.5	63.2	64.5	70.2
Black or African American only														
Below 100 percent	*5.0	*22.6	28.8	42.3	38.4	40.7	37.6	33.8	34.9	39.5	36.1	48.9	46.0	53.3
100 percent to 199 percent	7.8	*20.9	28.1	36.6	36.2	41.9	43.5	46.9	46.4	45.6	44.5	46.9	49.1	46.9
200 percent to 399 percent	*5.9	*21.7	35.5	41.6	40.0	48.7	44.5	49.3	51.8	54.2	54.1	49.4	47.9	44.1
400 percent or more	*	*	*32.6	44.6	*24.7	43.6	56.5	45.8	50.1	49.1	45.4	50.3	56.0	61.8
Any Basic Actions Difficulty or Complex Activity Limitation[7]														
Any basic actions difficulty or complex activity limitation	NA	NA	56.6	61.6	61.4	64.2	64.9	65.9	63.9	67.0	65.4	64.4	66.7	66.4
Any basic actions difficulty	NA	NA	56.8	61.6	61.6	64.4	65.1	66.0	64.2	67.3	66.0	64.9	66.7	66.6
Any complex activity limitation	NA	NA	58.0	63.3	61.6	63.9	67.0	67.8	65.2	66.7	65.7	66.1	67.6	67.1
No disability	NA	NA	47.9	47.8	50.0	47.0	53.4	53.1	53.3	55.6	53.2	53.1	53.7	59.4
Geographic Region														
Northeast	10.4	28.2	51.2	55.8	53.7	54.6	60.9	58.5	56.7	60.0	58.0	59.1	59.6	60.8
Midwest	13.7	31.0	52.6	58.5	61.5	60.6	63.8	58.4	61.2	65.6	63.8	62.3	65.4	68.3
South	14.9	35.9	51.3	57.4	55.7	58.5	59.8	61.9	60.9	63.2	59.5	59.3	60.9	62.3
West	17.9	41.1	59.7	51.4	57.2	55.6	55.4	63.0	58.9	59.5	58.2	58.3	59.3	63.7
Location of Residence														
Within MSA[8]	13.1	33.8	52.4	55.1	56.6	56.5	59.1	60.0	58.8	61.7	59.3	59.0	60.7	63.4
Outside MSA[8]	16.9	34.7	55.4	59.8	58.9	61.7	63.2	62.9	63.3	64.6	62.4	62.8	64.0	64.7

NA = Not available.
* = Estimates are considered unreliable. Data preceded by an asterisk have a relative standard error (RSE) of 20 percent to 30 percent. Data not shown have an RSE of greater than 30 percent.
[1] Respondents were asked, "Have you ever had a pneumonia shot? This shot is usually given only once or twice in a person's lifetime and is different from the flu shot. It is also called the pneumococcal vaccine."
[2] Estimates are age adjusted to the year 2000 standard population using four age groups: 18 to 44 years, 45 to 64 years, 65 to 74 years, and 75 years and over.
[3] Includes all other races not shown separately, unknown poverty level in 1989, and unknown disability status.
[4] High-risk group membership is based on recommendations of the Advisory Committee on Immunization Practices (ACIP). The high-risk group includes persons who reported diabetes, cancer, heart, lung, liver, or kidney disease. Starting with data year 2012, the survey questionnaire changed and now asks respondents if a health professional had ever told them they had chronic obstructive pulmonary disease (COPD), and this information was added to the list of lung diseases used to construct the high-risk category.
respondents if a health professional had ever told them they had chronic obstructive pulmonary disease (COPD), and this information was added to the list of lung diseases used to construct the high-risk category.
[5] The race groups White, Black, American Indian or Alaska Native, Asian, Native Hawaiian or Other Pacific Islander, and two or more races, include persons of Hispanic and non-Hispanic origin. Persons of Hispanic origin may be of any race.
[6] Percent of poverty level is based on family income and family size and composition using U.S. Census Bureau poverty thresholds. Poverty level was unknown for 11 percent of persons 18 years of age and over in 1989. Missing family income data were imputed for 1991 and beyond.
[7] Any basic actions difficulty or complex activity limitation is defined as having one or more of the following limitations or difficulties: movement difficulty, emotional difficulty, sensory (seeing or hearing) difficulty, cognitive difficulty, self-care (activities of daily living or instrumental activities of daily living) limitation, social limitation, or work limitation.
[8] MSA = metropolitan statistical area.

Table 3-40. Use of Mammography[1] Among Women 40 Years of Age and Over, by Selected Characteristics, Selected Years, 1987–2015

(Percent.)

Characteristic	1987	1990	1991	1993	1994	1998	1999	2000	2003	2005	2008	2010	2013	2015
40 years and over, age-adjusted[2,3]	29.0	51.7	54.7	59.7	61.0	67.0	70.3	70.4	69.5	66.6	67.1	66.5	65.7	64.0
40 years and over, crude[2]	28.7	51.4	54.6	59.7	60.9	66.9	70.3	70.4	69.7	66.8	67.6	67.1	66.8	65.3
50 years and over, age-adjusted[2,3]	27.3	49.8	54.3	59.7	60.9	69.0	72.1	73.7	72.4	68.2	70.3	68.8	69.1	67.2
50 years and over, crude[2]	27.4	49.7	54.1	59.7	60.6	68.9	71.9	73.6	72.4	68.4	70.5	69.2	69.5	67.8
Age														
40 to 49 years	31.9	55.1	55.6	59.9	61.3	63.4	67.2	64.3	64.4	63.5	61.5	62.3	59.6	58.3
50 to 64 years	31.7	56.0	60.3	65.1	66.5	73.7	76.5	78.7	76.2	71.8	74.2	72.6	71.4	71.3
65 years and over	22.8	43.4	48.1	54.2	55.0	63.8	66.8	67.9	67.7	63.8	65.5	64.4	66.9	63.3
65 to 74 years	26.6	48.7	55.7	64.2	63.0	69.4	73.9	74.0	74.6	72.5	72.6	71.9	75.3	72.2
75 years and over	17.3	35.8	37.8	41.0	44.6	57.2	58.9	61.3	60.6	54.7	57.9	55.7	56.5	51.5
Race[4]														
40 years and over, crude														
White only	29.6	52.2	55.6	60.0	60.6	67.4	70.6	71.4	70.1	67.4	67.9	67.4	66.8	65.3
Black or African American only	24.0	46.4	48.0	59.1	64.3	66.0	71.0	67.8	70.4	64.9	68.0	67.9	67.1	69.8
American Indian or Alaska Native only	*	43.2	54.5	49.8	65.8	45.2	63.0	47.4	63.1	72.8	62.7	71.2	62.6	51.5
Asian only	*	46.0	45.9	55.1	55.8	60.2	58.3	53.5	57.6	54.6	66.1	62.4	66.6	59.7
Native Hawaiian or Other Pacific Islander only	NA	NA	NA	NA	NA	NA	*	*	*	*	*	*	*	*
Two or more races	NA	NA	NA	NA	NA	NA	70.2	69.2	65.3	63.7	55.2	51.4	65.4	62.7
Hispanic Origin and Race[4]														
40 years and over, crude														
Hispanic or Latina	18.3	45.2	49.2	50.9	51.9	60.2	65.7	61.2	65.0	58.8	61.2	64.2	61.4	60.9
Not Hispanic or Latina	29.4	51.8	54.9	60.3	61.5	67.5	70.7	71.1	70.1	67.5	68.3	67.4	67.5	65.9
White only	30.3	52.7	56.0	60.6	61.3	68.0	71.1	72.2	70.5	68.3	68.7	67.8	67.6	65.8
Black or African American only	23.8	46.0	47.7	59.2	64.4	66.0	71.0	67.9	70.5	65.2	68.3	67.4	67.2	69.7
Age, Hispanic Origin, and Race[4]														
40 to 49 years														
Hispanic or Latina	*15.3	45.1	44.0	52.6	47.5	55.2	61.6	54.1	59.4	54.2	54.1	59.8	56.4	50.3
Not Hispanic or Latina														
White only	34.3	57.0	58.1	61.6	62.0	64.4	68.3	67.2	65.2	65.5	64.1	62.6	60.3	58.8
Black or African American only	27.8	48.4	48.0	55.6	67.2	65.0	69.2	60.9	68.2	62.1	59.5	63.5	59.4	67.8
50 to 64 years														
Hispanic or Latina	23.0	47.5	61.7	59.2	60.1	67.2	69.7	66.5	69.4	61.5	71.3	68.6	65.6	71.6
Not Hispanic or Latina														
White only	33.6	58.1	61.5	66.2	67.5	75.3	77.9	80.6	77.2	73.5	74.1	73.5	72.1	71.4
Black or African American only	26.4	48.4	52.4	65.5	63.6	71.2	75.0	77.7	76.2	71.6	76.7	74.0	71.7	73.5
65 years and over														
Hispanic or Latina														
Not Hispanic or Latina	*	41.1	40.9	*35.7	48.0	59.0	67.2	68.3	69.5	63.8	59.0	65.2	63.2	60.9
White only														
Black or African American only	24.0	43.8	49.1	54.7	54.9	64.3	66.8	68.3	68.1	64.7	66.1	65.0	67.3	63.9
Age and Percent of Poverty Level[5]														
40 years and over, crude														
Below 100 percent	14.6	30.8	35.2	41.1	44.2	50.1	57.4	54.8	55.4	48.5	51.4	51.4	49.9	52.2
100 percent to 199 percent	20.9	39.1	44.4	47.5	48.6	56.1	59.5	58.1	60.8	55.3	55.8	53.8	56.7	54.9
200 percent to 399 percent	29.7	53.3	57.5	63.2	65.0	67.4	69.1	68.8	69.9	67.2	64.4	66.2	66.0	63.4
400 percent or more	42.9	68.7	69.8	74.1	74.1	76.8	79.8	81.5	77.7	76.6	79.0	78.1	77.2	74.7
40 to 49 years														
Below 100 percent	18.6	32.2	33.0	36.1	43.0	44.8	51.3	47.4	50.6	42.5	46.6	48.1	43.3	45.8
100 percent to 199 percent	18.4	39.0	43.8	47.8	47.6	46.9	52.8	43.6	54.0	49.8	46.5	46.2	52.0	47.5
200 percent to 399 percent	31.2	55.2	56.3	63.0	64.5	61.8	63.0	60.2	63.0	61.8	56.8	59.2	58.5	55.6
400 percent or more	44.1	68.9	69.6	69.6	69.9	72.7	77.4	75.8	71.6	73.6	72.5	73.6	69.0	68.2
50 to 64 years														
Below 100 percent	14.6	29.9	37.3	47.3	46.2	52.7	63.3	61.7	58.3	50.4	57.5	54.7	55.0	56.9
100 percent to 199 percent	24.2	39.8	50.2	47.0	49.0	61.8	64.9	68.3	64.0	58.8	58.9	57.3	57.2	60.5
200 percent to 399 percent	29.7	56.2	60.2	66.1	69.6	71.1	74.8	75.1	74.1	70.7	69.8	70.7	69.5	69.0
400 percent or more	44.7	71.6	72.6	78.7	78.0	83.4	83.4	86.9	84.9	80.6	84.3	82.8	80.9	79.2
65 years and over														
Below 100 percent	13.1	30.8	35.2	40.4	43.9	51.9	57.6	54.8	57.0	52.3	49.1	50.6	49.8	52.7
100 percent to 199 percent	19.9	38.6	41.8	47.6	48.8	57.8	60.2	60.3	62.8	56.1	59.4	55.5	59.3	54.4
200 percent to 399 percent	27.7	47.4	55.9	60.3	61.0	69.5	70.0	71.1	72.3	68.6	65.0	67.2	68.1	63.3
400 percent or more	34.7	61.2	63.0	71.3	73.0	71.1	76.7	81.9	73.0	72.6	78.3	74.5	79.0	73.1
Health Insurance Status at the Time of Interview[6]														
40 to 64 years														
Insured	NA	NA	NA	66.2	68.3	72.3	75.5	76.0	75.1	72.5	73.4	74.1	72.1	69.7

NA = Not available.
* = Estimates are considered unreliable. Data preceded by an asterisk have a relative standard error (RSE) of 20 percent to 30 percent. Data not shown have an RSE of greater than 30 percent.
[1]Questions concerning use of mammography differed slightly on the National Health Interview Survey across the years for which data are shown.
[2]Includes all other races not shown separately, unknown poverty level in 1987, unknown health insurance status, unknown education level, and unknown disability status.
[3]Estimates for women 40 years of age and over are age-adjusted to the year 2000 standard population using four age groups: 40 to 49 years, 50 to 64 years, 65 to 74 years, and 75 years and over. Estimates for women 50 years of age and over are age-adjusted using three age groups.
[4]The race groups White, Black, American Indian or Alaska Native, Asian, Native Hawaiian or Other Pacific Islander, and two or more races, include persons of Hispanic and non-Hispanic origin. Persons of Hispanic origin may be of any race.
[5]Percent of poverty level is based on family income and family size and composition using U.S. Census Bureau poverty thresholds. Poverty level was unknown for 11 percent of women 40 years of age and over in 1987. Missing family income data were imputed for 1997 and beyond.
[6]Health insurance categories are mutually exclusive. Persons who reported both Medicaid and private coverage are classified as having private coverage. Medicaid includes other public assistance through 1996. Starting with 1997 data, state-sponsored health plan coverage is included as Medicaid coverage. Starting with 1999 data, coverage by the Children's Health Insurance Program (CHIP) is included with Medicaid coverage. Persons not covered by private insurance, Medicaid, CHIP, public assistance (through 1996), state-sponsored or other government-sponsored health plans (starting in 1997), Medicare, or military plans are considered to have no health insurance coverage. Persons with only Indian Health Service coverage are considered to have no health insurance coverage. Health insurance status was unknown for 8 to 9 percent of children in 1993-1996 and about 1 percent in 1997-2011.

Table 3-40. Use of Mammography[1] Among Women 40 Years of Age and Over, by Selected Characteristics, Selected Years, 1987–2015—Continued

(Percent.)

Characteristic	1987	1990	1991	1993	1994	1998	1999	2000	2003	2005	2008	2010	2013	2015
Private..	NA	NA	NA	67.1	69.4	73.4	76.3	77.1	76.3	74.5	74.2	75.6	73.4	72.2
Medicaid.....................................	NA	NA	NA	51.9	54.5	59.7	62.5	61.7	63.5	55.6	64.2	64.4	63.5	57.7
Uninsured...................................	NA	NA	NA	36.0	34.0	40.1	44.8	40.7	41.5	38.1	39.7	36.0	37.3	30.0
Health Insurance Status Prior to Interview[6]														
40 to 64 years														
Insured continuously all 12 months.................	NA	NA	NA	66.6	68.6	73.0	76.1	76.8	75.6	73.1	74.1	74.7	72.7	70.6
Uninsured for any period up to 12 months	NA	NA	NA	49.4	49.9	47.6	57.1	53.0	56.0	51.3	55.3	57.3	54.5	50.0
Uninsured more than 12 months	NA	NA	NA	28.4	26.6	36.3	38.9	34.0	37.0	32.9	34.6	30.0	32.8	23.9
Age and Education[7]														
40 years and over, crude														
No high school diploma or GED......................	17.8	36.4	40.0	46.4	48.2	54.5	56.7	57.7	58.1	52.8	53.8	53.0	53.6	51.7
High school diploma or GED...........................	31.3	52.7	55.8	59.0	61.0	66.7	69.2	69.7	67.8	64.9	65.2	64.4	63.4	60.1
Some college or more.....................................	37.7	62.8	65.2	69.5	69.7	72.8	77.3	76.2	75.1	72.7	73.4	72.1	71.6	70.5
40 to 49 years														
No high school diploma or GED......................	15.1	38.5	40.8	43.6	50.4	47.3	48.8	46.8	53.3	51.2	46.9	44.9	46.9	43.8
High school diploma or GED...........................	32.6	53.1	52.0	56.6	55.8	59.1	60.8	59.0	60.8	58.8	57.2	58.4	51.8	47.5
Some college or more.....................................	39.2	62.3	63.7	66.1	68.7	68.3	74.4	70.6	68.1	68.3	66.3	66.5	64.3	64.0
50 to 64 years														
No high school diploma or GED......................	21.2	41.0	43.6	51.4	51.6	58.8	62.3	66.5	63.4	56.9	64.9	56.7	58.2	58.1
High school diploma or GED...........................	33.8	56.5	60.8	62.4	67.8	73.3	77.2	76.6	71.8	70.1	70.4	69.9	66.9	67.0
Some college or more.....................................	40.5	68.0	72.7	78.5	74.7	79.8	81.2	84.2	82.7	77.0	78.5	77.0	75.7	75.3
65 years and over														
No high school diploma or GED......................	16.5	33.0	37.7	44.2	45.6	54.7	56.6	57.4	56.9	50.7	49.2	54.1	53.4	50.8
High school diploma or GED...........................	25.9	47.5	54.0	57.4	59.1	66.8	68.4	71.8	69.7	64.3	65.7	62.5	66.5	60.0
Some college or more.....................................	32.3	56.7	57.9	64.8	64.3	71.3	77.1	74.1	75.1	73.0	75.6	70.9	73.6	69.8
Disability Measure[8]														
40 years and over, crude														
Any basic actions difficulty or complex activity limitation..	NA	NA	NA	NA	NA	65.8	67.6	67.8	67.2	63.5	63.9	63.3	63.5	62.2
Any basic actions difficulty	NA	NA	NA	NA	NA	65.9	67.1	67.9	67.3	63.5	63.9	63.3	63.8	62.4
Any complex activity limitation	NA	NA	NA	NA	NA	61.8	64.8	64.1	62.3	59.9	60.2	58.2	58.4	56.1
No disability	NA	NA	NA	NA	NA	68.2	72.3	72.6	71.8	69.8	71.1	70.8	69.8	68.0

NA = Not available.

[1]Questions concerning use of mammography differed slightly on the National Health Interview Survey across the years for which data are shown.

[6]Health insurance categories are mutually exclusive. Persons who reported both Medicaid and private coverage are classified as having private coverage. Medicaid includes other public assistance through 1996. Starting with 1997 data, state-sponsored health plan coverage is included as Medicaid coverage. Starting with 1999 data, coverage by the Children's Health Insurance Program (CHIP) is included with Medicaid coverage. Persons not covered by private insurance, Medicaid, CHIP, public assistance (through 1996), state-sponsored or other government-sponsored health plans (starting in 1997), Medicare, or military plans are considered to have no health insurance coverage. Persons with only Indian Health Service coverage are considered to have no health insurance coverage. Health insurance status was unknown for 8 to 9 percent of children in 1993-1996 and about 1 percent in 1997-2011.

[7]Education categories shown are for 1998 and subsequent years. GED is General Educational Development high school equivalency diploma. In years prior to 1998, the following categories based on number of years in school completed were used: less than 12 years, 12 years, and 13 years or more.

[8]Any basic actions difficulty or complex activity limitation is defined as having one or more of the following limitations or difficulties: movement difficulty, emotional difficulty, sensory (seeing or hearing) difficulty, cognitive difficulty, self-care (activities of daily living or instrumental activities of daily living) limitation, social limitation, or work limitation.

Table 3-41. Percent of Women 18 Years of Age and Over Who Have Had a Pap Smear[1] Within the Last Three Years, by Selected Characteristics, Selected Years, 1987–2015

(Percent.)

Characteristic	1987	1993	1994	1998	1999	2000	2003	2005	2008	2010	2013	2015
18 years and over, age-adjusted[2,3]	74.1	77.7	76.8	79.3	80.8	81.3	79.2	77.9	75.6	73.7	70.4	70.2
18 years and over, crude[3]	74.4	77.7	76.8	79.1	80.8	81.2	79.0	77.7	75.1	73.2	69.4	69.0
Age												
18 to 44 years	83.3	84.6	82.8	84.4	86.8	84.9	83.9	83.6	81.8	80.4	77.2	76.1
18 to 20 years	59.4	66.8	62.9	59.5	65.3	59.8	63.7	61.1	57.5	52.0	38.6	34.0
21 to 44 years	86.1	86.2	84.7	87.1	89.2	87.8	86.1	86.3	84.8	84.0	81.6	81.1
21 to 24 years	85.3	86.1	85.4	84.2	85.3	84.1	82.7	84.0	80.2	81.1	74.6	69.7
25 to 44 years	86.3	86.3	84.6	87.6	89.9	88.5	86.8	86.8	85.7	84.6	83.2	83.5
45 to 64 years	70.5	77.2	77.4	81.4	81.7	84.6	81.3	80.6	78.8	76.9	73.9	75.5
45 to 54 years	75.7	82.1	81.9	83.7	83.8	86.3	83.6	83.4	81.0	79.9	78.6	79.7
55 to 64 years	65.2	70.6	71.0	78.0	78.4	82.0	77.8	76.8	76.0	73.2	68.6	71.1
65 years and over	50.8	57.6	57.3	59.8	61.0	64.5	60.8	54.9	50.0	47.1	42.7	42.3
65 to 74 years	57.9	64.7	64.9	67.0	70.0	71.6	70.1	66.3	61.6	58.0	54.5	52.9
75 years and over	40.4	48.0	47.3	51.2	50.8	56.7	51.1	42.7	37.5	34.6	27.9	28.1
Race[4]												
18 years and over, crude												
White only	74.1	77.3	76.2	78.9	80.6	81.3	78.7	77.7	74.9	72.8	68.7	68.4
Black or African American only	80.7	82.7	83.5	84.2	85.7	85.1	84.0	81.1	80.1	77.9	75.3	74.6
American Indian or Alaska Native only	85.4	78.1	73.5	74.6	92.2	76.8	84.8	75.2	69.4	73.4	70.1	60.9
Asian only	51.9	68.8	66.4	68.5	64.4	66.4	68.3	64.1	65.1	68.0	65.3	64.9
Native Hawaiian or Other Pacific Islander only	NA	NA	NA	NA	*	*	*	*	*	*	*	*
Two or more races	NA	NA	NA	NA	86.9	80.0	81.6	86.2	77.1	70.8	70.8	72.5
Hispanic Origin and Race[4]												
18 years and over, crude	67.6	77.2	74.4	75.2	76.3	77.0	75.4	75.5	75.4	73.6	70.5	68.6
Hispanic or Latina	74.9	77.8	77.0	79.6	81.3	81.7	79.5	78.0	75.1	73.1	69.2	69.0
Not Hispanic or Latina	74.7	77.3	76.5	79.3	81.0	81.8	79.3	78.1	74.9	72.8	68.4	68.4
White only	80.9	82.7	83.8	84.2	86.0	85.1	83.8	81.2	80.0	77.4	75.1	74.6
Black or African American only												
Age, Hispanic Origin, and Race[4]												
18 to 44 years												
Hispanic or Latina	73.9	80.9	80.6	76.4	77.0	78.1	75.9	76.5	77.9	75.9	72.3	70.2
Not Hispanic or Latina												
White only	84.5	85.3	82.9	85.7	88.7	86.6	85.8	85.8	83.8	82.1	79.0	78.2
Black or African American only	89.1	88.0	89.1	88.9	90.8	88.5	88.6	86.4	83.5	84.2	82.8	82.1
45 to 64 years												
Hispanic or Latina	57.7	75.8	70.1	78.3	79.5	77.8	77.9	78.4	78.2	75.4	74.4	74.0
Not Hispanic or Latina												
White only	71.2	77.2	77.5	81.7	81.9	85.9	81.4	81.4	79.0	77.2	73.6	75.5
Black or African American only	76.2	80.3	82.2	84.1	84.6	85.7	84.7	80.5	82.1	78.2	76.0	77.4
65 years and over												
Hispanic or Latina	41.7	57.1	43.8	59.8	63.7	66.8	64.6	60.0	52.6	54.2	49.4	46.2
Not Hispanic or Latina												
White only	51.8	57.1	58.2	59.7	60.5	64.2	60.7	54.1	49.0	46.5	41.4	41.9
Black or African American only	44.8	61.2	59.5	61.7	64.5	67.2	59.6	60.1	58.7	48.0	45.8	43.5
Age and Percent of Poverty Level[5]												
18 years and over, crude												
Below 100 percent	64.3	70.3	68.8	69.8	73.6	72.0	70.5	68.7	68.9	65.1	60.6	63.2
100 percent to 199 percent	68.2	71.2	68.8	70.6	72.5	73.4	71.4	69.0	65.0	64.3	59.8	60.3
200 percent to 399 percent	77.6	80.6	80.1	79.7	80.6	80.2	78.6	77.9	72.5	71.3	68.5	66.6
400 percent or more	83.6	85.1	85.4	87.0	87.6	89.1	86.6	85.7	84.4	83.1	79.4	77.6
18 to 44 years												
Below 100 percent	77.1	77.0	78.9	77.1	79.7	77.1	77.1	76.2	76.5	73.0	69.2	69.1
100 percent to 199 percent	80.4	81.9	78.2	79.2	84.0	79.4	79.5	78.1	75.5	75.7	72.6	73.5
200 percent to 399 percent	84.8	86.6	84.5	85.3	86.7	86.1	84.0	85.5	82.6	79.8	78.6	74.7
400 percent or more	88.9	91.3	88.7	89.8	91.1	89.8	89.5	88.7	87.0	88.9	84.5	83.2
45 to 64 years												
Below 100 percent	53.6	66.5	62.0	67.6	73.1	73.6	66.0	65.9	66.2	61.7	54.9	63.7
100 percent to 199 percent	60.4	64.8	66.2	69.9	70.4	76.1	71.4	69.6	65.6	63.2	61.2	64.2
200 percent to 399 percent	71.0	79.5	80.3	79.7	79.9	80.0	80.8	79.3	75.3	75.2	73.7	73.5
400 percent or more	79.1	83.9	84.0	88.2	87.4	91.5	87.5	87.4	87.1	85.7	82.8	82.9
65 years and over												
Below 100 percent	33.2	47.4	44.0	48.2	51.9	53.7	52.6	44.4	41.6	35.1	34.1	37.1
100 percent to 199 percent	50.4	55.7	51.5	55.1	54.7	61.0	55.4	49.5	43.5	40.7	33.0	31.9

NA = Not available.
* = Figure does not meet standards of reliability or precision. Data not shown have an RSE of greater than 30 percent.
[1]Questions concerning use of Pap smears differed slightly on the National Health Interview Survey across the years for which data are shown.
[2]Includes all other races not shown separately, unknown poverty level in 1987, unknown health insurance status, unknown education level, and unknown disability status.
[3]Estimates are age adjusted to the year 2000 standard population using five age groups: 18 to 44 years, 45 to 54 years, 55 to 64 years, 65 to 74 years, and 75 years and over.
[4]The race groups White, Black, American Indian or Alaska Native, Asian, Native Hawaiian or Other Pacific Islander, and two or more races, include persons of Hispanic and non-Hispanic origin. Persons of Hispanic origin may be of any race.
[5]Percent of poverty level is based on family income and family size and composition. Missing family income data were imputed for 1993 and beyond.

Table 3-41. Percent of Women 18 Years of Age and Over Who Have Had a Pap Smear[1] Within the Last Three Years, by Selected Characteristics, Selected Years, 1987–2015—*Continued*

(Percent.)

Characteristic	1987	1993	1994	1998	1999	2000	2003	2005	2008	2010	2013	2015
200 percent to 399 percent	58.0	59.7	63.7	64.2	64.0	65.1	62.4	56.8	45.8	47.1	39.6	41.5
400 percent or more	65.2	67.5	76.2	67.5	70.4	75.4	70.2	64.6	65.7	57.7	58.1	52.3
Health Insurance Status at the Time of Interview[6]												
18 to 64 years, crude												
Insured	NA	84.7	83.8	86.0	87.2	87.8	86.4	85.6	83.4	82.8	80.0	78.2
Private	NA	84.8	83.6	86.5	87.5	88.0	87.0	86.5	84.2	84.2	81.3	79.6
Medicaid	NA	82.7	86.2	83.0	84.2	85.8	82.8	80.9	80.3	78.0	75.7	72.6
Uninsured	NA	69.4	68.6	69.6	73.3	70.4	66.6	67.7	67.1	61.9	57.6	57.3
Health Insurance Status Prior to Interview[6]												
18 to 64 years, crude												
Insured continuously all 12 months	NA	84.8	83.7	86.3	87.3	88.0	86.6	85.8	83.7	83.2	80.4	78.5
Uninsured for any period up to 12 months	NA	81.8	83.4	81.7	83.5	83.7	81.8	81.3	78.9	78.3	72.3	72.0
Uninsured more than 12 months	NA	65.1	63.6	64.0	68.8	65.1	60.2	62.0	62.1	55.2	52.7	51.0
Age and Education[7]												
25 years and over, crude												
No high school diploma or GED	57.1	61.9	60.9	65.0	66.1	69.9	64.9	64.1	60.6	56.7	56.2	55.9
High school diploma or GED	76.4	78.2	76.0	77.4	79.3	79.8	75.9	73.8	69.5	66.8	62.0	62.0
Some college or more	84.0	84.4	85.2	86.9	87.8	88.0	86.2	84.6	82.6	80.7	77.1	76.9
25 to 44 years												
No high school diploma or GED	75.1	73.6	73.6	76.8	79.0	79.6	71.7	75.5	76.2	69.1	71.7	73.3
High school diploma or GED	85.6	85.4	82.4	83.9	87.6	86.2	84.3	83.1	80.0	79.0	79.5	75.1
Some college or more	90.1	89.8	89.1	91.5	93.0	91.4	90.8	90.5	89.3	89.0	86.1	87.2
45 to 64 years												
No high school diploma or GED	58.0	65.6	66.1	69.2	71.6	75.7	71.4	69.7	70.4	63.4	63.0	60.3
High school diploma or GED	72.3	77.6	75.9	81.0	79.8	81.8	77.6	79.0	73.9	72.4	67.0	70.7
Some college or more	80.1	83.0	84.7	85.5	85.7	89.1	86.2	84.1	83.0	81.5	78.7	79.9
65 years and over												
No high school diploma or GED	44.0	50.7	47.7	52.4	51.8	56.6	52.5	46.0	36.7	37.7	33.8	32.9
High school diploma or GED	55.4	61.6	61.2	60.7	63.7	66.9	61.2	52.5	49.3	42.6	38.8	39.0
Some college or more	59.4	62.3	66.5	67.9	68.8	69.8	67.8	63.8	59.0	54.9	49.7	47.5
Disability measure[8]												
18 years and over, crude												
Any basic actions difficulty or complex activity limitation	NA	NA	NA	72.7	74.4	75.4	72.7	69.1	66.1	63.8	59.3	59.9
Any basic actions difficulty	NA	NA	NA	72.4	74.3	75.1	72.6	69.1	66.2	63.6	59.2	59.9
Any complex activity limitation	NA	NA	NA	67.9	69.3	71.0	67.6	62.2	60.1	58.5	52.8	54.6
No disability	NA	NA	NA	82.5	83.8	84.1	82.5	82.6	80.4	78.9	75.2	74.5

NA = Not available.

* = Figure does not meet standards of reliability or precision. Data not shown have an RSE of greater than 30 percent.

[1] Questions concerning use of Pap smears differed slightly on the National Health Interview Survey across the years for which data are shown.

[6] Health insurance categories are mutually exclusive. Persons who reported both Medicaid and private coverage are classified as having private coverage. Medicaid includes other public assistance through 1996. Starting with 1997 data, state-sponsored health plan coverage is included as Medicaid coverage. Starting with 1999 data, coverage by the Children's Health Insurance Program (CHIP) is included with Medicaid coverage. Persons not covered by private insurance, Medicaid, CHIP, public assistance (through 1996), state-sponsored or other government-sponsored health plans (starting in 1997), Medicare, or military plans are considered to have no health insurance coverage. Persons with only Indian Health Service coverage are considered to have no health insurance coverage. Health insurance status was unknown for 8 to 9 percent of children in 1993-1996 and about 1 percent in 1997-2011.

[7] Education categories shown are for 1998 and subsequent years. GED is General Educational Development high school equivalency diploma. In years prior to 1998, the following categories based on number of years in school completed were used: less than 12 years, 12 years, and 13 years or more.

[8] Any basic actions difficulty or complex activity limitation is defined as having one or more of the following limitations or difficulties: movement difficulty, emotional difficulty, sensory (seeing or hearing) difficulty, cognitive difficulty, self-care (activities of daily living or instrumental activities of daily living) limitation, social limitation, or work limitation.

Table 3-42. Use of Colorectal Tests or Procedures Among Adults 50 to 75 Years of Age, by Selected Characteristics, Selected Years, 2000–2015

(Percent.)

Characteristic	Any colorectal test or procedure[1,2]					Colonoscopy[2,3]				
	2000	2003	2005	2008	2015	2000	2003	2005	2008	2015
All adults, 50 to 75 years[4]	33.9	39.1	44.3	51.6	62.4	19.1	29.2	37.6	46.7	59.2
Sex										
Male	33.1	40.1	44.4	51.4	61.6	19.5	30.2	37.9	46.9	58.4
Female	34.5	38.1	44.2	51.9	63.1	18.8	28.4	37.4	46.6	60.0
Race[5]										
White only	34.9	39.8	45.6	52.8	63.7	19.7	30.0	38.9	47.8	60.7
Black or African American only	29.6	35.2	38.1	46.9	59.6	17.4	24.8	32.2	43.1	56.3
American Indian or Alaska Native only	*35.2	*37.9	*33.9	28.5	48.9	*	*	*	*26.7	45.3
Asian only	20.4	26.7	30.8	47.1	52.3	*8.6	20.0	24.4	39.3	45.8
Native Hawaiian and Other Pacific Islander only	*	*	*	*	*	*	*	*	*	*
Two or more races	37.5	40.7	33.8	38.4	52.7	*25.1	29.7	29.6	37.4	49.8
Hispanic Origin and Race[5]										
Hispanic or Latino	21.7	27.2	28.5	34.0	47.4	13.3	19.8	23.1	29.3	44.0
Mexican	19.3	22.4	24.6	27.5	41.2	11.2	14.2	18.2	21.2	37.6
Not Hispanic or Latino	34.7	40.0	45.6	53.3	64.1	19.5	30.0	38.9	48.4	61.0
White only	35.7	41.0	47.4	54.8	65.6	20.0	30.9	40.5	49.8	62.8
Black or African American only	29.7	35.3	38.0	47.4	60.3	17.5	25.0	32.0	43.5	56.9
Percent of Poverty Level[6]										
Below 100 percent	26.5	29.7	28.7	33.9	45.6	16.3	22.0	23.6	28.5	42.8
100 percent to 199 percent	29.4	31.9	38.4	42.7	51.8	17.7	23.3	31.5	38.0	48.0
200 percent to 399 percent	33.7	38.8	43.6	49.9	61.3	18.6	29.4	37.0	44.3	58.6
400 percent or more	37.1	43.8	49.6	58.9	70.0	20.5	32.7	42.8	54.5	66.8
Hispanic Origin and Race and Percent of Poverty Level[5,6]										
Hispanic or Latino										
Below 100 percent	15.3	21.4	19.3	21.1	40.4	*9.3	15.2	13.1	17.9	37.0
100 percent to 199 percent	16.8	20.5	24.6	27.7	37.7	8.6	16.0	19.4	24.4	34.0
200 percent to 399 percent	23.6	29.0	28.3	39.3	48.9	*13.7	20.7	21.6	33.8	45.0
400 percent or more	31.1	37.9	42.1	43.9	61.5	22.4	27.1	39.3	37.6	58.7
Not Hispanic or Latino										
White only										
Below 100 percent	29.6	33.9	30.6	39.8	46.1	19.3	26.8	26.8	33.2	43.7
100 percent to 199 percent	32.1	34.7	42.4	46.0	55.1	19.7	25.7	35.0	40.7	51.6
200 percent to 399 percent	35.2	40.3	47.3	51.6	64.3	19.3	31.0	40.2	45.8	62.1
400 percent or more	37.9	44.3	50.6	60.5	71.3	20.7	32.9	43.8	56.3	68.3
Black or African American only										
Below 100 percent	27.5	27.4	29.0	35.1	49.1	14.5	17.6	23.5	30.1	44.8
100 percent to 199 percent	28.7	30.0	36.2	46.7	56.2	17.2	20.0	30.3	43.2	51.8
200 percent to 399 percent	27.7	36.8	35.8	48.5	60.2	16.5	25.6	31.8	44.7	58.2
400 percent or more	33.9	43.5	48.9	54.3	71.9	20.7	33.3	40.2	50.6	68.5
Education[7]										
No high school diploma or GED	25.9	28.9	34.5	36.2	46.6	14.9	21.2	29.0	31.8	43.7
High school diploma or GED	33.1	38.3	42.1	48.5	58.2	19.0	29.3	35.7	44.6	55.2
Some college or more	37.8	43.3	48.7	57.5	67.2	20.9	32.1	41.6	52.1	63.9
Disability Measure[8]										
Any basic actions difficulty or complex activity limitation	37.8	42.0	47.7	54.2	64.9	22.1	31.9	40.1	48.5	61.8
Any basic actions difficulty	38.1	41.9	47.9	54.6	65.1	22.5	31.9	40.6	48.9	62.0
Any complex activity limitation	37.4	41.5	48.1	52.4	62.9	22.6	31.3	39.7	46.7	59.5
No disability	30.9	36.9	41.6	50.0	60.7	16.6	27.1	35.6	45.8	57.5
Geographic Region										
Northeast	34.4	43.5	50.9	54.7	66.4	19.1	33.1	44.8	51.0	64.5
Midwest	35.2	40.4	43.5	52.5	63.1	19.8	30.6	36.6	47.8	61.7
South	32.5	36.7	43.9	51.6	60.4	20.0	28.5	38.1	47.4	57.8
West	34.1	37.0	39.6	48.2	61.8	16.3	24.3	31.3	41.1	54.9
Location of Residence										
Within MSA[9]	34.1	40.3	44.7	52.4	63.2	19.0	29.9	37.9	47.6	59.8
Outside MSA[9]	33.2	34.8	42.7	48.5	58.5	19.6	26.8	36.7	43.3	56.5

* = Figure does not meet standards of reliability or precision. Data preceded by an asterisk have a relative standard error (RSE) of 20 percent to 30 percent. Data not shown have an RSE of greater than 30 percent.

[1]Includes reports of home fecal occult blood test (FOBT) in the past year, sigmoidoscopy procedure in the past 5 years with FOBT in the past 3 years, or colonoscopy in the past 10 years. Colorectal procedures are performed for diagnostic and screening purposes.

[2]Questions differed slightly on the National Health Interview Survey across the years for which data are shown.

[3]Includes any colonoscopy in the past 10 years, alone or in addition to another type of colorectal test or procedure.

[4]Includes all other races not shown separately, unknown disability status, and unknown education level.

[5]The race groups White, Black, American Indian or Alaska Native, Asian, Native Hawaiian or Other Pacific Islander, and two or more races include persons of Hispanic and non-Hispanic origin. Persons of Hispanic origin may be of any race.

[6]Based on family income and family size and composition using U.S. Census Bureau poverty thresholds. Missing family income data were imputed.

[7]GED is General Educational Development high school equivalency diploma.

[8]Any basic actions difficulty or complex activity limitation is defined as having one or more of the following limitations or difficulties: movement difficulty, emotional difficulty, sensory (seeing or hearing) difficulty, cognitive difficulty, self-care (activities of daily living or instrumental activities of daily living) limitation, social limitation, or work limitation.

[9]MSA = metropolitan statistical area.

Table 3-43. Emergency Department Visits Within the Past 12 Months Among Children Under 18 Years of Age, by Selected Characteristics, Selected Years, 1997–2015

(Percent.)

Characteristic	Under 18 years					Under 6 years					6 to 17 years				
	1997	2000	2005	2010	2015	1997	2000	2005	2010	2015	1997	2000	2005	2010	2015
PERCENT OF CHILDREN WITH ONE OR MORE EMERGENCY DEPARTMENT VISITS[1]															
All children[2]	19.9	20.3	20.5	22.1	16.9	24.3	25.7	26.8	27.8	21.7	17.7	17.6	17.4	19.1	14.5
Sex															
Male	21.5	21.5	21.7	23.3	17.3	25.2	27.7	27.6	29.3	23.0	19.6	18.6	18.8	20.1	14.6
Female	18.3	19.0	19.2	20.9	16.3	23.3	23.7	25.9	26.3	20.4	15.7	16.6	15.9	18.2	14.4
Race[3]															
White only	19.4	19.9	19.8	21.2	16.3	22.6	24.8	25.3	26.6	20.9	17.8	17.6	17.1	18.4	14.1
Black or African American only	24.0	22.7	23.8	27.6	21.6	33.1	30.8	31.6	34.0	27.4	19.4	19.0	20.0	24.2	18.8
American Indian or Alaska Native only	*24.1	38.0	*32.1	20.9	23.3	*24.3	*	67.1	*35.4	*37.2	*24.0	*39.0	*	*	*17.5
Asian only	12.6	12.3	14.6	15.0	9.2	20.8	*16.7	20.2	18.4	13.9	8.6	9.8	12.3	13.3	*7.0
Native Hawaiian and Other Pacific Islander only	NA	*	*	*	*	NA	*	*	*	*	NA	*	*	*	*
Two or more races	NA	24.2	24.8	27.2	18.6	NA	31.7	38.3	34.9	23.1	NA	18.3	17.1	21.6	*15.8
Hispanic Origin and Race[3]															
Hispanic or Latino	21.1	18.6	19.5	23.6	18.8	25.7	23.9	28.0	30.2	25.9	18.1	15.6	14.5	19.4	15.2
Not Hispanic or Latino	19.7	20.6	20.7	21.7	16.2	24.0	26.2	26.5	27.0	20.3	17.6	18.0	18.0	19.0	14.3
White only	19.2	20.2	19.9	20.4	15.4	22.2	25.1	24.5	25.1	18.8	17.7	17.9	17.9	18.2	13.8
Black or African American only	23.6	22.7	23.8	27.2	21.3	32.7	30.9	31.8	34.4	27.2	19.2	19.0	20.0	23.3	18.4
Percent of Poverty Level[4]															
Below 100 percent	25.1	25.0	27.3	30.6	23.1	29.5	30.7	33.5	35.4	28.8	22.2	21.7	23.5	27.6	19.9
100 percent to 199 percent	22.0	22.4	21.8	25.7	18.7	28.0	27.4	30.8	31.6	24.0	19.0	19.9	17.4	22.3	16.2
200 percent to 399 percent	18.0	19.0	18.9	18.4	14.7	21.4	25.7	25.9	22.7	20.8	16.4	15.9	15.7	16.4	11.8
400 percent or more	16.3	17.0	16.8	15.9	12.9	19.1	20.3	19.1	21.7	14.7	15.1	15.6	15.8	13.3	12.0
Hispanic Origin and Race and Percent of Poverty Level[3,4]															
Hispanic or Latino															
Below 100 percent	21.9	19.9	21.8	27.0	21.7	25.0	25.7	28.4	32.0	27.9	19.6	16.4	17.4	23.4	18.2
100 percent to 199 percent	20.8	18.2	17.8	23.3	18.1	28.8	20.8	26.1	31.6	24.9	15.6	16.6	13.1	18.0	15.3
200 percent to 399 percent	21.4	17.9	20.2	19.5	17.0	24.6	26.1	31.7	25.2	28.2	19.6	13.3	14.3	16.1	11.0
400 percent or more	17.7	17.6	15.3	21.4	16.0	*20.2	*22.9	23.3	28.6	*18.0	16.4	15.4	*11.5	18.0	14.9
Not Hispanic or Latino															
White only															
Below 100 percent	25.5	26.5	34.1	33.7	24.7	27.2	35.6	37.3	37.4	26.8	24.4	21.2	32.2	31.6	23.6
100 percent to 199 percent	22.3	24.7	22.8	26.3	17.8	25.8	29.2	30.7	29.2	21.5	20.7	22.7	19.1	24.7	15.9
200 percent to 399 percent	17.8	19.5	17.9	17.6	13.9	20.9	26.0	22.9	21.2	18.3	16.3	16.6	15.7	15.9	11.8
400 percent or more	16.5	16.9	16.8	15.5	12.7	19.0	18.5	18.7	21.0	15.0	15.4	16.2	16.0	13.2	11.7
Black or African American only															
Below 100 percent	29.3	27.8	27.1	32.4	23.7	39.5	28.9	34.8	41.6	30.8	23.0	27.3	22.6	26.6	20.1
100 percent to 199 percent	22.5	20.8	24.1	27.5	23.5	31.7	35.3	33.3	34.5	29.3	18.5	13.8	20.3	23.7	20.6
200 percent to 399 percent	18.5	19.6	22.6	22.3	17.4	23.9	28.3	33.3	24.6	*27.1	16.3	16.2	17.8	21.4	13.8
400 percent or more	16.1	19.3	16.9	18.9	16.3	*18.8	32.8	*	*24.1	*	15.2	*13.9	17.4	16.1	*18.0
Health Insurance Status at the Time of Interview[5]															
Insured	19.8	20.7	20.7	22.3	16.9	24.4	25.8	26.8	28.1	21.7	17.5	18.2	17.7	19.2	14.6
Private	17.5	18.4	17.4	17.1	12.5	20.9	22.8	21.7	21.8	16.7	15.9	16.5	15.5	14.9	10.6
Medicaid	28.2	28.6	28.5	30.0	22.8	33.0	33.2	35.5	35.5	27.3	24.1	25.5	23.6	26.4	20.4
Uninsured	20.2	17.2	18.4	19.4	14.3	23.0	24.5	26.6	24.0	*19.4	18.9	13.9	15.4	17.6	12.7
Health Insurance Status Prior to Interview[5]															
Insured continuously all 12 months	19.6	20.2	20.5	22.2	16.8	24.1	25.3	26.7	28.1	21.4	17.3	17.8	17.3	19.1	14.6
Uninsured for any period up to 12 months	24.0	25.9	26.0	23.7	20.7	27.1	33.9	34.4	28.0	29.2	21.9	21.7	22.4	21.3	16.6
Uninsured more than 12 months	18.4	14.7	14.4	17.6	*10.4	19.3	19.1	*15.7	*21.3	*	18.1	13.1	14.0	16.7	*9.8
Geographic Region															
Northeast	18.5	19.7	20.9	22.3	16.5	20.7	21.6	26.3	27.8	22.4	17.4	18.8	18.5	19.6	13.7
Midwest	19.5	20.3	21.8	23.3	19.1	26.0	25.6	30.1	28.8	23.5	16.4	17.8	17.8	20.7	17.1
South	21.8	21.9	21.7	23.4	17.6	25.6	28.6	27.1	30.4	23.5	19.9	18.7	18.8	19.5	14.9
West	18.5	18.0	16.7	19.1	13.7	23.5	24.7	22.9	23.3	17.2	15.9	14.7	13.8	16.8	11.9
Location of Residence															
Within MSA[6]	19.7	19.9	20.0	21.8	16.4	23.9	24.5	25.7	27.7	21.1	17.4	17.6	17.2	18.6	14.0
Outside MSA[6]	20.8	21.9	22.4	24.2	20.0	26.2	31.3	31.8	28.6	25.6	18.6	17.8	18.2	22.1	17.3

NA = Not available.

* = Figure does not meet standards of reliability or precision. Data preceded by an asterisk have a relative standard error (RSE) of 20 percent to 30 percent. Data not shown have an RSE of greater than 30 percent.

[1]See Appendix II of Health, United States, 2016, for more information.

[2]Includes all other races not shown separately and unknown health insurance status.

[3]The race groups, White, Black, American Indian or Alaska Native, Asian, Native Hawaiian or Other Pacific Islander, and 2 or more races, include persons of Hispanic and non-Hispanic origin. Persons of Hispanic origin may be of any race.

[4]Percent of poverty level is based on family income and family size and composition using U.S. Census Bureau poverty thresholds. Missing family data were imputed for 1997 and beyond.

[5]Health insurance categories are mutually exclusive. Persons who reported both Medicaid and private coverage are classified as having private coverage. Medicaid includes other public assistance through 1996. Starting with 1997 data, state-sponsored health plan coverage is included as Medicaid coverage. Starting with 1999 data, coverage by the Children's Health Insurance Program (CHIP) is included with Medicaid coverage. Persons not covered by private insurance, Medicaid, CHIP, public assistance (through 1996), state-sponsored or other government-sponsored health plans (starting in 1997), Medicare, or military plans are considered to have no health insurance coverage. Persons with only Indian Health Service coverage are considered to have no health insurance coverage. Health insurance status was unknown for 8 to 9 percent of children in 1993-1996 and about 1 percent in 1997-2011.

[6]MSA = metropolitan statistical area.

Table 3-43. Emergency Department Visits Within the Past 12 Months Among Children Under 18 Years of Age, by Selected Characteristics, Selected Years, 1997–2015—*Continued*

(Percent.)

Characteristic	Under 18 years					Under 6 years					6 to 17 years				
	1997	2000	2005	2010	2015	1997	2000	2005	2010	2015	1997	2000	2005	2010	2015
PERCENT OF CHILDREN WITH TWO OR MORE EMERGENCY DEPARTMENT VISITS															
All children[2]	7.1	7.0	6.8	8.4	5.3	9.6	10.0	9.8	10.8	7.0	5.8	5.6	5.4	7.2	4.5
Sex															
Male	7.3	7.3	7.2	8.5	5.4	9.9	10.3	10.7	11.3	7.4	6.0	5.8	5.4	7.0	4.4
Female	6.9	6.7	6.5	8.3	5.3	9.4	9.6	8.9	10.3	6.5	5.7	5.3	5.3	7.3	4.7
Race[3]															
White only	6.6	6.4	6.3	7.6	4.9	8.4	8.7	9.1	10.1	6.0	5.7	5.4	4.9	6.3	4.3
Black or African American only	9.6	10.5	9.2	12.6	7.6	14.9	16.2	12.7	15.7	10.0	6.9	7.9	7.5	11.0	6.3
American Indian or Alaska Native only	*	*	*	*	*13.5	*	*	*	*	*	*	*	*	*	*
Asian only	*5.7	*3.1	*4.6	7.3	*2.6	*12.9	*	*	*	*	*	*	*3.9	*7.1	*
Native Hawaiian and Other Pacific Islander only	NA	*	*	*	*	NA	*	*	*	*	NA	*	*	*	*
Two or more races	NA	*8.7	*8.6	10.3	6.7	NA	*14.3	*13.2	*11.7	*10.2	NA	*	*	*9.2	*
Hispanic Origin and Race[3]															
Hispanic or Latino	8.9	7.0	7.7	8.6	6.2	11.8	9.4	12.1	11.7	8.6	7.0	5.6	5.2	6.6	5.0
Not Hispanic or Latino	6.8	7.0	6.6	8.4	5.0	9.2	10.1	9.2	10.5	6.4	5.7	5.6	5.4	7.3	4.3
White only	6.2	6.3	5.9	7.4	4.4	7.8	8.6	8.2	9.3	5.1	5.5	5.2	4.9	6.4	4.1
Black or African American only	9.3	10.6	9.1	12.3	7.4	14.6	16.6	12.4	15.8	9.8	6.8	7.9	7.5	10.4	6.2
Percent of Poverty Level[4]															
Below 100 percent	11.1	11.9	11.2	13.4	8.9	14.5	16.4	15.9	15.3	11.8	8.9	9.4	8.4	12.1	7.4
100 percent to 199 percent	8.3	8.0	7.9	10.3	7.2	12.2	11.8	12.7	13.4	9.7	6.3	6.1	5.5	8.4	6.0
200 percent to 399 percent	6.2	5.6	5.7	6.3	3.4	7.4	8.0	7.6	7.3	4.1	5.6	4.5	4.8	5.9	3.0
400 percent or more	4.0	4.7	4.4	5.0	3.0	5.0	5.8	5.1	7.3	*3.5	3.6	4.2	4.0	3.9	2.7
Hispanic Origin and Race and Percent of Poverty Level[3,4]															
Hispanic or Latino															
Below 100 percent	10.4	8.2	10.0	9.9	7.0	13.9	10.9	13.8	10.9	*9.1	8.0	6.6	7.4	9.2	5.9
100 percent to 199 percent	8.2	7.4	6.1	9.4	7.3	12.0	8.5	*8.7	15.4	11.7	5.7	6.7	*4.7	5.5	5.5
200 percent to 399 percent	8.5	6.2	7.7	5.9	*4.0	10.0	9.2	14.2	*8.0	*5.7	*7.6	*4.5	*4.4	*4.6	*3.1
400 percent or more	*5.0	*4.0	*5.4	*6.5	*5.6	*	*	*	*	*	*	*	*	*5.2	*
Not Hispanic or Latino															
White only															
Below 100 percent	10.7	12.8	13.5	14.0	9.6	12.2	18.4	18.6	15.5	*10.1	9.8	*9.5	10.4	13.1	*9.4
100 percent to 199 percent	8.0	8.0	8.2	10.4	7.7	11.2	11.8	13.7	12.3	*8.6	6.4	6.3	*5.5	9.4	7.3
200 percent to 399 percent	6.0	5.4	5.1	5.7	2.9	6.7	7.7	6.1	*6.5	*2.8	5.6	4.4	4.6	5.4	*3.0
400 percent or more	3.7	4.5	3.7	5.0	2.6	4.6	4.5	4.1	7.6	*3.5	3.3	4.5	3.5	3.9	*2.2
Black or African American only															
Below 100 percent	12.7	14.7	11.4	16.1	9.9	19.1	18.5	16.2	22.1	14.5	8.8	12.8	8.6	12.4	*7.5
100 percent to 199 percent	9.2	8.9	8.4	12.4	6.9	*13.5	17.5	*13.3	*14.6	*	*7.2	*4.8	*6.5	11.1	*6.5
200 percent to 399 percent	5.8	7.8	*7.6	9.9	*5.6	*8.9	*12.5	*	*10.2	*	*4.5	*6.0	*7.5	*9.8	*
400 percent or more	*	*8.9	*7.2	*3.7	*	*	*17.8	*	*	*	*	*	*	*	*
Health Insurance Status at the Time of Interview[5]															
Insured	7.0	7.0	6.8	8.5	5.4	9.6	9.6	9.7	11.0	7.1	5.7	5.7	5.3	7.1	4.6
Private	5.2	5.2	5.0	5.5	3.0	6.8	7.1	6.2	7.4	3.5	4.5	4.5	4.4	4.6	2.8
Medicaid	13.1	13.1	11.1	12.8	8.8	16.2	15.9	15.8	15.3	11.5	10.4	11.2	7.7	11.2	7.4
Uninsured	7.7	6.6	7.0	8.0	*3.5	9.8	11.3	11.5	*8.5	*	6.8	4.5	5.4	7.8	*3.5
Health Insurance Status Prior to Interview[5]															
Insured continuously all 12 months	6.9	6.7	6.7	8.4	5.3	9.4	9.2	9.7	10.8	6.9	5.7	5.5	5.2	7.1	4.5
Uninsured for any period up to 12 months	8.5	10.6	8.9	10.1	7.8	11.5	16.0	13.6	13.3	*10.1	6.6	7.7	6.9	8.4	*6.7
Uninsured more than 12 months	6.8	5.8	5.5	7.8	*	*8.6	8.9	*	*	*	6.2	4.7	5.3	*7.9	*
Geographic Region															
Northeast	6.2	6.4	6.2	7.8	4.6	7.6	7.9	8.9	10.3	7.5	5.4	5.6	5.0	6.6	3.2
Midwest	6.6	6.6	6.9	9.1	5.7	10.4	9.0	9.6	11.4	6.5	4.8	5.5	5.5	8.0	5.3
South	8.0	8.5	7.9	9.1	5.9	10.1	12.6	10.8	12.9	7.6	6.9	6.6	6.3	7.1	5.1
West	7.1	5.4	5.5	7.2	4.5	10.0	8.5	9.1	7.6	6.2	5.6	3.9	3.9	7.0	3.6
Location of Residence															
Within MSA[6]	7.2	6.6	6.7	8.3	5.0	9.6	8.9	9.5	10.6	6.6	5.9	5.5	5.2	7.0	4.2
Outside MSA[6]	6.8	8.6	7.5	9.3	7.2	9.7	15.0	11.2	12.2	9.5	5.6	5.8	5.9	7.9	6.2

NA = Not available.
* = Figure does not meet standards of reliability or precision. Data preceded by an asterisk have a relative standard error (RSE) of 20 percent to 30 percent. Data not shown have an RSE of greater than 30 percent.
[1]See Appendix II of Health, United States, 2016, for more information.
[2]Includes all other races not shown separately and unknown health insurance status.
[3]The race groups, White, Black, American Indian or Alaska Native, Asian, Native Hawaiian or Other Pacific Islander, and 2 or more races, include persons of Hispanic and non-Hispanic origin. Persons of Hispanic origin may be of any race.
[4]Percent of poverty level is based on family income and family size and composition using U.S. Census Bureau poverty thresholds. Missing family data were imputed for 1997 and beyond.
[5]Health insurance categories are mutually exclusive. Persons who reported both Medicaid and private coverage are classified as having private coverage. Medicaid includes other public assistance through 1996. Starting with 1997 data, state-sponsored health plan coverage is included as Medicaid coverage. Starting with 1999 data, coverage by the Children's Health Insurance Program (CHIP) is included with Medicaid coverage. Persons not covered by private insurance, Medicaid, CHIP, public assistance (through 1996), state-sponsored or other government-sponsored health plans (starting in 1997), Medicare, or military plans are considered to have no health insurance coverage. Persons with only Indian Health Service coverage are considered to have no health insurance coverage. Health insurance status was unknown for 8 to 9 percent of children in 1993-1996 and about 1 percent in 1997-2011.
[6]MSA = metropolitan statistical area.

Table 3-44. Emergency Department Visits Within the Past 12 Months Among Adults 18 Years of Age and Over, by Selected Characteristics, Selected Years, 1997–2015

(Percent.)

Characteristic	One or more emergency department visits					Two or more emergency department visits				
	1997	2000	2005	2010	2015	1997	2000	2005	2010	2015
18 years and over, age-adjusted[1,2]	19.6	20.2	20.5	21.4	18.8	6.7	6.9	7.1	7.8	6.9
18 years and over, crude[1]	19.6	20.1	20.4	21.3	18.8	6.7	6.8	7.0	7.7	6.9
Age										
18 to 44 years	20.7	20.5	20.8	22.0	18.6	6.8	7.0	7.1	8.4	6.9
18 to 24 years	26.3	25.7	25.3	25.4	20.5	9.1	8.8	8.9	9.6	7.5
25 to 44 years	19.0	18.8	19.2	20.7	17.9	6.2	6.4	6.5	8.0	6.7
45 to 64 years	16.2	17.6	18.2	19.2	17.4	5.6	5.6	6.4	6.7	6.1
45 to 54 years	15.7	17.9	17.6	18.6	16.4	5.5	5.8	6.1	6.6	6.0
55 to 64 years	16.9	17.0	19.0	19.8	18.4	5.7	5.3	6.8	6.8	6.2
65 years and over	22.0	23.7	23.7	23.7	21.8	8.1	8.6	8.2	7.7	8.2
65 to 74 years	20.3	21.6	20.8	20.7	18.3	7.1	7.4	7.4	6.4	6.9
75 years and over	24.3	26.2	27.1	27.4	26.7	9.3	10.0	9.1	9.4	10.0
Sex[2]										
Male	19.1	18.7	18.6	18.5	16.9	5.9	5.7	5.9	6.0	5.7
Female	20.2	21.6	22.3	24.3	20.6	7.5	7.9	8.2	9.6	8.1
Race[2,3]										
White only	19.0	19.4	19.8	20.7	18.0	6.2	6.4	6.5	7.2	6.4
Black or African American only	25.9	26.5	26.3	28.6	26.6	11.1	10.8	11.9	12.6	10.9
American Indian or Alaska Native only	24.8	30.3	31.0	22.6	28.3	13.1	*12.6	*11.1	*11.8	16.1
Asian only	11.6	13.6	15.4	13.3	9.4	*2.9	*3.8	*3.8	3.3	2.7
Native Hawaiian and Other Pacific Islander only	NA	*	*	*	*	NA	*	*	*	*
Two or more races	NA	32.5	25.7	29.7	27.1	NA	11.3	12.8	11.1	12.4
American Indian or Alaska Native; White	NA	33.9	29.3	31.1	29.0	NA	*9.4	*15.3	*15.2	*14.1
Hispanic Origin and Race[2,3]										
Hispanic or Latino	19.2	18.3	20.1	19.8	17.3	7.4	7.0	7.1	6.9	6.4
Mexican	17.8	17.4	17.2	18.1	16.0	6.4	7.1	5.8	6.1	6.0
Not Hispanic or Latino	19.7	20.6	20.7	21.9	19.2	6.7	6.9	7.1	8.1	7.0
White only	19.1	19.8	20.1	21.1	18.3	6.2	6.4	6.4	7.4	6.4
Black or African American only	25.9	26.5	26.2	29.0	26.5	11.0	10.8	11.9	12.7	10.8
Percent of Poverty Level[2,4]										
Below 100 percent	28.1	29.0	29.8	30.6	29.5	12.8	13.3	13.7	14.9	14.7
100 percent to 199 percent	23.8	23.9	23.2	25.6	24.1	9.3	9.6	9.6	10.5	9.9
200 percent to 399 percent	18.3	19.8	20.2	20.4	17.1	5.9	6.3	6.5	6.8	6.2
400 percent or more	15.9	16.8	16.9	17.0	14.3	3.9	4.5	4.5	4.7	3.6
Hispanic Origin and Race and Percent of Poverty Level[2,3,4]										
Hispanic or Latino										
Below 100 percent	22.1	22.4	24.0	23.6	22.6	9.8	9.7	9.2	11.5	11.5
100 percent to 199 percent	19.2	18.1	18.7	19.9	17.7	8.1	6.7	7.1	6.3	6.7
200 percent to 399 percent	18.5	17.3	18.9	18.1	13.3	6.0	7.4	5.9	5.2	4.1
400 percent or more	14.6	16.4	20.9	18.8	17.5	*3.8	*4.3	*6.9	*5.5	*4.4
Not Hispanic or Latino										
White only										
Below 100 percent	29.5	30.1	30.8	33.3	32.0	13.0	13.9	13.7	15.5	16.0
100 percent to 199 percent	24.3	25.5	24.3	26.8	26.0	9.1	10.4	9.8	11.2	10.5
200 percent to 399 percent	18.1	20.1	20.7	20.3	17.4	5.8	6.3	6.4	6.5	6.4
400 percent or more	15.8	16.3	16.2	16.9	14.0	3.8	4.1	4.0	4.9	3.5
Black or African American only										
Below 100 percent	34.6	35.4	35.4	36.9	35.8	17.5	17.4	18.3	20.2	17.1
100 percent to 199 percent	29.2	28.5	28.9	33.5	32.6	12.8	12.2	14.2	15.9	14.0
200 percent to 399 percent	20.8	23.2	21.5	25.7	22.2	8.1	8.0	8.7	10.2	8.3
400 percent or more	18.2	22.6	22.6	18.8	18.3	5.9	8.8	*9.2	*4.0	5.4
Health Insurance Status at the Time of Interview[5,6]										
18 to 64 years										
Insured	18.8	19.5	20.0	20.8	18.0	6.1	6.4	6.6	7.5	6.5
Private	16.9	17.6	17.3	17.4	14.1	4.7	5.1	4.8	5.2	3.9
Medicaid	37.6	42.2	40.1	40.2	34.9	19.7	21.0	20.1	21.1	18.0
Uninsured	20.0	19.3	19.5	21.3	18.0	7.5	6.9	8.0	8.9	6.9
Health Insurance Status Prior to Interview[5,6]										
18 to 64 years										
Insured continuously all 12 months	18.3	19.0	19.4	20.2	17.6	5.8	6.1	6.3	7.1	6.2

NA = Not available.

* = Figure does not meet standards of reliability or precision. Data preceded by an asterisk have a relative standard error (RSE) of 20 percent to 30 percent. Data not shown have an RSE of greater than 30 percent.

[1]Includes all other races not shown separately, unknown health insurance status, and unknown disability status.

[2]Estimates are for persons 18 years of age and over and are age adjusted to the year 2000 standard population using five age groups: 18 to 44 years, 45 to 54 years, 55 to 64 years, 65 to 74 years, and 75 years and over.

[3]The race groups White, Black, American Indian or Alaska Native, Asian, Native Hawaiian or Other Pacific Islander, and two or more races include persons of Hispanic and non-Hispanic origin. Persons of Hispanic origin may be of any race.

[4]Percent of poverty level is based on family income and family size and composition using U.S. Census Bureau poverty thresholds. Missing family income data were imputed for 1997 and beyond.

[5]Health insurance categories are mutually exclusive. Persons who reported both Medicaid and private coverage are classified as having private coverage. Medicaid includes other public assistance through 1996. Starting with 1997 data, state-sponsored health plan coverage is included as Medicaid coverage. Starting with 1999 data, coverage by the Children's Health Insurance Program (CHIP) is included with Medicaid coverage. Persons not covered by private insurance, Medicaid, CHIP, public assistance (through 1996), state-sponsored or other government-sponsored health plans (starting in 1997), Medicare, or military plans are considered to have no health insurance coverage. Persons with only Indian Health Service coverage are considered to have no health insurance coverage. Health insurance status was unknown for 8 to 9 percent of children in 1993-1996 and about 1 percent in 1997-2011.

Table 3-44. Emergency Department Visits Within the Past 12 Months Among Adults 18 Years of Age and Over, by Selected Characteristics, Selected Years, 1997–2015—*Continued*

(Percent.)

Characteristic	One or more emergency department visits					Two or more emergency department visits				
	1997	2000	2005	2010	2015	1997	2000	2005	2010	2015
Uninsured for any period up to 12 months	25.5	28.2	28.0	26.0	22.6	9.4	10.3	12.4	12.5	9.9
Uninsured more than 12 months	18.9	17.3	18.0	20.6	16.6	7.1	6.4	7.0	8.1	6.4
Percent of Poverty Level and Health Insurance Status Prior to Interview[4,5,6]										
18 to 64 years										
Below 100 percent										
Insured continuously all 12 months.................	30.2	31.6	33.6	35.2	31.7	14.7	15.4	15.3	18.3	16.7
Uninsured for any period up to 12 months	34.1	43.7	39.1	34.2	32.7	16.1	18.1	21.5	16.5	15.3
Uninsured more than 12 months	20.8	20.5	20.5	23.4	21.6	8.1	9.1	8.5	11.7	8.8
100 percent to 199 percent										
Insured continuously all 12 months.................	24.5	25.5	23.7	26.1	25.1	8.9	10.2	9.8	10.8	10.2
Uninsured for any period up to 12 months	28.7	27.7	28.4	29.7	26.7	12.3	11.7	12.7	15.6	13.8
Uninsured more than 12 months	19.0	17.4	18.5	21.2	17.4	8.3	6.4	7.7	7.8	6.6
200 to 399 percent..										
Insured continuously all 12 months.................	17.5	19.5	19.7	19.6	15.7	5.3	6.3	6.4	6.0	5.5
Uninsured for any period up to 12 months	21.6	24.6	26.8	25.4	18.9	6.6	7.3	10.6	12.2	7.3
Uninsured more than 12 months	16.8	15.6	14.7	17.6	12.4	5.9	4.5	4.5	5.7	*5.7
400 percent or more										
Insured continuously all 12 months.................	14.9	15.5	15.6	15.9	13.2	3.7	3.7	3.6	4.5	3.0
Uninsured for any period up to 12 months	18.0	20.1	20.2	12.5	*14.5	*3.1	6.4	7.2	*	*
Uninsured more than 12 months	19.1	15.8	17.9	19.4	*8.7	*	*5.2	*7.4	*	*
Disability Measure[2,7]										
Any basic actions difficulty or complex activity limitation	30.8	32.0	34.4	34.9	32.5	13.5	14.6	15.6	16.8	15.9
Any basic actions difficulty	30.5	32.4	34.9	35.0	32.8	13.5	14.9	15.8	17.2	16.4
Any complex activity limitation	39.7	41.5	42.3	43.8	41.0	19.9	21.2	22.4	24.5	22.4
No disability...	14.5	15.3	14.9	16.1	12.9	3.7	3.9	3.9	4.4	3.4
Geographic Region[2]										
Northeast	19.5	20.0	21.6	22.6	18.1	6.9	6.2	7.2	8.4	5.8
Midwest	19.3	20.1	21.6	22.3	20.5	6.2	6.9	7.2	8.2	8.1
South	20.9	21.2	20.7	22.1	19.5	7.3	7.6	7.6	8.0	7.0
West..	17.7	18.6	17.8	18.9	16.6	6.0	6.3	6.0	6.7	6.4
Location of Residence[2]										
Within MSA[8]	19.1	19.6	20.1	20.8	18.2	6.4	6.6	6.8	7.5	6.5
Outside MSA[8]..	21.5	22.5	22.3	25.5	22.8	7.8	7.8	8.1	9.8	9.6

NA = Not available.

* = Figure does not meet standards of reliability or precision. Data preceded by an asterisk have a relative standard error (RSE) of 20 percent to 30 percent. Data not shown have an RSE of greater than 30 percent.

[2]Estimates are for persons 18 years of age and over and are age adjusted to the year 2000 standard population using five age groups: 18 to 44 years, 45 to 54 years, 55 to 64 years, 65 to 74 years, and 75 years and over.

[4]Percent of poverty level is based on family income and family size and composition using U.S. Census Bureau poverty thresholds. Missing family income data were imputed for 1997 and beyond.

[5]Estimates for persons 18 to 64 years of age are age adjusted to the year 2000 standard population using three age groups: 18 to 44 years, 45 to 54 years, and 55 to 64 years.

[6]Health insurance categories are mutually exclusive. Persons who reported both Medicaid and private coverage are classified as having private coverage. Medicaid includes other public assistance through 1996. Starting with 1997 data, state-sponsored health plan coverage is included as Medicaid coverage. Starting with 1999 data, coverage by the Children's Health Insurance Program (CHIP) is included with Medicaid coverage. Persons not covered by private insurance, Medicaid, CHIP, public assistance (through 1996), state-sponsored or other government-sponsored health plans (starting in 1997), Medicare, or military plans are considered to have no health insurance coverage. Persons with only Indian Health Service coverage are considered to have no health insurance coverage. Health insurance status was unknown for 8 to 9 percent of children in 1993-1996 and about 1 percent in 1997-2011.

[7]Any basic actions difficulty or complex activity limitation is defined as having one or more of the following limitations or difficulties: movement difficulty, emotional difficulty, sensory (seeing or hearing) difficulty, cognitive difficulty, self-care (activities of daily living or instrumental activities of daily living) limitation, social limitation, or work limitation.

[8]MSA = metropolitan statistical area.

Table 3-45. Initial Injury-Related Visits to Hospital Emergency Departments, by Sex, Age, and Intent and Mechanism of Injury, Selected Annual Averages, 2005–2006 Through 2012–2013

(Numbers in thousands; rate per 10,000 population.)

Sex, age, and intent and mechanism of injury[1]	Initial injury-related visits in thousands							Initial injury-related visits per 10,000 persons						
	2005–2006	2007–2008	2008–2009	2009–2010	2010–2011	2011–2012	2012–2013	2005–2006	2007–2008	2008–2009	2009–2010	2010–2011	2011–2012	2012–2013
Both Sexes														
All ages, age-adjusted[2,3]	31,706	28,699	31,328	32,204	33,007	31,546	30,402	1,076.4	960.9	1,040.8	1,063.2	1,084.0	1,029.7	983.4
All ages, crude[2]	31,706	28,699	31,328	32,204	33,007	31,546	30,402	1,068.6	951.3	1,029.4	1,049.7	1,067.9	1,012.6	968.9
Unintentional injuries[4]	25,658	23,670	25,725	26,523	27,215	25,955	25,078	864.7	784.6	845.3	864.5	882.4	833.2	799.2
Falls	8,100	8,144	8,900	9,393	9,932	9,225	8,760	273.0	270.0	292.4	306.2	321.3	296.1	279.2
Struck by or against objects or persons	2,935	2,746	2,916	3,055	3,166	3,106	3,149	98.9	91.0	95.8	99.6	102.4	99.7	100.4
Motor vehicle traffic	3,714	3,387	3,508	3,622	3,557	3,199	3,207	125.2	112.3	115.3	118.1	115.1	102.7	102.2
Cut or pierce	2,145	1,944	2,008	1,829	1,922	1,941	1,699	72.3	64.4	66.0	59.6	62.2	62.3	54.1
Intentional injuries	1,977	1,888	2,313	2,418	2,446	2,119	1,692	66.6	62.6	76.0	78.8	79.1	68.0	53.9
Male														
All ages, age-adjusted[2,3]	16,966	15,332	16,640	17,124	17,483	16,474	15,184	1,166.1	1,039.7	1,118.0	1,143.0	1,164.5	1,094.6	1,000.4
All ages, crude[2]	16,966	15,332	16,640	17,124	17,483	16,474	15,184	1,164.2	1,033.8	1,111.8	1,133.8	1,150.5	1,077.8	985.9
Unintentional injuries[4]	13,736	12,611	13,590	14,083	14,451	13,503	12,447	942.5	850.3	908.0	932.4	951.0	883.4	808.1
Falls	3,685	3,581	3,944	4,285	4,689	4,205	3,649	252.9	241.4	263.5	283.7	308.6	275.1	236.9
Struck by or against objects or persons	1,833	1,771	1,863	1,931	2,008	1,903	1,781	125.8	119.4	124.4	127.8	132.2	124.5	115.6
Motor vehicle traffic	1,733	1,693	1,734	1,762	1,710	1,515	1,519	118.9	114.2	115.8	116.7	112.5	99.1	98.6
Cut or pierce	1,392	1,270	1,263	1,183	1,236	1,224	1,042	95.5	85.7	84.4	78.3	81.4	80.1	67.7
Intentional injuries	1,135	1,020	1,266	1,348	1,396	1,169	907	77.8	68.8	84.6	89.3	91.8	76.5	58.9
Under 18 years[2]	5,072	4,602	5,132	5,403	5,309	4,598	4,117	1,346.6	1,216.8	1,351.1	1,416.3	1,397.8	1,218.1	1,093.6
Unintentional injuries[4]	4,391	3,995	4,509	4,817	4,724	4,058	3,641	1,165.8	1,056.3	1,187.1	1,262.9	1,243.9	1,075.2	967.0
Falls	1,362	1,305	1,512	1,647	1,737	1,441	1,092	361.5	345.0	398.1	431.8	457.4	381.9	290.1
Struck by or against objects or persons	816	850	909	1,022	997	827	735	216.6	224.6	239.2	267.9	262.6	219.2	195.2
Motor vehicle traffic	357	265	305	309	301	239	198	94.8	70.0	80.3	81.0	79.1	63.2	52.6
Cut or pierce	291	264	284	248	238	273	265	77.3	69.8	74.8	64.9	62.7	72.4	70.5
Intentional injuries	190	198	194	173	167	125	*122	50.4	52.2	51.1	45.3	44.1	33.1	*32.5
18 to 24 years[2]	2,552	2,305	2,562	2,516	2,511	2,337	2,122	1,729.5	1,547.4	1,695.5	1,630.1	1,612.1	1,495.4	1,348.5
Unintentional injuries[4]	1,985	1,788	1,947	1,878	1,890	1,790	1,634	1,345.4	1,200.6	1,288.6	1,216.7	1,213.7	1,145.7	1,038.4
Falls	318	309	366	375	390	347	268	215.2	207.7	242.4	243.0	250.4	222.3	170.3
Struck by or against objects or persons	290	280	283	216	259	290	227	196.9	188.0	187.4	140.2	166.6	185.4	144.0
Motor vehicle traffic	386	366	373	406	357	331	343	261.6	245.8	247.0	263.2	229.3	211.6	217.9
Cut or pierce	265	190	215	187	192	179	152	179.5	127.8	142.6	121.4	123.5	114.5	96.8
Intentional injuries	273	308	381	389	403	318	216	185.2	206.9	252.2	252.2	258.7	203.2	137.3
25 to 44 years[2]	5,199	4,471	4,611	4,719	4,850	4,867	4,429	1,243.6	1,072.7	1,109.5	1,140.9	1,184.3	1,194.1	1,079.9
Unintentional injuries[4]	4,001	3,531	3,540	3,577	3,690	3,673	3,426	957.1	847.0	851.8	864.8	901.1	901.4	835.4
Falls	763	677	703	739	815	813	791	182.4	162.5	169.2	178.7	199.1	199.4	192.8
Struck by or against objects or persons	472	384	401	400	452	500	495	112.9	92.1	96.4	96.8	110.4	122.6	120.7
Motor vehicle traffic	629	638	578	585	591	501	509	150.5	153.0	139.1	141.5	144.3	122.8	124.1
Cut or pierce	480	426	401	380	423	464	354	114.8	102.2	96.5	91.9	103.2	113.9	86.4
Intentional injuries	436	350	495	586	589	528	424	104.4	83.9	119.2	141.6	143.8	129.5	103.4
45 to 64 years[2]	2,842	2,707	2,996	3,071	3,270	3,193	3,101	790.0	718.3	780.7	788.7	822.7	791.7	767.3
Unintentional injuries[4]	2,275	2,223	2,437	2,531	2,741	2,671	2,505	632.5	590.0	635.1	649.9	689.6	662.3	620.0
Falls	599	651	669	775	909	790	716	166.6	172.8	174.2	199.0	228.6	195.9	177.2
Struck by or against objects or persons	208	205	216	208	204	219	256	57.9	54.3	56.4	53.3	51.4	54.4	63.4
Motor vehicle traffic	262	331	375	334	334	350	389	72.9	87.9	97.7	85.9	84.0	86.7	96.3
Cut or pierce	285	309	306	297	294	231	190	79.2	81.9	79.7	76.2	73.9	57.4	47.1
Intentional injuries	205	145	168	180	219	170	130	57.1	38.4	43.9	46.2	55.2	42.1	32.1
65 years and over[2]	1,301	1,247	1,340	1,415	1,544	1,478	1,415	837.5	768.6	805.1	824.7	871.6	804.3	736.6
Unintentional injuries[4]	1,082	1,073	1,157	1,280	1,406	1,311	1,240	696.8	661.7	695.2	746.1	793.5	713.1	645.5
Falls	644	638	694	749	838	814	782	414.5	393.2	416.7	436.3	473.0	442.7	407.3
Struck by or against objects or persons	46	*52	*54	84	95	*66	*67	29.8	*32.3	*32.2	49.1	53.6	*36.1	*35.1
Motor vehicle traffic	98	93	103	127	128	*96	*79	63.4	57.4	61.7	74.1	72.1	*52.0	*41.4
Cut or pierce	70	81	*57	71	90	*76	*80	45.3	50.0	*34.0	41.1	50.6	*41.4	*41.7
Intentional injuries	*	*	*	*	*	*	*	*	*	*	*	*	*	*
Female														
All ages, age-adjusted[2,3]	14,740	13,367	14,688	15,080	15,524	15,072	15,218	980.5	874.2	955.6	976.8	997.2	958.5	959.0
All ages, crude[2]	14,740	13,367	14,688	15,080	15,524	15,072	15,218	976.3	871.6	949.7	968.2	988.0	949.9	952.6
Unintentional injuries[4]	11,922	11,060	12,134	12,439	12,824	12,451	12,632	789.7	721.1	784.6	798.6	816.1	784.7	790.7
Falls	4,415	4,564	4,956	5,109	5,243	5,020	5,111	292.4	297.6	320.4	328.0	333.6	316.4	319.9
Struck by or against objects or persons	1,102	976	1,053	1,124	1,158	1,204	1,368	73.0	63.6	68.1	72.2	73.7	75.9	85.7
Motor vehicle traffic	1,981	1,695	1,774	1,860	1,847	1,684	1,688	131.2	110.5	114.7	119.4	117.6	106.1	105.7

Note: An emergency department visit was considered injury related if the first-listed diagnosis was injury related (ICD-9-CM 800-909.2, 909.4, 909.9-994.9, 995.50-995.59, and 995.80-995.85) or the first-listed external cause code (E code) was injury related (ICD-9-CM E800-E869, E880-E929, and E950-E999).

* = Figure does not meet standards of reliability or precision. Data preceded by an asterisk have a relative standard error (RSE) of 20 percent to 30 percent. Data not shown have an RSE greater than 30 percent.

[1]Intent and mechanism of injury are based on the first-listed external cause of injury code (E code). Intentional injuries include suicide attempts and assaults.

[2]Includes all injury-related visits not shown separately in table, including those with undetermined intent (1 percent in 2012 to 2013) and insufficient or no information to code cause of injury (11 percent in 2012 to 2013).

[3]Rates are age adjusted to the year 2000 standard population using six age groups: under 18 years, 18 to 24 years, 25 to 44 years, 45 to 64 years, 65 to 74 years, and 75 years and over.

[4]Includes unintentional injury-related visits with mechanism of injury not shown in table.

Table 3-45. Initial Injury-Related Visits to Hospital Emergency Departments, by Sex, Age, and Intent and Mechanism of Injury, Selected Annual Averages, 2005–2006 Through 2012–2013—*Continued*

(Numbers in thousands; rate per 10,000 population.)

Sex, age, and intent and mechanism of injury[1]	Initial injury-related visits in thousands							Initial injury-related visits per 10,000 persons						
	2005–2006	2007–2008	2008–2009	2009–2010	2010–2011	2011–2012	2012–2013	2005–2006	2007–2008	2008–2009	2009–2010	2010–2011	2011–2012	2012–2013
Cut or pierce	753	673	745	646	685	717	657	49.9	43.9	48.2	41.5	43.6	45.2	41.1
Intentional injuries	843	867	1,048	1,070	1,050	951	785	55.8	56.5	67.7	68.7	66.8	59.9	49.1
Under 18 years[2]	3,625	3,062	3,508	3,645	3,673	3,643	3,602	1,008.7	848.2	967.5	1,001.6	1,013.2	1,009.5	1,000.4
Unintentional injuries[4]	3,058	2,690	3,008	3,115	3,120	3,096	3,105	851.1	745.3	829.5	855.9	860.7	857.9	862.2
Falls	1,039	1,014	1,096	1,144	1,138	1,093	1,047	289.1	280.9	302.3	314.3	314.0	302.8	290.9
Struck by or against objects or persons	419	391	439	454	425	473	522	116.7	108.3	121.1	124.7	117.2	131.0	145.0
Motor vehicle traffic	367	282	249	285	302	275	273	102.1	78.2	68.6	78.3	83.4	76.1	75.8
Cut or pierce	160	145	154	139	158	167	*148	44.4	40.1	42.4	38.2	43.7	46.2	*41.0
Intentional injuries	188	163	222	207	196	193	144	52.3	45.1	61.4	56.8	54.1	53.6	39.9
18 to 24 years[2]	1,882	1,698	1,736	1,854	1,936	1,790	1,769	1,329.3	1,186.5	1,194.5	1,259.9	1,297.1	1,180.1	1,160.3
Unintentional injuries[4]	1,431	1,318	1,325	1,437	1,530	1,370	1,367	1,010.5	921.0	911.7	976.4	1,025.0	903.7	896.7
Falls	290	301	307	299	305	288	326	205.0	210.5	210.9	203.5	204.5	190.0	214.2
Struck by or against objects or persons	146	106	110	135	171	142	129	103.4	74.0	75.4	91.6	114.7	93.9	84.4
Motor vehicle traffic	397	378	360	426	460	387	372	280.6	264.5	247.5	289.8	308.1	255.4	244.3
Cut or pierce	116	89	77	*81	*94	*81	81	82.2	61.9	53.2	*55.1	*63.3	*53.6	53.2
Intentional injuries	176	209	232	262	251	198	151	124.2	145.8	159.7	177.9	168.4	130.8	99.2
25 to 44 years[2]	4,173	3,733	4,087	4,152	4,233	3,956	3,914	1,004.2	905.4	996.6	1,016.6	1,034.6	962.1	947.8
Unintentional injuries[4]	3,266	2,865	3,179	3,244	3,308	3,123	3,105	785.8	694.7	775.1	794.2	808.5	759.5	751.8
Falls	873	900	1,004	986	941	908	921	210.1	218.2	244.7	241.4	229.9	220.8	223.0
Struck by or against objects or persons	309	216	198	250	284	251	326	74.3	52.4	48.3	61.2	69.4	60.9	79.0
Motor vehicle traffic	719	572	621	612	616	554	529	173.1	138.8	151.3	149.9	150.5	134.8	128.0
Cut or pierce	269	214	270	230	219	227	215	64.7	51.8	65.9	56.4	53.6	55.3	52.1
Intentional injuries	313	345	396	396	408	367	310	75.4	83.6	96.5	96.9	99.8	89.3	75.0
45 to 64 years[2]	2,904	2,681	3,061	3,106	3,101	3,106	3,173	767.8	677.5	760.0	759.3	741.9	732.3	746.6
Unintentional injuries[4]	2,278	2,209	2,539	2,536	2,519	2,521	2,538	602.2	558.3	630.4	619.9	602.7	594.4	597.4
Falls	865	886	1,012	1,067	1,075	1,005	993	228.7	223.9	251.2	260.8	257.1	237.0	233.7
Struck by or against objects or persons	160	171	216	205	197	227	246	42.2	43.2	53.5	50.0	47.2	53.6	58.0
Motor vehicle traffic	359	345	399	403	345	343	388	94.8	87.3	99.0	98.4	82.6	80.8	91.2
Cut or pierce	158	163	190	159	157	169	159	41.7	41.1	47.2	38.8	37.6	39.8	37.4
Intentional injuries	149	130	161	184	182	180	*171	39.4	32.9	39.9	45.0	43.5	42.5	*40.2
65 years and over[2]	2,155	2,193	2,294	2,322	2,582	2,577	2,760	1,002.9	989.9	1,016.3	1,014.2	1,110.7	1,078.8	1,116.8
Unintentional injuries[4]	1,889	1,978	2,083	2,108	2,348	2,341	2,517	879.1	892.5	922.8	920.4	1,009.8	980.0	1,018.2
Falls	1,347	1,463	1,538	1,612	1,784	1,726	1,823	626.9	660.1	681.2	704.1	767.2	722.4	737.7
Struck by or against objects or persons	69	91	91	81	81	*111	*145	31.9	41.2	40.4	35.5	34.7	*46.3	*58.6
Motor vehicle traffic	139	116	146	134	124	125	127	64.5	52.5	64.7	58.3	53.5	52.2	51.2
Cut or pierce	*50	*64	*54	*37	*56	*72	*54	*23.3	*28.8	*23.9	*16.3	*24.2	*30.1	*21.8
Intentional injuries	*	*	*	*	*	*	*	*	*	*	*	*	*	*

Note: An emergency department visit was considered injury related if the first-listed diagnosis was injury related (ICD-9-CM 800-909.2, 909.4, 909.9-994.9, 995.50-995.59, and 995.80-995.85) or the first-listed external cause code (E code) was injury related (ICD-9-CM E800-E869, E880-E929, and E950-E999).
* = Figure does not meet standards of reliability or precision. Data preceded by an asterisk have a relative standard error (RSE) of 20 percent to 30 percent. Data not shown have an RSE greater than 30 percent.
[1]Intent and mechanism of injury are based on the first-listed external cause of injury code (E code). Intentional injuries include suicide attempts and assaults.
[2]Includes all injury-related visits not shown separately in table, including those with undetermined intent (1 percent in 2012 to 2013) and insufficient or no information to code cause of injury (11 percent in 2012 to 2013).
[3]Rates are age adjusted to the year 2000 standard population using six age groups: under 18 years, 18 to 24 years, 25 to 44 years, 45 to 64 years, 65 to 74 years, and 75 years and over.
[4]Includes unintentional injury-related visits with mechanism of injury not shown in table.

Table 3-46. Visits to Physician Offices, Hospital Outpatient Departments, and Hospital Emergency Departments, by Age, Sex, and Race, Selected Years, 1995–2013

(Number; rate.)

Age, sex, and race	All places[1]					Physician offices				
	1995	2000	2009	2010	2013	1995	2000	2009	2010	2013
	Number of visits in thousands									
Age										
Total..........................	860,859	1,014,848	1,270,001	1,239,387	NA	697,082	823,542	1,037,796	1,008,802	922,596
Under 18 years..................	194,644	212,165	239,590	246,228	NA	150,351	163,459	183,999	191,500	151,036
18 to 44 years..................	285,184	315,774	341,209	342,797	NA	219,065	243,011	257,890	261,941	224,256
45 to 64 years..................	188,320	255,894	374,775	352,001	NA	159,531	216,783	316,395	296,385	282,109
45 to 54 years................	104,891	142,233	190,701	171,039	NA	88,266	119,474	158,120	140,819	131,013
55 to 64 years................	83,429	113,661	184,074	180,962	NA	71,264	97,309	158,275	155,566	151,096
65 years and over..............	192,712	231,014	314,428	298,362	NA	168,135	200,289	279,514	258,976	265,195
65 to 74 years................	102,605	116,505	153,884	151,075	NA	90,544	102,447	137,452	132,201	141,507
75 years and over.............	90,106	114,510	160,544	147,287	NA	77,591	97,842	142,062	126,775	123,688
	Number of visits per 100 persons									
Total, age-adjusted[2]...........	334	374	414	401	NA	271	304	337	325	285
Total, crude....................	329	370	421	408	NA	266	300	344	332	297
Under 18 years................	275	293	322	331	NA	213	226	247	257	206
18 to 44 years................	264	291	309	310	NA	203	224	234	237	201
45 to 64 years................	364	422	475	441	NA	309	358	401	371	343
45 to 54 years...............	339	385	431	388	NA	286	323	358	320	303
55 to 64 years...............	401	481	532	505	NA	343	412	457	434	387
65 years and over.............	612	706	829	767	NA	534	612	737	666	611
65 to 74 years...............	560	656	749	713	NA	494	577	669	624	566
75 years and over............	683	766	923	831	NA	588	654	817	715	672
Sex and Age										
Male, age-adjusted[2]...........	290	325	358	350	NA	232	261	290	283	250
Male, crude....................	277	314	356	350	NA	220	251	289	283	256
Under 18 years................	273	302	334	340	NA	209	231	257	262	206
18 to 44 years................	190	203	201	205	NA	139	148	145	151	137
45 to 54 years...............	275	316	361	324	NA	229	260	296	265	263
55 to 64 years...............	351	428	473	460	NA	300	367	403	396	359
65 to 74 years...............	508	614	731	680	NA	445	539	654	597	530
75 years and over............	711	771	907	871	NA	616	670	807	760	679
Female, age-adjusted[2].........	377	420	469	452	NA	309	345	383	367	318
Female, crude..................	378	424	483	464	NA	310	348	397	379	336
Under 18 years................	277	285	310	322	NA	217	221	237	252	206
18 to 44 years................	336	377	416	415	NA	265	298	322	323	263
45 to 54 years...............	400	451	499	450	NA	339	384	417	372	341
55 to 64 years...............	446	529	586	546	NA	382	453	507	469	413
65 to 74 years...............	603	692	764	741	NA	534	609	681	647	598
75 years and over............	666	763	934	804	NA	571	645	823	685	667
Race and Age[3]										
White, age-adjusted[2]..........	339	380	421	408	NA	282	315	351	336	304
White, crude...................	338	381	434	421	NA	281	316	365	349	323
Under 18 years................	295	306	339	341	NA	237	243	269	270	230
18 to 44 years................	267	301	312	319	NA	211	239	244	249	218
45 to 54 years...............	334	386	432	389	NA	286	330	369	326	318
55 to 64 years...............	397	480	531	505	NA	345	416	466	440	405
65 to 74 years...............	557	641	752	727	NA	496	568	678	642	582
75 years and over............	689	764	936	838	NA	598	658	835	723	701
Black or African American, age-adjusted[2]...........	309	353	459	439	NA	204	239	314	316	243
Black or African American, crude......................	281	324	438	425	NA	178	214	296	303	235
Under 18 years................	193	264	315	351	NA	100	167	198	241	158
18 to 44 years................	260	257	373	339	NA	158	149	228	222	170
45 to 54 years...............	387	383	486	466	NA	281	269	329	339	284
55 to 64 years...............	414	495	645	617	NA	294	373	478	481	339
65 to 74 years...............	553	656	821	715	NA	429	512	667	565	527
75 years and over............	534	745	908	845	NA	395	568	718	682	542

Note: In 2012 and 2013, data for all places and physician offices exclude visits to community health centers; in 2006–2011, data for all places and physician offices include visits to community health centers (2%–3% of visits to physician offices in 2006–2011 were to community health centers). Prior to 2006, visits to community health centers were not included in the survey.

NA = Not available.

* = Estimates are considered unreliable. Data preceded by an asterisk have a relative standard error (RSE) of 20 percent to 30 percent. Data not shown have an RSE greater than 30 percent.

[1] All places includes visits to physician offices and hospital outpatient and emergency departments.

[2] Estimates are age adjusted to the year 2000 standard population using six age groups: under 18 years, 18 to 44 years, 45 to 54 years, 55 to 64 years, 65 to 74 years, and 75 years and over.

[3] Estimates by racial group should be used with caution because information on race was collected from medical records and race is imputed for records missing that information. Information on the race imputation process used in each data year is available in the public-use file documentation. Starting with 1999 data, the instruction for the race item on the Patient Record Form was changed so that more than one race could be recorded. In previous years only one race could be recorded. Estimates for race in this table are for visits where only one race was recorded. Because of the small number of responses with more than one racial group recorded, estimates for visits with multiple races recorded are unreliable and are not presented.

Table 3-46. Visits to Physician Offices, Hospital Outpatient Departments, and Hospital Emergency Departments, by Age, Sex, and Race, Selected Years, 1995–2013—*Continued*

(Number; rate.)

Age, sex, and race	Hospital outpatient departments					Hospital emergency departments				
	1995	2000	2009	2010	2013	1995	2000	2009	2010	2013
	Number of visits in thousands									
Age										
Total	67,232	83,289	96,132	100,742	NA	96,545	83,289	96,132	100,742	NA
Under 18 years	17,636	21,076	22,418	24,913	NA	26,657	21,076	22,418	24,913	NA
18 to 44 years	24,299	26,947	29,535	28,159	NA	41,820	26,947	29,535	28,159	NA
45 to 64 years	14,811	20,772	29,083	27,739	NA	13,978	20,772	29,083	27,739	NA
45 to 54 years	8,029	11,558	15,310	13,639	NA	8,595	11,558	15,310	13,639	NA
55 to 64 years	6,782	9,214	13,774	14,100	NA	5,383	9,214	13,774	14,100	NA
65 years and over	10,486	14,494	15,096	19,932	NA	14,090	14,494	15,096	19,932	NA
65 to 74 years	6,004	7,515	8,036	10,675	NA	6,057	7,515	8,036	10,675	NA
75 years and over	4,482	6,979	7,060	9,257	NA	8,033	6,979	7,060	9,257	NA
	Number of visits per 100 persons									
Total, age-adjusted[2]	26	31	31	33	NA	37	40	46	43	42
Total, crude	26	30	32	33	NA	37	39	45	43	42
Under 18 years	25	29	30	33	NA	38	38	45	40	38
18 to 44 years	22	25	27	25	NA	39	42	49	48	46
45 to 64 years	29	34	37	35	NA	27	30	37	35	37
45 to 54 years	26	31	35	31	NA	28	30	39	38	40
55 to 64 years	33	39	40	39	NA	26	30	35	32	33
65 years and over	33	44	40	51	NA	45	50	52	50	48
65 to 74 years	33	42	39	50	NA	33	37	41	39	37
75 years and over	34	47	41	52	NA	61	65	66	64	62
Sex and Age										
Male, age-adjusted[2]	21	26	25	27	NA	37	38	42	40	38
Male, crude	21	25	26	27	NA	36	38	42	39	38
Under 18 years	25	29	30	34	NA	40	41	46	43	39
18 to 44 years	14	17	16	16	NA	37	38	40	38	37
45 to 54 years	20	26	28	24	NA	26	30	36	35	37
55 to 64 years	26	32	35	32	NA	25	30	34	32	34
65 to 74 years	29	38	37	47	NA	34	36	40	37	36
75 years and over	34	42	37	50	NA	61	59	63	60	55
Female, age-adjusted[2]	31	35	37	38	NA	37	41	49	47	47
Female, crude	31	35	38	39	NA	37	41	48	46	46
Under 18 years	25	29	30	33	NA	35	35	43	37	38
18 to 44 years	31	33	38	35	NA	40	46	57	57	55
45 to 54 years	32	36	41	37	NA	29	31	42	40	43
55 to 64 years	38	45	44	46	NA	26	31	35	31	33
65 to 74 years	36	46	41	54	NA	32	37	42	40	39
75 years and over	34	49	43	53	NA	61	69	68	66	67
Race and Age[3]										
White, age-adjusted[2]	23	28	29	31	NA	34	37	41	41	40
White, crude	23	28	29	32	NA	34	37	41	40	40
Under 18 years	23	27	29	33	NA	35	36	40	39	37
18 to 44 years	20	23	24	25	NA	36	39	43	45	43
45 to 54 years	23	28	30	28	NA	25	28	34	34	36
55 to 64 years	28	36	34	36	NA	24	28	30	29	31
65 to 74 years	29	38	35	48	NA	32	35	38	37	35
75 years and over	31	44	36	52	NA	60	63	64	62	63
Black or African American, age-adjusted[2]	48	51	59	51	NA	58	62	85	73	73
Black or African American, crude	45	48	58	50	NA	58	62	84	72	72
Under 18 years	39	40	42	48	NA	53	57	75	62	60
18 to 44 years	38	40	50	37	NA	64	68	94	81	83
45 to 54 years	55	61	74	54	NA	51	53	83	73	77
55 to 64 years	73	70	91	73	NA	47	52	76	62	64
65 to 74 years	*77	85	*81	*85	NA	47	59	73	66	63
75 years and over	66	85	*	*74	NA	73	92	95	89	69

Note: In 2012 and 2013, data for all places and physician offices exclude visits to community health centers; in 2006–2011, data for all places and physician offices include visits to community health centers (2%–3% of visits to physician offices in 2006–2011 were to community health centers). Prior to 2006, visits to community health centers were not included in the survey.
NA = Not available.
* = Estimates are considered unreliable. Data preceded by an asterisk have a relative standard error (RSE) of 20 percent to 30 percent. Data not shown have an RSE greater than 30 percent.
[2]Estimates are age adjusted to the year 2000 standard population using six age groups: under 18 years, 18 to 44 years, 45 to 54 years, 55 to 64 years, 65 to 74 years, and 75 years and over.
[3]Estimates by racial group should be used with caution because information on race was collected from medical records and race is imputed for records missing that information. Information on the race imputation process used in each data year is available in the public-use file documentation. Starting with 1999 data, the instruction for the race item on the Patient Record Form was changed so that more than one race could be recorded. In previous years only one race could be recorded. Estimates for race in this table are for visits where only one race was recorded. Because of the small number of responses with more than one racial group recorded, estimates for visits with multiple races recorded are unreliable and are not presented.

Table 3-47. Visits to Primary Care Generalist and Specialist Physicians, by Selected Characteristics and Type of Physician, Selected Years, 1980–2013

(Percent.)

Age, sex, and race	Type of primary care generalist physician[1]														
	All primary care generalists					General and family practice					Internal medicine				
	1980	1990	2000	2009	2013	1980	1990	2000	2009	2013	1980	1990	2000	2009	2013
Age															
Total	66.2	63.6	58.9	55.9	49.1	33.5	29.9	24.1	23.1	18.9	12.1	13.8	15.3	14.8	13.7
Under 18 years	77.8	79.5	79.7	78.8	74.1	26.1	26.5	19.9	16.3	12.4	2.0	2.9	*	*	*0.6
18 to 44 years	65.3	65.2	62.1	61.5	53.7	34.3	31.9	28.2	29.7	20.9	8.6	11.8	12.7	11.0	12.8
45 to 64 years	60.2	55.5	51.2	48.6	42.1	36.3	32.1	26.4	25.5	21.5	19.5	18.6	20.1	18.0	16.4
45 to 54 years	60.2	55.6	52.3	50.9	42.9	37.4	32.0	27.8	27.5	22.5	17.1	17.1	18.7	17.1	15.1
55 to 64 years	60.2	55.5	49.9	46.4	41.3	35.4	32.1	24.7	23.5	20.6	21.8	20.0	21.7	19.0	17.6
65 years and over	61.6	52.6	46.5	43.9	38.3	37.5	28.1	20.2	18.8	18.0	22.7	23.3	24.5	23.5	18.8
65 to 74 years	61.2	52.7	46.6	41.9	37.5	37.4	28.1	19.7	19.9	17.6	22.1	23.0	24.5	20.0	18.2
75 years and over	62.3	52.4	46.4	45.9	39.1	37.6	28.0	20.8	17.7	18.4	23.5	23.7	24.5	26.9	19.6
Sex and Age															
Male															
Under 18 years	77.3	78.1	77.7	77.6	73.8	25.6	24.1	18.3	15.2	12.1	2.0	3.0	*	*	*
18 to 44 years	50.8	51.8	51.5	52.4	41.5	38.0	35.9	34.2	36.6	24.9	11.5	15.0	14.4	14.1	14.9
45 to 64 years	55.6	50.6	49.4	45.2	38.9	34.4	31.0	28.7	26.4	21.4	20.5	19.2	19.8	18.7	17.4
65 years and over	58.2	51.2	43.1	38.6	34.1	35.6	27.7	19.3	18.3	16.3	22.3	23.3	23.8	20.1	17.7
Female															
Under 18 years	78.5	81.1	82.0	80.2	74.5	26.6	29.1	21.7	17.6	12.7	2.0	2.8	*	*	*0.6
18 to 44 years	72.1	71.3	67.2	65.6	59.9	32.5	30.0	25.3	26.6	18.9	7.3	10.3	11.9	9.6	11.8
45 to 64 years	63.4	58.8	52.5	51.1	44.6	37.7	32.8	24.9	24.9	21.6	18.9	18.2	20.2	17.6	15.7
65 years and over	63.9	53.5	48.9	47.8	41.3	38.7	28.3	20.9	19.2	19.2	22.9	23.3	25.0	26.0	19.7
Race and Age[2]															
White															
Under 18 years	77.6	79.2	78.5	78.1	74.5	26.4	27.1	21.2	16.3	13.0	2.0	2.3	*	*	*
18 to 44 years	64.8	64.4	61.4	60.4	52.4	34.5	31.9	29.2	30.3	21.5	8.6	10.6	11.0	10.1	12.7
45 to 64 years	59.6	54.2	49.3	47.6	41.5	36.0	31.5	27.3	25.9	22.1	19.2	17.6	17.1	17.0	15.4
65 years and over	61.4	51.9	45.1	43.2	38.1	36.6	27.5	20.3	18.7	18.2	23.3	23.1	23.0	22.9	18.5
Black or African American															
Under 18 years	79.9	85.5	87.3	80.8	73.2	23.7	20.2	*	*15.5	*10.3	*2.2	9.8	*	*	*
18 to 44 years	68.5	68.3	65.0	64.4	60.8	31.7	31.9	22.0	26.6	20.0	9.0	18.1	20.9	*15.2	11.8
45 to 64 years	66.1	61.6	61.7	50.0	45.7	38.6	31.2	23.3	23.4	19.4	22.6	26.9	35.9	*21.4	22.3
65 years and over	64.6	58.6	52.8	45.7	41.9	49.0	28.9	*18.5	*15.8	15.6	14.2	28.7	33.4	*28.6	24.8

Age, sex, and race	Type of primary care generalist physician[1]										Specialty care physicians				
	Obstetrics and gynecology					Pediatrics									
	1980	1990	2000	2009	2013	1980	1990	2000	2009	2013	1980	1990	2000	2009	2013
Age															
Total	9.6	8.7	7.8	7.0	6.3	10.9	11.2	11.7	11.1	10.2	33.8	36.4	41.1	44.1	50.9
Under 18 years	1.3	1.2	*1.1	0.8	*0.6	48.5	48.9	57.3	60.5	60.5	22.2	20.5	20.3	21.2	25.9
18 to 44 years	21.7	20.8	20.4	19.8	18.8	0.7	0.7	*0.9	*1.1	1.1	34.7	34.8	37.9	38.5	46.3
45 to 64 years	4.2	4.6	4.5	4.9	4.1	*	*	*	*	*	39.8	44.5	48.8	51.4	57.9
45 to 54 years	5.6	6.3	5.6	6.0	5.3	*	*	*	*	*	39.8	44.4	47.7	49.1	57.1
55 to 64 years	2.9	3.1	3.3	3.8	3.1	*	*	*	*	*	39.8	44.5	50.1	53.6	58.7
65 years and over	1.4	1.1	1.5	*1.5	1.4	*	*	*	*	*	38.4	47.4	53.5	56.1	61.7
65 to 74 years	1.7	1.6	2.0	*1.8	1.7	*	*	*	*	*	38.8	47.3	53.4	58.1	62.5
75 years and over	1.0	*0.6	*1.0	*1.1	1.1	*	*	*	*	*	37.7	47.6	53.6	54.1	60.9
Sex and Age															
Male															
Under 18 years	X	X	X	X	X	49.4	50.7	58.0	61.2	61.0	22.7	21.9	22.3	22.4	26.2
18 to 44 years	X	X	X	X	X	1.0	0.7	*1.7	*1.8	1.6	49.2	48.2	48.5	47.6	58.5
45 to 64 years	X	X	X	X	X	*	*	*	*	*	44.4	49.4	50.6	54.8	61.1
65 years and over	X	X	X	X	X	*	*	*	*	*	41.8	48.8	56.9	61.4	65.9
Female															
Under 18 years	2.5	2.3	2.1	1.7	*1.1	47.4	46.9	56.5	59.8	60.0	21.5	18.9	18.0	19.8	25.5
18 to 44 years	31.7	30.4	29.6	28.7	28.4	0.6	0.7	*	*	0.9	27.9	28.7	32.8	34.4	40.1
45 to 64 years	6.7	7.7	7.3	8.4	7.2	*	*	*	*	*	36.6	41.2	47.5	48.9	55.4
65 years and over	2.1	1.8	2.6	*2.5	2.4	*	*	*	*	*	36.1	46.5	51.1	52.2	58.7
Race and Age[2]															
White															
Under 18 years	1.1	1.0	*1.2	*0.7	*0.5	48.2	48.8	54.7	60.1	60.3	22.4	20.8	21.5	21.9	25.5
18 to 44 years	21.0	21.1	20.4	18.8	17.1	0.7	0.7	*0.8	*1.2	1.1	35.2	35.6	38.6	39.6	47.6
45 to 64 years	4.1	4.8	4.7	4.5	4.0	*	*	*	*	*	40.4	45.8	50.7	52.4	58.5
65 years and over	1.4	1.2	1.5	*1.4	1.4	*	*	*	*	*	38.6	48.1	54.9	56.8	61.9
Black or African American															
Under 18 years	2.8	*3.4	*	*	*	51.2	52.1	75.0	62.7	61.3	20.1	14.5	*12.7	*19.2	26.8
18 to 44 years	27.1	17.9	20.7	22.1	27.8	*	*	*	*	*1.2	31.5	31.7	35.0	35.6	39.2
45 to 64 years	4.8	3.5	*2.4	*5.1	*4.0	*	*	*	*	0.0	33.9	38.4	38.3	50.0	54.3
65 years and over	*	*	*	*	*	*	*	*	*	0.0	35.4	41.4	47.2	54.3	58.1

Note: This table presents data on visits to physician offices and excludes visits to other sites, such as hospital outpatient and emergency departments. In 2012 and 2013, data exclude visits to community health centers; in 2006–2011, data include visits to community health centers (2%–3% of visits to physician offices in 2006–2011 were to community health centers). Prior to 2006, visits to community health centers were not included in the survey.

X = Not applicable.

* = Figure does not meet standards of reliability or precision. Data preceded by an asterisk have a relative standard error (RSE) of 20 percent to 30 percent. Data not shown have a RSE greater than 30 percent.

[1]Type of physician is based on physician's self-designated primary area of practice. Primary care generalist physicians are defined as practitioners in the fields of general and family practice, general internal medicine, general obstetrics and gynecology, and general pediatrics and exclude primary care specialists. Primary care generalists in general and family practice exclude primary care specialties, such as sports medicine and geriatrics. Primary care internal medicine physicians exclude internal medicine specialists, such as allergists, cardiologists, and endocrinologists. Primary care obstetrics and gynecology physicians exclude obstetrics and gynecology specialties, such as gynecological oncology, maternal and fetal medicine, obstetrics and gynecology critical care medicine, and reproductive endocrinology. Primary care pediatricians exclude pediatric specialists, such as adolescent medicine specialists, neonatologists, pediatric allergists, and pediatric cardiologists.

[2]Estimates by racial group should be used with caution because information on race was collected from medical records. In 2013, race data were missing and imputed for 30 percent of visits.

Table 3-48. Dental Visits in the Past Year, by Selected Characteristics, Selected Years, 1997–2015

(Percent.)

Characteristic	2 years and over 1997	2000	2010	2015	2 to 17 years 1997	2000	2010	2015	18 to 64 years 1997	2000	2010	2015	65 years and over[1] 1997	2000	2010	2015
Total with Dental Visit[2,3]	65.1	66.2	64.7	68.2	72.7	74.1	78.9	84.7	64.1	65.1	61.1	64.0	54.8	56.6	57.7	62.7
Sex																
Male	62.9	63.5	61.7	66.0	72.3	73.7	78.3	84.2	60.4	60.7	56.8	60.5	55.4	56.1	56.2	62.1
Female	67.1	68.8	67.5	70.3	73.0	74.6	79.6	85.2	67.7	69.4	65.4	67.3	54.4	56.9	58.9	63.2
Race[4]																
White only	66.4	67.9	65.6	68.8	74.0	75.8	79.2	84.8	65.7	67.2	62.4	64.6	56.8	58.4	59.3	64.9
Black or African American only	58.9	59.5	58.8	64.3	68.8	70.0	79.0	85.1	57.0	57.1	53.1	59.4	35.4	38.2	40.6	46.3
American Indian or Alaska Native only	55.1	58.6	57.4	61.7	66.8	71.3	73.2	82.1	49.9	55.0	49.8	57.9	*	*	72.2	*36.1
Asian only	62.5	67.1	66.5	71.1	69.9	72.8	74.8	82.2	60.3	65.6	64.6	69.2	53.9	60.6	61.9	62.8
Native Hawaiian and Other Pacific Islander only	NA	*	*	*	NA	*	*	*	NA	*	*	*	NA	*	*	*
Two or more races	NA	65.1	65.2	68.1	NA	71.4	77.9	84.7	NA	60.5	54.7	58.3	NA	57.4	48.1	41.7
Black or African American; White	NA	63.5	72.5	71.6	NA	65.7	78.4	84.2	NA	60.7	62.1	50.7	NA	*	*	*
American Indian or Alaska Native; White	NA	61.7	54.7	56.9	NA	63.4	70.0	83.1	NA	61.6	49.0	51.5	NA	*57.8	*54.5	*41.9
Hispanic Origin and Race[4]																
Hispanic or Latino	54.0	52.3	56.5	62.2	61.0	60.6	74.8	83.8	50.8	48.6	48.5	53.2	47.8	44.5	42.1	52.2
Not Hispanic or Latino	66.4	68.2	66.2	69.5	74.7	76.8	80.1	85.0	65.7	67.5	63.4	66.2	55.2	57.2	59.0	63.6
White only	68.0	69.9	67.6	70.4	76.4	78.9	80.9	85.4	67.5	69.4	65.4	67.4	57.2	59.1	60.9	66.1
Black or African American only	58.8	59.4	58.7	64.3	68.8	70.0	79.2	85.1	56.9	57.2	53.1	59.4	35.3	38.0	40.5	46.8
Percent of Poverty Level[5]																
Below 100 percent	50.5	50.4	50.6	55.8	62.0	62.4	73.2	82.2	46.9	46.8	41.0	45.0	31.5	33.3	32.8	35.9
100 percent to 199 percent	50.8	52.2	51.6	55.4	62.5	66.1	73.4	81.2	48.4	48.4	44.1	47.1	40.3	43.8	44.0	44.0
200 percent to 399 percent	66.2	65.6	63.5	66.4	76.1	75.5	79.0	84.1	63.4	62.2	59.6	61.8	60.7	62.8	57.9	61.3
400 percent or more	78.9	79.5	79.3	81.2	85.7	85.9	88.0	90.1	77.7	78.5	77.5	79.2	74.7	73.8	77.2	80.8
Hispanic Origin and Race and Percent of Poverty Level[4,5]																
Hispanic or Latino																
Below 100 percent	45.7	43.4	50.8	58.5	55.9	54.2	74.3	85.2	39.2	36.8	34.7	40.8	33.6	31.3	32.4	41.3
100 percent to 199 percent	47.2	45.5	50.8	57.1	53.8	56.9	71.1	83.8	43.5	39.2	40.2	44.7	47.9	42.9	39.5	42.9
200 percent to 399 percent	61.2	57.2	59.1	61.8	70.5	65.6	76.5	79.1	57.5	53.7	54.1	56.4	57.0	54.8	46.0	54.2
400 percent or more	73.0	70.0	73.3	77.7	82.4	78.4	84.2	89.3	70.8	68.7	71.6	74.8	64.9	53.4	54.3	74.4
Not Hispanic or Latino																
White only																
Below 100 percent	51.7	53.6	49.3	52.6	64.4	65.0	69.1	78.5	50.6	53.3	44.4	46.9	32.0	37.2	36.4	35.4
100 percent to 199 percent	52.4	53.8	52.7	52.4	66.1	69.7	75.3	78.7	50.4	51.7	47.2	45.3	42.2	43.4	45.4	45.2
200 percent to 399 percent	67.5	67.6	64.7	67.5	77.1	78.3	79.6	85.1	65.0	64.4	61.4	62.9	61.9	63.9	59.8	63.7
400 percent or more	79.7	80.8	79.8	82.0	86.8	87.5	88.6	90.9	78.5	79.7	77.9	80.1	75.5	76.1	78.8	81.9
Black or African American only																
Below 100 percent	52.8	51.8	52.0	57.1	66.1	67.1	78.0	82.9	46.2	44.4	39.7	44.8	27.7	21.7	20.9	31.2
100 percent to 199 percent	48.7	52.4	50.0	58.7	61.2	67.3	75.9	84.0	46.3	48.0	41.5	52.3	26.9	35.2	33.6	36.7
200 percent to 399 percent	63.3	62.3	61.2	65.5	75.0	74.0	81.2	88.2	60.7	58.4	57.2	62.0	41.5	48.4	45.3	48.0
400 percent or more	74.6	72.8	77.2	77.3	81.8	74.2	87.2	88.2	73.4	73.3	75.9	75.8	66.1	60.5	69.8	72.4
Disability Measure[6]																
Any basic actions difficulty or complex activity limitation	X	X	X	X	X	X	X	X	55.1	57.3	53.5	55.1	49.0	50.7	50.7	56.0
Any basic actions difficulty	X	X	X	X	X	X	X	X	54.7	57.0	53.2	55.1	48.7	50.7	50.5	55.7
Any complex activity limitation	X	X	X	X	X	X	X	X	51.0	52.5	47.4	48.4	44.6	44.4	43.1	49.1
No disability	X	X	X	X	X	X	X	X	67.4	67.7	64.2	67.2	64.2	65.7	68.8	73.3
Geographic Region																
Northeast	69.6	72.3	70.1	72.6	77.5	81.1	83.8	86.8	69.6	72.1	67.9	70.9	55.5	58.1	61.5	62.8
Midwest	68.4	69.9	67.3	69.3	76.4	77.2	80.8	83.8	67.4	69.2	64.3	65.3	57.6	58.6	58.2	64.8
South	60.2	61.0	60.9	64.9	68.0	69.5	77.4	84.7	59.4	59.8	56.5	59.2	49.0	50.8	54.1	60.1
West	65.0	65.3	63.9	69.3	71.5	72.0	76.1	84.2	62.9	63.0	60.2	65.1	61.9	63.1	59.8	65.4
Location of Residence																
Within MSA[7]	66.7	67.5	65.9	69.4	73.6	74.3	79.3	84.9	65.7	66.5	62.4	65.3	57.6	58.9	59.4	64.6
Outside MSA[7]	59.1	61.2	58.4	60.8	69.3	73.3	76.4	83.3	58.0	59.7	53.8	55.0	46.1	49.3	51.3	54.2

NA = Not available.
X = Not applicable.
* = Estimates do not meet the standards of reliability and precision.
[1]Based on the 1997-2015 National Health Interview Surveys, about 19 to 30 percent of persons 65 years and over were edentulous (having lost all their natural teeth). In 1997-2015, about 69 to 73 percent of older dentate persons, compared with 17 to 24 percent of older edentate persons, had a dental visit in the past year.
[2]Respondents were asked, "About how long has it been since you last saw or talked to a dentist?"
[3]Includes all other races not shown separately and unknown disability status.
[4]The race groups White, Black, American Indian or Alaska Native, Asian, Native Hawaiian or Other Pacific Islander, and two or more races include persons of Hispanic and non-Hispanic origin. Persons of Hispanic origin may be of any race.
[5]Percent of poverty level is based on family income and family size and composition using U.S. Census Bureau poverty thresholds. Missing family income data were imputed for 1997 and beyond.
[6]Any basic actions difficulty or complex activity limitation is defined as having one or more of the following limitations or difficulties: movement difficulty, emotional difficulty, sensory (seeing or hearing) difficulty, cognitive difficulty, self-care (activities of daily living or instrumental activities of daily living) limitation, social limitation, or work limitation.
[7]MSA = metropolitan statistical area.

Table 3-49. Prescription Drug Use in the Past 30 Days, by Sex, Age, Race and Hispanic Origin, Selected Years, 1988–1994 Through 2011–2014

(Percent.)

Sex, race, Hispanic origin, and age[1]	At least one prescription drug in past 30 days				Three or more prescription drugs in past 30 days				Five or more prescription drugs in past 30 days			
	1988–1994	1999–2002	2007–2010	2011–2014	1988–1994	1999–2002	2007–2010	2011–2014	1988–1994	1999–2002	2007–2010	2011–2014
All ages, age-adjusted[2]												
Both sexes[3]	39.1	45.2	47.5	46.9	11.8	17.8	20.8	21.5	4.0	7.5	10.1	10.9
Male	32.7	39.8	42.8	42.6	9.4	14.8	19.1	19.7	2.9	6.1	9.2	9.7
Female	45.0	50.3	52.0	51.2	13.9	20.4	22.5	23.2	4.9	8.7	11.0	12.0
Not Hispanic or Latino												
White only	41.1	48.7	52.8	51.9	12.4	18.9	22.4	23.1	4.2	7.8	10.7	11.5
White only, male	34.2	43.0	47.5	46.8	9.9	15.9	20.6	21.0	3.1	6.3	9.8	10.2
White only, female	47.6	54.3	57.9	57.0	14.6	21.8	24.3	25.1	5.1	9.2	11.6	12.8
Black or African American only	36.9	40.1	42.3	44.2	12.6	16.5	20.7	22.5	3.8	7.7	10.8	12.1
Black or African American only, male	31.1	35.4	36.7	38.3	10.2	14.5	17.7	19.4	2.9	6.4	9.1	10.1
Black or African American only, female	41.4	43.8	46.8	49.0	14.3	18.1	22.9	24.9	4.5	8.7	12.0	13.7
Asian only	NA	NA	NA	34.3	NA	NA	NA	14.3	NA	NA	NA	6.2
Asian only, male	NA	NA	NA	31.9	NA	NA	NA	14.1	NA	NA	NA	6.2
Asian only, female	NA	NA	NA	36.3	NA	NA	NA	14.6	NA	NA	NA	6.1
Hispanic or Latino	NA	NA	35.2	35.7	NA	NA	15.7	16.0	NA	NA	8.4	8.4
Hispanic or Latino, male	NA	NA	31.7	32.1	NA	NA	14.0	15.0	NA	NA	7.3	7.9
Hispanic or Latina, female	NA	NA	38.8	39.2	NA	NA	17.4	17.1	NA	NA	9.5	8.8
Mexican origin	31.7	31.7	33.9	34.2	9.0	11.2	15.0	15.9	2.9	4.4	7.9	8.7
Mexican origin, male	27.5	25.8	31.0	31.8	7.0	9.5	13.4	14.9	2.0	3.5	7.2	8.2
Mexican origin, female	36.0	37.8	37.0	36.9	11.0	12.8	16.6	17.0	3.7	5.2	8.7	9.2
All ages, crude												
Both sexes[3]	37.8	45.0	48.5	48.9	11.0	17.6	21.7	23.1	3.6	7.4	10.6	11.9
Male	30.6	38.6	43.0	43.7	8.3	13.9	19.0	20.4	2.5	5.6	9.1	10.0
Female	44.6	51.1	53.8	53.9	13.6	21.1	24.2	25.8	4.7	9.1	12.1	13.6
Not Hispanic or Latino												
White only	41.4	50.7	56.2	57.0	12.5	20.6	25.8	27.7	4.2	8.7	12.6	14.3
White only, male	33.5	43.8	50.3	51.4	9.5	16.5	22.9	24.6	2.9	6.6	11.0	12.1
White only, female	48.9	57.5	61.8	62.4	15.4	24.5	28.6	30.7	5.4	10.8	14.2	16.4
Black or African American only	31.2	36.0	40.2	42.8	9.2	13.5	18.6	21.1	2.6	6.2	9.4	11.2
Black or African American only, male	25.5	30.7	33.9	36.3	7.0	10.9	15.0	17.5	1.8	4.8	7.5	8.9
Black or African American only, female	36.2	40.6	45.7	48.5	11.1	15.7	21.7	24.2	3.3	7.4	11.1	13.1
Asian only	NA	NA	NA	34.0	NA	NA	NA	13.6	NA	NA	NA	5.7
Asian only, male	NA	NA	NA	30.5	NA	NA	NA	12.6	NA	NA	NA	5.5
Asian only, female	NA	NA	NA	37.1	NA	NA	NA	14.5	NA	NA	NA	6.0
Hispanic or Latino	NA	NA	28.6	29.5	NA	NA	10.3	10.9	NA	NA	5.0	5.3
Hispanic or Latino, male	NA	NA	24.9	25.4	NA	NA	8.4	9.3	NA	NA	3.8	4.6
Hispanic or Latina, female	NA	NA	32.5	33.5	NA	NA	12.3	12.6	NA	NA	6.2	6.0
Mexican origin	24.0	23.6	26.4	27.0	4.8	6.1	9.0	9.8	1.4	2.1	4.1	4.9
Mexican origin, male	20.1	18.8	23.7	24.9	3.4	4.8	7.6	9.0	0.9	1.6	3.4	4.6
Mexican origin, female	28.1	28.9	29.4	29.3	6.4	7.5	10.6	10.8	1.9	2.7	4.9	5.4
Both sexes												
Under 18 years	20.5	23.8	24.0	21.5	2.4	4.1	3.8	3.9	*	*0.8	0.8	0.8
18-44 years	31.3	35.9	38.7	37.1	5.7	8.4	9.7	10.1	1.2	2.3	3.1	3.9
45-64 years	54.8	64.1	66.2	69.0	20.0	30.8	34.4	36.4	7.4	13.3	16.8	18.3
65 years and over	73.6	84.7	89.7	90.6	35.3	51.8	66.6	66.8	13.8	27.1	39.7	40.7
Male												
Under 18 years	20.4	25.7	24.5	21.1	2.6	4.3	4.4	4.3	*	*	0.8	0.9
18-44 years	21.5	27.1	29.5	28.8	3.6	6.7	7.1	7.5	*0.8	1.7	2.1	3.0
45-64 years	47.2	55.6	61.3	65.6	15.1	23.6	30.4	33.0	4.8	9.5	14.4	15.7
65 years and over	67.2	80.1	88.8	88.7	31.3	46.3	66.8	65.2	11.3	24.7	39.5	38.4
Female												
Under 18 years	20.6	21.7	23.5	22.0	2.3	3.9	3.1	3.5	*	*0.8	*0.7	*
18-44 years	40.7	44.6	47.6	45.3	7.6	10.2	12.2	12.6	1.7	2.8	4.0	4.8
45-64 years	62.0	72.0	70.8	72.1	24.7	37.5	38.1	39.4	9.7	16.8	19.1	20.7
65 years and over	78.3	88.1	90.4	92.1	38.2	55.9	66.4	68.1	15.6	28.9	39.8	42.6

NA = Not available.

* = Figure does not meet standards of reliability or precision. Data preceded by an asterisk have a relative standard error (RSE) of 20 to 30 percent. Data not shown have an RSE of greater than 30 percent.

[1] Persons of Hispanic and Mexican origin may be of any race. Starting with 1999 data, race-specific estimates are tabulated according to the 1997 Revisions to the Standards for the Classification of Federal Data on Race and Ethnicity and are not strictly comparable with estimates for earlier years. The non-Hispanic race categories shown in the table conform to the 1997 Standards. Starting with 1999 data, race-specific estimates are for persons who reported only one racial group. Prior to data year 1999, estimates were tabulated according to the 1977 Standards. Estimates for single-race categories prior to 1999 included persons who reported one race or, if they reported more than one race, identified one race as best representing their race.

[2] Estimates are age-adjusted to the year 2000 standard population using four age groups: under 18 years, 18–44 years, 45–64 years, and 65 years and over. Age-adjusted estimates in this table may differ from other age-adjusted estimates based on the same data and presented elsewhere if different age groups are used in the adjustment procedure.

[3] Includes persons of all races and Hispanic origins, not just those shown separately.

Table 3-50. Selected Prescription Drug Classes Used in the Past 30 Days, by Sex and Age, Selected Years, 1988–1994 Through 2011–2014

(Percent.)

Age group and Multum Lexicon Plus therapeutic class[1] (common indications for use)	Total 1988–1994	Total 1999–2002	Total 2011–2014	Male 1988–1994	Male 1999–2002	Male 2011–2014	Female 1988–1994	Female 1999–2002	Female 2011–2014
All Ages									
Antihyperlipidemic agents (high cholesterol)	1.7	6.5	14.3	1.5	7.1	15.0	1.8	5.8	13.7
Analgesics (pain relief)	7.2	9.4	9.1	5.4	7.3	7.6	9.0	11.3	10.5
Antidepressants (depression and related disorders)	1.8	6.4	10.7	1.2	4.4	7.3	2.3	8.3	13.9
Proton pump inhibitors (gastrointestinal reflux, ulcers)[2]	2.8	5.3	8.5	2.4	4.7	7.5	3.0	5.9	9.4
Beta-adrenergic blocking agents (high blood pressure, heart disease)	3.1	4.4	7.7	2.7	4.1	7.1	3.5	4.6	8.4
ACE inhibitors (high blood pressure, heart disease)	2.4	4.6	7.3	2.4	4.7	8.1	2.4	4.5	6.6
Antidiabetic agents (diabetes)	2.6	3.7	6.6	2.5	3.7	6.8	2.6	3.8	6.3
Diuretics (high blood pressure, heart disease, kidney disease)[3]	3.4	4.1	5.6	2.3	3.1	4.4	4.4	5.1	6.7
Thyroid hormones (hypothyroidism)	2.3	3.9	5.1	0.8	1.5	1.9	3.7	6.2	8.0
Bronchodilators (asthma, breathing)	2.6	3.5	4.6	2.5	3.1	4.5	2.7	3.8	4.6
Sex hormones (contraceptives, menopause, hot flashes)[4]	X	X	X	X	X	X	X	X	X
Anxiolytics, sedatives, and hypnotics (anxiety, insomnia, and related disorders)	2.8	3.3	5.3	1.9	2.6	4.4	3.6	4.0	6.2
Antihypertensive combinations (high blood pressure)	2.4	2.9	4.1	1.4	1.9	3.3	3.3	3.8	4.8
Anticonvulsants (epilepsy, seizure, and related disorders)	1.4	2.4	4.9	1.2	2.1	4.3	1.6	2.7	5.5
Calcium channel blocking agents (high blood pressure, heart disease)	3.6	4.2	4.7	3.4	3.5	4.6	3.8	4.8	4.7
Under 18 Years									
Bronchodilators (asthma, breathing)	3.0	4.0	4.4	3.3	4.4	4.9	2.7	3.6	3.9
CNS stimulants (attention deficit disorder, hyperactivity)	*0.8	2.9	3.4	*1.2	4.4	5.0	*	1.4	1.7
Penicillins (bacterial infections)	6.1	5.1	2.6	5.9	5.2	2.0	6.4	5.0	3.2
Leukotriene modifiers (asthma, allergies)	X	0.7	2.1	X	*0.9	2.5	X	*	1.7
Antihistamines (allergies)	2.0	4.4	2.0	2.1	4.9	2.3	1.9	3.9	1.8
Respiratory inhalant products (asthma, chronic obstructive pulmonary disease, and related disorders)	*0.7	1.5	1.9	*	1.7	2.4	*	1.3	*1.3
Adrenal cortical steroids (anti-inflammatory)	*0.5	0.8	1.0	*	*0.7	*1.0	*0.5	0.9	*1.1
Nasal preparations (nose symptoms)	*	1.1	1.7	*	*1.3	2.2	*	1.0	*
Antidepressants (depression and related disorders)	*	1.8	*1.3	*	2.2	*0.7	*	*1.5	*
Upper respiratory combinations (cough and cold, congestion)	2.3	2.3	*	2.6	*2.4	*	2.0	*2.2	*
Analgesics (pain relief)	1.2	1.4	1.1	*1.2	1.3	*1.0	1.4	1.6	*1.3
Dermatological agents (skin symptoms)	0.7	1.1	1.1	*	1.1	*0.9	*1.0	*1.1	1.4
18 to 44 Years									
Analgesics (pain relief)	7.2	8.0	7.0	5.1	6.0	5.3	9.1	9.9	8.8
Antidepressants (depression and related disorders)	1.6	6.0	8.8	*1.0	3.6	6.4	2.3	8.5	11.2
Sex hormones (contraceptives, menopause, hot flashes)[4]	X	X	X	X	X	X	11.5	13.5	13.4
Proton pump inhibitors (gastrointestinal reflux, ulcers)[2]	2.0	3.0	3.8	1.6	3.0	4.2	2.4	3.0	3.4
Anxiolytics, sedatives, and hypnotics (generalized anxiety and related disorders)	1.4	2.1	4.2	*1.0	*1.7	3.5	1.9	2.5	5.0
Anticonvulsants (epilepsy, seizure, and related disorders)	0.8	1.6	4.1	*0.6	1.6	4.0	1.0	*1.5	4.2
Bronchodilators (asthma, breathing)	1.4	2.2	2.9	*1.1	1.6	2.6	*1.8	2.8	3.2
Antihyperlipidemic agents (high cholesterol)	*0.4	1.3	2.3	*	2.0	2.9	*	*	1.8
Antihistamines (allergies)	2.5	3.9	1.8	1.8	3.6	*1.6	3.2	4.2	*2.0
Thyroid hormones (hypothyroidism)	1.3	1.6	2.2	*	*	*0.7	2.1	2.8	3.6
ACE inhibitors (high blood pressure, heart disease)	0.7	1.4	2.1	*0.9	1.5	2.1	*0.6	*1.2	2.2
Antidiabetic agents (diabetes)	*1.0	1.5	2.5	*	*1.5	2.1	*1.0	*1.6	2.9
Muscle relaxants (muscle spasm and related disorders)	1.0	1.3	1.7	*1.3	*1.1	1.4	*0.7	*1.4	2.1
Beta-adrenergic blocking agents (high blood pressure, heart disease)	1.1	*1.2	1.6	*0.9	*1.3	1.2	1.3	*	2.0
Nasal preparations (nose symptoms)	*0.6	1.5	1.4	*	*1.2	*0.8	*0.7	1.7	2.1
45 to 64 Years									
Antihyperlipidemic agents (high cholesterol)	4.3	13.8	25.6	4.4	17.2	28.2	4.2	10.7	23.1
Proton pump inhibitors (gastrointestinal reflux, ulcers)[2]	5.2	9.9	14.1	5.3	8.4	12.7	5.2	11.3	15.4
Antidepressants (depression and related disorders)	3.5	10.5	17.5	*2.3	7.0	12.5	4.6	13.8	22.2
Sex hormones (contraceptives, menopause, hot flashes)[4]	X	X	X	X	X	X	X	X	X
Analgesics (pain relief)	11.9	16.0	15.5	9.2	13.5	14.3	14.3	18.3	16.7
Beta-adrenergic blocking agents (high blood pressure, heart disease)	6.6	8.7	11.5	7.0	7.8	10.8	6.2	9.5	12.1
ACE inhibitors (high blood pressure, heart disease)	5.2	8.8	12.5	5.7	9.8	14.9	4.6	7.9	10.2
Antidiabetic agents (diabetes)	5.5	7.0	11.3	5.9	7.8	12.5	5.1	6.3	10.2
Thyroid hormones (hypothyroidism)	4.7	6.6	8.1	*1.2	*2.7	*2.6	8.1	10.1	13.2
Antihypertensive combinations (high blood pressure)	5.3	5.6	7.9	3.3	*3.7	7.4	7.1	7.3	8.3
Anxiolytics, sedatives, and hypnotics (generalized anxiety and related disorders)	6.0	6.2	8.6	4.3	4.9	7.7	7.5	7.4	9.4
Diuretics (high blood pressure, heart disease, kidney disease)[3]	6.1	6.6	8.6	4.8	4.8	7.2	7.3	8.3	9.9
Anticonvulsants (epilepsy, seizure, and related disorders)	2.7	4.3	7.5	*2.5	3.5	6.3	2.9	5.1	8.6
Bronchodilators (asthma, breathing)	3.4	3.8	5.2	2.9	3.1	*4.6	3.8	4.5	5.8
Calcium channel blocking agents (high blood pressure, heart disease)	7.0	6.7	6.6	8.2	5.9	7.9	5.9	7.5	5.4
65 Years and Over									
Antihyperlipidemic agents (high cholesterol)	5.9	23.4	50.3	5.3	24.3	54.4	6.4	22.7	47.1
Beta-adrenergic blocking agents (high blood pressure, heart disease)	11.8	15.9	30.5	10.4	17.5	31.4	12.8	14.8	29.8

X = Not applicable.

* = Figure does not meet standards of reliability or precision. Data preceded by an asterisk have a relative standard error (RSE) of 20 to 30 percent. Data not shown have an RSE of greater than 30 percent.

[1]The drug therapeutic class is based on the December 2014 Lexicon Plus, a proprietary database of Cerner Multum, Inc. Lexicon Plus is a comprehensive database of all prescription and some nonprescription drug products available in the U.S. drug market. Data on prescription drug use are collected by the National Health and Nutrition Examination Survey. Respondents were asked if they had taken a prescription drug in the past 30 days. Those who answered "yes" were asked to show the interviewer the medication containers for all prescriptions. If no container was available, the respondent was asked to verbally report the name of the medication. Each drug's complete name was recorded and classified. Data presented are based on the second level classification of prescription drugs. Up to four classes are assigned to each drug. Drugs classified into more than one class were counted in each class. Some drug classes were not available in 1988–1994 and are coded as not applicable.

[2]The drugs classes proton pump inhibitors (272) and H2 antagonists (94) have been combined because of their similar indications for use.

[3]This category includes carbonic anhydrase inhibitors which are primarily used to treat glaucoma.

[4]Although sex hormones may be used by males, most are used by females. Therefore, data for sex hormones are only presented for females.

Table 3-50. Selected Prescription Drug Classes Used in the Past 30 Days, by Sex and Age, Selected Years, 1988–1994 Through 2011–2014—*Continued*

(Percent.)

Age group and Multum Lexicon Plus therapeutic class[1] (common indications for use)	Total			Male			Female		
	1988–1994	1999–2002	2011–2014	1988–1994	1999–2002	2011–2014	1988–1994	1999–2002	2011–2014
Diuretics (high blood pressure, heart disease, kidney disease)[3]	16.2	19.2	21.1	12.2	17.1	19.0	19.1	20.7	22.7
ACE inhibitors (high blood pressure, heart disease)									
Proton pump inhibitors (gastrointestinal reflux, ulcers)[2]	7.5	14.6	23.2	7.2	14.1	19.8	7.7	15.0	25.9
Antidiabetic agents (diabetes)	9.0	12.4	19.5	9.0	12.9	22.6	9.0	12.0	17.1
Anticoagulants or antiplatelet agents (blood clot prevention)[5]	6.1	9.1	14.6	6.8	11.5	17.8	5.6	7.4	12.1
Analgesics (pain relief)	13.8	18.4	16.4	11.4	15.0	14.2	15.6	20.9	18.2
Calcium channel blocking agents (high blood pressure, heart disease)	16.1	19.1	17.8	14.5	17.4	16.7	17.3	20.4	18.7
Thyroid hormones (hypothyroidism)	7.0	14.3	15.5	3.3	6.7	7.7	9.7	19.8	21.7
Antihypertensive combinations (high blood pressure)	9.6	9.8	11.7	6.0	7.4	8.0	12.2	11.6	14.6
Antidepressants (depression and related disorders)	3.0	9.3	18.9	*2.3	7.2	12.0	3.5	10.8	24.4
Angiotensin II inhibitors (high blood pressure, heart disease)	X	4.8	12.2	...	4.1	11.8	...	5.3	12.6
Antiarrhythmic agents (heart rhythm irregularities)	23.1	16.6	8.8	21.6	17.9	8.4	24.3	15.6	9.0
65 to 74 Years									
Antihyperlipidemic agents (high cholesterol)	7.3	26.2	49.1	6.2	26.6	51.9	8.1	25.9	46.7
Beta-adrenergic blocking agents (high blood pressure, heart disease)	11.3	14.8	25.8	10.6	16.0	27.9	11.9	13.9	24.1
ACE inhibitors (high blood pressure, heart disease)	9.6	17.2	23.5	10.6	18.1	28.9	8.9	16.4	18.9
Proton pump inhibitors (gastrointestinal reflux, ulcers)[2]	7.0	14.7	20.7	6.3	13.4	18.3	7.5	15.8	22.8
Antidiabetic agents (diabetes)	8.8	12.9	19.9	8.0	13.8	22.5	9.4	12.0	17.7
Diuretics (high blood pressure, heart disease, kidney disease)[3]	14.2	15.9	17.2	10.8	14.6	14.6	17.0	16.9	19.4
Analgesics (pain relief)	13.0	18.5	16.8	10.5	14.9	15.3	15.0	21.4	18.0
Antihypertensive combinations (high blood pressure)	8.1	8.0	11.8	4.8	*6.7	8.5	10.8	9.0	14.5
Anticoagulants or antiplatelet agents (blood clot prevention)[5]	5.4	6.7	10.7	6.3	9.8	*13.8	4.6	*4.2	8.1
Antidepressants (depression and related disorders)	2.8	9.3	18.7	*2.3	5.8	12.6	3.1	12.1	23.9
Calcium channel blocking agents (high blood pressure, heart disease)	15.0	16.1	14.4	14.0	15.3	15.0	15.8	16.8	13.9
Thyroid hormones (hypothyroidism)	6.4	13.0	14.6	*3.4	*5.0	*7.3	8.9	19.7	20.8
Angiotensin II inhibitors (high blood pressure, heart disease)	X	4.2	11.1	...	*3.5	9.5	X	4.9	12.4
Antiarrhythmic agents (heart rhythm irregularities)	20.2	13.0	6.4	19.0	15.5	*5.8	21.1	10.8	6.9
75 Years and Over									
Antihyperlipidemic agents (high cholesterol)	3.8	19.9	52.1	*3.5	21.1	58.4	4.0	19.2	47.6
Beta-adrenergic blocking agents (high blood pressure, heart disease)	12.5	17.3	37.0	9.8	19.6	36.8	14.1	15.8	37.1
Diuretics (high blood pressure, heart disease, kidney disease)[3]	19.2	23.2	26.5	14.7	20.5	26.0	21.9	24.9	26.9
ACE inhibitors (high blood pressure, heart disease)	9.3	16.4	25.0	8.5	17.7	27.0	9.8	15.6	23.7
Anticoagulants or antiplatelet agents (blood clot prevention)[5]	7.2	12.0	20.1	7.8	13.9	24.1	6.9	10.9	17.4
Proton pump inhibitors (gastrointestinal reflux, ulcers)[2]	8.3	14.6	26.8	9.0	15.3	22.3	7.9	14.2	30.0
Calcium channel blocking agents (high blood pressure, heart disease)	17.8	22.8	22.6	15.3	20.5	19.4	19.2	24.2	24.9
Thyroid hormones (hypothyroidism)	7.9	15.8	16.8	3.0	9.2	8.2	10.9	20.0	22.9
Analgesics (pain relief)	15.1	18.4	16.0	13.0	15.1	12.6	16.3	20.4	18.3
Antidiabetic agents (diabetes)	9.3	11.8	18.9	10.7	11.5	22.8	8.5	12.0	16.3
Antihypertensive combinations (high blood pressure)	11.9	12.0	11.5	8.3	*8.2	7.1	14.0	14.4	14.6
Antiarrhythmic agents (heart rhythm irregularities)	27.7	21.0	12.1	26.3	21.3	12.6	28.6	20.7	11.7
Angiotensin II inhibitors (high blood pressure, heart disease)	X	5.4	13.9	X	*4.9	15.2	X	5.8	12.9
Antidepressants (depression and related disorders)	3.4	9.3	19.2	*2.3	9.2	11.0	4.0	9.4	X

X = Not applicable.

* = Figure does not meet standards of reliability or precision. Data preceded by an asterisk have a relative standard error (RSE) of 20 to 30 percent. Data not shown have an RSE of greater than 30 percent.

[1] The drug therapeutic class is based on the December 2014 Lexicon Plus, a proprietary database of Cerner Multum, Inc. Lexicon Plus is a comprehensive database of all prescription and some nonprescription drug products available in the U.S. drug market. Data on prescription drug use are collected by the National Health and Nutrition Examination Survey. Respondents were asked if they had taken a prescription drug in the past 30 days. Those who answered "yes" were asked to show the interviewer the medication containers for all prescriptions. If no container was available, the respondent was asked to verbally report the name of the medication. Each drug's complete name was recorded and classified. Data presented are based on the second level classification of prescription drugs. Up to four classes are assigned to each drug. Drugs classified into more than one class were counted in each class. Some drug classes were not available in 1988-1994 and are coded as not applicable.

[2] The drugs classes proton pump inhibitors (272) and H2 antagonists (94) have been combined because of their similar indications for use.

[3] This category includes carbonic anhydrase inhibitors which are primarily used to treat glaucoma.

[5] The drugs classes anticoagulants (82) and antiplatelet agents (83) have been combined because of their similar indications for use.

INPATIENT CARE

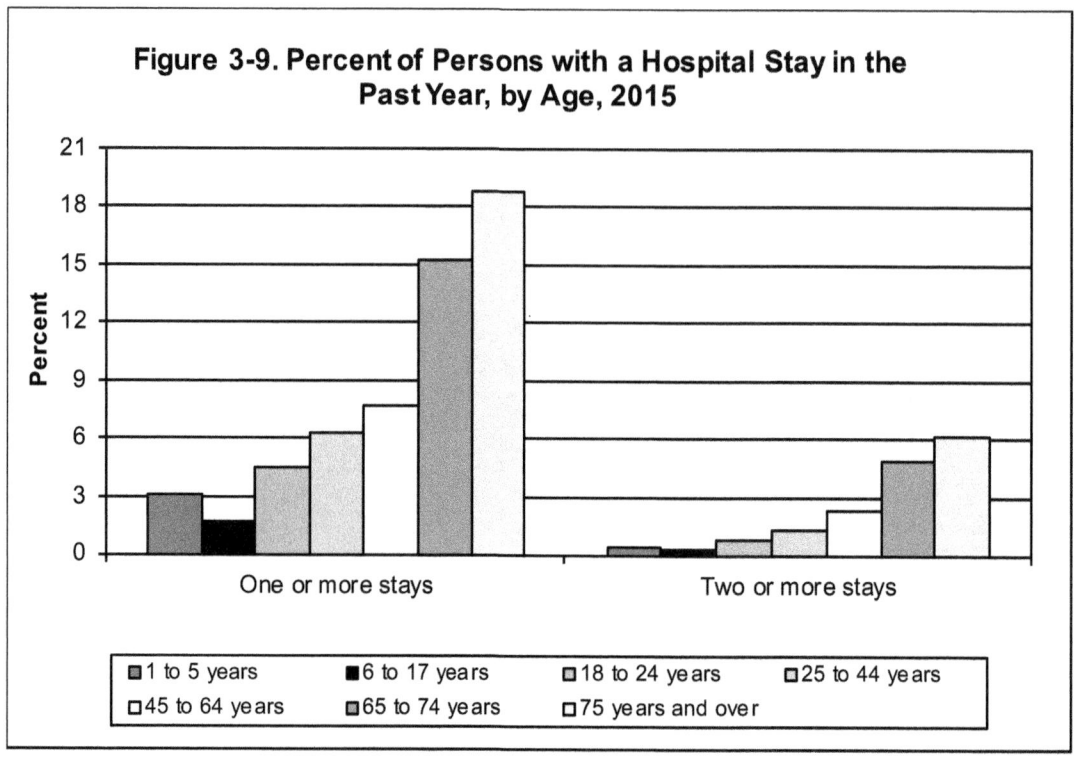

Table 3-51. Persons with Hospital Stays in the Past Year, by Selected Characteristics, Selected Years, 1997–2015

(Percent.)

Characteristic	One or more hospital stays[1]					Two or more hospital stays[1]				
	1997	2000	2005	2010	2015	1997	2000	2005	2010	2015
1 year and over, age-adjusted[2,3]	7.8	7.6	7.4	7.0	6.5	1.8	1.8	1.7	1.8	1.7
1 year and over, crude[2]	7.7	7.5	7.4	7.2	6.9	1.7	1.8	1.8	1.9	1.8
Age										
1 to 17 years	2.8	2.5	2.5	2.4	2.1	0.5	0.4	0.4	0.5	0.3
1 to 5 years	3.9	3.8	3.7	3.4	3.1	0.7	0.7	0.8	0.6	*0.4
6 to 17 years	2.3	1.9	2.0	1.9	1.7	0.4	0.3	0.3	0.5	0.3
18 to 44 years	7.4	7.0	6.7	6.3	5.8	1.2	1.1	1.1	1.3	1.2
18 to 24 years	7.9	7.0	6.3	5.7	4.5	1.3	1.1	1.0	1.1	0.8
25 to 44 years	7.3	7.0	6.9	6.6	6.3	1.2	1.2	1.2	1.3	1.3
45 to 64 years	8.2	8.4	8.2	8.3	7.7	2.2	2.2	2.2	2.5	2.3
45 to 54 years	6.9	7.3	7.1	7.3	6.4	1.7	1.8	1.8	2.1	1.8
55 to 64 years	10.2	10.0	9.8	9.5	9.2	2.9	2.8	2.9	2.9	2.7
65 years and over	18.0	18.2	17.8	16.1	15.2	5.4	5.8	5.4	4.9	4.9
65 to 74 years	16.1	16.1	14.5	13.6	12.8	4.8	4.9	4.5	3.8	4.0
75 years and over	20.4	20.7	21.4	19.0	18.8	6.2	6.8	6.4	6.2	6.2
75 to 84 years	19.8	20.1	19.9	18.3	17.3	6.1	6.2	6.1	6.1	5.7
85 years and over	22.8	23.4	26.6	20.8	22.5	6.2	9.0	7.4	6.6	7.3
1 to 64 Years										
Total, 1 to 64 years[2,4]	6.3	6.1	5.9	5.7	5.2	1.3	1.2	1.2	1.3	1.2
Sex										
Male, crude	4.4	4.2	4.5	4.2	4.2	0.9	1.0	1.1	1.1	1.2
1 to 17 years	2.9	2.4	2.8	2.4	2.1	0.6	0.4	0.5	0.5	0.4
18 to 44 years	3.6	3.1	3.2	2.9	3.1	0.6	0.6	0.7	0.7	0.9
45 to 64 years	6.0	7.0	6.6	6.4	5.9	1.4	1.8	1.9	1.9	1.7
65 years and over	11.1	10.2	10.3	9.3	9.7	3.0	3.0	3.4	2.8	2.9
Female, crude	8.0	7.9	7.5	7.6	6.6	1.6	1.5	1.4	1.7	1.4
1 to 17 years	2.6	2.5	2.2	2.3	2.1	0.5	0.4	0.4	0.5	0.3
18 to 44 years	11.2	10.8	10.2	9.8	8.5	1.8	1.7	1.6	1.9	1.5
45 to 64 years	7.6	7.6	7.6	8.3	6.8	2.0	1.9	1.7	2.3	2.0
65 years and over	9.4	9.8	9.3	9.7	8.8	2.9	2.7	2.4	2.9	2.4
Race[4,5]										
White only	6.2	5.9	5.9	5.6	5.1	1.2	1.1	1.1	1.3	1.1
Black or African American only	7.6	7.4	6.6	6.7	6.4	1.9	1.9	1.8	1.9	2.0
American Indian or Alaska Native only	7.6	7.0	6.9	*7.6	5.7	*	*	*2.5	*2.4	*
Asian only	3.9	3.9	3.9	3.6	3.3	*0.5	*0.6	*0.5	*0.4	0.8
Native Hawaiian and Other Pacific Islander only	NA	*	*	*	*	NA	*	*	*	*
Two or more races	NA	8.8	6.0	7.7	5.7	NA	*1.6	*1.9	*2.4	*1.6
Hispanic Origin and Race[4,5]										
Hispanic or Latino	6.8	5.5	5.4	5.2	4.8	1.3	0.9	1.2	1.1	1.2
Not Hispanic or Latino	6.2	6.1	6.0	5.8	5.3	1.3	1.3	1.2	1.4	1.2
White only	6.1	6.0	6.0	5.7	5.3	1.2	1.2	1.1	1.3	1.1
Black or African American only	7.5	7.4	6.6	6.7	6.4	1.9	1.9	1.7	1.9	2.0
Percent of Poverty Level[4,6]										
Below 100 percent	10.3	9.1	8.8	8.3	8.3	2.8	2.6	2.5	2.7	2.9
100 percent to 199 percent	7.3	7.3	7.4	7.0	6.1	1.7	1.9	1.9	1.9	1.7
200 percent to 399 percent	6.0	6.0	5.4	5.2	4.9	1.2	1.1	1.1	1.1	1.1
400 percent or more	4.7	5.0	4.8	4.5	4.1	0.7	0.8	0.8	0.8	0.6
Hispanic Origin and Race and Percent of Poverty Level[4,5,6]										
Hispanic or Latino										
Below 100 percent	9.1	7.4	7.6	7.3	6.7	2.0	1.6	2.0	2.0	2.1
100 percent to 199 percent	5.9	5.4	5.9	4.8	4.8	1.0	0.8	1.4	1.1	1.1
200 percent to 399 percent	5.9	4.6	4.4	4.3	3.7	1.1	0.7	0.8	0.7	0.9
400 percent or more	5.5	4.7	3.8	4.4	4.6	*1.1	*0.6	*0.6	*0.8	*0.8
Not Hispanic or Latino										
White only										
Below 100 percent	10.7	9.6	9.3	8.8	9.1	3.2	2.7	2.5	2.9	3.3
100 percent to 199 percent	7.7	7.8	8.2	7.8	7.0	1.8	2.2	2.0	2.2	1.8

NA = Not available.
* = Figure does not meet standards of reliability or precision. Data preceded by an asterisk have a relative standard error (RSE) of 20 to 30 percent. Data not shown have an RSE of greater than 30 percent.
[1] These estimates exclude hospitalizations for institutionalized persons and those who died while hospitalized.
[2] Includes all other races not shown separately, unknown health insurance status, and unknown disability status.
[3] Estimates are for persons 1 year of age and over and are age adjusted to the year 2000 standard population using six age groups: 1 to 17 years, 18 to 44 years, 45 to 54 years, 55 to 64 years, 65 to 74 years, and 75 years and over.
[4] Estimates are for persons 1 to 64 years of age and are age adjusted to the year 2000 standard population using four age groups: 1 to 17 years, 18 to 44 years, 45 to 54 years, and 55 to 64 years. The disability measure is age adjusted using the three adult age groups.
[5] The race groups White, Black, American Indian or Alaska Native, Asian, Native Hawaiian or Other Pacific Islander, and two or more races include persons of Hispanic and non-Hispanic origin. Persons of Hispanic origin may be of any race.
[6] Percent of poverty level is based on family income and family size and composition using U.S. Census Bureau poverty thresholds. Missing family data were imputed for 1997 and beyond.

Table 3-51. Persons with Hospital Stays in the Past Year, by Selected Characteristics, Selected Years, 1997–2015—*Continued*

(Percent.)

Characteristic	One or more hospital stays[1]					Two or more hospital stays[1]				
	1997	2000	2005	2010	2015	1997	2000	2005	2010	2015
200 percent to 399 percent	6.1	6.1	5.8	5.5	5.2	1.2	1.1	1.1	1.2	1.0
400 percent or more	4.7	5.0	4.9	4.6	4.2	0.7	0.8	0.7	0.8	0.6
Black or African American only										
Below 100 percent	11.4	10.8	9.4	9.4	9.4	3.3	3.4	3.1	3.1	3.1
100 percent to 199 percent	8.0	8.5	7.7	7.7	6.8	2.1	2.3	2.0	2.3	2.6
200 percent to 399 percent	6.2	6.1	5.2	5.3	5.7	1.5	1.3	1.3	1.4	1.7
400 percent or more	4.7	5.8	5.1	4.5	4.0	*0.9	*1.3	*1.2	*1.0	*1.0
Health Insurance Status at the Time of Interview[4,7]										
Insured	6.6	6.4	6.3	6.2	5.4	1.3	1.3	1.3	1.4	1.2
Private	5.6	5.5	5.2	5.0	4.3	1.0	1.0	0.9	0.9	0.7
Medicaid	16.1	15.9	14.6	12.7	10.3	4.9	4.7	4.1	4.5	3.4
Uninsured	4.8	4.5	4.4	4.0	3.7	1.0	0.9	0.9	0.9	1.0
Disability Measure Among Adults 18 to 64 Years[4,8]										
Any basic actions difficulty or complex activity limitation	14.1	15.1	15.2	14.3	12.9	4.1	4.4	4.9	5.2	4.4
Any basic actions difficulty	13.9	15.1	15.1	14.2	12.8	4.1	4.4	4.9	5.1	4.6
Any complex activity limitation	21.5	22.6	23.2	21.2	19.0	7.7	8.8	8.6	8.6	7.5
No disability	5.8	5.6	5.4	5.4	4.6	0.6	0.7	0.6	0.8	0.6
Geographic Region[4]										
Northeast	6.0	5.5	5.8	5.2	5.3	1.2	1.0	1.1	1.2	1.2
Midwest	6.5	6.3	6.3	6.3	5.8	1.5	1.3	1.3	1.5	1.3
South	6.8	6.6	6.3	6.0	5.3	1.4	1.5	1.4	1.5	1.3
West	5.4	5.2	4.8	4.9	4.3	0.8	0.9	0.8	1.1	0.9
Location of Residence[4]										
Within MSA[9]	6.1	5.8	5.7	5.5	5.1	1.2	1.1	1.2	1.3	1.2
Outside MSA[9]	7.0	6.9	6.8	6.9	5.7	1.6	1.5	1.4	1.6	1.4
65 Years and Over										
Total, 65 years and over[2,10]	18.1	18.3	17.8	16.2	15.6	5.4	5.8	5.4	4.9	5.0
65 to 74 years	16.1	16.1	14.5	13.6	12.8	4.8	4.9	4.5	3.8	4.0
75 years and over	20.4	20.7	21.4	19.0	18.8	6.2	6.8	6.4	6.2	6.2
Sex[10]										
Male	19.0	19.5	18.6	16.2	17.0	5.8	5.8	6.0	5.4	5.6
Female	17.5	17.4	17.3	16.2	14.6	5.1	5.7	4.9	4.6	4.6
Hispanic Origin and Race[5,10]										
Hispanic or Latino	17.3	16.6	17.7	13.9	14.7	6.2	6.4	5.7	5.0	5.2
Not Hispanic or Latino	18.2	18.4	17.9	16.4	15.7	5.4	5.8	5.4	4.9	5.0
White only	18.3	18.4	17.9	16.5	15.8	5.4	5.7	5.4	4.9	5.0
Black or African American only	18.9	19.8	19.0	16.9	16.2	5.5	7.5	6.3	5.5	5.5
Percent of Poverty Level[6,10]										
Below 100 percent	20.9	20.9	22.1	18.8	18.0	6.4	7.5	7.9	5.1	8.1
100 percent to 199 percent	19.6	19.2	19.2	17.2	17.7	6.5	6.6	5.9	5.2	5.9
200 percent to 399 percent	17.3	18.1	17.2	16.0	15.9	4.9	5.8	4.8	5.5	5.0
400 percent or more	16.6	16.0	16.1	15.0	13.7	4.7	4.2	5.1	4.1	3.9
Disability Measure[8,10]										
Any basic actions difficulty or complex activity limitation	22.6	24.7	24.1	20.2	21.9	7.2	8.6	8.3	6.4	7.9
Any basic actions difficulty	22.7	24.7	24.2	20.4	22.0	7.2	8.7	8.5	6.6	8.0
Any complex activity limitation	29.0	31.5	29.3	25.4	28.2	10.8	12.2	11.1	9.2	11.1
No disability	7.8	9.7	8.3	10.6	7.8	1.1	1.9	*1.6	*1.6	*1.8
Geographic Region[10]										
Northeast	17.2	16.6	16.1	16.5	14.2	5.1	4.5	4.5	6.1	4.5
Midwest	18.2	19.5	18.9	16.4	17.9	5.6	7.2	5.8	4.7	6.6
South	19.4	19.5	19.7	16.4	15.6	6.1	6.3	6.3	4.7	4.8
West	16.5	16.4	15.0	15.3	14.6	4.4	4.4	4.3	4.5	4.3
Location of Residence[10]										
Within MSA[9]	17.8	17.8	17.4	15.9	15.5	5.2	5.4	5.2	4.8	5.1
Outside MSA[9]	19.1	19.6	19.2	17.3	16.2	6.3	6.9	6.2	5.6	4.8

NA = Not available.

* = Figure does not meet standards of reliability or precision. Data preceded by an asterisk have a relative standard error (RSE) of 20 to 30 percent. Data not shown have an RSE of greater than 30 percent.

[1]These estimates exclude hospitalizations for institutionalized persons and those who died while hospitalized.

[4]Estimates are for persons 1 to 64 years of age and are age adjusted to the year 2000 standard population using four age groups: 1 to 17 years, 18 to 44 years, 45 to 54 years, and 55 to 64 years. The disability measure is age adjusted using the three adult age groups.

[5]The race groups White, Black, American Indian or Alaska Native, Asian, Native Hawaiian or Other Pacific Islander, and two or more races include persons of Hispanic and non-Hispanic origin. Persons of Hispanic origin may be of any race.

[6]Percent of poverty level is based on family income and family size and composition using U.S. Census Bureau poverty thresholds. Missing family data were imputed for 1997 and beyond.

[7]Health insurance categories are mutually exclusive. Persons who reported both Medicaid and private coverage are classified as having private coverage. Medicaid includes other public assistance through 1996. Starting with 1997 data, state-sponsored health plan coverage is included as Medicaid coverage. Starting with 1999 data, coverage by the Children's Health Insurance Program (CHIP) is included with Medicaid coverage. Persons not covered by private insurance, Medicaid, CHIP, public assistance (through 1996), state-sponsored or other government-sponsored health plans (starting in 1997), Medicare, or military plans are considered to have no health insurance coverage. Persons with only Indian Health Service coverage are considered to have no health insurance coverage. Health insurance status was unknown for 8 to 9 percent of children in 1993-1996 and about 1 percent in 1997-2011.

[8]Any basic actions difficulty or complex activity limitation is defined as having one or more of the following limitations or difficulties: movement difficulty, emotional difficulty, sensory (seeing or hearing) difficulty, cognitive difficulty, self–care (activities of daily living or instrumental activities of daily living) limitation, social limitation, or work limitation.

[9]MSA = metropolitan statistical area.

[10]Estimates are for persons 65 years of age and over and are age adjusted to the standard population using two age groups: 65 to 74 years and 75 years and over.

Table 3-52. Discharges, Days of Care, and Average Length of Stay in Nonfederal Short-Stay Hospitals, by Selected Characteristics, Selected Years, 1980 Through 2009–2010

(Rate per 10,000 population, number.)

Characteristic	1980[1]	1985[1]	1990	1995	2000	2005	2006	2007	2008[2]	2009[2]	2009–2010[2]
DISCHARGES PER 10,000 POPULATION											
Total, age-adjusted[3]	1,744.5	1,522.3	1,252.4	1,180.2	1,132.8	1,162.4	1,153.1	1,124.0	1,150.3	1,149.3	1,125.1
Total, crude	1,676.8	1,484.1	1,222.7	1,157.4	1,128.3	1,174.4	1,168.7	1,143.9	1,178.6	1,181.2	1,160.3
Age											
Under 18 years	756.5	614.0	463.5	423.7	402.6	411.0	393.9	376.7	343.3	340.2	336.2
Under 1 year	2,317.6	2,137.9	1,915.3	1,977.6	2,027.6	1,949.3	1,818.4	1,639.3	1,657.5	1,550.7	1,542.6
1 to 4 years	864.6	650.2	466.9	457.1	458.0	429.7	418.8	389.9	337.1	335.2	340.8
5 to 17 years	609.3	477.4	334.1	290.2	268.6	286.5	276.0	271.5	238.2	244.9	239.5
18 to 44 years	1,578.8	1,301.2	1,026.6	914.3	849.4	898.0	906.7	888.8	884.6	886.7	867.3
18 to 24 years	1,570.3	1,297.8	1,065.3	928.9	854.1	862.4	870.4	846.1	817.0	811.8	789.0
25 to 44 years	1,582.8	1,302.5	1,013.8	909.9	847.9	910.3	919.3	903.8	908.6	914.0	896.0
25 to 34 years	1,682.9	1,416.9	1,140.3	1,015.0	942.5	1,007.8	1,011.2	1,003.5	1,003.8	998.1	981.9
35 to 44 years	1,438.3	1,153.1	868.8	808.0	764.8	821.5	834.6	810.4	817.4	830.2	809.3
45 to 64 years	1,947.6	1,707.8	1,354.5	1,185.4	1,114.2	1,147.0	1,161.2	1,143.9	1,197.6	1,221.3	1,200.5
45 to 54 years	1,750.2	1,470.7	1,123.9	984.7	920.8	964.3	970.5	959.3	1,033.3	1,021.8	999.3
55 to 64 years	2,153.6	1,948.0	1,632.6	1,483.4	1,415.0	1,402.4	1,422.1	1,391.2	1,413.8	1,476.6	1,453.1
65 years and over	3,836.9	3,698.0	3,341.2	3,477.4	3,533.6	3,595.6	3,507.9	3,395.1	3,576.5	3,521.5	3,436.1
65 to 74 years	3,158.4	2,972.6	2,616.3	2,600.0	2,546.0	2,628.9	2,533.6	2,439.9	2,531.3	2,554.9	2,487.1
75 years and over	4,893.0	4,756.1	4,340.3	4,590.7	4,619.6	4,588.4	4,512.6	4,392.4	4,698.4	4,591.7	4,493.8
75 to 84 years	4,638.6	4,464.2	3,957.0	4,155.7	4,124.4	4,131.7	4,025.9	3,983.3	4,213.1	4,068.0	3,982.8
85 years and over	5,764.6	5,728.9	5,606.3	5,925.1	6,050.9	5,758.1	5,711.4	5,358.9	5,803.2	5,814.6	5,667.7
Sex[3]											
Male	1,543.9	1,382.5	1,130.0	1,048.5	990.8	1,013.0	1,000.5	973.8	997.3	1,004.3	975.3
Female	1,951.9	1,675.6	1,389.5	1,317.3	1,277.3	1,319.6	1,312.3	1,280.6	1,311.8	1,303.4	1,283.5
Sex and Age											
Male, all ages	1,390.4	1,240.2	1,002.2	941.7	910.6	959.0	954.9	936.7	964.9	978.8	957.4
Under 18 years	762.6	626.4	463.1	431.3	408.6	412.2	401.5	385.6	353.1	348.0	343.1
18 to 44 years	950.9	776.9	579.2	507.2	450.0	471.1	476.8	460.8	439.3	456.0	434.0
45 to 64 years	1,953.1	1,775.6	1,402.7	1,212.0	1,127.4	1,148.8	1,175.7	1,156.6	1,214.1	1,235.4	1,209.8
65 to 74 years	3,474.1	3,255.2	2,877.6	2,762.2	2,649.1	2,742.6	2,584.3	2,559.3	2,601.6	2,678.2	2,598.5
75 to 84 years	5,093.5	5,031.8	4,417.3	4,361.1	4,294.1	4,388.1	4,220.3	4,162.6	4,498.4	4,242.3	4,137.3
85 years and over	6,372.3	6,406.9	6,420.9	6,387.9	6,166.6	5,984.1	5,983.5	5,440.6	6,003.9	6,425.5	6,193.4
Female, all ages	1,944.0	1,712.2	1,431.7	1,362.9	1,336.6	1,382.2	1,375.3	1,344.0	1,385.2	1,377.2	1,357.1
Under 18 years	750.2	601.0	464.1	415.7	396.2	409.8	385.9	367.3	333.1	332.0	329.0
18 to 44 years	2,180.2	1,808.3	1,468.0	1,318.0	1,248.1	1,330.9	1,343.5	1,324.5	1,338.7	1,326.4	1,310.2
45 to 64 years	1,942.5	1,645.9	1,309.7	1,160.5	1,101.7	1,145.3	1,147.3	1,131.7	1,182.0	1,207.8	1,191.6
65 to 74 years	2,916.6	2,754.8	2,411.2	2,469.4	2,461.0	2,533.1	2,490.7	2,338.4	2,471.3	2,449.3	2,391.0
75 to 84 years	4,370.4	4,130.4	3,678.9	4,024.1	4,013.5	3,957.7	3,893.0	3,859.8	4,015.1	3,944.7	3,871.9
85 years and over	5,500.3	5,458.0	5,289.6	5,743.7	6,003.3	5,654.4	5,584.1	5,320.0	5,706.2	5,531.7	5,415.6
Geographic Region[3]											
Northeast	1,622.9	1,428.7	1,332.2	1,335.3	1,274.8	1,245.9	1,261.4	1,274.6	1,283.7	1,361.0	1,299.6
Midwest	1,925.2	1,584.7	1,287.5	1,132.8	1,109.2	1,174.9	1,168.0	1,125.5	1,172.1	1,153.7	1,146.8
South	1,814.1	1,569.4	1,325.0	1,252.4	1,209.2	1,202.5	1,198.8	1,139.9	1,179.0	1,149.3	1,136.1
West	1,519.7	1,469.6	1,006.6	967.4	894.0	1,005.9	964.1	966.0	960.2	959.2	932.7
DAYS OF CARE PER 10,000 POPULATION											
Total, age-adjusted[3]	13,027.0	10,017.9	8,189.3	6,386.2	5,576.8	5,541.7	5,474.7	5,404.1	5,577.2	5,536.3	5,369.2
Total, crude	12,166.8	9,576.6	7,840.5	6,201.7	5,546.5	5,620.9	5,577.8	5,539.4	5,773.9	5,748.1	5,598.7
Age											
Under 18 years	3,415.1	2,812.3	2,263.1	1,846.7	1,789.7	1,918.3	1,857.6	1,785.0	1,482.8	1,491.6	1,479.5
Under 1 year	13,213.9	14,141.2	11,484.7	10,834.5	11,524.0	12,131.6	11,624.2	8,466.7	9,401.0	9,277.7	9,170.4
1 to 4 years	3,333.5	2,280.4	1,700.1	1,525.6	1,482.2	1,355.3	1,405.4	1,280.3	1,018.8	1,041.0	1,111.0
5 to 17 years	2,698.5	2,049.8	1,633.2	1,240.3	1,172.1	1,300.9	1,239.1	1,406.4	984.0	1,012.6	990.5
18 to 44 years	8,323.6	6,294.7	4,676.7	3,517.2	3,093.8	3,305.0	3,360.6	3,258.0	3,180.3	3,268.3	3,147.4
18 to 24 years	7,174.6	5,287.2	4,015.9	2,987.4	2,679.5	2,819.9	2,889.4	2,738.7	2,606.0	2,755.3	2,687.1
25 to 44 years	8,861.4	6,685.2	4,895.5	3,676.4	3,225.5	3,472.8	3,524.5	3,439.7	3,383.8	3,454.9	3,316.3
25 to 34 years	8,497.5	6,688.9	4,939.7	3,536.1	3,161.7	3,434.3	3,462.0	3,423.1	3,462.0	3,482.0	3,342.6
35 to 44 years	9,386.6	6,680.4	4,844.8	3,812.3	3,281.5	3,507.9	3,581.9	3,455.2	3,308.9	3,428.0	3,289.7
45 to 64 years	15,969.5	12,015.9	9,139.3	6,574.5	5,515.4	5,717.3	5,793.0	5,868.2	6,284.3	6,184.5	6,058.0
45 to 54 years	13,167.2	9,692.8	6,996.6	5,162.0	4,374.2	4,711.2	4,667.4	4,745.9	5,185.7	4,772.0	4,719.7
55 to 64 years	18,895.4	14,369.5	11,722.6	8,671.6	7,290.8	7,124.0	7,333.6	7,371.8	7,729.7	7,993.0	7,739.0
65 years and over	40,983.5	32,279.7	28,956.1	23,736.5	21,118.9	19,882.8	19,197.5	18,951.7	20,391.2	19,933.0	19,225.8
65 to 74 years	31,470.3	24,373.3	20,878.2	16,847.0	14,389.7	13,985.0	13,170.2	13,274.8	13,911.2	13,888.2	13,504.6
75 years and over	55,788.2	43,812.7	40,090.8	32,478.1	28,518.6	25,939.4	25,413.1	24,878.5	27,347.0	26,625.9	25,602.5
75 to 84 years	51,836.2	40,521.6	35,995.1	28,947.5	25,397.8	23,155.3	22,671.7	22,658.1	24,400.0	23,644.1	22,884.1
85 years and over	69,332.0	54,782.4	53,616.9	43,305.9	37,537.8	33,071.5	32,165.5	30,124.5	34,055.6	33,588.7	31,848.6
Sex[3]											
Male	12,475.8	9,792.1	8,057.8	6,239.0	5,358.8	5,301.3	5,208.8	5,157.4	5,376.4	5,342.4	5,158.3
Female	13,662.9	10,340.4	8,404.5	6,548.8	5,809.7	5,828.7	5,764.2	5,685.1	5,832.4	5,784.1	5,630.6
Sex and Age											
Male, all ages	10,674.1	8,518.8	6,943.0	5,507.5	4,860.8	4,979.7	4,947.3	4,937.6	5,176.0	5,178.1	5,043.5
Under 18 years	3,473.1	2,942.7	2,335.7	1,998.0	1,955.7	2,006.2	1,968.0	1,858.1	1,646.9	1,526.4	1,555.6

[1]Comparisons of data from 1980–1985 with data from subsequent years should be made with caution because estimates of change may reflect improvements in the survey design rather than true changes in hospital use.
[2]Starting with 2008 data, the sample of nonfederal short-stay hospitals was cut in half. This smaller sample size has increased standard errors. Therefore, caution should be exercised in interpreting trends in these data.
[3]Estimates are age adjusted to the year 2000 standard population using six age groups: under 18 years, 18 to 44 years, 45 to 54 years, 55 to 64 years, 65 to 74 years, and 75 years and over.

Table 3-52. Discharges, Days of Care, and Average Length of Stay in Nonfederal Short-Stay Hospitals, by Selected Characteristics, Selected Years, 1980 Through 2009–2010—*Continued*

(Rate per 10,000 population, number.)

Characteristic	1980[1]	1985[1]	1990	1995	2000	2005	2006	2007	2008[2]	2009[2]	2009–2010[a]
18 to 44 years	6,102.4	4,746.6	3,517.4	2,729.7	2,175.0	2,282.7	2,375.6	2,241.8	2,045.7	2,203.9	2,036.6
45 to 64 years	15,894.9	12,290.1	9,434.2	6,822.7	5,704.4	5,773.5	6,004.3	6,103.5	6,553.3	6,443.8	6,327.1
65 to 74 years	33,697.6	26,220.5	22,515.5	17,697.4	14,897.4	14,502.6	13,262.1	13,666.7	14,473.2	14,915.8	14,462.9
75 to 84 years	54,723.3	44,087.4	38,257.8	29,642.6	26,616.7	25,106.9	23,972.7	23,894.6	26,208.6	24,959.5	24,184.6
85 years and over	77,013.1	58,609.5	60,347.3	45,263.6	37,765.3	35,179.0	32,604.0	31,480.6	37,292.7	37,649.7	35,211.1
Female, all ages	13,560.1	10,566.3	8,691.1	6,863.4	6,202.7	6,239.5	6,186.8	6,121.1	6,352.3	6,300.0	6,137.1
Under 18 years	3,354.5	2,675.5	2,186.8	1,687.9	1,615.1	1,826.1	1,741.8	1,708.3	1,310.9	1,455.1	1,399.7
18 to 44 years	10,450.7	7,792.0	5,820.3	4,297.9	4,010.8	4,341.8	4,361.5	4,292.3	4,337.0	4,354.8	4,283.0
45 to 64 years	16,037.1	11,765.5	8,865.1	6,341.7	5,336.4	5,663.9	5,592.2	5,644.3	6,028.1	5,937.5	5,801.9
65 to 74 years	29,764.7	22,949.2	19,592.7	16,162.0	13,971.3	13,549.0	13,092.4	12,942.1	13,431.6	13,007.9	12,678.4
75 to 84 years	50,133.3	38,424.7	34,628.3	28,502.5	24,601.0	21,830.1	21,782.1	21,806.2	23,144.7	22,713.5	21,949.6
85 years and over	65,990.5	53,253.6	51,000.5	42,538.6	37,444.4	32,103.5	31,960.3	29,479.5	32,492.0	31,707.4	30,236.0
Geographic Region[a]											
Northeast	14,024.4	11,143.1	10,266.8	8,389.7	7,185.9	6,636.5	6,608.5	7,284.4	7,055.4	7,512.7	7,072.6
Midwest	14,871.9	10,803.6	8,306.5	5,908.8	5,005.3	4,954.3	4,893.5	4,775.3	5,176.9	4,990.1	4,932.7
South	12,713.5	9,642.6	8,204.1	6,659.9	5,925.1	5,830.4	5,844.8	5,555.7	5,667.9	5,610.4	5,514.2
West	9,635.2	8,300.7	5,755.1	4,510.6	4,082.0	4,690.3	4,451.6	4,184.5	4,528.7	4,241.2	4,084.4
AVERAGE LENGTH OF STAY IN DAYS											
Total, age-adjusted[a]	7.5	6.6	6.5	5.4	4.9	4.8	4.7	4.8	4.8	4.8	4.8
Total, crude	7.3	6.5	6.4	5.4	4.9	4.8	4.8	4.8	4.9	4.9	4.8
Age											
Under 18 years	4.5	4.6	4.9	4.4	4.4	4.7	4.7	4.7	4.3	4.4	4.4
Under 1 year	5.7	6.6	6.0	5.5	5.7	6.2	6.4	5.2	5.7	6.0	5.9
1 to 4 years	3.9	3.5	3.6	3.3	3.2	3.2	3.4	3.3	3.0	3.1	3.3
5 to 17 years	4.4	4.3	4.9	4.3	4.4	4.5	4.5	5.2	4.1	4.1	4.1
18 to 44 years	5.3	4.8	4.6	3.8	3.6	3.7	3.7	3.7	3.6	3.7	3.6
18 to 24 years	4.6	4.1	3.8	3.2	3.1	3.3	3.3	3.2	3.2	3.4	3.4
25 to 44 years	5.6	5.1	4.8	4.0	3.8	3.8	3.8	3.8	3.7	3.8	3.7
25 to 34 years	5.0	4.7	4.3	3.5	3.4	3.4	3.4	3.4	3.4	3.5	3.4
35 to 44 years	6.5	5.8	5.6	4.7	4.3	4.3	4.3	4.3	4.0	4.1	4.1
45 to 64 years	8.2	7.0	6.7	5.5	5.0	5.0	5.0	5.1	5.2	5.1	5.0
45 to 54 years	7.5	6.6	6.2	5.2	4.8	4.9	4.8	4.9	5.0	4.7	4.7
55 to 64 years	8.8	7.4	7.2	5.8	5.2	5.1	5.2	5.3	5.5	5.4	5.3
65 years and over	10.7	8.7	8.7	6.8	6.0	5.5	5.5	5.6	5.7	5.7	5.6
65 to 74 years	10.0	8.2	8.0	6.5	5.7	5.3	5.2	5.4	5.5	5.4	5.4
75 years and over	11.4	9.2	9.2	7.1	6.2	5.7	5.6	5.7	5.8	5.8	5.7
75 to 84 years	11.2	9.1	9.1	7.0	6.2	5.6	5.6	5.7	5.8	5.8	5.7
85 years and over	12.0	9.6	9.6	7.3	6.2	5.7	5.6	5.6	5.9	5.8	5.6
Sex[a]											
Male	8.1	7.1	7.1	6.0	5.4	5.2	5.2	5.3	5.4	5.3	5.3
Female	7.0	6.2	6.0	5.0	4.5	4.4	4.4	4.4	4.4	4.4	4.4
Sex and Age											
Male, all ages	7.7	6.9	6.9	5.8	5.3	5.2	5.2	5.3	5.4	5.3	5.3
Under 18 years	4.6	4.7	5.0	4.6	4.8	4.9	4.9	4.8	4.7	4.4	4.5
18 to 44 years	6.4	6.1	6.1	5.4	4.8	4.8	5.0	4.9	4.7	4.8	4.7
45 to 64 years	8.1	6.9	6.7	5.6	5.1	5.0	5.1	5.3	5.4	5.2	5.2
65 to 74 years	9.7	8.1	7.8	6.4	5.6	5.3	5.1	5.3	5.6	5.6	5.6
75 to 84 years	10.7	8.8	8.7	6.8	6.2	5.7	5.7	5.7	5.8	5.9	5.8
85 years and over	12.1	9.1	9.4	7.1	6.1	5.9	5.4	5.8	6.2	5.9	5.7
Female, all ages	7.0	6.2	6.1	5.0	4.6	4.5	4.5	4.6	4.6	4.6	4.5
Under 18 years	4.5	4.5	4.7	4.1	4.1	4.5	4.5	4.7	3.9	4.4	4.3
18 to 44 years	4.8	4.3	4.0	3.3	3.2	3.3	3.2	3.2	3.2	3.3	3.3
45 to 64 years	8.3	7.1	6.8	5.5	4.8	4.9	4.9	5.0	5.1	4.9	4.9
65 to 74 years	10.2	8.3	8.1	6.5	5.7	5.3	5.3	5.5	5.4	5.3	5.3
75 to 84 years	11.5	9.3	9.4	7.1	6.1	5.5	5.6	5.6	5.8	5.8	5.7
85 years and over	12.0	9.8	9.6	7.4	6.2	5.7	5.7	5.5	5.7	5.7	5.6
Geographic Region[a]											
Northeast	8.6	7.8	7.7	6.3	5.6	5.3	5.2	5.7	5.5	5.5	5.4
Midwest	7.7	6.8	6.5	5.2	4.5	4.2	4.2	4.2	4.4	4.3	4.3
South	7.0	6.1	6.2	5.3	4.9	4.8	4.9	4.9	4.8	4.9	4.9
West	6.3	5.6	5.7	4.7	4.6	4.7	4.6	4.3	4.3	4.7	4.4

[1]Comparisons of data from 1980–1985 with data from subsequent years should be made with caution because estimates of change may reflect improvements in the survey design rather than true changes in hospital use.
[2]Starting with 2008 data, the sample of nonfederal short-stay hospitals was cut in half. This smaller sample size has increased standard errors. Therefore, caution should be exercised in interpreting trends in these data.
[a]Estimates are age adjusted to the year 2000 standard population using six age groups: under 18 years, 18 to 44 years, 45 to 54 years, 55 to 64 years, 65 to 74 years, and 75 years and over.

Table 3-53. Discharges in Nonfederal Short-Stay Hospitals, by Sex, Age, and Selected First-Listed Diagnosis, Selected Years, 1990 Through 2009–2010

(Numbers in thousands.)

Age and first-listed diagnosis	Both sexes 1990	Both sexes 1995	Both sexes 2009[1]	Both sexes 2009–2010[1]	Male 1990	Male 1995	Male 2009[1]	Male 2009–2010[1]	Female 1990	Female 1995	Female 2009[1]	Female 2009–2010[1]
ALL AGES[2]	30,788	30,722	36,120	35,599	12,280	12,198	14,721	14,461	18,508	18,525	21,398	21,139
Under 18 Years[2]	3,072	3,002	*2,536	*2,506	1,572	1,565	*1,327	*1,309	1,500	1,437	*1,209	*1,197
Dehydration	63	106	*73	*64	32	59	*39	*35	31	47	*34	*29
Acute bronchitis and bronchiolitis	114	170	*109	*119	67	109	*70	*73	47	61	*40	*46
Pneumonia	221	250	170	*167	126	143	*86	*84	95	107	*84	*83
Asthma	182	227	*143	*140	111	137	*92	*88	71	90	*50	*52
Appendicitis	83	69	*76	*72	50	41	*47	*45	34	28	29	*26
Injury	329	286	161	*173	210	171	*96	*104	119	115	*65	*69
Fracture	117	102	*67	*76	76	66	*42	*48	42	36	*25	*28
Complications of care and adverse effects	41	46	*43	*39	22	25	*23	*21	19	*21	*20	*18
18 to 44 Years[2]	11,138	9,996	9,963	9,746	3,120	2,761	2,588	2,465	8,018	7,235	7,375	7,280
HIV/AIDS	*20	88	23	24	*15	66	*17	17	*	22	*6	*7
Cancer, all	181	150	113	114	64	47	*35	40	116	102	77	74
Childbirth	X	X	X	X	X	X	X	X	3,815	3,574	3,862	3,851
Uterine fibroids	X	X	X	X	X	X	X	X	110	115	81	84
Diabetes	105	102	159	159	61	52	79	79	44	50	80	81
Alcohol and drug	284	363	224	215	199	255	152	147	84	107	71	69
Schizophrenia, mood disorders, delusional disorders, nonorganic psychoses	384	551	544	541	184	262	268	271	200	289	276	271
Schizophrenia	145	*181	148	140	88	*118	88	84	57	63	*61	56
Mood disorders	211	324	359	368	83	121	160	166	128	203	199	202
Heart disease	236	265	239	228	163	157	144	140	73	108	95	88
Ischemic heart disease	129	130	72	68	95	90	48	47	34	39	*25	21
Pneumonia	136	149	126	107	69	74	59	51	67	75	67	56
Asthma	106	119	90	85	27	30	*28	26	79	89	62	59
Intervertebral disc disorders	222	157	105	96	138	94	53	49	84	62	52	47
Injury	935	688	555	503	641	465	359	316	294	223	196	187
Fracture	302	250	221	203	217	176	162	142	85	74	59	61
Poisoning and toxic effects	124	118	134	125	54	59	58	55	70	59	76	70
Complications of care and adverse effects	135	146	195	187	63	64	81	74	72	82	114	113
45 to 64 Years[2]	6,244	6,168	9,686	9,585	3,115	3,053	4,781	4,710	3,129	3,115	4,906	4,874
HIV/AIDS	*3	20	*16	16	*3	15	*12	12	*	*5	*4	*4
Cancer, all	545	461	525	497	236	193	255	244	309	268	269	253
Colorectal cancer	59	29	66	60	33	17	32	30	26	13	34	29
Lung/bronchus/tracheal cancer	101	76	68	62	60	37	31	28	41	39	*37	34
Breast cancer[3]	X	X	X	X	X	X	X	X	69	61	48	47
Prostate cancer	X	X	X	X	19	32	*57	*53	X	X	X	X
Uterine fibroids	X	X	X	X	X	X	X	X	70	74	93	95
Diabetes	134	172	256	255	65	86	124	128	70	86	132	127
Alcohol and drug	100	128	191	194	77	100	138	142	23	28	53	52
Schizophrenia, mood disorders, delusional disorders, nonorganic psychoses	152	194	384	379	56	75	177	169	95	118	207	210
Schizophrenia	47	*67	119	115	19	*	*66	61	28	36	54	54
Mood disorders	91	112	241	242	32	37	98	97	58	74	142	146
Heart disease	1,100	1,152	1,204	1,162	704	749	756	730	397	403	448	432
Ischemic heart disease	739	762	579	544	502	537	393	371	237	225	187	173
Heart attack	233	256	205	210	165	188	144	147	68	68	61	63
Arrhythmias	131	131	186	197	79	75	115	121	53	56	71	76
Heart failure	122	143	271	254	68	75	161	145	54	68	111	109
Hypertension	75	82	155	143	38	37	76	69	37	45	80	74
Stroke	162	182	275	288	91	96	149	160	72	86	126	127
Pneumonia	154	163	264	261	76	75	141	135	79	88	122	126
Chronic obstructive pulmonary disease	73	154	236	231	39	72	95	94	34	82	141	137
Asthma	86	87	132	125	26	21	40	34	59	66	93	92
Osteoarthritis	87	110	476	491	36	47	211	211	51	64	265	280
Intervertebral disc disorders	145	115	167	162	82	65	85	82	63	51	81	79
Injury	334	296	441	450	178	165	229	242	157	131	211	208
Fracture	149	147	211	233	74	74	109	122	75	72	102	111
Poisoning and toxic effects	29	30	101	95	10	13	44	43	19	17	57	52
Internal organ injury	36	38	64	56	23	27	36	35	14	11	*28	*21
Complications of care and adverse effects	148	186	402	398	79	92	204	199	69	94	198	199
65 to 74 Years[2]	4,689	4,832	5,312	5,251	2,268	2,290	2,569	2,540	2,421	2,542	2,743	2,711
Septicemia	49	65	139	150	27	27	67	76	21	38	72	74
Cancer, all	436	416	326	311	222	203	178	171	214	212	147	140
Colorectal cancer	48	46	43	35	24	22	*23	20	24	24	*20	15
Lung/bronchus/tracheal cancer	77	73	61	58	50	44	*34	33	26	29	27	25
Breast cancer[3]	X	X	X	X	X	X	X	X	42	35	*21	19
Prostate cancer	X	X	X	X	40	41	*34	29	X	X	X	X
Diabetes	93	93	107	96	34	44	45	45	59	49	61	51
Schizophrenia, mood disorders, delusional disorders, nonorganic psychoses	59	80	*65	*62	20	20	*26	*21	39	60	*38	*41
Dementia and Alzheimer's disease	10	18	*14	*18	4	11	*	*	*6	7	*	*9
Heart disease	1,000	1,115	888	860	547	618	514	498	453	497	375	363
Ischemic heart disease	576	614	389	359	331	365	241	229	245	250	148	131

X = Not applicable.
* = Figure does not meet standards of reliability or precision. Data preceded by an asterisk have a relative standard error (RSE) of 20 to 30 percent. Data not shown have an RSE of greater than 30 percent.
[1]Starting with 2008 data, the sample of nonfederal short-stay hospitals was cut in half. This smaller sample size has increased standard errors. Therefore, caution should be exercised in interpreting trends in these data.
[2]Includes discharges with first-listed diagnoses not shown in table.
[3]Shown for women only.

Table 3-53. Discharges in Nonfederal Short-Stay Hospitals, by Sex, Age, and Selected First-Listed Diagnosis, Selected Years, 1990 Through 2009–2010—*Continued*

(Numbers in thousands.)

Age and first-listed diagnosis	Both sexes 1990	1995	2009[1]	2009–2010[1]	Male 1990	1995	2009[1]	2009–2010[1]	Female 1990	1995	2009[1]	2009–2010[1]
Heart attack	185	210	138	131	110	129	83	81	75	82	54	50
Arrhythmias	124	153	176	180	67	74	97	97	57	79	79	82
Heart failure	188	233	209	198	93	126	114	110	95	107	95	88
Hypertension	39	42	*77	61	13	14	*32	*24	26	28	*45	38
Stroke	222	250	225	231	108	141	125	124	114	109	100	107
Pneumonia	176	214	174	177	90	105	79	85	86	109	95	92
Chronic obstructive pulmonary disease	81	191	211	208	41	83	96	91	40	107	115	117
Gallstones	79	78	49	47	30	31	25	23	49	46	23	24
Kidney disease	18	31	121	121	9	16	65	70	9	15	56	51
Urinary tract infection	54	50	82	80	17	20	29	25	37	30	53	56
Hyperplasia of the prostate	X	X	X	X	113	62	*23	21	X	X	X	X
Osteoarthritis	122	154	308	339	44	53	115	133	78	101	193	206
Injury	193	176	201	203	71	67	80	75	122	109	121	128
Fracture	120	109	121	126	36	36	37	37	85	72	84	88
Hip fracture	48	44	40	39	12	15	12	12	36	29	*28	27
Complications of care and adverse effects	125	144	204	203	68	66	107	102	57	78	97	101
75 to 84 Years[2]	3,949	4,590	5,349	5,257	1,660	1,880	2,311	2,283	2,289	2,710	3,038	2,973
Septicemia	54	87	171	183	24	38	81	84	30	50	90	99
Cancer, all	300	281	236	227	158	131	108	109	142	150	128	119
Colorectal cancer	50	46	39	39	20	22	*15	17	29	24	24	22
Lung/bronchus/tracheal cancer	36	32	44	44	22	17	*21	22	*15	15	23	22
Breast cancer[3]	X	X	X	X	X	X	X	X	24	24	*10	13
Prostate cancer	X	X	X	X	37	18	*5	*6	X	X	X	X
Diabetes	44	73	100	88	17	30	39	37	27	43	*60	51
Schizophrenia, mood disorders, delusional disorders, nonorganic psychoses	39	44	*	*	*10	10	*	*	28	35	*23	*24
Dementia and Alzheimer's disease	20	46	53	58	9	19	*29	26	11	26	*25	33
Heart disease	865	1,057	1,025	976	377	471	480	466	488	585	545	510
Ischemic heart disease	382	479	358	328	177	228	189	173	205	251	169	156
Heart attack	156	188	165	149	83	91	79	70	73	97	86	78
Arrhythmias	133	175	241	223	58	83	99	92	76	92	143	131
Heart failure	261	290	296	291	108	116	132	137	153	174	164	154
Hypertension	23	31	64	50	*	*11	*21	*17	19	20	43	33
Stroke	258	297	258	260	104	129	123	116	154	169	135	144
Pneumonia	224	282	234	237	112	142	109	107	112	140	124	130
Chronic obstructive pulmonary disease	55	143	181	173	34	63	86	83	22	80	94	91
Gallstones	48	55	51	52	20	22	20	22	28	33	*31	30
Kidney disease	24	28	143	145	10	17	70	68	*14	12	73	77
Urinary tract infection	86	99	158	162	25	35	46	48	61	64	112	114
Hyperplasia of the prostate	X	X	X	X	69	41	*21	21	X	X	X	X
Osteoarthritis	69	115	205	213	25	34	80	84	44	80	125	129
Injury	259	270	306	313	58	77	104	104	201	193	202	208
Fracture	195	208	211	219	35	53	60	62	161	154	151	158
Hip fracture	115	122	83	92	20	29	20	25	95	93	63	66
Complications of care and adverse effects	81	108	159	162	38	40	81	83	43	68	78	79
85 Years and Over[2]	1,694	2,134	3,274	3,256	543	648	1,145	1,153	1,151	1,486	2,129	2,102
Septicemia	41	57	134	150	12	17	52	60	29	40	82	90
Cancer, all	77	77	94	83	31	32	43	39	45	45	51	44
Colorectal cancer	14	17	*12	10	*5	*	*	*4	9	11	*7	*6
Lung/bronchus/tracheal cancer	*6	*4	*13	*14	*	*2	*	*	*	*	*	*6
Breast cancer[3]	X	X	X	X	X	X	X	X	*9	8	*	*5
Prostate cancer	X	X	X	X	*7	*	*	*4	X	X	X	X
Diabetes	16	22	*34	34	*5	*	*13	13	11	15	*21	*21
Schizophrenia, mood disorders, delusional disorders, nonorganic psychoses	*8	16	*	*	*	*	*	*8	*7	*12	*	*
Dementia and Alzheimer's disease	15	28	42	44	*2	*6	16	18	13	22	26	26
Heart disease	335	446	611	606	112	135	236	228	223	311	376	378
Ischemic heart disease	128	144	139	142	49	48	62	60	79	96	76	82
Heart attack	60	73	88	92	23	28	37	37	37	44	51	56
Arrhythmias	51	72	127	122	16	20	37	40	35	51	90	82
Heart failure	126	181	263	259	39	52	101	98	87	129	162	161
Hypertension	*5	8	37	28	*	*	*12	*9	*4	*6	*25	19
Stroke	129	156	162	163	35	42	48	52	95	114	114	111
Pneumonia	151	194	207	204	64	73	74	80	88	121	134	124
Chronic obstructive pulmonary disease	13	39	81	83	*6	18	*28	32	*7	21	53	50
Gallstones	18	21	*24	23	*6	*7	*7	*8	13	15	*17	15
Kidney disease	14	16	90	96	8	*8	36	43	*6	*9	54	53
Urinary tract infection	65	74	195	185	20	*18	46	40	45	56	149	144
Hyperplasia of the prostate	X	X	X	X	13	9	*6	*6	X	X	X	X
Osteoarthritis	13	20	36	40	*	*6	*10	*10	8	14	26	30
Injury	164	216	300	302	37	47	78	80	127	169	223	222
Fracture	133	172	227	228	28	32	54	51	104	140	173	177
Hip fracture	82	108	123	122	19	19	29	29	63	88	94	93
Complications of care and adverse effects	29	29	75	73	11	*10	*27	30	18	19	48	43

X = Not applicable.
* = Figure does not meet standards of reliability or precision. Data preceded by an asterisk have a relative standard error (RSE) of 20 to 30 percent. Data not shown have an RSE of greater than 30 percent.
[1]Starting with 2008 data, the sample of nonfederal short-stay hospitals was cut in half. This smaller sample size has increased standard errors. Therefore, caution should be exercised in interpreting trends in these data.
[2]Includes discharges with first-listed diagnoses not shown in table.
[3]Shown for women only.

Table 3-54. Discharge Rate in Nonfederal Short-Stay Hospitals, by Sex, Age, and Selected First-Listed Diagnosis, Selected Years 1990 Through 2009–2010

(Number per 10,000 population.)

Age and first-listed diagnosis	Both sexes				Male				Female			
	1990	2000	2009¹	2009–2010¹	1990	2000	2009¹	2009–2010¹	1990	2000	2009¹	2009–2010¹
All Ages, Age-Adjusted²,³	1,252.4	1,132.8	1,149.3	1,125.1	1,130.0	990.8	1,004.3	975.3	1,389.5	1,277.3	1,303.4	1,283.5
All Ages, Crude³	1,222.7	1,128.3	1,181.2	1,160.3	1,002.2	910.6	978.8	957.4	1,431.7	1,336.6	1,377.2	1,357.1
Under 18 Years³	463.5	402.6	*340.2	*336.2	463.1	408.6	*348.0	*343.1	464.1	396.2	*332.0	*329.0
Dehydration	9.5	15.7	*9.8	*8.6	9.4	17.2	*10.4	*9.1	9.7	14.2	*9.2	*8.0
Acute bronchitis and bronchiolitis	17.2	27.8	*14.7	*16.0	19.6	31.4	*18.3	*19.1	14.6	24.1	*10.9	*12.7
Pneumonia	33.3	25.2	22.7	*22.4	37.0	25.7	*22.5	*22.0	29.5	24.6	*23.0	*22.7
Asthma	27.5	29.6	*19.1	*18.7	32.7	34.8	*24.2	*23.1	22.0	24.0	*13.8	*14.2
Appendicitis	12.6	11.9	*10.2	*9.6	14.6	13.0	*12.2	*11.9	10.5	10.8	8.1	*7.2
Injury	49.7	33.6	21.6	*23.2	62.0	42.0	*25.1	*27.2	36.8	24.8	*17.9	*19.1
Fracture	17.7	13.8	*8.9	*10.2	22.3	18.3	*10.9	*12.6	12.9	9.0	*6.9	*7.8
Complications of care and adverse effects	6.2	*7.3	*5.8	*5.2	6.5	*7.9	*6.0	*5.5	5.9	*6.6	*5.5	*4.9
18 to 44 Years³	1,026.6	849.4	886.7	867.3	579.2	450.0	456.0	434.0	1,468.0	1,248.1	1,326.4	1,310.2
HIV/AIDS	*1.8	4.3	2.1	2.2	*2.8	5.8	*3.0	3.1	*	2.8	*1.1	*1.2
Cancer, all	16.6	10.5	10.0	10.1	11.9	7.3	*6.2	7.0	21.3	13.9	13.3	13.3
Childbirth	X	X	X	X	X	X	X	X	698.6	645.2	694.5	693.1
Uterine fibroids	X	X	X	X	X	X	X	X	20.2	21.7	14.6	15.2
Diabetes	9.7	11.5	14.1	14.2	11.3	13.0	13.9	13.9	8.1	9.9	14.4	14.5
Alcohol and drug	26.2	29.7	19.9	19.2	37.0	39.1	26.9	25.8	15.5	*20.2	12.8	12.4
Schizophrenia, mood disorders, delusional disorders, nonorganic psychoses	35.4	*53.6	48.5	48.2	34.1	*53.2	47.3	47.6	36.7	*53.9	49.7	48.7
Schizophrenia	13.4	*14.4	13.2	12.4	16.4	*18.6	15.5	14.8	10.5	*10.1	*10.9	10.0
Mood disorders	19.4	*35.9	31.9	32.8	15.4	*31.0	28.2	29.3	23.4	*40.9	35.8	36.3
Heart disease	21.7	21.8	21.3	20.3	30.2	26.6	25.4	24.6	13.4	17.0	17.1	15.8
Ischemic heart disease	11.9	9.9	6.4	6.0	17.7	14.2	8.4	8.3	6.3	5.6	*4.5	3.7
Pneumonia	12.5	10.9	11.2	9.5	12.8	10.0	10.4	8.9	12.2	11.9	12.0	10.1
Asthma	9.8	9.0	8.0	7.6	5.1	5.4	*4.9	4.6	14.4	12.6	11.1	10.7
Intervertebral disc disorders	20.5	12.5	9.3	8.5	25.6	14.5	9.4	8.6	15.4	10.4	9.3	8.4
Injury	86.2	45.8	49.4	44.8	119.0	62.3	63.2	55.7	53.8	29.4	35.3	33.6
Fracture	27.8	17.8	19.7	18.1	40.2	25.4	28.5	25.0	15.5	10.2	10.6	11.0
Poisoning and toxic effects	11.4	8.5	11.9	11.2	10.0	6.7	10.2	9.7	12.7	10.3	13.7	12.6
Complications of care and adverse effects	12.5	12.2	17.4	16.6	11.7	11.2	14.3	13.1	13.3	13.1	20.5	20.3
45 to 64 Years³	1,354.5	1,114.2	1,221.3	1,200.5	1,402.7	1,127.4	1,235.4	1,209.8	1,309.7	1,101.7	1,207.8	1,191.6
HIV/AIDS	*0.6	*3.2	*2.0	2.0	*1.2	*4.9	*3.0	3.0	*	*	*1.0	*1.1
Cancer, all	118.3	62.9	66.1	62.2	106.3	62.1	65.9	62.6	129.5	63.6	66.3	61.8
Colorectal cancer	12.7	7.9	8.3	7.5	14.8	8.9	8.2	7.8	10.8	6.9	8.3	7.2
Lung/bronchus/tracheal cancer	21.8	6.9	8.6	7.8	26.8	8.6	8.1	7.2	17.2	5.2	*9.2	8.3
Breast cancer⁴	X	X	X	X	X	X	X	X	29.0	14.2	11.8	11.5
Prostate cancer	X	X	X	X	8.5	9.6	*14.6	*13.5	X	X	X	X
Uterine fibroids	X	X	X	X	X	X	X	X	29.3	35.6	22.9	23.3
Diabetes	29.1	33.1	32.3	32.0	29.1	37.4	32.0	32.9	29.2	29.0	32.6	31.1
Alcohol and drug	21.7	23.3	24.1	24.2	34.6	33.5	35.6	36.4	9.6	13.7	13.0	12.7
Schizophrenia, mood disorders, delusional disorders, nonorganic psychoses	32.9	42.7	48.4	47.5	25.4	*39.6	45.7	43.5	39.8	45.6	50.9	51.3
Schizophrenia	10.1	12.8	15.1	14.4	8.4	*14.4	*17.0	15.7	11.7	11.3	13.2	13.2
Mood disorders	19.6	*26.9	30.3	30.4	14.5	*21.6	25.4	24.9	24.4	*32.0	35.1	35.6
Heart disease	238.7	203.6	151.8	145.6	316.8	264.0	195.3	187.5	166.1	146.4	110.3	105.6
Ischemic heart disease	160.3	126.4	73.1	68.2	226.1	177.3	101.4	95.4	99.2	78.2	46.0	42.3
Heart attack	50.6	38.8	25.9	26.4	74.4	58.7	37.3	37.8	28.4	19.9	15.0	15.4
Arrhythmias	28.5	25.1	23.5	24.7	35.5	31.8	29.8	31.1	22.1	18.7	17.5	18.6
Heart failure	26.4	31.4	34.2	31.8	30.7	33.5	41.5	37.3	22.4	29.3	27.3	26.6
Hypertension	16.3	19.0	19.6	17.9	16.9	17.6	19.6	17.6	15.6	20.3	19.6	18.2
Stroke	35.2	36.7	34.7	36.0	40.8	38.3	38.6	41.2	30.1	35.2	31.0	31.1
Pneumonia	33.5	35.3	33.2	32.6	34.0	34.2	36.5	34.7	33.0	36.4	30.2	30.7
Chronic obstructive pulmonary disease	15.8	30.8	29.7	28.9	17.4	30.8	24.5	24.1	14.3	30.8	34.8	33.5
Asthma	18.6	13.4	16.7	15.7	11.8	6.2	10.3	8.7	24.9	20.2	22.8	22.4
Osteoarthritis	18.9	24.0	60.0	61.5	16.3	20.8	54.6	54.1	21.2	27.0	65.1	68.4
Intervertebral disc disorders	31.5	21.2	21.0	20.3	36.8	22.5	22.1	21.2	26.5	20.0	20.0	19.4
Injury	72.5	47.9	55.6	56.4	79.9	51.2	59.3	62.2	65.6	44.7	52.0	50.8
Fracture	32.4	26.2	26.6	29.2	33.4	25.3	28.2	31.3	31.5	27.0	25.0	27.2
Poisoning and toxic effects	6.3	6.3	12.7	11.9	4.5	5.5	11.3	11.0	8.0	7.1	14.1	12.7
Internal organ injury	7.9	4.5	8.1	7.1	10.2	5.9	9.3	9.1	5.7	3.2	*6.8	*5.1
Complications of care and adverse effects	32.0	34.5	50.7	49.8	35.6	36.3	52.8	51.0	28.7	32.7	48.8	48.7
65 to 74 Years³	2,616.3	2,546.0	2,554.9	2,487.1	2,877.6	2,649.1	2,678.2	2,598.5	2,411.2	2,461.0	2,449.3	2,391.0
Septicemia	27.2	35.6	66.9	71.3	34.9	40.1	69.7	77.9	21.2	32.0	65.5	65.5
Cancer, all	243.1	159.0	156.6	147.5	281.4	176.4	186.0	175.3	213.0	144.7	131.4	123.6
Colorectal cancer	27.0	22.8	20.5	16.6	30.6	29.9	*24.1	20.1	24.1	16.9	*17.4	13.5
Lung/bronchus/tracheal cancer	42.9	26.1	29.2	27.3	63.9	28.2	*35.2	33.6	26.4	24.5	24.0	21.9
Breast cancer⁴	X	X	X	X	X	X	X	X	42.3	31.2	*18.8	16.7
Prostate cancer	X	X	X	X	50.6	37.1	*35.9	30.1	X	X	X	X
Diabetes	51.8	46.4	51.3	45.4	43.6	46.8	47.1	45.7	58.3	46.2	54.9	45.2
Schizophrenia, mood disorders, delusional disorders, nonorganic psychoses	32.7	37.1	*31.0	*29.2	25.3	*34.2	*27.5	*21.6	38.6	39.6	*34.0	*35.7
Dementia and Alzheimer's disease	5.6	*11.2	*6.9	*8.3	4.9	*16.2	*	*	*6.1	*7.0	*	*7.6
Heart disease	558.1	604.8	427.2	407.4	694.2	706.4	535.4	509.0	451.3	521.0	334.4	319.8
Ischemic heart disease	321.3	307.0	187.0	170.2	419.9	396.5	251.4	233.9	243.9	233.2	131.8	115.2

X = Not applicable.
* = Figure does not meet standards of reliability or precision. Data preceded by an asterisk have a relative standard error (RSE) of 20 to 30 percent. Data not shown have an RSE of greater than 30 percent.
¹Starting with 2008 data, the sample of nonfederal short-stay hospitals was cut in half. This smaller sample size has increased standard errors. Therefore, caution should be exercised in interpreting trends in these data.
²Estimates are age adjusted to the year 2000 standard population using six age groups: under 18 years, 18 to 44 years, 45 to 54 years, 55 to 64 years, 65 to 74 years, and 75 years and over.
³Includes discharges with first-listed diagnoses not shown in table.
⁴Shown for women only.

Table 3-54. Discharge Rate in Nonfederal Short-Stay Hospitals, by Sex, Age, and Selected First-Listed Diagnosis, Selected Years 1990 Through 2009–2010—Continued

(Number per 10,000 population.)

Age and first-listed diagnosis	Both sexes				Male				Female			
	1990	2000	2009¹	2009–2010¹	1990	2000	2009¹	2009–2010¹	1990	2000	2009¹	2009–2010¹
Heart attack	103.3	100.3	66.3	62.0	139.8	124.7	86.9	82.8	74.6	80.2	48.6	44.1
Arrhythmias	69.1	102.6	84.6	85.1	84.7	108.3	101.4	99.4	56.9	97.9	70.2	72.7
Heart failure	105.2	131.6	100.6	93.9	118.0	136.4	119.3	112.3	95.1	127.6	84.6	78.0
Hypertension	21.8	21.5	*37.0	29.1	16.2	16.5	*33.0	*24.3	26.2	25.5	*40.4	33.2
Stroke	123.9	127.1	108.1	109.5	137.5	131.8	129.9	126.6	113.1	123.2	89.4	94.7
Pneumonia	98.1	121.3	83.5	83.8	113.6	127.7	81.9	86.8	85.9	116.1	84.9	81.2
Chronic obstructive pulmonary disease	45.3	102.3	101.5	98.5	52.6	102.6	100.1	92.8	39.6	102.0	102.7	103.4
Gallstones	44.2	33.4	23.4	22.2	38.2	30.2	26.4	23.6	48.9	36.0	20.9	21.1
Kidney disease	9.9	19.1	58.2	57.1	11.0	21.0	67.9	71.3	9.0	17.5	49.9	44.9
Urinary tract infection	30.2	25.5	39.4	38.0	21.7	19.7	29.8	25.4	36.9	30.3	47.6	49.0
Hyperplasia of the prostate	X	X	X	X	143.5	53.6	*23.7	21.6	X	X	X	X
Osteoarthritis	68.0	101.4	148.0	160.7	55.2	103.1	119.9	136.4	78.0	100.1	172.0	181.7
Injury	107.7	101.5	96.8	96.4	90.7	83.8	83.4	77.1	121.1	116.2	108.3	112.9
Fracture	67.2	63.3	58.2	59.5	45.2	46.8	38.8	38.0	84.4	76.9	74.8	77.9
Hip fracture	26.7	26.4	19.2	18.3	15.3	*20.0	12.4	12.2	35.7	31.7	*25.0	23.6
Complications of care and adverse effects	69.7	80.0	98.3	96.3	85.7	95.7	112.0	104.5	57.2	67.1	86.4	89.3
75 to 84 Years³	3,957.0	4,124.4	4,068.0	3,982.8	4,417.3	4,294.1	4,242.3	4,137.3	3,678.9	4,013.5	3,944.7	3,871.9
Septicemia	53.9	68.3	129.9	138.7	63.8	78.1	148.5	151.6	47.9	61.9	116.7	129.3
Cancer, all	300.3	194.0	179.8	172.3	420.8	211.0	198.9	197.3	227.6	182.9	166.3	154.3
Colorectal cancer	49.8	33.0	29.8	29.8	54.0	37.5	*27.4	30.8	47.3	30.1	31.4	29.1
Lung/bronchus/tracheal cancer	36.5	27.0	33.4	33.5	57.2	32.2	*38.4	40.5	*24.0	23.6	29.8	28.5
Breast cancer⁴	X	X	X	X	X	X	X	X	38.7	30.8	*12.5	16.5
Prostate cancer	X	X	X	X	99.2	27.4	*9.4	*11.1	X	X	X	X
Diabetes	44.3	63.4	75.7	66.9	44.8	68.1	72.0	67.5	44.0	60.3	*78.3	66.5
Schizophrenia, mood disorders, delusional disorders, nonorganic psychoses	38.8	41.4	*	*	*27.3	*30.6	*	*	45.7	48.5	*29.7	*31.3
Dementia and Alzheimer's disease	20.0	36.5	40.7	44.0	22.8	36.8	*52.4	46.2	18.3	36.3	*32.4	42.3
Heart disease	866.6	954.8	779.8	739.5	1,003.8	1,062.5	881.6	844.7	783.7	884.3	707.7	663.8
Ischemic heart disease	382.4	416.7	272.1	248.7	470.5	528.5	346.4	312.9	329.1	343.6	219.5	202.7
Heart attack	155.9	166.9	125.5	112.8	220.9	212.8	144.2	127.7	116.7	136.9	112.2	102.2
Arrhythmias	133.4	176.8	183.6	168.7	153.3	174.4	181.6	165.9	121.4	178.3	185.1	170.7
Heart failure	261.4	263.1	225.1	220.7	286.2	271.1	242.9	248.3	246.4	257.9	212.5	200.9
Hypertension	22.6	39.7	48.9	38.0	*	*28.4	*38.9	*31.7	30.7	47.1	56.0	42.5
Stroke	259.0	255.5	196.5	196.9	277.7	278.4	225.7	210.6	247.7	240.6	175.8	187.1
Pneumonia	224.6	263.5	177.7	179.3	297.8	310.8	201.0	193.3	180.4	232.6	161.3	169.3
Chronic obstructive pulmonary disease	55.4	146.2	137.5	131.4	89.4	179.6	158.7	149.9	34.8	124.3	122.5	118.0
Gallstones	47.6	39.6	38.7	39.1	51.9	41.4	36.5	39.0	45.0	38.5	*40.2	39.1
Kidney disease	24.5	37.6	108.9	110.2	27.6	48.7	129.1	123.9	*22.6	30.4	94.6	100.3
Urinary tract infection	86.0	85.6	120.1	123.0	66.6	72.5	84.6	87.6	97.8	94.2	145.2	148.5
Hyperplasia of the prostate	X	X	X	X	183.3	67.2	*39.1	38.5	X	X	X	X
Osteoarthritis	68.6	100.6	156.0	161.4	65.2	76.5	147.5	152.6	70.7	116.4	162.1	167.8
Injury	259.1	229.1	232.8	237.0	153.4	171.7	190.3	189.0	323.0	266.6	262.9	271.5
Fracture	195.8	170.2	160.4	166.2	92.6	116.4	110.4	111.8	258.1	205.4	195.7	205.3
Hip fracture	115.2	99.0	63.2	69.4	53.7	68.6	36.0	45.6	152.4	118.8	82.3	86.5
Complications of care and adverse effects	81.5	101.4	121.1	123.1	101.4	136.0	149.4	150.8	69.4	78.8	101.1	103.2
85 Years and Over³	5,606.3	6,050.9	5,814.6	5,667.7	6,420.9	6,166.6	6,425.5	6,193.4	5,289.6	6,003.3	5,531.7	5,415.6
Septicemia	135.6	153.9	237.5	261.4	139.0	207.3	292.9	320.8	134.3	131.9	211.8	232.8
Cancer, all	254.0	194.5	167.7	144.0	370.6	250.5	241.0	209.0	208.7	171.5	133.7	112.8
Colorectal cancer	47.6	49.7	*21.8	17.0	*59.1	*58.8	*	*20.7	43.2	45.9	*18.3	*15.2
Lung/bronchus/tracheal cancer	*19.1	12.1	*23.1	*25.0	*	*20.9	*	*	*	*8.5	*	*15.2
Breast cancer⁴	X	X	X	X	X	X	X	X	*41.7	*20.5	*	*12.0
Prostate cancer	X	X	X	X	*87.8	*49.3	*	*20.0	X	X	X	X
Diabetes	53.0	65.6	*59.8	58.7	*53.5	*54.2	*70.1	69.4	52.8	70.3	*55.1	*53.6
Schizophrenia, mood disorders, delusional disorders, nonorganic psychoses	*27.9	*37.3	*	*	*	*	*	*40.6	*30.7	*43.0	*	*
Dementia and Alzheimer's disease	49.7	107.0	73.8	77.2	*28.9	94.3	88.7	96.2	57.7	112.2	66.9	68.0
Heart disease	1,107.0	1,298.2	1,085.8	1,054.7	1,320.3	1,407.4	1,323.1	1,224.2	1,024.1	1,253.4	975.9	973.4
Ischemic heart disease	423.0	427.2	246.1	246.9	581.6	534.4	349.8	323.5	361.3	383.2	198.1	210.2
Heart attack	199.8	251.1	155.6	161.0	274.2	296.0	205.0	197.1	170.9	232.7	132.7	143.6
Arrhythmias	167.2	232.4	225.0	212.3	189.6	247.1	207.0	213.2	158.5	226.4	233.3	211.9
Heart failure	416.7	480.4	466.6	451.7	460.5	455.7	565.1	528.8	399.7	490.5	421.0	414.7
Hypertension	*17.9	41.1	66.2	49.1	*	*18.3	*69.3	*47.6	*19.3	50.4	*64.8	49.8
Stroke	427.2	373.8	288.3	284.1	408.2	396.7	270.7	278.5	434.6	364.3	296.4	286.8
Pneumonia	501.0	514.9	367.9	355.3	753.7	607.8	412.7	429.2	402.8	476.8	347.1	319.9
Chronic obstructive pulmonary disease	44.1	130.9	144.3	144.0	*72.9	150.4	*157.2	173.4	*32.9	123.0	138.4	129.8
Gallstones	60.7	39.2	*42.4	39.7	*68.2	*29.7	*40.4	*40.6	57.8	*43.1	*43.3	39.3
Kidney disease	47.1	49.5	160.2	167.4	92.4	*68.1	202.1	230.5	*29.4	*41.9	140.8	137.1
Urinary tract infection	216.5	191.5	346.0	321.9	239.3	153.1	259.5	217.0	207.6	207.2	386.1	372.1
Hyperplasia of the prostate	X	X	X	X	158.6	*69.9	*33.5	*31.8	X	X	X	X
Osteoarthritis	44.5	56.0	64.5	70.2	*	*	*57.3	*54.9	35.8	57.3	67.8	77.6
Injury	542.0	545.5	533.3	525.3	435.4	355.6	435.1	428.4	583.4	623.5	578.9	571.7
Fracture	439.0	450.9	403.5	396.6	335.7	252.4	302.1	275.7	479.2	532.4	450.4	454.6
Hip fracture	272.3	275.1	218.2	211.6	224.4	146.5	160.6	155.4	291.0	327.9	244.9	238.6
Complications of care and adverse effects	96.6	79.1	132.8	127.1	132.3	90.5	*151.7	160.0	82.7	74.4	124.1	111.4

X = Not applicable.
* = Figure does not meet standards of reliability or precision. Data preceded by an asterisk have a relative standard error (RSE) of 20 to 30 percent. Data not shown have an RSE of greater than 30 percent.
¹Starting with 2008 data, the sample of nonfederal short-stay hospitals was cut in half. This smaller sample size has increased standard errors. Therefore, caution should be exercised in interpreting trends in these data.
²Estimates are age adjusted to the year 2000 standard population using six age groups: under 18 years, 18 to 44 years, 45 to 54 years, 55 to 64 years, 65 to 74 years, and 75 years and over.
³Includes discharges with first-listed diagnoses not shown in table.
⁴Shown for women only.

Table 3-55. Discharges with at Least One Procedure in Nonfederal Short-Stay Hospitals, by Sex, Age, and Selected Procedures, Selected Years, 1990 Through 2009–2010

(Percent; rate per 10,000 population.)

Age and procedure (any listed)	Both sexes 1990	2000	2005	2009¹	2009-2010¹	Male 1990	2000	2005	2009¹	2009-2010¹	Female 1990	2000	2005	2009¹	2009-2010¹
18 Years and Over															
Hospital discharges with at least one procedure, crude (percent)²	67.4	62.1	62.6	63.3	63.2	65.2	59.2	59.4	60.0	59.9	68.7	63.9	64.7	65.5	65.3
Hospital discharges with at least one procedure, age-adjusted²,³	1,020.1	859.9	893.5	908.8		882.2	701.4	722.0	733.7		1,176.4	1,026.2	1,078.1	1,098.0	
Hospital discharges with at least one procedure, crude²	1,006.4	856.8	893.8	920.0	900.0	788.1	648.4	683.9	716.3	697.8	1,205.9	1,049.8	1,090.9	1,112.3	1,091.3
Operations on vessels of heart	28.3	41.2	41.2	36.0	33.1	41.9	56.9	58.5	50.2	46.7	15.8	26.7	25.0	22.6	20.2
Coronary angioplasty or arthrectomy	14.0	26.2	28.5	25.6	23.2	20.5	34.9	40.5	34.8	31.7	8.0	18.1	17.3	17.0	15.1
Coronary artery stent insertion	X	21.7	27.0	22.6	20.5	X	28.7	38.5	30.4	28.0	X	15.3	16.2	15.2	13.5
Drug-eluting stent insertion	X	X	23.9	15.8	15.0	X	X	34.1	21.0	20.4	X	X	14.4	10.9	9.9
Coronary artery bypass graft (CABG)	14.1	15.0	11.8	10.5	9.9	21.2	21.8	16.6	15.6	15.0	7.7	8.7	7.2	5.7	5.1
Cardiac catheterization	52.1	57.8	53.9	46.1	43.1	68.3	72.1	68.5	55.1	53.0	37.4	44.6	40.2	37.5	33.7
Pacemaker	8.6	8.5	9.6	9.2	8.7	10.1	8.5	10.5	9.0	9.0	7.1	8.5	8.8	9.4	8.4
Carotid (neck arteries) endarterectomy	3.6	5.9	4.6	4.0	4.1	4.1	6.6	5.7	4.6	4.7	3.1	5.3	3.6	3.5	3.5
Endoscopy of small intestine	40.8	42.5	45.8	45.7	44.6	38.6	39.1	42.3	42.3	40.7	42.8	45.6	49.1	48.9	48.3
Endoscopy of large intestine	27.9	25.0	24.0	21.9	20.6	22.5	20.2	19.7	19.1	18.0	32.8	29.4	28.0	24.4	23.1
Gall bladder removal	27.9	19.6	17.7	18.4	18.2	16.5	13.3	13.2	14.5	13.1	38.2	25.5	21.9	22.2	23.0
Laparoscopic gall bladder removal	X	14.8	13.5	14.7	14.8	X	9.2	8.8	10.4	9.6	X	20.1	17.9	18.7	19.7
Treatment of intra-abdominal scar tissue	17.0	14.4	15.3	15.1	14.7	6.5	5.7	6.5	7.8	7.8	26.6	22.4	23.5	22.0	21.3
Reduction of fracture	27.6	24.9	23.2	22.8	23.2	27.3	22.0	21.1	20.5	20.0	27.8	27.7	25.2	25.0	26.3
Excision of intervertebral disc and spinal fusion	18.7	18.2	18.4	22.3	21.8	22.3	20.0	18.8	22.5	21.4	15.4	16.4	18.0	22.2	22.1
Total hip replacement	6.4	7.3	10.5	13.8	13.9	5.4	6.8	10.1	14.0	13.6	7.3	7.7	10.9	13.5	14.1
Partial hip replacement	4.8	5.0	10.2	13.3	13.1	2.0	2.3	7.8	*11.3	10.9	7.3	7.6	12.3	15.2	15.1
Total knee replacement	6.7	13.8	23.1	28.0	28.8	4.9	11.0	16.4	20.2	21.6	8.4	16.4	29.3	35.4	35.6
CT scan	68.4	29.2	27.9	*17.1	*17.0	68.6	27.4	26.1	16.0	15.7	68.2	30.9	29.7	*18.1	*18.2
Arteriography and angiocardiography with contrast	59.7	63.0	59.9	56.4	53.8	75.6	76.2	72.1	64.9	63.4	45.2	50.7	48.5	48.3	44.8
Diagnostic ultrasound	72.3	36.9	36.0	34.7	34.9	62.1	33.1	35.2	34.0	33.9	81.7	40.4	36.7	35.4	35.9
Magnetic resonance imaging	9.5	9.2	11.2	*10.1	9.8	9.4	8.2	10.3	*9.4	9.0	9.6	10.2	12.1	*10.7	*10.6
Mechanical ventilation	17.6	23.0	27.0	32.9	32.4	18.8	23.9	29.5	34.9	34.0	16.4	22.1	24.7	31.1	30.9
18 to 44 Years															
Hospital discharges with at least one procedure, crude (percent)²	73.0	71.7	71.7	71.9	72.4	62.6	55.9	54.0	53.6	53.7	77.0	77.4	78.1	78.4	78.7
Hospital discharges with at least one procedure²	749.3	609.1	644.0	638.0	627.6	362.8	251.6	254.4	244.3	233.3	1,130.6	965.9	1,039.0	1,039.7	1,030.6
Operations on vessels of heart	3.0	3.9	4.1	*3.1	2.8	4.9	5.5	5.7	4.5	4.1	*1.2	2.3	2.4	*	*1.5
Coronary angioplasty or arthrectomy	1.9	3.0	3.0	*2.5	*2.3	3.0	4.3	4.3	*3.5	3.4	*0.8	1.6	*1.7	*	*1.2
Coronary artery stent insertion	X	2.5	3.1	*2.3	*2.0	X	3.6	4.3	*3.1	*2.9	X	1.4	*1.8	*	*1.1
Drug-eluting stent insertion	X	X	2.6	*	*1.5	X	X	3.4	*	*2.1	X	X	*1.8	*	*
Coronary artery bypass graft (CABG)	1.0	0.9	0.8	*	*0.5	*1.8	1.1	*1.1	*	*0.8	*	*0.7	*	*	*
Cardiac catheterization	9.0	8.5	7.6	7.1	6.3	12.5	11.0	9.6	8.7	8.3	5.5	5.9	5.6	5.5	4.3
Endoscopy of small intestine	13.1	10.3	13.3	15.7	14.7	13.2	10.4	11.7	12.2	11.4	13.0	10.2	14.9	19.3	18.0
Endoscopy of large intestine	6.9	5.5	6.5	7.2	6.2	5.6	4.7	5.5	*6.2	5.3	8.1	6.3	7.5	8.3	7.0
Gall bladder removal	18.7	11.9	11.5	13.5	12.8	6.2	4.3	5.1	6.5	5.1	31.0	19.4	17.9	20.6	20.7
Laparoscopic gall bladder removal	X	9.9	9.9	11.0	11.0	X	3.0	4.1	4.5	3.7	X	16.8	15.8	17.7	18.4
Treatment of intra-abdominal scar tissue	14.1	10.8	11.7	11.1	10.5	2.0	1.5	*1.8	*2.9	*2.5	26.0	20.1	21.7	19.4	18.6
Hysterectomy	X	X	X	X	X	X	X	X	X	X	63.3	55.7	51.2	37.4	38.0
Abdominal hysterectomy	X	X	X	X	X	X	X	X	X	X	47.1	34.6	31.5	22.8	21.3
Vaginal hysterectomy	X	X	X	X	X	X	X	X	X	X	15.8	19.1	15.6	*10.6	*12.3
Forceps, vacuum, and breech delivery	X	X	X	X	X	X	X	X	X	X	77.5	59.9	51.1	*45.0	*43.9
Episiotomy	X	X	X	X	X	X	X	X	X	X	293.3	160.8	90.9	52.3	53.6
Other procedures inducing or assisting delivery	X	X	X	X	X	X	X	X	X	X	387.9	384.2	396.7	418.5	422.6
Medical induction of labor	X	X	X	X	X	X	X	X	X	X	41.1	77.7	107.5	120.5	125.9
Cesarean section	X	X	X	X	X	X	X	X	X	X	167.1	149.5	220.7	232.5	233.5
Reduction of fracture	19.1	13.7	13.2	12.0	11.6	27.9	19.0	18.9	17.2	15.3	10.4	8.4	7.5	6.8	7.9
Excision of intervertebral disc and spinal fusion	17.0	14.1	11.7	11.9	10.7	21.5	16.2	13.1	11.7	10.3	12.6	12.1	10.3	12.1	11.0
CT scan	27.5	10.6	12.6	*6.5	*6.6	32.3	11.0	12.3	5.8	*6.1	22.7	10.3	12.8	*7.2	*7.1
Arteriography and angiocardiography with contrast	12.5	10.3	10.5	9.7	9.1	17.4	12.9	12.2	9.7	9.9	7.6	7.7	8.7	9.7	8.2
Diagnostic ultrasound	34.2	11.6	12.3	9.8	10.0	19.3	8.3	9.5	*7.3	7.2	48.9	14.9	15.1	12.3	12.8
Magnetic resonance imaging	4.9	3.8	4.3	*4.4	*4.1	4.9	3.6	3.8	*	*2.9	4.9	*4.0	4.8	*5.6	*5.4
Mechanical ventilation	4.6	7.0	8.8	11.0	9.9	5.4	8.2	10.1	11.9	11.2	3.8	5.8	7.5	10.1	8.6
45 to 64 Years															
Hospital discharges with at least one procedure, crude (percent)²	68.2	62.3	62.6	63.2	63.0	68.9	63.4	63.3	63.5	63.3	67.6	61.3	61.8	62.9	62.8
Hospital discharges with at least one procedure²	924.2	694.6	717.4	771.7	756.7	965.9	714.4	727.3	784.1	766.2	885.4	675.9	708.1	759.9	747.7
Operations on vessels of heart	53.0	57.7	53.5	42.5	40.0	83.2	88.5	83.5	62.8	59.5	24.8	28.4	24.9	23.1	21.4
Coronary angioplasty or arthrectomy	29.4	37.5	38.4	31.2	28.9	45.3	55.9	59.4	46.1	42.7	14.5	20.0	18.3	17.1	15.8

X = Not applicable.

* = Figure does not meet standards of reliability or precision. Data preceded by an asterisk have a relative standard error (RSE) of 20 to 30 percent. Data not shown have an RSE of greater than 30 percent.

¹Starting with 2008 data, the sample of nonfederal short-stay hospitals was cut in half. This smaller sample size has increased standard errors. Therefore, caution should be exercised in interpreting trends in these data.

²Includes discharges for procedures not shown separately.

³Estimates are age-adjusted to the year 2000 standard population using five age groups: 18 to 44 years, 45 to 54 years, 55 to 64 years, 65 to 74 years, and 75 years and over.

Table 3-55. Discharges with at Least One Procedure in Nonfederal Short-Stay Hospitals, by Sex, Age, and Selected Procedures, Selected Years, 1990 Through 2009–2010—Continued

(Percent; rate per 10,000 population.)

Age and procedure (any listed)	Both sexes 1990	2000	2005	2009¹	2009-2010¹	Male 1990	2000	2005	2009¹	2009-2010¹	Female 1990	2000	2005	2009¹	2009-2010¹
Coronary artery stent insertion	X	31.1	36.7	26.9	25.4	X	46.5	57.7	39.9	37.5	X	16.5	16.7	14.6	13.8
Drug-eluting stent insertion	X	X	33.0	18.7	18.7	X	X	51.8	28.1	27.5	X	X	15.1	*9.8	10.2
Coronary artery bypass graft (CABG)	23.4	20.3	14.0	11.5	11.1	37.5	32.5	21.9	17.1	16.9	10.3	8.6	6.4	*6.1	*5.5
Cardiac catheterization	98.2	83.0	69.7	56.6	54.4	136.8	113.9	95.6	75.7	72.3	62.3	53.7	45.1	38.4	37.2
Pacemaker	7.8	4.0	3.9	3.2	3.2	10.9	5.2	4.6	*4.5	4.2	*4.9	2.8	3.2	*2.0	*2.3
Carotid (neck arteries) endarterectomy	4.0	5.2	2.9	2.6	3.1	5.2	5.2	3.7	*3.1	3.6	3.0	*5.2	2.2	*2.1	*2.7
Endoscopy of small intestine	45.0	36.4	42.5	43.5	43.2	46.3	40.7	44.7	45.3	42.2	43.8	32.3	40.3	41.9	44.2
Endoscopy of large intestine	28.5	19.3	19.4	18.9	18.0	25.4	18.1	17.4	16.7	15.9	31.4	20.4	21.2	21.0	20.0
Gall bladder removal	36.4	20.6	17.6	18.4	18.0	22.3	16.3	14.0	15.6	13.8	49.5	24.6	20.9	21.0	21.9
Laparoscopic gall bladder removal	X	15.3	13.0	15.0	14.6	X	12.1	9.0	11.8	10.6	X	18.5	16.8	18.0	18.5
Treatment of intra-abdominal scar tissue	17.1	15.0	15.6	14.6	13.8	9.5	7.0	6.2	8.5	8.2	24.2	22.6	24.5	20.4	19.1
Removal of prostate	X	X	X	X	X	35.8	15.6	14.4	*17.9	16.9	X	X	X	X	X
Transurethral prostatectomy	X	X	X	X	X	30.4	7.0	4.6	*2.7	3.3	X	X	X	X	X
Hysterectomy	X	X	X	X	X	X	X	X	X	X	76.4	78.2	63.8	54.5	54.1
Abdominal hysterectomy	X	X	X	X	X	X	X	X	X	X	58.4	53.2	39.7	33.9	32.1
Vaginal hysterectomy	X	X	X	X	X	X	X	X	X	X	17.6	21.6	19.3	14.4	15.4
Reduction of fracture	20.3	18.5	16.5	17.0	18.2	19.5	17.6	17.9	16.7	18.1	21.0	19.3	15.3	17.3	18.3
Excision of intervertebral disc and spinal fusion	26.1	25.7	26.9	31.1	30.8	29.4	27.1	27.0	30.6	31.3	23.1	24.4	26.8	31.7	30.2
Total hip replacement	6.2	8.1	10.9	18.3	18.0	5.7	9.1	12.3	20.8	19.0	6.5	7.2	9.6	15.8	17.1
Partial hip replacement	*	*1.3	9.1	*14.0	*13.8	*	*0.8	8.8	*14.1	*13.7	*	*1.7	9.5	*13.9	*13.8
Total knee replacement	6.7	12.7	25.4	36.5	37.1	5.8	8.7	17.7	27.0	27.8	*7.4	16.4	32.7	45.5	46.0
Mastectomy	X	X	X	.	X	X	X	X	X	X	21.2	10.6	8.1	8.5	9.3
CT scan	65.4	25.2	26.1	17.0	*17.1	69.9	25.9	26.7	18.0	17.4	61.2	24.5	25.5	*16.1	*16.9
Arteriography and angiocardiography with contrast	105.4	85.3	73.2	66.3	64.3	138.5	111.4	94.6	86.7	83.3	74.6	60.7	52.8	46.9	46.3
Diagnostic ultrasound	69.5	34.3	33.5	30.9	31.8	73.8	38.0	39.4	35.9	36.3	65.5	30.9	27.9	26.2	27.5
Magnetic resonance imaging	10.9	8.9	11.6	8.9	9.2	10.7	9.4	12.4	9.2	9.2	11.0	8.4	11.0	*8.6	9.2
Mechanical ventilation	17.6	21.2	24.7	32.2	32.9	18.6	22.9	28.0	33.5	34.4	16.7	19.6	21.6	30.8	31.5

65 to 74 Years

Age and procedure (any listed)	Both sexes 1990	2000	2005	2009¹	2009-2010¹	Male 1990	2000	2005	2009¹	2009-2010¹	Female 1990	2000	2005	2009¹	2009-2010¹
Hospital discharges with at least one procedure, crude (percent)²	66.5	61.3	62.9	63.9	63.2	69.3	63.9	65.0	64.4	64.6	63.8	58.9	60.9	63.4	62.0
Hospital discharges with at least one procedure²	1,739.4	1,559.8	1,653.0	1,632.6	1,573.0	1,994.1	1,692.3	1,783.2	1,725.0	1,678.0	1,539.4	1,450.6	1,543.1	1,553.5	1,482.5
Operations on vessels of heart	97.0	139.8	142.1	117.4	104.2	148.9	195.3	211.0	165.8	152.6	56.3	94.1	84.0	75.9	62.4
Coronary angioplasty or arthrectomy	44.1	86.3	91.2	83.2	69.4	64.9	116.0	138.2	113.2	96.6	27.8	61.9	51.5	57.4	45.9
Coronary artery stent insertion	X	71.7	86.2	73.6	61.1	X	94.9	129.4	97.3	83.3	X	52.5	49.8	53.2	42.0
Drug-eluting stent insertion	X	X	76.8	53.5	46.1	X	X	115.7	69.1	62.5	X	X	44.0	*40.2	32.1
Coronary artery bypass graft (CABG)	52.1	53.9	47.4	34.4	34.7	83.1	79.7	68.1	52.9	55.9	27.7	32.6	30.0	*18.6	16.5
Cardiac catheterization	164.0	174.2	170.3	130.9	120.4	213.8	222.7	230.4	159.3	153.7	124.9	134.2	119.6	106.6	91.7
Pacemaker	24.6	22.5	23.7	19.6	18.6	32.1	22.8	29.0	*17.3	18.1	18.7	22.3	19.1	*21.5	19.0
Carotid (neck arteries) endarterectomy	14.6	24.1	24.0	*17.8	15.6	18.0	29.5	31.2	*21.8	21.8	11.9	19.6	18.0	*14.3	*10.3
Endoscopy of small intestine	92.8	106.6	102.5	99.4	93.2	91.5	102.4	102.6	106.7	99.0	93.7	110.0	102.4	93.2	88.2
Endoscopy of large intestine	70.3	64.8	58.3	45.7	44.3	62.5	59.7	52.1	44.9	41.6	76.5	69.0	63.6	46.4	46.7
Gall bladder removal	45.0	42.1	34.4	31.3	30.0	42.0	37.9	34.0	33.7	31.9	47.4	45.5	34.8	29.3	28.3
Laparoscopic gall bladder removal	X	29.5	23.6	21.9	22.0	X	24.4	22.4	*20.3	21.2	X	33.7	24.6	23.2	22.6
Treatment of intra-abdominal scar tissue	23.1	21.4	23.5	27.4	29.0	17.1	14.5	19.6	*20.5	24.3	27.7	27.1	26.8	*33.2	33.0
Removal of prostate	X	X	X	X	X	201.1	83.7	65.3	56.9	50.8	X	X	X	X	X
Transurethral prostatectomy	X	X	X	X	X	180.9	59.4	39.5	*23.7	24.1	X	X	X	X	X
Hysterectomy	X	X	X	X	X	X	X	X	X	X	37.4	35.9	28.0	*29.3	30.2
Abdominal hysterectomy	X	X	X	X	X	X	X	X	X	X	20.8	20.5	12.8	*12.2	15.0
Vaginal hysterectomy	X	X	X	X	X	X	X	X	X	X	16.5	14.7	14.1	*15.0	*14.1
Reduction of fracture	36.2	36.4	38.0	34.8	32.9	24.3	26.2	25.8	19.0	18.4	45.5	44.8	48.3	48.3	45.5
Excision of intervertebral disc and spinal fusion	16.3	21.1	31.1	41.7	42.1	14.2	22.5	27.6	*45.9	39.2	18.0	20.0	34.1	*38.0	*44.5
Total hip replacement	24.0	25.4	36.6	37.4	39.3	23.0	26.4	36.2	34.6	37.1	24.9	24.5	37.0	39.9	41.2
Partial hip replacement	8.9	7.6	20.1	*24.7	*25.3	*4.0	*	15.4	*20.8	*19.1	*12.7	10.5	24.1	*27.9	*30.7
Total knee replacement	33.2	65.4	99.5	104.6	108.3	26.4	64.5	71.8	76.2	84.0	38.6	66.0	122.8	128.9	129.3
Mastectomy	X	X	X	X	X	X	X	X	X	X	30.7	22.7	*11.5	*15.5	*12.9
CT scan	153.7	64.3	53.7	*30.9	*29.4	163.4	65.7	53.6	*32.6	*31.1	146.1	63.1	53.7	*29.5	*27.9
Arteriography and angiocardiography with contrast	184.5	186.2	180.8	153.6	146.5	239.0	231.9	233.2	191.5	186.7	141.7	148.5	136.6	121.2	111.9
Diagnostic ultrasound	155.2	92.7	80.9	82.7	79.8	165.2	94.1	87.0	*93.0	85.6	147.4	91.6	75.8	73.9	74.8
Magnetic resonance imaging	20.6	17.2	24.4	*18.1	*18.3	19.2	*14.6	19.9	*19.2	18.9	21.7	*19.3	28.3	*	*17.8
Mechanical ventilation	48.6	60.0	70.1	79.5	79.9	58.7	70.3	83.0	86.0	90.7	40.6	51.6	59.3	73.9	70.7

75 to 84 Years

Age and procedure (any listed)	Both sexes 1990	2000	2005	2009¹	2009-2010¹	Male 1990	2000	2005	2009¹	2009-2010¹	Female 1990	2000	2005	2009¹	2009-2010¹
Hospital discharges with at least one procedure, crude (percent)²	59.0	53.6	54.9	57.1	56.4	61.7	56.3	58.1	59.6	59.0	57.0	51.8	52.5	55.2	54.5
Hospital discharges with at least one procedure²	2,332.9	2,212.3	2,269.1	2,322.2	2,247.8	2,723.9	2,416.5	2,549.4	2,528.1	2,441.4	2,096.7	2,078.8	2,078.7	2,176.6	2,108.7
Operations on vessels of heart	69.1	143.2	142.3	138.6	126.0	107.6	202.5	199.6	208.3	189.8	45.8	104.5	103.4	89.2	80.2
Coronary angioplasty or arthrectomy	22.4	84.7	97.3	87.3	82.7	33.7	109.3	134.8	121.2	116.8	15.7	68.7	71.9	63.3	58.2
Coronary artery stent insertion	X	69.8	88.2	79.6	75.3	X	86.5	122.2	111.4	107.5	X	58.8	65.2	57.1	52.2

X = Not applicable.

* = Figure does not meet standards of reliability or precision. Data preceded by an asterisk have a relative standard error (RSE) of 20 to 30 percent. Data not shown have an RSE of greater than 30 percent.

¹Starting with 2008 data, the sample of nonfederal short-stay hospitals was cut in half. This smaller sample size has increased standard errors. Therefore, caution should be exercised in interpreting trends in these data.

²Includes discharges for procedures not shown separately.

Table 3-55. Discharges with at Least One Procedure in Nonfederal Short-Stay Hospitals, by Sex, Age, and Selected Procedures, Selected Years, 1990 Through 2009–2010—*Continued*

(Percent; rate per 10,000 population.)

Age and procedure (any listed)	Both sexes					Male					Female				
	1990	2000	2005	2009¹	2009-2010¹	1990	2000	2005	2009¹	2009-2010¹	1990	2000	2005	2009¹	2009-2010¹
Drug-eluting stent insertion	X	X	75.5	55.6	54.7	X	X	104.9	77.5	77.5	X	X	55.6	*40.2	38.2
Coronary artery bypass graft (CABG)	47.0	57.7	44.4	*50.7	42.7	74.7	90.5	62.6	*86.2	*72.3	30.3	36.2	32.0	*25.7	*21.5
Cardiac catheterization	116.6	190.2	183.9	159.3	149.3	166.0	236.9	238.1	179.6	179.9	86.8	159.6	147.1	144.8	127.4
Pacemaker	50.8	58.1	67.9	59.9	60.0	70.6	72.2	91.0	79.6	84.9	38.8	48.9	52.2	46.0	42.1
Carotid (neck arteries) endarterectomy	19.8	32.8	24.4	23.3	23.7	24.2	45.5	34.1	31.6	29.6	*17.1	24.5	17.7	*17.5	19.5
Endoscopy of small intestine	171.4	189.7	182.2	167.4	166.0	188.9	193.8	202.0	162.5	164.2	160.8	187.0	168.7	170.9	167.3
Endoscopy of large intestine	131.1	123.7	106.4	93.7	87.9	126.1	113.8	109.3	89.5	83.9	134.1	130.1	104.3	96.7	90.7
Gall bladder removal	51.8	43.4	43.3	38.2	43.6	64.4	46.7	48.9	50.7	50.5	44.2	41.3	39.4	29.3	38.7
Laparoscopic gall bladder removal	X	28.9	30.5	32.3	35.9	X	29.6	30.4	40.7	39.2	X	28.5	30.5	26.4	33.6
Treatment of intra-abdominal scar tissue	34.0	28.6	27.9	28.1	30.2	28.2	26.3	*34.5	*30.0	28.7	37.5	30.2	23.4	26.7	31.3
Removal of prostate	X	X	X	X	X	273.5	98.0	65.4	*47.0	41.2	X	X	X	X	X
Transurethral prostatectomy	X	X	X	X	X	257.5	89.0	58.6	*44.0	36.6	X	X	X	X	X
Hysterectomy	X	X	X	X	X	X	X	X	X	X	28.5	25.5	16.1	*23.2	18.5
Abdominal hysterectomy	X	X	X	X	X	X	X	X	X	X	18.8	16.2	8.6	*14.7	*11.1
Vaginal hysterectomy	X	X	X	X	X	X	X	X	X	X	*9.4	8.1	7.1	*	*5.6
Reduction of fracture	86.2	80.1	70.7	61.9	68.1	43.4	57.2	41.5	*41.9	46.0	112.1	95.0	90.6	76.0	84.0
Excision of intervertebral disc and spinal fusion	12.0	17.4	16.4	36.1	36.5	*13.2	*20.4	14.3	*42.8	*39.9	11.3	15.3	17.8	31.3	34.0
Total hip replacement	30.7	26.3	44.4	47.3	49.4	*26.9	*21.3	36.6	*44.4	47.2	33.1	29.6	49.7	49.4	51.1
Partial hip replacement	43.6	36.6	39.9	41.2	37.9	*14.3	20.0	27.4	*29.9	*29.9	61.2	47.5	48.3	49.1	43.7
Total knee replacement	28.4	59.3	90.4	89.8	86.2	*19.5	48.7	83.6	80.4	80.4	33.9	66.3	95.0	96.5	90.4
Mastectomy	X	X	X	X	X	X	X	X	X	X	29.2	22.0	16.2	*8.7	*11.3
CT scan	279.7	119.2	95.8	*56.8	*55.2	307.2	127.9	92.3	*58.3	*51.0	263.0	113.5	98.1	*55.8	*58.3
Arteriography and angiocardiography with contrast	141.0	219.2	212.4	198.1	187.8	192.3	287.9	269.9	219.0	223.3	109.9	174.3	173.3	183.4	162.2
Diagnostic ultrasound	273.5	134.1	133.0	122.4	122.0	315.7	142.8	148.3	135.8	137.7	248.0	128.4	122.6	113.0	110.8
Magnetic resonance imaging	30.5	*37.3	38.4	*38.5	*37.6	43.0	*33.6	41.3	*47.9	*44.0	*23.0	*39.8	36.5	*31.9	*33.0
Mechanical ventilation	79.8	91.1	102.6	105.3	102.0	110.3	106.5	119.4	139.7	119.5	61.3	80.9	91.1	81.1	89.5
85 Years and Over															
Hospital discharges with at least one procedure, crude (percent)²	49.3	44.6	45.4	47.0	46.8	52.4	45.4	47.7	51.4	50.5	47.8	44.3	44.2	44.6	44.7
Hospital discharges with at least one procedure²	2,762.1	2,700.5	2,612.5	2,731.1	2,650.6	3,367.3	2,797.9	2,857.1	3,301.9	3,125.0	2,526.8	2,660.6	2,500.2	2,466.7	2,423.0
Operations on vessels of heart	*14.0	51.1	53.9	60.9	55.5	*	83.0	86.2	*124.2	98.6	*	38.0	39.1	*31.6	34.8
Coronary angioplasty or arthrectomy	*	36.3	45.0	*51.7	44.6	*	*52.9	*64.6	*101.8	74.6	*	29.5	35.9	*28.4	*30.2
Coronary artery stent insertion	X	31.6	43.2	45.5	40.0	X	*48.9	*62.3	*83.9	66.6	X	*24.4	34.4	*27.7	*27.2
Drug-eluting stent insertion	X	X	38.4	*27.2	22.7	X	X	*55.8	*	*36.9	X	X	30.4	*19.6	*15.8
Coronary artery bypass graft (CABG)	*	*15.1	*	*	*10.1	*	*30.1	*	*	*22.5	*	*9.0	*3.0	*	*4.2
Cardiac catheterization	*23.7	87.7	88.8	*96.7	78.5	*	122.8	122.5	*145.1	111.7	*19.0	73.2	73.3	*74.4	62.6
Pacemaker	79.5	82.9	92.7	105.3	89.3	120.4	104.3	122.7	*121.0	100.6	63.5	74.2	78.9	*98.0	84.0
Carotid (neck arteries) endarterectomy	*	*12.0	*9.2	*	*	*	*	*	*	*7.1	*	*4.8	*	*	*
Endoscopy of small intestine	228.8	262.4	251.8	192.1	192.2	288.7	245.1	217.8	224.3	228.5	205.5	269.5	267.3	177.2	174.7
Endoscopy of large intestine	180.8	158.1	139.4	99.2	98.1	188.0	133.3	104.3	131.1	128.9	178.0	168.3	155.6	84.4	83.4
Gall bladder removal	46.4	40.9	29.1	*24.7	23.0	*68.4	*42.9	*48.4	*	*30.2	37.8	*40.1	20.3	*22.7	*19.5
Laparoscopic gall bladder removal	X	*30.4	18.6	*15.6	15.4	X	*	*28.2	*	*	X	*30.5	*14.2	*13.5	*14.0
Treatment of intra-abdominal scar tissue	29.6	24.3	29.0	*28.9	23.0	*	*16.4	*20.6	*	*13.9	33.7	*27.5	*32.8	*35.2	*27.4
Removal of prostate	X	X	X	X	X	257.2	*113.0	73.0	*39.7	42.7	X	X	X	X	X
Transurethral prostatectomy	X	X	X	X	X	247.1	*110.0	67.1	*39.7	41.8	X	X	X	X	X
Hysterectomy	X	X	X	X	X	X	X	X	X	X	*	*	*5.9	*	*
Abdominal hysterectomy	X	X	X	X	X	X	X	X	X	X	*	*	*4.3	*	*
Vaginal hysterectomy	X	X	X	X	X	X	X	X	X	X	*	*	*	*	*
Reduction of fracture	196.2	200.5	160.6	182.9	180.3	150.6	93.8	75.4	147.5	132.8	213.9	244.3	199.7	199.4	203.0
Excision of intervertebral disc and spinal fusion	*	*2.3	*	*	*6.2	*	*	*	*	*	*	*	*	*	*
Total hip replacement	*27.8	*20.7	*24.8	*31.6	*25.5	*	*	*	*	*	*23.2	*26.3	*23.6	*	*21.6
Partial hip replacement	67.4	82.2	71.2	78.1	77.1	*52.9	*44.1	56.4	67.0	66.2	73.1	97.9	78.0	83.3	82.3
Total knee replacement	*12.4	*22.9	*30.2	*26.7	34.0	*	*	*27.0	*	*31.3	*	*16.2	*31.7	*31.1	35.3
Mastectomy	X	X	X	X	X	X	X	X	X	X	*28.9	*15.7	*	*	*
CT scan	378.4	158.7	123.7	*86.2	*84.9	401.2	141.4	*131.8	*79.2	*84.8	369.5	165.9	119.9	*	*85.0
Arteriography and angiocardiography with contrast	50.6	120.8	126.6	156.8	135.6	*87.6	164.4	175.2	197.2	161.9	36.2	102.8	104.3	138.2	123.0
Diagnostic ultrasound	327.7	208.5	179.3	203.3	200.6	394.5	181.4	200.7	215.6	216.3	301.7	219.6	169.6	*197.6	193.1
Magnetic resonance imaging	*18.5	*40.4	40.5	*	*35.7	*	*	*40.8	*	*35.9	*16.2	*	*40.5	*	*
Mechanical ventilation	91.5	106.0	110.0	139.1	130.3	97.9	116.5	166.1	199.1	172.2	89.1	101.7	84.3	111.3	110.2

X = Not applicable.
* = Figure does not meet standards of reliability or precision. Data preceded by an asterisk have a relative standard error (RSE) of 20 to 30 percent. Data not shown have an RSE of greater than 30 percent.
¹Starting with 2008 data, the sample of nonfederal short-stay hospitals was cut in half. This smaller sample size has increased standard errors. Therefore, caution should be exercised in interpreting trends in these data.
²Includes discharges for procedures not shown separately.
³Estimates are age-adjusted to the year 2000 standard population using five age groups: 18 to 44 years, 45 to 54 years, 55 to 64 years, 65 to 74 years, and 75 years and over.

HEALTH PERSONNEL

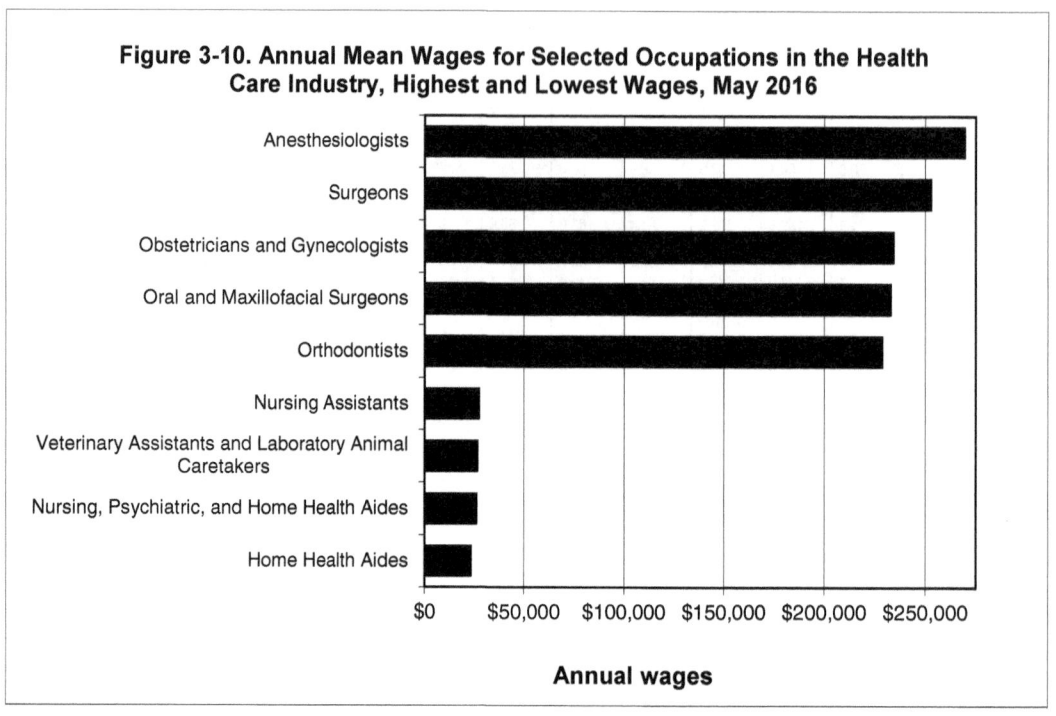

Figure 3-10. Annual Mean Wages for Selected Occupations in the Health Care Industry, Highest and Lowest Wages, May 2016

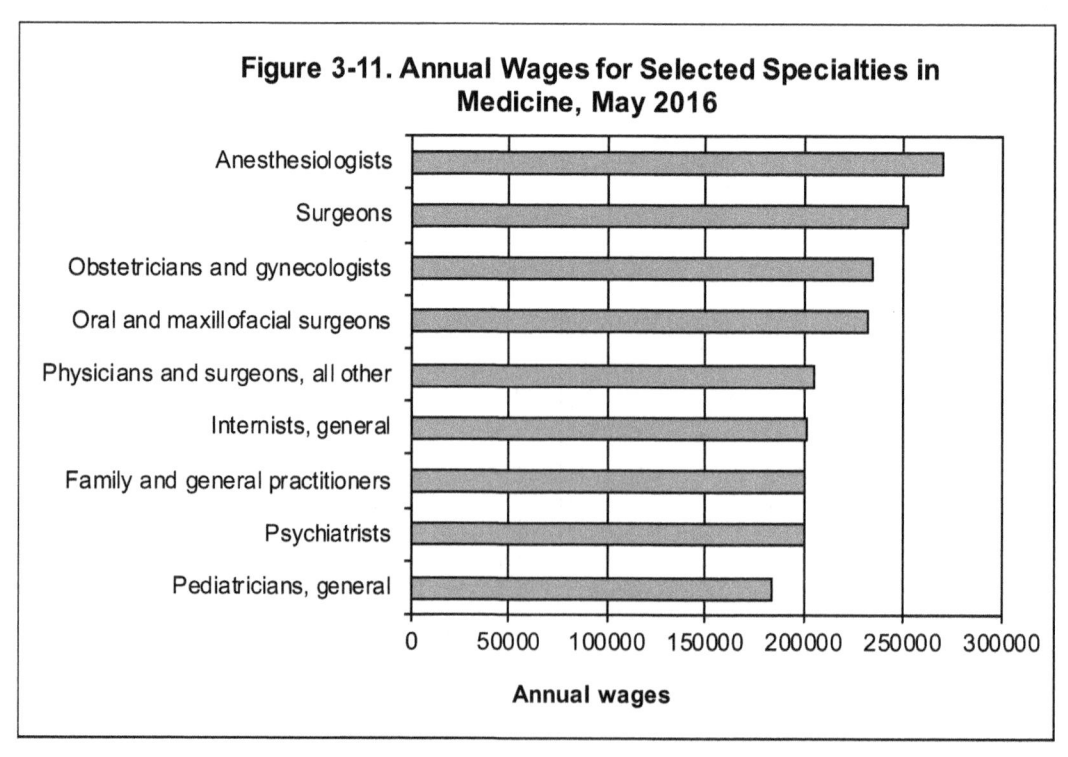

Figure 3-11. Annual Wages for Selected Specialties in Medicine, May 2016

Table 3-56. Health Care Employment and Wages, by Selected Occupations, Selected Years, 2001–2015

(Number; dollars.)

Occupation title	Employment[1]					Mean hourly wage (dollars)[2]				
	2001	2005	2009	2012	2015	2001	2005	2009	2012	2015
Health Care Practitioners and Technical Occupations										
Audiologists	11,040	10,030	12,590	12,060	12,070	$23.89	$27.72	$32.14	$35.04	$37.22
Cardiovascular technologists and technicians	40,990	43,560	48,070	50,530	51,400	17.55	19.99	23.91	25.51	26.97
Dental hygienists	149,880	161,140	173,900	190,290	200,550	27.30	29.15	32.63	33.99	34.96
Diagnostic medical sonographers	32,990	43,590	51,630	57,700	61,250	23.08	26.65	30.60	31.90	34.08
Dietetic technicians	28,940	23,780	24,510	24,660	28,950	11.23	12.20	13.72	13.79	14.03
Dietitians and nutritionists	43,200	48,850	53,220	58,240	59,740	19.74	22.09	25.59	27.00	28.08
Emergency medical technicians and paramedics	170,690	196,880	217,920	232,860	236,890	12.24	13.68	15.88	16.53	17.04
Licensed practical and licensed vocational nurses	683,790	710,020	728,670	718,800	697,250	15.14	17.41	19.66	20.39	21.17
Magnetic resonance imaging technologists	NA	NA	NA	29,560	33,460	NA	NA	NA	31.45	32.86
Medical and clinical laboratory technicians	146,920	142,330	152,420	157,920	157,610	14.52	15.95	18.20	18.91	19.91
Medical and clinincal laboratory technologists	145,400	155,250	166,860	160,700	162,950	20.70	23.37	26.74	28.19	29.74
Medical records and health information technicians	142,170	160,450	170,580	182,370	189,930	12.20	13.81	16.29	17.68	19.44
Nuclear medicine technologists	17,360	18,280	21,670	20,480	19,740	24.65	29.10	32.91	34.06	36.06
Nurse anesthetists	NA	NA	NA	34,180	39,410	NA	NA	NA	74.22	77.04
Nurse midwives	NA	NA	NA	5,710	7,430	NA	NA	NA	43.78	45.01
Nurse practitioners	NA	NA	NA	105,780	136,060	NA	NA	NA	43.97	48.68
Occupational therapists	77,080	87,430	97,840	105,540	114,660	25.10	28.41	33.98	36.73	39.27
Opticians, dispensing	63,120	70,090	60,840	64,930	73,520	13.49	14.80	16.73	16.83	17.70
Pharmacists	223,630	229,740	267,860	281,560	295,620	35.02	42.62	51.27	55.27	57.34
Pharmacy technicians	207,140	266,790	331,890	353,340	379,430	10.82	12.19	13.92	14.63	15.23
Physical therapists	126,450	151,280	174,490	191,460	209,690	28.43	31.42	36.64	38.99	41.25
Physician assistants	56,200	63,350	76,900	83,640	98,470	30.00	34.17	40.78	44.45	47.73
Psychiatric technicians	59,750	62,040	70,730	67,760	58,450	12.94	14.04	14.77	15.93	17.44
Radiation therapists	13,460	14,120	15,570	18,230	16,930	25.71	30.59	37.18	38.66	40.61
Radiologic technologists[3]	168,240	184,580	213,560	194,790	195,590	18.68	22.60	26.05	27.14	28.13
Recreational therapists	26,830	23,260	21,960	19,180	17,880	14.92	16.90	19.84	21.29	22.98
Registered nurses[4]	2,217,990	2,368,070	2,583,770	2,633,980	2,745,910	23.19	27.35	31.99	32.66	34.14
Respiratory therapists	82,930	95,320	107,270	116,960	120,330	19.17	22.24	26.06	27.50	28.67
Respiratory therapy technicians	28,700	22,060	15,100	13,460	10,000	16.93	18.57	21.96	22.84	23.90
Speech-language pathologists	83,110	94,660	111,640	121,690	131,450	24.20	27.89	32.86	34.97	36.97
Health Care Support Occupations										
Dental assistants	267,840	270,720	294,020	300,160	323,110	13.29	14.41	16.35	16.86	17.75
Home health aides	560,190	663,280	955,220	839,930	820,630	8.90	9.34	10.39	10.49	11.00
Massage therapists	26,440	37,670	55,920	71,040	92,090	15.93	19.33	19.13	19.40	20.76
Medical assistants	345,930	382,720	495,970	553,140	601,240	11.71	12.58	14.16	14.69	15.34
Medical equipment preparers	33,540	41,790	47,070	50,230	50,330	11.29	12.42	14.32	15.51	16.80
Medical transcriptionists	94,090	90,380	82,810	74,810	57,830	12.99	14.36	16.03	16.66	17.17
Nursing assistants[5]	1,307,600	1,391,430	1,438,010	1,420,020	1,420,570	9.54	10.67	12.01	12.32	12.89
Occupational therapy aides	7,560	6,220	8,040	7,950	7,570	11.70	13.20	13.89	14.36	14.95
Occupational therapy assistants	17,520	22,160	26,680	29,500	35,460	17.39	19.13	24.44	25.52	28.05
Orderlies	NA	NA	NA	53,920	52,660	NA	NA	NA	12.35	13.26
Pharmacy aides	58,130	46,610	52,230	42,600	38,040	9.22	9.76	10.74	11.28	13.20
Physical therapist aides	35,250	41,930	44,160	48,700	50,540	10.45	11.01	12.01	12.22	13.19
Physical therapist assistants	47,810	58,670	63,750	69,810	81,230	17.18	18.98	23.36	25.15	26.56
Psychiatric aides	59,640	56,150	62,610	77,880	69,550	11.42	11.47	13.19	12.83	13.55

Note: This table excludes occupations such as dentists, physicians, and chiropractors, which have a large percentage of workers who are self-employed.

[1]Employment is the number of filled positions. This table includes both full-time and part-time wage and salary positions. Estimates do not include business establishments where persons are self-employed, owners and partners in unincorporated firms, household workers, or unpaid family workers and were rounded to the nearest 10.

[2]The mean hourly wage rate for an occupation is the total wages that all workers in the occupation earn in an hour divided by the total employment of the occupation. More information is available from: http://www.bls.gov/oes/current/oes_tec.htm.

[3]Starting with 2012 data, the radiologic technologists and technicians occupation category was split into two occupations as part of the 2010 Standard Occupational Classifcation (SOC) revision: Radiologic technologists (29-2034) and Magnetic resonance imaging technologists (29-2035). Thus, data prior to 2012 include radiologic technologists as well as magnetic resonance imaging technologists and are not comparable with 2012–2015 data.

[4]Starting with 2012 data, the registered nurses occupation category was split into four occupations as part of the 2010 SOC revision: Registered nurses (29-1141), plus three advanced practice nursing occupations: Nurse anesthetists (29-1151), Nurse midwives (29-1161), and Nurse practitioners (29-1171). Thus, data prior to 2012 include registered nurses as well as nurse anesthetists, nurse midwives, and nurse practitioners and are not comparable with 2012–2015 data.

[5]Starting with 2012 data, the nursing aides, orderlies, and attendants occupation category was split into two occupations as part of the 2010 SOC revision: Nursing assistants (31-1014) and Orderlies (31-1015). Thus, data prior to 2012 include nursing assistants as well as orderlies and are not comparable with 2012–2015 data.

Table 3-57. Employment and Wages in the Health Care Industry, by Selected Occupation, May 2016

(Number; dollars.)

Occupation	Employment	Median hourly wage (dollars)	Mean hourly wage (dollars)	Annual mean wage (dollars)
Healthcare Practitioners and Technical Occupations	8,318,500	30.49	38.06	79,160
Chiropractors	32,960	32.46	39.04	81,210
Dentists, General	105,620	73.99	83.59	173,860
Oral and Maxillofacial Surgeons	5,380	#	111.96	232,870
Orthodontists	5,200	#	109.99	228,780
Prosthodontists	750	60.60	80.84	168,140
Dentists, All Other Specialists	5,380	83.17	82.64	171,900
Dietitians and Nutritionists	61,430	28.33	28.69	59,670
Optometrists	36,430	51.03	56.53	117,580
Pharmacists	305,510	58.77	57.82	120,270
Anesthesiologists	30,190	#	129.62	269,600
Family and General Practitioners	122,970	91.58	96.54	200,810
Internists, General	45,290	94.42	97.04	201,840
Obstetricians and Gynecologists	19,800	#	112.65	234,310
Pediatricians, General	26,960	81.24	88.58	184,240
Psychiatrists	24,820	93.63	96.26	200,220
Surgeons	41,190	#	121.59	252,910
Physicians and Surgeons, All Other	338,620	99.48	98.83	205,560
Physician Assistants	104,050	48.79	49.08	102,090
Podiatrists	9,800	60.01	69.28	144,110
Therapists	651,500	36.07	37.28	77,540
Occupational Therapists	118,070	39.38	40.25	83,730
Physical Therapists	216,920	41.06	41.93	87,220
Radiation Therapists	17,450	38.54	40.86	84,980
Recreational Therapists	18,100	22.31	23.17	48,190
Respiratory Therapists	126,770	28.21	29.15	60,640
Speech-Language Pathologists	135,980	35.90	37.60	78,210
Therapists, All Other	11,320	27.26	29.13	60,590
Veterinarians	67,650	42.68	48.34	100,560
Registered Nurses	2,857,180	32.91	34.70	72,180
Nurse Anesthetists	39,860	77.05	78.86	164,030
Nurse Midwives	6,270	47.97	49.23	102,390
Nurse Practitioners	150,230	48.52	50.30	104,610
Audiologists	12,310	36.53	38.12	79,290
Miscellaneous Health Diagnosing and Treating Practitioners	36,280	35.83	40.77	84,800
Health Technologists and Technicians	3,018,820	20.55	22.34	46,460
Clinical Laboratory Technologists and Technicians	326,920	24.48	25.13	52,280
Medical and Clinical Laboratory Technologists	166,730	29.36	30.02	62,440
Medical and Clinical Laboratory Technicians	160,190	18.73	20.05	41,700
Dental Hygienists	204,990	35.05	35.31	73,440
Diagnostic Related Technologists and Technicians	375,690	29.40	30.27	62,960
Cardiovascular Technologists and Technicians	53,760	26.71	27.45	57,100
Diagnostic Medical Sonographers	65,790	33.49	34.49	71,750
Nuclear Medicine Technologists	19,650	35.75	36.52	75,960
Radiologic Technologists	200,650	27.62	28.49	59,260
Emergency Medical Technicians and Paramedics	244,960	15.71	17.36	36,110
Health Practitioner Support Technologists and Technicians	752,050	15.93	16.91	35,180
Dietetic Technicians	32,240	12.67	14.12	29,360
Pharmacy Technicians	398,390	14.86	15.47	32,170
Psychiatric Technicians	61,720	14.89	17.25	35,870
Respiratory Therapy Technicians	10,600	23.93	24.29	50,520
Surgical Technologists	105,720	21.71	22.50	46,800
Veterinary Technologists and Technicians	99,390	15.62	16.29	33,870
Licensed Practical and Licensed Vocational Nurses	702,400	21.20	21.56	44,840
Medical Records and Health Information Technicians	200,140	18.29	19.93	41,460
Opticians, Dispensing	75,270	17.08	18.20	37,860
Orthotists and Prosthetists	7,500	31.55	33.62	69,920
Hearing Aid Specialists	6,740	24.16	25.48	53,000
Health Technologists and Technicians, All Other	122,170	19.75	22.13	46,020
Other Healthcare Practitioners and Technical Occupations	156,040	28.49	30.41	63,250
Occupational Health and Safety Specialists and Technicians	93,190	32.13	33.14	68,930
Occupational Health and Safety Specialists	76,630	34.09	34.85	72,480
Occupational Health and Safety Technicians	16,560	23.47	25.25	52,520
Athletic Trainers	24,130	*	*	47,880
Genetic Counselors	2,720	35.64	36.04	74,960
Healthcare Practitioners and Technical Workers, All Other	36,000	23.47	27.87	57,960
Healthcare Support Occupations	4,043,480	13.42	14.65	30,470
Home Health Aides	814,300	10.87	11.35	23,600
Psychiatric Aides	67,410	12.85	13.83	28,770

= This wage is equal to or greater than $90.00 per hour or $187,199 per year.
* = Wages for some occupations that do not generally work year-round, full time, are reported either as hourly wages or annual salaries depending on how they are typically paid.

Table 3-57. Employment and Wages in the Health Care Industry, by Selected Occupation, May 2016—*Continued*

(Number; dollars.)

Occupation	Employment	Median hourly wage (dollars)	Mean hourly wage (dollars)	Annual mean wage (dollars)
Nursing assistants	1,443,150	12.78	13.29	27,650
Orderlies	52,940	12.83	13.73	28,550
Occupational Therapy Assistants	38,170	28.37	28.62	59,530
Occupational Therapy Aides	7,210	13.62	15.31	31,840
Physical Therapist Assistants	85,580	27.21	27.33	56,850
Physical Therapist Aides	50,030	12.35	13.41	27,890
Massage Therapists	95,830	19.17	21.39	44,480
Dental Assistants	327,290	17.76	18.22	37,890
Medical Assistants	623,560	15.17	15.79	32,850
Medical Equipment Preparers	52,500	16.54	17.29	35,960
Medical Transcriptionists	54,070	17.17	17.86	37,150
Pharmacy Aides	36,660	12.14	13.66	28,420
Veterinary Assistants and Laboratory Animal Caretakers	79,990	12.14	12.89	26,810
Phlebotomists	120,970	15.72	16.22	33,750
Healthcare Support Workers, All Other	93,830	17.46	18.13	37,720

Table 3-58. Employment and Wages for the Highest- and Lowest-Paying Detailed Health Sector Occupations, by Annual Mean Wage, May 2016

(Dollars; number.)

Occupation title	Annual mean wage (dollars)[1]	Median hourly wage (dollars)	Employment
Highest-Paying Positions			
Anesthesiologists	269,600	129.62	30,190
Surgeons	252,910	121.60	41,190
Obstetricians and Gynecologists	234,310	112.65	19,800
Oral and Maxillofacial Surgeons	232,870	111.96	5,380
Orthodontists	228,780	109.99	5,200
Physicians and Surgeons	210,170	101.05	649,850
Physicians and Surgeons, All Other	205,560	99.48	338,620
Internists, General	201,840	94.42	45,290
Family and General Practitioners	200,810	91.58	122,970
Psychiatrists	200,220	93.63	24,820
Lowest-Paying Positions			
Home Health Aides	23,600	10.87	814,300
Nursing, Psychiatric, and Home Health Aides	26,320	11.93	2,377,790
Veterinary Assistants and Laboratory Animal Caretakers	26,810	12.14	79,990
Nursing Assistants	27,650	12.78	1,443,150
Physical Therapist Aides	27,890	12.35	50,030
Pharmacy Aides	28,420	12.14	36,660
Orderlies	28,550	12.83	52,940
Psychiatric Aides	28,770	12.85	67,410
Dietetic Technicians	29,360	12.67	32,240

[1]Annual wages have been calculated by multiplying the hourly mean wage by a "year-round, full-time" hours figure of 2,080 hours; for those occupations where there is not an hourly mean wage published, the annual wage has been directly calculated from the reported survey data.

Table 3-59. Industries with the Highest Levels of Employment and Highest Concentration of Employment in Health Care and Practitioner and Technical Occupations, May 2016

(Number; dollars.)

Industry	Employment[1]	Percent of industry employment	Hourly mean wage (dollars)	Annual mean wage (dollars)[2]
Industries with the Highest Levels of Employment in Health Care and Practitioner and Technical Occupations				
Health Diagnosing and Treating Practitioners	4,236,060	65.04	47.83	99,490
Healthcare Support Occupations	3,582,650	55.01	14.52	30,200
Office and Administrative Support Occupations	2,785,270	42.77	17.43	36,260
Registered Nurses	2,510,810	38.55	34.72	72,210
Health Technologists and Technicians	2,233,760	34.30	23.78	49,460
Industries with the Highest Concentration of Employment in Health Care and Practitioner and Technical Occupations				
Registered Nurses	2,510,810	38.55	34.72	72,210
Health Technologists and Technicians	2,233,760	34.30	23.78	49,460
Nursing, Psychiatric, and Home Health Aides	2,205,250	33.86	12.54	26,080
Personal Care and Service Occupations	2,030,900	31.18	11.31	23,530
Other Personal Care and Service Workers	1,939,040	29.77	11.02	22,920

[1]Estimates for detailed occupations do not sum to the totals because the totals include occupations not shown separately. Estimates do not include self-employed workers.
[2]Annual wages have been calculated by multiplying the hourly mean wage by a "year-round, full-time" hours figure of 2,080 hours; for those occupations where there is not an hourly mean wage published, the annual wage has been directly calculated from the reported survey data.

Table 3-60. States with the Highest Level of Employment and Highest Concentration of Jobs in Health Care Practitioner and Technical Occupations, May 2016

(Number, dollar.)

State	Employment[1]	Employment per thousand jobs	Location quotient[2]	Hourly mean wage (dollars)	Annual mean wage (dollars)[3]
States with the Highest Employment Level in This Occupation					
California	799,030	50.04	0.84	$45.42	$92,480
Texas	645,920	54.99	0.93	36.30	75,500
New York	528,800	58.12	.98	42.50	88,390
Florida	512,580	62.34	1.05	35.97	74,820
Pennsylvania	386,050	67.17	1.13	35.86	74,590
States with the Highest Concentration of Jobs and Location Quotients in This Occupation					
West Virginia	58,860	84.4	1.42	$32.24	$67,070
South Dakota	29,800	71.37	1.20	33.29	69,230
Mississippi	77,970	69.78	1.18	30.87	64,210
Massachusetts	240,340	69.46	1.17	44.29	92,130
Delaware	30,160	68.43	1.15	40.18	83,570

[1]Estimates for detailed occupations do not sum to the totals because the totals include occupations not shown separately. Estimates do not include self-employed workers.
[2]The location quotient is the ratio of the area concentration of occupational employment to the national average concentration. A location quotient greater than one indicates the occupation has a higher share of employment than average, and a location quotient less than one indicates the occupation is less prevalent in the area than average.
[3]Annual wages have been calculated by multiplying the hourly mean wage by a "year-round, full-time" hours figure of 2,080 hours; for those occupations where there is not an hourly mean wage published, the annual wage has been directly calculated from the reported survey data.

Table 3-61. Top Paying Metropolitan Areas for Health Care Practitioner and Technical Occupations, May 2016

(Number, dollar.)

Metropolitan area	Employment[1]	Employment per thousand jobs	Location quotient[2]	Hourly mean wage (dollars)	Annual mean wage (dollars)[3]
San Jose-Sunnyvale-Santa Clara, CA	42,390	40.55	0.68	$54.57	$113,510
San Francisco-Redwood City-South San Francisco, CA Metropolitan Division	42,850	40.15	0.68	53.91	112,140
Napa, CA	4,180	59.07	1.00	51.76	107,670
San Rafael, CA Metropolitan Division	5,220	46.75	0.79	51.44	107,000
Salinas, CA	6,580	39.94	0.67	50.87	105,810
Oakland-Hayward-Berkeley, CA Metropolitan Division	56,660	52.25	0.88	50.15	104,310
Vallejo-Fairfield, CA	9,100	1.04	1.19	49.91	103,810
Santa Maria-Santa Barbara, CA	8,270	45.36	0.77	49.10	102,140
Sacramento--Roseville--Arden-Arcade, CA	49,760	54.50	0.92	48.87	101,650
Silver Spring-Frederick-Rockville, MD Metropolitan Division	40,770	70.12	1.18	48.51	100,900

[1]Estimates for detailed occupations do not sum to the totals because the totals include occupations not shown separately. Estimates do not include self-employed workers.
[2]The location quotient is the ratio of the area concentration of occupational employment to the national average concentration. A location quotient greater than one indicates the occupation has a higher share of employment than average, and a location quotient less than one indicates the occupation is less prevalent in the area than average.
[3]Annual wages have been calculated by multiplying the hourly mean wage by a "year-round, full-time" hours figure of 2,080 hours; for those occupations where there is not an hourly mean wage published, the annual wage has been directly calculated from the reported survey data.

Table 3-62. Top Paying Nonmetropolitan Areas for Health Care Practitioner and Technical Occupations, May 2016

(Number, dollar.)

Metropolitan area	Employment[1]	Employment per thousand jobs	Location quotient[2]	Hourly mean wage (dollars)	Annual mean wage (dollars)[3]
Balance of Alaska nonmetropolitan area	2,930	39.74	0.67	$51.31	$106,720
Southeast Alaska nonmetropolitan area	1,550	43.97	0.74	49.03	101,980
West Central New Hampshire nonmetropolitan area	6,160	95.86	1.62	46.30	96,310
Los Alamos County, New Mexico nonmetropolitan area	490	32.16	0.54	44.56	92,690
Northwest Washington nonmetropolitan area	2,880	57.96	0.98	43.79	91,090

[1]Estimates for detailed occupations do not sum to the totals because the totals include occupations not shown separately. Estimates do not include self-employed workers.
[2]The location quotient is the ratio of the area concentration of occupational employment to the national average concentration. A location quotient greater than one indicates the occupation has a higher share of employment than average, and a location quotient less than one indicates the occupation is less prevalent in the area than average.
[3]Annual wages have been calculated by multiplying the hourly mean wage by a "year-round, full-time" hours figure of 2,080 hours; for those occupations where there is not an hourly mean wage published, the annual wage has been directly calculated from the reported survey data.

HEALTH EXPENDITURES

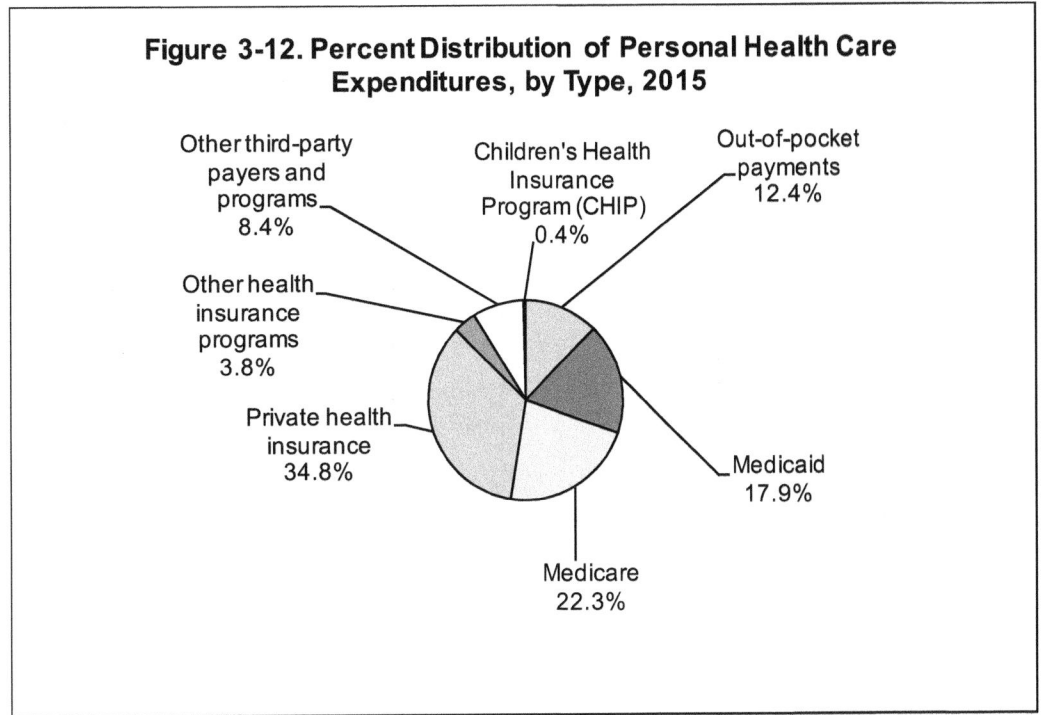

Figure 3-12. Percent Distribution of Personal Health Care Expenditures, by Type, 2015

Table 3-63. Gross Domestic Product, National Health Expenditures, Per Capita Amounts, Percent Distribution, and Average Annual Percent Change, Selected Years, 1960–2015

(Number; dollars.)

Gross domestic product and national health expenditures	1960	1970	1980	1990	2000	2009	2014	2015
Gross domestic product (GDP), in billions	$543	$1,076	$2,863	$5,980	$10,285	$14,419	$17,393	$18,037
Price deflator for GDP[1]	17.5	22.8	44.5	66.8	81.9	100.0	108.8	110.0
Amount (in Billions)								
National health expenditures	$27.2	$74.6	$255.3	$721.4	$1,369.7	$2,494.7	$3,029.3	$3,205.6
Health consumption expenditures	24.7	67.0	235.5	674.1	1,286.4	2,355.7	2,878.4	3,050.8
Personal health care	23.3	63.1	217.0	615.3	1,162.0	2,114.2	2,562.8	2,717.2
Administration and net cost of private health insurance	1.1	2.6	12.1	38.7	81.3	167.4	236.6	252.7
Public health	0.4	1.4	6.4	20.0	43.0	74.1	79.0	80.9
Investment[2]	2.5	7.5	19.9	47.3	83.3	139.0	150.9	154.7
Chain-weighted national health expenditure deflator[1]	NA	NA	NA	NA	NA	100.0	110.2	111.5
Per Capita Amount (in Dollars)								
National health expenditures	$146	$355	$1,108	$2,843	$4,857	$8,141	$9,515	$9,990
Health consumption expenditures	133	319	1,022	2,657	4,562	7,687	9,041	9,508
Personal health care	125	300	942	2,425	4,121	6,899	8,050	8,468
Administration and net cost of private health insurance	6	13	52	153	288	546	743	787
Public health	2	6	28	79	153	242	248	252
Investment[2]	13	36	86	187	295	453	474	482
Percent								
National health expenditures as percent of GDP	5.0	6.9	8.9	12.1	13.3	17.3	17.4	17.8
Percent Distribution								
National health expenditures	100.0	100.0	100.0	100.0	100.0	100.0	100.0	100.0
Health consumption expenditures	90.8	89.9	92.2	93.4	93.9	94.4	95.0	95.2
Personal health care	85.5	84.6	85.0	85.3	84.8	84.7	84.6	84.8
Administration and net cost of private health insurance	3.9	3.5	4.7	5.4	5.9	6.7	7.8	7.9
Public health	1.4	1.8	2.5	2.8	3.1	3.0	2.6	2.5
Investment[2]	9.2	10.1	7.8	6.6	6.1	5.6	5.0	4.8
Average Annual Percent Change from Previous Year Shown								
GDP	X	7.1	11.1	7.6	5.6	3.8	3.8	3.7
National health expenditures	X	10.6	13.9	10.9	6.6	6.9	4.0	5.8
Health consumption expenditures	X	10.5	14.2	11.1	6.7	7.0	4.1	6.0
Personal health care	X	10.5	13.9	11.0	6.6	6.9	3.9	6.0
Administration and net cost of private health insurance	X	9.4	19.6	12.4	7.7	8.4	7.2	6.8
Public health	X	13.8	16.8	12.0	8.0	6.2	1.3	2.4
Investment[2]	X	11.6	10.3	9.1	5.8	5.8	1.7	2.6
National health expenditures	X	9.3	12.9	9.9	5.5	5.9	3.2	5.0
Health consumption expenditures	X	9.1	13.2	10.0	5.6	6.0	3.3	5.2
Personal health care	X	9.1	12.9	9.9	5.4	5.9	3.1	5.2
Administration and net cost of private health insurance	X	8.0	18.8	11.4	6.5	7.4	6.4	5.9
Public health	X	11.6	16.6	10.9	6.8	5.2	0.5	1.6
Investment[2]	X	10.7	9.4	8.1	4.7	4.9	0.9	1.7

Note: Dollar amounts are in current dollars. The data reflect preliminary annual estimates of the resident population for the United States, as of July 1, 2010, excluding the Armed Forces overseas.
NA = Not available.
X = Not applicable.
[1]Year 2009 = 100.
[2]Investment consists of research and structures and equipment.

Table 3-64. National Health Expenditures, Average Annual Percent Change and Percent Distribution, by Type of Expenditure, Selected Years, 1960–2015

(Dollars; percent.)

Type of national health expenditure	1960	1970	1980	1990	2000	2009	2014	2015
Amount (in Billions of Dollars)								
National health expenditures	$27.2	$74.6	$255.3	$721.4	$1,369.7	$2,494.7	$3,029.3	$3,205.6
Health consumption expenditures	24.7	67.0	235.5	674.1	1,286.4	2,355.7	2,878.4	3,050.8
Personal health care	23.3	63.1	217.0	615.3	1162.0	2114.2	2562.8	2717.2
Hospital care	9.0	27.2	100.5	250.4	415.5	779.7	981.0	1036.1
Professional services	7.9	19.8	64.5	207.3	387.5	668.2	792.8	840.2
Physician and clinical services	5.6	14.3	47.7	158.4	288.7	498.7	597.1	634.9
Other professional services	0.4	0.7	3.5	17.3	36.6	67.2	82.8	87.7
Dental services	2.0	4.7	13.3	31.6	62.1	102.3	112.8	117.5
Other health, residential, and personal care	0.4	1.3	8.4	23.8	63.9	123.4	151.5	163.3
Home health care[1]	0.1	0.2	2.4	12.5	32.3	67.3	83.6	88.8
Nursing care facilities and continuing care retirement communities[1]	0.8	4.0	15.3	44.7	85.0	134.9	152.6	156.8
Retail outlet sales of medical products	5.0	10.6	25.9	76.5	177.8	340.8	401.4	432.0
Prescription drugs	2.7	5.5	12.0	40.3	121.0	252.7	297.9	324.6
Durable medical equipment	0.7	1.7	4.1	13.8	25.2	37.8	46.6	48.5
Other nondurable medical products	1.6	3.3	9.8	22.4	31.6	50.3	56.9	59.0
Government administration[2]	0.1	0.7	2.8	7.2	17.1	29.6	41.2	42.6
Net cost of health insurance[3]	1.0	1.9	9.3	31.6	64.2	137.9	195.3	210.1
Government public health activities[4]	0.4	1.4	6.4	20.0	43.1	74.1	79.0	80.9
Investment	2.5	7.5	19.9	47.3	83.3	139.0	150.9	154.7
Research[5]	0.7	2.0	5.4	12.7	25.5	45.4	45.9	46.7
Structures and equipment	1.8	5.6	14.4	34.6	57.8	93.6	105.0	108.0
Average Annual Percent Change from Previous Year Shown								
National health expenditures	X	10.6	13.9	10.9	6.6	6.9	4.0	5.8
Health consumption expenditures	X	10.5	14.2	11.1	6.7	7.0	4.1	6.0
Personal health care	X	10.5	13.9	11.0	6.6	6.9	3.9	6.0
Hospital care	X	11.7	14.4	9.6	5.2	7.2	4.7	5.6
Professional services	X	9.6	13.2	12.4	6.5	6.2	3.5	6.0
Physician and clinical services	X	9.9	13.5	12.7	6.2	6.3	3.7	6.3
Other professional services	X	6.3	21.1	17.4	7.8	7.0	4.3	5.9
Dental services	X	9.0	10.7	9.0	7.0	5.7	2.0	4.2
Other health, residential, and personal care	X	11.5	23.9	11.0	10.4	7.6	4.2	7.8
Home health care[1]	X	14.5	30.7	18.1	9.9	8.5	4.4	6.3
Nursing care facilities and continuing care retirement communities[1]	X	17.4	13.7	11.4	6.6	5.3	2.5	2.7
Retail outlet sales of medical products	X	7.7	10.4	11.4	8.8	7.5	3.3	7.6
Prescription drugs	X	7.5	8.4	12.8	11.6	8.5	3.3	9.0
Durable medical equipment	X	9.0	7.7	13.0	6.2	4.6	4.3	3.9
Other nondurable medical products	X	7.4	14.6	8.6	3.5	5.3	2.5	3.7
Government administration[2]	X	30.0	13.2	10.0	9.0	6.3	6.9	3.2
Net cost of health insurance[3]	X	6.4	22.0	13.0	7.4	8.9	7.2	7.6
Government public health activities[4]	X	13.8	16.8	12.0	8.0	6.2	1.3	2.4
Investment	X	11.6	10.3	9.1	5.8	5.8	1.7	2.6
Research[5]	X	10.9	10.0	8.9	7.2	6.6	0.2	1.8
Structures and equipment	X	11.9	10.4	9.2	5.3	5.5	2.3	2.9
Percent Distribution								
National health expenditures	100.0	100.0	100.0	100.0	100.0	100.0	100.0	100.0
Health consumption expenditures	90.8	89.9	92.2	93.4	93.9	94.4	95.0	95.2
Personal health care	85.5	84.6	85.0	85.3	84.8	84.7	84.6	84.8
Hospital care	33.0	36.4	39.4	34.7	30.3	31.3	32.4	32.3
Professional services	29.1	26.5	25.3	28.7	28.3	26.8	26.2	26.2
Physician and clinical services	20.4	19.2	18.7	22.0	21.1	20.0	19.7	19.8
Other professional services	1.4	1.0	1.4	2.4	2.7	2.7	2.7	2.7
Dental services	7.3	6.3	5.2	4.4	4.5	4.1	3.7	3.7
Other health, residential, and personal care	1.6	1.7	3.3	3.3	4.7	4.9	5.0	5.1
Home health care[1]	0.2	0.3	0.9	1.7	2.4	2.7	2.8	2.8
Nursing care facilities and continuing care retirement communities[1]	3.0	5.4	6.0	6.2	6.2	5.4	5.0	4.9
Retail outlet sales of medical products	18.5	14.2	10.1	10.6	13.0	13.7	13.3	13.5
Prescription drugs	9.8	7.4	4.7	5.6	8.8	10.1	9.8	10.1
Durable medical equipment	2.7	2.3	1.6	1.9	1.8	1.5	1.5	1.5
Other nondurable medical products	6.0	4.5	3.8	3.1	2.3	2.0	1.9	1.8
Government administration[2]	0.2	1.0	1.1	1.0	1.2	1.2	1.4	1.3
Net cost of health insurance[3]	3.7	2.5	3.6	4.4	4.7	5.5	6.4	6.6
Government public health activities[4]	1.4	1.8	2.5	2.8	3.1	3.0	2.6	2.5
Investment	9.2	10.1	7.8	6.6	6.1	5.6	5.0	4.8
Research[5]	2.6	2.6	2.1	1.8	1.9	1.8	1.5	1.5
Structures and equipment	6.7	7.5	5.7	4.8	4.2	3.8	3.5	3.4
Percent Distribution								
Personal health care	100.0	100.0	100.0	100.0	100.0	100.0	100.0	100.0
Hospital care	38.6	43.1	46.3	40.7	35.8	36.9	38.3	38.1
Professional services	34.1	31.3	29.7	33.7	33.3	31.6	30.9	30.9
Physician and clinical services	23.9	22.7	22.0	25.7	24.8	23.6	23.3	23.4
Other professional services	1.7	1.2	1.6	2.8	3.2	3.2	3.2	3.2
Dental services	8.5	7.5	6.1	5.1	5.3	4.8	4.4	4.3
Other health, residential, and personal care	1.9	2.1	3.9	3.9	5.5	5.8	5.9	6.0
Home health care[1]	0.2	0.3	1.1	2.0	2.8	3.2	3.3	3.3
Nursing care facilities and continuing care retirement communities[1]	3.5	6.4	7.0	7.3	7.3	6.4	6.0	5.8
Retail outlet sales of medical products	21.7	16.8	11.9	12.4	15.3	16.1	15.7	15.9
Prescription drugs	11.5	8.7	5.6	6.5	10.4	12.0	11.6	11.9
Durable medical equipment	3.2	2.8	1.9	2.2	2.2	1.8	1.8	1.8
Other nondurable medical products	7.0	5.3	4.5	3.6	2.7	2.4	2.2	2.2

X = Not applicable.

[1] Includes expenditures for care in freestanding facilities only. Additional services of this type are provided in hospital-based facilities and are considered hospital care.

[2] Includes all administrative costs (federal and state and local employees' salaries; contracted employees, including fiscal intermediaries; rent and building costs; computer systems and programs; other materials and supplies; and other miscellaneous expenses) associated with insuring individuals enrolled in the following health insurance programs: Medicare, Medicaid, Children's Health Insurance Program, Department of Defense, Department of Veterans Affairs, Indian Health Service, workers' compensation, maternal and child health, vocational rehabilitation, Substance Abuse and Mental Health Services Administration, and other federal programs.

[3] Net cost of health insurance is calculated as the difference between calendar year incurred premiums earned and benefits incurred for private health insurance. This includes administrative costs, and in some cases additions to reserves, rate credits and dividends, premium taxes, and net underwriting gains or losses. Also included in this category is the difference between premiums earned and benefits incurred for the private health insurance companies that insure the enrollees of the following programs: Medicare, Medicaid, Children's Health Insurance Program, and workers' compensation (health portion only).

[4] Includes personal care services delivered by government public health agencies.

[5] Research and development expenditures of drug companies and other manufacturers and providers of medical equipment and supplies are excluded. These are included in the expenditure class in which the product falls because such expenditures are covered by the payment received for that product.

Table 3-65. Personal Health Care Expenditures, by Source of Funds and Type of Expenditure, Selected Years, 1960–2015

(Number; percent.)

Type of personal health care expenditures and source of funds	1960	1970	1980	1990	2000	2009	2014	2015
Amount in Billions								
Per capita	$125	$300	$942	$2,425	$4,121	$6,899	$8,050	$8,468
Amount in Billions								
All personal health care expenditures[1]	$23.3	$63.1	$217.0	$615.3	$1,162.0	$2,114.2	$2,562.8	$2,717.2
Out-of-pocket payments	12.9	25.0	58.1	137.9	199.0	293.1	329.7	338.1
Health insurance	6.6	29.7	132.1	402.9	844.2	1,636.7	2,009.4	2,151.2
Private health insurance	5.0	14.1	61.5	204.8	406.1	734.4	875.2	944.7
Medicare	X	7.3	36.3	107.3	216.3	470.3	580.6	605.0
Medicaid	X	5.0	24.7	69.7	186.9	346.2	446.7	486.5
Federal	X	2.7	13.7	40.3	109.3	230.6	274.4	306.2
State and local	X	2.3	11.0	29.4	77.6	115.6	172.3	180.3
CHIP[2]	X	X	X	X	2.5	9.5	10.8	12.0
Federal	X	X	X	X	1.8	6.7	7.6	9.0
State and local	X	X	X	X	0.8	2.8	3.3	3.0
Other health insurance programs[3]	1.7	3.3	9.6	21.2	32.3	76.2	96.2	103.0
Other third-party payers and programs[4]	3.7	8.5	26.7	74.5	118.9	184.4	223.7	227.8
Amount in Billions								
Chain-weighted personal health care deflator (2009 = 100.0)[5]	9.3	13.5	28.5	56.3	75.7	100.0	109.9	111.0
Percent Distribution								
All sources of funds	100.0	100.0	100.0	100.0	100.0	100.0	100.0	100.0
Out-of-pocket payments	55.7	39.6	26.8	22.4	17.1	13.9	12.9	12.4
Health insurance	28.5	47.0	60.9	65.5	72.6	77.4	78.4	79.2
Private health insurance	21.3	22.3	28.4	33.3	34.9	34.7	34.1	34.8
Medicare	X	11.5	16.7	17.4	18.6	22.2	22.7	22.3
Medicaid	X	8.0	11.4	11.3	16.1	16.4	17.4	17.9
Federal	X	4.3	6.3	6.6	9.4	10.9	10.7	11.3
State and local	X	3.7	5.1	4.8	6.7	5.5	6.7	6.6
CHIP[2]	X	X	X	X	0.2	0.5	0.4	0.4
Federal	X	X	X	X	0.2	0.3	0.3	0.3
State and local	X	X	X	X	0.1	0.1	0.1	0.1
Other health insurance programs[3]	7.2	5.2	4.4	3.4	2.8	3.6	3.8	3.8
Other third-party payers and programs[4]	15.8	13.4	12.3	12.1	10.2	8.7	8.7	8.4
Amount in Billions								
Hospital expenditures[6]	$9.0	$27.2	$100.5	$250.4	$415.5	$779.7	$981.0	$1,036.1
Percent Distribution								
All sources of funds	100.0	100.0	100.0	100.0	100.0	100.0	100.0	100.0
Out-of-pocket payments	20.6	9.0	5.4	4.5	3.2	3.3	3.4	3.1
Health insurance	50.7	71.5	79.7	82.6	86.2	87.4	86.8	87.7
Private health insurance	35.6	32.5	36.6	38.5	33.9	36.6	37.7	39.0
Medicare	X	19.7	26.1	26.9	29.7	27.5	25.8	24.8
Medicaid	X	9.7	9.2	10.6	17.1	17.1	17.2	17.9
Federal	X	5.2	5.0	6.3	10.3	11.3	10.7	11.5
State and local	X	4.5	4.2	4.3	6.8	5.8	6.5	6.3
CHIP[2]	X	X	X	X	0.2	0.4	0.3	0.4
Federal	X	X	X	X	0.2	0.3	0.2	0.3
State and local	X	X	X	X	0.1	0.1	0.1	0.1
Other health insurance programs[3]	15.2	9.6	7.8	6.5	5.3	5.8	5.8	5.8
Other third-party payers and programs[4]	28.6	19.5	15.0	12.9	10.6	9.3	9.8	9.2
Amount in Billions								
Physician and clinical expenditures	$5.6	$14.3	$47.7	$158.4	$288.7	$498.7	$597.1	$634.9
Percent Distribution								
All sources of funds	100.0	100.0	100.0	100.0	100.0	100.0	100.0	100.0
Out-of-pocket payments	59.5	45.1	29.8	18.9	11.1	9.1	9.0	8.9
Health insurance	33.1	48.8	59.8	67.8	76.4	80.5	80.9	81.1
Private health insurance	28.7	29.4	34.8	42.1	47.1	45.9	42.8	42.9
Medicare	X	11.5	17.4	19.2	20.3	22.5	23.1	22.7
Medicaid	X	4.5	5.1	4.4	6.7	8.1	10.7	11.0
Federal	X	2.4	2.9	2.6	3.9	5.6	7.4	7.7
State and local	X	2.1	2.2	1.8	2.7	2.5	3.3	3.3
CHIP[2]	X	X	X	X	0.3	0.6	0.5	0.5
Federal	X	X	X	X	0.2	0.4	0.4	0.4
State and local	X	X	X	X	0.1	0.2	0.2	0.1
Other health insurance programs[3]	4.4	3.4	2.4	2.1	2.1	3.5	3.9	3.9
Other third-party payers and programs[4]	7.4	6.1	10.4	13.3	12.5	10.4	10.0	10.0
Amount in Billions								
Home health care expenditures[7]	$2.0	$4.7	$13.3	$31.6	$62.1	$102.3	$112.8	$117.5
Percent Distribution								
All sources of funds	100.0	100.0	100.0	100.0	100.0	100.0	100.0	100.0
Out-of-pocket payments	96.0	90.0	65.8	48.3	44.2	41.6	40.8	39.9
Health insurance	3.2	9.5	33.4	51.2	55.3	57.9	58.8	59.7

X = Not applicable.

0.0 = Quantity more than zero but less than 0.05.

[1]Includes all expenditures for specified health services and supplies other than expenses for government administration, net cost of health insurance, public health activities, research, and structures and equipment.

[2]Children's Health Insurance Program (CHIP). Medicaid CHIP expansions are included.

[3]Includes Department of Defense and Department of Veterans Affairs.

[4]Includes worksite health care, other private revenues, Indian Health Service, workers' compensation, general assistance, maternal and child health, vocational rehabilitation, other federal programs, Substance Abuse and Mental Health Services Administration, other state and local programs, and school health.

[5]The personal health care deflator is calculated as a chain-weighted price index using the Producer Price Indexes for hospitals, offices of physicians, medical and diagnostic laboratories, home health care services, and nursing care facilities; and Consumer Price Indices specific to each of the remaining personal health care components.

[6]Includes expenditures for hospital-based nursing home and home health agency care.

[7]Includes expenditures for care in freestanding nursing homes. Expenditures for care in hospital-based nursing homes are included with hospital care.

Table 3-65. Personal Health Care Expenditures, by Source of Funds and Type of Expenditure, Selected Years, 1960–2015 —*Continued*

(Number; percent.)

Type of personal health care expenditures and source of funds	1960	1970	1980	1990	2000	2009	2014	2015
Private health insurance...	1.9	4.5	28.4	47.9	50.3	48.3	47.1	46.5
Medicare	X	X	X	X	0.1	0.3	0.4	0.4
Medicaid	X	3.4	3.8	2.4	3.9	7.5	8.8	9.8
Federal	X	1.8	2.1	1.3	2.2	5.1	5.5	6.5
State and local	X	1.6	1.7	1.0	1.7	2.4	3.3	3.3
CHIP[2]	X	X	X	X	0.4	0.7	1.3	1.4
Federal	X	X	X	X	0.3	0.5	0.9	1.0
State and local	X	X	X	X	0.1	0.2	0.4	0.3
Other health insurance programs[3]	1.3	1.6	1.2	0.9	0.6	1.1	1.3	1.6
Other third-party payers and programs[4]	0.8	0.4	0.8	0.6	0.6	0.5	0.4	0.4

Amount in Billions

Nursing care facilities and continuing care retirement communities expenditures[7]	$0.1	$0.2	$2.4	$12.5	$32.3	$67.3	$83.6	$88.8

Percent Distribution

All sources of funds	100.0	100.0	100.0	100.0	100.0	100.0	100.0	100.0
Out-of-pocket payments	12.3	9.5	15.3	17.8	19.2	8.3	9.4	9.9
Health insurance	5.3	37.7	53.7	66.2	71.8	88.4	87.4	87.0
Private health insurance	1.8	3.2	14.7	22.8	24.0	7.3	9.8	10.6
Medicare	X	26.8	26.8	26.0	26.5	45.0	41.0	39.6
Medicaid	X	6.8	11.6	17.1	20.9	35.6	36.1	36.1
Federal	X	3.2	6.2	9.2	11.3	23.2	20.4	20.6
State and local	X	3.2	5.4	8.0	9.6	12.4	15.7	15.4
CHIP[2]	X	X	X	X	0.0	0.0	0.0	0.1
Federal	X	X	X	X	0.0	0.0	0.0	0.0
State and local	X	X	X	X	0.0	0.0	0.0	0.0
Other health insurance programs[3]	3.5	1.4	0.5	0.3	0.3	0.4	0.5	0.7
Other third-party payers and programs[4]	80.7	52.7	31.1	16.0	9.0	3.3	3.2	3.1

Amount in Billions

Prescription drug expenditures	$0.8	$4.0	$15.3	$44.7	$85.0	$134.9	$152.6	$156.8

Percent Distribution

All sources of funds	100.0	100.0	100.0	100.0	100.0	100.0	100.0	100.0
Out-of-pocket payments	74.4	49.2	40.5	40.3	31.9	27.3	26.0	25.6
Health insurance	X	28.5	51.9	49.0	61.2	66.2	66.7	67.4
Private health insurance	X	0.2	1.3	6.2	8.8	7.3	8.0	8.6
Medicare	X	3.5	2.0	3.8	12.7	22.3	23.3	24.0
Medicaid	X	23.3	46.2	36.7	37.5	33.7	32.2	31.7
Federal	X	12.5	26.1	20.7	21.8	22.5	18.4	18.2
State and local	X	10.8	20.1	16.1	15.7	11.2	13.8	13.5
CHIP[2]	X	X	X	X	0.0	0.0	0.0	0.0
Federal	X	X	X	X	0.0	0.0	0.0	0.0
State and local	X	X	X	X	0.0	0.0	0.0	0.0
Other health insurance programs[3]	X	1.5	2.4	2.2	2.2	2.9	3.1	3.2
Other third-party payers and programs[4]	25.5	22.3	7.6	10.8	6.9	6.5	7.3	7.0

Amount in Billions

Dental services expenditures	$2.7	$5.5	$12.0	$40.3	$121.0	$252.7	$297.9	$324.6

Percent Distribution

All sources of funds	100.0	100.0	100.0	100.0	100.0	100.0	100.0	100.0
Out-of-pocket payments	96.0	82.4	71.3	56.8	27.8	19.4	15.0	14.0
Health insurance	1.5	16.5	26.9	40.3	70.3	79.2	84.3	85.4
Private health insurance	1.3	8.8	15.0	27.0	50.5	45.9	43.0	43.1
Medicare	X	X	X	0.5	1.7	21.6	28.5	29.0
Medicaid	X	7.6	11.7	12.6	16.3	8.1	9.4	9.8
Federal	X	4.1	6.8	7.2	9.3	5.4	6.0	6.5
State and local	X	3.5	4.9	5.4	7.0	2.7	3.3	3.3
CHIP[2]	X	X	X	X	0.2	0.5	0.5	0.5
Federal	X	X	X	X	0.2	0.4	0.3	0.3
State and local	X	X	X	X	0.1	0.2	0.1	0.1
Other health insurance programs[3]	0.1	0.1	0.2	0.2	1.5	3.1	2.9	3.0
Other third-party payers and programs[4]	2.5	1.1	1.8	3.0	1.9	1.4	0.7	0.6

Amount in Billions

All other personal health care expenditures[8]	$3.2	$7.1	$25.7	$77.3	$157.3	$278.7	$337.8	$358.5

Percent Distribution

All sources of funds	100.0	100.0	100.0	100.0	100.0	100.0	100.0	100.0
Out-of-pocket payments	84.6	74.2	56.9	49.7	37.6	31.6	30.8	30.2
Health insurance	4.1	9.1	25.7	33.7	45.0	52.2	53.9	55.0
Private health insurance	3.1	4.6	7.8	13.0	13.7	14.3	14.2	14.4
Medicare	X	1.0	2.8	5.5	8.1	10.3	10.3	10.1
Medicaid	X	3.0	14.8	15.0	22.8	27.0	28.7	29.7
Federal	X	1.6	8.1	8.5	13.0	18.0	16.6	17.4
State and local	X	1.4	6.7	6.4	9.8	9.0	12.1	12.4
CHIP[2]	X	X	X	X	0.2	0.4	0.4	0.5
Federal	X	X	X	X	0.1	0.3	0.3	0.4
State and local	X	X	X	X	0.1	0.1	0.1	0.1
Other health insurance programs[3]	1.1	0.5	0.3	0.2	0.2	0.2	0.3	0.3
Other third-party payers and programs[4]	11.2	16.7	17.4	16.6	17.4	16.2	15.3	14.8

X = Not applicable.
0.0 = Quantity more than zero but less than 0.05.
[1]Includes all expenditures for specified health services and supplies other than expenses for government administration, net cost of health insurance, public health activities, research, and structures and equipment.
[2]Children's Health Insurance Program (CHIP). Medicaid CHIP expansions are included.
[3]Includes Department of Defense and Department of Veterans Affairs.
[4]Includes worksite health care, other private revenues, Indian Health Service, workers' compensation, general assistance, maternal and child health, vocational rehabilitation, other federal programs, Substance Abuse and Mental Health Services Administration, other state and local programs, and school health.
[7]Includes expenditures for care in freestanding nursing homes. Expenditures for care in hospital-based nursing homes are included with hospital care.
[8]Includes expenditures for other professional services, other nondurable medical products, durable medical equipment, and other health, residential, and personal care, not shown separately.

Table 3-66. Cost of Hospital Discharges with Common Hospital Operating Room Procedures in Nonfederal Community Hospitals, by Age and Selected Principal Procedure, Selected Years, 2000–2014

(Dollars.)

Age and principal operating room procedure[1]	Mean inflation-adjusted cost per hospitalization: 2014 dollars[2]			Number of discharges with operating room principal procedure			Total inflation-adjusted national costs: 2014 dollars (in millions of dollars)[2]		
	2000	2010	2014	2000	2010	2014	2000	2010	2014
All Ages									
Hospital discharges with an operating room principal procedure[3]	$13,782	$19,186	$19,266	8,743,631	9,637,687	8,308,949	$119,757	$184,725	$159,951
Laminectomy (back surgery)	8,493	11,920	14,883	285,636	204,786	151,705	2,436	2,440	2,268
Heart valve procedures	44,609	56,426	51,896	79,719	98,101	110,915	3,550	5,541	5,756
Coronary artery bypass graft (CABG)	32,520	41,897	41,932	337,972	164,801	160,240	11,028	6,907	6,717
Percutaneous coronary angioplasty (PTCA) (balloon angioplasty of heart)	15,587	20,957	21,448	581,183	488,521	377,475	9,057	10,240	8,104
Insertion, revision, replacement, removal of cardiac pacemaker or cardioverter/defibrillator	28,757	38,023	34,974	66,286	122,847	78,970	1,921	4,667	2,762
Colorectal resection (removal of part of the bowel)	20,241	25,560	23,616	253,780	261,401	234,290	5,244	6,678	5,529
Appendectomy	7,616	9,934	10,657	269,089	273,753	177,550	2,027	2,719	1,897
Cholecystectomy (gall bladder removal)	10,811	13,767	13,327	389,079	379,753	300,245	4,170	5,232	4,006
Hysterectomy	6,790	9,617	10,394	580,019	354,313	184,950	3,910	3,411	1,923
Cesarean section	5,646	6,313	6,150	898,859	1,226,435	1,142,680	4,956	7,750	7,032
Treatment, fracture or dislocation of hip and femur	13,072	18,814	17,286	237,615	248,777	246,135	3,159	4,678	4,255
Arthroplasty knee (knee replacement)	14,357	17,592	16,292	318,854	693,086	723,086	4,551	12,198	11,783
Hip replacement	15,568	18,820	17,079	295,940	437,380	487,625	4,664	8,229	8,328
Spinal fusion	18,119	30,933	28,949	204,320	444,508	413,206	3,614	13,755	11,970
Under 18 Years									
Hospital discharges with an operating room principal procedure[3]	13,831	21,126	28,582	382,455	413,852	297,290	5,112	8,759	8,457
Incision and excision of CNS (a type of brain surgery)	30,026	44,269	47,633	6,352	8,925	7,870	184	396	372
Tonsillectomy and/or adenoidectomy	4,597	6,465	7,897	12,045	13,000	8,635	57	85	69
Small bowel resection (removal of part of the small bowel)	37,710	44,954	60,727	1,712	2,694	1,855	64	120	112
Appendectomy	6,833	9,206	10,336	75,481	79,575	46,745	502	733	483
Cesarean section	6,269	6,718	6,594	23,690	22,582	12,090	134	152	80
Spinal fusion	30,463	56,100	60,000	7,463	10,628	10,995	224	596	658
18 to 44 Years									
Hospital discharges with an operating room principal procedure[3]	9,107	12,588	12,289	2,806,078	2,842,807	2,339,211	25,005	35,784	28,735
Incision and excision of CNS (a type of brain surgery)	26,477	39,120	37,330	19,510	22,908	18,660	497	902	699
Laminectomy	7,643	11,222	14,038	95,687	44,303	27,800	736	498	392
Appendectomy	7,014	9,112	9,519	133,662	116,699	71,470	924	1,064	683
Cholecystectomy (gall bladder removal)	8,855	10,939	10,747	132,538	139,244	102,825	1,127	1,526	1,108
Oophorectomy (removal of one or both ovaries)	6,602	9,584	10,800	38,252	32,130	17,915	255	308	193
Ligation of fallopian tubes ("tying" of fallopian tubes)	4,882	5,546	7,516	75,221	44,524	31,045	346	247	230
Hysterectomy	6,296	8,729	9,481	291,704	149,442	72,870	1,811	1,306	691
Cesarean section	5,628	6,300	6,141	873,231	1,198,961	1,126,890	4,809	7,561	6,925
Treatment, fracture or dislocation of lower extremity (other than hip or femur)	9,702	15,136	17,248	68,015	59,800	45,040	648	904	776
Spinal fusion	17,033	29,044	27,341	73,228	89,655	64,600	1,206	2,605	1,768
45 to 64 Years									
Hospital discharges with an operating room principal procedure[3]	$15,076	$21,513	$21,420	2,435,212	3,085,028	2,636,652	$36,552	$66,262	$56,404
Laminectomy	8,567	12,311	15,482	107,720	80,487	59,585	924	990	927
Heart valve procedures	41,898	54,544	50,655	22,849	28,546	28,045	951	1,558	1,421
Coronary artery bypass graft (CABG)	30,385	40,362	39,934	139,897	73,265	67,165	4,271	2,958	2,682
Percutaneous coronary angioplasty (PTCA)	15,086	20,557	20,751	252,151	224,713	170,935	3,796	4,620	3,550
Insertion, revision, replacement, removal of cardiac pacemaker or cardioverter/defibrillator	35,219	40,063	37,584	15,957	36,456	23,770	558	1,460	893
Colorectal resection	18,207	23,500	22,622	76,604	99,837	90,725	1,422	2,349	2,050
Cholecystectomy	10,197	13,874	13,322	117,432	120,321	97,220	1,198	1,670	1,297
Oophorectomy	7,903	10,736	13,172	21,232	37,253	22,565	168	400	297
Hysterectomy	6,926	9,742	10,369	231,498	164,344	88,465	1,601	1,603	918
Arthroplasty knee (knee replacement)	14,687	17,632	16,404	95,902	291,502	303,150	1,402	5,141	4,973
Hip replacement	16,180	18,471	16,915	65,118	150,253	176,055	1,061	2,774	2,976
Spinal fusion	17,391	29,546	27,210	87,388	218,349	193,710	1,480	6,454	5,272
65 to 74 Years									
Hospital discharges with an operating room principal procedure[3]	16,890	22,719	22,079	1,511,467	1,648,763	1,623,736	25,661	37,391	35,822
Laminectomy	8,975	11,479	14,571	45,976	43,879	36,780	413	503	538
Heart valve procedures	45,656	56,733	50,565	23,236	26,078	29,145	1,052	1,481	1,473
Coronary artery bypass graft (CABG)	33,093	41,966	42,230	112,652	53,818	56,070	3,726	2,258	2,367
Percutaneous coronary angioplasty (PTCA)	15,519	21,035	21,929	166,497	125,005	99,675	2,579	2,629	2,189
Insertion, revision, replacement, removal of cardiac pacemaker or cardioverter/defibrillator	31,418	39,604	36,477	19,096	32,601	20,425	603	1,290	746
Endarterectomy (plaque removal from artery lining of brain, head, neck)	9,044	10,830	10,809	51,292	34,638	30,055	476	375	325
Colorectal resection	20,355	26,106	23,350	63,693	59,112	58,000	1,336	1,539	1,354
Cholecystectomy	11,945	15,967	15,122	65,953	52,412	48,435	801	836	733
Arthroplasty knee	14,623	17,438	16,075	110,961	232,195	264,425	1,607	4,053	4,253
Hip replacement	15,508	18,526	16,729	71,986	106,955	135,840	1,133	1,981	2,273
Spinal fusion	19,151	32,385	29,609	23,419	84,861	100,785	446	2,748	2,986
75 to 84 Years									
Hospital discharges with an operating room principal procedure[3]	17,144	22,844	22,152	1,224,573	1,189,769	1,010,816	21,299	27,126	22,392
Laminectomy	9,684	11,627	14,173	31,059	28,311	21,510	304	329	307
Heart valve procedures	47,093	58,243	52,058	21,004	26,690	30,675	1,001	1,555	1,597
Coronary artery bypass graft (CABG)	35,880	44,789	45,596	68,750	29,874	29,395	2,486	1,339	1,340
Percutaneous coronary angioplasty (PTCA)	16,431	21,714	22,467	111,169	87,441	63,865	1,838	1,899	1,437
Insertion, revision, replacement, removal of cardiac pacemaker or cardioverter/defibrillator	25,771	36,946	33,177	19,975	33,287	19,725	524	1,228	654

Note: Excludes newborn infants.

[1]Data are based on valid operating room procedures. Operating room procedures were identified using the Centers for Medicare & Medicaid Services' Diagnosis Related Groups (DRGs). For DRGs, physician panels identified International Classification of Diseases (ICD-9-CM) procedure codes, which would be performed in operating rooms in most hospitals. Operating room procedures, as defined by DRGs, are classified by the Clinical Classifications Software (CCS) into 1 of 231 clinically meaningful categories. Mean costs per hospitalization are based on the principal procedure as determined by the CCS. The number of discharges is based on the first-listed (principal) major procedure.

[2]Charges (the amount billed by the hospital) were converted to costs using cost-charge ratios from the Centers for Medicare & Medicaid Services. Costs are for the entire hospitalization including the principal procedure. Costs were adjusted to 2010 dollars for inflation using the gross domestic product deflator.

[3]Includes discharges for operating room principal procedures not shown separately.

Table 3-66. Cost of Hospital Discharges with Common Hospital Operating Room Procedures in Nonfederal Community Hospitals, by Age and Selected Principal Procedure, Selected Years, 2000–2014—*Continued*

(Dollars.)

Age and principal operating room procedure[1]	Mean inflation-adjusted cost per hospitalization: 2014 dollars[2]			Number of discharges with operating room principal procedure			Total inflation-adjusted national costs: 2014 dollars (in millions of dollars)[2]		
	2000	2010	2014	2000	2010	2014	2000	2010	2014
Endarterectomy (plaque removal from artery lining of brain, head, neck)	9,395	11,012	11,049	45,337	28,078	23,495	439	309	260
Colorectal resection	22,198	28,167	24,861	62,096	48,800	39,230	1,416	1,372	975
Cholecystectomy	13,689	18,110	16,705	52,448	42,922	33,660	733	777	563
Treatment, fracture or dislocation of hip and femur	12,310	17,392	16,203	73,332	66,038	63,765	930	1,150	1,034
Arthroplasty knee	14,615	17,530	16,188	79,138	133,319	123,855	1,158	2,338	2,006
Hip replacement	15,321	19,155	17,336	92,715	102,563	100,695	1,443	1,964	1,746
Spinal fusion	19,927	32,830	29,844	11,770	36,462	39,065	233	1,197	1,166
85 Years and Over									
Hospital discharges with an operating room principal procedure[3]	$15,718	$20,752	$20,304	382,341	445,658	399,570	$6,104	$9,247	$8,120
Heart valve procedures	49,507	52,561	50,551	2,985	5,639	13,005	147	297	658
Coronary artery bypass graft (CABG)	40,365	52,110	48,287	5,280	2,955	3,170	211	154	153
Percutaneous coronary angioplasty (PTCA)	18,647	22,360	22,746	16,682	23,538	20,930	308	527	476
Insertion, revision, replacement, removal of cardiac pacemaker or cardioverter/defibrillator	15,294	28,712	25,877	7,071	11,702	8,845	111	335	229
Colorectal resection	23,987	30,829	25,933	20,729	18,420	15,005	508	568	389
Cholecystectomy	16,660	19,751	18,071	15,698	16,524	13,485	265	326	243
Treatment, fracture or dislocation of hip and femur	11,986	16,550	15,737	76,900	76,798	77,365	949	1,273	1,219
Arthroplasty knee	14,819	18,543	17,068	10,122	18,713	17,250	151	347	294
Hip replacement	14,899	19,487	17,855	50,005	57,878	56,850	757	1,128	1,015
Amputation of lower extremity (amputation of leg, foot or toe)	13,752	18,157	18,145	12,855	8,243	8,315	179	150	151

Note: Excludes newborn infants.

[1]Data are based on valid operating room procedures. Operating room procedures were identified using the Centers for Medicare & Medicaid Services' Diagnosis Related Groups (DRGs). For DRGs, physician panels identified International Classification of Diseases (ICD-9-CM) procedure codes, which would be performed in operating rooms in most hospitals. Operating room procedures, as defined by DRGs, are classified by the Clinical Classifications Software (CCS) into 1 of 231 clinically meaningful categories. Mean costs per hospitalization are based on the principal procedure as determined by the CCS. The number of discharges is based on the first-listed (principal) major procedure.

[2]Charges (the amount billed by the hospital) were converted to costs using cost-charge ratios from the Centers for Medicare & Medicaid Services. Costs are for the entire hospitalization including the principal procedure. Costs were adjusted to 2010 dollars for inflation using the gross domestic product deflator.

[3]Includes discharges for operating room principal procedures not shown separately.

Table 3-67. Expenses[1] for Health Care and Prescribed Medicine, by Selected Population Characteristics, Selected Years, 1987–2013

(Number, percent, dollars.)

Characteristic	Total expenses[1] Population in millions[3]				Percent of persons with expense				Mean annual expense per person with expense (dollars)[3]			
	1997	2000	2005	2013	1987	2000	2005	2013	1987	2000	2005	2013
All Ages	271.3	278.4	296.2	315.7	84.5	83.5	84.7	84.4	$3,193	$3,653	$4,869	$5,256
Under 65 Years												
Total	237.1	243.6	258.7	269.3	83.2	81.8	82.9	82.5	2,482	2,877	3,864	4,282
Under 6 years....................	23.8	24.1	23.8	23.9	88.9	86.7	88.9	90.3	2,118	1,520	1,851	2,850
6 to 17 years.....................	48.1	48.4	49.7	50.1	80.2	80.0	83.0	85.4	1,380	1,512	1,955	2,044
18 to 44 years...................	108.9	109.0	111.1	112.1	81.5	77.7	77.1	75.4	2,180	2,577	3,436	3,655
45 to 64 years...................	56.3	62.1	74.1	83.2	87.0	88.5	89.7	88.0	4,231	4,819	6,242	6,737
Sex												
Male....................................	118.0	120.9	129.2	133.7	78.8	76.6	77.5	77.6	2,345	2,754	3,489	3,835
Female	119.1	122.7	129.6	135.6	87.5	87.0	88.4	87.3	2,601	2,984	4,191	4,673
Hispanic Origin and Race[4]												
Hispanic or Latino..............	29.4	32.0	41.1	51.0	71.0	69.0	69.3	72.2	1,986	1,960	2,624	2,995
Not Hispanic or Latino												
White.................................	166.2	169.2	166.5	160.4	86.9	86.6	88.1	87.7	2,488	3,011	4,190	4,712
Black or African American.............	31.3	32.1	32.8	34.0	72.2	71.3	76.4	77.2	3,016	3,056	3,935	4,332
Asian.................................	X	X	11.3	14.8	X	X	75.5	73.5	X	X	2,385	2,912
American Indian, Alaska Native, Native Hawaiian, Other Pacific Islander, and multiple race.........	X	X	7.0	9.1	X	X	82.0	83.0	X	X	3,561	4,347
Insurance Status[5]												
Any private insurance.......................	174.0	181.6	180.1	174.3	86.5	85.9	87.9	88.0	2,379	2,741	3,892	4,401
Public insurance only.......................	29.8	29.7	42.2	54.6	82.4	83.6	84.2	85.2	4,006	4,368	4,698	4,777
Uninsured all year..........................	33.3	32.3	36.4	40.3	61.8	57.3	56.8	54.9	1,529	2,029	2,214	2,416
65 Years and Over												
Total....................................	34.2	34.8	37.5	46.5	93.7	95.5	96.7	95.6	7,902	8,306	10,824	10,125
Sex												
Male....................................	14.6	15.0	16.0	20.4	92.0	93.4	95.9	94.6	8,085	8,907	10,591	10,471
Female	19.6	19.8	21.5	26.0	94.9	97.1	97.2	96.4	7,776	7,870	10,994	9,859
Hispanic Origin and Race[4]												
Hispanic or Latino..............	1.7	1.9	2.4	3.6	82.5	92.5	92.0	92.1	7,516	7,454	9,370	8,247
Not Hispanic or Latino												
White.................................	28.8	28.9	30.0	36.1	94.9	95.9	97.3	96.1	7,777	8,432	10,948	10,354
Black or African American.............	2.8	2.9	3.1	4.0	88.5	94.0	94.9	94.6	9,551	7,988	12,968	10,357
Asian.................................	X	X	1.3	1.9	X	X	94.4	93.5	X	X	6,356	6,585
American Indian, Alaska Native, Native Hawaiian, Other Pacific Islander, and multiple race.........	X	X	*	*	X	X	*	*	X	X	*	*
Insurance Status												
Medicare only	8.8	12.0	10.9	16.9	85.9	94.8	96.2	93.3	6,221	7,131	10,465	9,271
Medicare and private insurance	21.7	19.2	20.7	21.9	95.4	96.0	97.8	97.3	7,818	8,517	10,398	9,980
Medicare and other public coverage ...	3.2	3.2	5.5	6.8	94.4	96.3	95.5	96.8	12,154	11,398	13,297	13,176

X = Not applicable.

* = Estimates are considered unreliable. Data preceded by an asterisk have a relative standard error equal to or greater than 30%. Data not shown if based on fewer than 100 sample cases.

[1]Includes expenses for inpatient hospital and physician services, ambulatory physician and nonphysician services, prescribed medicines, home health services, dental services, and other medical equipment, supplies, and services that were purchased or rented during the year. Excludes expenses for over-the-counter medications, phone contacts with health providers, and premiums for health insurance.

[3]Estimates of expenses were converted to 2013 dollars using the Consumer Price Index (all items).

[4]Persons of Hispanic origin may be of any race. Estimates for Asian persons as well as for American Indian, Alaska Native, Native Hawaiian, Other Pacifc Islander, and Multiple Race persons are not available for years prior to 2002 because Asian persons could not be distinguished separately and multiple race information was not collected.

[5]Any private insurance includes individuals with insurance that provided coverage for hospital and physician care at any time during the year, other than Medicare, Medicaid, or other public coverage for hospital or physician services. Public insurance only includes individuals who were not covered by private insurance at any time during the year but were covered by Medicare, Medicaid, other public coverage for hospital or physician services, and/or CHAMPUS/CHAMPVA (TRICARE) at any point during the year. Uninsured includes persons not covered by either private or public insurance throughout the entire year or period of eligibility for the survey. Individuals with Indian Health Service coverage only are considered uninsured.

Table 3-67. Expenses[1] for Health Care and Prescribed Medicine, by Selected Population Characteristics, Selected Years, 1987–2013—*Continued*

(Number, percent, dollars.)

	Prescribed medicine expenses[2]							
	Percent of persons with expense				Mean annual expense per person with expense (dollars)[3]			
	1987	2000	2005	2013	1987	2000	2005	2013
All Ages	57.3	62.3	63.1	60.7	$189	$371	$528	$265
Under 65 Years								
Total..	54.0	58.5	59.1	55.6	139	269	392	217
Under 6 years.................................	61.8	56.9	54.5	48.6	49	50	72	28
6 to 17 years.................................	44.3	46.2	47.1	43.2	93	95	118	84
18 to 44 years...............................	51.3	56.0	54.9	50.6	109	205	275	155
45 to 64 years...............................	65.3	73.3	74.8	71.8	265	508	712	361
Sex								
Male..	46.5	51.3	52.0	49.5	129	236	362	214
Female...	61.4	65.6	66.1	61.6	147	295	416	220
Hispanic Origin and Race[4]								
Hispanic or Latino..........................	41.6	45.0	44.2	42.9	101	198	275	142
Not Hispanic or Latino								
White	57.7	63.8	65.5	61.9	146	289	427	248
Black or African American..............	44.1	47.6	51.1	52.0	124	222	329	160
Asian..	X	X	42.0	40.6	X	X	221	193
American Indian, Alaska Native, Native Hawaiian, Other Pacific Islander, and multiple race.........	X	X	59.7	52.2	X	X	422	160
Insurance Status[5]								
Any private insurance......................	56.5	61.6	63.4	59.6	144	231	370	224
Public insurance only......................	56.5	62.4	59.4	56.9	96	385	378	114
Uninsured all year	35.1	37.6	37.3	36.1	153	446	604	388
65 Years and Over								
Total..	81.6	88.3	91.1	90.3	434	843	1,135	434
Sex								
Male..	78.0	83.9	89.8	89.8	404	632	885	438
Female...	84.0	91.5	92.1	90.7	453	989	1,316	432
Hispanic Origin and Race[4]								
Hispanic or Latino..........................	74.7	83.9	85.8	84.4	*575	710	966	246
Not Hispanic or Latino								
White	82.3	89.0	91.9	91.3	443	874	1,179	468
Black or African American..............	79.5	85.3	90.2	89.5	340	720	1,069	355
Asian..	X	X	84.8	84.4	X	X	617	247
American Indian, Alaska Native, Native Hawaiian, Other Pacific Islander, and multiple race.........	X	X	*	*	X	X	*	*
Insurance Status								
Medicare only	70.6	87.7	90.0	88.6	480	1,007	1,471	423
Medicare and private insurance	83.4	89.0	92.6	91.9	452	780	1,085	518
Medicare and other public coverage	88.2	88.5	90.3	91.9	163	668	681	211

X = Not applicable.

* = Estimates are considered unreliable. Data preceded by an asterisk have a relative standard error equal to or greater than 30%. Data not shown if based on fewer than 100 sample cases.

[1]Includes expenses for inpatient hospital and physician services, ambulatory physician and nonphysician services, prescribed medicines, home health services, dental services, and other medical equipment, supplies, and services that were purchased or rented during the year. Excludes expenses for over-the-counter medications, phone contacts with health providers, and premiums for health insurance.

[2]Includes persons in the civilian noninstitutionalized population for all or part of the year. Expenditures for persons in this population for only part of the year are restricted to those incurred during periods of eligibility (e.g., expenses incurred during periods of institu- tionalization and military service are not included in estimates).

[3]Estimates of expenses were converted to 2013 dollars using the Consumer Price Index (all items).

[4]Persons of Hispanic origin may be of any race. Estimates for Asian persons as well as for American Indian, Alaska Native, Native Hawaiian, Other Pacifc Islander, and Multiple Race persons are not available for years prior to 2002 because Asian persons could not be distinguished separately and multiple race information was not collected.

[5]Any private insurance includes individuals with insurance that provided coverage for hospital and physician care at any time during the year, other than Medicare, Medicaid, or other public coverage for hospital or physician services. Public insurance only includes indi- viduals who were not covered by private insurance at any time during the year but were covered by Medicare, Medicaid, other public coverage for hospital or physician services, and/or CHAMPUS/CHAMPVA (TRICARE) at any point during the year. Uninsured includes persons not covered by either private or public insurance throughout the entire year or period of eligibility for the survey. Individuals with Indian Health Service coverage only are considered uninsured.

Table 3-68. Out-of-Pocket Health Care Expenses Among Persons with Medical Expenses, by Age, Selected Years 1987–2013

(Percent.)

Age and year	Percent of persons with expenses	Amount paid out of pocket among persons with expenses[1]						
		Total	$0	$1 to 99	$100 to 499	$500 to 999	$1,000 to 1,999	$2,000+
All Ages								
1987	84.5	100.0	10.4	19.9	36.6	15.3	10.0	7.7
1997	84.1	100.0	8.5	26.1	35.1	14.3	9.4	6.6
1998	83.8	100.0	7.7	26.6	35.6	14.0	9.5	6.5
1999	84.3	100.0	7.4	27.1	34.2	14.5	9.5	7.3
2000	83.5	100.0	6.9	26.6	34.4	14.4	9.8	7.8
2001	85.4	100.0	7.1	24.6	33.8	14.6	11.0	8.8
2002	85.2	100.0	7.8	23.4	32.5	15.1	11.9	9.4
2003	85.6	100.0	7.6	21.9	32.1	15.8	12.1	10.4
2004	84.7	100.0	8.8	22.1	31.2	14.9	12.0	11.1
2005	84.7	100.0	8.7	21.2	31.5	15.8	11.9	10.8
2006	84.6	100.0	8.7	21.4	31.6	15.8	12.2	10.2
2007	84.9	100.0	9.8	22.6	31.6	15.3	11.5	9.2
2008	84.4	100.0	9.9	22.9	32.1	14.8	11.2	9.1
2009	84.6	100.0	11.0	22.3	31.3	15.4	11.2	8.7
2010	84.6	100.0	12.6	22.7	31.0	14.2	10.8	8.7
2011	84.6	100.0	12.1	22.2	31.8	14.8	11.0	8.2
2012	84.7	100.0	12.2	23.3	31.4	13.9	10.6	8.6
2013	84.4	100.0	13.4	22.0	31.7	14.0	10.3	8.7
Under 6 Years								
1987	88.9	100.0	19.2	28.0	39.8	8.5	2.5	2.0
1997	88.0	100.0	20.0	44.5	28.7	4.0	2.2	0.7
1998	87.6	100.0	17.4	48.0	28.7	4.0	1.5	0.3
1999	87.9	100.0	17.7	50.7	26.0	4.2	0.7	0.7
2000	86.7	100.0	16.7	51.4	25.9	4.1	1.4	0.5
2001	88.8	100.0	18.5	49.0	27.9	3.0	1.3	0.3
2002	88.8	100.0	21.5	42.8	28.8	4.9	1.4	0.5
2003	91.3	100.0	20.6	42.4	29.6	5.4	1.4	0.6
2004	90.0	100.0	26.0	40.5	26.0	4.8	2.1	0.7
2005	88.9	100.0	27.2	36.6	27.5	6.1	1.9	0.7
2006	89.2	100.0	27.1	39.3	26.4	4.3	1.9	1.0
2007	88.7	100.0	30.2	36.5	24.7	5.1	2.0	1.4
2008	88.8	100.0	31.4	36.1	25.9	3.9	1.9	0.8
2009	88.7	100.0	34.2	33.7	24.1	5.3	1.9	*0.8
2010	88.9	100.0	40.0	33.8	21.1	3.2	1.5	*0.5
2011	89.6	100.0	40.1	31.5	22.5	3.9	1.4	*0.7
2012	88.8	100.0	38.4	35.1	19.8	3.9	2.4	*0.4
2013	90.3	100.0	41.4	29.6	21.1	3.4	2.6	2.0
6 to 17 Years								
1987	80.2	100.0	15.5	27.4	37.4	9.0	5.7	5.0
1997	81.7	100.0	16.5	36.2	32.1	7.5	3.6	4.1
1998	80.6	100.0	16.3	36.3	32.7	7.9	3.9	3.0
1999	81.5	100.0	15.0	38.0	31.6	7.9	3.8	3.8
2000	80.0	100.0	14.7	37.2	33.0	6.5	4.1	4.5
2001	83.2	100.0	15.0	36.5	32.3	7.3	3.8	5.2
2002	83.6	100.0	16.6	35.8	31.8	7.9	3.7	4.3
2003	84.1	100.0	16.1	32.8	33.1	8.9	5.4	3.8
2004	83.9	100.0	18.7	33.8	30.2	8.3	4.7	4.4
2005	83.0	100.0	18.6	32.4	31.1	9.2	4.6	4.0
2006	83.6	100.0	19.2	32.8	29.9	8.7	4.1	5.3
2007	84.0	100.0	21.6	33.0	29.4	7.6	4.2	4.1
2008	82.5	100.0	22.4	33.0	28.3	7.4	4.0	4.9
2009	85.3	100.0	24.5	30.4	28.5	7.6	4.9	4.1
2010	84.4	100.0	28.4	29.8	26.7	7.3	3.3	4.4
2011	84.9	100.0	28.5	30.2	26.1	7.1	3.7	4.4
2012	85.7	100.0	29.0	28.2	26.8	6.4	3.7	6.0
2013	85.4	100.0	30.8	26.9	26.2	7.8	3.9	4.4
18 to 44 Years								
1987	81.5	100.0	10.1	22.0	39.4	14.9	8.3	5.4
1997	78.3	100.0	7.3	28.4	39.4	14.0	6.9	3.9
1998	78.0	100.0	6.4	29.1	40.3	13.1	7.0	4.1
1999	78.9	100.0	6.4	29.6	39.2	13.3	7.1	4.4
2000	77.7	100.0	5.8	29.4	39.8	13.8	6.9	4.4
2001	79.3	100.0	6.0	26.4	39.7	15.1	8.4	4.5
2002	78.5	100.0	6.7	26.3	38.3	14.6	8.8	5.3
2003	79.0	100.0	6.4	24.5	38.8	15.4	9.2	5.7
2004	77.0	100.0	7.2	24.8	37.6	14.8	9.4	6.2
2005	77.1	100.0	7.0	24.8	37.9	15.0	9.0	6.2
2006	76.9	100.0	6.8	24.2	38.3	15.2	8.9	6.5

*Estimates are considered unreliable. Data preceded by an asterisk have a relative standard error equal to or greater than 30 percent.
[1]Estimates of expenses were converted to 2013 dollars using the Consumer Price Index (all items).

Table 3-68. Out-of-Pocket Health Care Expenses Among Persons with Medical Expenses, by Age, Selected Years 1987–2013—Continued

(Percent.)

Age and year	Percent of persons with expenses	Amount paid out of pocket among persons with expenses[1]						
		Total	$0	$1 to 99	$100 to 499	$500 to 999	$1,000 to 1,999	$2,000+
2007	77.3	100.0	7.7	26.7	37.1	14.2	8.8	5.5
2008	76.5	100.0	7.9	27.1	36.6	14.0	8.3	6.1
2009	76.2	100.0	8.5	25.8	35.9	15.1	8.8	5.9
2010	76.0	100.0	9.5	28.0	36.2	13.1	7.9	5.4
2011	75.6	100.0	8.7	26.7	37.6	13.2	8.1	5.6
2012	75.5	100.0	9.6	28.5	35.1	12.5	8.3	6.0
2013	75.4	100.0	10.6	27.3	36.7	11.8	8.1	5.5
45 to 64 Years								
1987	87.0	100.0	5.7	12.5	35.7	20.9	14.7	10.5
1997	89.2	100.0	3.4	16.8	36.3	19.6	14.8	9.2
1998	89.2	100.0	2.9	17.2	36.3	19.7	14.5	9.5
1999	88.9	100.0	2.7	16.6	35.9	20.2	14.7	9.9
2000	88.5	100.0	2.6	15.7	35.2	20.4	15.1	11.0
2001	89.9	100.0	2.4	14.3	33.8	19.9	17.2	12.4
2002	90.0	100.0	2.3	14.0	31.2	21.1	18.3	13.1
2003	89.6	100.0	2.4	12.9	29.9	21.2	18.1	15.6
2004	88.9	100.0	2.7	13.1	30.8	20.8	17.3	15.2
2005	89.7	100.0	2.4	12.9	29.5	21.7	18.6	14.8
2006	89.2	100.0	2.7	12.9	30.4	21.1	17.9	15.0
2007	89.2	100.0	2.9	14.3	30.6	21.2	17.0	14.1
2008	89.1	100.0	2.8	15.2	33.2	20.0	16.4	12.3
2009	88.4	100.0	3.4	15.9	32.5	19.0	16.6	12.6
2010	89.2	100.0	4.0	16.3	32.1	18.9	15.6	13.1
2011	88.8	100.0	3.7	16.6	32.2	19.4	16.2	11.9
2012	88.9	100.0	3.8	17.7	33.3	17.8	15.4	11.9
2013	88.0	100.0	4.4	17.5	32.4	18.0	14.9	12.8
65 to 74 Years								
1987	92.8	100.0	5.3	10.0	27.3	21.8	19.4	16.2
1997	94.6	100.0	3.2	10.7	31.6	23.6	17.0	14.0
1998	94.3	100.0	2.0	9.8	33.6	21.6	19.5	13.6
1999	95.3	100.0	1.4	10.0	27.4	23.8	19.4	17.9
2000	94.7	100.0	1.5	10.0	27.2	22.1	21.0	18.3
2001	95.6	100.0	1.5	9.9	27.0	21.5	20.6	19.5
2002	96.1	100.0	1.8	6.3	25.4	21.4	24.1	21.1
2003	95.3	100.0	1.7	6.5	21.0	23.8	23.3	23.8
2004	96.6	100.0	1.5	8.0	23.2	19.3	20.6	27.3
2005	95.9	100.0	1.7	6.5	24.8	20.8	21.5	24.6
2006	95.7	100.0	1.7	7.3	23.7	22.0	25.6	19.7
2007	95.8	100.0	2.7	8.8	28.9	23.0	20.8	15.9
2008	95.8	100.0	1.5	9.6	28.8	22.0	20.4	17.7
2009	95.7	100.0	2.0	11.6	28.3	24.2	18.7	15.2
2010	95.8	100.0	2.4	9.1	28.8	22.5	21.3	15.8
2011	96.2	100.0	2.6	9.8	30.1	23.9	20.0	13.6
2012	95.5	100.0	1.9	12.0	32.0	21.6	17.8	14.6
2013	94.9	100.0	2.8	11.3	31.1	22.6	18.0	14.2
75 Years and Over								
1987	95.1	100.0	5.6	7.6	24.7	20.0	19.7	22.4
1997	95.8	100.0	2.4	9.8	27.5	19.5	21.2	19.7
1998	96.3	100.0	3.0	9.6	26.6	20.3	21.0	19.4
1999	95.3	100.0	2.7	8.9	26.3	22.4	19.7	20.0
2000	96.5	100.0	2.6	10.0	25.2	21.5	19.8	20.9
2001	97.0	100.0	1.7	7.0	22.1	19.5	23.0	26.7
2002	96.5	100.0	2.2	6.2	20.1	18.5	24.9	28.2
2003	97.5	100.0	1.9	6.2	19.0	19.5	23.5	29.9
2004	97.7	100.0	1.8	6.1	19.2	16.9	24.8	31.1
2005	97.4	100.0	1.6	6.3	21.2	19.7	19.7	31.4
2006	97.6	100.0	1.7	6.8	22.1	22.8	24.0	22.6
2007	97.3	100.0	1.9	8.7	25.9	19.8	21.8	21.9
2008	97.6	100.0	1.9	10.0	25.9	20.5	22.0	19.7
2009	97.5	100.0	2.7	10.1	24.3	23.4	19.7	19.9
2010	97.0	100.0	3.0	9.7	27.6	19.9	22.1	17.7
2011	96.7	100.0	2.4	11.1	29.7	22.1	19.3	15.5
2012	97.4	100.0	2.3	11.6	30.0	22.8	18.1	15.2
2013	96.5	100.0	3.4	10.2	31.5	22.6	15.3	17.0

*Estimates are considered unreliable. Data preceded by an asterisk have a relative standard error equal to or greater than 30 percent.
[1]Estimates of expenses were converted to 2013 dollars using the Consumer Price Index (all items).

Table 3-69. Expenditures for Health Services and Supplies and Percent Distribution, by Sponsor, Selected Years, 1987–2013

(Dollars, percent.)

Type of sponsor	1987	1990	1995	2000	2009	2010	2012	2013
NATIONAL HEALTH EXPENDITURES (AMOUNT IN BILLIONS)	$519.1	$724.3	$1,027.4	$1,378.0	$2,505.8	$2,604.1	$2,817.3	$2,919.1
Business, Households, and Other Private Revenues	354.0	488.2	642.3	888.4	1,415.2			
Private business	122.3	178.3	243.7	346.5	530.3	533.7	587.3	610.9
Employer contribution to private health insurance premiums[1]	84.3	129.5	176.3	255.1	411.8	413.5	453.9	471.1
Employer contribution to Medicare hospital insurance trust fund[2]	24.6	29.4	43.1	62.3	77.9	79.7	88.0	91.7
Workers compensation and temporary disability insurance and worksite health care	13.4	19.3	24.3	29.1	40.6	40.5	45.4	48.2
Household	189.9	253.0	318.9	434.0	717.3	738.3	801.5	823.8
Employee contribution to private health insurance premiums and individual policy premiums[3]	44.0	68.5	100.3	133.6	260.7	270.8	293.8	300.2
Employee and self-employment contributions and voluntary premiums paid to Medicare hospital insurance trust fund[4]	29.5	35.7	56.0	82.6	108.4	112.1	125.5	124.8
Premiums paid by individuals to Medicare supplementary medical insurance trust fund[5]	6.2	10.2	16.4	16.3	47.2	49.2	53.4	59.4
Out-of-pocket health spending	110.2	138.6	146.2	201.5	300.9	306.2	328.8	339.4
Other private revenues	41.9	56.9	79.7	107.9	167.6	174.6	203.9	218.1
Governments	165.1	236.1	385.2	489.6	1,090.6	1,157.5	1,224.6	1,266.3
Federal government	86.2	125.3	217.3	261.9	682.8	733.1	731.5	757.5
Employer contributions to private health insurance premiums	4.9	9.9	11.4	14.3	26.8	28.5	31.0	32.4
Employer contributions to Medicare hospital insurance trust fund	1.7	2.0	2.3	2.7	3.9	4.1	4.1	4.0
Adjusted Medicare[6]	17.4	27.7	57.6	49.2	236.0	250.2	266.2	274.0
Health program expenditures (excluding Medicare)	62.2	85.8	146.0	195.8	416.1	450.3	430.2	447.1
Medicaid[7]	28.2	43.3	87.9	119.4	255.5	275.9	251.5	267.1
Other programs[8]	34.0	42.5	58.1	76.4	160.6	174.5	178.8	180.0
State and local government	78.9	110.8	167.9	227.7	407.9	424.5	493.1	508.8
Employer contributions to private health insurance premiums[9]	16.0	26.4	38.9	56.9	127.8	142.9	153.5	156.0
Employer contributions to Medicare hospital insurance trust fund	3.1	4.1	5.6	7.5	11.3	11.2	11.3	11.4
Health expenditures by program	59.8	80.3	123.3	163.4	268.8	270.4	328.3	341.5
Medicaid[7]	22.7	31.5	60.3	85.3	130.8	135.0	185.5	196.3
Other programs[10]	37.1	48.8	63.1	78.0	138.0	135.3	142.8	145.2
PERCENT DISTRIBUTION								
NATIONAL HEALTH EXPENDITURES	100.0	100.0	100.0	100.0	100.0	100.0	100.0	100.0
Business, Households, and Other Private Revenues	68.2	67.4	62.5	64.5	56.5	55.6	56.5	56.6
Private business	23.6	24.6	23.7	25.1	21.2	20.5	20.8	20.9
Employer contribution to private health insurance premiums[1]	16.2	17.9	17.2	18.5	16.4	15.9	16.1	16.1
Employer contribution to Medicare hospital insurance trust fund[2]	4.7	4.1	4.2	4.5	3.1	3.1	3.1	3.1
Workers compensation and temporary disability insurance and worksite health care	2.6	2.7	2.4	2.1	1.6	1.6	1.6	1.7
Household	36.6	34.9	31.0	31.5	28.6	28.4	28.4	28.2
Employee contribution to private health insurance premiums and individual policy premiums[3]	8.5	9.5	9.8	9.7	10.4	10.4	10.4	10.3
Employee and self-employment contributions and voluntary premiums paid to Medicare hospital insurance trust fund[4]	5.7	4.9	5.5	6.0	4.3	4.3	4.5	4.3
Premiums paid by individuals to Medicare supplementary medical insurance trust fund[5]	1.2	1.4	1.6	1.2	1.9	1.9	1.9	2.0
Out-of-pocket health spending	21.2	19.1	14.2	14.6	12.0	11.8	11.7	11.6
Other private revenues	8.1	7.9	7.8	7.8	6.7	6.7	7.2	7.5
Governments	31.8	32.6	37.5	35.5	43.5	44.4	43.5	43.4
Federal government	16.6	17.3	21.2	19.0	27.2	28.2	26.0	25.9
Employer contributions to private health insurance premiums	0.9	1.4	1.1	1.0	1.1	1.1	1.1	1.1
Employer contributions to Medicare hospital insurance trust fund	0.3	0.3	0.2	0.2	0.2	0.2	0.1	0.1
Adjusted Medicare[6]	3.4	3.8	5.6	3.6	9.4	9.6	9.4	9.4
Health program expenditures (excluding Medicare)	12.0	11.8	14.2	14.2	16.6	17.3	15.3	15.3
Medicaid[7]	5.4	6.0	8.6	8.7	10.2	10.6	8.9	9.2
Other programs[8]	6.5	5.9	5.7	5.5	6.4	6.7	6.3	6.2
State and local government	15.2	15.3	16.3	16.5	16.3	16.3	17.5	17.4
Employer contributions to private health insurance premiums[9]	3.1	3.6	3.8	4.1	5.1	5.5	5.4	5.3
Employer contributions to Medicare hospital insurance trust fund	0.6	0.6	0.5	0.5	0.5	0.4	0.4	0.4
Health expenditures by program								
Medicaid[7]	4.4	4.3	5.9	6.2	5.2	5.2	6.6	6.7
Other programs[10]	7.1	6.7	6.1	5.7	5.5	5.2	5.1	5.0

[1]Excludes Medicare Retiree Drug Subsidy (RDS) payments to private plans beginning in 2006, small-business tax credits beginning in 2010 and Early Retirement Reinsurance Program (ERRP) payments for 2010–2011.
[2]Includes one-half of self-employment contribution to the Medicare Hospital Insurance (HI) Trust Fund.
[3]Excludes government-subsidized Consolidated Omnibus Budget Reconciliation Act (COBRA) payments in 2009–2011.
[4]Includes one-half of self-employment contribution to Medicare HI Trust Fund and trust fund revenues from the income taxation of Social Security benefits.
[5]Includes premiums paid for the Pre-Existing Condition Insurance Plan (PCIP) beginning in 2010.
[6]Federal government Medicare expenditures equal Trust Fund interest income and Federal general revenue contributions to Medicare less the net change in Trust Fund balances. Includes Medicare RDS paid to private and state and local government employer plans beginning in 2006. Excludes Part D state phase-down payments to Medicare beginning in 2006 and Medicare premium buy-in programs by Medicaid for people eligible for both Medicaid and Medicare (dual eligibles).
[7]Includes Medicare Premium buy-in programs by Medicaid for people eligible for both Medicaid and Medicare.
[8]Includes maternal and child health, vocational rehabilitation, Substance Abuse and Mental Health Services Administration, Indian Health Service, federal workers' compensation, and other federal programs, public health activities, Department of Defense, Department of Veterans Affairs, Children's Health Insurance Program (CHIP), and investment (research, structures and equipment). Also includes government-subsidized COBRA payments in 2009–2011, small business tax credits beginning in 2006, and ERRP payments in 2010–2011. Excludes premiums paid for the Pre-Existing Condition Insurance Plan (PCIP) premiums beginning in 2010.
[9]Excludes Medicare RDS payments to state and local government employer plans beginning in 2006 and ERRP payments in 2010–2011.
[10]Includes maternal and child health, vocational rehabilitation, general assistance, school health, CHIP, public health activities, other state and local programs, investment (research, structures and equipment). Also includes Part D state phase-down payments to Medicare beginning in 2006.

Table 3-70. Department of Veterans Affairs Health Care Expenditures and Use, and Persons Treated, by Selected Characteristics, Selected Fiscal Years, 2000–2015

(Dollars; numbers in thousands; percent.)

Type of expenditure and use	2000	2003	2005	2006	2007	2008	2009	2010	2011	2012	2013	2014	2015
All Expenditures (Amount in Millions)[1]	$19,327	$25,647	$30,291	$31,909	$34,025	$38,282	$42,955	$47,280	$50,575	$51,880	$54,738	$58,010	$64,688
Percent Distribution													
All services	100.0	100.0	100.0	100.0	100.0	100.0	100.0	100.0	100.0	100.0	100.0	100.0	100.0
Inpatient hospital	37.3	32.2	24.3	24.0	24.0	23.5	22.7	21.4	20.6	20.1	19.8	19.8	18.4
Outpatient care	45.7	49.5	53.4	55.2	53.5	53.2	53.5	52.5	52.6	53.8	53.2	55.5	59.6
Nursing home care	8.2	8.1	8.4	8.2	8.3	8.1	7.8	7.4	7.2	7.3	7.0	7.0	6.4
All other[2]	8.8	10.2	13.9	12.6	14.2	15.2	16.0	18.8	19.6	18.8	20.0	17.7	15.6
Health Care Use													
Inpatient hospital discharges[3]	579	588	614	601	607	622	640	656	653	646	632	619	592
Outpatient visits[4]	38,370	49,760	57,169	59,132	62,234	66,484	73,969	79,457	83,146	87,370	90,226	93,852	101,791
Nursing home discharges[5]	91	93	61	59	63	64	65	67	63	67	69	68	68
Inpatients[6]	417	443	488	467	477	492	512	532	540	546	545	558	566
Percent Distribution													
Total	100.0	100.0	100.0	100.0	100.0	100.0	100.0	100.0	100.0	100.0	100.0	100.0	100.0
Veterans with service-connected disability	34.4	36.2	37.6	38.8	39.9	41.1	42.6	43.5	44.9	46.5	48.3	50.0	52.0
Veterans without service-connected disability	64.7	62.9	61.5	60.2	59.1	58.0	56.4	55.6	54.3	52.6	50.8	49.1	47.2
Low income	41.7	40.8	39.9	37.9	36.9	35.4	34.8	34.6	33.4	32.1	30.4	28.8	28.2
Veterans receiving aid and attendance or housebound benefits or who are catastrophically disabled	16.0	13.5	12.1	11.6	11.3	11.1	10.5	10.1	9.8	9.6	9.4	9.0	8.3
Veterans receiving medical care subject to copayments[7]	5.2	8.0	8.6	9.7	9.8	10.0	9.5	9.3	9.3	9.2	9.3	9.6	9.1
Other and unknown[8]	1.8	0.6	1.0	1.0	1.0	1.6	1.6	1.6	1.7	1.7	1.7	1.6	1.5
Nonveterans	0.9	0.8	0.9	0.9	0.9	0.9	1.0	0.9	0.9	0.9	0.9	0.9	0.9
Outpatients[6]	3,657	4,715	5,077	5,180	5,221	5,291	5,439	5,631	5,789	5,903	6,009	6,176	6,296
Percent Distribution													
Total	100.0	100.0	100.0	100.0	100.0	100.0	100.0	100.0	100.0	100.0	100.0	100.0	100.0
Veterans with service-connected disability	30.7	30.3	31.6	32.4	33.8	34.7	37.1	38.6	39.8	41.7	44.0	45.8	47.6
Veterans without service-connected disability	60.8	63.4	62.7	62.0	60.8	59.7	57.2	56.4	55.1	53.3	51.1	49.0	46.9
Low income	37.6	32.7	31.8	30.3	28.9	27.2	25.9	25.7	24.9	24.0	22.6	21.3	21.0
Veterans receiving aid and attendance or housebound benefits or who are catastrophically disabled	3.8	3.4	3.5	3.4	3.5	3.5	3.4	3.4	3.3	3.2	3.2	3.1	2.9
Veterans receiving medical care subject to copayments[7]	15.4	26.1	25.4	25.7	25.5	25.2	23.8	23.0	22.3	21.4	20.7	20.1	18.8
Other and unknown[8]	4.0	1.1	2.0	2.6	3.0	3.8	4.0	4.3	4.6	4.6	4.6	4.5	4.2
Nonveterans	8.5	6.3	5.7	5.6	5.4	5.7	5.7	5.1	5.1	5.1	4.9	5.3	5.5

[1]Health care expenditures exclude construction, medical administration, and miscellaneous operating expenses at Department of Veterans Affairs headquarters.
[2]Includes miscellaneous benefits and services, contract hospitals, education and training, subsidies to state veterans hospitals, nursing homes and residential rehabilitation treatment programs (formerly domiciliaries), and the Civilian Health and Medical Program of the Department of Veterans Affairs.
[3]Discharges from medicine, surgery, psychiatry, rehabilitation medicine, spinal cord, and neurology units. Starting with FY2005 data, includes domiciliary care. Does not include long-term stays.
[4]Hospital outpatient care. Includes the following services: physicians, laboratory tests, home-based primary care, or outpatient fee-basis care.
[5]Includes VA-covered state nursing home veteran patients.
[6]Individuals receiving services. Individuals with multiple discharges or visits are only counted once in the inpatient or outpatient category. The inpatient and outpatient totals are not additive because most inpatients are also treated as outpatients.
[7]Includes veterans who receive medical care subject to copayments according to income level, based on financial means testing.
[8]Includes expenditures for services for veterans who were prisoners of war, exposed to Agent Orange, and other. Veterans reporting Agent Orange exposure but not treated for it were means tested and placed in the low income or other group depending on income.

HEALTH INSURANCE

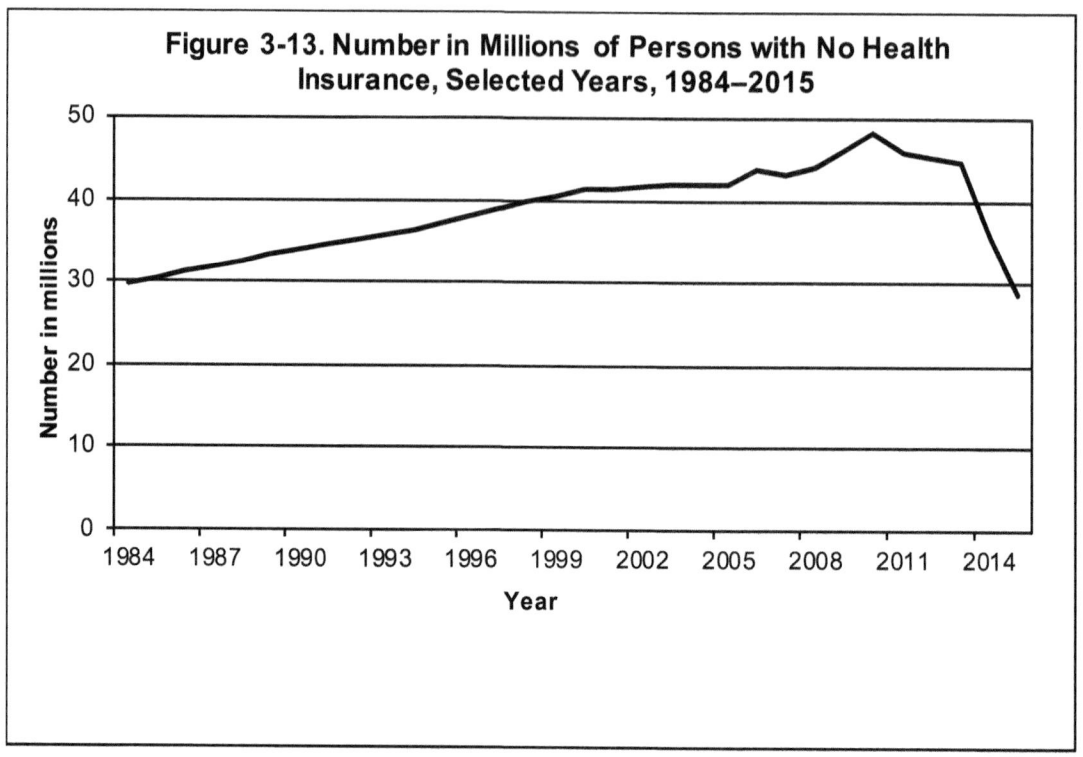

Figure 3-13. Number in Millions of Persons with No Health Insurance, Selected Years, 1984–2015

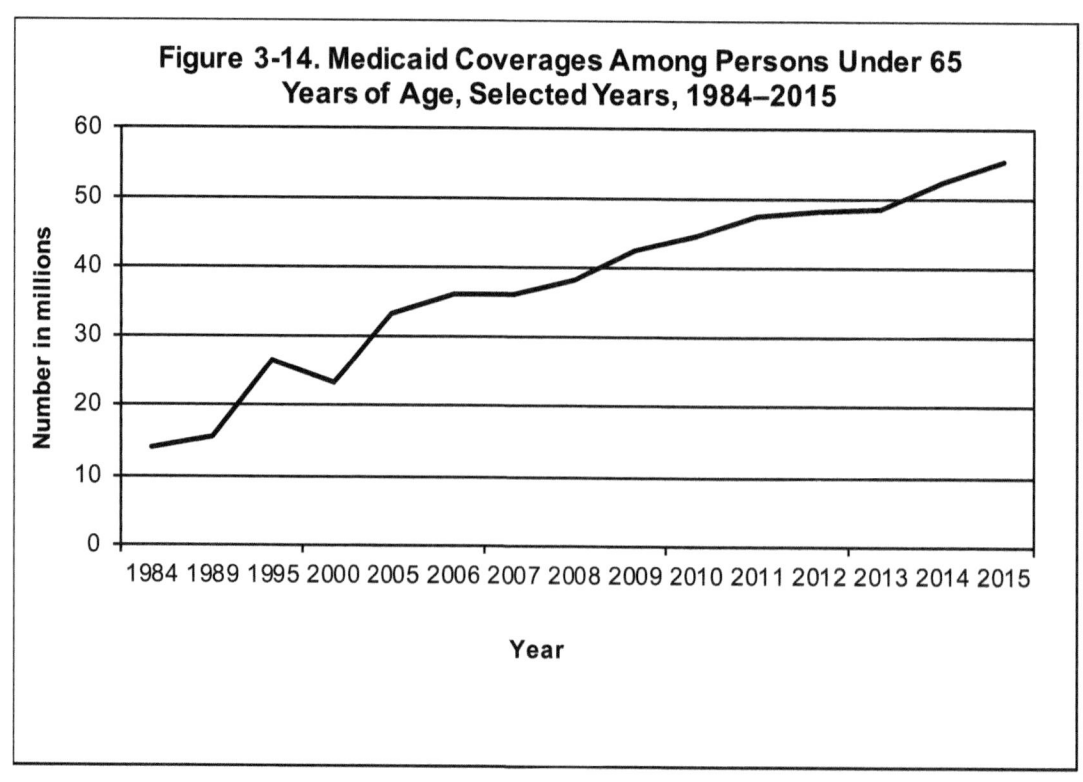

Figure 3-14. Medicaid Coverages Among Persons Under 65 Years of Age, Selected Years, 1984–2015

Table 3-71. Private Health Insurance[1] Coverage Among Persons Under 65 Years of Age, by Selected Characteristics, Selected Years, 1984–2015

(Numbers in millions; percent.)

Characteristic	1984[2]	1989[2]	1995[2]	2000[3]	2005	2006	2007	2008	2009	2010	2011	2012	2013	2014	2015
Total (number in millions)[4]	157.5	162.7	164.2	174.0	174.7	171.2	174.1	171.9	166.7	163.9	164.5	164.9	165.3	170.7	176.6
Total (percent of population)[4]	76.8	75.9	71.3	71.5	68.2	66.3	66.8	65.6	63.3	61.7	61.8	61.8	61.8	63.7	65.5
Age															
Under 19 years	72.6	71.9	65.4	66.7	62.3	59.5	59.9	58.6	56.1	54.3	53.9	53.6	53.5	54.1	55.0
Under 6 years	68.1	67.9	59.5	62.7	56.6	54.7	54.1	53.2	50.1	48.3	47.8	48.4	47.3	50.2	51.0
6 to 18 years	74.8	73.9	68.3	68.5	64.9	61.7	62.6	61.1	59.0	57.2	56.9	56.0	56.3	55.9	56.7
Under 18 years	72.6	71.8	65.2	66.6	62.1	59.4	59.8	58.4	55.8	54.1	53.7	53.4	53.2	53.7	54.6
6 to 17 years	74.9	74.0	68.3	68.5	64.7	61.7	62.6	61.1	58.8	57.2	56.7	55.8	56.0	55.4	56.2
18 to 64 years	78.6	77.6	73.9	73.5	70.7	69.1	69.5	68.5	66.2	64.7	65.0	65.1	65.1	67.4	69.7
18 to 44 years	76.5	75.5	70.9	70.5	66.6	65.0	65.5	64.4	61.7	60.0	60.9	61.4	61.8	64.3	66.8
18 to 24 years	67.4	64.5	60.8	60.3	58.0	57.0	59.0	56.2	54.4	52.3	57.2	58.1	59.0	62.0	64.8
19 to 25 years	67.4	63.8	60.1	59.1	56.3	56.1	57.9	55.8	53.0	51.8	56.9	58.1	58.9	62.2	65.5
25 to 34 years	77.4	75.9	70.1	70.1	65.1	63.0	63.5	62.7	60.0	58.7	58.6	58.7	59.0	62.0	65.1
35 to 44 years	83.9	82.7	77.7	77.0	73.7	72.0	71.7	71.7	68.4	66.9	66.0	66.7	67.0	68.6	70.0
45 to 64 years	83.3	82.5	80.1	78.7	76.9	75.2	75.5	74.3	72.6	71.3	70.6	70.0	69.5	71.7	73.6
45 to 54 years	83.3	83.4	80.9	80.0	77.4	75.1	75.4	74.8	72.6	70.9	70.1	69.6	69.8	71.6	74.1
55 to 64 years	83.3	81.6	79.0	76.7	76.2	75.4	75.5	73.6	72.6	71.8	71.2	70.4	69.1	71.7	73.1
Sex															
Male	77.3	76.1	71.6	71.6	68.0	65.9	66.4	65.3	62.9	61.1	61.4	61.8	61.9	63.8	65.4
Female	76.2	75.7	70.9	71.3	68.4	66.7	67.1	65.9	63.7	62.4	62.2	61.9	61.7	63.5	65.6
Sex and Marital Status[5]															
Male															
Married	85.0	84.2	80.2	81.5	79.6	78.1	78.1	77.7	75.8	75.1	74.5	74.9	74.8	77.1	78.3
Divorced, separated, widowed	65.5	64.6	62.4	62.2	56.7	55.4	55.8	56.0	52.9	50.6	50.5	51.0	50.9	54.0	56.6
Never married	71.3	68.3	65.4	63.8	60.2	57.8	59.8	57.9	54.9	52.5	55.1	54.7	55.8	58.2	60.6
Female															
Married	83.8	83.5	79.3	81.0	79.3	78.6	78.4	77.7	76.7	75.6	75.1	75.0	74.3	75.9	78.0
Divorced, separated, widowed	63.1	63.6	61.7	63.2	59.9	56.3	57.0	56.3	54.2	53.9	52.6	51.8	52.1	55.1	58.1
Never married	72.2	70.0	66.2	64.2	61.5	59.0	60.8	58.8	56.4	54.1	55.9	56.2	56.2	58.4	60.4
Race[6]															
White only	79.9	79.1	74.5	75.7	70.9	69.1	69.7	68.5	66.3	64.9	64.9	64.8	64.7	66.6	68.2
Black or African American only	58.1	57.7	53.0	55.9	52.9	51.3	51.8	50.0	47.4	44.8	45.9	45.8	45.4	47.1	50.6
American Indian or Alaska Native only	49.1	45.5	45.3	43.7	43.0	36.3	36.4	30.7	35.9	31.7	33.7	34.9	36.0	34.7	41.1
Asian only	69.9	71.9	68.4	72.1	72.2	72.1	73.2	74.3	71.3	68.1	65.9	67.6	69.4	72.5	73.8
Native Hawaiian or Other Pacific Islander only	NA	NA	NA	*	*	*	*	*	*	*	*	*	*	*	*
Two or more races	NA	NA	NA	61.4	57.6	54.0	52.7	58.0	47.8	52.4	52.3	52.9	50.0	55.4	55.3
Hispanic Origin and Race[6]															
Hispanic or Latino	55.7	51.5	46.4	47.8	42.4	40.0	41.7	39.9	37.3	36.8	36.4	36.7	37.3	41.2	43.8
Mexican	53.3	46.8	42.6	45.4	39.7	36.5	37.9	36.8	34.7	33.4	33.9	34.1	34.9	39.0	40.9
Puerto Rican	48.4	45.6	47.6	51.1	48.5	46.1	54.2	48.2	46.2	46.0	45.5	43.7	42.1	46.8	48.0
Cuban	72.5	70.3	63.6	63.9	58.1	63.4	64.8	57.9	54.3	53.8	51.1	49.1	45.3	56.6	61.7
Other Hispanic or Latino	61.6	61.0	51.4	50.7	45.6	44.3	44.3	43.5	39.7	40.9	38.1	39.5	41.2	43.1	47.8
Not Hispanic or Latino	78.7	78.5	74.4	75.2	73.0	71.3	71.7	70.8	68.6	67.0	67.3	67.5	67.4	68.9	70.7
White only	82.4	82.5	78.6	79.5	77.3	75.6	76.2	75.3	73.3	72.0	72.2	72.6	72.4	73.7	75.2
Black or African American only	58.2	57.7	53.4	56.0	53.1	52.2	52.3	50.6	48.0	45.1	46.5	46.4	45.7	48.0	51.2
Age and Percent of Poverty Level[7]															
Under 65 years															
Below 100 percent	32.2	27.0	22.6	25.2	21.4	21.4	21.4	19.2	15.3	16.0	17.2	16.5	15.5	17.4	18.6
100 percent to 199 percent	70.3	64.3	55.3	50.1	44.7	42.8	40.0	38.1	37.4	34.8	35.1	36.7	35.1	38.2	39.8
100 percent to 133 percent	59.4	52.8	41.7	39.3	36.0	33.6	29.5	27.3	26.1	24.4	24.1	26.9	25.3	26.5	30.6
134 percent to 199 percent	75.2	69.5	62.7	55.3	49.4	47.8	45.4	43.7	43.3	40.3	41.1	42.4	40.8	45.1	45.1
200 percent to 399 percent	89.3	89.2	86.4	78.1	74.8	74.9	73.2	72.3	70.6	70.7	71.1	71.3	71.3	73.6	73.4
400 percent or more	95.4	94.6	93.2	91.9	90.6	89.8	91.0	90.1	90.2	89.9	90.7	90.6	90.4	91.5	91.9
Under 19 years															
Below 100 percent	29.6	24.1	19.0	20.3	15.0	15.0	14.1	12.4	9.7	9.8	10.6	10.0	9.3	9.5	10.6
100 percent to 199 percent	73.6	68.5	55.8	49.5	41.6	38.5	35.7	34.1	34.0	31.5	31.2	32.4	29.2	30.4	30.3
100 percent to 133 percent	63.8	56.9	42.5	37.1	32.6	29.0	25.4	23.2	21.3	20.1	19.1	22.3	18.3	18.2	22.3
134 percent to 199 percent	78.4	74.0	64.4	56.1	47.0	44.6	41.7	40.1	41.3	38.1	38.0	38.4	36.2	38.6	35.5
200 percent to 399 percent	91.1	92.1	89.1	80.8	76.6	77.1	75.8	73.7	73.2	72.6	72.4	72.5	71.8	73.5	71.1
400 percent or more	96.2	96.2	93.3	93.0	92.5	91.4	93.2	92.0	91.8	91.2	92.7	91.2	92.3	92.5	92.7
Under 18 years															
Below 100 percent	28.5	22.3	16.9	19.5	14.2	14.0	12.7	11.3	9.3	9.2	9.7	9.1	8.4	8.6	9.3
100 percent to 199 percent	73.9	68.9	56.1	49.4	41.4	38.3	35.6	34.1	34.0	31.5	31.0	32.1	28.5	30.2	30.1
100 percent to 133 percent	63.9	57.3	42.3	36.8	32.0	29.0	25.4	23.2	21.1	19.9	19.0	21.6	17.8	18.2	21.9

NA = Not available.

* = Figure does not meet standards of reliability or precision. Data not shown have a relative standard error of greater than 30 percent.

[1]Any private insurance at the time of interview that was originally obtained through a present or former employer or union, or, starting with 1997 data, through the workplace, self-employment, or a professional association; includes those who also had another type of coverage.

[2]Data prior to 1997 are not strictly comparable with data for later years due to the 1997 questionnaire redesign.

[3]Estimates for 2000–2002 were calculated using 2000-based sample weights and may differ from estimates in other reports that used 1990-based sample weights for 2000-2002 estimates.

[4]Includes all other races not shown separately, those with unknown marital status, unknown disability status, and, in 1984 and 1989, persons with unknown poverty level.

[5]Includes persons 14 to 64 years of age.

[6]The race groups White, Black, American Indian or Alaska Native, Asian, Native Hawaiian or Other Pacific Islander, and two or more races include persons of Hispanic and non-Hispanic origin. Persons of Hispanic origin may be of any race.

[7]Percent of poverty level is based on family income and family size and composition using U.S. Census Bureau poverty thresholds. Poverty level was unknown for 10 to 11 percent of persons under 65 years of age in 1984 and 1989. Missing family income data were imputed for 1995 and beyond.

Table 3-71. Private Health Insurance[1] Coverage Among Persons Under 65 Years of Age, by Selected Characteristics, Selected Years, 1984–2015—Continued

(Numbers in millions; percent.)

Characteristic	1984[2]	1989[2]	1995[2]	2000[3]	2005	2006	2007	2008	2009	2010	2011	2012	2013	2014	2015
134 percent to 199 percent	78.6	74.5	64.9	56.2	47.0	44.4	41.5	40.1	41.3	38.3	37.7	38.4	35.3	38.3	35.3
200 percent to 399 percent	91.3	92.3	89.2	81.1	76.6	77.3	76.0	73.8	73.0	72.6	72.5	72.5	71.9	73.2	71.1
400 percent or more	96.1	96.5	93.1	93.1	92.5	91.6	93.4	92.2	91.8	91.4	92.8	91.4	92.2	92.6	92.7
18 to 64 years															
Below 100 percent	35.0	30.8	27.0	29.1	25.9	26.1	26.8	24.0	19.2	20.4	21.8	20.9	19.9	22.7	24.3
100 percent to 199 percent	68.3	61.5	54.8	50.5	46.5	45.1	42.5	40.2	39.1	36.4	37.2	38.9	38.2	42.1	44.6
100 percent to 133 percent	56.6	50.0	41.4	40.9	38.3	36.4	32.1	29.6	28.8	26.9	26.7	29.6	29.2	31.1	35.4
134 percent to 199 percent	73.3	66.6	61.5	54.9	50.7	49.4	47.5	45.7	44.3	41.3	42.8	44.2	43.2	48.2	49.8
200 percent to 399 percent	88.3	87.6	85.0	76.7	74.0	73.9	72.0	71.7	69.6	70.0	70.5	70.8	71.1	73.7	74.3
400 percent or more	95.2	94.4	93.2	91.6	90.1	89.3	90.4	89.6	89.8	89.5	90.2	90.4	89.9	91.2	91.8
Disability Measure among Adults 18 to 64 Years[5]															
Any basic actions difficulty or complex activity limitation	NA	NA	NA	63.1	58.1	56.4	56.4	53.2	51.6	53.0	49.3	50.8	48.6	51.1	53.6
Any basic actions difficulty	NA	NA	NA	63.9	58.8	57.1	56.9	54.3	52.3	53.8	49.6	51.7	49.2	51.8	54.0
Any complex activity limitation	NA	NA	NA	48.4	44.0	41.7	40.3	37.0	36.0	38.6	35.7	36.0	34.8	34.7	38.3
No disability	NA	NA	NA	77.2	73.7	72.5	72.9	73.3	70.4	69.3	70.5	70.2	70.7	72.5	75.3
Geographic Region															
Northeast	80.5	82.0	75.4	76.3	74.0	70.8	72.2	71.3	69.7	68.2	66.8	67.2	66.1	67.7	70.2
Midwest	80.6	81.5	77.3	78.8	74.6	71.7	72.0	69.9	67.5	66.7	67.9	68.4	68.0	68.7	70.1
South	74.3	71.4	66.9	66.8	62.5	61.8	62.6	62.1	59.3	57.5	57.8	57.3	57.4	59.4	62.5
West	71.9	71.2	67.5	66.5	65.6	64.6	64.0	62.8	60.6	58.9	58.4	58.5	59.6	62.9	62.6
Location of Residence															
Within MSA[6]	77.5	76.5	72.1	72.3	69.0	67.5	67.8	66.5	64.6	62.9	63.2	63.0	63.0	64.8	66.7
Outside MSA[6]	75.2	73.8	67.9	67.8	64.6	60.3	61.0	61.1	56.2	55.1	54.1	55.3	54.7	56.2	57.8

NA = Not available.

* = Figure does not meet standards of reliability or precision. Data not shown have a relative standard error of greater than 30 percent.

[1]Any private insurance at the time of interview that was originally obtained through a present or former employer or union, or, starting with 1997 data, through the workplace, self-employment, or a professional association; includes those who also had another type of coverage.

[2]Data prior to 1997 are not strictly comparable with data for later years due to the 1997 questionnaire redesign.

[3]Estimates for 2000–2002 were calculated using 2000-based sample weights and may differ from estimates in other reports that used 1990-based sample weights for 2000-2002 estimates.

[5]Any basic actions difficulty or complex activity limitation is defined as having one or more of the following limitations or difficulties: movement difficulty, emotional difficulty, sensory (seeing or hearing) difficulty, cognitive difficulty, self-care (activities of daily living or instrumental activities of daily living) limitation, social limitation, or work limitation.

[6]MSA = metropolitan statistical area.

Table 3-72. Private Health Insurance¹ Coverage Obtained Through the Workplace Among Persons Under 65 Years of Age, by Selected Characteristics, Selected Years, 1984–2015

(Numbers in millions; percent.)

Characteristic	1984²	1989²	1995²	2000³	2005	2006	2007	2008	2009	2010	2011	2012	2013	2014	2015
Total Population (in Millions)⁴	141.8	146.3	150.7	160.8	160.1	155.8	157.9	155.6	150.2	147.6	146.4	148.6	148.3	146.4	151.2
Age															
Under 19 years	66.4	65.6	60.5	63.1	58.7	55.6	55.8	54.5	52.0	50.9	49.9	50.1	49.6	49.6	49.8
Under 6 years	62.1	62.3	55.1	58.9	53.4	50.8	50.8	49.6	46.3	44.9	44.3	45.0	44.2	45.7	46.6
6 to 18 years	68.4	67.3	63.1	64.9	61.1	57.8	58.1	56.9	54.8	53.8	52.5	52.4	52.0	51.3	51.2
Under 18 years	66.5	65.8	60.4	63.0	58.6	55.5	55.8	54.4	51.8	50.7	49.7	49.9	49.3	49.3	49.6
6 to 17 years	68.7	67.7	63.3	65.0	61.1	57.8	58.3	56.9	54.7	53.8	52.4	52.3	51.8	51.1	51.0
18 to 64 years	70.3	69.4	67.6	68.8	65.7	63.9	63.9	62.9	60.4	58.9	59.1	59.6	59.5	59.2	60.4
18 to 44 years	69.6	68.4	65.3	66.5	62.2	60.6	60.3	59.4	56.6	54.6	55.6	56.7	56.9	57.0	58.6
18 to 24 years	58.7	55.3	53.5	55.5	52.1	51.7	52.3	49.5	47.4	45.3	51.0	52.7	53.1	53.9	55.8
19 to 25 years	59.0	55.0	53.0	54.2	50.6	50.7	51.4	48.9	45.9	44.1	50.5	52.7	53.0	54.0	56.7
25 to 34 years	71.2	69.5	65.0	66.4	61.1	59.3	59.0	58.4	55.5	53.3	53.0	53.8	53.8	54.2	56.9
35 to 44 years	77.4	76.2	72.7	73.2	69.9	67.5	67.0	67.0	64.3	62.8	61.6	62.7	63.1	62.2	62.4
45 to 64 years	71.8	71.6	72.2	72.9	70.9	68.9	69.2	68.0	65.7	64.8	63.9	63.6	62.9	62.2	62.8
45 to 54 years	74.6	74.4	74.7	75.6	72.6	70.2	70.4	69.5	67.1	65.9	64.7	64.4	64.3	63.8	65.0
55 to 64 years	69.0	68.3	68.4	68.6	68.6	67.2	67.7	66.2	64.0	63.4	63.0	62.6	61.3	60.4	60.5
Sex															
Male	69.8	68.7	65.9	67.3	63.6	61.2	61.3	60.3	57.6	56.1	56.1	57.1	56.9	56.9	57.6
Female	68.4	67.9	64.9	66.9	63.6	61.8	61.9	60.8	58.4	57.1	56.7	56.8	56.4	56.0	57.3
Sex and Marital Status⁵															
Male															
Married	77.9	76.9	74.9	77.5	75.3	73.3	73.3	72.7	70.6	70.1	69.3	69.9	69.8	69.6	70.3
Divorced, separated, widowed	58.0	57.3	56.4	57.4	51.9	51.0	50.8	51.0	48.0	45.3	45.0	46.2	45.3	45.7	45.3
Never married	61.5	58.8	58.2	58.8	54.9	52.6	53.5	51.9	48.8	46.2	48.4	49.6	50.0	50.1	51.6
Female															
Married	76.1	75.5	73.2	76.3	74.2	73.1	72.7	72.2	70.7	69.8	69.2	69.3	68.5	67.7	69.2
Divorced, separated, widowed	51.9	54.9	54.6	57.8	54.3	51.5	51.3	51.4	48.6	48.1	46.5	46.3	46.3	45.8	46.2
Never married	63.5	60.9	59.2	60.1	56.3	54.2	55.1	53.0	50.6	50.2	50.0	50.9	50.6	50.7	51.7
Race⁶															
White only	72.0	71.2	68.4	71.0	66.1	64.0	64.2	63.0	60.6	59.3	59.0	59.6	59.2	59.2	59.9
Black or African American only	52.4	52.8	49.3	53.4	50.6	48.5	49.1	47.7	45.3	42.3	43.5	43.2	42.9	42.0	44.8
American Indian or Alaska Native only	45.8	40.9	40.2	41.7	39.9	33.7	35.1	29.4	33.6	*29.4	32.4	34.0	34.2	30.9	35.9
Asian only	59.0	61.1	59.6	65.8	64.4	64.5	64.6	66.2	62.5	60.6	58.7	60.1	61.4	61.4	62.2
Native Hawaiian or Other Pacific Islander only	NA	NA	NA	*	*	*	*	*	*	*	*	*	*	*	*
Two or more races	NA	NA	NA	59.8	54.8	50.6	49.7	54.3	45.0	49.5	48.3	48.8	46.9	50.9	47.8
Hispanic Origin and Race⁶															
Hispanic or Latino	52.0	47.3	43.4	45.3	40.0	37.7	38.8	37.6	34.9	34.6	34.1	34.6	34.9	36.5	37.4
Mexican	50.5	44.2	40.9	43.6	37.6	34.9	35.7	35.2	32.6	31.6	32.0	32.5	32.5	35.1	36.2
Puerto Rican	45.9	42.3	44.5	49.4	46.2	43.5	51.2	45.9	42.9	42.8	41.6	40.8	42.6	42.7	41.6
Cuban	57.4	56.5	54.0	53.6	53.5	56.9	54.7	49.2	46.4	47.4	45.0	42.8	41.2	42.7	40.6
Other Hispanic or Latino	57.4	54.7	46.7	47.3	42.6	40.9	40.8	39.8	36.9	37.8	35.1	36.7	38.6	37.3	38.8
Not Hispanic or Latino	70.7	70.5	68.2	70.6	68.0	66.0	66.1	65.2	62.8	62.3	61.3	62.0	61.7	61.7	62.2
White only	74.0	74.1	72.1	74.5	71.9	69.9	70.2	69.0	66.8	66.5	65.7	65.5	66.6	66.1	66.3
Black or African American only	52.5	52.8	49.8	53.6	50.9	49.5	49.5	48.2	45.9	45.9	42.6	44.1	43.6	43.2	45.4
Age and Percent of Poverty Level⁷															
Under 65 years															
Below 100 percent	24.1	19.8	17.5	21.0	17.8	17.6	17.4	15.5	11.9	12.4	13.6	13.6	12.2	12.2	12.7
100 percent to 199 percent	61.7	56.1	49.3	45.4	40.1	38.3	35.5	33.8	33.3	30.2	30.4	32.2	31.0	31.0	30.2
100 percent to 133 percent	50.0	44.3	36.0	35.0	31.3	30.0	25.3	23.8	22.6	20.6	19.7	23.0	21.7	20.5	22.7
134 percent to 199 percent	66.9	61.5	56.6	50.5	44.8	42.9	40.7	39.1	39.0	35.3	36.2	37.5	36.3	37.3	34.5
200 percent to 399 percent	82.8	82.2	80.5	73.4	69.8	69.7	67.7	66.8	64.7	65.3	65.0	65.9	65.6	65.4	64.0
400 percent or more	88.8	87.8	86.7	87.9	86.1	84.7	85.5	84.6	84.1	84.2	85.0	85.1	84.6	84.5	84.8
Under 19 years															
Below 100 percent	23.6	18.6	15.1	17.1	13.3	12.7	12.1	11.3	7.9	8.2	9.1	8.7	7.8	7.2	7.8
100 percent to 199 percent	67.0	62.1	50.5	45.8	38.3	35.5	32.7	31.4	31.9	28.8	27.9	29.7	26.6	26.8	26.1
100 percent to 133 percent	56.1	49.9	37.4	33.6	29.1	27.0	22.4	21.0	19.8	17.9	16.3	20.5	16.4	15.6	19.7
134 percent to 199 percent	72.3	67.9	58.8	52.2	43.7	41.0	38.6	37.1	38.9	35.1	34.4	35.2	33.1	34.4	30.3
200 percent to 399 percent	85.7	86.0	83.9	76.9	72.4	72.5	71.2	68.3	67.7	68.7	67.0	68.0	66.7	67.6	64.4
400 percent or more	90.8	90.3	87.5	89.5	88.3	86.3	87.5	86.9	86.0	86.5	87.5	86.3	86.9	87.1	86.9
Under 18 years															
Below 100 percent	23.0	17.5	13.6	16.6	12.5	11.8	11.2	10.3	7.5	7.8	8.4	8.1	7.2	6.7	6.9
100 percent to 199 percent	67.5	62.5	50.9	45.8	38.2	35.4	32.7	31.4	32.0	28.8	27.7	29.4	26.0	26.7	26.0
100 percent to 133 percent	56.3	50.3	37.2	33.5	28.6	27.1	22.5	21.0	19.8	17.8	16.1	19.8	16.0	15.6	19.7
134 percent to 199 percent	72.8	68.4	59.6	52.4	43.9	40.8	38.5	37.1	38.9	35.2	34.1	35.2	32.4	34.3	30.1

NA = Not available.

* = Figure does not meet standards of reliability or precision. Data not shown have a relative standard error of greater than 30 percent.

¹Any private insurance at the time of interview that was originally obtained through a present or former employer or union, or, starting with 1997 data, through the workplace, self-employment, or a professional association; includes those who also had another type of coverage.

²Data prior to 1997 are not strictly comparable with data for later years due to the 1997 questionnaire redesign.

³Estimates for 2000–2002 were calculated using 2000-based sample weights and may differ from estimates in other reports that used 1990-based sample weights for 2000-2002 estimates.

⁴Includes all other races not shown separately, those with unknown marital status, unknown disability status, and, in 1984 and 1989, persons with unknown poverty level.

⁵Includes persons 14 to 64 years of age.

⁶The race groups White, Black, American Indian or Alaska Native, Asian, Native Hawaiian or Other Pacific Islander, and two or more races include persons of Hispanic and non-Hispanic origin. Persons of Hispanic origin may be of any race.

⁷Percent of poverty level is based on family income and family size and composition using U.S. Census Bureau poverty thresholds. Poverty level was unknown for 10 to 11 percent of persons under 65 years of age in 1984 and 1989. Missing family income data were imputed for 1995 and beyond.

Table 3-72. Private Health Insurance[1] Coverage Obtained Through the Workplace Among Persons Under 65 Years of Age, by Selected Characteristics, Selected Years, 1984–2015—Continued

(Numbers in millions; percent.)

Characteristic	1984[2]	1989[2]	1995[2]	2000[3]	2005	2006	2007	2008	2009	2010	2011	2012	2013	2014	2015
200 percent to 399 percent	85.9	86.4	84.1	77.1	72.4	72.7	71.5	68.4	67.6	68.7	67.0	68.1	66.8	67.5	64.4
400 percent or more	90.7	90.5	87.1	89.7	88.5	86.4	87.7	87.1	86.0	86.6	87.7	86.4	86.8	87.2	87.0
18 to 64 years															
Below 100 percent	24.8	21.8	20.5	24.0	21.2	21.3	21.2	18.7	14.8	15.4	16.8	16.9	15.2	15.6	16.3
100 percent to 199 percent	58.3	52.3	48.4	45.2	41.1	39.9	37.0	35.1	34.0	30.9	31.8	33.6	33.3	33.1	32.2
100 percent to 133 percent	46.0	40.4	35.3	35.9	32.9	31.8	27.0	25.5	24.2	22.1	21.5	24.6	24.7	23.2	24.4
134 percent to 199 percent	63.6	57.5	55.0	49.5	45.3	43.9	41.8	40.1	39.0	35.3	37.2	38.7	38.0	38.6	36.6
200 percent to 399 percent	81.4	80.2	78.8	71.7	68.7	68.4	66.2	66.1	63.6	63.9	64.3	65.0	65.2	64.7	63.8
400 percent or more	88.5	87.5	86.7	87.5	85.4	84.3	84.9	83.9	83.6	83.6	84.2	84.7	84.0	83.8	84.3
Disability Measure among Adults 18 to 64 Years[8]															
Any basic actions difficulty or complex activity limitation	NA	NA	NA	58.5	53.3	52.0	51.5	49.1	46.7	48.0	44.4	45.8	44.0	43.0	44.6
Any basic actions difficulty	NA	NA	NA	59.1	54.0	52.6	52.1	49.9	47.4	48.9	44.9	46.7	44.6	43.8	45.0
Any complex activity limitation	NA	NA	NA	43.5	38.9	37.2	35.4	33.5	31.1	32.8	30.3	30.5	29.6	26.1	29.3
No disability	NA	NA	NA	72.5	68.5	67.3	67.1	67.5	64.8	63.5	64.6	64.7	64.7	64.2	65.8
Geographic Region															
Northeast	74.0	75.0	69.8	72.5	70.6	67.5	68.2	68.0	65.3	64.4	63.0	63.4	62.3	61.5	62.9
Midwest	72.0	73.3	71.2	74.9	70.1	67.0	68.0	64.7	62.0	61.8	62.2	63.8	62.6	61.5	62.7
South	66.2	63.6	61.8	62.5	58.0	57.2	57.2	56.7	54.1	52.2	52.3	52.3	52.2	52.4	54.3
West	64.7	63.9	60.4	61.1	59.7	58.1	57.3	56.8	54.5	52.7	52.2	52.8	53.6	54.7	53.5
Location of Residence															
Within MSA[9]	70.9	69.6	66.6	68.2	64.5	62.7	62.7	61.5	59.3	57.9	57.8	58.1	57.8	57.8	58.6
Outside MSA[9]	65.3	63.5	60.7	62.6	59.6	55.4	55.7	55.1	50.8	49.4	48.7	50.3	49.4	48.0	50.0

NA = Not available.

* = Figure does not meet standards of reliability or precision. Data not shown have a relative standard error of greater than 30 percent.

[1]Any private insurance at the time of interview that was originally obtained through a present or former employer or union, or, starting with 1997 data, through the workplace, self-employment, or a professional association; includes those who also had another type of coverage.

[2]Data prior to 1997 are not strictly comparable with data for later years due to the 1997 questionnaire redesign.

[3]Estimates for 2000–2002 were calculated using 2000-based sample weights and may differ from estimates in other reports that used 1990-based sample weights for 2000-2002 estimates.

[8]Any basic actions difficulty or complex activity limitation is defined as having one or more of the following limitations or difficulties: movement difficulty, emotional difficulty, sensory (seeing or hearing) difficulty, cognitive difficulty, self-care (activities of daily living or instrumental activities of daily living) limitation, social limitation, or work limitation.

[9]MSA = metropolitan statistical area.

Table 3-73. No Health Insurance Coverage Among Persons Under 65 Years of Age, by Selected Characteristics, Selected Years, 1984–2015

(Numbers in millions; percent.)

Characteristic	1984[1]	1989[1]	1995[1]	2000[2]	2005[3]	2006[3]	2007[3]	2008[3]	2009[3]	2010[3]	2011[3]	2012[3]	2013[3]	2014[3]	2015[3]
Total (number in millions)[4]	29.8	33.4	37.1	41.4	42.1	43.9	43.3	44.1	46.2	48.3	45.8	45.2	44.6	35.7	28.7
Total (percent of population)[4]	14.5	15.6	16.1	17.0	16.4	17.0	16.6	16.8	17.5	18.2	17.2	16.9	16.7	13.3	10.6
Age															
Under 19 years	14.1	15.0	13.7	12.9	9.7	9.8	9.4	9.5	8.5	8.3	7.4	7.0	7.1	5.7	4.8
Under 6 years	14.9	15.1	11.8	11.8	7.7	7.5	7.3	7.6	6.6	6.3	5.0	4.6	5.0	4.1	3.3
6 to 18 years	13.8	15.0	14.6	13.4	10.6	10.9	10.4	10.5	9.4	9.2	8.5	8.1	8.0	6.5	5.5
Under 18 years	13.9	14.7	13.4	12.6	9.3	9.5	9.0	9.0	8.2	7.8	7.0	6.6	6.6	5.4	4.5
6 to 17 years	13.4	14.5	14.3	13.0	10.1	10.5	9.9	9.8	9.0	8.6	8.0	7.6	7.4	6.1	5.1
18 to 64 years	14.8	16.0	17.3	18.9	19.3	20.0	19.6	19.9	21.2	22.3	21.2	20.9	20.5	16.3	13.0
18 to 44 years	17.1	18.4	20.4	22.4	23.5	24.6	23.9	24.4	25.9	27.1	25.4	24.8	24.2	19.7	15.9
18 to 24 years	25.0	27.1	28.0	30.4	29.1	29.9	27.9	29.0	29.6	31.4	25.9	24.5	24.6	18.1	14.6
19 to 25 years	25.1	27.9	28.8	32.3	31.7	32.4	30.5	31.1	32.8	33.8	27.9	26.3	26.7	19.7	16.0
25 to 34 years	16.2	18.3	21.1	23.3	25.6	27.2	26.1	26.6	27.8	28.3	28.1	28.1	27.1	22.7	18.0
35 to 44 years	11.2	12.3	15.1	16.9	17.9	18.8	19.1	19.1	21.4	22.6	22.2	21.7	21.0	17.7	14.6
45 to 64 years	9.6	10.5	10.9	12.6	12.9	13.2	13.5	13.6	14.6	15.7	15.4	15.6	15.4	11.8	9.0
45 to 54 years	10.5	11.0	11.6	12.8	14.2	15.0	14.9	14.9	16.5	17.9	17.4	17.7	17.1	13.7	10.2
55 to 64 years	8.7	10.0	9.9	12.4	11.1	10.8	11.6	11.8	12.2	12.8	13.0	13.2	13.5	9.7	7.7
Sex															
Male	15.3	16.8	17.4	18.1	17.9	18.8	18.2	18.3	19.4	20.3	18.8	18.5	18.1	14.7	12.0
Female	13.8	14.4	14.8	15.9	15.0	15.3	15.1	15.4	15.7	16.1	15.6	15.4	15.2	11.9	9.3
Sex and Marital Status[5]															
Male															
Married	11.1	12.5	15.0	14.1	14.4	15.3	15.3	15.4	16.3	17.2	16.5	16.2	15.9	12.6	10.6
Divorced, separated, widowed	24.9	25.0	24.0	25.8	28.6	29.1	28.1	27.0	29.8	31.4	30.0	29.3	28.1	23.2	20.0
Never married	22.4	25.0	25.6	27.2	27.6	28.6	27.0	27.6	29.4	31.1	28.0	27.5	26.9	21.9	17.4
Female															
Married	11.2	11.8	13.6	13.3	13.0	13.5	13.5	13.5	14.2	14.7	14.4	14.6	14.6	11.6	8.8
Divorced, separated, widowed	19.2	19.1	18.1	21.3	22.1	23.0	22.6	22.1	22.8	23.6	24.0	24.2	22.8	17.7	13.4
Never married	16.3	18.0	17.5	21.1	20.0	20.4	19.5	20.7	21.0	21.9	20.5	19.6	19.6	15.1	12.1
Race[6]															
White only	13.6	14.5	15.5	15.4	15.9	16.7	16.3	16.7	17.1	17.6	16.7	16.7	16.3	13.3	10.7
Black or African American only	19.9	21.6	18.0	19.5	18.4	18.1	17.0	18.0	18.9	20.6	19.0	18.0	18.9	13.7	11.3
American Indian or Alaska Native only	22.5	28.4	34.3	38.4	32.2	38.0	38.8	28.4	32.5	44.0	34.2	27.0	29.4	28.3	21.4
Asian only	18.5	16.9	18.6	17.6	17.1	15.0	15.4	13.9	16.2	17.1	16.5	16.8	14.2	10.8	7.5
Native Hawaiian or Other Pacific Islander only	NA	NA	NA	*	*	*	*	*	*	*	*	*	*	*	*
Two or more races	NA	NA	NA	16.8	16.5	18.4	15.0	15.8	18.2	15.8	16.0	14.5	15.3	10.1	9.5
Hispanic Origin and Race[6]															
Hispanic or Latino	29.5	33.7	31.4	35.6	33.0	35.0	31.8	33.3	32.9	32.0	31.1	30.4	30.7	25.5	21.1
Mexican	33.8	39.9	35.6	39.9	36.0	38.6	34.7	36.1	35.0	34.8	33.0	33.2	33.4	27.2	23.5
Puerto Rican	18.3	24.7	17.6	16.4	16.3	16.8	12.8	16.8	18.0	17.8	13.7	15.8	14.4	15.6	9.6
Cuban	21.6	20.6	22.3	25.4	23.2	22.8	20.7	28.1	27.8	26.5	28.1	24.3	26.6	19.4	14.2
Other Hispanic or Latino	27.4	25.8	30.2	33.4	32.6	33.2	32.7	32.5	33.4	32.4	31.8	30.1	28.8	26.2	19.7
Not Hispanic or Latino	13.2	13.7	14.2	14.0	13.4	13.6	13.7	13.5	14.4	15.2	14.2	13.9	13.4	10.5	8.2
White only	11.9	12.1	13.0	12.5	12.0	12.5	12.6	12.5	13.2	13.7	12.9	12.7	12.2	9.7	7.5
Black or African American only	19.7	21.5	17.9	19.5	18.3	17.5	16.8	17.9	18.8	20.7	18.8	17.8	18.8	13.5	11.2
Age and Percent of Poverty Level[7]															
Under 65 years															
Below 100 percent	33.9	35.2	29.6	34.2	30.6	30.2	28.4	29.0	30.4	30.3	28.4	28.2	28.0	23.0	18.2
100 percent to 199 percent	21.8	25.6	28.3	31.0	28.6	29.6	30.0	30.6	29.8	32.4	30.0	29.3	29.3	23.4	18.3
100 percent to 133 percent	28.8	32.3	34.1	35.7	30.1	31.3	32.0	32.8	30.1	34.9	32.0	31.1	30.4	25.0	18.4
134 percent to 199 percent	18.7	22.6	25.1	28.7	27.8	28.7	29.0	29.5	29.6	31.0	28.9	28.4	28.6	22.4	18.1
200 percent to 399 percent	7.6	8.3	10.0	15.4	15.7	15.5	16.9	16.6	17.8	17.4	16.5	16.2	16.1	12.6	11.1
400 percent or more	3.2	4.2	5.4	5.9	6.3	6.5	5.6	6.2	5.8	5.6	5.2	4.9	4.8	3.8	3.3
Under 19 years															
Below 100 percent	29.0	31.7	20.4	22.6	15.2	14.2	12.7	14.0	12.2	11.3	9.4	8.3	8.9	6.7	5.4
100 percent to 199 percent	18.0	20.7	22.6	22.1	15.6	16.4	16.4	16.3	13.0	13.5	12.1	11.1	11.7	9.3	7.4
100 percent to 133 percent	24.4	27.6	26.4	26.5	15.6	17.9	17.4	17.3	12.9	15.9	12.5	9.6	11.6	9.4	7.7
134 percent to 199 percent	14.9	17.4	20.1	19.7	15.6	15.5	15.9	15.8	13.1	12.0	11.9	12.0	11.7	9.3	7.2
200 percent to 399 percent	5.1	4.9	6.7	9.6	8.2	7.8	8.5	8.0	8.0	7.4	6.8	6.8	6.7	5.7	5.4
400 percent or more	1.8	2.1	4.4	3.5	3.3	3.4	2.3	2.8	2.4	2.3	2.1	2.2	1.9	1.7	1.6
Under 18 years															
Below 100 percent	28.9	31.6	20.0	22.0	14.3	13.9	11.9	13.3	11.8	10.6	8.8	7.6	8.2	6.4	4.9
100 percent to 199 percent	17.5	20.2	22.0	21.7	15.0	16.0	15.7	15.5	12.3	12.7	11.4	10.4	11.1	8.7	6.9
100 percent to 133 percent	24.0	27.1	26.1	26.4	15.1	17.5	16.5	16.4	11.8	15.1	11.5	9.0	11.2	8.9	7.3

NA = Not available.

* = Figure does not meet standards of reliability or precision. Data not shown have a relative standard error of greater than 30 percent.

[1] Data prior to 1997 are not strictly comparable with data for later years due to the 1997 questionnaire redesign.

[2] Estimates for 2000-2002 were calculated using 2000-based sample weights and may differ from estimates in other reports that used 1990-based sample weights for 2000-2002 estimates.

[3] Beginning in quarter 3 of the 2004 NHIS, persons under 65 years of age with no reported coverage were asked explicitly about Medicaid coverage. Estimates were calculated without and with the additional information from this question in the columns labeled 2004(1) and 2004(2), respectively, and estimates were calculated with the additional information starting with 2005 data.

[4] Includes all other races not shown separately, those with unknown marital status, unknown disability status, and, in 1984 and 1989, persons with unknown poverty level.

[5] Includes persons 14 to 64 years of age.

[6] The race groups White, Black, American Indian or Alaska Native, Asian, Native Hawaiian or Other Pacific Islander, and two or more races include persons of Hispanic and non-Hispanic origin. Persons of Hispanic origin may be of any race.

[7] Percent of poverty level is based on family income and family size and composition using U.S. Census Bureau poverty thresholds. Poverty level was unknown for 10 to 11 percent of persons under 65 years of age in 1984 and 1989. Missing family income data were imputed for 1995 and beyond.

Table 3-73. No Health Insurance Coverage Among Persons Under 65 Years of Age, by Selected Characteristics, Selected Years, 1984–2015—*Continued*

(Numbers in millions; percent.)

Characteristic	1984[1]	1989[1]	1995[1]	2000[2]	2005[3]	2006[3]	2007[3]	2008[3]	2009[3]	2010[3]	2011[3]	2012[3]	2013[3]	2014[3]	2015[3]
134 percent to 199 percent	14.4	16.9	19.5	19.1	15.0	15.1	15.3	15.0	12.6	11.3	11.3	11.3	11.1	8.5	6.7
200 percent to 399 percent	4.9	4.7	6.6	9.3	7.8	7.4	8.2	7.5	7.8	7.0	6.4	6.7	6.3	5.5	5.2
400 percent or more	1.8	1.9	4.6	3.3	3.2	3.1	2.2	2.7	2.3	2.1	2.0	2.1	1.8	*1.6	1.6
18 to 64 years															
Below 100 percent	37.6	38.2	37.0	42.4	40.9	40.7	38.6	38.6	42.5	42.7	40.4	40.5	40.0	32.9	26.2
100 percent to 199 percent	24.4	28.8	32.0	36.4	35.9	36.7	37.9	38.9	38.9	42.1	39.3	38.6	37.8	30.5	23.9
100 percent to 133 percent	31.9	35.6	39.7	41.7	38.9	39.8	41.7	42.1	40.4	45.7	42.5	42.2	40.4	33.9	24.5
134 percent to 199 percent	21.1	25.9	28.2	34.0	34.4	35.1	36.1	37.3	38.1	40.3	37.6	36.5	36.4	28.7	23.6
200 percent to 399 percent	8.9	10.0	11.7	18.2	19.0	18.8	20.5	20.2	21.7	21.3	20.4	19.8	19.7	15.3	13.3
400 percent or more	3.4	4.4	5.5	6.6	7.1	7.4	6.5	7.1	6.7	6.5	6.1	5.6	5.6	4.3	3.8
Disability Measure among Adults 18 to 64 Years[6]															
Any basic actions difficulty or complex activity limitation	NA	NA	NA	17.6	19.6	20.0	19.6	19.5	21.4	20.8	22.0	20.4	20.4	16.2	11.6
Any basic actions difficulty	NA	NA	NA	17.6	19.8	20.0	19.6	19.4	21.2	20.9	22.3	20.3	20.4	16.3	11.8
Any complex activity limitation	NA	NA	NA	16.1	16.9	17.3	18.3	15.8	19.2	17.2	18.2	18.3	17.1	12.5	9.2
No disability	NA	NA	NA	18.5	19.5	20.5	19.9	19.8	21.2	21.6	20.2	20.4	19.9	16.3	13.1
Geographic Region															
Northeast	10.2	10.9	13.3	12.2	11.3	11.2	11.0	11.4	11.4	12.4	11.8	11.5	11.2	9.3	6.8
Midwest	11.3	10.7	12.2	12.3	11.9	13.4	13.0	13.9	14.6	14.1	13.4	13.6	13.1	10.3	8.2
South	17.7	19.7	19.4	20.5	21.0	21.1	20.1	20.1	21.2	21.9	20.4	20.3	19.9	16.9	14.2
West	18.2	18.8	17.9	20.7	18.4	18.8	18.9	18.8	19.4	20.6	20.0	19.0	18.9	13.3	10.1
Location of Residence															
Within MSA[9]	13.6	15.2	15.5	16.6	16.1	16.6	16.1	16.4	17.1	17.8	16.7	16.4	16.2	13.0	10.3
Outside MSA[9]	16.6	17.0	18.6	18.6	17.8	19.3	19.4	19.1	20.2	20.4	19.8	19.9	19.3	15.2	12.8

NA = Not available.

* = Figure does not meet standards of reliability or precision. Data not shown have a relative standard error of greater than 30 percent.

[1]Data prior to 1997 are not strictly comparable with data for later years due to the 1997 questionnaire redesign.

[2]Estimates for 2000-2002 were calculated using 2000-based sample weights and may differ from estimates in other reports that used 1990-based sample weights for 2000-2002 estimates.

[3]Beginning in quarter 3 of the 2004 NHIS, persons under 65 years of age with no reported coverage were asked explicitly about Medicaid coverage. Estimates were calculated without and with the additional information from this question in the columns labeled 2004(1) and 2004(2), respectively, and estimates were calculated with the additional information starting with 2005 data.

[6]Any basic actions difficulty or complex activity limitation is defined as having one or more of the following limitations or difficulties: movement difficulty, emotional difficulty, sensory (seeing or hearing) difficulty, cognitive difficulty, self-care (activities of daily living or instrumental activities of daily living) limitation, social limitation, or work limitation.

[9]MSA = metropolitan statistical area.

Table 3-74. Health Insurance Coverage of Noninstitutionalized Medicare Beneficiaries 65 Years of Age and Over, by Type of Coverage and Selected Characteristics, Selected Years, 1992–2013

(Numbers in millions; percent.)

Characteristic	Medicare Advantage Plan[1]						Medicaid[2]					
	1992	1995	2000	2005	2010	2013	1992	1995	2000	2005	2010	2013
Age												
65 years and over (number in millions)	1.1	2.6	5.9	4.6	10.3	13.8	2.7	2.8	2.7	3.2	3.2	3.6
65 years and over (percent of population)	3.9	8.9	19.3	14.5	26.7	31.2	9.4	9.6	9.0	10.1	8.4	8.1
65 to 74 years	4.2	9.5	20.6	13.9	26.9	30.3	7.9	8.8	8.5	9.9	7.7	7.2
75 to 84 years	3.7	8.3	18.5	15.3	27.6	33.8	10.6	9.6	8.9	9.9	9.1	8.6
85 years and over	*	7.3	16.3	13.9	23.7	29.4	16.6	13.6	11.2	11.9	9.5	11.4
Sex												
Male	4.6	9.2	19.3	13.5	25.4	30.0	6.3	6.2	6.3	7.2	6.3	5.7
Female	3.4	8.6	19.3	15.2	27.8	32.3	11.6	12.0	10.9	12.3	10.1	10.1
Race and Hispanic Origin												
White, not Hispanic or Latino	3.6	8.4	18.4	13.2	23.9	29.1	5.6	5.4	5.1	6.1	5.4	4.9
Black, not Hispanic or Latino	*	7.9	20.7	17.1	34.3	33.4	28.5	30.3	23.6	23.6	16.8	17.8
Hispanic	*	15.5	27.5	27.2	47.2	46.7	39.0	40.5	28.7	29.2	18.8	20.1
Percent of Poverty Level[3]												
Below 100 percent	3.6	7.7	18.4	NA	NA	NA	22.3	17.2	15.9	NA	NA	NA
100 percent to less than 200 percent	3.7	9.5	23.4	NA	NA	NA	6.7	6.3	8.4	NA	NA	NA
200 percent or more	4.2	10.1	18.0	NA	NA	NA	*	*	*	NA	NA	NA
Marital Status												
Married	4.6	9.5	18.7	13.8	27.1	30.2	4.0	4.3	4.3	5.4	3.6	3.5
Widowed	2.3	7.7	19.4	15.0	25.4	31.2	14.9	15.0	13.6	14.9	12.6	12.5
Divorced	*	9.7	24.4	17.1	29.1	35.2	23.4	24.5	20.2	20.0	16.9	16.0
Never married	*	*	15.8	13.9	23.1	32.1	19.2	19.0	17.0	21.3	19.8	17.9

Characteristic	Employer-sponsored plan[4]						Medigap[5]					
	1992	1995	2000	2005	2010	2013	1992	1995	2000	2005	2010	2013
Age												
65 years and over (number in millions)	12.5	11.3	10.7	11.6	11.9	12.1	9.9	9.5	7.6	8.2	7.6	8.2
65 years and over (percent of population)	42.8	38.6	35.2	36.4	30.6	27.4	33.9	32.5	25.0	25.7	19.6	18.7
65 to 74 years	46.9	41.1	36.6	38.1	32.5	29.5	31.4	29.9	21.7	23.2	17.4	17.5
75 to 84 years	38.2	37.1	35.0	35.5	28.4	24.4	37.5	35.2	27.8	27.3	21.3	19.8
85 years and over	31.6	30.2	29.4	31.8	28.5	24.9	38.3	37.6	31.1	30.8	24.7	21.1
Sex												
Male	46.3	42.1	37.7	39.4	32.9	29.1	30.6	30.0	23.4	23.8	18.2	17.2
Female	40.4	36.0	33.4	34.2	28.9	25.9	36.2	34.4	26.2	27.1	20.8	19.9
Race and Hispanic Origin												
White, not Hispanic or Latino	45.9	41.3	38.6	39.5	33.5	29.5	37.2	36.2	28.3	29.1	23.0	22.1
Black, not Hispanic or Latino	25.9	26.7	22.0	27.9	23.7	26.7	13.6	10.2	7.5	9.5	6.7	5.3
Hispanic	20.7	16.9	15.8	18.6	14.8	13.9	15.8	10.1	11.3	11.1	6.4	5.6
Percent of Poverty Level[3]												
Below 100 percent	29.0	32.1	28.1	NA	NA	NA	30.8	29.8	22.6	NA	NA	NA
100 percent to less than 200 percent	37.5	32.0	27.0	NA	NA	NA	39.3	39.1	28.4	NA	NA	NA
200 percent or more	58.4	52.8	49.0	NA	NA	NA	32.8	32.2	26.2	NA	NA	NA
Marital Status												
Married	49.9	44.6	41.0	41.7	35.9	33.0	33.0	32.6	25.6	27.0	19.6	19.6
Widowed	34.1	30.3	28.7	30.4	26.3	21.3	37.5	35.2	26.7	26.2	22.0	19.9
Divorced	27.3	26.6	22.4	25.1	18.9	17.2	27.9	24.1	16.9	19.8	15.3	14.8
Never married	38.0	35.1	28.5	29.1	25.2	21.5	29.1	26.2	21.9	15.4	17.5	13.1

NA = Not available.

* = Figure does not meet standards of reliability or precision. Estimates are considered unreliable if the sample cell size is 50 or fewer.

[1]Enrollee has a Medicare Advantage plan regardless of other insurance. Medicare Advantage plans include health maintenance organizations, preferred provider organizations, private fee-for-service plans, special needs plans, and Medicare medical savings account plans. Starting with 2013 data, the term Medicare Risk Health Maintenance Organization was replaced with Medicare Advantage plan.

[2]Enrolled in Medicaid and not enrolled in a Medicare Advantage plan.

[3]Percent of poverty level is based on family income and family size and composition using U.S. Census Bureau poverty thresholds.

[4]Private insurance plans purchased through employers (own, current, or former employer, family business, union, or former employer or union of spouse) and not enrolled in a Medicare risk HMO or Medicaid.

[5]Supplemental insurance purchased privately or through organizations such as American Association of Retired Persons or professional organizations, and not enrolled in a Medicare risk HMO, Medicaid, or employer-sponsored plan.

Table 3-74. Health Insurance Coverage of Noninstitutionalized Medicare Beneficiaries 65 Years of Age and Over, by Type of Coverage and Selected Characteristics, Selected Years, 1992–2013—*Continued*

(Numbers in millions; percent.)

Characteristic	Medicare fee-for-service only or other[e]					
	1992	1995	2000	2005	2010	2013
Age						
65 years and over (number in millions)	2.9	3.1	3.5	4.3	5.7	6.4
65 years and over (percent of population)	9.9	10.5	11.5	13.3	14.6	14.6
65 to 74 years	9.7	10.7	12.6	14.9	15.5	15.5
75 to 84 years	10.1	9.9	9.9	11.9	13.5	13.5
85 years and over	10.8	11.3	12.1	11.6	13.6	13.3
Sex						
Male	12.2	12.6	13.3	16.2	17.3	18.0
Female	8.3	8.9	10.2	11.2	12.5	11.9
Race and Hispanic Origin						
White, not Hispanic or Latino	7.7	8.7	9.6	12.2	14.2	14.3
Black, not Hispanic or Latino	26.7	25.0	26.1	21.9	18.6	16.8
Hispanic	18.3	17.1	16.7	13.9	12.7	13.7
Percent of Poverty Level[3]						
Below 100 percent	14.3	13.3	15.1	NA	NA	NA
100 percent to less than 200 percent	12.9	13.1	12.7	NA	NA	NA
200 percent or more	4.0	4.5	6.3	NA	NA	NA
Marital Status						
Married	8.5	9.0	10.5	12.1	13.9	13.8
Widowed	11.2	11.9	11.6	13.5	13.7	15.2
Divorced	15.7	15.1	16.1	17.9	19.8	16.9

NA = Not available.
* = Figure does not meet standards of reliability or precision. Estimates are considered unreliable if the sample cell size is 50 or fewer.
[3]Percent of poverty level is based on family income and family size and composition using U.S. Census Bureau poverty thresholds.
[e]Medicare fee-for-service only or other public plans (except Medicaid).

Table 3-75. Persons Under 65 Years of Age Without Health Insurance Coverage, by State, Territory, and Age, 2009–2015

(Percent.)

Characteristic	2009	2010	2011	2012	2013	2014	2015
Under 65 Years							
United States[1]	17.2	17.6	17.2	16.9	16.7	13.4	10.9
Alabama	16.0	16.9	16.3	15.4	15.9	14.0	11.9
Alaska	22.0	19.4	21.7	22.0	20.3	19.2	16.0
Arizona	19.8	19.5	19.9	20.3	20.3	16.0	13.1
Arkansas	19.3	20.2	19.7	19.0	18.8	13.8	11.0
California	20.1	20.7	20.3	20.0	19.3	14.0	9.6
Colorado	17.4	17.6	17.0	16.3	15.7	11.9	9.2
Connecticut	10.1	10.3	9.8	10.6	10.8	8.0	7.0
Delaware	11.9	11.5	10.2	9.9	11.7	8.7	6.5
District of Columbia	7.8	8.4	8.3	6.1	7.1	6.1	4.0
Florida	24.8	25.4	25.0	24.0	24.2	20.1	16.2
Georgia	21.0	21.9	21.8	20.8	21.1	17.8	15.7
Hawaii	7.9	8.7	8.4	7.7	8.3	5.7	4.5
Idaho	19.1	20.3	17.8	18.3	18.5	15.4	13.1
Illinois	14.9	15.7	14.5	14.6	14.4	11.2	8.1
Indiana	15.8	17.0	16.6	16.6	16.2	13.8	11.4
Iowa	10.1	10.8	10.4	9.7	10.2	6.7	5.7
Kansas	14.5	15.6	14.4	14.6	14.3	12.2	10.8
Kentucky	16.5	17.5	16.6	15.8	16.8	10.2	7.1
Louisiana	19.5	20.1	19.9	19.0	19.2	16.6	13.9
Maine	11.9	12.5	13.1	12.4	13.3	11.8	10.4
Maryland	12.5	12.7	11.5	11.5	11.4	9.0	7.6
Massachusetts	4.9	4.9	4.8	4.5	4.4	3.9	3.2
Michigan	14.1	14.3	13.6	13.4	12.8	9.8	7.1
Minnesota	10.2	10.1	9.9	9.4	9.5	6.8	5.2
Mississippi	20.0	20.7	20.2	19.7	19.6	16.8	14.7
Missouri	15.3	15.2	15.7	16.1	15.2	13.5	11.3
Montana	21.9	19.6	21.8	21.4	19.7	16.2	13.8
Nebraska	13.1	13.4	13.6	12.7	12.2	10.8	9.1
Nevada	24.6	25.4	24.7	25.0	23.4	17.5	14.1
New Hampshire	12.0	12.7	11.4	12.8	12.6	10.9	8.1
New Jersey	14.2	15.0	14.7	14.5	15.3	12.6	10.1
New Mexico	23.1	22.8	22.8	21.6	22.2	17.3	12.7
New York	13.0	13.5	13.0	12.5	12.4	9.9	8.1
North Carolina	18.2	19.2	18.7	18.9	18.0	15.2	13.1
North Dakota	11.4	11.5	11.5	12.4	11.9	9.2	9.4
Ohio	14.0	14.1	13.9	13.4	12.8	9.7	7.5
Oklahoma	21.3	22.0	21.3	21.1	20.4	17.7	16.5
Oregon	19.8	19.7	18.0	16.9	17.4	11.5	8.3
Pennsylvania	11.3	11.9	11.8	11.3	11.3	10.1	7.4
Rhode Island	12.8	13.7	12.6	13.3	13.9	8.3	6.1
South Carolina	19.2	20.2	19.4	19.3	18.4	16.0	12.8
South Dakota	15.6	13.6	13.4	12.3	14.3	11.6	13.1
Tennessee	16.3	16.4	17.0	16.1	16.2	13.9	12.0
Texas	26.3	26.3	25.5	24.8	24.5	21.2	19.0
Utah	15.7	17.0	16.5	15.3	14.7	13.6	11.7
Vermont	9.9	9.0	8.3	7.7	8.1	5.4	5.0
Virginia	13.3	14.5	14.1	14.2	14.1	12.4	10.7
Washington	15.3	16.1	16.0	15.7	16.1	10.5	7.5
West Virginia	16.7	17.2	18.2	16.9	16.1	10.7	6.6
Wisconsin	10.4	10.9	10.6	10.6	10.4	8.7	6.7
Wyoming	17.5	16.6	17.5	18.3	14.6	14.1	12.0
Puerto Rico[2]	9.4	9.4	8.9	8.5	7.7	7.2	6.7
Under 18 Years							
United States[1]	8.5	8.0	7.5	7.1	7.1	6.0	4.8
Alabama	6.1	5.9	5.2	4.0	4.5	3.7	2.7
Alaska	12.8	9.3	13.9	13.3	11.7	12.3	9.2
Arizona	12.1	13.0	12.8	12.8	12.1	10.0	8.7
Arkansas	6.2	6.3	5.5	5.4	5.7	4.5	4.9
California	9.4	9.0	8.0	8.0	7.3	5.4	3.3
Colorado	9.8	9.8	9.3	8.1	8.4	6.0	4.1
Connecticut	3.9	2.9	2.5	3.7	4.1	3.9	3.5

[1]Excludes data for Puerto Rico.

[2]Data for Puerto Rico are collected in the Puerto Rico Community Survey. Data are not collected for the other territories.

Table 3-75. Persons Under 65 Years of Age Without Health Insurance Coverage, by State, Territory, and Age, 2009–2015—*Continued*

(Percent.)

Characteristic	2009	2010	2011	2012	2013	2014	2015
Delaware	5.7	5.6	3.5	3.6	5.1	*5.0	*2.7
District of Columbia	*	*2.0	*4.1	*	*2.2	*2.6	*1.5
Florida	14.7	12.7	11.9	10.8	11.0	9.2	6.8
Georgia	10.7	9.8	9.5	8.9	9.5	7.5	7.0
Hawaii	2.4	3.7	3.9	2.9	3.2	2.0	*1.4
Idaho	10.7	10.6	8.5	7.6	8.3	7.2	6.0
Illinois	4.4	4.8	3.4	3.2	4.3	3.8	2.5
Indiana	8.5	8.9	8.4	8.0	8.4	7.2	7.1
Iowa	4.4	4.3	4.6	4.3	4.8	3.2	3.3
Kansas	8.1	7.7	6.1	6.9	6.6	6.1	5.2
Kentucky	5.8	5.8	5.9	5.9	5.9	4.3	4.4
Louisiana	6.4	5.6	5.7	5.3	5.6	5.0	3.5
Maine	5.7	3.8	5.5	4.2	5.1	6.1	6.2
Maryland	4.7	4.9	4.5	3.8	4.3	3.4	4.2
Massachusetts	1.7	1.4	1.6	1.3	1.5	1.6	1.2
Michigan	4.3	4.2	3.9	4.2	4.2	3.6	3.3
Minnesota	7.0	6.3	6.1	5.7	6.1	3.5	3.2
Mississippi	10.1	8.2	7.4	7.2	7.3	5.4	4.0
Missouri	7.2	6.3	6.7	7.2	7.3	6.8	5.8
Montana	13.4	12.7	12.8	10.9	10.4	8.6	7.4
Nebraska	6.3	5.2	7.3	5.4	5.9	5.0	4.7
Nevada	18.0	17.9	16.1	16.5	13.9	9.7	7.6
New Hampshire	4.6	4.9	3.2	4.2	3.5	5.2	3.2
New Jersey	6.2	6.0	5.2	5.1	5.7	4.5	3.8
New Mexico	12.0	9.9	9.1	8.1	9.0	7.6	4.4
New York	4.8	4.8	4.4	4.0	4.1	3.4	2.5
North Carolina	7.9	8.1	7.8	7.3	5.9	5.3	4.5
North Dakota	6.3	6.6	7.6	7.4	7.7	6.7	8.5
Ohio	6.4	5.9	6.1	5.4	5.1	4.9	4.3
Oklahoma	11.1	10.4	10.9	9.9	10.5	8.7	8.1
Oregon	10.8	8.8	7.0	5.6	6.3	4.3	3.4
Pennsylvania	5.0	5.2	5.4	5.1	5.0	5.4	4.0
Rhode Island	4.9	4.8	3.9	5.1	6.0	3.3	3.2
South Carolina	9.5	9.8	8.7	7.8	7.0	5.2	4.2
South Dakota	6.8	7.2	5.6	3.9	7.2	7.2	7.2
Tennessee	5.7	5.3	5.8	5.6	5.7	5.2	4.3
Texas	16.3	14.7	13.3	12.3	12.5	11.2	9.4
Utah	10.2	11.1	11.1	9.3	9.0	9.2	7.6
Vermont	*3.3	*2.7	*	*3.0	*	*	*
Virginia	6.7	6.4	5.8	5.6	5.7	5.9	4.9
Washington	7.0	6.4	6.1	5.5	6.3	4.4	2.8
West Virginia	5.4	4.7	5.0	3.9	4.0	3.0	2.6
Wisconsin	4.6	5.2	4.6	4.7	4.4	4.9	3.6
Wyoming	9.0	7.4	8.7	9.9	6.3	6.7	6.2
Puerto Rico[2]	4.2	4.5	4.0	4.3	3.5	3.1	2.7
18 to 64 Years							
United States[1]	20.6	21.4	21.0	20.6	20.3	16.2	13.1
Alabama	19.8	21.2	20.5	19.7	20.2	17.9	15.4
Alaska	25.8	23.6	24.8	25.5	23.9	22.0	18.8
Arizona	23.3	22.3	22.8	23.4	23.7	18.5	14.8
Arkansas	24.6	25.8	25.4	24.5	24.0	17.6	13.5
California	24.5	25.3	25.1	24.7	23.8	17.3	12.0
Colorado	20.3	20.5	19.9	19.4	18.5	14.0	11.0
Connecticut	12.4	13.0	12.4	13.1	13.1	9.4	8.2
Delaware	14.3	13.7	12.7	12.2	14.1	10.1	7.9
District of Columbia	9.2	9.9	9.3	7.1	8.3	7.0	4.6
Florida	28.6	29.9	29.5	28.6	28.8	23.8	19.5
Georgia	25.4	26.9	26.8	25.6	25.8	21.9	19.2
Hawaii	9.9	10.5	10.1	9.4	10.1	7.1	5.7
Idaho	22.8	24.7	22.0	23.1	23.1	19.2	16.3
Illinois	19.0	20.0	18.8	19.0	18.1	13.9	10.1
Indiana	18.8	20.3	19.8	20.0	19.2	16.4	13.1
Iowa	12.2	13.3	12.6	11.8	12.3	8.0	6.6
Kansas	17.1	18.9	17.9	17.8	17.4	14.8	13.1

*Estimates are considered unreliable. Data preceded by an asterisk have a relative standard error of 20 percent to 30 percent. Data not shown have an RSE greater than 30 percent.
[1]Excludes data for Puerto Rico.
[2]Data for Puerto Rico are collected in the Puerto Rico Community Survey. Data are not collected for the other territories.

Table 3-75. Persons Under 65 Years of Age Without Health Insurance Coverage, by State, Territory, and Age, 2009–2015—*Continued*

(Percent.)

Characteristic	2009	2010	2011	2012	2013	2014	2015
Kentucky	20.6	22.0	20.7	19.5	20.8	12.4	8.2
Louisiana	24.8	25.8	25.6	24.4	24.5	21.2	18.0
Maine	14.0	15.4	15.5	15.1	15.8	13.7	11.8
Maryland	15.4	15.5	14.0	14.3	14.0	11.0	8.8
Massachusetts	5.9	6.1	5.8	5.5	5.3	4.6	3.9
Michigan	17.8	18.1	17.3	16.8	16.0	12.1	8.5
Minnesota	11.4	11.6	11.3	10.9	10.8	8.1	5.9
Mississippi	24.3	26.0	25.6	25.0	24.6	21.4	19.0
Missouri	18.4	18.7	19.2	19.5	18.2	16.0	13.4
Montana	25.0	22.1	25.0	25.1	23.0	18.9	16.1
Nebraska	15.9	16.8	16.2	15.7	14.8	13.1	10.9
Nevada	27.3	28.4	28.1	28.4	27.1	20.4	16.5
New Hampshire	14.4	15.3	14.1	15.6	15.6	12.6	9.6
New Jersey	17.2	18.3	18.2	17.9	18.7	15.5	12.3
New Mexico	27.8	28.2	28.5	27.2	27.6	21.1	16.1
New York	16.0	16.6	16.0	15.4	15.2	12.1	10.0
North Carolina	22.2	23.5	22.9	23.3	22.6	19.0	16.3
North Dakota	13.2	13.3	12.9	14.1	13.4	10.1	9.7
Ohio	16.9	17.2	16.8	16.4	15.6	11.5	8.7
Oklahoma	25.6	26.8	25.6	25.6	24.5	21.4	19.9
Oregon	23.1	23.6	21.9	20.9	21.2	14.0	9.9
Pennsylvania	13.6	14.2	14.0	13.4	13.5	11.7	8.6
Rhode Island	15.5	16.7	15.5	16.0	16.4	9.8	7.0
South Carolina	23.0	24.2	23.5	23.6	22.5	19.9	15.9
South Dakota	19.1	16.3	16.6	15.7	17.2	13.4	15.5
Tennessee	20.4	20.7	21.2	20.0	20.1	17.1	14.9
Texas	30.9	31.5	30.9	30.4	29.7	25.6	23.1
Utah	18.6	20.1	19.3	18.4	17.7	16.0	13.8
Vermont	12.0	11.1	10.3	9.2	9.6	6.8	6.2
Virginia	15.8	17.4	17.1	17.3	17.1	14.7	12.8
Washington	18.4	19.7	19.6	19.4	19.8	12.7	9.2
West Virginia	20.5	21.5	22.7	21.2	20.2	13.3	8.0
Wisconsin	12.5	13.1	12.8	12.8	12.7	10.1	7.8
Wyoming	20.7	20.2	20.7	21.5	17.8	16.9	14.2
Puerto Rico[a]	11.5	11.3	10.9	10.0	9.2	8.7	8.2

[a]Data for Puerto Rico are collected in the Puerto Rico Community Survey. Data are not collected for the other territories.

Table 3-76. Medicaid Coverage Among Persons Under 65 Years of Age, by Selected Characteristics, Selected Years, 1984–2015

(Percent.)

Characteristic	1984[1]	1989[1]	1995[1]	2000[2]	2005[3]	2006[3]	2007[3]	2008[3]	2009[3]	2010[3]	2011[3]	2012[3]	2013[3]	2014[3]	2015[3]
Total (number in millions)[4]	14.0	15.4	26.6	23.2	33.2	36.2	36.2	38.4	42.4	44.8	47.4	48.1	48.5	52.6	55.4
Total (percent of population)[4]	6.8	7.2	11.5	9.5	12.9	14.0	13.9	14.7	16.1	16.9	17.8	18.0	18.1	19.6	20.6
Age															
Under 19 years	11.7	12.2	21.1	19.2	26.6	29.4	29.3	30.6	33.9	35.7	37.5	38.1	38.1	38.6	39.2
Under 6 years	15.5	15.7	29.3	24.7	34.0	36.6	36.6	38.1	41.4	43.7	46.1	45.7	45.9	43.8	44.2
6 to 18 years	9.8	10.5	17.0	16.8	23.3	26.1	25.9	27.1	30.3	31.8	33.4	34.7	34.6	36.3	36.9
Under 18 years	11.9	12.6	21.5	19.6	27.2	29.9	29.8	31.3	34.5	36.4	38.2	38.9	38.9	39.4	39.9
6 to 17 years	10.1	10.9	17.4	17.2	23.9	26.7	26.4	27.9	30.9	32.5	34.1	35.5	35.5	37.3	37.9
18 to 64 years	4.5	4.9	7.1	5.2	7.2	7.7	7.5	8.1	8.9	9.2	9.9	10.0	10.2	12.1	13.2
18 to 44 years	5.1	5.2	7.8	5.6	8.3	8.6	8.7	9.2	10.3	10.9	11.6	11.6	11.6	13.8	15.0
18 to 24 years	6.4	6.8	10.4	8.1	11.3	11.4	11.4	12.2	14.0	14.5	15.2	15.4	14.2	17.9	18.5
19 to 25 years	6.3	6.6	10.2	7.3	10.3	9.7	9.9	10.6	12.2	12.6	13.4	13.4	12.1	16.1	16.3
25 to 34 years	5.3	5.2	8.2	5.5	8.0	8.3	8.5	9.3	10.1	11.1	11.5	11.4	11.7	13.3	14.7
35 to 44 years	3.5	4.0	5.9	4.3	6.6	7.1	7.0	7.1	7.7	8.1	9.0	8.8	9.6	11.3	12.8
45 to 64 years	3.4	4.3	5.6	4.5	5.5	6.3	5.9	6.4	6.9	6.8	7.5	8.0	8.4	9.9	10.8
45 to 54 years	3.2	3.8	5.1	4.2	5.2	6.4	6.0	6.2	7.0	7.0	8.0	8.2	8.6	9.8	11.2
55 to 64 years	3.6	4.9	6.4	4.9	5.8	6.1	5.7	6.8	6.8	6.6	6.9	7.7	8.2	9.9	10.4
Sex															
Male	5.4	5.7	9.6	8.2	11.6	12.6	12.5	13.4	14.4	15.2	16.3	16.3	16.5	17.8	19.1
Female	8.1	8.6	13.4	10.8	14.3	15.5	15.2	15.9	17.8	18.5	19.3	19.7	19.8	21.4	22.0
Sex and Marital Status[5]															
Male															
Married	1.9	1.8	2.9	2.2	3.5	3.7	3.5	3.6	4.1	4.0	4.9	4.8	5.3	6.2	7.0
Divorced, separated, widowed	4.9	5.4	7.7	6.1	7.0	7.9	7.8	8.1	8.3	9.3	9.8	9.7	10.3	12.0	12.6
Never married	4.8	5.6	8.1	7.2	10.4	11.6	11.3	12.1	13.1	13.5	14.5	15.1	14.8	17.6	19.6
Female															
Married	2.6	3.0	5.2	3.1	4.7	4.6	4.7	5.2	5.3	5.7	6.4	6.2	6.9	8.1	8.8
Divorced, separated, widowed	16.0	16.1	19.0	12.7	14.6	16.2	16.3	17.2	18.7	17.6	18.0	18.8	18.8	21.6	23.3
Never married	10.7	11.9	16.5	13.2	17.3	19.0	18.1	18.7	20.9	22.2	21.9	22.6	22.2	24.9	25.7
Race[6]															
White only	4.6	5.1	8.9	7.1	11.0	11.8	11.4	12.1	13.7	14.5	15.4	15.5	15.6	16.9	17.9
Black or African American only	20.5	19.0	28.5	21.2	24.9	26.6	27.7	28.3	29.5	30.4	30.9	31.6	31.6	34.1	34.3
American Indian or Alaska Native only	*28.2	29.7	19.0	15.1	24.2	24.3	21.2	37.0	29.7	21.6	29.0	36.5	32.0	35.5	34.3
Asian only	*8.7	*8.8	10.5	7.5	8.2	9.7	8.7	9.2	9.9	12.0	14.7	13.0	13.2	14.7	16.5
Native Hawaiian or Other Pacific Islander only	NA	NA	NA	*	*	*	*	*	*	*	*	*	*	*	*
Two or more races	NA	NA	NA	19.1	22.0	24.0	27.9	24.7	30.1	27.4	27.2	29.1	30.4	30.2	31.5
Hispanic Origin and Race[6]															
Hispanic or Latino	13.3	13.5	21.9	15.5	22.9	23.1	24.7	24.9	27.6	28.6	30.1	30.5	29.5	31.3	33.5
Mexican	12.2	12.4	21.6	14.0	23.0	23.0	25.9	25.4	28.4	29.5	31.0	31.0	29.8	32.1	34.2
Puerto Rican	31.5	27.3	33.4	29.4	31.9	35.7	28.0	31.0	32.1	35.7	33.0	35.3	36.9	35.7	38.9
Cuban	*4.8	*7.7	13.4	9.2	17.7	*11.3	13.3	13.0	16.7	17.3	20.0	22.9	23.3	22.4	22.8
Other Hispanic or Latino	7.9	11.1	18.2	14.5	19.7	20.2	21.4	22.3	24.6	24.5	27.7	28.3	27.0	28.6	30.7
Not Hispanic or Latino	6.2	6.5	10.2	8.5	11.1	12.3	11.7	12.6	13.7	14.4	15.2	15.2	15.5	16.9	17.5
White only	3.7	4.1	7.1	6.1	8.5	9.5	8.5	9.2	10.4	11.0	11.8	11.5	11.9	13.0	13.6
Black or African American only	20.7	19.0	28.1	21.0	24.8	26.2	27.3	27.9	29.1	30.0	30.5	31.3	31.3	33.4	33.6
Age and Percent of Poverty Level[7]															
Under 65 years															
Below 100 percent	33.0	37.6	48.4	38.4	45.7	45.8	47.6	49.1	51.2	50.8	51.4	52.5	53.7	56.5	60.6
100 percent to 199 percent	5.3	7.5	14.4	16.2	23.4	23.8	26.1	27.4	29.0	28.5	30.6	30.1	30.8	34.0	38.1
100 percent to 133 percent	8.7	11.9	23.1	22.4	30.6	30.8	34.8	36.1	39.3	36.3	38.8	38.0	38.8	43.9	47.6
134 percent to 199 percent	3.7	5.6	9.7	13.1	19.5	20.0	21.7	22.9	23.6	24.4	26.1	25.5	26.2	28.1	32.6
200 percent to 399 percent	0.8	1.3	2.3	4.0	6.6	7.0	6.8	7.8	8.0	8.4	8.9	9.0	9.0	9.9	11.3
400 percent or more	0.2	0.5	0.4	0.9	1.5	1.7	1.5	1.6	1.7	2.0	1.7	1.7	1.9	2.2	2.2
Under 19 years															
Below 100 percent	42.0	45.8	63.5	56.9	69.4	70.4	72.7	73.4	77.5	78.4	79.9	82.1	82.1	83.3	84.8
100 percent to 199 percent	6.5	8.6	21.3	27.8	41.7	44.1	47.2	48.5	52.7	53.5	56.7	56.3	58.9	59.1	61.9
100 percent to 133 percent	10.3	13.4	32.4	36.4	51.0	51.3	57.5	60.0	65.6	63.5	69.1	68.8	70.3	71.7	70.9
134 percent to 199 percent	4.7	6.3	14.3	23.3	36.2	39.4	41.3	42.3	45.3	47.7	49.9	48.8	51.6	50.6	55.9
200 percent to 399 percent	1.0	1.7	3.5	7.6	13.0	13.5	13.3	16.4	16.4	17.7	18.3	18.8	19.1	18.5	20.9
400 percent or more	*	*1.2	*	2.1	2.9	3.5	3.0	3.5	3.6	4.3	3.5	3.6	3.2	3.8	4.3
Under 18 years															
Below 100 percent	43.3	47.8	66.0	58.5	71.2	72.0	75.0	75.3	78.3	79.8	81.4	83.7	83.9	84.7	86.7
100 percent to 199 percent	6.6	8.7	21.6	28.4	42.5	44.7	48.1	49.5	53.5	54.3	57.6	57.3	60.1	60.0	62.6
100 percent to 133 percent	10.4	13.5	32.9	36.9	52.0	51.7	58.4	61.1	66.9	64.6	70.1	70.1	71.2	72.3	72.0
134 percent to 199 percent	4.8	6.4	14.4	23.8	36.9	40.1	42.2	43.2	45.9	48.2	50.6	49.6	52.9	51.6	56.5

NA = Not available.
* = Figure does not meet standards of reliability or precision. Data not shown have a relative standard error of greater than 30 percent.
[1] Data prior to 1997 are not strictly comparable with data for later years due to the 1997 questionnaire redesign.
[2] Estimates for 2000-2002 were calculated using 2000-based sample weights and may differ from estimates in other reports that used 1990-based sample weights for 2000-2002 estimates.
[3] Beginning in quarter 3 of the 2004 NHIS, persons under 65 years of age with no reported coverage were asked explicitly about Medicaid coverage. Estimates were calculated with the additional information starting with 2005 data.
[4] Includes all other races not shown separately, those with unknown marital status, unknown disability status, and, in 1984 and 1989, persons with unknown poverty level.
[5] Includes persons 14 to 64 years of age.
[6] The race groups White, Black, American Indian or Alaska Native, Asian, Native Hawaiian or Other Pacific Islander, and two or more races include persons of Hispanic and non-Hispanic origin. Persons of Hispanic origin may be of any race.
[7] Percent of poverty level is based on family income and family size and composition using U.S. Census Bureau poverty thresholds. Poverty level was unknown for 10 to 11 percent of persons under 65 years of age in 1984 and 1989. Missing family income data were imputed for 1995 and beyond.

Table 3-76. Medicaid Coverage Among Persons Under 65 Years of Age, by Selected Characteristics, Selected Years, 1984–2015—*Continued*

(Percent.)

Characteristic	1984[1]	1989[1]	1995[1]	2000[2]	2005[3]	2006[3]	2007[3]	2008[3]	2009[3]	2010[3]	2011[3]	2012[3]	2013[3]	2014[3]	2015[3]
200 percent to 399 percent	1.0	1.7	3.5	7.6	13.3	13.8	13.3	16.8	16.8	18.0	18.6	19.1	19.5	18.9	21.2
400 percent or more	*	*1.1	*	2.2	2.9	3.4	3.0	3.6	3.7	4.3	3.6	3.6	3.3	4.0	4.3
18 to 64 years															
Below 100 percent	25.3	29.1	34.8	24.9	29.6	28.9	30.6	33.0	33.6	32.4	33.0	34.0	35.4	39.7	44.8
100 percent to 199 percent	4.5	6.8	10.2	9.1	13.1	13.0	14.0	15.3	16.2	15.7	17.1	16.8	17.1	21.4	25.9
100 percent to 133 percent	7.6	10.8	16.3	13.2	17.9	17.8	20.2	21.9	23.7	21.0	22.7	21.8	22.0	28.3	34.2
134 percent to 199 percent	3.1	5.1	7.2	7.2	10.7	10.5	11.0	11.8	12.4	13.0	14.1	13.9	14.4	17.6	21.3
200 percent to 399 percent	0.7	1.1	1.7	2.4	3.8	4.2	4.0	4.1	4.6	4.8	5.2	5.1	5.1	6.7	7.6
400 percent or more	0.2	0.4	0.4	0.6	1.1	1.2	1.1	1.1	1.2	1.3	1.2	1.2	1.6	1.7	1.7
Disability Measure among Adults 18 to 64 Years[6]															
Any basic actions difficulty or complex activity limitation	NA	NA	NA	12.8	16.4	16.2	16.5	18.6	18.2	17.8	19.6	19.3	21.1	22.9	25.1
Any basic actions difficulty	NA	NA	NA	12.2	15.5	15.3	15.9	17.7	17.8	16.7	19.1	18.4	20.6	22.0	24.6
Any complex activity limitation	NA	NA	NA	23.2	28.5	28.7	28.7	31.0	30.2	30.0	30.8	30.8	32.3	35.6	36.9
No disability	NA	NA	NA	3.0	4.9	5.1	5.2	4.9	6.4	6.8	6.9	7.0	6.8	8.7	9.2
Geographic Region															
Northeast	8.6	6.6	11.7	10.6	13.3	16.8	15.4	16.1	17.3	17.9	19.6	19.3	20.8	21.4	21.6
Midwest	7.4	7.6	10.5	8.0	12.3	13.9	13.7	14.5	16.4	17.3	16.7	16.3	16.9	18.6	19.8
South	5.1	6.5	11.3	9.4	12.7	12.9	12.9	13.5	14.8	16.0	17.3	17.8	17.8	18.7	18.4
West	7.0	8.5	12.9	10.4	13.8	13.8	14.5	15.7	16.8	17.1	18.4	19.1	18.0	20.9	24.0
Location of Residence															
Within MSA[9]	7.1	7.0	11.3	8.9	12.4	13.3	13.3	14.2	15.2	16.1	17.0	17.4	17.4	18.9	19.8
Outside MSA[9]	6.1	7.9	12.3	11.9	15.5	17.7	17.1	17.2	20.8	21.4	22.1	21.4	22.5	24.4	25.4

NA = Not available.

* = Figure does not meet standards of reliability or precision. Data not shown have a relative standard error of greater than 30 percent.

[1]Data prior to 1997 are not strictly comparable with data for later years due to the 1997 questionnaire redesign.

[2]Estimates for 2000-2002 were calculated using 2000-based sample weights and may differ from estimates in other reports that used 1990-based sample weights for 2000-2002 estimates.

[3]Beginning in quarter 3 of the 2004 NHIS, persons under 65 years of age with no reported coverage were asked explicitly about Medicaid coverage. Estimates were calculated with the additional information starting with 2005 data.

[7]Percent of poverty level is based on family income and family size and composition using U.S. Census Bureau poverty thresholds. Poverty level was unknown for 10 to 11 percent of persons under 65 years of age in 1984 and 1989. Missing family income data were imputed for 1995 and beyond.

[8]Any basic actions difficulty or complex activity limitation is defined as having one or more of the following limitations or difficulties: movement difficulty, emotional difficulty, sensory (seeing or hearing) difficulty, cognitive difficulty, self-care (activities of daily living or instrumental activities of daily living) limitation, social limitation, or work limitation.

[9]MSA = metropolitan statistical area.

Table 3-77. Medicaid Beneficiaries and Payments, by Basis of Eligibility, and Race and Hispanic Origin, Selected Fiscal Years, 1999–2013

(Number, percent, dollar.)

Characteristic	1999	2000	2005	2007	2008	2009	2010	2011[1]	2012[1]	2013[1]
Beneficiaries (Number in Millions)[2]										
All beneficiaries	40.1	42.8	57.7	56.8	58.8	62.6	65.7	71.4	71.6	73.7
Percent of Beneficiaries										
Basis of eligibility										
Aged (65 years and over)	9.4	8.7	7.6	7.1	7.1	6.7	6.5	5.7	5.7	5.6
Blind and disabled	16.7	16.1	14.2	14.8	14.8	14.4	14.3	13.1	13.2	13.0
Adults in families with dependent children[3]	18.7	20.5	21.8	21.8	22.0	23.1	23.7	18.9	19.5	19.0
Children under age 21[4]	46.9	46.1	47.2	48.4	47.8	47.7	48.3	40.5	40.6	40.4
Other Title XIX[5]	8.4	8.6	9.1	7.8	8.4	8.1	7.2	9.6	8.7	9.8
Separate CHIP[6]	NA	NA	NA	NA	NA	NA	NA	12.2	12.3	12.1
Race and Hispanic Origin[7]										
White	NA	NA	39.3	38.6	38.1	38.2	38.9	37.2	37.2	36.1
Black or African American	NA	NA	21.5	21.6	21.1	20.7	20.6	19.8	20.1	19.5
American Indian or Alaska Native	NA	NA	1.2	1.2	1.3	1.2	1.2	1.1	1.1	1.1
Asian or Pacific Islander	NA	NA	3.5	3.5	3.5	3.6	3.6	3.6	3.8	3.8
Asian	NA	NA	2.5	2.6	2.6	2.7	2.7	2.8	2.9	3.0
Pacific Islander	NA	NA	0.9	0.9	0.9	0.9	0.9	0.9	0.8	0.8
Hispanic or Latino	NA	NA	20.6	21.6	21.7	22.3	22.3	17.4	17.4	17.4
Multiple race or unknown	NA	NA	13.9	13.5	14.3	14.0	13.3	20.9	20.4	22.0
Payments (Billions of Dollars)[8]										
All payments	$153.5	$168.3	$274.9	$276.2	$296.8	$326.0	$339.0	$368.6	$363.9	$375.3
Percent Distribution	100.0	100.0	100.0	100.0	100.0	100.0	100.0	100.0	100.0	100.0
Basis of eligibility										
Aged (65 years and over)	27.7	26.4	23.1	20.7	20.6	19.7	19.4	16.6	16.7	16.7
Blind and disabled	42.9	43.2	43.4	43.3	43.5	43.4	43.4	40.8	41.2	41.0
Adults in families with dependent children[3]	10.3	10.6	11.8	12.4	12.7	13.9	14.2	12.6	13.3	13.1
Children under age 21[4]	15.7	15.9	17.2	19.4	19.2	19.6	19.8	18.1	18.2	18.4
Other Title XIX[5]	3.4	3.9	4.6	4.2	4.0	3.3	3.1	4.5	3.5	3.5
Separate CHIP[6]	NA	NA	NA	NA	NA	NA	NA	7.4	7.2	7.4
Race and Hispanic Origin[5]										
White	NA	NA	53.0	50.7	50.2	50.0	50.2	48.1	48.3	47.5
Black or African American	NA	NA	19.8	20.8	20.6	20.7	20.5	20.3	20.8	20.3
American Indian or Alaska Native	NA	NA	1.2	1.2	1.3	1.2	1.3	1.2	1.3	1.3
Asian or Pacific Islander	NA	NA	2.7	2.8	2.9	3.1	3.0	3.1	3.2	3.5
Asian	NA	NA	1.9	2.0	2.1	2.3	2.3	2.4	2.5	2.7
Pacific Islander	NA	NA	0.8	0.8	0.8	0.8	0.7	0.7	0.7	0.7
Hispanic or Latino	NA	NA	12.2	13.1	13.7	14.2	14.2	9.9	9.7	10.1
Multiple race or unknown	NA	NA	11.1	11.4	11.4	10.8	10.8	17.4	16.7	17.4
Payments per Beneficiary (Dollars)[6]										
All beneficiaries	$3,819	$3,936	$4,768	$4,862	$5,051	$5,209	$5,160	$5,159	$5,082	$5,094
Basis of eligibility										
Aged (65 years and over)	11,268	11,929	14,427	14,141	14,742	15,337	15,286	15,073	14,862	15,194
Blind and disabled	9,832	10,559	14,531	14,194	14,843	15,670	15,695	16,104	15,825	16,115
Adults in families with dependent children[3]	2,104	2,030	2,583	2,753	2,912	3,144	3,095	3,443	3,460	3,503
Children under age 21[4]	1,282	1,358	1,732	1,951	2,035	2,145	2,122	2,300	2,281	2,315
Other Title XIX[5]	1,532	1,778	2,380	2,622	2,407	2,104	2,219	2,402	2,030	1,803
Separate CHIP[6]	NA	NA	NA	NA	NA	NA	NA	3,125	2,979	3,083
Race and Hispanic Origin[7]										
White	NA	NA	6,422	6,390	6,657	6,809	6,663	6,677	6,598	6,691
Black or African American	NA	NA	4,397	4,669	4,928	5,216	5,142	5,308	5,266	5,314
American Indian or Alaska Native	NA	NA	4,626	4,826	5,218	5,382	5,421	5,461	5,649	5,824
Asian or Pacific Islander	NA	NA	3,710	3,863	4,133	4,402	4,300	4,483	4,365	4,585
Asian	NA	NA	3,624	3,847	4,123	4,386	4,307	4,482	4,383	4,575
Pacific Islander	NA	NA	3,947	3,907	4,161	4,448	4,275	4,484	4,302	4,624
Hispanic or Latino	NA	NA	2,822	2,960	3,175	3,322	3,276	2,944	2,821	2,958
Multiple race or unknown	NA	NA	3,816	4,106	4,014	4,025	4,173	4,298	4,161	4,025

Note: Data are for fiscal years ending September 30.

NA = Not available.

[1]Starting with 2011, a new tabular methodology was used. Therefore, estimates may not be comparable to earlier data and caution should be used with trend analysis.

[2]Beneficiaries include those who were enrolled or received services through Medicaid or the Children's Health Insurance Program (CHIP). Beneficiary counts for 2011 and subsequent years were derived from MSIS claims files. Separate CHIP beneficiaries are included for 2011 and subsequent years.

[3]Includes adults who meet the requirements for the Aid to Families with Dependent Children (AFDC) program that were in effect in their state on July 16, 1996, or, at state option, meet more liberal criteria (with some exceptions). Includes adults in the Temporary Assistance for Needy Families (TANF) program. Starting with 2001 data, includes women in the Breast and Cervical Cancer Prevention and Treatment Program and unemployed adults.

[4]Includes children (including those in the foster care system) in the TANF program.

[5]Includes some participants in the Supplemental Security Income program and other people deemed medically needy in participating states. Prior to 2001, includes unemployed adults. Excludes foster care children and includes unknown eligibility.

[6]CHIP is Children's Health Insurance Program. CHIP provides federal funds for states to provide health care coverage to eligible low-income, uninsured children who do not qualify for Medicaid. Some states use CHIP funds to expand Medicaid. For 2012 data, all states except Colorado and Idaho had separate CHIP beneficiaries.

[7]Race and Hispanic origin are as determined on initial Medicaid application. Categories are mutually exclusive. Starting with 2001 data, the Hispanic category included Hispanic persons, regardless of race. Persons indicating more than one race were included in the multiple race category.

[8]Medicaid payments exclude disproportionate share hospital (DSH) payments ($14.7 billion in FY2010) and DSH mental health facility payments ($2.9 billion in FY2010).

Table 3-78. Medicaid Beneficiaries and Payments, by Type of Service, Selected Fiscal Years, 1999–2013

(Number; percent.)

Type of service	1999	2000	2005	2007	2008	2009	2010	2011[1]	2012[1]	2013[1]
Beneficiaries (Number in Millions)[2]										
All beneficiaries	40.2	42.8	57.7	56.8	58.8	62.6	65.7	71.4	71.6	73.7
Percent										
Inpatient hospital	11.2	11.5	9.5	9.0	8.9	8.7	6.9	11.4	11.8	12.5
Mental health facility	0.2	0.2	0.2	0.2	0.2	0.2	0.2	0.2	0.2	0.2
Intermediate care facility for individuals with intellectual disabilities[3]	0.3	0.3	0.2	0.2	0.2	0.2	0.2	0.1	0.1	0.1
Nursing facility	4.0	4.0	3.0	2.9	2.7	2.6	2.4	2.5	2.3	2.3
Physician	45.7	44.7	42.0	38.8	36.9	36.9	36.9	62.6	64.4	65.5
Dental	14.0	13.8	16.2	16.8	16.7	17.8	19.1	26.6	27.4	28.3
Other practitioner	9.9	11.1	10.2	9.5	8.8	8.8	9.2	13.6	14.2	14.3
Outpatient hospital	30.9	30.9	28.2	26.2	25.2	26.4	24.2	38.8	39.5	40.1
Clinic	16.8	17.9	20.7	20.6	20.2	20.6	20.7	24.4	23.6	23.9
Laboratory and radiological	25.4	26.6	27.7	27.8	26.6	26.2	25.8	41.6	42.0	42.5
Home health	2.0	2.3	2.1	2.1	1.9	1.7	1.7	2.4	2.5	2.4
Prescribed drugs	49.4	48.0	49.2	42.1	41.8	42.6	44.7	56.8	57.2	57.5
Capitated care	51.5	49.7	58.1	64.5	64.9	66.6	70.8	93.6	86.9	88.4
Primary care case management	9.7	13.0	15.1	12.5	14.9	13.1	13.3	13.3	13.6	11.4
Personal support	10.1	10.6	11.8	11.6	10.8	10.7	11.0	1.7	1.7	1.6
Other care[4]	21.6	21.4	21.9	21.5	21.3	20.6	19.9	47.6	47.9	49.3
Payments (Billions of Dollars)[3]										
All payments	$153.5	$168.3	$274.9	$276.2	$296.8	$326.0	$339.0	$368.6	$363.9	$375.3
Percent Distribution	100.0	100.0	100.0	100.0	100.0	100.0	100.0	100.0	100.0	100.0
Inpatient hospital	14.5	14.4	12.8	13.4	12.5	11.8	9.9	10.7	10.3	9.5
Mental health facility	1.1	1.1	0.8	0.9	0.8	0.8	0.7	0.7	0.6	0.6
Intermediate care facility for individuals with intellectual disabilities[3]	6.1	5.6	4.3	4.3	4.2	3.9	3.7	3.6	3.3	3.1
Nursing facility	21.7	20.5	16.3	16.8	16.1	14.9	14.4	13.1	13.0	12.5
Physician	4.3	4.0	4.1	3.6	3.5	3.5	3.5	3.3	3.0	2.8
Dental	0.8	0.8	1.1	1.2	1.3	1.4	1.6	1.6	1.3	1.0
Other practitioner	0.3	0.4	0.4	0.3	0.3	0.3	0.3	0.5	0.5	0.5
Outpatient hospital	4.0	4.2	3.6	3.7	3.7	3.7	3.8	3.5	3.5	3.3
Clinic	3.8	3.7	3.2	3.1	3.1	3.1	3.2	3.4	3.2	3.3
Laboratory and radiological	0.8	0.8	1.1	1.1	1.0	1.0	1.0	1.0	0.8	0.8
Home health	1.9	1.9	2.0	2.3	2.2	2.2	2.1	2.0	1.8	1.7
Prescribed drugs	10.8	11.9	15.6	8.0	7.9	7.8	8.0	7.9	6.1	4.9
Capitated care	14.0	14.5	16.9	21.2	23.0	25.5	27.2	29.5	33.6	37.8
Primary care case management	0.3	0.1	0.1	0.1	0.1	0.1	0.1	0.1	0.1	0.1
Personal support	6.9	6.9	7.5	8.4	8.3	8.0	7.7	3.3	3.3	3.0
Other care[4]	8.6	8.8	10.2	11.6	12.0	11.9	12.7	15.9	15.6	15.0
Payments per Beneficiary (Dollars)[3]										
All beneficiaries	$3,819	$3,936	$4,768	$4,862	$5,051	$5,209	$5,160	$5,159	$5,082	$5,094
Inpatient hospital	4,943	4,919	6,411	7,191	7,083	7,070	7,347	4,858	4,437	3,885
Mental health facility	18,094	17,800	19,252	21,407	21,975	21,404	20,782	14,557	13,221	12,691
Intermediate care facility for individuals with intellectual disabilities[3]	76,443	79,330	107,028	113,735	123,053	127,837	125,851	129,806	119,903	120,995
Nursing facility	20,568	20,220	26,185	28,282	29,533	29,551	31,617	26,995	28,060	27,808
Physician	357	356	465	457	485	496	492	271	238	219
Dental	214	238	326	340	389	423	432	301	245	181
Other practitioner	118	139	200	170	171	171	190	186	183	173
Outpatient hospital	491	533	617	695	736	735	803	470	454	424
Clinic	860	805	749	741	772	792	791	712	680	709
Laboratory and radiological	114	113	183	185	188	198	205	119	102	91
Home health	3,571	3,135	4,487	5,334	5,789	6,628	6,375	4,286	3,565	3,581
Prescribed drugs	837	975	1,509	926	957	951	926	719	540	432
Capitated care	1,040	1,148	1,386	1,598	1,786	1,991	1,983	1,627	1,964	2,178
Primary care case management	119	30	27	33	32	41	49	45	47	50
Personal support	2,583	2,543	3,035	3,534	3,852	3,903	3,593	9,959	9,619	9,588
Other care[4]	1,508	1,600	2,228	2,611	2,856	3,015	3,289	1,724	1,653	1,554

[1]Starting with 2011, a new tabular methodology was used. Therefore, estimates may not be comparable to earlier data and caution should be used with trend analysis.
[2]Beneficiaries include those who were enrolled or received services through Medicaid or the Children's Health Insurance Program (CHIP). Separate CHIP beneficiaries are included for 2011 and subsequent years.
[3]This category was previously known as Intermediate care facility for the mentally retarded. This is a change in terminology only and not measurement.
[4]Estimates for 2010 and earlier include unknown services and payments with Other care.

Table 3-79. Medicaid Beneficiaries, Beneficiaries in Managed Care, and Payments Per Beneficiary, by State, Selected Fiscal Years, 2000–2011

(Number.)

State	Beneficiaries (in thousands)[1]		Percent of beneficiaries in managed care[2]		Payments Per Beneficiary[3]	
	2000	2011	2000	2011	2000	2011
United States	42,763	68,850	56	74	$3,936	$5,304
Alabama	619	938	60	61	3,860	4,457
Alaska	96	135	-	-	4,876	9,693
Arizona	681	1,990	92	89	3,100	4,743
Arkansas	489	784	57	78	3,086	4,647
California	7,915	11,501	50	60	2,155	3,266
Colorado	381	737	90	95	4,747	4,717
Connecticut	420	730	72	69	6,762	8,001
Delaware	115	229	79	81	4,584	6,445
District of Columbia	139	236	66	67	5,715	9,028
Florida	2,360	3,829	60	64	3,114	4,507
Georgia	1,290	2,143	96	91	2,774	3,908
Hawaii	204	314	74	99	2,626	4,674
Idaho[4]	131	261	30	100	4,530	5,533
Illinois	1,516	2,917	10	68	5,150	4,072
Indiana	705	1,212	67	70	4,224	4,756
Iowa	314	545	90	91	4,707	6,023
Kansas	263	404	56	87	4,670	6,362
Kentucky	771	1,086	81	89	3,780	5,192
Louisiana	761	1,298	6	65	3,456	4,241
Maine	192	NA	35	NA	6,820	NA
Maryland	665	1,004	81	75	5,396	7,160
Massachusetts	1,047	1,720	64	53	5,153	6,584
Michigan	1,352	2,304	100	88	3,611	5,158
Minnesota	559	993	63	66	5,857	7,998
Mississippi	605	820	39	87	2,987	4,514
Missouri	890	1,151	40	98	3,673	5,465
Montana	104	137	61	76	4,173	5,838
Nebraska	229	284	77	85	4,185	5,666
Nevada	138	363	39	84	3,733	3,843
New Hampshire	97	152	6	-	6,712	6,769
New Jersey	822	1,310	59	78	5,724	6,789
New Mexico	376	572	64	73	3,325	4,513
New York	3,420	5,421	25	77	7,646	9,445
North Carolina	1,209	1,901	68	83	3,996	5,059
North Dakota	61	89	55	64	5,852	8,279
Ohio	1,305	2,527	21	75	5,434	6,262
Oklahoma	507	957	69	86	3,163	3,949
Oregon	542	749	83	98	3,135	4,782
Pennsylvania	1,492	2,444	73	82	4,266	7,242
Rhode Island	179	221	69	69	5,982	7,265
South Carolina	685	979	6	100	3,900	5,263
South Dakota	102	135	93	76	3,935	5,687
Tennessee	1,568	1,488	100	100	2,226	7,532
Texas	2,603	4,996	34	71	3,487	4,487
Utah	224	435	90	100	4,277	4,946
Vermont	139	187	47	58	3,451	5,622
Virginia	627	1,019	59	58	3,960	5,860
Washington	895	1,396	100	88	2,717	4,491
West Virginia	335	411	35	51	4,154	7,119
Wisconsin	577	1,319	44	64	5,039	4,353
Wyoming	46	76	-	-	4,609	7,550

NA = Not available.
- = Quantity zero.
[1]Beneficiaries include those who received services through Medicaid.
[2]Medicaid managed care enrollment data include individuals in state health care reform programs that expand eligibility beyond traditional Medicaid eligibility standards. The managed care enrollment data include enrollees receiving comprehensive and limited benefits. Managed care enrollment as of June 30 of year shown. Starting with 2001 data, U.S. total excludes Puerto Rico and Virgin Islands. Managed care enrollment data may change year to year due to a variety of factors, including changes in waiver programs, outreach efforts, and data reporting practices. For more information, see: http://www.medicaid.gov.
[3]Medicaid payments exclude disproportionate share hospital (DSH) payments ($14.3 billion in FY2011) and DSH mental health facility payments ($2.9 billion in FY2011). Available from: http://medicaid.gov/Medicaid-CHIP-Program-Information/By-Topics/Data-and-Systems/MBES/CMS-64-Quarterly-Expense-Report.html.
[4]In 2010, Idaho implemented a new Medicaid management information system. This system assigned new identification numbers to enrollees and redesigned Idaho's Medicaid Statistical Information System. These changes may have affected Idaho's Medicaid data. Therefore, trends of data for Idaho should be interpreted with caution.

Table 3-80. Medicare Enrollees and Expenditures and Percent Distribution, by Medicare Program and Type of Service, Selected Years, 1970–2015

(Number; dollars; percent.)

Medicare program and type of service	1970	1980	1990	1995	2000	2005	2008	2009	2010	2011	2012	2013	2014	2015[1]
Enrollees (Numbers in Millions)														
Total Medicare[2]	20.4	28.4	34.3	37.6	39.7	42.6	45.5	46.6	47.7	48.9	50.9	52.5	54.1	55.3
Hospital insurance	20.1	28.0	33.7	37.2	39.3	42.2	45.1	46.3	47.4	48.5	50.5	52.1	53.7	54.9
Supplementary medical insurance (SMI)[3]	19.5	27.3	32.6	35.6	37.3	NA	NA	NA	NA	NA	NA	NA	NA	NA
Part B	19.5	27.3	32.6	35.6	37.3	39.8	42.0	42.9	43.9	44.9	46.5	48.0	49.4	50.7
Part D[4]	NA	NA	NA	NA	NA	1.8	32.6	33.6	34.8	35.7	37.4	39.1	40.5	41.8
Expenditures (Dollars in Billions)	$7.5	$36.8	$111.0	$184.2	$221.8	$336.4	$468.2	$509.0	$522.9	$549.1	$574.2	$582.9	$613.3	$647.6
Total Medicare	5.3	25.6	67.0	117.6	131.1	182.9	235.6	242.5	247.9	256.7	266.8	266.2	269.3	278.9
Total hospital insurance (HI)	NA	0.0	2.7	6.7	21.4	24.9	50.6	59.4	60.7	64.6	70.2	73.1	74.0	78.5
HI payments to managed care organizations[5]	5.1	25.0	63.4	109.5	105.1	156.6	172.8	179.5	183.3	186.9	189.2	184.7	186.4	191.5
HI payments for fee-for-service utilization	4.8	24.1	56.9	82.3	87.1	123.3	130.5	134.1	136.1	133.9	138.9	134.2	136.2	139.2
Inpatient hospital	0.2	0.4	2.5	9.1	11.1	19.3	24.3	26.1	27.0	31.9	28.4	28.4	28.5	29.7
Skilled nursing facility	0.1	0.5	3.7	16.2	4.0	6.0	6.6	7.0	7.1	7.1	6.8	6.8	6.5	6.6
Home health agency	NA	NA	0.3	1.9	2.9	8.0	11.4	12.3	13.1	14.0	15.0	15.2	15.2	15.9
Hospice	NA	NA	NA	NA	NA	NA	NA	NA	NA	0.9	2.8	3.5	3.7	2.6
Other programs[6]	NA	NA	NA	NA	1.7	NA	NA	NA	NA	NA	NA	NA	NA	NA
Home health agency transfer[7]	NA	NA	NA	NA	NA	0.1	0.1	0.2	0.2	0.2	0.3	0.3	0.3
Medicare Advantage premiums[8]	NA	NA	NA	NA	NA	-1.9	8.5	NA	NA	NA	NA	NA	NA	NA
Accounting error (CY 2005-2008)[9]	0.2	0.5	0.9	1.4	2.9	3.3	3.6	3.5	3.8	4.0	4.3	4.7	4.9	5.9
Administrative expenses[10]	2.2	11.2	44.0	66.6	90.7	153.5	232.6	266.5	274.9	292.5	307.4	316.7	344.0	368.8
Total supplementary medical insurance (SMI)[3]	2.2	11.2	44.0	66.6	90.7	152.4	183.3	205.7	212.9	225.3	240.5	247.1	265.9	279.0
Total Part B	0.0	0.2	2.8	6.6	18.4	22.0	48.1	53.4	55.2	59.1	66.0	72.7	85.7	93.8
Part B payments to managed care organizations[5]	1.9	10.4	39.6	58.4	72.2	125.0	140.5	149.0	154.3	162.3	170.3	170.8	175.8	181.5
Part B payments for fee-for-service utilization[11]	1.8	8.2	29.6	NA	NA	NA	NA	NA	NA	NA	NA	NA	NA	NA
Physician/supplies[12]	0.1	1.9	8.5	NA	NA	NA	NA	NA	NA	NA	NA	NA	NA	NA
Outpatient hospital[13]	0.0	0.1	1.5	NA	NA	NA	NA	NA	NA	NA	NA	NA	NA	NA
Independent laboratory[14]	NA	NA	NA	31.7	37.0	57.7	60.6	61.8	63.9	67.5	69.5	68.6	69.2	70.3
Physician fee schedule	NA	NA	NA	3.7	4.7	8.0	8.6	8.2	8.3	8.2	8.2	7.2	6.3	6.8
Durable medical equipment	NA	NA	NA	4.3	4.4	6.9	7.9	8.2	8.4	8.4	9.2	9.1	8.2	8.5
Laboratory[15]	NA	NA	NA	9.9	13.6	26.7	29.6	33.1	34.2	36.0	38.4	38.3	39.5	41.1
Other[16]	NA	NA	NA	8.7	8.1	18.7	23.6	26.0	27.6	30.2	33.6	36.2	41.5	43.7
Hospital[17]	0.0	0.2	0.1	0.2	4.5	7.1	10.3	11.7	12.0	12.1	11.4	11.4	11.1	11.1
Home health agency	NA	NA	NA	NA	-1.7	NA	NA	NA	NA	NA	NA	NA	NA	NA
Home health agency transfer[7]	NA	NA	NA	NA	NA	0.1	0.1	0.2	0.2	0.2	0.3	0.3	0.4
Medicare Advantage premiums[8]	NA	NA	NA	NA	NA	1.9	-8.5	NA	NA	NA	NA	NA	NA	NA
Accounting error (CY 2005-2008)[9]	0.2	0.6	1.5	1.6	1.8	2.8	3.1	3.2	3.2	3.7	4.0	3.4	4.1	3.3
Administrative expenses[10]	NA	NA	NA	NA	NA	0.7	0.0	NA	NA	NA	NA	NA	NA	NA
Part D start-up costs[18]	NA	NA	NA	NA	NA	1.1	49.3	60.8	62.1	67.1	66.9	69.7	78.1	89.8
Total Part D[4]														
Percent Distribution of Expenditures														
Total hospital insurance (HI)	100.0	100.0	100.0	100.0	100.0	100.0	100.0	100.0	100.0	100.0	100.0	100.0	100.0	100.0
HI payments to managed care organizations[5]	NA	0.0	4.0	5.7	16.3	13.6	21.5	24.5	24.5	25.2	26.3	27.5	27.5	28.2
HI payments for fee-for-service utilization	97.0	97.9	94.6	93.1	80.2	85.6	73.4	74.0	73.9	72.8	70.9	69.4	69.2	68.6
Inpatient hospital	91.4	94.3	85.0	70.0	66.4	67.4	55.4	55.3	54.9	52.2	52.1	50.4	50.6	49.9
Skilled nursing facility	4.7	1.5	3.7	7.8	8.5	10.6	10.3	10.8	10.9	12.4	10.7	10.7	10.6	10.7
Home health agency	1.0	2.1	5.5	13.8	3.1	3.3	2.8	2.9	2.9	2.8	2.6	2.6	2.4	2.4
Hospice	NA	NA	0.5	1.6	2.2	4.4	4.8	5.1	5.3	5.5	5.6	5.7	5.6	5.7
Other programs[6]	NA	NA	NA	NA	NA	NA	NA	NA	NA	0.3	1.1	1.3	1.4	0.9
Home health agency transfer[7]	NA	NA	NA	NA	1.3	NA	NA	NA	NA	NA	NA	NA	NA	NA
Medicare Advantage premiums[8]	NA	NA	NA	NA	NA	NA	0.0	0.1	0.1	0.1	0.1	0.1	0.1	0.1
Accounting error (CY 2005-2008)[9]	NA	NA	NA	NA	NA	3.6	NA	NA	NA	NA	NA	NA	NA
Administrative expenses[10]	3.0	2.1	1.4	1.2	2.2	1.8	1.5	1.4	1.5	1.6	1.6	1.8	1.8	2.1
Total supplementary medical insurance (SMI)[3]	100.0	100.0	100.0	100.0	100.0	100.0	100.0	100.0	100.0	100.0	100.0	100.0	100.0	100.0
Total Part B	100.0	100.0	100.0	100.0	100.0	99.3	78.8	77.2	77.4	77.1	78.2	78.0	77.3	75.6
Part B payments to managed care organizations[5]	1.2	1.8	6.4	9.9	20.2	14.3	20.7	20.0	20.1	20.2	21.5	22.9	24.9	25.4
Part B payments for fee-for-service utilization[11]	88.1	92.8	90.1	87.6	79.6	81.5	60.4	55.9	56.1	55.5	55.4	53.9	51.1	49.2

NA = Not available.

0.0 = Quantity more than zero but less than 0.05.

[1] Preliminary estimates.

[2] Average number enrolled in the hospital insurance (HI) and/or supplementary medical insurance (SMI) programs for the period.

[3] Starting with 2004 data, the SMI trust fund consists of two separate accounts: Part B (which pays for a portion of the costs of physicians' services, outpatient hospital services, and other related medical and health services for voluntarily enrolled individuals) and Part D (Medicare Prescription Drug Account, which pays private plans to provide prescription drug coverage).

[4] The Medicare Modernization Act, enacted on December 8, 2003, established within SMI two Part D accounts related to prescription drug benefits: the Medicare Prescription Drug Account and the Transitional Assistance Account.

[5] Medicare-approved managed care organizations.

[6] Includes Community-Based Care Transitions Program ($0.1 billion in each of 2011–2015) and Electronic Health Records Incentive Program ($0.7 billion in 2011, $2.7 billion in 2012, $3.4 billion in 2013, $3.6 billion in 2014, and $2.5 billion in 2015).

[7] For 1998 to 2003 data, reflects annual home health HI to SMI transfer amounts.

[8] When a beneficiary chooses a Medicare Advantage plan whose monthly premium exceeds the benchmark amount, the additional premiums (that is, amounts beyond those paid by Medicare to the plan) are the responsibility of the beneficiary.

[9] Represents misallocation of benefit payments between the HI trust fund and the Part B account of the SMI trust fund from May 2005 to September 2007, and the transfer made in June 2008 to correct the misallocation.

[10] Includes expenditures for research, experiments and demonstration projects, peer review activity (performed by Peer Review Organizations from 1983 to 2001 and by Quality Review Organizations from 2002 to present), and to combat and prevent fraud and abuse.

[11] Type-of-service reporting categories for fee-for-service reimbursement differ before and after 1991.

[12] Includes payment for physicians, practitioners, durable medical equipment, and all suppliers other than independent laboratory through 1990. Starting with 1991 data, physician services subject to the physician fee schedule are shown. Payments for laboratory services paid under the laboratory fee schedule and performed in a physician office are included under Laboratory beginning in 1991.

[13] Includes payments for hospital outpatient department services, skilled nursing facility outpatient services, Part B services received as an inpatient in a hospital or skilled nursing facility setting, and other types of outpatient facilities.

[14] Starting with 1991 data, those independent laboratory services that were paid under the laboratory fee schedule (most of the independent laboratory category) are included in the Laboratory line; the remaining services are included in the Physician fee schedule and Other lines.

[15] Payments for laboratory services paid under the laboratory fee schedule performed in a physician office, independent laboratory, or in a hospital outpatient department.

[16] Includes payments for physician-administered drugs; freestanding ambulatory surgical center facility services; ambulance services; supplies; freestanding end-stage renal disease (ESRD) dialysis facility services; rural health clinics; outpatient rehabilitation facilities; psychiatric hospitals; and federally qualified health centers.

[17] Includes the hospital facility costs for Medicare Part B services that are predominantly in the outpatient department, with the exception of hospital outpatient laboratory services, which are included on the Laboratory line. Physician reimbursement is included on the Physician fee schedule line.

[18] Part D start-up costs were funded through the SMI Part B account in 2004-2008.

Table 3-80. Medicare Enrollees and Expenditures and Percent Distribution, by Medicare Program and Type of Service, Selected Years, 1970–2015—*Continued*

(Number; dollars; percent.)

Medicare program and type of service	1970	1980	1990	1995	2000	2005	2008	2009	2010	2011	2012	2013	2014	2015[1]
Physician/supplies[12]	80.9	72.8	67.3	NA	NA	NA	NA	NA	NA	NA	NA	NA	NA	NA
Outpatient hospital[13]	5.2	16.9	19.3	NA	NA	NA	NA	NA	NA	NA	NA	NA	NA	NA
Independent laboratory[14]	0.5	1.0	3.4	NA	NA	NA	NA	NA	NA	NA	NA	NA	NA	NA
Physician fee schedule	NA	NA	NA	47.5	40.8	37.6	26.0	23.2	23.2	23.1	22.6	21.7	20.1	19.1
Durable medical equipment	NA	NA	NA	5.5	5.2	5.2	3.7	3.1	3.0	2.8	2.7	2.3	1.8	1.8
Laboratory[15]	NA	NA	NA	6.4	4.8	4.5	3.4	3.1	3.1	2.9	3.0	2.9	2.4	2.3
Other[16]	NA	NA	NA	14.8	15.0	17.4	12.7	12.4	12.4	12.3	12.5	12.1	11.5	11.1
Hospital[17]	NA	NA	NA	13.0	8.9	12.2	10.1	9.7	10.0	10.3	10.9	11.4	12.1	11.9
Home health agency	1.5	2.1	0.2	0.3	4.9	4.6	4.4	4.4	4.4	4.1	3.7	3.6	3.2	3.0
Home health agency transfer[7]	NA	NA	NA	NA	-1.9	NA	NA	NA	NA	NA	NA	NA	NA	NA
Medicare Advantage premiums[8]	NA	NA	NA	NA	NA	NA	0.0	0.0	0.1	0.1	0.1	0.1	0.1	0.1
Accounting error (CY 2005-2008)[9]	NA	NA	NA	NA	NA	1.2	-3.6	NA	NA	NA	NA	NA	NA	NA
Administrative expenses[10]	10.7	5.4	3.5	2.4	2.0	1.8	1.3	1.2	1.2	1.3	1.3	1.1	1.2	0.9
Part D start-up costs[18]	NA	NA	NA	NA	NA	0.4	0.0	NA	NA	NA	NA	NA	NA	NA
Total Part D[4]	NA	NA	NA	NA	NA	0.7	21.2	22.8	22.6	22.9	21.8	22.0	22.7	24.4

NA = Not available.
0.0 = Quantity more than zero but less than 0.05.
[1]Preliminary estimates.
[4]The Medicare Modernization Act, enacted on December 8, 2003, established within SMI two Part D accounts related to prescription drug benefits: the Medicare Prescription Drug Account and the Transitional Assistance Account.
[7]For 1998 to 2003 data, reflects annual home health HI to SMI transfer amounts.
[8]When a beneficiary chooses a Medicare Advantage plan whose monthly premium exceeds the benchmark amount, the additional premiums (that is, amounts beyond those paid by Medicare to the plan) are the responsibility of the beneficiary.
[9]Represents misallocation of benefit payments between the HI trust fund and the Part B account of the SMI trust fund from May 2005 to September 2007, and the transfer made in June 2008 to correct the misallocation.
[10]Includes expenditures for research, experiments and demonstration projects, peer review activity (performed by Peer Review Organizations from 1983 to 2001 and by Quality Review Organizations from 2002 to present), and to combat and prevent fraud and abuse.
[12]Includes payment for physicians, practitioners, durable medical equipment, and all suppliers other than independent laboratory through 1990. Starting with 1991 data, physician services subject to the physician fee schedule are shown. Payments for laboratory services paid under the laboratory fee schedule and performed in a physician office are included under Laboratory beginning in 1991.
[13]Includes payments for hospital outpatient department services, skilled nursing facility outpatient services, Part B services received as an inpatient in a hospital or skilled nursing facility setting, and other types of outpatient facilities.
[14]Starting with 1991 data, those independent laboratory services that were paid under the laboratory fee schedule (most of the independent laboratory category) are included in the Laboratory line; the remaining services are included in the Physician fee schedule and Other lines.
[15]Payments for laboratory services paid under the laboratory fee schedule performed in a physician office, independent laboratory, or in a hospital outpatient department.
[16]Includes payments for physician-administered drugs; freestanding ambulatory surgical center facility services; ambulance services; supplies; freestanding end-stage renal disease (ESRD) dialysis facility services; rural health clinics; outpatient rehabilitation facilities; psychiatric hospitals; and federally qualified health centers.
[17]Includes the hospital facility costs for Medicare Part B services that are predominantly in the outpatient department, with the exception of hospital outpatient laboratory services, which are included on the Laboratory line. Physician reimbursement is included on the Physician fee schedule line.
[18]Part D start-up costs were funded through the SMI Part B account in 2004-2008.

Table 3-81. Medicare Enrollees, Enrollees in Managed Care, Payment Per Fee-for-Service Enrollee, and Short-Stay Hospital Utilization, by State, 1994 and 2015

(Number; percent; dollars; rate per 1,000 enrollees.)

| | Enrollment in thousands[1] | | Percent of enrollees in managed care | | Average payment per fee-for-service enrollee | | Short-stay hospital utilization | | | |
| | | | | | | | Discharges per 1,000 enrollees[2] | | Average length of stay in days[2] | |
State	1994	2015	1994	2015	1994	2015	1994	2015	1994	2015
United States[3]	36,190	54,286	7.9	31.3	$4,375	$9,635	345	282	7.5	5.3
Alabama	633	968	0.8	25.3	4,454	8,611	413	313	7.0	5.5
Alaska	33	84	0.6	1.0	3,687	8,301	269	181	6.3	6.0
Arizona	578	1,140	24.8	38.1	4,442	8,728	292	228	5.9	4.9
Arkansas	416	594	0.2	20.1	3,719	8,360	366	288	7.0	5.3
California	3,582	5,645	30.0	40.5	5,219	10,294	366	242	6.1	5.4
Colorado	413	786	17.2	36.9	3,935	7,914	302	218	6.0	4.7
Connecticut	497	630	2.6	25.6	4,426	10,636	287	293	8.1	5.7
Delaware	99	181	0.2	8.3	4,712	9,803	326	278	8.1	5.5
District of Columbia	80	88	3.9	13.1	5,655	10,058	376	320	10.1	6.3
Florida	2,584	4,040	13.8	39.8	5,027	10,715	326	324	7.1	5.3
Georgia	819	1,521	0.4	31.5	4,402	9,042	378	275	6.9	5.4
Hawaii	146	244	29.8	45.8	3,069	6,459	301	162	9.1	6.4
Idaho	146	283	2.5	32.6	3,045	7,706	274	181	5.2	4.6
Illinois	1,605	2,063	5.5	21.0	4,324	9,910	374	308	7.3	5.1
Indiana	805	1,151	2.6	23.8	3,945	9,332	345	293	6.9	5.1
Iowa	470	572	3.1	14.9	3,080	8,286	322	235	6.6	5.1
Kansas	378	487	3.3	13.7	3,847	8,652	348	261	6.5	4.9
Kentucky	578	863	2.3	26.2	3,862	9,012	396	315	7.2	5.2
Louisiana	572	793	0.4	30.1	5,468	10,047	399	301	7.2	5.4
Maine	198	306	0.1	22.9	3,464	8,232	322	218	7.6	5.3
Maryland	596	930	1.4	8.7	4,997	11,010	362	293	7.5	5.5
Massachusetts	924	1,217	6.1	20.9	5,147	10,394	350	295	7.6	5.2
Michigan	1,331	1,894	0.7	33.3	4,307	10,381	328	336	7.6	5.2
Minnesota	625	912	19.6	53.8	3,394	12,904	334	405	5.7	4.9
Mississippi	391	560	0.1	14.7	4,189	9,659	423	319	7.4	5.6
Missouri	821	1,136	3.4	28.3	4,191	9,042	349	306	7.3	5.1
Montana	128	201	0.4	18.3	3,114	7,277	306	185	5.9	4.9
Nebraska	247	314	2.2	12.3	2,926	8,948	281	239	6.3	5.0
Nevada	187	455	19.0	33.1	4,306	9,216	291	248	7.0	5.7
New Hampshire	152	266	0.2	7.5	3,414	8,374	281	218	7.6	5.4
New Jersey	1,158	1,489	2.6	15.4	4,531	10,898	354	294	10.2	5.8
New Mexico	205	373	13.6	31.7	3,110	7,680	301	208	6.0	5.6
New York	2,601	3,339	6.2	37.0	4,855	10,572	334	290	11.2	6.7
North Carolina	1,001	1,771	0.5	29.8	3,465	8,858	314	277	8.0	5.3
North Dakota	101	119	0.6	16.9	3,218	8,723	327	247	6.3	5.4
Ohio	1,649	2,153	2.4	41.0	3,982	9,613	350	309	7.1	5.0
Oklahoma	481	679	2.5	16.9	4,098	9,348	355	295	7.0	5.3
Oregon	469	756	27.7	43.8	3,285	7,842	305	191	5.2	4.8
Pennsylvania	2,053	2,531	3.3	39.9	5,212	9,687	379	304	8.0	5.3
Rhode Island	166	203	7.0	35.1	4,148	9,224	312	296	8.1	5.3
South Carolina	497	943	0.1	23.2	3,777	8,635	319	265	8.3	5.4
South Dakota	114	156	0.1	19.0	2,952	8,969	356	258	6.1	4.9
Tennessee	754	1,236	0.3	34.3	4,441	8,963	375	300	7.1	5.3
Texas	2,029	3,636	4.1	31.8	4,703	10,603	333	289	7.2	5.3
Utah	182	346	9.4	33.8	3,443	8,187	238	207	5.4	4.3
Vermont	82	131	0.1	7.5	3,182	7,917	283	179	7.6	5.5
Virginia	803	1,349	1.5	18.1	3,748	8,280	348	273	7.3	5.1
Washington	676	1,192	12.5	30.0	3,401	7,920	269	207	5.3	4.9
West Virginia	326	416	8.3	26.8	3,798	8,641	420	312	7.1	5.4
Wisconsin	752	1,050	2.0	37.9	3,246	8,746	310	253	6.8	4.9
Wyoming	58	95	3.3	3.9	3,537	8,235	315	205	5.6	4.8

[1] Total persons enrolled in hospital insurance, supplementary medical insurance, or both, as of July 1. Includes fee-for-service and managed care enrollees.
[2] Data are for fee-for-service enrollees only.
[3] Includes residents of any of the 50 states and the District of Columbia.

NOTES AND DEFINITIONS

Sources of Data

The principal source for data presented in this part is from National Center for Health Statistics. *Health, United States, 2016: with Chartbook on Long-Term Trends in Health*, Hyattsville, MD. 2017. This is an annual report on trends in health statistics compiled by the National Center of Health Statistics (NCHS), a component of the Centers for Disease Control and Prevention (CDC). Updated tables for this publication can be found at https://www.cdc.gov/nchs/hus/contents2016.htm#110.

The data for Tables 3-57 through 3-62 are from the Bureau of Labor Statistics (BLS), Occupational Employment Statistics. For more detailed information, see Occupational Employment and Wages news release. OES can be accessed at https://www.bls.gov/oes/home.htm.

Concepts and Definitions

Age-adjustment—used to compare risks of two or more populations at one point in time or one population at two or more points in time. Age-adjusted rates are computed by the direct method by applying age-specific rates in a population of interest to a standardized age distribution, to eliminate differences in observed rates that result from age differences in population composition. Age-adjusted rates should be viewed as relative indexes rather than actual measures of risk. Age-adjusted estimates from other age-adjusted estimates based on the same data and presented elsewhere if different age groups are used in the adjustment procedure.

Body mass index (BMI)—a measure that adjusts bodyweight for height. It is calculated as weight in kilograms divided by height in meters squared. Overweight for children and adolescents is defined as BMI at or above the sex- and age-specific 95th percentile BMI cut points from the 2000 CDC Growth Charts. Healthy weight for adults is defined as a BMI of 18.5 to less than 25; overweight, as greater than or equal to a BMI of 25; and obesity, as greater than or equal to a BMI of 30.

Cholesterol, serum—a measure of the total blood cholesterol. Elevated total blood cholesterol—a combination of high-density lipoproteins (HDL), low-density lipoproteins (LDL), and very-low density lipoproteins (VLDL)—is a risk factor for cardiovascular disease. According to the National Cholesterol Education Program, high serum cholesterol is defined as greater than or equal to 240 mg/dL (6.20 mmol/L). Borderline high serum cholesterol is defined as greater than or equal to 200 mg/dL and less than 240 mg/dL. Assessments of the components of total cholesterol or lower thresholds for high total cholesterol may be used for individuals with other risk factors for cardiovascular disease.

Condition—A health condition is a departure from a state of physical or mental well being. In the National Health Interview Survey, each condition reported as a cause of an individual's activity limitation has been classified as chronic, not chronic, or unknown if chronic, based on the nature and duration of the condition.

Dental caries—evidence of tooth decay on any surface of the tooth. Untreated dental caries are determined by an oral examination conducted by a trained dentist.

Diagnosis—the act or process of identifying or determining the nature and cause of a disease or injury through evaluation of patient history, examination, and review of laboratory data.

Gross domestic product (GDP)—the market value of the goods and services produced by labor and property located in the United States. As long as the labor and property are located in the United States, the suppliers (i.e., the workers and, for property, the owners) may be U.S. residents or residents of other countries.

Health expenditures, national—estimated by the Centers for Medicare & Medicaid Services (CMS) it measures spending for health care in the United States by type of service delivered (e.g., hospital care, physician services, nursing home care) and source of funding for those services (e.g., private health insurance, Medicare, Medicaid, out-of-pocket spending). CMS produces both historical and projected estimates of health expenditures by category.

Health insurance coverage—broadly defined to include both public and private payers who cover medical expenditures incurred by a defined population in a variety of settings.

Health maintenance organization (HMO)—a health care system that assumes or shares both the financial risks and the delivery risks associated with providing comprehensive medical services to a voluntarily enrolled population in a particular geographic area, usually in return for a fixed, prepaid fee. Pure HMO enrollees use only the prepaid capitated health services of the HMO panel of medical care providers. Open-ended HMO enrollees use the prepaid HMO health services but, in addition, may receive medical care from providers who are not part of the HMO panel. There is usually a substantial deductible, co-payment, or co-insurance associated with use of non-panel providers.

Hispanic origin—includes persons of Mexican, Puerto Rican, Cuban, Central and South American, and other or unknown Latin American or Spanish origins. Persons of Hispanic origin may be of any race.

Hypertension—elevated blood pressure or hypertension is defined as having an average systolic blood pressure reading of at least 140mmHg or diastolic pressure of at least 90 mmHg, which is consistent with the Seventh Report of the Joint National Committee on Prevention, Detection, Evaluation, and Treatment of High Blood Pressure. People are also considered to have hypertension if they report that they are taking a prescription medicine for high blood pressure, even if their blood pressure readings are within normal range.

Incidence—the number of cases of disease having their onset during a prescribed period of time. It is often expressed as a rate (e.g., the incidence of measles per 1,000 children 5–15 years of age during a specified year). Incidence is a measure of morbidity or other events that occur within a specified period of time. Measuring incidence may be complicated because the population at risk for the disease may change during the period of interest, for example, due to births, deaths, or migration. In addition, determining that a case is new—that is, that its onset occurred during the prescribed period of time—may be difficult. Because of these difficulties in measuring incidence, many health statistics are measured using prevalence.

Instrumental activities of daily living (IADL)—activities related to independent living and include preparing meals, managing money, shopping for groceries or personal items, performing light or heavy housework, and using a telephone. In the National Health Interview Survey (NHIS) respondents are asked whether they or family members 18 years of age and over need the help of another person for handling routine IADL needs because of a physical, mental, or emotional problem. Persons are considered to have an IADL limitation in the NHIS if any causal condition is chronic.

Limitation of activity—may be defined different ways, depending on the conceptual framework. In the National Health Interview Survey, limitation of activity refers to a long-term reduction in a person's capacity to perform the usual kind or amount of activities associated with his or her age group as a result of a chronic condition. Limitation of activity is assessed by asking persons a series of questions about limitations in their or household members' ability to perform activities usual for their age group because of a physical, mental, or emotional problem. Persons are asked about limitations in activities of daily living, instrumental activities of daily living, play, school, work, difficulty walking or remembering, and any other activity limitations. For reported limitations, the causal health conditions are determined, and persons are considered limited if one or more of these conditions is chronic. Children under 18 years of age who receive special education or early intervention services are considered to have a limitation of activity.

Mammography—an x-ray image of the breast used to detect irregularities of the breast tissue.

Managed care—a term originally used to refer to the prepaid health care sector (health maintenance organizations or HMOs) where care is provided under a fixed budget and costs are therein capable of being managed. Increasingly, the term is being used to include preferred provider organizations (PPOs) and even forms of indemnity.

Medicare—the federal program which helps pay health care costs for people 65 and older and for certain people under 65 with long-term disabilities.

Medicaid—a program authorized by the Social Security Act in 1965 as a jointly funded cooperative venture between the federal and state governments to assist states in the provision of adequate medical care to eligible needy persons. Families with dependent children, the aged, blind, and disabled who are in financial need are eligible for Medicaid.

Notifiable disease—a disease, that when diagnosed, health providers are required, usually by law, to report to state or local public health officials. Notifiable diseases are those of public interest by reason of their contagiousness, severity, or frequency.

Pap smear—a microscopic examination of cells scraped from the cervix that is used to detect cancerous or precancerous conditions of the cervix or other medical conditions.

Physical activity, leisure-time—starting with 1998 data, leisure-time physical activity is assessed in the National Health Interview Survey by asking adults a series of questions about how often they do vigorous or light/moderate physical activity of at least 10 minutes duration and for about how long these sessions generally last. Vigorous physical activity is described as causing heavy sweating or a large increase in breathing or heart rate and light/moderate as causing light sweating or a slight to moderate increase in breathing or heart rate. Adults classified as inactive did not report any sessions of light/moderate or vigorous leisure-time physical activity of at least 10 minutes duration or reported they were unable to perform leisure-time physical activity. Adults classified with some leisure-time activity reported at least one session of light/moderate or vigorous activity of at least 10 minutes duration but did not meet the requirement for regular leisure-time activity. Adults classified with regular leisure-time activity reported at least three sessions per week of vigorous leisure-time physical activity lasting at least 20 minutes in duration or at least five sessions per week of light/moderate physical activity lasting at least 30 minutes in duration.

Poverty—based on definitions originally developed by the Social Security Administration. These include a set of money income thresholds that vary by family size and composition. Families or individuals with income below their appropriate thresholds are classified as below poverty. These thresholds are updated annually by the U.S. Census Bureau to reflect changes in the Consumer Price Index for all urban consumers (CPI-U). For example, the average poverty threshold for a family of four was $24,563 in 2016, $22,314 in 2010, $17,603 in 2000, and $13,359 in 1990.

Preferred provider organization (PPO)—a type of medical plan where coverage is provided to participants through a network of selected health care providers (such as hospitals and physicians). The enrollees may go outside the network, but they would pay a greater percentage of the cost of coverage than within the network.

Prevalence—the number of cases of a disease, infected persons, or persons with some other attribute present during a particular interval of time. It is often expressed as a rate (e.g., the prevalence of diabetes per 1,000 persons during a year).

Short-stay hospital—hospitals that provide general (rather than specialized) care and have an average length of stay of less than 30 days.

Specialty hospital—hospitals that provide a particular type of service to the majority of their patients such as psychiatric, tuberculosis, chronic disease, rehabilitation, maternity, and alcoholic or narcotic.

State Children's Health Insurance Program (SCHIP)—Title XXI of the Social Security Act, known as the State Children's Health Insurance Program (SCHIP), is a program initiated by the Balanced Budget Act of 1997 (BBA). SCHIP provides more federal funds for states to provide health care coverage to low-income, uninsured children. SCHIP gives states broad flexibility in program design while protecting beneficiaries through federal standards. Funds from SCHIP may be used to expand Medicaid or to provide medical assistance to children during a presumptive eligibility period for Medicaid. This is one of several options from which states may select to provide health care coverage for more children, as prescribed within the BBA's Title XXI program.

Substance use—the use of selected substances including alcohol, tobacco products, drugs, inhalants, and other substances that can be consumed, inhaled, injected, or otherwise absorbed into the body with possible detrimental effects.

Suicidal ideation—having thoughts of suicide or of taking action to end one's own life. Suicidal ideation includes all thoughts of suicide, both when the thoughts include a plan to commit suicide and when they do not include a plan. Suicidal ideation is measured in the Youth Risk Behavior Survey by the question "During the past 12 months, did you ever seriously consider attempting suicide?"

Uninsured—in the Current Population Survey (CPS) persons are considered uninsured if they do not have coverage through private health insurance, Medicare, Medicaid, State Children's Health Insurance Program, military or Veterans coverage, another government program, a plan of someone outside the household, or other insurance. Persons with only Indian Health Service coverage are considered uninsured. In addition, if the respondent has missing Medicaid information but has income from certain low-income public programs, then Medicaid coverage is imputed. The questions on health insurance are administered in March and refer to the previous calendar year.

PART IV:
MARRIAGE AND DIVORCE

PART IV: MARRIAGE AND DIVORCE

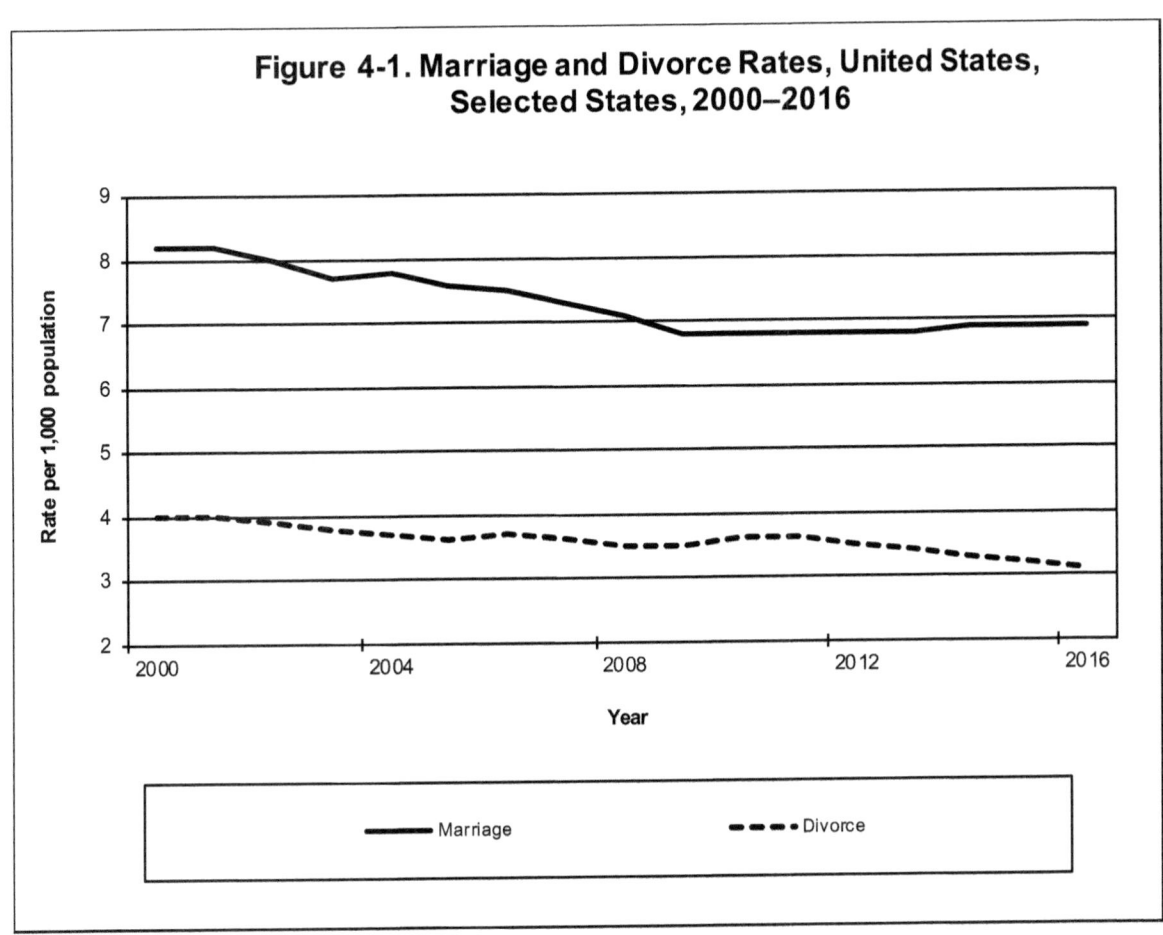

Figure 4-1. Marriage and Divorce Rates, United States, Selected States, 2000–2016

HIGHLIGHTS

- In 2016, Nevada had the highest rate of marriage per 1,000 resident population at 28.4, significantly greater than the next-highest states (Hawaii, 15.6; Arkansas, 9.9; and Utah, 9.0). Illinois had the lowest marriage rate, at 5.4, followed by Connecticut, Delaware, Wisconsin, and Minnesota at 5.6 each and New Jersey at 5.7. (Table 4-1)

- Among reporting states in 2016, (California, Georgia, Hawaii, Indiana, Minnesota, and New Mexico did not have available information), Iowa had the lowest divorce rate, at 1.3 per 1,000 resident population, followed by Illinois and Louisiana (2.0 each), Massachusetts (2.3), and South Carolina (2.5 each). Oklahoma had the highest divorce rate at 4.4, followed by Nevada (the state with the highest marriage rate) at 4.3, and Texas and Wyoming (4.2 each). (Table 4-2)

- The median age at first marriage for all races and origins in the United States was 29.9 years for males and 27.9 years for females in 2016. Male median ages ranged from 28.2 for Native Hawaiian and Other Pacific Islanders to 31.8 for Black or African American alone males. Ages for females ranged from 26.3 for Native Hawaiian and Other Pacific Islanders alone to 31.2 for Black or African American alone. (Table 4-6)

- In the United States, the median duration of current marriages was 19.7 years in 2016. The District of Columbia had the shortest median duration, at 10.6 years, while Maine had the longest median duration, at 22.4 years. (Table 4-10)

Table 4-1. Marriage Rates, by State, Selected Years, 1990–2016

(Rate per 1,000 total population residing in area.)

State	Marriage rate															
	1990	1995	1999	2000	2005	2006	2007	2008	2009	2010	2011	2012	2013	2014	2015	2016
Alabama	10.6	9.8	10.8	10.1	9.2	9.2	8.9	8.6	8.3	8.2	8.4	8.2	7.8	7.8	7.4	7.1
Alaska	10.2	9.0	8.6	8.9	8.2	8.2	8.5	8.4	7.8	8.0	7.8	7.2	7.3	7.5	7.4	7.1
Arizona	10.0	8.8	8.2	7.5	6.6	6.5	6.4	6.0	5.6	5.9	5.7	5.6	5.4	5.8	5.9	5.9
Arkansas	15.3	14.4	14.8	15.4	12.9	12.4	12.0	10.6	10.7	10.8	10.4	10.9	9.8	10.1	10.0	9.9
California[1]	7.9	6.3	6.4	5.8	6.4	6.3	6.2	6.7	5.8	5.8	5.8	6.0	6.5	6.4	6.2	6.5
Colorado	9.8	9.0	8.2	8.3	7.6	7.2	7.1	7.4	6.9	6.9	7.0	6.8	6.5	7.1	6.8	7.4
Connecticut	7.9	6.6	5.8	5.7	5.8	5.5	5.5	5.4	5.9	5.6	5.5	5.2	5.0	5.4	5.3	5.6
Delaware	8.4	7.3	6.7	6.5	5.9	5.9	5.7	5.5	5.5	5.2	5.2	5.8	6.6	6.0	5.7	5.6
District of Columbia	8.2	6.1	6.6	4.9	4.1	4.0	4.2	4.1	4.7	7.6	8.7	8.4	10.8	11.8	8.2	8.1
Florida	10.9	9.9	8.7	8.9	8.9	8.6	8.5	8.0	7.5	7.3	7.4	7.2	7.0	7.3	8.2	8.1
Georgia	10.3	8.4	7.8	6.8	7.0	7.3	6.8	6.0	6.6	7.3	6.6	6.5	NA	NA	6.2	6.8
Hawaii	16.4	15.7	18.9	20.6	22.6	21.9	20.8	19.1	17.2	17.6	17.6	17.5	16.3	17.7	15.9	15.6
Idaho	13.9	13.1	12.1	10.8	10.5	10.1	10.0	9.5	8.9	8.8	8.6	8.2	8.2	8.4	8.2	8.1
Illinois	8.8	6.9	7.0	6.9	5.9	6.2	6.1	5.9	5.7	5.7	5.6	5.8	5.4	6.2	5.9	5.4
Indiana	9.6	8.6	8.1	7.9	6.9	7.0	7.0	8.0	7.9	6.3	6.8	6.7	6.6	7.1	6.9	6.9
Iowa	9.0	7.7	7.9	6.9	6.9	6.7	6.6	6.5	7.0	6.9	6.7	6.8	7.4	6.9	6.3	6.1
Kansas	9.2	8.5	7.1	8.3	6.8	6.8	6.8	6.7	6.4	6.4	6.3	6.3	6.0	6.1	5.9	6.2
Kentucky	13.5	12.2	10.9	9.8	8.7	8.4	7.8	7.9	7.6	7.4	7.5	7.2	7.3	6.9	7.2	7.4
Louisiana	9.6	9.3	9.1	9.1	8.0	NA	7.5	6.8	7.1	6.9	6.4	5.7	6.4	6.9	6.8	6.1
Maine	9.7	8.7	8.6	8.8	8.2	7.8	7.4	7.4	7.1	7.1	7.2	7.3	8.3	7.7	7.6	7.6
Maryland	9.7	8.4	7.5	7.5	6.9	6.6	6.5	5.9	5.8	5.7	5.8	5.6	6.8	6.5	6.2	6.3
Massachusetts	7.9	7.1	6.2	5.8	6.2	5.9	5.9	5.7	5.6	5.6	5.5	5.5	5.5	5.6	5.5	5.8
Michigan	8.2	7.3	6.8	6.7	6.1	5.9	5.7	5.6	5.4	5.5	5.7	5.6	5.8	5.8	6.0	5.9
Minnesota	7.7	7.0	6.8	6.8	6.0	6.0	5.8	5.4	5.3	5.3	5.6	5.6	6.0	5.9	5.6	5.6
Mississippi	9.4	7.9	7.8	6.9	5.8	5.7	5.4	5.1	4.8	4.9	4.9	5.8	6.7	6.9	7.0	7.0
Missouri	9.6	8.3	8.1	7.8	7.0	6.9	6.9	6.8	6.5	6.5	6.6	6.5	6.4	6.7	6.2	6.9
Montana	8.6	7.6	7.4	7.3	7.4	7.4	7.5	7.6	7.3	7.4	7.8	7.8	7.4	7.9	8.0	7.8
Nebraska	8.0	7.3	7.5	7.6	7.0	6.8	6.8	6.9	6.6	6.6	6.6	6.7	6.3	6.4	6.4	6.5
Nevada	99.0	85.2	82.3	72.2	57.4	52.1	48.6	42.3	40.3	38.3	36.9	35.1	32.3	31.9	31.0	28.4
New Hampshire	9.5	8.3	7.9	9.4	7.3	7.2	7.1	6.8	6.5	7.3	7.1	6.8	6.9	7.2	6.9	7.0
New Jersey	7.6	6.5	5.9	6.0	5.7	5.5	5.4	5.4	5.0	5.1	4.8	4.9	5.1	5.4	5.6	5.7
New Mexico	8.8	8.8	8.0	8.0	6.6	6.8	5.6	4.0	5.0	7.7	8.0	6.9	7.3	8.1	6.2	6.4
New York	8.6	8.0	7.3	7.1	6.8	6.9	6.8	6.6	6.5	6.5	6.9	7.0	6.9	6.7	7.1	7.5
North Carolina	7.8	8.4	8.5	8.2	7.3	7.3	7.0	6.9	6.6	6.6	6.7	6.6	6.5	6.9	7.0	7.0
North Dakota	7.5	7.1	6.6	7.2	6.8	6.7	6.6	6.5	6.4	6.5	6.7	6.6	6.3	6.3	6.2	6.0
Ohio	9.0	8.0	7.8	7.8	6.5	6.3	6.1	6.0	5.8	5.8	5.9	5.8	5.7	5.8	5.9	6.0
Oklahoma	10.6	8.6	6.8	NA	7.3	7.3	7.3	7.1	6.9	7.2	6.9	6.9	7.1	7.1	7.4	6.7
Oregon	8.9	8.1	7.6	7.6	7.3	7.3	7.2	6.9	6.6	6.5	6.6	6.6	6.3	6.8	6.9	6.9
Pennsylvania	7.1	6.2	6.1	6.0	5.8	5.7	5.7	5.5	5.3	5.3	5.3	5.5	5.4	5.8	5.7	5.8
Rhode Island	8.1	7.3	7.5	7.6	7.0	6.6	6.4	6.1	5.9	5.8	6.0	6.1	6.2	6.7	6.4	6.7
South Carolina	15.9	11.9	10.2	10.6	8.3	7.8	7.9	7.3	7.3	7.4	7.2	7.4	7.1	7.6	7.5	6.6
South Dakota	11.1	9.9	9.1	9.4	8.4	8.0	7.8	7.7	7.3	7.3	7.5	7.5	7.0	7.1	7.2	7.2
Tennessee	13.9	15.5	14.7	15.5	10.9	10.6	10.1	9.4	8.4	8.8	9.0	8.8	8.4	8.4	8.5	8.6
Texas	10.5	9.9	9.1	9.4	7.8	7.6	7.4	7.3	7.1	7.1	7.1	7.3	7.0	6.9	7.2	7.1
Utah	11.2	10.7	9.6	10.8	9.8	9.2	9.6	9.0	8.4	8.5	8.6	8.4	7.5	7.3	8.1	9.0
Vermont	10.9	10.3	10.0	10.0	8.9	8.6	8.5	7.9	8.7	9.3	8.3	8.2	9.2	8.7	8.1	8.3
Virginia	11.4	10.2	9.2	8.8	8.2	7.8	7.5	7.2	6.9	6.8	6.8	6.8	6.7	6.7	7.0	7.0
Washington	9.5	7.7	7.2	6.9	6.5	6.5	6.4	6.3	6.0	6.0	6.1	6.3	7.1	7.0	6.2	6.2
West Virginia	7.2	6.1	7.5	8.7	7.4	7.3	7.3	7.1	6.7	6.7	7.2	7.0	6.6	6.7	6.6	6.4
Wisconsin	7.9	7.0	6.7	6.7	6.1	6.0	5.7	5.6	5.3	5.3	5.3	5.4	5.2	5.7	5.6	5.6
Wyoming	10.7	10.6	9.9	10.0	9.3	9.3	9.0	8.6	8.0	7.6	7.8	7.6	7.5	7.7	7.3	7.1

NA = Not available.

[1] Marriage data includes nonlicensed marriages registered.

Table 4-2. Divorce Rates, by State, Selected Years, 1990–2016

(Rate per 1,000 total population residing in area.)

State	Divorce rate[1]															
	1990	1995	1999	2000	2005	2006	2007	2008	2009	2010	2011	2012	2013	2014	2015	2016
Alabama	6.1	6.0	5.7	5.5	4.9	4.9	4.5	4.3	4.4	4.4	4.3	3.6	3.7	3.8	3.9	3.8
Alaska	5.5	5.0	5.0	3.9	4.3	4.2	4.3	4.4	4.4	4.7	4.8	4.5	4.5	4.0	4.1	3.9
Arizona	6.9	6.2	4.6	4.6	4.2	4.0	4.0	3.8	3.6	3.5	3.9	4.3	3.9	3.9	3.6	3.4
Arkansas	6.9	6.3	6.2	6.4	6.0	5.8	5.9	5.5	5.7	5.7	5.3	5.3	5.0	4.8	4.8	3.9
California	4.3	NA	NA	NA	NA	NA	NA	NA	NA	NA	NA	NA	NA	NA	NA	NA
Colorado	5.5	NA	4.8	4.7	4.4	4.5	4.4	4.3	4.3	4.3	4.4	4.3	4.1	3.9	3.7	3.6
Connecticut	3.2	2.9	3.0	3.3	3.0	3.1	3.2	3.4	3.0	2.9	3.1	2.7	2.8	2.6	3.1	3.2
Delaware	4.4	5.0	4.5	3.9	3.8	3.8	3.7	3.5	3.6	3.5	3.6	3.5	3.4	3.3	3.1	3.1
District of Columbia	4.5	3.2	3.6	3.2	2.0	2.1	1.7	2.7	2.7	2.8	2.9	2.9	2.8	2.6	2.8	2.7
Florida	6.3	5.5	5.1	5.1	4.6	4.7	4.6	4.3	4.2	4.4	4.5	4.2	4.1	4.0	4.0	3.9
Georgia	5.5	5.1	4.1	3.3	NA	NA	NA	NA	NA	NA	NA	NA	NA	NA	NA	NA
Hawaii	4.6	4.6	3.8	3.9	NA	NA	NA	NA	NA	NA	NA	NA	NA	NA	NA	NA
Idaho	6.5	5.8	5.4	5.5	5.0	5.0	4.9	4.8	5.0	5.2	4.9	4.7	4.5	4.2	4.1	4.0
Illinois	3.8	3.2	3.3	3.2	2.6	2.5	2.6	2.5	2.5	2.6	2.6	2.4	2.3	2.2	2.2	2.0
Indiana	NA	NA	NA	NA	NA	NA	NA	NA	NA	NA	NA	NA	NA	NA	NA	NA
Iowa	3.9	3.7	3.3	3.3	2.7	2.7	2.5	2.6	2.4	2.4	2.4	2.2	1.9	1.5	1.2	1.3
Kansas	5.0	4.1	3.4	3.6	3.1	3.1	3.4	3.5	3.6	3.7	3.9	3.4	3.0	3.0	2.8	2.7
Kentucky	5.8	5.9	5.5	5.1	4.6	5.0	4.6	4.6	4.6	4.5	4.4	4.1	4.2	2.2	2.3	2.8
Louisiana	NA	NA	NA	NA	NA	NA	NA	NA	NA	NA	NA	NA	NA	NA	NA	2.0
Maine	4.3	4.4	5.1	5.0	4.1	4.2	4.2	4.2	4.1	4.2	4.2	3.9	4.0	3.6	3.4	3.4
Maryland	3.4	3.0	3.2	3.3	3.1	3.0	2.9	2.8	2.8	2.8	2.9	2.8	2.5	2.5	2.6	2.7
Massachusetts	2.8	2.2	2.5	2.5	2.2	2.3	2.3	2.0	2.2	2.5	2.7	2.7	2.6	2.7	2.6	2.3
Michigan	4.3	4.1	3.8	3.9	3.4	3.5	3.4	3.4	3.3	3.5	3.4	3.3	3.3	3.0	3.0	2.9
Minnesota	3.5	3.4	3.2	3.2	NA	NA	NA	NA	NA	NA	NA	NA	NA	NA	NA	NA
Mississippi	5.5	4.8	5.0	5.0	4.4	4.8	4.5	4.3	4.1	4.3	4.0	4.0	3.6	3.4	3.4	3.2
Missouri	5.1	5.0	4.4	4.5	3.6	3.8	3.8	3.7	3.8	3.9	3.9	3.7	3.4	3.3	3.2	3.3
Montana	5.1	4.8	2.8	4.2	4.5	4.4	4.0	4.1	4.0	3.9	4.0	3.9	3.4	3.4	3.4	3.1
Nebraska	4.0	3.8	3.7	3.7	3.3	3.4	3.4	3.3	3.4	3.6	3.5	3.4	3.3	3.1	3.2	3.1
Nevada	11.4	7.8	7.8	9.9	7.4	6.7	6.4	6.4	6.6	5.9	5.6	5.5	5.1	5.3	4.6	4.3
New Hampshire	4.7	4.2	5.1	4.8	3.9	4.1	3.8	3.9	3.7	3.8	3.8	3.6	3.7	3.5	3.3	3.4
New Jersey	3.0	3.0	3.0	3.0	2.9	3.0	3.0	3.0	2.7	3.0	2.9	2.8	2.8	2.8	2.8	2.7
New Mexico	4.9	6.6	4.6	5.1	4.6	4.3	4.2	4.1	3.9	4.0	3.3	3.0	3.4	3.6	3.3	NA
New York	3.2	3.0	3.3	3.0	2.9	3.1	2.9	2.8	2.6	2.9	2.9	2.9	2.7	2.8	2.7	2.7
North Carolina	5.1	5.0	4.6	4.5	4.1	4.0	4.0	3.8	3.8	3.8	3.7	3.7	3.4	3.4	3.1	3.2
North Dakota	3.6	3.4	4.4	3.4	2.9	3.0	2.9	2.9	2.8	3.1	2.7	3.1	2.9	2.8	2.8	2.6
Ohio	4.7	4.3	3.9	4.2	3.5	3.5	3.4	3.3	3.3	3.4	3.4	3.4	3.3	3.2	3.1	3.0
Oklahoma	7.7	6.6	NA	NA	5.6	5.3	5.2	5.3	4.8	5.2	5.2	4.8	4.5	4.5	4.4	4.4
Oregon	5.5	4.7	4.6	4.8	4.2	4.0	3.9	3.9	3.9	4.0	3.8	3.8	3.6	3.4	3.4	3.4
Pennsylvania	3.3	3.2	3.1	3.1	2.3	2.8	2.8	2.7	2.7	2.7	2.8	2.8	2.7	2.7	2.6	2.6
Rhode Island	3.7	3.6	2.7	2.9	3.0	3.0	2.8	2.7	3.0	3.2	3.2	3.2	3.1	2.8	3.0	2.8
South Carolina	4.5	3.9	3.8	3.8	2.9	2.9	3.0	2.8	3.0	3.1	3.2	3.2	3.2	2.9	2.8	2.5
South Dakota	3.7	3.9	3.7	3.5	2.8	3.2	3.1	3.1	3.3	3.4	3.3	3.0	2.9	2.8	2.6	2.8
Tennessee	6.5	6.2	5.8	5.9	4.6	4.6	4.3	4.2	3.9	4.2	4.3	4.2	4.1	3.8	3.7	3.8
Texas	5.5	5.2	3.8	4.0	3.3	3.4	3.3	3.3	3.3	3.3	3.2	3.0	2.9	2.7	2.6	4.2
Utah	5.1	4.4	4.0	4.3	4.1	3.9	3.7	3.8	3.7	3.7	3.7	3.3	3.1	3.1	3.6	3.6
Vermont	4.5	4.7	4.4	4.1	3.6	3.8	3.6	3.6	3.5	3.8	3.6	3.5	3.5	3.5	3.1	3.1
Virginia	4.4	4.3	4.4	4.3	4.0	4.0	3.8	3.8	3.7	3.8	3.8	3.7	3.6	3.5	3.3	3.4
Washington	5.9	5.4	5.0	4.6	4.3	4.1	4.0	3.9	3.9	4.2	4.1	3.9	3.8	3.6	3.4	3.5
West Virginia	5.3	5.2	4.9	5.1	5.1	5.0	5.1	4.8	5.1	5.1	5.2	4.7	4.6	4.2	4.0	3.8
Wisconsin	3.6	3.4	3.2	3.2	2.9	3.0	2.9	3.0	2.9	3.0	2.9	2.9	2.8	2.7	2.6	2.6
Wyoming	6.6	6.6	5.7	5.8	5.2	5.1	4.9	4.9	4.9	5.1	5.1	4.8	4.4	4.3	4.6	4.2

Note. Rates for 2001-2009 have been revised and are based on intercensal population estimates from the 2000 and 2010 censuses.

NA = Not available.

[1]Includes annulments. Includes divorce petitions filed or legal separations for some counties or states.

Table 4-3. Marital Status, United States, American Community Survey 1-Year Estimates, by Age, Sex, Race and Hispanic Origin, Place of Birth, and Labor Force Status, 2016

(Number; percent.)

Characteristic	Total	Now married (except separated)	Widowed	Divorced	Separated	Never married
Total Population, 15 Years and Over	262,140,054	47.5	5.8	11.0	2.0	33.7
Age and Sex						
Males, 15 years and over	127,863,548	49.1	2.6	9.7	1.7	36.9
15 to 19 years	10,991,723	0.9	0.0	0.0	0.1	99.0
20 to 34 years	33,804,063	26.1	0.1	2.8	1.0	70.0
35 to 44 years	20,215,641	60.0	0.4	10.6	2.6	26.5
45 to 54 years	21,101,370	63.4	1.1	15.7	2.7	17.2
55 to 64 years	19,990,313	66.0	2.6	16.9	2.2	12.2
65 years and over	21,760,438	69.5	11.6	11.9	1.4	5.6
Females, 15 years and over	134,276,506	46.0	8.8	12.3	2.3	30.6
15 to 19 years	10,500,178	1.3	0.0	0.1	0.1	98.5
20 to 34 years	32,758,858	33.1	0.2	4.0	1.8	60.8
35 to 44 years	20,439,951	61.1	0.9	13.0	3.8	21.2
45 to 54 years	21,654,220	61.6	2.8	18.6	3.6	13.5
55 to 64 years	21,468,572	60.1	7.4	20.0	2.7	9.8
65 years and over	27,454,727	43.9	34.2	15.1	1.2	5.6
Race and Hispanic Origin						
One race	255,869,928	47.8	5.9	11.0	2.0	33.3
White	194,105,615	50.8	6.2	11.5	1.7	29.8
Black or African American	32,390,126	28.8	5.6	12.0	3.7	49.9
American Indian and Alaska Native	2,069,594	36.1	5.1	12.9	2.8	43.2
Asian	14,617,774	58.0	4.5	5.2	1.2	31.2
Native Hawaiian and Other Pacific Islander	465,879	43.3	5.0	8.2	2.3	41.1
Some other race	12,220,940	41.8	2.9	7.5	3.4	44.4
Two or more races	6,270,126	33.5	3.0	9.7	2.3	51.5
Hispanic or Latino (of any race)	41,992,584	42.7	3.4	8.5	3.1	42.3
White, not Hispanic or Latino	166,743,034	51.9	6.7	11.9	1.5	28.1
Labor Force Participation						
Males, 16 years and over	125,723,528	49.9	2.7	9.8	1.7	35.8
In labor force	85,906,484	53.1	0.9	9.1	1.7	35.2
Females, 16 years and over	132,227,193	46.7	9.0	12.4	2.3	29.6
In labor force	76,985,559	47.3	2.8	13.4	2.6	33.9

Table 4-4. Marital Status, United States, American Community Survey 1-Year Estimates, by State, 2016

(Number; percent.)

State	Total population, 15 years and over	Now married (except separated)	Widowed	Divorced	Separated	Never married
United States..	257,770,670	47.7	5.9	11	2.1	33.3
Alabama...	3,962,122	46.9	7.2	12.6	2.3	31.0
Alaska...	584,670	47.5	3.5	11.2	1.8	36.0
Arizona..	5,579,306	46.8	5.7	12.5	1.7	33.3
Arkansas..	2,400,908	48.9	6.9	13.5	2.6	28.1
California..	31,696,515	46.5	5.0	9.4	2.1	37.0
Colorado...	4,490,574	50.4	4.4	11.8	1.4	32.0
Connecticut.......................................	2,966,525	46.9	5.8	10.8	1.3	35.2
Delaware..	782,833	46.6	6.0	11.2	1.7	34.4
District of Columbia	576,040	28.3	4.3	8.9	2.0	56.6
Florida...	17,195,240	45.8	6.9	13.1	2.4	31.8
Georgia..	8,232,061	46.6	5.6	11.5	2.3	34.1
Hawaii...	1,168,033	49.3	6.5	9.1	1.4	33.8
Idaho..	1,320,797	53.9	4.9	12.4	1.2	27.6
Illinois...	10,394,067	47.1	5.9	10.0	1.6	35.5
Indiana..	5,331,071	48.6	5.9	12.6	1.4	31.5
Iowa...	2,529,447	52.2	6.1	10.8	1.1	29.8
Kansas..	2,310,304	51.0	6.0	11.6	1.3	30.1
Kentucky..	3,600,690	48.2	6.7	13.2	2.2	29.7
Louisiana..	3,751,715	42.5	6.2	12.3	2.6	36.4
Maine..	1,123,728	48.7	6.5	14.6	1.1	29.1
Maryland..	4,902,314	46.4	5.5	10.1	2.2	35.8
Massachusetts....................................	5,683,233	45.8	5.5	9.5	1.7	37.5
Michigan..	8,138,464	47.5	6.0	11.8	1.3	33.4
Minnesota...	4,446,706	51.3	5.2	10.3	1.0	32.2
Mississippi..	2,388,158	44.3	7.1	11.4	3.0	34.2
Missouri...	4,943,723	48.8	6.5	12.1	1.8	30.8
Montana...	852,293	51.6	5.7	12.4	1.1	29.2
Nebraska..	1,509,438	51.7	6.1	10.6	1.1	30.5
Nevada..	2,376,250	44.3	5.3	14.2	2.3	33.9
New Hampshire...................................	1,123,706	51.3	5.7	12.1	1.1	29.8
New Jersey..	7,313,609	48.6	5.9	8.6	2.0	34.9
New Mexico.......................................	1,676,659	44.2	6.1	13.2	1.7	34.8
New York..	16,287,464	44.1	5.9	8.8	2.5	38.8
North Carolina....................................	8,250,416	48.4	6.1	10.8	2.7	31.9
North Dakota......................................	608,512	52.0	5.5	9.8	0.9	31.8
Ohio...	9,469,520	47.4	6.3	12.2	1.6	32.5
Oklahoma...	3,117,282	48.9	6.4	13.3	2.2	29.2
Oregon..	3,374,727	48.9	5.5	13.1	1.6	31.0
Pennsylvania......................................	10,585,604	47.1	6.7	9.9	2.1	34.2
Rhode Island......................................	886,433	42.7	6.2	12.4	1.6	37.2
South Carolina	4,046,525	46.2	7.0	11.1	3.0	32.7
South Dakota	684,721	50.5	6.1	10.5	1.1	31.8
Tennessee	5,405,690	48.4	6.3	12.7	2.3	30.3
Texas	21,772,944	48.7	5.1	10.6	2.5	33.1
Utah	2,276,760	54.9	3.6	9.1	1.6	30.7
Vermont	527,074	47.9	6.3	13.2	1.0	31.6
Virginia..	6,860,841	49.4	5.5	10.1	2.4	32.5
Washington..	5,929,275	50.4	4.9	11.9	1.5	31.4
West Virginia......................................	1,519,860	48.7	7.7	13.9	1.6	28.1
Wisconsin	4,718,806	50.0	5.6	10.9	1.0	32.5
Wyoming	466,401	53.0	5.1	12.9	1.5	27.5

Table 4-5. Median Age at First Marriage, American Community Survey 1-Year Estimates, by Sex and State, 2016

(Number.)

State	Male median age at first marriage	Female median age at first marriage
United States...	29.9	27.9
Alabama	28.3	26.3
Alaska	30.6	26.8
Arizona	29.8	28.0
Arkansas	27.2	25.6
California	30.6	28.7
Colorado	29.3	27.3
Connecticut..	31.6	29.5
Delaware	30.6	28.6
District of Columbia	30.9	30.3
Florida	30.7	29.0
Georgia	29.3	27.1
Hawaii	28.9	27.7
Idaho	27.0	25.1
Illinois	30.4	28.8
Indiana	28.9	26.9
Iowa	28.6	26.8
Kansas	27.5	26.0
Kentucky	28.4	26.3
Louisiana	29.8	27.5
Maine	30.0	27.0
Maryland..	30.5	28.9
Massachusetts...	31.2	29.8
Michigan	29.9	27.9
Minnesota	29.6	27.6
Mississippi	28.6	26.6
Missouri..	28.7	27.3
Montana	29.6	26.4
Nebraska	28.7	26.2
Nevada	29.7	28.2
New Hampshire..	30.6	28.4
New Jersey	30.9	29.3
New Mexico	28.5	26.8
New York..	31.0	29.8
North Carolina	29.2	27.7
North Dakota	28.1	26.7
Ohio	29.5	27.8
Oklahoma..	27.7	25.7
Oregon	29.7	27.6
Pennsylvania..	30.4	28.9
Rhode Island	30.9	30.0
South Carolina	29.9	28.4
South Dakota	28.0	26.0
Tennessee	28.4	27.0
Texas..	28.9	26.9
Utah	26.3	24.7
Vermont...	30.7	28.4
Virginia..	29.9	27.4
Washington..	29.5	27.0
West Virginia..	28.8	26.5
Wisconsin	29.8	28.1
Wyoming	28.8	26.0

Table 4-6. Median Age at First Marriage, American Community Survey 1-Year Estimates, by Sex and Race, United States, 2016

(Number.)

Race and origin	Male median age at first marriage	Female median age at first marriage
Median, Total, United States..	29.9	27.9
White alone...	29.5	27.5
Black or African American alone..	31.8	31.2
American Indian and Alaska Native alone..	30.8	29.1
Asian alone	30.2	27.6
Native Hawaiian or Other Pacific Islander alone	28.2	26.3
Some other race alone	29.9	27.3
Two or more races	30.2	28.7
Hispanic or Latino (of any race)...	29.6	27.5
White alone, not Hispanic or Latino	29.5	27.5

Table 4-7. Marriages in the Last Year for the Population Age 15 Years and Over, American Community Survey 1-Year Estimates, by Sex and State, 2016

(Number.)

State	Total, age 15 years and over	Male					Female				
		Total	Never married	Total, ever married	Married last year	Not married last year	Total	Never married	Total, ever married	Married last year	Not married last year
United States............	262,140,054	127,863,548	47,194,876	80,668,672	2,321,487	78,347,185	134,276,506	41,142,530	93,133,976	2,286,230	90,847,746
Alabama..............	3,962,122	1,894,579	645,555	1,249,024	31,627	1,217,397	2,067,543	583,215	1,484,328	32,805	1,451,523
Alaska...............	584,670	307,284	124,922	182,362	6,923	175,439	277,386	85,832	191,554	7,117	184,437
Arizona..............	5,579,306	2,754,161	1,021,830	1,732,331	45,572	1,686,759	2,825,145	838,293	1,986,852	47,773	1,939,079
Arkansas............	2,400,908	1,164,988	365,387	799,601	25,865	773,736	1,235,920	308,549	927,371	25,879	901,492
California............	31,696,515	15,633,439	6,342,454	9,290,985	284,900	9,006,085	16,063,076	5,400,492	10,662,584	265,834	10,396,750
Colorado............	4,490,574	2,251,218	802,589	1,448,629	50,869	1,397,760	2,239,356	633,684	1,605,672	52,706	1,552,966
Connecticut..........	2,966,525	1,433,885	554,927	878,958	22,824	856,134	1,532,640	489,942	1,042,698	24,404	1,018,294
Delaware............	782,833	374,374	140,011	234,363	5,294	229,069	408,459	129,018	279,441	5,395	274,046
District of Columbia...	576,040	270,633	155,103	115,530	7,533	107,997	305,407	170,936	134,471	7,163	127,308
Florida..............	17,195,240	8,325,278	2,929,277	5,396,001	140,597	5,255,404	8,869,962	2,541,569	6,328,393	128,836	6,199,557
Georgia.............	8,232,061	3,957,018	1,458,472	2,498,546	80,280	2,418,266	4,275,043	1,344,777	2,930,266	75,814	2,854,452
Hawaii..............	1,168,033	583,715	223,677	360,038	12,484	347,554	584,318	170,598	413,720	11,632	402,088
Idaho...............	1,320,797	655,592	201,696	453,896	12,753	441,143	665,205	162,455	502,750	13,773	488,977
Illinois..............	10,394,067	5,056,969	1,940,750	3,116,219	85,551	3,030,668	5,337,098	1,747,773	3,589,325	81,248	3,508,077
Indiana.............	5,331,071	2,600,798	901,195	1,699,603	51,671	1,647,932	2,730,273	778,923	1,951,350	54,557	1,896,793
Iowa................	2,529,447	1,245,027	415,556	829,471	20,132	809,339	1,284,420	337,782	946,638	20,392	926,246
Kansas.............	2,310,304	1,142,169	386,511	755,658	22,911	732,747	1,168,135	308,531	859,604	22,520	837,084
Kentucky............	3,600,690	1,752,576	579,303	1,173,273	33,197	1,140,076	1,848,114	488,955	1,359,159	33,408	1,325,751
Louisiana...........	3,751,715	1,815,491	725,764	1,089,727	26,759	1,062,968	1,936,224	641,451	1,294,773	29,134	1,265,639
Maine...............	1,123,728	544,729	177,638	367,091	6,840	360,251	578,999	149,838	429,161	8,999	420,162
Maryland............	4,902,314	2,346,134	903,101	1,443,033	41,310	1,401,723	2,556,180	850,257	1,705,923	42,786	1,663,137
Massachusetts.......	5,683,233	2,728,402	1,099,367	1,629,035	45,224	1,583,811	2,954,831	1,029,325	1,925,506	44,540	1,880,966
Michigan............	8,138,464	3,967,891	1,449,488	2,518,403	65,284	2,453,119	4,170,573	1,269,324	2,901,249	68,218	2,833,031
Minnesota...........	4,446,706	2,197,537	784,388	1,413,149	37,915	1,375,234	2,249,169	647,681	1,601,488	38,653	1,562,835
Mississippi..........	2,388,158	1,137,123	419,901	717,222	24,894	692,328	1,251,035	396,965	854,070	24,636	829,434
Missouri............	4,943,723	2,402,847	820,274	1,582,573	41,600	1,540,973	2,540,876	703,563	1,837,313	42,806	1,794,507
Montana............	852,293	427,876	142,314	285,562	7,724	277,838	424,417	106,666	317,751	7,669	310,082
Nebraska...........	1,509,438	747,768	253,630	494,138	13,476	480,662	761,670	206,641	555,029	13,288	541,741
Nevada.............	2,376,250	1,185,734	450,143	735,591	23,112	712,479	1,190,516	355,858	834,658	21,796	812,862
New Hampshire......	1,123,706	555,109	182,984	372,125	9,019	363,106	568,597	151,594	417,003	8,831	408,172
New Jersey..........	7,313,609	3,537,022	1,345,377	2,191,645	54,404	2,137,241	3,776,587	1,207,560	2,569,027	49,605	2,519,422
New Mexico.........	1,676,659	824,879	313,853	511,026	12,648	498,378	851,780	269,035	582,745	11,609	571,136
New York...........	16,287,464	7,816,473	3,234,830	4,581,643	126,195	4,455,448	8,470,991	3,084,457	5,386,534	120,614	5,265,920
North Carolina.......	8,250,416	3,961,788	1,377,377	2,584,411	72,878	2,511,533	4,288,628	1,254,842	3,033,786	75,970	2,957,816
North Dakota........	608,512	311,519	112,971	198,548	6,457	192,091	296,993	80,687	216,306	5,551	210,755
Ohio................	9,469,520	4,597,677	1,639,270	2,958,407	77,650	2,880,757	4,871,843	1,438,290	3,433,553	77,819	3,355,734
Oklahoma...........	3,117,282	1,528,795	501,814	1,026,981	32,274	994,707	1,588,487	408,475	1,180,012	31,639	1,148,373
Oregon.............	3,374,727	1,657,986	567,475	1,090,511	30,581	1,059,930	1,716,741	478,351	1,238,390	30,041	1,208,349
Pennsylvania........	10,585,604	5,138,564	1,916,471	3,222,093	80,432	3,141,661	5,447,040	1,702,435	3,744,605	77,976	3,666,629
Rhode Island........	886,433	424,571	170,386	254,185	6,560	247,625	461,862	159,423	302,439	6,450	295,989
South Carolina.......	4,046,525	1,937,011	690,100	1,246,911	37,504	1,209,407	2,109,514	633,057	1,476,457	37,256	1,439,201
South Dakota........	684,721	342,764	122,174	220,590	6,554	214,036	341,957	95,725	246,232	6,402	239,830
Tennessee..........	5,405,690	2,608,425	870,117	1,738,308	54,868	1,683,440	2,797,265	769,930	2,027,335	54,559	1,972,776
Texas...............	21,772,944	10,719,917	3,890,744	6,829,173	225,770	6,603,403	11,053,027	3,325,891	7,727,136	227,975	7,499,161
Utah................	2,276,760	1,139,070	386,824	752,246	30,733	721,513	1,137,690	312,644	825,046	30,358	794,688
Vermont............	527,074	257,638	89,531	168,107	3,120	164,987	269,436	76,869	192,567	3,816	188,751
Virginia.............	6,860,841	3,344,431	1,190,041	2,154,390	67,707	2,086,683	3,516,410	1,042,315	2,474,095	64,157	2,409,938
Washington..........	5,929,275	2,943,737	1,033,508	1,910,229	56,912	1,853,317	2,985,538	825,474	2,160,064	56,794	2,103,270
West Virginia........	1,519,860	742,920	240,042	502,878	10,018	492,860	776,940	186,715	590,225	10,796	579,429
Wisconsin...........	4,718,806	2,330,764	832,052	1,498,712	38,459	1,460,253	2,388,042	703,306	1,684,736	39,057	1,645,679
Wyoming............	466,401	237,253	71,712	165,541	5,623	159,918	229,148	56,562	172,586	5,174	167,412

Table 4-8. Marriages Ending in Widowhood for the Population Age 15 Years and Over, American Community Survey 1-Year Estimates, by Sex and State, 2016

(Number.)

State	Total, age 15 years and over	Male					Female				
		Total	Never married	Ever married			Total	Never married	Ever married		
				Total, ever married	Widowed last year	Not widowed last year			Total, ever married	Widowed last year	Not widowed last year
United States	262,140,054	127,863,548	47,194,876	80,668,672	463,022	80,205,650	134,276,506	41,142,530	93,133,976	997,298	92,136,678
Alabama	3,962,122	1,894,579	645,555	1,249,024	9,063	1,239,961	2,067,543	583,215	1,484,328	17,718	1,466,610
Alaska	584,670	307,284	124,922	182,362	496	181,866	277,386	85,832	191,554	1,448	190,106
Arizona	5,579,306	2,754,161	1,021,830	1,732,331	9,244	1,723,087	2,825,145	838,293	1,986,852	21,747	1,965,105
Arkansas	2,400,908	1,164,988	365,387	799,601	5,999	793,602	1,235,920	308,549	927,371	10,998	916,373
California	31,696,515	15,633,439	6,342,454	9,290,985	47,639	9,243,346	16,063,076	5,400,492	10,662,584	101,894	10,560,690
Colorado	4,490,574	2,251,218	802,589	1,448,629	5,715	1,442,914	2,239,356	633,684	1,605,672	12,910	1,592,762
Connecticut	2,966,525	1,433,885	554,927	878,958	5,847	873,111	1,532,640	489,942	1,042,698	10,608	1,032,090
Delaware	782,833	374,374	140,011	234,363	837	233,526	408,459	129,018	279,441	2,808	276,633
District of Columbia	576,040	270,633	155,103	115,530	519	115,011	305,407	170,936	134,471	1,859	132,612
Florida	17,195,240	8,325,278	2,929,277	5,396,001	33,469	5,362,532	8,869,962	2,541,569	6,328,393	72,386	6,256,007
Georgia	8,232,061	3,957,018	1,458,472	2,498,546	12,347	2,486,199	4,275,043	1,344,777	2,930,266	33,053	2,897,213
Hawaii	1,168,033	583,715	223,677	360,038	1,443	358,595	584,318	170,598	413,720	5,321	408,399
Idaho	1,320,797	655,592	201,696	453,896	3,203	450,693	665,205	162,455	502,750	4,819	497,931
Illinois	10,394,067	5,056,969	1,940,750	3,116,219	16,782	3,099,437	5,337,098	1,747,773	3,589,325	39,434	3,549,891
Indiana	5,331,071	2,600,798	901,195	1,699,603	9,503	1,690,100	2,730,273	778,923	1,951,350	24,406	1,926,944
Iowa	2,529,447	1,245,027	415,556	829,471	5,385	824,086	1,284,420	337,782	946,638	8,798	937,840
Kansas	2,310,304	1,142,169	386,511	755,658	4,907	750,751	1,168,135	308,531	859,604	9,121	850,483
Kentucky	3,600,690	1,752,576	579,303	1,173,273	7,484	1,165,789	1,848,114	488,955	1,359,159	17,973	1,341,186
Louisiana	3,751,715	1,815,491	725,764	1,089,727	7,589	1,082,138	1,936,224	641,451	1,294,773	13,384	1,281,389
Maine	1,123,728	544,729	177,638	367,091	2,850	364,241	578,999	149,838	429,161	4,155	425,006
Maryland	4,902,314	2,346,134	903,101	1,443,033	7,965	1,435,068	2,556,180	850,257	1,705,923	17,417	1,688,506
Massachusetts	5,683,233	2,728,402	1,099,367	1,629,035	9,354	1,619,681	2,954,831	1,029,325	1,925,506	20,235	1,905,271
Michigan	8,138,464	3,967,891	1,449,488	2,518,403	17,397	2,501,006	4,170,573	1,269,324	2,901,249	32,628	2,868,621
Minnesota	4,446,706	2,197,537	784,388	1,413,149	8,434	1,404,715	2,249,169	647,681	1,601,488	15,589	1,585,899
Mississippi	2,388,158	1,137,123	419,901	717,222	5,040	712,182	1,251,035	396,965	854,070	10,315	843,755
Missouri	4,943,723	2,402,847	820,274	1,582,573	9,344	1,573,229	2,540,876	703,563	1,837,313	20,061	1,817,252
Montana	852,293	427,876	142,314	285,562	1,549	284,013	424,417	106,666	317,751	2,987	314,764
Nebraska	1,509,438	747,768	253,630	494,138	2,520	491,618	761,670	206,641	555,029	6,422	548,607
Nevada	2,376,250	1,185,734	450,143	735,591	5,026	730,565	1,190,516	355,858	834,658	7,938	826,720
New Hampshire	1,123,706	555,109	182,984	372,125	1,470	370,655	568,597	151,594	417,003	3,459	413,544
New Jersey	7,313,609	3,537,022	1,345,377	2,191,645	9,006	2,182,639	3,776,587	1,207,560	2,569,027	26,840	2,542,187
New Mexico	1,676,659	824,879	313,853	511,026	2,503	508,523	851,780	269,035	582,745	7,347	575,398
New York	16,287,464	7,816,473	3,234,830	4,581,643	21,843	4,559,800	8,470,991	3,084,457	5,386,534	55,132	5,331,402
North Carolina	8,250,416	3,961,788	1,377,377	2,584,411	15,356	2,569,055	4,288,628	1,254,842	3,033,786	38,042	2,995,744
North Dakota	608,512	311,519	112,971	198,548	950	197,598	296,993	80,687	216,306	2,410	213,896
Ohio	9,469,520	4,597,677	1,639,270	2,958,407	21,167	2,937,240	4,871,843	1,438,290	3,433,553	38,336	3,395,217
Oklahoma	3,117,282	1,528,795	501,814	1,026,981	6,252	1,020,729	1,588,487	408,475	1,180,012	14,556	1,165,456
Oregon	3,374,727	1,657,986	567,475	1,090,511	6,520	1,083,991	1,716,741	478,351	1,238,390	10,685	1,227,705
Pennsylvania	10,585,604	5,138,564	1,916,471	3,222,093	22,301	3,199,792	5,447,040	1,702,435	3,744,605	42,921	3,701,684
Rhode Island	886,433	424,571	170,386	254,185	1,735	252,450	461,862	159,423	302,439	3,428	299,011
South Carolina	4,046,525	1,937,011	690,100	1,246,911	8,526	1,238,385	2,109,514	633,057	1,476,457	19,352	1,457,105
South Dakota	684,721	342,764	122,174	220,590	1,818	218,772	341,957	95,725	246,232	3,145	243,087
Tennessee	5,405,690	2,608,425	870,117	1,738,308	12,380	1,725,928	2,797,265	769,930	2,027,335	21,851	2,005,484
Texas	21,772,944	10,719,917	3,890,744	6,829,173	35,311	6,793,862	11,053,027	3,325,891	7,727,136	76,290	7,650,846
Utah	2,276,760	1,139,070	386,824	752,246	2,906	749,340	1,137,690	312,644	825,046	6,854	818,192
Vermont	527,074	257,638	89,531	168,107	968	167,139	269,436	76,869	192,567	2,158	190,409
Virginia	6,860,841	3,344,431	1,190,041	2,154,390	11,223	2,143,167	3,516,410	1,042,315	2,474,095	28,338	2,445,757
Washington	5,929,275	2,943,737	1,033,508	1,910,229	10,948	1,899,281	2,985,538	825,474	2,160,064	20,658	2,139,406
West Virginia	1,519,860	742,920	240,042	502,878	4,184	498,694	776,940	186,715	590,225	8,624	581,601
Wisconsin	4,718,806	2,330,764	832,052	1,498,712	8,023	1,490,689	2,388,042	703,306	1,684,736	16,996	1,667,740
Wyoming	466,401	237,253	71,712	165,541	682	164,859	229,148	56,562	172,586	1,444	171,142

Table 4-9. Divorces in the Last Year for the Population Age 15 Years and Over, American Community Survey 1-Year Estimates, by Sex and State, 2016

(Number.)

State	Total, age 15 years and over	Male					Female				
		Total	Never married	Ever married			Total	Never married	Ever married		
				Total, ever married	Divorced last year	Not divorced last year			Total, ever married	Divorced last year	Not divorced last year
United States........................	262,140,054	127,863,548	47,194,876	80,668,672	994,183	79,674,489	134,276,506	41,142,530	93,133,976	1,098,805	92,035,171
Alabama........................	3,962,122	1,894,579	645,555	1,249,024	16,436	1,232,588	2,067,543	583,215	1,484,328	19,366	1,464,962
Alaska........................	584,670	307,284	124,922	182,362	2,841	179,521	277,386	85,832	191,554	2,398	189,156
Arizona........................	5,579,306	2,754,161	1,021,830	1,732,331	19,857	1,712,474	2,825,145	838,293	1,986,852	28,034	1,958,818
Arkansas........................	2,400,908	1,164,988	365,387	799,601	13,141	786,460	1,235,920	308,549	927,371	16,103	911,268
California........................	31,696,515	15,633,439	6,342,454	9,290,985	102,730	9,188,255	16,063,076	5,400,492	10,662,584	116,989	10,545,595
Colorado........................	4,490,574	2,251,218	802,589	1,448,629	19,731	1,428,898	2,239,356	633,684	1,605,672	18,067	1,587,605
Connecticut........................	2,966,525	1,433,885	554,927	878,958	8,699	870,259	1,532,640	489,942	1,042,698	14,426	1,028,272
Delaware........................	782,833	374,374	140,011	234,363	2,652	231,711	408,459	129,018	279,441	3,581	275,860
District of Columbia........................	576,040	270,633	155,103	115,530	1,811	113,719	305,407	170,936	134,471	1,762	132,709
Florida........................	17,195,240	8,325,278	2,929,277	5,396,001	70,478	5,325,523	8,869,962	2,541,569	6,328,393	74,969	6,253,424
Georgia........................	8,232,061	3,957,018	1,458,472	2,498,546	32,512	2,466,034	4,275,043	1,344,777	2,930,266	42,224	2,888,042
Hawaii........................	1,168,033	583,715	223,677	360,038	3,279	356,759	584,318	170,598	413,720	4,193	409,527
Idaho........................	1,320,797	655,592	201,696	453,896	8,159	445,737	665,205	162,455	502,750	7,366	495,384
Illinois........................	10,394,067	5,056,969	1,940,750	3,116,219	34,858	3,081,361	5,337,098	1,747,773	3,589,325	36,296	3,553,029
Indiana........................	5,331,071	2,600,798	901,195	1,699,603	24,845	1,674,758	2,730,273	778,923	1,951,350	26,983	1,924,367
Iowa........................	2,529,447	1,245,027	415,556	829,471	9,119	820,352	1,284,420	337,782	946,638	9,838	936,800
Kansas........................	2,310,304	1,142,169	386,511	755,658	11,953	743,705	1,168,135	308,531	859,604	10,636	848,968
Kentucky........................	3,600,690	1,752,576	579,303	1,173,273	16,093	1,157,180	1,848,114	488,955	1,359,159	18,400	1,340,759
Louisiana........................	3,751,715	1,815,491	725,764	1,089,727	16,142	1,073,585	1,936,224	641,451	1,294,773	19,307	1,275,466
Maine........................	1,123,728	544,729	177,638	367,091	4,316	362,775	578,999	149,838	429,161	5,371	423,790
Maryland........................	4,902,314	2,346,134	903,101	1,443,033	18,945	1,424,088	2,556,180	850,257	1,705,923	20,920	1,685,003
Massachusetts........................	5,683,233	2,728,402	1,099,367	1,629,035	16,250	1,612,785	2,954,831	1,029,325	1,925,506	16,596	1,908,910
Michigan........................	8,138,464	3,967,891	1,449,488	2,518,403	33,036	2,485,367	4,170,573	1,269,324	2,901,249	31,926	2,869,323
Minnesota........................	4,446,706	2,197,537	784,388	1,413,149	14,617	1,398,532	2,249,169	647,681	1,601,488	15,299	1,586,189
Mississippi........................	2,388,158	1,137,123	419,901	717,222	8,572	708,650	1,251,035	396,965	854,070	10,914	843,156
Missouri........................	4,943,723	2,402,847	820,274	1,582,573	23,083	1,559,490	2,540,876	703,563	1,837,313	20,852	1,816,461
Montana........................	852,293	427,876	142,314	285,562	4,189	281,373	424,417	106,666	317,751	4,307	313,444
Nebraska........................	1,509,438	747,768	253,630	494,138	5,450	488,688	761,670	206,641	555,029	6,023	549,006
Nevada........................	2,376,250	1,185,734	450,143	735,591	12,187	723,404	1,190,516	355,858	834,658	11,180	823,478
New Hampshire........................	1,123,706	555,109	182,984	372,125	4,531	367,594	568,597	151,594	417,003	4,140	412,863
New Jersey........................	7,313,609	3,537,022	1,345,377	2,191,645	23,939	2,167,706	3,776,587	1,207,560	2,569,027	23,119	2,545,908
New Mexico........................	1,676,659	824,879	313,853	511,026	6,310	504,716	851,780	269,035	582,745	6,906	575,839
New York........................	16,287,464	7,816,473	3,234,830	4,581,643	44,658	4,536,985	8,470,991	3,084,457	5,386,534	52,254	5,334,280
North Carolina........................	8,250,416	3,961,788	1,377,377	2,584,411	31,067	2,553,344	4,288,628	1,254,842	3,033,786	33,865	2,999,921
North Dakota........................	608,512	311,519	112,971	198,548	2,666	195,882	296,993	80,687	216,306	2,603	213,703
Ohio........................	9,469,520	4,597,677	1,639,270	2,958,407	35,462	2,922,945	4,871,843	1,438,290	3,433,553	37,373	3,396,180
Oklahoma........................	3,117,282	1,528,795	501,814	1,026,981	15,837	1,011,144	1,588,487	408,475	1,180,012	16,900	1,163,112
Oregon........................	3,374,727	1,657,986	567,475	1,090,511	13,265	1,077,246	1,716,741	478,351	1,238,390	17,595	1,220,795
Pennsylvania........................	10,585,604	5,138,564	1,916,471	3,222,093	38,892	3,183,201	5,447,040	1,702,435	3,744,605	41,269	3,703,336
Rhode Island........................	886,433	424,571	170,386	254,185	2,701	251,484	461,862	159,423	302,439	3,231	299,208
South Carolina........................	4,046,525	1,937,011	690,100	1,246,911	16,672	1,230,239	2,109,514	633,057	1,476,457	18,085	1,458,372
South Dakota........................	684,721	342,764	122,174	220,590	2,295	218,295	341,957	95,725	246,232	2,392	243,840
Tennessee........................	5,405,690	2,608,425	870,117	1,738,308	23,805	1,714,503	2,797,265	769,930	2,027,335	27,960	1,999,375
Texas........................	21,772,944	10,719,917	3,890,744	6,829,173	87,327	6,741,846	11,053,027	3,325,891	7,727,136	101,725	7,625,411
Utah........................	2,276,760	1,139,070	386,824	752,246	8,092	744,154	1,137,690	312,644	825,046	12,575	812,471
Vermont........................	527,074	257,638	89,531	168,107	1,741	166,366	269,436	76,869	192,567	1,763	190,804
Virginia........................	6,860,841	3,344,431	1,190,041	2,154,390	27,279	2,127,111	3,516,410	1,042,315	2,474,095	26,038	2,448,057
Washington........................	5,929,275	2,943,737	1,033,508	1,910,229	25,128	1,885,101	2,985,538	825,474	2,160,064	27,494	2,132,570
West Virginia........................	1,519,860	742,920	240,042	502,878	7,778	495,100	776,940	186,715	590,225	7,022	583,203
Wisconsin........................	4,718,806	2,330,764	832,052	1,498,712	17,152	1,481,560	2,388,042	703,306	1,684,736	16,817	1,667,919
Wyoming........................	466,401	237,253	71,712	165,541	1,605	163,936	229,148	56,562	172,586	3,353	169,233

Table 4-10. Median Duration of Current Marriage in Years for the Population Age 15 Years and Over, American Community Survey 1-Year Estimates, by Sex, Marital Status, and State, 2016

(Years.)

State	Total, age 15 years and over	Male				Female			
		Total	Married, spouse present	Married, spouse absent	Separated	Total	Married, spouse present	Married, spouse absent	Separated
United States	19.7	19.6	20.2	12.2	16.0	19.7	20.3	12.8	16.3
Alabama	19.9	20.0	20.9	11.9	14.4	19.8	20.7	12.4	13.7
Alaska	16.7	16.5	17.2	12.2	15.7	16.9	17.1	10.3	17.1
Arizona	19.9	19.8	20.5	11.8	14.5	19.9	20.6	11.2	17.6
Arkansas	19.5	19.3	20.2	9.5	13.0	19.7	20.5	8.8	14.2
California	18.7	18.6	19.1	12.0	17.3	18.9	19.2	14.1	18.6
Colorado	17.4	17.5	18.0	9.9	14.7	17.4	17.8	11.0	14.6
Connecticut	21.4	21.4	21.7	16.4	20.3	21.4	21.7	16.2	17.3
Delaware	21.1	21.7	22.2	11.4	22.3	20.7	22.1	8.2	16.1
District of Columbia	10.6	10.4	9.7	13.6	13.8	10.9	10.5	7.1	19.7
Florida	20.7	20.6	21.6	12.6	15.4	20.8	21.6	14.5	16.4
Georgia	18.1	18.2	18.7	10.7	15.4	18.1	18.8	11.7	14.5
Hawaii	17.9	17.8	18.5	12.4	16.8	18.1	18.7	13.8	16.1
Idaho	18.9	19.2	19.8	11.5	16.5	18.7	19.3	10.0	12.6
Illinois	20.4	20.3	20.7	13.6	16.5	20.5	20.9	14.7	16.5
Indiana	20.3	20.4	20.9	11.7	15.1	20.1	20.7	10.1	13.0
Iowa	21.5	21.6	22.0	15.8	11.4	21.4	21.8	18.0	12.4
Kansas	19.6	19.8	20.2	15.1	14.6	19.5	20.1	9.9	15.0
Kentucky	20.2	20.2	20.8	10.5	16.0	20.1	20.9	15.7	12.7
Louisiana	19.3	19.2	20.3	12.0	13.9	19.4	20.5	11.4	13.6
Maine	22.4	22.8	22.9	22.3	19.2	21.9	22.1	18.9	19.3
Maryland	18.9	18.9	19.4	12.8	15.7	18.9	19.4	11.5	17.0
Massachusetts	20.6	20.7	21.1	12.2	19.2	20.6	21.0	13.2	18.8
Michigan	21.8	21.6	22.2	12.8	15.3	21.9	22.3	16.6	16.9
Minnesota	21.1	21.2	21.5	16.9	15.3	21.1	21.4	16.6	16.0
Mississippi	19.0	19.1	20.1	9.3	14.1	19.0	20.0	8.9	15.7
Missouri	20.2	20.4	20.8	13.2	16.4	20.0	20.6	13.3	14.9
Montana	21.2	21.1	21.6	18.9	12.3	21.2	21.8	14.4	16.2
Nebraska	20.6	20.7	21.0	15.4	15.6	20.4	20.9	15.3	12.1
Nevada	17.4	17.4	17.8	11.4	16.4	17.3	17.8	10.1	17.1
New Hampshire	21.9	21.9	22.6	9.5	14.5	21.8	22.2	11.7	16.9
New Jersey	20.4	20.3	20.8	13.8	17.7	20.5	20.9	14.5	18.6
New Mexico	20.2	20.2	20.6	15.8	15.1	20.2	20.9	11.9	17.0
New York	20.3	20.2	20.9	11.5	18.3	20.5	21.1	13.6	20.3
North Carolina	19.4	19.4	20.0	13.2	14.9	19.3	20.1	12.1	14.6
North Dakota	20.5	20.2	20.8	14.5	14.2	20.8	21.0	15.5	10.4
Ohio	21.1	21.1	21.6	12.2	16.5	21.2	21.7	15.2	16.4
Oklahoma	18.7	18.8	19.5	11.4	15.0	18.6	19.5	11.5	13.2
Oregon	19.1	19.2	19.5	13.3	14.1	19.0	19.3	13.6	16.2
Pennsylvania	22.2	22.2	22.8	15.1	17.5	22.2	22.9	16.1	17.1
Rhode Island	20.9	21.2	21.8	10.6	17.9	20.7	21.4	13.4	17.3
South Carolina	20.6	20.6	21.2	12.7	16.3	20.6	21.6	10.9	15.9
South Dakota	21.6	22.0	22.3	19.0	11.9	21.2	21.6	17.7	15.6
Tennessee	19.3	19.3	20.1	8.4	14.3	19.3	20.0	10.5	16.1
Texas	17.5	17.4	18.0	10.9	15.4	17.5	18.1	10.4	15.0
Utah	17.2	17.2	17.8	7.5	13.1	17.2	17.8	9.6	12.5
Vermont	21.6	21.8	22.1	19.4	17.4	21.5	21.7	16.7	15.6
Virginia	18.9	18.9	19.5	11.4	14.8	18.9	19.6	11.2	14.8
Washington	18.4	18.5	18.9	11.7	15.2	18.2	18.5	11.4	16.9
West Virginia	21.6	21.7	22.4	14.8	13.9	21.5	22.1	19.7	14.6
Wisconsin	22.2	22.3	22.6	16.5	16.3	22.1	22.4	16.2	17.9
Wyoming	19.1	18.8	19.3	15.8	14.6	19.6	20.1	16.5	13.5

Table 4-11. Number of Times Married for the Population Age 15 Years and Over, American Community Survey 1-Year Estimates, by Sex, Marital Status, and State, 2016

(Number.)

State	Total, age 15 years and over	Male Total	Male Never married	Male Ever married Total	Male Ever married Once	Male Ever married Twice	Male Ever married Three or more times	Female Total	Female Never married	Female Ever married Total	Female Ever married Once	Female Ever married Twice	Female Ever married Three or more times
United States	262,140,054	127,863,548	47,194,876	80,668,672	60,897,524	15,438,326	4,332,822	134,276,506	41,142,530	93,133,976	70,419,493	17,838,290	4,876,193
Alabama	3,962,122	1,894,579	645,555	1,249,024	861,689	281,558	105,777	2,067,543	583,215	1,484,328	1,011,541	346,161	126,626
Alaska	584,670	307,284	124,922	182,362	135,137	36,356	10,869	277,386	85,832	191,554	141,804	35,386	14,364
Arizona	5,579,306	2,754,161	1,021,830	1,732,331	1,237,183	377,573	117,575	2,825,145	838,293	1,986,852	1,420,449	429,400	137,003
Arkansas	2,400,908	1,164,988	365,387	799,601	518,847	192,135	88,619	1,235,920	308,549	927,371	602,823	224,749	99,799
California	31,696,515	15,633,439	6,342,454	9,290,985	7,473,263	1,474,152	343,570	16,063,076	5,400,492	10,662,584	8,568,058	1,720,035	374,491
Colorado	4,490,574	2,251,218	802,589	1,448,629	1,094,994	277,541	76,094	2,239,356	633,684	1,605,672	1,193,662	326,641	85,369
Connecticut	2,966,525	1,433,885	554,927	878,958	707,494	148,500	22,964	1,532,640	489,942	1,042,698	851,465	164,099	27,134
Delaware	782,833	374,374	140,011	234,363	177,858	44,122	12,383	408,459	129,018	279,441	215,156	50,837	13,448
District of Columbia	576,040	270,633	155,103	115,530	95,536	17,045	2,949	305,407	170,936	134,471	114,531	17,894	2,046
Florida	17,195,240	8,325,278	2,929,277	5,396,001	3,759,962	1,238,745	397,294	8,869,962	2,541,569	6,328,393	4,476,124	1,423,196	429,073
Georgia	8,232,061	3,957,018	1,458,472	2,498,546	1,798,367	530,904	169,275	4,275,043	1,344,777	2,930,266	2,120,180	616,927	193,159
Hawaii	1,168,033	583,715	223,677	360,038	288,761	56,464	14,813	584,318	170,598	413,720	335,966	65,188	12,566
Idaho	1,320,797	655,592	201,696	453,896	316,871	99,840	37,185	665,205	162,455	502,750	345,941	113,861	42,948
Illinois	10,394,067	5,056,969	1,940,750	3,116,219	2,466,036	531,446	118,737	5,337,098	1,747,773	3,589,325	2,839,504	609,104	140,717
Indiana	5,331,071	2,600,798	901,195	1,699,603	1,213,263	361,511	124,829	2,730,273	778,923	1,951,350	1,391,525	416,578	143,247
Iowa	2,529,447	1,245,027	415,556	829,471	638,558	150,331	40,582	1,284,420	337,782	946,638	723,166	179,274	44,198
Kansas	2,310,304	1,142,169	386,511	755,658	559,687	142,791	53,180	1,168,135	308,531	859,604	622,963	178,520	58,121
Kentucky	3,600,690	1,752,576	579,303	1,173,273	816,522	259,409	97,342	1,848,114	488,955	1,359,159	951,272	299,033	108,854
Louisiana	3,751,715	1,815,491	725,764	1,089,727	788,189	228,740	72,798	1,936,224	641,451	1,294,773	945,699	266,186	82,888
Maine	1,123,728	544,729	177,638	367,091	266,002	78,676	22,413	578,999	149,838	429,161	309,988	93,868	25,305
Maryland	4,902,314	2,346,134	903,101	1,443,033	1,121,633	268,700	52,700	2,556,180	850,257	1,705,923	1,337,923	308,676	59,324
Massachusetts	5,683,233	2,728,402	1,099,367	1,629,035	1,348,946	242,006	38,083	2,954,831	1,029,325	1,925,506	1,613,072	277,344	35,090
Michigan	8,138,464	3,967,891	1,449,488	2,518,403	1,899,977	489,231	129,195	4,170,573	1,269,324	2,901,249	2,191,826	566,217	143,206
Minnesota	4,446,706	2,197,537	784,388	1,413,149	1,143,800	226,006	43,343	2,249,169	647,681	1,601,488	1,299,623	254,595	47,270
Mississippi	2,388,158	1,137,123	419,901	717,222	488,578	168,883	59,761	1,251,035	396,965	854,070	601,478	187,491	65,101
Missouri	4,943,723	2,402,847	820,274	1,582,573	1,121,353	343,324	117,896	2,540,876	703,563	1,837,313	1,282,125	415,203	139,985
Montana	852,392	427,876	142,314	285,562	206,426	59,875	19,261	424,417	106,666	317,751	222,887	73,036	21,828
Nebraska	1,509,438	747,768	253,630	494,138	385,947	86,151	22,040	761,670	206,641	555,029	430,900	97,125	27,004
Nevada	2,376,250	1,185,734	450,143	735,591	521,124	155,813	58,654	1,190,516	355,858	834,658	580,549	190,409	63,700
New Hampshire	1,123,706	555,109	182,984	372,125	276,501	76,263	19,361	568,597	151,594	417,003	314,700	83,999	18,304
New Jersey	7,313,609	3,537,022	1,345,377	2,191,645	1,824,089	322,352	45,204	3,776,587	1,207,560	2,569,027	2,162,804	362,718	43,505
New Mexico	1,676,659	824,879	313,853	511,026	379,403	101,609	30,014	851,780	269,035	582,745	432,566	116,565	33,614
New York	16,287,464	7,816,473	3,234,830	4,581,643	3,802,155	667,262	112,226	8,470,991	3,084,455	5,386,534	4,532,264	747,451	106,819
North Carolina	8,250,416	3,961,788	1,377,377	2,584,411	1,872,469	554,034	157,908	4,288,628	1,254,842	3,033,786	2,207,653	646,590	179,543
North Dakota	608,512	311,519	112,971	198,548	163,008	29,293	6,247	296,993	80,687	216,306	176,068	32,898	7,340
Ohio	9,469,520	4,597,677	1,639,270	2,958,407	2,177,539	603,744	177,124	4,871,843	1,438,290	3,433,553	2,546,113	693,859	193,581
Oklahoma	3,117,282	1,528,795	501,814	1,026,981	684,083	244,910	97,988	1,588,487	408,475	1,180,012	777,346	281,769	120,897
Oregon	3,374,727	1,657,986	567,475	1,090,511	780,049	233,927	76,535	1,716,741	478,351	1,238,390	867,469	278,471	92,450
Pennsylvania	10,585,604	5,138,564	1,916,471	3,222,093	2,540,003	573,033	109,057	5,447,040	1,702,435	3,744,605	2,980,960	639,672	123,973
Rhode Island	886,433	424,571	170,386	254,185	203,849	42,329	8,007	461,862	159,423	302,439	244,850	49,704	7,885
South Carolina	4,046,525	1,937,011	690,100	1,246,911	889,993	279,833	77,085	2,109,514	633,057	1,476,457	1,069,251	316,023	91,183
South Dakota	684,721	342,764	122,174	220,590	171,554	39,648	9,388	341,957	95,725	246,232	188,743	45,282	12,207
Tennessee	5,405,690	2,608,425	870,117	1,738,308	1,195,081	394,906	148,321	2,797,265	769,930	2,027,335	1,391,460	461,111	174,764
Texas	21,772,944	10,719,917	3,890,744	6,829,173	5,088,488	1,316,370	424,315	11,053,027	3,325,891	7,727,136	5,719,182	1,536,377	471,577
Utah	2,276,760	1,139,070	386,824	752,246	588,707	122,383	41,156	1,137,690	312,644	825,046	630,492	147,861	46,693
Vermont	527,074	257,638	89,531	168,107	126,846	33,341	7,920	269,436	76,869	192,567	143,220	39,988	9,359
Virginia	6,860,841	3,344,431	1,190,041	2,154,390	1,613,535	438,521	102,334	3,516,410	1,042,315	2,474,095	1,868,358	485,944	119,793
Washington	5,929,275	2,943,737	1,033,508	1,910,229	1,408,762	387,983	113,484	2,985,538	825,474	2,160,064	1,575,072	446,752	138,240
West Virginia	1,519,860	742,920	240,042	502,878	345,265	119,346	38,267	776,940	186,715	590,225	408,345	139,112	42,768
Wisconsin	4,718,806	2,330,764	832,052	1,498,712	1,198,411	252,358	47,943	2,388,042	703,306	1,684,736	1,322,755	299,092	62,889
Wyoming	466,401	237,253	71,712	165,541	115,731	37,053	12,757	229,148	56,562	172,586	117,622	40,019	14,945

SOURCES OF DATA

Tables 4-1 and 4-2 are from the Centers for Disease Control and Prevention's National Vital Statistics System. Detailed state tables can be found at http://www.cdc.gov/nchs/mardiv. htm#state_tables. Rates for 2001 to 2009 have been revised and are based on intercensal population estimates from the 2000 and 2010 censuses.

Tables 4-3 through 4-11 are from the 1-year estimates from the 2016 American Community Survey, which is conducted by the U.S. Census Bureau. Although the American Community Survey (ACS) produces population, demographic and housing unit estimates, it is the Census Bureau's Population Estimates Program that produces and disseminates the official estimates of the population for the nation, states, counties, cities and towns and estimates of housing units for states and counties.

NOTES AND DEFINITIONS

Accuracy of the data—Data are based on a sample and are subject to sampling variability. The degree of uncertainty for an estimate arising from sampling variability is represented through the use of a margin of error. The margin of error can be interpreted roughly as providing a 90 percent probability that the interval defined by the estimate minus the margin of error and the estimate plus the margin of error (the lower and upper confidence bounds) contains the true value. In addition to sampling variability, the ACS estimates are subject to nonsampling error. The effect of nonsampling error is not represented in these tables.

Foreign born—Foreign born excludes people born outside the United States to a parent who is a U.S. citizen.

Population—ACS population comprises individuals age 15 to 54 years.

Widowhood—Widowhood estimates may vary from the mortality data released by the National Center for Health Statistics (NCHS) because of differences in methodology and data collection. NCHS uses information collected on death certificates from each state that record the current marital status of the decedent at the time of death. From these administrative records, NCHS then publishes information about men and women who died in that calendar year by their marital status. By inference, people who were married at their time of death were survived by a widowed spouse. In contrast, the ACS collects survey-based reports from individuals as to whether or not they were widowed in the last 12 months. We recommend using caution when comparing the NCHS estimates to the ACS estimates of widowhood.

INDEX